MW01269096

Vera Pyle's Current Medical Terminology

10th Edition

by Health Professions Institute

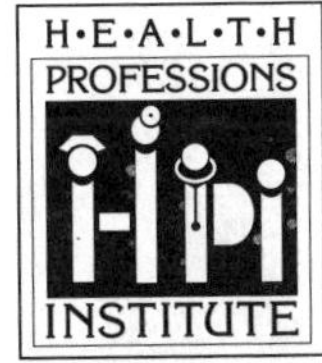

Health Professions Institute • Modesto, California • 2005

Vera Pyle's Current Medical Terminology
10th Edition
by Health Professions Institute

Published by:

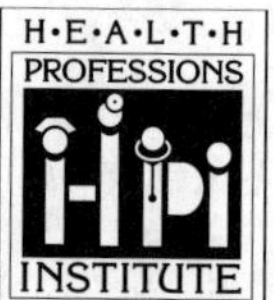

Health Professions Institute
P. O. Box 801
Modesto, California 95353-0801
Phone (209) 551-2112
Fax (209) 551-0404
Web site: http://www.hpisum.com
E-mail: hpi@hpisum.com
Sally Crenshaw Pitman
Editor & Publisher

Printed by:
Parks Printing & Lithograph
Modesto, California

ISBN: 0-934385-82-3
Last digit is the print number: 9 8 7 6 5 4 3 2 1

To those who have contributed to this book,
To those who read it and find it useful,
To all who love words.

and

To Dan Pae, who passed through life—
and made a difference.

Preface to the 10th Edition

The 10th edition of *Vera Pyle's Current Medical Terminology* includes over 150 pages of new material drawn from research in print and electronic medical references. At the same time that we added new material, we pruned many outdated drugs older than three years from the text. Every term retained has been reexamined and reconfirmed. In this way, we were able to retain important terms from past research, add hundreds of new entries, and reduce the number of pages to make the book a manageable size. We hope you will find that the new glossary meets your needs for new, difficult, and hard-to-find terms.

A special feature of this edition is hundreds of genetics and stem cell research terms provided by John H. Dirckx, M.D. Examples of other new terms include Brugada syndrome, Kousseff syndrome, Sedlackova syndrome, Allgower-Donati technique, Antia-Buch chondrocutaneous advancement flap, Enteryx endoscopic procedure, acquired long QT syndrome, acute flaccid paralysis (AFP) syndrome, anosognostic syndrome, EMS (endolymphatic mastoid shunt), and complex regional pain syndrome (CRPS).

We also added many new cross-reference lists to make it easier to find terms. In past editions we listed many medical devices under the catchall term *device* when we did not have enough similar entries to justify a main category, such as *catheter* and *laser*. In the 10th edition we accumulated enough devices in the same category to justify new cross-reference lists. We pulled various therapies out of the *operation or procedure* list and made *endoscopic procedures, radiotherapy,* and *therapy* main entries.

We have many more phonetic entries in this edition to help students and practitioners interpret and spell difficult terms. For example, "air-sahzh" (hersage), "alfa-thal-trate" (alpha thalassemia trait), "first-lipped" (pursed lipped breathing), "mobes" (mobilizations), "nick-yoo" (NICU, Neonatal Intensive Care Unit), "rat" (WRAT, Wide Range Achievement Test), "seb kers" (seborrheic keratoses), "to be to a" (IIb-IIa platelet inhibitor), "fem-la" (FMLA, Family Medical Leave Act), "homo-2" (home O_2), "eff-pies" (FPIES, food protein-induced enterocolitis syndrome), "ten-ten" (specific gravity value, 1.010), "sonameter" (cm, centimeter), and "zo-med" (Xomed).

Physician dictation is characterized by medical jargon and slang terms which the medical transcriptionist must translate and expand before entering into medical reports, and the 10th edition provides scores of them with appropriate translations; for example, "beetle" (BTL, bilateral tubal ligation), "gents" (gentamicins), "at U" (at the level of the umbilicus), "moxi" (amoxicillin), "L&L panel" (liver and lipids panel). Other odd terms heard in dictation are defined: anchovy, banana bag, cookie, peanut, marshmallow, sweetheart, angry brain, hostile neck, candy-cane stirrups, cracker test, duck waddle test, jelling, and soft-pass.

The 10th edition of *Vera Pyle's Current Medical Terminology* represents primarily the research and editing efforts of Ellen Drake, CMT; Linda Campbell, CMT; and Sally C. Pitman; and the brilliant medical editing of John H. Dirckx, M.D. A special thanks to many others who provided entries for this edition, especially Stacy Brown, Georgia Green, Ann Ragle, Gail Everett, and Nola Pinkstaff. Research of new terms is an ongoing effort between editions of the book, with new terms posted on the HPI Web site (**http://www. hpisum.com**) under "Current Terms." These terms and others are gathered periodically for publication in "What's New in Medicine" in *e-Perspectives on the Medical Transcription Profession* at HPI's Web site. Even so, we performed a great deal of additional research in order to cull new terms from medical references to complete the 10th edition.

Our success in identifying hundreds of drugs that are no longer new or on the market was achieved by the hard work and professional expertise of HPI Development Editor Ellen Drake, co-author with Randy Drake of the annual *Saunders Pharmaceutical Word Book*. With access to the Drake and Drake database of pharmaceuticals, she identified medications for deletion from the previous edition and verified the accuracy of new drugs. We are greatly in her debt.

In spite of all the additions, deletions, and changes we've made over the years, Vera Pyle's favorite quote from Lewis Carroll's *Alice in Wonderland* ("What good is a book without pictures or conversations?") characterizes the 10th edition of *Vera Pyle's Current Medical Terminology*. Vera Pyle's stories about words and her word pictures set the style and tone of the book. Those of us who have worked on the book feel her spirit as we work and try to remain true to her style and her voice. She has long been our mentor.

As always, we are deeply grateful to medical transcriptionists everywhere who call and write to us with their questions and examples from medical dictation. Many tell us what they don't know and need to know, and we make every effort to research their questions and provide new terms as we find them.

Sally Crenshaw Pitman
Editor & Publisher

Contents

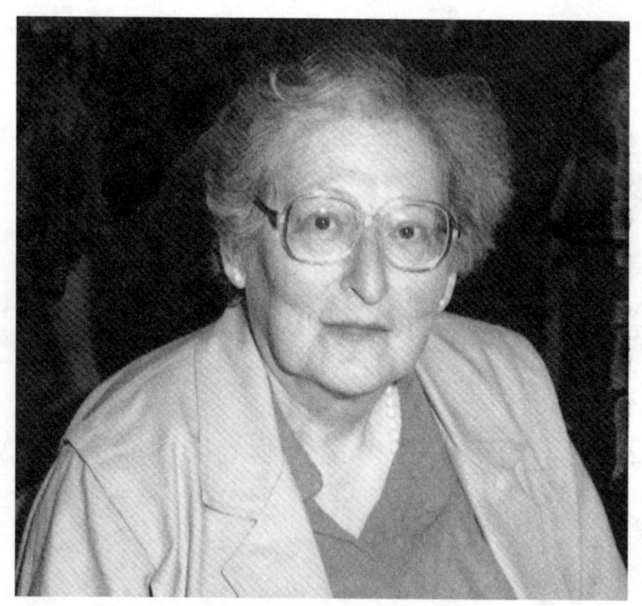

Vera Pyle, 1917-1998

Savoring Vera Pyle

One of the pivotal events in my life was meeting Vera Pyle in 1976. She taught medical transcription at City College of San Francisco and was supervisor of medical transcription at University of California Medical Center in San Francisco, and I owned a medical transcription business two hours away in Modesto, where medical transcriptionists formed a professional association. One of the inquiry letters sent to teaching hospitals in California reached Vera Pyle. She carried it back and forth from her office to her home for several weeks, planning to write an encouraging response. When her letter finally arrived, we were excited by her enthusiastic support and invited her to Modesto to speak at our November 1976 meeting. She visited my home, and that was the beginning of the beautiful friendship and mutually rewarding professional association that shaped our lives.

Vera Pyle and I worked together over the years to accomplish many things, some of them even great things. Helping to found the American Association for Medical Transcription (AAMT) in 1978, we served as national directors for two three-year terms (Vera's membership number is 12 and mine is 9). Each of us received the Distinguished Member Award, and our publishing company was the first corporate member. We have written and edited many publications and educational materials for medical transcription audiences, and we have worked together to set a professional tone and the highest professional standards for medical transcriptionists. Our leadership roles in the medical transcription profession were an essential part of the 23-year history we shared.

One of the important truths about history is that it doesn't deal just with the past, but with the present and the future. That's apparent when I think of the most valuable tangible result of our professional relationship—Vera Pyle's book, *Current Medical Terminology*. The past, the present, and the future are very much a part of this book and its importance to us as friends and professional colleagues.

Life is to be savored—an important lesson we learned from Vera Pyle. She believed life is to be lived to the fullest and then remembered and shared with fondness and joy. It isn't that she had more treasured moments than the rest of us, but that she *savored* special times and experiences and shared them with friends and family with such obvious delight. She taught us to recognize the wonders of even ordinary life. Her generosity of spirit was reflected in her enjoyment of life, which she approached with keen insight and understanding, with hope and love and kindness.

A natural storyteller, Vera had the capacity to distill simple experiences into special moments to be re-created over and over and shared with friends. Perhaps a trivial example, but the "pat of butter" story comes to mind every time I think of the word *savor* in connection with her. A few years ago she was told by her doctor to reduce her fat intake to practically zilch, so she learned to spread only a tiny bit of butter on bread and then to gingerly place a bite of bread, butter side down, on her tongue and savor the taste. So even though she couldn't eat butter the way she liked, she made sure she received the maximum benefit of what she had. Who among us is so philosophical about our self-imposed culinary deprivations?

She went to a great deal of effort to provide special treats for her friends. For weeks before Christmas she baked persimmon puddings (little rich, moist individual cakes with walnuts), and carefully packed and mailed them to friends all over the world. She gave walking *sticks* (not *canes*, she emphasized) to elderly friends and silver spoons to newborns. She believed that every child deserves to be born with a silver spoon in its mouth, and she brought silver spoons from England for each of my six grandchildren (and for other friends as well). They were not ordinary spoons, but antique silver spoons purchased from an out-of-the-way antique dealer in London. She apologized that the one she bought most recently for my granddaughter was not as old as the others; it was made as recently as 1856. She took popcorn to friends in England, and a can of Spam to a friend who wondered if it would taste as good now as it did during World War II. And she brought me "worry beads" from Greece.

She savored friends and family. She never tried to impose her own desires or prejudices on anyone else, firmly believing that intelligent people should make their own choices, and she maintained that spirit of independence up until her death of cancer on July 24, 1998. What she said of her friend and mentor Dan Pae applies even more to her. "She passed through life—and made a difference." Her life has immeasurably enriched ours.

Sally Crenshaw Pitman

Adapted from editorial comments by Sally Pitman in *Perspectives on the Medical Transcription Profession*, "Our History" (Winter-Spring 1997-98), and "Savoring Life" (Summer 1998), published by Health Professions Institute.

Vera Pyle's Silver Book

I can see the handwriting on the wall—and it is misspelled.

One thing I have learned is that this is proving a bigger project than I had anticipated.

This is a continuing learning process, and one of the things I've learned is this: There is more than one right way.

How far should we go in trying to verify a word? One can spend hours researching a word, but in my book, that's artsy-craftsy, not professional.

What I am finding in medical word research is that nothing is gospel, nothing is graven on the tablet. It just depends on which tablet you check. This shakes your confidence, for how can you be as perfect as humanly possible when there are so many chances for error?

Medical transcriptionists don't dictate, physicians do.

Praise and credit rise to the highest person on the totem pole, criticism and blame fall on the lowest.

Collectively we could come up with many other quotable quotes from Vera Pyle. Her emphasis on quality medical transcription and the highest professional standards made her one of the most respected members of our profession. She provided an eloquent voice for medical transcriptionists. "Let me tell you a story" prefaced many of her favorite anecdotes, and they invariably ended with "Now you know all I know." And if you asked, "Are you sure?" she would inhale and launch another story.

Vera Pyle's love of *words* characterized her professional life. "How do you spell it and what is your source?" introduced her first column of new, difficult, and hard-to-find medical terms in November 1979, when she first began writing for medical transcriptionists. *Vera Pyle's Current Medical Terminology* is the first edition released since her death in 1998. It continues the professional traditions she established over twenty years ago.

Every book in its eighth edition has a history. What is apparent in the proud owners of the previous editions of *Current Medical Terminology* is that their fondness of the book is inextricably linked with their affection and respect for its author. For over twenty years Vera Pyle was associated with the best in medical transcription. To those who know and love this book and its author, it is often known as "the silver bullet," "my Vera," "Pyle," or "my bible."

Current Medical Terminology was written *by* medical transcriptionists especially *for* medical transcriptionists, although physicians and other health-care professionals find it useful as well. The unique qualities of the book are immediately apparent to anyone who gives more than a cursory glance at the words and phrases defined. First of all, the definitions are interesting, some even chatty, a few humorous or ironic, and many have quotations to show how the terms are used in medical dictation. Extensive cross-references help the reader on a word-search.

Vera Pyle always thought we are all word freaks. Long ago she wrote, "If I were cast away on a desert island, the book I would probably want to take with me is an *Unabridged Webster's* and I could be happy for years. Couldn't you? We get lost in a dictionary. We look up a word and we see something else that is exciting, and we look up another word, and so on. It's a common symptom among medical transcriptionists. I myself would rather have a dozen new medical words, researched and defined, than a five-pound box of candy. And I bet you would too."

As a lexicographer, Pyle never took her responsibility lightly, nor did she consider herself a self-appointed expert on medical language. Researching new medical terms and writing definitions proved to be a bigger challenge than she anticipated when she volunteered in 1979 to compile a list of new terms for bimonthly issues of *The AAMT Newsletter*. She spent hundreds of hours doing research in medical journals, dictionaries, equipment catalogs, and textbooks; corresponding with medical transcriptionists in all work settings; questioning physicians, nurses, pharmacists, surgical technicians, and lab technologists; and persuading friends in Central Supply to read her exactly how the name of an instrument was written on the package. That was many years before the Internet provided instant access to medical references.

Despite endless efforts to be correct in her findings, she admitted regretfully, "There has been a time or two—or three—that I have rushed to press, triumphantly, with a word hot out of the operating room, newly born, nowhere else to be found, a real scoop—only to find it in print at a later date, and to learn that it had been given us—wrong."

Editing a word list for medical transcriptionists is not a job for the faint-hearted. Medical transcriptionists are necessarily perfectionists and can be ruthless in their criticism of anyone who makes an *error* in spelling or defining a new medical term. Criticism, lots of it, is to be expected and borne with equanimity. Over the years Vera Pyle necessarily developed a thick skin.

When she first began writing, her task was to provide a *reliable* and *immediate* source of information to tens of thousands of medical transcriptionists. She recognized that medical transcriptionists need the words as soon as they are used in dictation; they cannot wait until they appear in dictionaries and reference books updated every five to ten years.

When she published spellings that were later proved incorrect, she was flooded with mail from irate readers. She was sure her mailman thought she was giving away gold bricks. One reader chastised her: "We need to 'know' when the dictator 'knows,' not after the fact. . . . If we knew the 'new' words by preview, the time and effort saved could be tremendous!" Pyle responded to the criticism with a marvelous fantasy of a modern-day Paul Revere who would ride through the countryside, shouting out the new terms that medical transcriptionists would need in the next day's dictation.

She tried to provide something for everybody. Deciding which words were worthy of inclusion in a word list was the first challenge. How could she be sure a word new to her was new to others in the field? She tried to determine if new terms will stand the test of time and not be merely faddish, trendy, highly personal, or regional among certain doctors. "My own criteria for using new words or slang would be (1) need for the word or term, (2) broad understanding of the term, and (3) potential for survival." Good judgment and a wealth of experience in medical transcription served her well.

Writing for a national audience of medical transcriptionists means that terms might be commonly used in certain regions of the country and not yet in circulation elsewhere. Doctors' in-language and jargon in one setting might not be accepted in other settings. Pyle often had to translate examples of abbreviations, acronyms, and brief forms that hospital residents and interns sprinkled in their dictation—a kind of medical "short-tongue" she thought made them feel professional. They often coined terms like *CABG* ("cabbage") and *COWS*, and she translated, defined, and illustrated how they are used in dictation.

COWS (cold to the opposite, warm to the same)—a mnemonic device to help remember the Hallpike caloric stimulation response. "Caloric testing produced COWS." See *caloric testing*.

Understanding new procedures and explaining them to someone else in an interesting way, without being too technical, is always a challenge. Pyle's wonder and fascination with new techniques and her ability to describe them to a nontechnical audience are apparent in this definition:

subtraction films (Radiol)—a method to visualize the arteries and veins on x-ray. A scout film is taken first, before the dye is injected. The scout negative is made into a positive (darkens it). Then the angiogram is taken (this is a negative). Then a scout positive is taken and put under the dye-injected negative (the patient, not the film, has had the dye injection), which screens out the bone, so all that is then visible are the arteries and veins.

She believed that a picture was worth a thousand words, and she often used examples from dictation in order to provide a context and a word picture for an unusual phrase:

palmar beak ligament (Ortho)—"It has been suggested that instability resulting from incompetence of the palmar beak ligament is responsible for initiating the progression of degenerative joint disease."

She made a special effort to explain terms used commonly in medical dictation but not defined elsewhere. Students and trainees in medical transcription found such definitions as the following particularly helpful:

pack-year smoking history—the packs per day multiplied by the number of years of smoking; the cumulative result is the important factor. Usage: "The patient has a 50-pack-year smoking history." The patient has smoked a pack a day for 50 years, or two packs a day for 25 years, or five packs a day for ten years (or ten packs a day for five years!).

One of Vera Pyle's most treasured compliments came from a physician who was chair of the medical record committee in the teaching hospital where she supervised the medical transcription department: "The medical transcriptionists make my residents appear to be better dictators than I know them to be." She always had enormous respect for physicians who were as conscientious in their dictation practices as in their medical practice. She taught us not to accept a doctor's spelling as definitive, but to appreciate the effort of a thoughtful physician giving a hint on the spelling of an unfamiliar new term or test.

She encouraged us to transcribe with accuracy and sensitivity what the dictators *mean*, not just what they *say*. Too medically sophisticated to insist on verbatim transcription, she nevertheless believed it's important not to tamper with a physician's dictating style, not to impose our own style and preferences on medical reports. The dictation is to represent their style, not ours. A physician's style may need judicious editing, of course, but not *tampering*.

In the early years of producing word lists, somebody wrote to her, "Why don't you have *your staff* research the words more carefully?" "I am 'the staff'," she replied. But she enlisted the help of medical transcriptionists everywhere to contribute new terms they had encountered in dictation. "You're all medical word researchers on your own, on your jobs," she wrote. "New medical words tend to surface at university teaching hospitals, but a lot of you out there know things I don't know that haven't yet surfaced here. If you know enough to pick up on these things after we print them, why don't you tell me about them early on, before I fall on my face?"

Over the years Pyle's "staff" has grown to include many medical transcriptionists and others who have provided examples of new terms encountered in dictation. HPI staff and associates—Linda Campbell, Ellen Drake, Diane Heath, Georgia Green, Kathy Cameron, and John H. Dirckx, M.D.—have provided primary research, editing, and proofreading skills in production of each edition of the book.

In the early and mid-1980s, Bron Taylor of San Francisco contributed extensive lists of new AIDS terminology, when AIDS awareness was just beginning. Susan Turley provided scores of chemotherapy protocols and specialized nursing terms in the 1980s and early 1990s.

Of special help in this eighth edition were the many contributions of Arleen McGovern and Toni Mercandante from the popular Web site, *MT Desk.com.*

Now you know all I know. . . . I wish.

Sally Crenshaw Pitman
Editor & Publisher

Adapted from Sally Pitman, "Vera Pyle's Silver Book," *Perspectives on the Medical Transcription Profession* (Winter-Spring 1997-98, pp. 22-23), published by Health Professions Institute.

Preface

Words are a large part of the stock-in-trade of the medical transcriptionist, and we encounter new ones every day. There is the usual flurry of identifying the new word: "What do you hear? Yes, that's what I heard. What is it? What does it mean? How do you spell it? What's your source?"

Much has happened in medicine in the last ten years—monoclonal antibodies, magnetic resonance imaging (MRI), DNA recombinant method of producing biosynthetic hormones and other products, breakthroughs in our knowledge of cell function and reproduction, new methods of treatment without resorting to surgery, investigational drugs for treatment of AIDS and cancer. With all of these innovations, there are thousands of new words which, if you haven't yet heard, you soon will. In medicine, we can hardly say "current" for very long; thus, it is necessary to update *Current Medical Terminology* every two years.

New features include definitions of many specialized terms used in surgery and radiology. Under the entry *medication* is a quick-reference list of all the pharmaceuticals defined in main entries throughout the book, including drugs used in treating AIDS patients, chemicals, chemotherapy drugs and protocols, classes of drugs, contrast media, investigational drugs, natural substances, prescription and over-the-counter drugs, monoclonal antibodies, orphan drugs, radioisotopes, and solutions. In most cases we have listed both generic and brand name, the latter with capitalization where needed. Other lengthy quick-reference lists include those under main entries *device, disease, MRI terms, operation, pathogen, syndrome,* and *test*.

Extensive cross-referencing has been done. In most cases, the definition will appear with the form of the word most often used in dictation. That is, if the acronym, abbreviation, or brief form of the word is that most often dictated, then the definition will appear under that term, with a cross-reference to the other form. Sometimes a medical transcriptionist can hear or understand only one word of a phrase dictated by a physician; thus, cross-referencing under other important words of a phrase is provided.

I hope you will find this book even more useful than the earlier editions, which I know you all took to your hearts.

Vera Pyle, CMT
March 1998

Introduction

This book is intended primarily for medical transcriptionists, but now I find that it is also being used by court reporters, health information management professionals, coders, legal secretaries, nurses, and students in the allied health professions. Also, with the continued importance of the patient's medical record in reimbursement systems, insurance claims examiners and Medicare evaluators refer to it as well. The recent increase in medicolegal cases has driven court reporters to expand their medical knowledge and reference libraries, and many have found this book to be a valuable tool. So it now becomes necessary to keep a diverse group of readers in mind.

Most medical transcriptionists are either hospital-based or work for offsite transcription services. They transcribe and edit the very detailed and highly technical medical and surgical reports that are used in the delivery of medical care. These written reports assure that everyone involved in that care knows the patient's medical history, what was found on physical examination and on laboratory examinations, the pathology discovered, the treatment given, the medications administered, and the response to therapy noted.

These reports are of importance medically and legally, and in research. They are valued by everyone who uses them (they are often the only legible documents in a patient's record), but the people who transcribe them are largely unknown, individually and as a profession.

New medical terms crop up daily—new medications, new operative procedures, new instruments, new equipment, new techniques, new research terms, new laboratory tests, new abbreviations—many of them—and with little documentation except for a physician's occasional attempt at spelling. It therefore becomes necessary to provide a reliable and immediate source of information to tens of thousands of medical transcriptionists.

References are made throughout the book to "the dictator." These definitions were originally written for an "in-group" of medical transcriptionists who know that "the dictator" refers to the physician or medical student or other healthcare professional who dictates the medical and surgical reports.

Perhaps an explanation is in order at this time to help familiarize new readers with how I research terms, and how I arrive at conclusions (or decisions) when research fails.

Many years ago when my younger daughter was five or six, I overheard an argument she was having with one of her playmates. I don't now recall what it was all about, but I do remember my daughter's clinching argument—"My mother says . . ." Her friend was not prepared to challenge Taffy's mother; end of argument.

No one since then has appointed me The Higher Authority, and the self-appointed are setting themselves up for being leaders with no followers. So I feel that ours must be a collaborative venture. We give our opinions, our reasons for them, and our sources. Our readers may evaluate our conclusions, discuss their differences of opinion, and decide to accept them or not. I hasten to add that we all have a strong instinct for self-preservation and try to make certain that our sources are generally respected and accepted and that our conclusions are those we can defend.

Where do we find entries for *Current Medical Terminology*? From words encountered in medical transcription, from questions from medical transcriptionists, from dozens of medical journals we read regularly. We consult medical textbooks, talk to physicians, and have friends in central supply. Over the years we have learned to be less trusting of the written, as well as the spoken, word.

Of all sources, dictionaries are perhaps my most trusted, although I have found errors in even the most respected. Next are books, although I am finding that they, too, often have errors; apparently proofreading is considered an expendable luxury. I should mention that books do have the disadvantage of being dated, even when newly published. Somewhere at the top of the list would be the trusted person in central supply who will read the label on the equipment, instrument, or medication container, although there are times when there may be more than one spelling, as in *Tycron* and *Ti-Cron*. Next are journals, in which I find the most current information available, but I do find errors in even the most prestigious.

A close tie for last place on my list of trusted sources would be catalogs of instrument manufacturers and the spelling given us by physicians. An old newspaperman once told me that typesetters were given instructions to "follow the copy, even if it goes out the window." There are a few physicians whose spelling is impeccable and whose dictation I *would* "follow out the window," but, unfortunately, they are all too few.

In researching words, sometimes hunches and the educated guess based on experience and the knowledge of analogous words or terms are all one has to go on and are useful. Here is an example: I came across the word *Versatex* as a cardiac pacemaker. I should tell you that it is fatal in this situation to trust; it is *essential* that one question—everything and always. At any rate I felt uncomfortable with that spelling (it was guilty until proven innocent), and I decided to pursue it further. Unable to document it, but finding analogous terms (Activitrax and Spectrax), I felt quite comfortable with the spelling *Versatrax*.

A reader inquired about *Angiocath PRN* and wanted to know the meaning of *PRN*. My first information about Angiocath PRN, trade name of a catheter manufactured by Siemens Medical Systems, came from the *Journal of Neurosurgery*. I can only hazard a more-or-less educated guess as to what is meant. As you know, *p.r.n.* (L. *pro re nata*) means "as circumstances may require." This catheter has many different uses and the PRN may *perhaps* make reference to that.

Medical equipment manufacturers and pharmaceutical companies are most imaginative in creating names for their products. They are so clever, and running these things to earth is so frustrating. Sometimes they provide clues, e.g., Cefobid is a third-generation cephalosporin medication (which accounts for the first syllable) and is to be taken twice a day (b.i.d.), which accounts for the last syllable.

Sometimes there is no clue; one has to know what the device or medication is used for to know what the abbreviation means, e.g., the EID percutaneous central venous large-bore catheter manufactured by Arrow International, Inc. The *EID* turns out to mean *e*mergency *i*nfusion *d*evice! Or how about the SRT vaginal speculum by Amko Manufacturing Company? The *SRT* is from *s*moke *r*emoval *t*ube; the device has a supplementary tube used when smoke evacuation is necessary in laser-induced tissue vaporization.

A few years ago I searched for the definitive spelling of a needle we've been spelling *Verres* for many years. I got a letter from a medical transcriptionist who said she had been told by a physician that that spelling was in error, that it should be *Veress*. She said that she had looked in a dozen different textbooks and the spelling she found was indeed *Veress*, and she also sent me a photocopy of an article about this needle, written by the physician who had developed it, a Dr. Veress. We must assume that Dr. Veress knows how to spell his name, so we have now changed our spelling of this instrument to *Veress*.

In the medical field we don't have to look far or wait long for new words, abbreviations, and acronyms to appear. Just stand still for a couple of hours and a dozen new ones will have been born!

Vera Pyle, CMT
July 1992

A Medical Transcriptionist's Fantasy

A letter from a reader came in yesterday's mail. I thought about it during a sleepless night and at 3 a.m. arose from my bed, sat down in front of the typewriter, and ventilated.

Prices on many things have gone through the roof; dinner out, a play, even a film, are now rare treats. But there is something we can still afford—fantasy.

First, let me quote from the letter:

> *I will again bring to your attention an item I mentioned in a previous survey, to which I have never received a response either directly or indirectly. That is—the providing of information, be it names of newly approved drugs, newly developed prostheses, etc. I recently noted a reprint in one of the local newsletters from another professional journal. It contained "new" items. Although our present Notebook is terrific, it is just too limited to provide us with the information we require; that is, we need to "know" when the dictator "knows," not after the fact. Every time a "new" word is dictated, it involves excessive time and effort not only on the part of the transcriptionists, but on the part of the people they ask for help in listening, only to determine in the end that the spelling is not available to them because it is a "new" item, at which point either the word is researched or left blank for fill-in. If we knew the "new" words by preview, the time and effort saved could be tremendous!*

Now, let us fantasize. Wouldn't it be marvelous if we had a modern-day Paul Revere who would ride through the countryside shouting, not "The British are coming!" but instead "lithotriptor!—a new extracorporeal stone-disintegrating machine! First used in Europe, now being brought to the United States! Generates shock that breaks up kidney stones! Lowercase 'L'!"—as he rides off into the cold, starry night. Or how about "Kim-Ray Greenfield filter—used in prevention of pulmonary emboli! Kim-Ray is capitalized and hyphenated!" as he gallops, on his panting, snorting, sweating horse, to the next darkened village.

Let's fantasize further. Wouldn't it be wonderful if Dr. Andreas Grüntzig had called us and said: "Just wanted to let you know that I'm inventing a new balloon catheter; it will be a very nice thing to use in transluminal dilatation and in performing angioplasties. And, by the way, my name is spelled

G-r-ü-n-t-z-i-g, in which case don't forget the umlaut over the *u*; or else, you can spell it *Gruentzig*, but in that case, don't use the umlaut. However, I will answer to either."

Or—if Dr. Richard Osgood had written, "You may be interested in being among the first to know that my colleague, Dr. Carl Schlatter (that's spelled S-c-h-l-a-t-t-e-r; don't forget the *c*, and remember there are two *t*'s), and I have just identified a new disease entity—osteochondrosis of the tuberosity of the tibia; also called apophysitis tibialis adolescentium, which we are going to call 'Osgood-Schlatter disease.' If he should call you and tell you about this and tells you it is 'Schlatter-Osgood' disease, remember you heard it from me first, and correctly!"

There has been the time or two—or three—that I have rushed to press, triumphantly, with a word hot out of the operating room, newly born, nowhere else to be found, a real scoop—only to find it in print at a later date, and to learn that it had been given us—wrong.

Paul Revere, where are you now that we need you?

Adapted from Vera Pyle, "A Medical Transcriptionist's Fantasy," *Journal of the American Association for Medical Transcription*, Winter 1983-84, p. 3.

In Defense of "Sterilely"

A question from a medical transcriptionist about the word *sterilely* prompted the following responses. They are quoted here to illustrate the dilemma medical transcriptionists face in striving for accuracy, and a warning about what might happen if they forget that *physicians dictate and medical transcriptionists transcribe.*

The question was how to spell the adverb form of the word *sterile*. The inquirer wrote:

> *I say that if you use this word as an adverb, you retain the original form of the word and add "-ly," making the spelling* sterilely, *as it is in* futile, puerile, hostile, *etc. My colleagues see no point in dragging grammar into this and spell the word* sterilly, *as in* "Sterilly *we roll along."*

This is one of the questions to which I can say, with confidence, there is one and only one correct answer. The word is *sterilely*. I refer you to *Webster's Third International Dictionary, Unabridged* (1981), and to the *Random House Dictionary of the English Language, Unabridged,* 2nd ed. (1987); this is the only spelling given for this word.

I have just finished reading a book (in the nonmedical part of my life) about the people who colonized New England in the early 1600s, the Pilgrims and Puritans. Much of the journal written by Governor William Bradford of Plymouth was quoted, as well as letters written by many of the other men involved in the affairs of the Colony. Many of them were men of education, men who had studied at Cambridge. It was most interesting to see their spelling. In Elizabethan times there were no hard and fast spelling rules, and each person spelled as the spirit moved him, not even consistently with any individual. Shakespeare himself spelled his name a number of different ways. In those days this was not considered flouting of rules, since there were few if any rules. But that was then, and this is now.

Now there are dictionaries and rules. Sometimes there is more than one spelling of a word, and dictionaries will give preferred ones and acceptable ones. However, now, if one were to spell in a very personal manner, disregarding the rules, one would be open to criticism. And here I might give you Pyle's observation: Praise and credit rise to the highest person on the totem pole; criticism and blame fall on the lowest. So you see, we can ill afford to be cavalier about such things as correct spelling and grammar. Remember, we are judged and evaluated by people who know the rules and play by them, and they expect us to observe them as well.

A few months later I received the following comment, and apparently it struck a nerve; hence, the following response:

> *It was interesting to read the debate on the spelling of the word* sterilely. *Occasionally, due to progress in the English language, certain words or versions of certain words become outdated.* Sterilely *is one of them. I feel that proper grammar would dictate that we transcriptionists use the present-day terminology "in a sterile manner."*

Sterilely is not among my very favorite words. "I love you" and "I love your book" are higher on my list. Not too far behind comes ". . . the patient was taken to the recovery room in good condition." But I rise to the defense of *sterilely* for several reasons. First of all, there is nothing wrong with the word. Where has it been decreed that it is "outdated"? Words die when they are no longer viable and therefore no longer used. *Sterilely* is very much alive. If you don't believe it, transcribe operative reports in any hospital. If you don't want to believe it, just tell every surgeon in the country that it may no longer be used, that it is a forbidden word.

Imagine the unleashed fury of fifty thousand surgeons when they are told they may no longer say the WORD. I can see the backlash now—thousands of angry surgeons under the cover of night surging into the streets, chalking on fences and spray-painting on walls the naughty word—STERILELY, or possibly even (perish the thought) *sterilly*.

Carried to its logical conclusion, this stance puts us in the position of saying that physicians are permitted to use only those words that all transcriptionists can spell. Carried further there will then be no need for dictionaries, for drug books, for word books. Sounds like a dream, doesn't it? Now comes the alarm clock, shrilling the end of the dream. *Medical transcriptionists don't dictate, physicians do.*

I urge you—cease and desist. Don't type "The patient was draped in a sterile manner" when the surgeon dictates "The patient was sterilely draped," or the fence-chalking, spray-painting surgeons are likely to burn us in effigy.

Adapted from Vera Pyle, "A Question of Style," *Journal of the American Association for Medical Transcription*, Winter 1984-85, Fall 1985.

Medical Slang—Its Use and Abuse

The language of medicine is an "in-language." It is the means of communication for a comparatively small, select group in a world divided into "us" and "them." Its use makes one feel part of that group of "us's." Medical abbreviations and medical slang are subspecies of this language (slanguage?) and are particularly dear to the hearts of the newest members of the in-group.

Its use makes medical students feel that they sound "professional." It has much the same effect as wearing a stethoscope. To only a slightly lesser degree, this applies also to the intern and resident. I once asked a resident in surgery the reason for this. He thought about it for a while, grinned, and replied, "Well, when you've just learned all these new long words, it's a pity not to use them, and you must admit that some of them *are* pretty impressive." Interestingly enough, the truly impressive people in medicine speak simply, almost in lay language.

Language changes. It is far from static. The English we speak now is far from the English of Chaucer or Shakespeare. The language of medicine also changes. Many of these changes fill a real need, in which case they are likely to last. Some of this change is frivolous, "trendy," highly personal, and likely to be understood by few. Much of this language is not yet found in dictionaries for these reasons. Dictionaries, after all, are *de*scriptive, not *pre*scriptive, and many of these words are too new, too ephemeral, too localized to make their way into dictionaries. And for these same reasons, we cannot be certain that we can use them safely in reports which are considered legal documents.

I think we must take a long look at what is now being dictated, and we may find it necessary to accept terms that have been frowned on in the past, that have not yet been accepted in dictionaries but are used constantly by physicians because they fill a need.

Some twenty years ago, we began hearing the word "bovied" but were told, "You can't make a verb of a noun." So we would type, "Bleeders were electrocoagulated with the Bovie unit." All these years later, I find "bovied" still used a great deal—a useful term, succinct, and universally understood. Another such word is "saucerize," which refers to creation of a saucer-shaped excavation surgically.

I believe 20/20 hindsight might well be the determining factor in knowing what is a needed term, likely to survive and ultimately enter the language, and what is for the moment "flip," likely to have only narrow, local application, and short survival. My own criteria for using new words or slang would be (1) need for the word or term, (2) broad understanding of the term, and (3) potential for survival.

A new slang expression I have encountered only occasionally is "romied" and it may or may not last. Although it may fill a need, it is not commonly understood. I am not prepared to use it. It is a verb coined from the acronym ROMI, *r*ule *o*ut *m*yocardial *i*nfarction, and used thus: "The patient was admitted with severe precordial pain and cardiac arrhythmias, and was romied." My guess is that it is one of those terms that will not have wide circulation and will not survive because too few will know the acronym from which it is derived. It is an example of a sub-subspecies of an in-language, and may be known to some cardiologists (probably the newest of them only) and hence will not be a viable means of communication to a broader spectrum of the medical population.

It should also be remembered that our spoken language differs from our written (more formal) language, and that terms used in the operating room or on the ward are not necessarily what should be written in a report.

The following are other examples of acronyms that have become words: CABG (coronary artery bypass graft) and pronounced "cabbage," as in "The patient was given a CABG," or even "The patient was CABG'd." These evoke rather interesting images. (We have the option of using the acronyms or writing out the terms in full.) You may be astonished to hear a physician dictate, "Caloric testing produced COWS." "COWS" stands for "cold to the opposite, warm to the same" and is a mnemonic device used in otolaryngology to help remember the Hallpike caloric stimulation response.

It may be interesting to enter the arcane world of the operating room and discover the slang peculiar to it. For example, a "peanut" is a small gauze sponge used in surgery. This word is in widespread use, but some operating room personnel have their own terms for it. Cotton pledgets are small cotton balls (sponges) which are rolled so that they have somewhat pointed ends. They are used to absorb blood or other fluids from the operative site. In some parts of the country they are known as "pollywogs." The term "stick-tie" means different things to different people in different operating rooms. In some operating rooms it refers to a suture ligature, or transfixion suture; in others it refers to a long strand of suture clamped on a hemostat. If a surgeon asks the scrub nurse for "Mets" (or "Metz"), Metzenbaum scissors are wanted. It is understandable that under the time pressures in surgery, "OR shorthand" would be used, but in a formal document the word should be transcribed "Metzenbaum scissors."

In the dim, distant past, some words originated as medical slang and are now firmly rooted in our language. "Gurney" is one such. I do not know its origin; it may well have been a trade name. It may also have been the brainchild of someone in one hospital and traveled with surgeons or nurses to others across the country. None of the references I have consulted gives a derivation. It is, however, such a commonly used word that it would be absurd now to say, "The patient was placed on a high wheeled cart for moving patients in a hospital and taken to the operating room."

So you see, we are dealing with not only the present but also the past and the future. We can, to some degree, judge from the kinds of words that have been accepted and have survived over the years which ones will have currency in the future. A surgical word we hear all the time is "prepped." Most attending surgeons with whose dictation I am familiar use "prepared." "Prepped" is, however, universally understood, and my inclination is to type whatever the dictator says; if residents feel that they are being "professional" by using it, I won't argue the point. It seems a lost cause anyhow. Perhaps I am getting too old to fight for lost causes; perhaps my sense of proportion tells me it's not worth it, or perhaps I am saving my ammunition for more important issues.

The purpose in dictating all this material, and the purpose in transcribing it, is communication—with other physicians, with nurses, with other healthcare professionals and paraprofessionals; with quality assurance, billing, risk management people; with insurance companies; with lawyers. If we are not successful in this communication, if we are "playing doctor" by being exclusionary with our in-language, if we are obfuscating rather than clarifying, what then is the point in all this effort?

Actually, I have more questions than I have answers. But these are questions that must be raised. I do want to be clear, to be understandable. It is *not*, I repeat, *not* our role to force doctors to do anything our way. This is not in any way a crusade. Doctors like us to be right, but they do resent our being righteous!

Adapted from Vera Pyle, "Medical Slang—Its Use and Abuse," *Journal of the American Association for Medical Transcription*, Fall 1983, pp. 38-39.

Notes

Sequence. Entries are alphabetized letter by letter, without regard to periods, spaces, and hyphens in main entries and subentries; the *'s* and *s'* of possessives are ignored in alphabetizing. Initial numbers are alphabetized as if they were written out, although subscript and superscript numbers are ignored.

Medical specialties. To provide a context in which a term is likely to be encountered in medical transcription, one or more medical specialties may appear in parentheses in an entry. Medical specialties are not listed when they are obvious in context.

Anes	Anesthesiology
Cardio	Cardiology; Cardiac Surgery
Derm	Dermatology
ENT	Ear, Nose, and Throat
GI	Gastroenterology
Lab	Laboratory Medicine
Neonat	Neonatology
Nuclear Med	Nuclear Medicine
Neuro	Neurology; Neurosurgery
Ob-Gyn	Obstetrics-Gynecology
Oph	Ophthalmology
Oncol	Oncology
Oral Surg	Oral Surgery
Ortho	Orthopedics; Orthopedic Surgery
Path	Pathology
Peds	Pediatrics
Phys Ther	Physical Therapy
Plas Surg	Plastic Surgery
Pod	Podiatric Surgery
Psych	Psychiatry
Pulm	Pulmonary Medicine
Radiol	Radiology
Rad Oncol	Radiation Oncology
Rehab	Rehabilitation; Physical Medicine
Resp Ther	Respiratory Therapy
Thor Surg	Thoracic Surgery
Urol	Urology
Vasc Surg	Vascular Surgery

A, a

AA (acetabular anteversion).

AAA (abdominal aortic aneurysm, "triple A")—medical slang.

AAA (anterior apical aneurysm). Cf. AAA (abdominal aortic aneurysm).

AAI (axial acetabular index).

AAMI (age-associated memory impairment).

AAMT (American Association for Medical Transcription)—a membership organization for medical transcriptionists. See *Certified Medical Transcriptionist*.

A&W—jargon for *alive and well,* usually referring to parents and siblings in the family history. Expand when encountered in dictation.

Aaron sign—pain on pressure over McBurney point in a patient with appendicitis.

Aarskog syndrome—characterized by shawl scrotum, long philtrum, short stature, downward eye slant, and thoracic deformity.

ab, Ab, AB (abortion or miscarriage; abortus) (Ob-Gyn)—common abbreviations used in dictation. *AB 2* (or *Ab 2*, *ab 2*) means that the patient has had two abortions or miscarriages. Cf. *GPMAL*.

abacavir sulfate, lamivudine, and zidovudine—see *Epzicom*.

ABBA (axillobilateral breast approach) —an approach used in endoscopic thyroid surgery.

Abbe-McIndoe vaginal construction—uses split-thickness skin grafts.

ABBI (advanced breast biopsy instrumentation) **system**—a device used to perform breast biopsies. In a one-step process, the ABBI device removes the entire specimen for biopsy. May also be referred to as the *ABBI procedure*.

Abbott-Rawson tube—a long gastrointestinal double-lumen tube.

Abbreviated Injury Scale (AIS).

ABC (Adriamycin, BCNU, cyclophosphamide)—chemotherapy protocol.

ABC (airway, breathing, circulation).

ABC (argon beam coagulator).

ABCD (amphotericin B colloid dispersion)—a drug used to treat cryptococcal meningitis in AIDS patients.

ABCD rule of dermatoscopy—diagnostic method of identifying malig-

ABCD *(cont.)*
nant melanoma with the use of a microscope. The parameters are asymmetry, border, color, and differential structure. See *dermatoscope.*

abdominal compartment syndrome (ACS)—a sustained increase in intra-abdominal pressure due to alterations in respiratory mechanics, cardiovascular hemodynamics, and renal function. The syndrome may follow laparotomy for severe abdominal trauma, ruptured abdominal aortic aneurysm, and intra-abdominal infection. Only recently recognized, it carries a death rate of over 50%.

abdominal cutaneous nerve entrapment syndrome—a common source of unexplained severe abdominal pain. The cause is believed to be compression of the rectus muscle channel, creating ischemia of the ninth thoracolumbar nerve.

abdominal-sacral colpoperineopexy—a modified version of the abdominal sacrocolpopexy to correct posterior compartment defects and perineal descent associated with vaginal vault prolapse.

abdominal sacrocolpopexy—uses a strip of fascia or inorganic mesh to repair uterine prolapse via the abdominal route.

abduct—to draw away from a position parallel to the median axis. Cf. *adduct*.

"a-b-duction"—dictated by a physician to clarify that **ab**duction, not **ad**duction, is intended.

abduction and external rotation (ABER) **position**.

ABER (abduction and external rotation) **position**—a technique used in MRI scan for improved detection of a horizontal component in partial-thickness tears of the rotator cuff.

Aberdeen knot (Surg)—a crochet knot popularized by Cushieri, used in laparoscopic suturing procedures. See *convertible slip knot*.

aberrant—wandering or deviating from the normal; abnormal. Cf. *apparent*.

aberrant crypt foci (ACF)—microscopic lesions of the colonic mucosa suspected of being preneoplastic.

aberrant ribonucleic acid—halts the production of the EAAT2 protein. A new test is being developed to detect this aberrant ribonucleic acid in the hopes of early detection of amyotrophic lateral sclerosis (Lou Gehrig disease).

ab-externo laser sclerotomy.

ABGs (arterial blood gases)—refer to PO_2, PCO_2, and oxygen saturation. From these data and the serum pH, the bicarbonate (or base excess) can be calculated.

ABI—see *ankle-brachial index*.

Abilify (aripiprazole)—a medication used in the treatment of acute bipolar mania, including manic and mixed episodes associated with bipolar disorder.

ab-interno laser sclerotomy.

AbioCor implantable replacement heart.

abirritant—a soothing agent.

ABI Vest airway clearance system (the "Vest")—a portable device consisting of an inflatable vest connected by hose to an air-pulse generator which rapidly inflates and deflates the vest, compressing and releasing the chest wall, moving mucus toward the larger airways where it can be cleared by coughing or suctioning. Used by cystic fibrosis patients. Commonly referred to as *high*

ABI *(cont.)* *frequency chest wall oscillation* (HFCWO). See also *ThAIRapy Vest.*

Ablatherm HIFU system—uses high-intensity focused ultrasound (HIFU) for endorectal treatment of localized prostate cancer. The procedure provides a nonsurgical alternative to surgical excision and radioactive seed implantation.

ablation—separation, eradication, extirpation, as in cryoablation, radiofrequency ablation.

ablation catheter—a long thin flexible tube that sends radiofrequency (RF) energy to the inside of the heart to destroy abnormal conduction pathways responsible for some cardiac arrhythmias.

ablation planner topography—see *Humphrey Systems ablation planner topography.*

ablative therapy with bone marrow rescue—an acceptable mode of therapy for many types of cancer.

ablepharon macrostomia syndrome (AMS)—inherited disorder in which the face, head, genitals, and abdomen do not develop normally. Children with AMS may experience delays in language development and, in some cases, mental retardation.

ABMT (autologous bone marrow transplantation).

abnormal bowel wall enhancement—a finding on CT possibly indicative of ischemia (also seen in hypotensive shock bowel).

abnormal uterine bleeding (AUB).

abortus (ab, Ab, AB)—miscarriage(s). See *ab, Ab, AB.*

ABPA (allergic bronchopulmonary aspergillosis).

ABPM (ambulatory blood pressure monitoring).

ABR (auditory brain stem response)—an audiometric technique to test for sensorineural hearing loss.

Abraxane (albumin nanoparticle paclitaxel)—a medication for treatment of metastatic breast cancer.

abreaction (Psych)—the reliving of an experience in such a way that previously repressed emotions associated with it are released.

abscess—circumscribed, localized collection of pus, usually caused by infection, and by the decomposition of tissue. Example: collar button abscess. See *Brodie abscess.* Cf. *aphthous.*

Abscession—biliary drainage catheter.

absence seizures—pronounced "ab-sahnz."

absent bow-tie sign—used to identify bucket-handle tears of the knee menisci on MR imaging. Cf. *bow-tie sign of cervical fracture.*

absent breath sounds—jargon term substituted for "absence of" in awkward expressions such as "auscultation revealed absent breath sounds."

Absolok extra absorbable ligating clips.

absolute neutrophil count (ANC).

absorbent—agent or material that takes up or soaks up another material (usually a liquid). Cf. *adsorbent.*

ACA (anticentromere antibody).

ACAD (atherosclerotic carotid artery disease).

acamprosate calcium—see *Campral.*

***Acanthamoeba* keratitis**—an inflammation of the cornea caused by *Acanthamoeba.*

acanthosis—diffuse hyperplasia and thickening of the prickle-cell layer of the epidermis, as in psoriasis.

acanthosis nigricans (AN)—a marker of insulin resistance and diabetes

acanthosis *(cont.)* mellitus, more common in people of African descent. It is often associated with malignancy.

Acapella chest physical therapy device—combines the benefits of positive-pressure therapy and airway vibrations to mobilize pulmonary secretions. It is intended for patients with lung disease and associated secretory problems.

ACAT (automated computerized axial tomography).

ACB test—an albumin cobalt binding test for the rapid detection of myocardial infarction, developed for use in the emergency department.

ACC/AHA/ESC (American College of Cardiology, American Heart Association, and the European Society of Cardiology) guidelines for the management of patients with atrial fibrillation.

accelerated idioventricular rhythm (AIVR).

accelerometer—an instrument used to measure acceleration of gait.

Accellon Combi biosampler—a cervical cytology collecting device that simplifies Pap smear process so that its fibers contact both exo- and endocervical mucosal surfaces.

Accel stopcock—used with high-flow percutaneous catheter introducer.

Ac'cents—permanent lash liner applied by plastic surgeon.

access—admittance. Usage: "This gave easy access to the abdominal cavity." Cf. *axis, excess*.

Access AFP immunoassay system—a quantitative test for serum alpha fetoprotein.

Access MV system—a beating-heart bypass system which creates easier access and facilitates multiple vessel procedures.

Access Ostase—serum-based test for assessment of osteoporosis and Paget disease of bone.

ACCLAIM (Advanced Chronic Heart Failure Clinical Assessment of Immune Modulation Therapy) **trial**.

Accolade—a brand name for orthopedic hip implants, components, and surgical instrumentation, including the TMZF femoral component.

accommodation—adjustment, as of the eye for distance.

accordion sign—a finding indicative of pseudomembranous colitis on CT scans in patients who received oral contrast material. The accordion appearance depends on the degree of edema of the haustral folds and the amount of contrast material trapped between the folds.

Accu-Chek InstantPlus system—small monitor that uses a test strip and a fingerstick blood sample to provide a total cholesterol value in three minutes or a blood glucose value in 12 seconds.

Accu-Chek II Freedom—self-monitoring blood glucose system for visually impaired diabetics. It talks users through self-blood-testing with clearly spoken cues.

Accucore II—core biopsy needle with echo-enhanced tip for ultrasound guidance and precise depth markings.

accuDEXA—a bone mineral density assessment device. See *DEXAscan*.

Accuform nasal splint—for immobilization of bony segments after surgery or trauma.

AccuGuide injection monitor—a lightweight BMG monitor with auditory and BMG feedback to improve the efficiency of injecting small muscle groups.

AccuLase excimer laser—for use in transmyocardial revascularization.

AccuLength arthroplasty measuring system—an intraoperative hip length measuring device for use during total hip arthroplasty.

Accu-Line knee instrumentation—to assist in total knee arthroplasty. Includes tibial resector, distal femoral resection instrument, dual pivot, chamfer resection guide, and patellar instruments.

Acculink self-expanding stent—for revascularization of stenotic carotid arteries secondary to atherosclerotic disease. The stent is advanced through a small incision in the femoral artery to the area of carotid occlusion. Once in place, the stent is deployed to maintain patency and prevent atherosclerotic plaque from becoming displaced. Carotid stenting offers a less invasive alternative to carotid endarterectomy procedures.

AccuNet embolic protection system—a device designed to trap particles of atherosclerotic plaque during the endovascular stenting procedure.

AccuPoint hCG Pregnancy Test Disc—for quick diagnosis.

AccuProbe—a DNA probe for the rapid diagnosis of *Histoplasma capsulatum*.

Accura hemofiltration system—delivers continuous renal replacement and plasma therapies in critical care settings.

Accurate Surgical and Scientific Instruments (ASSI)—a trade name, not a comment on quality.

AccuSet introducer catheter—used for the delivery of EndoFit aortic endovascular grafts.

AccuSharp instrument—used in carpal tunnel release.

AccuSpan tissue expander. Also, *PMT AccuSpan*.

AccuSway balance measurement system—used to measure balance and sway in physical and rehabilitation therapy.

Accutome—low-speed diamond saw.

Accu-Vu sizing catheter—combines a soft, highly radiopaque catheter tip with a choice of platinum radiopaque catheter marker patterns along the shaft of the catheter.

Accuzyme—enzymatic debriding agent.

ACD (active compression-decompression) **resuscitator**—a suction device for cardiopulmonary resuscitation (CPR). The two researchers who developed it after hearing of a heart attack victim who had been resuscitated with a bathroom plunger (a.k.a. plumber's friend). It is easier to use than standard CPR—a simple push-pull action—and studies have shown that the device pumps more blood through the heart and draws more air into the lungs.

ACD (allergic contact dermatitis).

ACE (adverse cardiac event).

ACE (angiotensin-converting enzyme) **inhibitor**—used to treat hypertension.

ACE (antegrade continence enema).

acentric (Genetics)—referring to an incomplete chromosome that lacks a centromere.

acetabular angle of Sharp.

acetabular anteversion (AA)—hip dysplasia measurement in children with cerebral palsy.

acetabular cages—implants classified as roof rings or anti-protrusio devices and used in hip surgery.

acetabular limbectomy—partial or complete excision of the rim or margin of the acetabulum for congenital hip dislocation. Although the procedure seems beneficial in the short-

acetabular *(cont.)* term, long-term (a decade or more) outcomes result in failure of the acetabular epiphysis to appear. Limbus-sparing procedures, on the other hand, resulted in improvement of the acetabular covering.

acetabular dysplasia—shallow hip socket leading to hip dislocation, maldirection, insufficiency, and incongruence.

acetabular head index (AHI).

acetabular roof-obliquity angle—a measurement used in the assessment of developmental dysplasia of the hip.

acetabuloplasty—a variety of pelvic osteotomy procedures performed in children or young adults in whom hip pain or instability of the hip is present. The aim is to obtain concentric reduction of the hip joint and fashion a stable acetabular roof.

acetabulum—cup-shaped, dish-shaped, egg-shaped congruous, saucer-shaped.

acetowhite test—acetic acid applied to affected area (such as warts or a dysplastic area of the cervix), causing the area to become whitish and more conspicuous.

acetylator—an agent capable of metabolic acetylation.

acetylcholine receptor antibody (AChRAb)—found in the sera of patients with myasthenia gravis.

ACF (aberrant crypt foci).

ACG knee (Ortho)—for tricompartmental knee arthroplasty.

Achieve off-pump system—enables physicians to perform beating-heart CABG procedures. The system is composed of a stabilization platform that steadies portions of the heart being treated and an access device that provides the surgeon easy exposure of otherwise difficult-to-reach vessels.

Achiever balloon dilatation catheter.

Achilles reflex—response to a tap on the heel of the foot. On percussion of the Achilles tendon just above the calcaneus, contraction of the muscles of the leg produces plantar flexion of the foot. Also, *gastrocnemius reflex, ankle jerk.*

Achilles tendon (English form), **tendo Achillis** (Latin form).

achondroplastic dwarfism—a disorder of connective tissue metabolism; the patient is normal except for bone growth and development.

Achromobacter lwoffi—see *Acinetobacter lwoffi.*

acidemia—see *isovaleric acidemia.*

acidic—having the characteristics of an acid. Cf. *ascitic.*

acid-related disorders (ARDs)—include dyspepsia, gastritis, GERD (gastroesophageal reflux disease), and PUD (peptic ulcer disease).

Acier stainless steel suture—nonabsorbable suture for use in abdominal wound closure, hernia repair, sternal closure, and certain orthopedic procedures including cerclage and tendon repair.

Acinetobacter lwoffi—normal flora of skin, mouth, and external genitalia, isolated from sputum and urine. Associated with conjunctivitis, keratitis, and chronic ear infections. Also, *Achromobacter lwoffi, Mima polymorpha, Moraxella lwoffi.*

AC-IOL (anterior chamber intraocular lens).

ACIS (adenocarcinoma in situ).

ACIS (automated cellular imaging system)—immunohistochemical staining method used to diagnose or

ACIS *(cont.)*
monitor numerous conditions, including cancer and infectious disease.

ACIS-assisted ("ay-siss" or "a-sis")—the use of the Automated Cellular Imaging System in areas such as human papillomavirus (HPV) and cancer screening.

ACL, ACA (anticardiolipin antibody).

Acland-Banis arteriotomy set—used for end-to-side microvascular anastomosis.

Acland microvascular clamps—used in hand surgery.

ACL (anterior cruciate ligament) **drill guide; ACL repair**.

ACLS (advanced cardiac life support).

ACMI Martin endoscopy forceps.

ACM (automated cardiac flow measurement) **technology**—measures left ventricular outflow tract pressure ultrasonically and thus noninvasively.

acne rosacea—affects facial skin and may affect eyes (ocular rosacea), causing mild blepharoconjunctivitis or vision-impairing corneal involvement.

ACNM (American College of Nurse Midwives)—confers the credential CNM (Certified Nurse Midwife).

ACNU—an acronym for the chemical formulation for nimustine hydrochloride.

Acolysis—an ultrasound intravascular thrombolysis system.

Acorn cardiac support device (ACSD)—a ventricular containment device designed to treat heart failure by mechanically preventing further ventricular dilation.

acoustical shadowing—a term used in ultrasonography. It refers to reflection of large amounts of ultrasonic waves from the surface of structures or materials that are physically incompressible (bone, gallstones), with blockage of further transmission.

acoustic stimulation test (AST)—an alternative to the standard nonstress test in managing high-risk pregnancies and identifying normal patterns of fetal activity and heart rate. The AST uses a sound-generating vibrator (also used by laryngectomy patients to generate a monotone quality of speech) which is applied to the abdomen over the position of the fetal head. Sound is produced for three one-second intervals. The test is considered normal if the fetal heart rate increases at least 15 beats per minute for at least 15 seconds.

acquired anterior ocular melanocytosis—may develop as a result of cataract extraction and posterior chamber lens implantation, which can induce episcleral/scleral hyperpigmentation and iris hyperchromia.

acquired immunodeficiency syndrome (AIDS). See *AIDS*.

acquired long QT syndrome (aLQTS)—a disorder that puts patients at risk for life-threatening arrhythmias. Patients on hERG-blocking drugs have a higher risk of developing acquired long QT syndrome. See *long QT syndrome* and *left cardiac sympathetic denervation.*

acquired perforating dermatosis—umbilicated keratotic papules with a central keratotic plug.

acquired von Willebrand disease (AvWD)—a rare complication of an autoimmune or neoplastic disease, associated mostly with a lymphoid or plasma cell proliferative disorder.

acquisition time—MRI term.

Acra-Cut Spiral craniotome blade—a cranial blade with spiral geometric design.

ACRES (amplification created restriction enzyme site)—a reliable and efficient method for detecting gene mutations and less expensive than sequencing.

acrocallosal syndrome, Schinzel type—rare disorder inherited as an autosomal recessive genetic trait and characterized by craniofacial abnormalities, absence or underdevelopment of the mass of white matter that unites the two halves of the brain, additional fingers and/or toes, loss of muscle tone, and mental retardation.

acrocentric (Genetics)—referring to a chromosome whose centromere is near one end.

acrochordon (Derm)—a skin tag.

acrodysostosis—characterized by abnormally short and malformed bones of the hands and feet, nasal hypoplasia, and mental retardation. Some researchers believe acrodysostosis occurs randomly for no apparent reason; others believe it is a form of pseudohypoparathyroidism.

AcroFlex-100 artificial disk—flexible artificial disk intended as an alternative to spinal fusion.

acromesomelic dysplasia—a rare inherited progressive disorder characterized by premature fusion of metaphyses where the shafts of certain long bones meet their epiphyses. As a result, affected individuals exhibit unusually short forearms, abnormal shortening of bones of the lower legs, and short-limbed dwarfism.

AcryDerm border island dressing—a composite, or multilayered, dressing for the management of wound exudate moisture from acute and chronic wounds (not for use in third-degree burns). The island component is a highly absorbent hydrogel matrix placed on the adhesive side of a medical grade polyurethane transparent thin film.

AcryDerm Strands—absorbent wound dressing.

acrylic cement—very strong glue used to cement orthopedic joint replacements in place.

acrylic wafer TMJ (temporomandibular joint) **splint**—for TMJ pain and dysfunction. It is worn between the upper and lower teeth all the time until the patient's pain improves, and then only at night.

Acryl-X-II bone cement removal system—for separation and simultaneous removal of acrylic bone cement, reducing risk of injury to bone.

AcrySof acrylic foldable intraocular lens—acrylic foldable lens allowing smaller incision in implant surgery.

AcrySof ReSTOR—an intraocular lens (IOL) that can restore a cataract patient's ability to see both near and distant objects without the aid of reading glasses or bifocals.

ACS (abdominal compartment syndrome).

ACS (advanced cardiovascular system).

ACS anchor exchange device—used to exchange devices during interventional procedures such as PTCA, atherectomy, or stenting.

ACS Concorde—an over-the-wire catheter system for use in opening blocked coronary arteries. It allows for a minimal entry diameter and provides for easier advancement of catheter through tight or tortuous lesions.

ACSD (Acorn cardiac support device).

ACS Endura—coronary dilation catheter used in heart-related operations.

ACS Hi-Torque Balance—middleweight guidewire.

ACS OTW (over-the-wire) **HP** (high pressure) **coronary stent**.

ACS OTW Lifestream coronary dilatation catheter—a perfusion catheter for treatment of blocked arteries in the heart.

ACS OTW (over-the-wire) **Photon**—coronary dilatation catheter.

ACS RX (rapid exchange) **Comet**—coronary dilatation catheter.

ACS RX Multi-Link stent—an expandable coronary stent with multiple linked rings that allows for flexibility and conformity.

ACS Tourguide II guiding catheter.

ACT (activated coagulation time).

ACT (adaptive cellular therapy)—see *RIGS/ACT*.

Actalyke—an activated clotting time (ACT) test performed at the bedside to monitor heparin anticoagulation therapy. It can provide test results within minutes.

ACTG (AIDS Clinical Trials Group).

ActHIB (*H. influenzae* type B vaccine).

Acticoat—silver-based antimicrobial burn barrier. Removes two of the greatest obstacles to wound healing: invasive infections and frequent dressing changes.

Acticon Neosphincter—implantable prosthesis for the treatment of severe fecal incontinence. The device consists of a cuff (placed around the anal canal), a pressure-regulating balloon (placed in the abdomen), and a control pump (placed in the labium or scrotum).

ACTID (analgesic cell therapy implantable device)—cell-containing biocompatible pain-control implant.

Actifier—a high-tech pacifier that is used as a diagnostic and treatment tool for premature infants. Designed to train babies to suck at the right time and in the right way, it may allow them to feed, thrive, and leave intensive care units earlier. The pacifier also may reduce the incidence or severity of certain developmental disabilities that appear in early childhood and beyond, as well as possibly boost IQ.

ActiPatch therapy—therapeutic electromagnetic field in an inexpensive, easily applied patch that enhances healing, marketed especially to plastic surgeons.

Actisorb silver 220 dressing.

Actis venous flow controller (VFC)—placed in tourniquet fashion at the base of the penis to control erectile dysfunction caused by venous leak syndrome. It creates enough pressure to prevent venous drainage but does not interfere with arterial inflow or ejaculatory function.

Activa dystonia therapy stimulator—a totally implanted brain stimulator to treat long-term primary dystonia (disordered muscle tone) that is not responsive to drug therapy.

Activa Parkinson control therapy—utilizes bilateral brain stimulation to treat symptoms of advanced, levodopa-responsive Parkinson disease.

activated charcoal—used as an antidote in some kinds of poisoning; it is an *adsorbent*, not an *absorbent*.

activated partial thromboplastin time (APTT).

active compression-decompression (ACD) **resuscitator**.

active movement scale (AMS)—a tool for assessing motor function in infants with obstetrical brachial plexus palsy.

Activskin—support pantyhose for men, euphemistically called performance wear. Soldiers in bug-infested parts of the world are using Activskin to protect themselves from insect bites. It reportedly also prevents chafing under the uniform and provides thermal insulation.

Activent—antimicrobial ventilation tubes for myringotomy.

active phase arrest (Ob-Gyn) (*not* "of rest")—during labor, when the cervix stops dilating and no progress is being made toward delivery.

active specific immunotherapy (ASI).

activities of daily living (ADLs).

Activitrax pacemaker—specialized cardiac pacemaker containing a microphone that senses muscle activity during exercise. It can be programmed to increase the rate of a ventricle 5 to 10 beats per increment of sensed muscle tone.

ACT MicroCoil—delivery system for minimally invasive treatment of intracranial aneurysms.

actocardiotocograph—a fetal monitor that displays a tracing of the fetal heart rate and simultaneously records fetal movements and uterine contractions. Used to monitor pregnancies with multiple fetuses.

Acucise—retrograde procedure for incision of ureteral stricture and ureteropelvic junction obstruction.

Acu-Derm I.V./TPN dressing—provides a moisture- and vapor-permeable covering that reduces the risk of catheter movement.

Acufex (*not* Acuflex) **arthroscopic instruments**—rotary punch, straight and curved basket forceps.

Acufex bioabsorbable suture anchor—used in orthopedic surgery.

AcuFix anterior cervical plate system—multisegment plating system designed for fusing the anterior cervical spine. Also, *SC-AcuFix*.

AcuMatch A series—acetabular component. Also, AcuMatch L and M series modular femoral hip prosthesis.

AcuNav—ultrasound catheter designed to capture images from inside the heart.

AcuPressor myotherapy tool—used in physical therapy.

acupressure—stimulation of acupuncture points performed with fingers or an instrument with a hard, ball-shaped head. Another variation is reflexology, or zone therapy, where soles of feet and posteroinferior regions of the ankle joints are stimulated.

acupuncture lasers—helium-neon (He-Ne), gallium-arsenide (GaA).

Acuson computed sonography—for Doppler and color Doppler imaging.

Acuson V5M—multiplanar TEE (transesophageal echocardiographic) monitor.

Acusyst Xcell—monoclonal antibody culturing system.

acute abdomen—an abdomen showing signs of acute inflammation.

acute cellular xenograft rejection—acute rejection reaction to transplantation of tissue of animal origin, addressed by the induction of T-cell tolerance.

acute compartment syndrome (Ortho)—found in tibial diaphyseal fractures. Delay in treatment can lead to contracture, infection, and occasionally amputation.

acute flaccid paralysis (AFP) **syndrome**—a condition now believed to be associated with West Nile virus infection in some children.

acute inflammatory demyelinating polyradiculoneuropathy (AIDP).

acute macular neuroretinopathy—teardrop-shaped scotomas noted on Amsler grid testing, corresponding to dark red wedge-shaped areas around the fovea seen on funduscopic examination. The lesions are highlighted by red-free light. The visual deficit is irreversible.

acute mountain sickness (AMS)—a group of symptoms that may occur in some people who ascend rapidly to altitudes higher than 8200 feet. Major symptoms include headaches, nausea, vomiting, and insomnia.

acute multifocal placoid pigment epitheliopathy (AMPPE, "amp-pee") —an acute disease involving rapid loss of vision and multifocal off-white, plaque-like spots of the retinal pigment epithelium of uncertain etiology but believed to be associated with a viral infection. Eventually resolves with restoration of vision. May be treated with topical or systemic steroids and, if associated with infection, an antibiotic. May be accompanied by vitreous floaters.

Acute Physiology and Chronic Health Evaluation (APACHE).

acute promyelocytic leukemia (APML).

acute repetitive seizure (ARS) **disorder**.

acute stroke team (AST)—staffed by specially trained physicians and/or nurses who respond immediately to cases of suspected stroke, either in patients already in the hospital or newly arrived in the emergency department.

ACUTENS—transcutaneous nerve stimulator that includes elements of acupuncture or acupressure, for control of pain. It is typed in all capital letters, as in TENS unit. See *TENS, PENS*.

acute zonal occult outer retinopathy (AZOOR).

AcuTrainer—an electronic bladder retraining device for children and adults. It's a noninvasive option for voiding dysfunction and many types of urinary incontinence.

Acutrak fusion system—for fusion of interphalangeal and distal interphalangeal joints of hand and first toe. It is a small-bone fixation system using compression screw fixation with tapering variable pitch screw designs.

A.D., AD (*auris dextra*)—right ear.

Adamkiewicz artery—supplies blood to the thoracolumbar spinal cord. Injury to this artery may be a cause of cauda equina syndrome.

Adams test—a forward-bending test for scoliosis in which the observer is positioned posterior to the patient, who slowly bends forward, imitating a diver, to approximately 90° of lumbar flexion. The purpose is to detect rib asymmetry or prominence, which is indicative of scoliosis.

Adaptar—a no-line contact lens that can accommodate all stages of presbyopia.

adaptive cellular therapy (ACT)—see *RIGS/ACT*.

adaptive focusing technology (AFT) —uses hyperthermia, or focused heat, to improve the results of both radiation and chemotherapy in cancer patients.

ADAS (Alzheimer Disease Assessment Scale)—evaluates memory, language, and praxis in Alzheimer patients. It notes changes in cognition and in activities of daily living.

ADAS-cog—see *Alzheimer Disease Assessment Scale cognitive subscale*.

ADCA (autosomal-dominant cerebellar ataxia) **type II**—a neurodegenerative disorder presenting with cerebellar ataxia and retinal degeneration.

ADC (analog-to-digital) **conversion quantization error**—MRI term.

Adcon-L—an antiadhesion barrier to prevent postlaminectomy scarring and adhesions.

Adcon-P—a proprietary resorbable carbohydrate polymer liquid that is designed to inhibit scarring and adhesions following pelvic and gynecological surgery.

ADD (attention-deficit disorder).

Add-On Bucky digital x-ray image acquisition system.

adduct—to draw toward a position near or parallel to the median axis. Cf. *abduct*.

"a-d-duction"—dictated by a physician to clarify that **ad**duction, not **ab**duction, is intended.

AddVent atrioventricular pacemaker.

adenine—a purine (symbol A), one of the four bases found in DNA and RNA; in the formation of a double-stranded nucleic acid, it always pairs with the purine guanine (G).

adenocarcinoma in situ (AIS) **of the cervix**—much less common than carcinoma in situ (CIS) but recently increasing in frequency. AIS is premalignant and highly curable.

adenocyst—adenocystoma (adenoma in which there is cyst formation). Cf. *adenosis*.

adenoma—see *carcinoma ex pleomorphic adenoma*.

adenomatous hyperplasia (AH)—parenchymal nodule of the liver containing portal and biliary elements and considered a regenerative, limited overgrowth. Some AH nodules grow gradually and finally progress to hepatocellular carcinoma (HCC), suggesting that an AH nodule may be premalignant. Distinguishing AH from HCC is important.

adenomyomatosis—a proliferation of epithelium with gland-like formations and outpouchings of the mucosa into or through the hypertrophied muscular layer. These hyperplastic mucosal diverticula in the gallbladder are also called *Rokitansky-Aschoff sinuses*.

adenosine echocardiography—a study in which the antiarrhythmic agent adenosine is given intravenously to assess patients with suspected coronary artery disease. It causes the coronary arteries to constrict, thus producing ischemic symptoms without a stress test. Even if the drug produces coronary artery constriction and exacerbates patient symptoms, its effect is extremely brief for it has a half-life of only 10 seconds.

adenosine triphosphate (ATP)**-sensitive potassium channel openers.**

adenosis—disease of the glands or abnormal development of glandular tissue. Types: blunt duct, florid, sclerosing. Cf. *adenocyst*.

adenovirus—a virus genetically engineered so that the virus is harmless but able to carry desirable genes into a variety of types of brain cells. Though years away from use in humans, scientists are working on developing such viruses for potential use in such debilitating conditions as Alzheimer, Huntington, and Parkinson diseases.

adenovirus test kit—for the detection of adenovirus in stool samples. The enzyme immunoassay uses a combination of antibodies to directly test for the virus and reduces the time required by traditional cell-culture isolation.

ADEPT (Advanced Elements of Pacing Trial).

Adept (icodextrin)—nonviscous solution for prevention of postoperative adhesions.

AD/FHD (ratio of acetabular depth to femoral head diameter).

adhese, adhesed—back-formations from the noun *adhesion*. The correct terms are *adhere* and *adhered*, but *adhese* and *adhesed* are widely used in dictation.

adhesion preventative
- Adcon-L
- Adcon-P
- Adept solution
- Hylagel-Nuro
- HylaSine
- Incert sponge
- Interceed adhesion barrier
- Intergel solution
- Parietex
- Repel film
- Seprafilm
- SprayGel adhesion barrier system

adhesive (see also *bandage, dressing*)
- Aron Alpha
- autologous fibrin tissue (AFTA)
- BA (bioactive) bone cement
- BEMA (bioerodible mucoadhesive)
- Beriplast P fibrin tissue glue
- bioactive glass
- Biobrane
- Bioerodible Mucoadhesive (BEMA)
- BioGlue surgical
- biologically-active apatite
- Body Glue
- bone cement
- CarraSmart foam
- Cica-Care topical gel sheeting
- Coe-pak paste
- CoSeal resorbable synthetic sealant
- Coverlet
- Cover-Roll gauze
- Cover-Strip wound closure strips

adhesive *(cont.)*
- cyanoacrylate
- Dermabond
- Durapore surgical tape
- EMLA anesthetic disc
- fibrin glue
- fibrin sealant
- FloSeal matrix hemostatic sealant
- FocalSeal-L sealant
- FocalSeal-S surgical sealant
- gelatin-resorcin-formalin tissue glue
- Hemaseel HMN biological tissue glue
- Histoacryl tissue glue
- Howmedica Osteonics bone cement
- hydroxyapatite (HA)
- Hypafix
- Implast bone cement
- Indermil topical tissue
- iodophor-impregnated adhesive drape
- isobutyl 2-cyanoacrylate (IBC)
- Kling
- LPPS hydroxyapatite
- MCW cement
- methylmethacrylate cement
- n-butyl cyanoacrylate (n-BCA)
- Omiderm transparent adhesive film
- OpSite Flexigrid transparent adhesive film
- Orthoset radiopaque bone cement
- Palacos cement
- Proceed hemostatic surgical sealant
- Pro-Clude transparent adhesive film
- ProCyte transparent adhesive film
- Quixil
- Simplex cement
- Simplex P radiopaque bone cement
- SiteGuard MVP transparent adhesive film
- Soothe-N-Seal
- Superglue
- Suresite transparent adhesive film
- Surfit
- Surgical Simplex P radiopaque
- Tisseel surgical glue

adhesive *(cont.)*
Tissucol
transparent adhesive film
Uniflex polyurethane adhesive surgical
Transeal transparent adhesive film
VersaBond
Vitex tissue
weld
Zimmer low viscosity

adiabatic fast passage—MRI term.

adiposis dolorosa—rare disorder of fat metabolism of unknown cause; fat accumulates in painful lumps over the body. Also called *Dercum disease.*

adjustable leg and ankle repositioning mechanism (ALARM).

adjuvant therapy—auxiliary therapy.

Adkins strut—used to retract the third rib to facilitate exposure to LIMA (left internal mammary artery) in MIDCAB (minimally invasive direct coronary artery bypass) procedures.

ADLs (activities of daily living) (Rehab). Usage: "Plan: Improve the patient's ADLs."

admix—to mingle, mix, or blend; a back-formation from the obsolete term *admixt*. This is a term you will likely hear in pathology dictation.

adnexa (Ob-Gyn)—the uterine appendages including the ovary and fallopian tube on each side. Adnexa is plural and always takes a plural verb. Usage: "The adnexa were unremarkable." Also, *ocular adnexa.*

Adolescent and Pediatric Pain Tool—see *APPT.*

adolescent idiopathic scoliosis (AIS).

adrenergic antagonist—a drug which blocks the action of naturally produced neurotransmitters on adrenergic receptors of sympathetic nervous system.

adRP (autosomal-dominant retinitis pigmentosa).

ADR Ultramark 4 ultrasound—portable microprocessor based on electrocardiography system.

AD7C—test that aids in diagnosis of Alzheimer disease. Results are significantly elevated in patients with the disease and correlate with severity of dementia symptoms.

Adson maneuver—to rule in or rule out scalenus anticus syndrome.

adsorbent—an agent that attracts other molecules to, or maintains them on, a surface. Cf. *absorbent.*

ADTRA—composite external fixator ring (Ortho).

adult chronic immune thrombocytopenic purpura (ITP)—a disorder more commonly known as *idiopathic thrombocytopenic purpura.*

adult respiratory distress syndrome (ARDS).

adult stem cell—an undifferentiated precursor cell, found in small numbers in the differentiated tissues of an adult, that can either divide so as to continue the line of such cells or differentiate into a specific cell type.

Adult Treatment Panel III (ATP III)—new guidelines issued by NIH's Expert Panel of the National Cholesterol Education Program. The guidelines recommend some significant changes from those outlined in step 1 (ATP I) and step 2 (ATP II) in the approach to detection, evaluation, and treatment of high blood cholesterol in adults.

advanced breast biopsy instrumentation (ABBI) **system**—permits sampling of a mammographic lesion while preserving the lesion's histologic architecture for complete pathologic analysis.

advanced cardiac life support (ACLS).

advanced cardiac mapping—multi-electrode catheter is guided into the heart chamber, showing the heart's electrical activity, locating any points of arrhythmia, and targeting sites for curative catheter procedures.

Advanced Care cholesterol test—self-administered test for checking cholesterol. It measures total serum cholesterol levels in approximately 15 minutes.

Advanced Chronic Heart Failure Clinical Assessment of Immune Modulation Therapy (ACCLAIM).

Advanced Elements of Pacing Trial (ADEPT)

advanced glycation end-products (AGE).

advanced real time motion analysis (ARTMA).

Advanta SST PTFE, Advanta VS, Advanta VXT, Advanta Super-Soft, Advanta V12—PTFE vascular grafts.

AdvanTeq II TENS unit.

Advantim revision knee system—using Ortholoc instrumentation.

Advantx LC+—cardiovascular imaging system.

adverse cardiac event (ACE).

adverse events (AEs)—a term used in clinical trials and surgical procedures to designate serious untoward consequences of treatment.

Advexin (p53 adenoviral gene)—a proprietary orphan drug used in the treatment of head and neck cancer, and currently on the FDA Fast Track for lung cancer and other advanced cancers.

Advia 120 hematology system—an automated cerebrospinal fluid assay.

AE (angiographic embolization)

AED (automatic external defibrillator) —device used by emergency medical technicians in the field or by families trained in its use for patients at risk for sudden death.

AE (aryepiglottic) **fold**.

Aegis aortic cannula—a cannula used during cardiac bypass surgery to prevent cerebral embolization.

Ae-H interval (anterograde conduction) —a term used in electrophysiologic studies of supraventricular tachycardia.

aeroallergens—see *pathogen*.

Aerochamber—a face mask which attaches to a bronchial inhaler device. The metered-dose aerosol can be breathed over several seconds by patients who have difficulty using inhaler devices.

aerogenous—descriptive term for bacteria which produce gas. Cf. *erogenous zones*.

Aeromonas sobria—a pathogen associated with left-sided segmental colitis. Chronic colitis frequently follows *Aeromonas* infection.

AeroTech II nebulizer—for administration of aerosolized drugs such as pentamidine.

AERx electronic inhaler—pulmonary drug delivery system creating an aerosol from a liquid drug and delivering it locally to the lung or into the bloodstream via the lung. It allows people with diabetes to control meal-time glucose levels by inhaling insulin. Also used to deliver morphine for pain control.

AEs (adverse events).

Aescula left ventricular (LV) **lead**—cardiac lead for use with left-ventricle-based cardiac stimulation systems.

Aesop 2000—a surgical robot capable of maneuvering and positioning a laparoscope in response to a surgeon's voice commands. Aesop is an

Aesop *(cont.)* acronym for automated endoscopic system for optimal positioning.

aesthetic—artistic or beautiful in appearance. Cf. *asthenic.*

Aestiva/5 MRI anesthesia machine—authorized for use on patients undergoing MRI exams.

A-FAIR (arrhythmia-insensitive flow-sensitive alternating inversion recovery) imaging.

AFBG (aortofemoral bypass graft).

affect—(verb) to change; to produce an effect, as "This should not affect the outcome"; (noun) outward appearance of an inner emotion (Neuro, Psych), as "The patient demonstrated a flat affect" (or "flattened affect"). Cf. *effect.*

afferent—moving towards the center, as in an afferent defect in ophthalmology. Cf. *efferent.*

Affinitac—antisense drug for treatment of non-small-cell lung carcinoma.

Affinity (trademarked with all capitals) **cage system**—a system of screws and surgical tools used to help make the cervical spine more stable and relieve pressure on spinal nerves. The screws, which are hollow and have holes in their sides, are implanted into the vertebrae, causing them to grow together.

affinity chromatography.

Affirm—a one-step pregnancy test that detects chorionic gonadotropin in human urine. The test is said to be 99% accurate and effective as early as the first day of a missed period and may be taken at any time of the day, giving visual results in one to two minutes.

AFFIRM (Atrial Fibrillation Follow-up Investigation of Rhythm Management) study.

Affymetrix GeneChip system—for lab analysis of genes associated with cancer. It provides rapid genetic analysis using miniaturized, high-density arrays of DNA probes and proprietary software to analyze and manage genetic information.

afib—slang for *atrial fibrillation.*

AFIP (Armed Forces Institute of Pathology). Pathologists often send specimens to AFIP for consultation.

Afipia felis—a bacterium found in the-lymph nodes of a patient with cat-scratch disease. First identified by AFIP (Armed Forces Institute of Pathology). Not currently regarded as a cause of cat-scratch disease. See *Bartonella henselae.*

AFM (atomic force microscopy).

AFO (ankle-foot orthosis).

AFP (acute flaccid paralysis) **syndrome**.

AFP (alpha-fetoprotein) **lab test**.

AFT (Adaptive Focusing Technology).

after-depolarizations (Cardiol)—used in study of cardiac arrhythmias by electrophysiology.

afterloading—see *RAB* (remote afterloading brachytherapy).

afterload reduction—the use of systemic vasodilators and other agents to reduce excessive left ventriculare-jection load in congestive heart failure and aortic regurgitation. Not "after load production."

Aftermath—a nutritional supplement claiming to be a total relaxation and rejuvenation formula.

"af-thus"—phonetic for *aphthous.*

Agar-IF (immunofixation in agar) of blood serum.

agarose gel electrophoresis (AGE).

Agatston score—quantifies calcium in coronary arteries as a risk factor for coronary artery disease.

AGC (anatomic graduated components).

AGC (atypical glandular cells)—formerly AGUS or AGCUS (atypical glandular cells of undetermined significance).

AGE (advanced glycation end-products)—used in ophthalmology.

AGE (agarose gel electrophoresis).

age-associated memory impairment (AAMI)—used in the context of senile dementia and Alzheimer disease workup. Alzheimer disease is not an age-associated memory impairment, while senile dementia is.

Agee carpal tunnel release system—a one-portal system used in endoscopic carpal tunnel release.

Agee-WristJack fracture reduction system—multiplanar ligamentotaxis to restore palmar tilt in distal radial fractures.

age-related cognitive decline (ARCD)—newer term replacing such terms as age-associated memory impairment (AAMI) and benign senescent forgetfulness.

age-related macular degeneration (AMD or ARMD). See *dry age-related macular degeneration* and *wet age-related macular degeneration.*

age-related maculopathy (ARM).

AGF (angle of greatest flexion).

AGF (autologous growth factors).

aggregate—a mass or cluster of material, as aggregate measurements.

aggregated human IgG.

aggressive angiomyxoma—a rare variant of myxoid tumor with a vascular component. It is a slow-growing soft-tissue tumor that occurs mostly in the female pelvis and perineum, primarily in young premenopausal women. These tumors tend to infiltrate surrounding tissue, are locally aggressive, and have recurrence rates of up to 70%. No metastases have been reported. The tumor can resemble a Bartholin gland abscess or can be misdiagnosed as angiomyofibroblastoma.

agminated atypical (dysplastic) **nevi.**

agminated lentiginosis (AL)—characterized by numerous brown macules or café au lait macules confined to a body segment, with a sharp demarcation at the midline.

agonist—a drug that stimulates activity of a receptor in the way it would be stimulated by naturally produced substances. Cf. *antagonist.*

Agris-Dingman submammary dissector—used for a transaxillary approach to breast augmentation.

Agrylin (anagrelide HCl) (previously marketed as Agrelin)—drug used as treatment for thrombocytosis.

AGUS (atypical glandular cells of undetermined significance).

aGvHD (acute graft-versus-host disease).

AH (adenomatous hyperplasia).

ahaustral—without haustra, the bands running circumferentially around the large bowel.

AHI (acetabular head index).

AHI (apnea/hypopnea index).

AHIMA (American Health Information Management Association)—a professional association for health information management professionals who have credentials of the Registered Health Information Administrator (RHIA), Registered Health Information Technician (RHIT), Certified Coding Specialist (CCS), and Certified Coding Specialist–Physician-based (CCS-P).

"ahn block" or **"on block"**—see *en bloc.*

Ahn thrombectomy catheter—for the treatment of thromboemboli. Named

Ahn *(cont.)*
for Samuel Ahn, M.D., the catheter incorporates a distal dual balloon design to more effectively remove thromboemboli, as well as a proximal-indicator safety balloon that allows the surgeon to visually determine inflation volume. The distal dual balloon traps blood clots more effectively and prevents contamination caused by blood spurting into the operator's face and eyes.

AH 1 gene—the newly discovered gene for a form of Joubert ("zhoobear") syndrome, a condition present before birth that affects an area of the brain controlling balance and coordination in about 1 in 10,000 individuals.

AHR (airway hyperreactivity).

AI (acetabular index)—hip dysplasia measurement in children with cerebral palsy.

AICA (pronounced "i'-ka") (anterior inferior communicating artery).

AICD (automatic implantable cardioverter-defibrillator).

AID (artificial insemination-donor).

AIDP (acute inflammatory demyelinating polyradicular) neuropathy.

AIDS (acquired immunodeficiency syndrome)—a lethal impairment of T lymphocyte function caused by the human immunodeficiency virus (HIV), leaving the body susceptible to such opportunistic infections as *Pneumocystis carinii* pneumonia, candidiasis, and cancers like Kaposi sarcoma. AIDS is transmitted almost exclusively by sexual contact or by contaminated hypodermic needles. See related entries: *AIDS virus, ARV, cytokines, HIV, HTLV/III,* and *Kaposi sarcoma.*

AIDS-associated ophthalmic *Pneumocystis* (Oph).

AIDS dementia complex—a progressive primary encephalopathy caused by HIV type 1 infection involving principally the subcortical white matter and deep gray nuclei, manifested by a variety of cognitive, motor, and behavior abnormalities. Also called *AIDS encephalopathy, HIV dementia complex,* and *HIV encephalitis.*

AIDS encephalopathy—see *AIDS dementia complex.*

AIDS-KS (AIDS-related Kaposi sarcoma).

AIDS-related complex (ARC)—a term used to describe a variety of symptoms and signs found in some persons infected with HIV, including decrease in CD4 cells, recurrent fevers, unexplained weight loss, swollen lymph nodes, and/or fungus infections of mouth and throat. Most clinical findings formerly denoted as ARC are now in groups 3 or 4 of the CDC AIDS classification system, although the term *ARC* is still used to describe these symptoms and diagnoses. ARC is also commonly described as symptomatic HIV infection.

AIDS virus—a retrovirus of the cytopathic lentivirus group that invades and inactivates helper/T-cells of the immune system. See *helper cell; HIV; pathogen.*

AIH (artificial insemination–husband).

AILD (angioimmunoblastic lymphadenopathy with dysproteinemia).

Ailee sutures and needles.

AIM CPM (continuous passive motion) **for hand**.

AIMS (Abnormal Involuntary Movement Scale)—a scale for rating tardive dyskinesia.

AIOD (aortoiliac obstructive disease).

AIP (acute intermittent porphyria).

air-bone gap—in audiology testing. (*Not* "ear-bone gap" or "air-borne gap.")

Aircast Swivel-Strap—ankle brace to treat ankle instability.

AirCom—compression-molded polyethylene used in modular components.

air conduction (*not* ear conduction)—refers to the transmission of sound through the ear canal, tympanic membrane, and ossicular chain to the cochlea and auditory nerve. Air conduction is tested by holding a vibrating tuning fork near the external auditory meatus. Cf. *bone conduction, Rinne test, Weber test.*

air contrast barium enema—radiology procedure.

air entrainment device—a device consisting of a jet orifice (to which the oxygen supply is connected) adjacent to a series of air entrainment ports, the distal end of the device being designed for connection to an oxygen delivery system supplying a patient.

AirFlex carpal tunnel splint. Also, AirFlex Plus.

air-fluid level (Radiol)—a line representing the level of a collection of fluid seen in profile, with air or gas above it. Cf. *free air.*

air hunger—in patients with chronic extreme anemia, uremia, and diabetic acidosis who have great difficulty struggling to breathe; long, deep, or panting breathing.

Airlift balloon retractor—used in Laparolift system for gasless laparoscopy.

Air-Limb—designed to provide protection and edema control for a patient's leg following amputation.

"air oximeter"—see *ear oximeter.*

Airprene hinged knee prosthesis—with breathable lining support, reportedly offers more comfort than ordinary material, superior compression and muscle stability, and hinged stainless steel side bars to provide increased support.

"air-SAHZH"—phonetic for *hersage.*

air-space disease (Radiol)—disease or abnormality of lung tissue that encroaches on space normally filled by air, as seen on chest x-ray.

air splint (also *inflatable splint*)—blown up like a balloon and usually used to immobilize the foot and ankle. There are other such splints used for the arm or the whole leg. Usage: "This is an acute ankle sprain, so she will be placed in an air splint and should keep her foot elevated."

Air Supply—a wearable air purifier to reduce exposure to a variety of germs, pollen, dust, and other airborne hazards, so that patients can breathe cleaner, healthier air.

air trousers—medical (or military) antishock trousers. See *MAST trousers.*

airway, breathing, circulation (ABC)—must be assessed immediately on trauma patients before anything else is done.

airway hyperreactivity (AHR)—found on helical CT scan following methacholine bronchoprovocation in asthmatics.

AIS (Abbreviated Injury Scale)—a system of scoring trauma injuries to each anatomic system.

AIS (adenocarcinoma in situ).

AIS (adolescent idiopathic scoliosis).

AIVR (accelerated idioventricular rhythm).

AJ (ankle jerk) (Neuro)—Usage: "He has preserved reflexes throughout, evaluated at 2+ AJs, 3+ KJs, trace brachioradialis, and 1+ biceps." (Note: *KJ* is *knee jerk*.)

akathisia—motor restlessness often localized in the muscles, resulting in inability to sit or lie quietly; a side effect of some antipsychotic drugs. Usage: "A protracted akathisia-like dystonic-type reaction to this medication is very remote." Cf. *extrapyramidal signs, pyramidal signs, tardive dyskinesia.*

A-K diamond knife—precalibrated.

akinesia—see *Nadbath*.

Akros extended care mattress—for pressure relief.

AL (agminated lentiginosis).

Alamar Blue—an oxidation-reduction indicator used in laboratory tests to assess sensitivity of fungi to antifungal agents.

alanine aminotransferase (ALT)—liver function test. See *ALT*.

alar flaring—flaring (dilatation) of the nostrils on inspiration, sometimes the only sign of dyspnea in a small child. Also called *nasal flaring*.

ALARM (adjustable leg and ankle repositioning mechanism)—used in orthopedic surgery.

AlaSTAT latex allergy test—measures IgE antibodies specific to latex in blood samples. According to the FDA, at least 15 deaths and 1,000 reactions due to latex allergy have been reported. The American Academy of Allergy and Immunology recommends testing healthcare and latex industry workers, spina bifida children, and people who have such risk factors as multiple surgeries, unexplained anaphylaxis, or oral itching after eating avocados, bananas, kiwi, or chestnuts.

Alatest latex-specific IgE allergen test kit—used to measure the circulating levels of immunoglobulin E (IgE) specific to latex. Although only about 1% of the general population is thought to have type I latex allergy, in healthcare workers and others in occupations exposing them to latex, this allergy may affect more than 14%.

Albarran deflecting level (Urol)—attached to a cystoscope, allowing slow water irrigation during prostate resection for benign prostatic hypertrophy.

Albert Famous Faces Test—neurological test.

Albert-Lembert method—a two-layer technique for anastomosis of gastrointestinal structures. Usage: "The distal end of the jejunum was anastomosed end to end by hand to the stump of the distal remnant stomach in two layers, using the Albert-Lembert method."

Albizzia procedure—leg-lengthening procedure that uses the gradual elongation intramedullary nailing technique. Also, Albizzia nail.

albumen—the white of the egg; it contains protein and not cholesterol. Cf. *albumin*.

albumin—the major plasma protein present in human serum. Cf. *albumen*.

albumin cobalt binding (ACB) **test**—see *ACB test*.

albumin nanoparticle paclitaxel (Abraxane).

albuminocytologic dissociation—cerebrospinal fluid protein elevation.

albuterol sulfate inhalation solution—for use in patients with reversible obstructive airway disease and acute attacks of bronchospasm.

ALC (argon laser coagulation).

Alcaligenes xylosoxidans—a pathogen changed to *Achromobacter xylosoxidans*, the type species of gram-negative, aerobic bacteria in the genus *Achromobacter*. Previously in the genus *Alcaligenes*, the classification and nomenclature of this species has been emended. The two subspecies, *Achromobacter xylosoxidans* subsp. *denitrificans* and *Achromobacter xylosoxidans* subsp. *xylosoxidans*, are associated with infections.

ALCAPA (anomalous origin of left coronary artery from the pulmonary artery) **syndrome**—a condition resulting in infarction with myocardial necrosis in affected neonates with almost entirely collateral circulation-dependent perfusion of the left ventricle and poor global left ventricular function. In the past infants rarely survived because of severe left heart failure, but revascularization with good functional recovery is improving the clinical outcomes for these infants. Also called *Bland-Garland-White syndrome.*

Alcian blue—a stain used in testing for mucopolysaccharides.

alcohol ablation—surgical technique to treat cardiomyopathy. A catheter is threaded into the heart and pure alcohol is injected to induce a controlled heart attack, killing part of the overgrown heart muscle that blocks the flow of blood.

alcohol epilepsy—seizures as a complication of chronic alcohol dependence.

alcohol, ethanol, EtOH—used interchangeably when referring to the consumption of alcohol.

alcoholic blackout—anterograde amnesia experienced by alcoholics during episodes of drinking, even when not fully intoxicated. Indicative of early but still reversible brain damage.

alcohol-related seizures (ARS).

Alcon crescent blade (Oph).

Alcon MA 60 BM lens (Oph).

Alcon pocket blade (Oph).

Alcon SA60AT intraocular lens implant. Note: There are many additional IOLs listed by model number, including SA30AT, SA30AL, MA30AC, MA60AC, MA30BA, MA60BM, MA60MA.

Alder-Reilly morphological abnormality.

aldesleukin—recombinant interleukin-2 product used as an antineoplastic and biological response modifier in the treatment of metastatic renal cell carcinoma. Administered IV.

aldosterone-producing adenoma (APA).

Alert catheter—an electrophysiology catheter used in tandem with the Alert Companion to deliver a biphasic low-energy waveform to convert atrial fibrillation to a normal sinus heart rhythm. See *Alert Companion II*.

Alert Companion II—a touch screen biphasic defibrillator for use with the Alert catheter to treat atrial fibrillation. See *Alert catheter.*

Alert internal cardioversion system—a device used to treat atrial fibrillation by shocking the inside of the heart. The system consists of a catheter and the Alert Companion II biphasic defibrillator. The catheter is a thin tube with 2 narrow bands of electrodes (used to deliver the shocks). The Companion is a computer-controlled heart monitor and

Alert *(cont.)*
defibrillator that provides the energy for the shock. The Alert system is an alternative to external defibrillation (cardioversion) for patients with atrial fibrillation.

Alexagram—breast lesion diagnostictest. See *Alexa 1000 system.*

alexandrite (solid-state) **laser.**

Alexa 1000 system—noninvasive diagnostic system for determining whether a breast lesion is malignant or benign (reportedly 95% accurate), as an alternative to more invasive surgical breast biopsy procedures. Immediate diagnostic results are provided by the Alexagram test.

AlexLAZR—an alexandrite laser used for the removal of tattoo pigments and pigmented lesions, with reduced risk of scarring and tissue damage.

alfa—international spelling for *alpha*. The pharmaceutical nomenclature committees in several countries are moving toward a common spelling of new generic drugs. Since many languages that use the Roman alphabet have replaced the digraph *ph* with *f*, the United States Adopted Name (USAN) council has agreed to use this spelling in newly approved generic names. This change does not retroactively affect current drug names, however. Thus, "alpha" becomes "alfa" in *interferon alfa* and *dornase alfa*, but not in *alpha tocopherol* or *alpha amylase*.

"alfa-thal-trate"—phonetic brief form of alpha thalassemia trait.

Alfieri mitral valve procedure—in which the surgeon joins the two leaflets of the mitral valve with a single stitch. The valve can still open on both sides of the stitch, allowing adequate blood flow through the valve. Named for Dr. Ottavio Alfieri; also called *bow tie procedure. Also, Jatene-Alfieri.*

AlgiDERM—alginate wound dressing.

Algidex—a wound dressing that combines the benefits of moisture and absorption while also lessening the patient's dependence on antibiotics.

alginate wound dressing—made from soft, nonwoven fiber derived from seaweed and usually produced in pad, rope, or ribbon form. It absorbs wound exudate and forms a gel-like covering over the wound. Most alginate dressings absorb many times their own weight. See *dressing*.

AlgiSite—alginate wound dressing.

algorithm—a problem-solving procedure, step-by-step, as with a computer; e.g., "We discussed the following: Should he not improve, there would be two more stools for ova and parasites and for culture. If these are normal, and should he still have symptomatology, he would have a barium enema. If this is normal and symptomatology still persists, he would have flexible sigmoidoscopy, and finally, if his symptomatology still persists, then an upper GI with small bowel series. I told him that there is no urgency in approaching this algorithm." See *DRC (dynamic range control) algorithm.*

Algosteril—alginate wound dressing.

ALHE (angiolymphoid hyperplasia with eosinophilia).

ALI (acute lung injury).

aliasing artifact (wrap-around ghosting)—MRI term.

alien hand sign (Neuro)—sequela of an extensive stroke in the medial frontal cortex. The hand opposite the affected side of the brain (the

alien *(cont.)* alien hand) instinctively grasps and does other purposeful behaviors that cannot be controlled by the patient. Often the patient must use the unaffected hand to hold and restrain the "alien hand."

ALIF (anterior lumbar interbody fusion)—see *PLIF, TLIF.*

AliMed positioner—one of many medical home care and rehabilitation products from AliMed.

Alinia (nitazoxanide) **oral suspension** —drug for treatment of children with diarrhea caused by *Cryptosporidium parvum* and *Giardia lamblia.*

aliquot ("al'-e-kwat")—an equal part of a whole, as in a solution. Usage: "The patient was then given 5 mg of Valium in 2.5 mg aliquots to minimize the artifact in this EEG."

Alista (alprostadil)—drug for treatment of female sexual arousal disorder (FSAD). It is a proprietary formulation which is used to treat male erectile dysfunction. The drug is applied locally to the female genitalia, increasing blood flow and thereby promoting engorgement and other natural processes that occur during sexual stimulation.

A listening—see *A, P, T, M.*

AlitraQ—a nutritionally complete formula for patients with impaired GI function.

alive and well (A&W).

alkaline phosphatase antialkaline phosphatase (APAAP) **antibody test**—venous blood test technique for determining CD4, CD3, CD8, CD22, and other factors.

alkylating (*not* alkalating) **agent**.

ALL (acute lymphoblastic leukemia)—seen primarily in children.

ALL (acute lymphocytic leukemia).

Allegra-D—nonsedating antihistamine drug with decongestant.

Allegretto Wave excimer laser system —a refractive (heatless) excimer laser system. It uses invisible ultraviolet light pulses to remove precise amounts of tissue from the cornea (the transparent medium at the front of the eyeball that helps focus light to create an image) to reduce or eliminate farsightedness and astigmatism (distorted vision).

allele (Genetics)—one of at least two alternative forms that may be taken by a gene at any given locus.

Allen-Brown shunt—a vascular access shunt, used in performing dialysis.

Allen picture test (Oph)—used to test visual acuity, especially in young children who can identify pictures better than they can read Snellen letters.

Allen test—for diagnosing occlusion of the ulnar and radial arteries.

allergic bronchopulmonary aspergillosis (ABPA)—characterized by asthma, recurrent lung infiltration, recurrent episodes of purulent cough with or without fever, sputum plugs containing *Aspergillus fumigatus*, wheezing, peripheral blood eosinophilia, and immunologic evidence of hypersensitivity to *A. fumigatus*.

allergic contact dermatitis (ACD).

allergic salute—repeated rubbing of the nose upward to scratch an itchy nose and open the obstructed airway, seen in patients with allergies.

allergic shiners—darkening of the skin around the eyes, resembling periorbital hematomas, as a symptom of allergic rhinitis.

Allevyn dressing—nonadherent dressing material that is absorbent even under pressure.

Allgower-Donati technique—a suturing technique used in orthopedic procedures.

ALLHAT (Antihypertensive and Lipid-Lowering Treatment to Prevent Heart Attack Trial) **trial**.

alligator grasper/forceps.

Allis sign—a sign of fracture of the femoral neck, when the fascia between the crest of the ilium and the greater trochanter relaxes.

Alliston procedure—used in the correction of gastroesophageal reflux.

AlloAnchor RC—allograft machined from cortical bone and used in soft tissue reattachment for rotator cuff repair.

AlloDerm processed tissue graft—cadaveric dermal matrix from which all cellular components have been removed. It is used in plastic surgery for facial contouring.

allodynia—pain resulting from a nonnoxious stimulus to normal skin.

allogeneic transplantation—the transplantation of cells, tissues, or organs from one individual to another of the same species.

allograft—a graft in which donor and host are members of the same species but not genetically identical.

AlloMatrix graft.

AlloMatrix injectable putty—bone graft substitute that combines bioassayed demineralized bone matrix, surgical-grad e calcium sulfate, and a biocompatible plasticizing agent, creating a moldable putty with osteoconductive and osteoinductive properties.

Allon thermoregulation system—enables physicians to maintain normal body temperature in patients undergoing surgery. In addition to preventing hypothermia, it allows a physician to lower brain temperature in order to improve patient outcome. Also, *Allon ThermoWrap*.

allos—slang for *allograft transplant patients*.

Allovectin-7—DNA plasma-lipid complex containing the human gene encoding the HLA-B7 antigen. It is injected directly into a tumor, where it is absorbed by the malignant cells and the HLA-B7 antigen expressed, alerting the immune system to the presence of foreign tissue. This induces the type of powerful immune response seen in organ transplant rejection.

all-trans retinoic acid (ATRA; tretinoin; Vesanoid). See also *Retin-A*.

allusion—an indirect reference to something. Usage: "He made allusion to a history of some kind of tropical disease." Cf. *elusion, illusion*.

allylamines—class of antifungal drugs.

Alm self-retaining retractor.

Aloka color Doppler system—provides real-time, two-dimensional blood flow imaging with Cine Memory. Also, *Aloka 650*.

Aloka SSD—ultrasound system and probes.

alopecia androgenetica—male pattern baldness.

alosetron ("a-LOW-se-tron")—see *Lotronex*.

Aloxi (palonosetron)—an antiemetic agent for the treatment of cancer-induced nausea and vomiting.

alphabet exercises—an exercise regimen in which the patient is asked to move the ankle in multiple planes of motion by drawing letters of the alphabet (in lower case and upper case).

alpha-BSM (bone substitute material) —a calcium phosphate bone substitute material used to repair or replace autologous bone.

AlphaCor synthetic cornea—a biocompatible one-piece synthetic cornea of Hydrogel poly (2-hydroxyethyl methacrylate). See *synthetic cornea.*

alpha-fetoprotein (AFP)—a globulin produced by the liver and other tissues of the fetus and newborn. Its level normally declines after one year of age. Normal value in amniotic fluid, less than 20; an elevated value (over 100,000) indicates the presence of an embryonal tumor, spina bifida, or Down syndrome.

alpha Gal antibody—anti-pig antibody, the source of hyperacute rejection of a porcine xenograft.

alpha interferon—see *alfa.*

Alpha 1 penile implant—with a new design that the manufacturer claims "eliminates the annoying and embarrassing problem of spontaneous inflation and involuntary erections."

$alpha_1$-proteinase inhibitor (A_1PI)—an intravenous drug for patients with emphysema due to $alpha_1$-antitrypsin deficiency.

Alphastar—a flexible, modular, lightweight operating room table.

Alphatec mini lag-screw system (MLS) for forefoot surgery.

Alphatec small fragment system (SFS) for extremity fractures.

alpha-2 antiplasmin functional assay —blood test to diagnose dysantiplasminemia, a rare inherited cause of a bleeding disorder.

ALPS (anterior locking plate system).

ALPS (autologous leukapheresis, processing, and storage)—collection and cryogenic storage of a patient's own peripheral (circulating) blood stem cells, increasing disease management options available to cancer patients and oncologists.

aLQTS (acquired long QT syndrome).

ALS Bluemax BM500—alternative light source to Wood lamp, for the detection of semen in emergency department evaluations of sexual assault.

ALS Functional Rating Scale (ALS-FRS)—an instrument for evaluation of functional status and functional change in patients with ALS (amyotrophic lateral sclerosis). May be used as a screening measure in situations where muscle strength cannot be measured directly, or as an adjunct to myometry.

Alström disease—a symptom complex including pigmentary retinopathy, diabetes, renal disease, and obesity, with sensorineural deafness and with severe visual loss in the first decade after diagnosis.

ALSVs (arm and lesser saphenous veins).

ALT (alanine aminotransferase) (newer name for *SGPT*)—an enzyme whose level in the serum is elevated in hepatitis, cirrhosis, and other liver diseases.

ALT (argon laser trabeculoplasty).

Altaire—high-field-performance open MR imaging system.

Alta reconstruction rod—a titanium alloy rod used to provide rotational stability and reduce interference with endosteal revascularization to promote fracture healing.

Altastaph (*Staphylococcus aureus* immune globulin [human])—a medication used for immediate protection against *Staphylococcus aureus* infections in low birth-weight infants.

Altastaph *(cont.)*
Altastaph is produced by vaccinating healthy volunteers with StaphVAX and then harvesting the antistaphylococcal antibodies.

ALTE (apparent life-threatening event).

Altemeier procedure—perineal rectosigmoidectomy for rectal prolapse.

alternans test—noninvasive cardiac diagnostic test designed to identify certain patients at risk for sudden life-threatening arrhythmias (cardiac arrest) and sudden cardiac death. The test works like a "super stress test," measuring extremely subtle beat-to-beat fluctuations in the heartbeat called *T-wave alternans*.

Alternaria—an inhalant antigen.

Alteromonas putrefaciens—gram-negative organism.

Altmann classification of congenital aural atresia.

Altocor (lovastatin)—extended-release drug for hypercholesterolemia.

ALTK (automated lamellar therapeutic keratoplasty system).

ALT-RCC (autolymphocyte-based treatment for renal cell carcinoma)—a treatment in which a small number of the patient's WBCs are removed, activated in the laboratory, and then returned to the patient to combat the cancer cells. This procedure, done on an outpatient basis (two visits per month for six months), has been shown to increase survival time.

alumina-alumina (this is *not* a stutter) —total hip replacement prosthesis.

alumina bioceramic joint replacement material.

aluminum chloride [hexahydrate] **20% in anhydrous ethyl alcohol**—see*Hypercare*.

ALVAD (abdominal left ventricular assist device).

ALVD (asymptomatic left ventricular dysfunction).

alveolar ridge—upper flattened surface of the mandible and lower flattened surface of the maxilla, in the sockets of which the teeth are rooted.

Alvesco (ciclesonide)—a medication used for the treatment of persistent asthma (regardless of severity) in adults, adolescents, and children four years of age and older.

alvimopan—see *Entereg*.

Alzate catheter.

ALZ-50—a protein found in the central nervous system of patients with Alzheimer disease. This may prove to be a good clinical marker in the diagnosis of this disease. Cf. *A68*.

AlzheimAlert—a test that measures neural thread protein, a premier marker molecule for Alzheimer disease.

Alzheimer disease—presenile dementia characterized by cortical atrophy and ventricular dilatation.

Alzheimer Disease Assessment Scale (ADAS)—notes changes in cognition and in activities of daily living.

Alzheimer Disease Assessment Scale cognitive subscale (ADAS-cog)—a battery of brief individual tests (word recall, naming, commands, praxis, orientation, word recognition, spoken language and comprehension, word-finding, recall of test instructions) used in most clinical trials, rather than for diagnosis in the community.

Alzhemed—a disease-modifying drug used in treating Alzheimer disease. It is aimed at preventing the buildup of protein in the brain that disrupts its message system.

Amadeus microkeratome—combines computer monitoring unit, one-

Amadeus *(cont.)*
handed operation, vacuum system, and integrated blade-loading system.

Amazr catheter—used to perform radiofrequency ablation of the inner atrial wall in treatment of refractory atrial fibrillation.

amblyopia—dimness of vision not due to refractive error or organic lesion in the eye.

ambrisentan—a medication for the treatment of pulmonary arterial hypertension; formerly AMB-220.

Ambu bag—a low-tech resuscitation tool in the emergency room.

Ambulator shoe—used in management of hyperkeratotic lesions of the foot.

ambulatory blood pressure monitoring (ABPM).

Ambulette—a paratransit van.

AMD or **ARMD** (age-related macular degeneration).

AMD-Fab—see *Lucentis (ranibizumab)*.

AME bone growth stimulators—noninvasive; can be used over casted or noncasted fracture sites for treatment of nonunion secondary to trauma. See *PEMF*.

Amelogen—composite dental restorative.

AME PinSite Shields—for protection of the site (soft skin) into which are inserted halo pins, external fixation pins, Ilizarov fixation, and traction pins. Made by AME (American Medical Electronics).

American Association for Medical Transcription—see *AAMT*.

American College of Cardiology, American Heart Association, and the European Society of Cardiology (ACC/AHA/ESC) **guidelines**—for the management of patients with atrial fibrillation.

American College of Nurse Midwives (ACNM).

American Health Information Management Association—see *AHIMA*.

American Liver Foundation (ALF)—offers free hepatitis B and C screening in 100 cities in the U.S. Intron (interferon alfa-2b) is now available as a treatment.

American Thoracic Society classification of dyspnea:

grade I—can keep pace walking on level ground with a normal person of similar age and body build, but not on hills or stairs.

grade II—can walk a mile at own pace without dyspnea but cannot keep pace with a normal person.

grade III—becomes breathless after walking about 100 yards or for a few minutes on level ground.

grade IV—becomes breathless while dressing or talking.

AMI (acute myocardial infarction).

Amicus separator—a blood collection device that separates and removes the white blood cells to provide a "leuko-reduced" platelet product for transfusion. White blood cells have been associated with a variety of transfusion reactions.

Amin-Aid—a special formula nutritional supplement usually used by patients with chronic renal failure.

amine precursor uptake and decarboxylation (APUD) **cells**—neural crest cells which are derived from gut endoderm and give rise to carcinoid tumors, usually in the GI tract.

aminobiphosphonates—a class of drugs used for treatment of postmenopausal syndrome.

aminoglycoside ototoxicity—toxicity of the ear attributed to the use of aminoglycosides (neomycin, streptomycin, and kanamycin), affecting mainly the inner and outer hair cells.

aminosterols—a class of naturally occurring pharmacologically active small molecules with potential to treat a number of diseases.

amino acid—any of 20 simple organic acids containing the amino group (-NH2); they serve as the building blocks of peptides and proteins, in which their arrangement is directed by DNA and RNA.

AMI panel—a group of laboratory tests (CK-MB, CK, myoglobin, troponin I) performed to diagnose acute myocardial infarction.

Amis 2000 respiratory mass spectrometer.

AMK (anatomic modular knee) **total knee system**.

AML (acute myeloblastic leukemia)—seen at any age, but mostly in adults.

AML (anatomic medullary locking) **total hip system**.

AML (angiomyolipoma)—solid renal tumor.

AMMOL (acute myelomonoblastic leukemia)—seen at all ages but somewhat more often in adults.

amniocentesis—the aspiration of amniotic fluid from the amniotic sac through a needle puncture of the abdominal wall at or after the 14th week of gestation; provides fluid for testing for biochemical markers of inherited diseases and fetal cells for karyotyping and DNA analysis.

amnioinfusion—a treatment that replenishes depleted amniotic fluid via an intrauterine infusion of saline solution. Used in post-term pregnancies to decrease the incidence of cord compression, variable heart rate decelerations, meconium aspiration, and resultant morbidities.

amnion—the innermost of the membranes enveloping the embryo and containing the amniotic fluid.

amniotic fluid—fluid that fills the the amniotic sac, providing a protective medium for the developing embryo and fetus.

amniotic fluid index (AFI) (Ob-Gyn)—a means of estimating amniotic fluid volume by using ultrasound and taking measurements of the largest pocket of fluid in each of the four quadrants of the uterus. Abnormally low AFI values correlate with the development of fetal distress, intrauterine passage of meconium, and the need for cesarean section.

amniotic membrane transplantation—a graft placed over the cornea for persistent corneal epithelial defect or stromal ulcer and covered by a bandage contact lens. The graft dissolves under the bandage contact lens over a period of 2 weeks.

AMO Array—foldable intraocular lens that can be implanted through small-incision cataract surgery.

AMOL (acute monoblastic leukemia)—seen at all ages, but a higher proportion of patients are adults.

amorphous silicon filmless digital x-ray detection technology—used in the fields of appendicular bone mass measurement and computer-assisted arthritis detection.

amp—brief form for *ampule*.

"ampanclaf"—a phonetic spelling for *amp and claf*, slang for *ampicillin* and *Claforan*.

amphotericin B colloid dispersion (ABCD)—drug treatment for cryptococcal meningitis.

Amplatzer ductal occluder—a device that enables closure of a patent ductus arteriosus defect, obviating the need for surgery.

Amplatzer septal occluder (ASO)—used for the occlusion of atrial septal defects.

Amplatz Super Stiff guidewire.

Amplatz ventricular septal defect device—two woven disks made of nitinol, a biocompatible shape-memory alloy, connected via a woven waist, all braided with polyester fibers to enhance thrombogenicity. The waist matches the diameter of the VSD and the thickness of the ventricular septum. The outer surfaces of the disks become slightly concave rather than bulging after deployment. A microscrew at one end for attachment to the delivery cable was designed to collapse before introduction into the delivery catheter.

AMPLE history—an acronym used by paramedics for the review of allergies, medications, past medical history, last meal, and existing circumstances.

Amplicor—see *COBAS Amplicor HBV monitor test*.

Amplicor Chlamydia Assay—a highly sensitive lab test for *Chlamydia* that can detect the infection in four hours, even in difficult samples such as male urine, compared to the cell culture method that takes several days to a week. It uses polymerase chain reaction technology. See *polymerase chain reaction*.

Amplicor CT/NG test—screening test for chlamydia and gonorrhea that uses polymerase chain reaction technology to check for both diseases simultaneously.

Amplicor *Mycobacterium tuberculosis* test—a PCR (polymerase chain reaction) assay for the direct detection of *Mycobacterium tuberculosis*.

amplification (Genetics)—the production of many copies of a region of DNA.

amplification created restriction enzyme site (ACRES)—a reliable and efficient method for detecting gene mutations and less expensive than sequencing.

Amplified *Mycobacterium tuberculosis* direct (MTD) **test**—a saliva test for tuberculosis that provides results in four to five hours instead of days, with 95.5% accuracy.

amplified perversity—epidemiological term referring to the tendency for harmful trends such as improvement in treating drug-sensitive disease leading to increase in severity of an epidemic, i.e., even more intractable drug-resistant strains.

amplified restriction fragment length polymorphisms (ARFLP) —a DNA fingerprinting technique based on amplification of DNA fragments known as restriction fragment length polymorphisms (RFLPs). Although these DNA sequences are not involved in the transmission of heritable traits or abnormalities, they are more distinctive than DNA sequences that encode proteins, and hence are particularly useful in confirming that two DNA specimens have come from the same subject.

AMPPE ("amp-pee")—see *acute multifocal placoid pigment epitheliopathy*.

AMS—see *ablepharon macrostomia syndrome*.

AMS—see *Active Movement Scale*.

AMS—see *acute mountain sickness*.

AMS (American Medical Systems) **700 CX inflatable penile prosthesis**.

AMS (automatic mode switching)—used in cardiac pacemakers.

AMS Sphincter 800 urinary prosthesis—a hydraulic saline-filled device consisting of an inflatable cuff placed around the urethra, a pressure-regulating balloon placed abdominally, and a control pump placed in the scrotum. The cuff is implanted around the urethra at the bladder neck in the female or around the bulbous urethra in the male, closing off the urethra. To urinate, the patient squeezes the pump to move fluid out of the cuff into the balloon, opening the urethra. The fluid then automatically returns from the balloon to the cuff, restoring continence.

Amset ALPS (anterior locking plate system)—provides anterior decompression and stabilization of the thoracolumbar and lumbar spine.

Amsler grid—a grid with a small dot in the middle; it tests for irregularities in the central 20° of the visual field.

AMT-25-enhanced MR images—MRI term.

amygdala—general term for an almond-shaped structure; specifically a nucleus of the basal ganglia.

AN (acanthosis nigricans).

ANA (antinuclear antibody)—detected by immunofluorescence in patients with rheumatoid arthritis, lupus erythematosus, and other autoimmune diseases.

anabaseine—an ant pheromone considered a possible drug candidate to slow deterioration of memory function in Alzheimer patients.

anabolic steroids—used illegally as street drugs and by body builders and other athletes to build muscle mass, but they are useful in AIDS treatment for patients with wasting syndrome.

anagen—the phase in which hair grows. See *telogen*.

anagrelide—see *Agrylin*.

anakmesis—arrest of maturation of leukocytes, resulting in smaller proportions of mature granular cells in the bone marrow, as observed in agranulocytosis.

anal EMG PerryMeter sensor—used for biofeedback in incontinence training.

analog-to-digital (ADC) **conversion quantization error**—MRI term.

analog-to-digital converter—MRI.

anal wink (or *anal reflex*)—contraction of the anal sphincter when the area around the anus is stroked. Loss of this response is indicative of a neurologic problem.

anaphase—the stage of mitosis or meiosis at which the chromosomes move to the opposite poles of the cell.

anaplastic—referring to tumor tissue containing primitive, undifferentiated cells, unlike the structurally differentiated cells of normal tissue.

Ana-Sal—saliva-based HIV test.

Anastaflo intravascular shunt—inserted into both ends of a severed coronary artery, preventing excessive blood loss. An interior channel within the Anastaflo conveys blood to the heart muscles beyond the grafting site while the replacement artery is sutured.

anastomoser—a coined word for an anastomosis stapler.

anatomical snuffbox—shallow depression between two tendons in the wrist, just proximal to the base of the thumb.

anatomic graduated components (AGC)—used in joint replacements.

ANCA (antineutrophil cytoplasmic antibody)—associated with cases of the syndrome of lung hemorrhage and

ANCA *(cont.)* nephritis. Also, *c-ANCA* and *p-ANCA*.

ancestral organs—five organs identified in acupuncture (brain/spinal cord, liver/gallbladder, bone marrow, uterus, and blood system).

Anchorlok soft-tissue anchor.

anchovy—a term used in microsurgery and hand surgery and refers to a rolled-up piece of fascia lata (that looks like an anchovy). Usage: "Operation: Carpal/metacarpal joint arthroplasty, with tensor fasciae latae anchovy." Also: "The fascia lata was initially rolled into an anchovy and tied together with corner chromic sutures. This anchovy would not adequately fill the irregular joint cavity. The anchovy was then unraveled and the fascia lata divided into three strips. These were carefully inserted into the joint space with the joint opened and distracted."

anconeus arthroplasty—a new procedure for reconstruction of the radio-humeral joint.

AnCore anuloplasty system—for mitral and tricuspid repair. Note preferred spelling of *anuloplasty* with one *n*.

Ancure system—minimally invasive endovascular repair of abdominal aortic aneurysm.

Andes virus—variation of hantavirus pulmonary syndrome found in Argentina and Chile.

Andractim (dihydrotestosterone gel)—drug used to treat male hormone deficiency in men, a condition also known as geriatric hypogonadism, or "male menopause." May also be used to treat benign prostatic hypertrophy.

Andrews spinal frame/table (Neuro)—frame attaches to an operating table and is used like the Hastings frame to keep the patient in a flexed knee-chest position. With the patient in the prone kneeling position for spinal surgery, the abdomen is kept from contact with the table, reducing vena caval pressure and bleeding intraoperatively. It distributes the patient's weight and relieves pressure on the knees. Also, *Andrews SST-3000*. See also *Hastings table*.

Androflo monitor—a device using Androsonix technology that continuously measures pulmonary ventilation and breathing regularity. It is useful in monitoring sleep disorders and patients suffering from respiratory pathologies. See also *Androsonix*.

androgen receptor mutation assay—a laboratory test used in evaluating prostate carcinoma.

Androgram—a noninvasive tool for monitoring pulmonary artery pressure.

Androscope Stethos, Androscope i-Stethos—a new type of stethoscope; the i-Stethos can be interfaced to a PDA (personal digital assistant) device.

Androsonix biological sound monitor—a disposable adhesive device affixed to the patient's skin that continuously captures and transmits changes in pressure due to cardiac and pulmonary sounds and vibrations. These sound signals are amplified and filtered before being converted to digital signals to be transmitted to a doctor performing auscultation from a remote location. See also *Androflo monitor*.

anechoic—in echocardiography, an area not generating echoes.

anecortave acetate—drug used to treat wet form of age-related macular degeneration. It is designed to prevent severe vision loss and inhibit lesion growth in the retina. It is delivered by an injection around and behind the sclera (a juxtascleral injection) once every 6 months.

anembryonic pregnancy—pregnancy in which the embryo has aborted but other products of conception are present.

anesthesia—see *medications*.
- BMX (Benadryl, Maalox, and Xylocaine) mouthwash
- EMLA (eutectic mixture of local anesthetics [lidocaine and prilocaine])
- MAC (bupivacaine [Marcaine], adrenaline, and cocaine)
- MAC (minimum alveolar concentration)
- MAC (monitored anesthesia care)
- LET (lidocaine, epinephrine, and tetracaine)
- LMA (laryngeal mask airway)
- TAC (tetracaine, adrenaline [epinephrine], and cocaine)

anesthetic vs. anesthesia—*anesthetic* is the drug that is *administered*; *anesthesia* (the state of unconsciousness) is *induced*.

aneuploid (Genetics)—having an abnormal number of chromosomes (in human beings, a number other than 46, or 23 pairs).

AneuRx stent-graft system—for treatment of abdominal aortic aneurysm. Also called *AneuRx tube graft*.

AngeCool RF (radiofrequency)—catheter ablation system used in the treatment of atrial arrhythmias.

AngeFlex leads—used with Sentinel implantable cardioverter-defibrillator.

Angelchik antireflux prosthesis—used in repair of sliding hiatal hernia and gastroesophageal reflux. The abdomen is entered and the stomach and a small portion of the esophagus pulled down below the diaphragm. The small C-shaped silicone prosthesis is placed around the esophagus and tied and the abdomen closed. The prosthesis then lies around the esophagus, below the diaphragm, and above the stomach, reinforcing the esophageal sphincter.

angel wing—a figurative term for a portion of a bevel resection guide, shaped like an angel wing, used in joint replacement surgery. Also may refer to a *Miller resection guide*.

angina pectoris triggers—see *four E's*.

Angiocath PRN—a flexible catheter.

angiographic embolization (AE)—an alternative modality for treatment of splenic injuries.

angiographically occult intracranial vascular malformation (AOIVM).

angiography, arteriography—the radiographic study of arteries into which radiopaque medium has been injected. Still pictures may be taken immediately after injection, or motion pictures may be made showing the flow of blood and contrast medium through vessels. See *digital subtraction angiography; fluorescein angiography; indocyanine green angiography; multi-slab and cine techniques for single breath-hold cardiac-synchronized angiography.*

angioimmunoblastic lymphadenopathy with dysproteinemia (AILD).

AngioJet Rheolytic thrombectomy system—a device to treat peripheral blood clots. It is a minimally inva-

AngioJet *(cont.)*
sive catheter system which allows rapid and safe removal of intravascular blood clots from leg and arm arteries and bypass grafts and would be an alternative to current methods, drug or surgery therapy.

angiolymphoid hyperplasia with eosinophilia—uncommon smooth-surfaced nodules, consisting of lymphocytes and eosinophils involving dermis and subcutaneous tissue.

angioma—see *cherry angioma*.

AngioMark—MRI contrast agent for noninvasive breast imaging.

angiomyolipoma (AML).

angioplasty, laser—used to ablate obstructing tissue. Causes less subintimal hemorrhage than balloon dilatation.

AngiOptic microcatheter—used for angiographic diagnosis of the peripheral vascular system.

Angio-Seal—a hemostatic puncture closure device. See *HPCD*.

AngioStent—balloon-expandable stent and delivery system for the treatment of malignant strictures in the biliary tree.

angiotensin-converting enzyme (ACE) **inhibitor**. See *ACE inhibitor.*

angiotensin II—a vasoconstrictor associated with primary aldosteronism and secretion of large amounts of renin in the blood in some hypertensive patients.

angle
acetabular angle of Sharp
acetabular roof-obliquity
antegonial
Baumann
blunted costophrenic angle
Boehler (Böhler)
center-edge angle (CE) of Wiberg
central collodiaphyseal (CCD)

angle *(cont.)*
cerebellopontile
cerebellopontine
Cobb
costophrenic (CP, CPA)
costosternal
distal articular set (DASA)
flip
gonial
Lovibond
neck-shaft angle (NSA) of femur
proximal articular set (PASA)
Wiberg center edge (CE)

angle of Hiss.

Angle's class III malocclusion.

angry—inflamed, as a descriptor for various tissues, such as the brain, breast, colon, and synovium in the following examples. Usage: (1) "The brain was quite soft at this point and was pulsating in a normal fashion.The brain itself did not appear contused or 'angry'." (2) "There are 'angry' looking red streaks near the sore area (of the breast)." (3) On a pathology specimen of resected colon: "(This) demonstrates not only the angry red mucosa but also the tendency for the inflamed tissue to throw itself up into inflammatory pseudopolyps." (4) "Normally (the synovium) is very thin and stops the natural fluid lubrication of the joint from leaking out. However, when inflamed it becomes very swollen, red and angry."

Angstrom MD—an implantable single-lead cardioverter-defibrillator.

angular frequency; **angular momentum**—MRI terms.

anhedonia (Psych)—loss of feelings of pleasure in things that usually give pleasure. Usage: "The patient describes anhedonia and low energy."

anhidrosis—see *congenital insensitivity to pain and anhidrosis* (CIPA); *congenital sensory neuropathy with anhidrosis* (CSNA).

animal-assisted therapy (AAT)—used in treating autistic children, stroke victims, nursing home patients, and others who respond to animals, when it is difficult for human therapists to make contact.

anion gap ("an-eye-on")—referring to electrolytes.

aniseikonia—inequality in size and shape of an object, as seen by each eye.

anisocoria—inequality of diameter of the pupils. Cf. *anisophoria.*

anisophoria—condition in which the visual lines of the pupils are not on the same horizontal plane; caused by unequal pull on the muscles of the eyes. Cf. *anisocoria.*

anisoylated plasminogen streptokinase activator complex (APSAC).

ankle air stirrup.

ankle-brachial index (ABI)—painless test to help determine if a patient has peripheral vascular disease. A regular blood pressure cuff and a special ultrasound stethoscope, using the Doppler-echo technique, check the blood pressure in the arm and in the inferior limbs. The pressure in the arm is compared to the pressure in the inferior limbs to determine how well blood flows. If atherosclerotic narrowing is present in the arteries of the inferior limbs, the blood pressure at that level might be lower than that found in the arm.

AnkleCiser exerciser (Phys Ther).

ankle jerk—see *Achilles reflex.*

ankle mortise—the normal articulation between the talus and the distal tibia and fibula. See *mortise.*

anlage (pl., anlagen)—a primordial structure in the developing embryo.

ANLL (acute nonlymphoid leukemia).

ANNs (artificial neural networks).

anomaly
  cervical aortic arch
  cervical rib
  cor triatriatum dexter
  DiGeorge (DGA)
  Ebstein cardiac
  Pelger-Huët
  Taussig-Bing

anorexia—see *reversed anorexia syndrome.*

anorexia nervosa—severe caloric restriction due to distortion of body image, with dangerous nutritional deficiency. See *bulimorexia.*

anosognostic—pertaining to a lack of knowledge, awareness, or recognition of one's own disease. *Not* anosmic agnostic.

anosognostic syndrome—a neuropsychiatric syndrome seen in paraplegia due to lesions of the superior parietal lobe; characterized by unawareness of paralysis, neglect of the paralyzed part, and sometimes visual or tactile hallucinations. Usage: "He became more alert and responsive, but he is impulsive, noncompliant, confused, disoriented, anosognostic, delusional, and paranoid."

ANP (atrial natriuretic peptide).

ANP-A (atrial natriuretic peptide [A-type]).

Anscore health management system—measures heart rate variability, which can be used as an indicator of autonomic nervous system dysfunction.

anserine bursitis syndrome—associated with pes anserine bursitis.

Anspach—neurosurgical and orthopedic surgery instruments, including

Anspach *(cont.)*
craniotomes, cranial perforators, and diamond dissecting cutters.

Antabuse (disulfiram)—drug given to recovering alcoholics to thwart their consumption of alcohol. This drug is often misspelled "Antiabuse" because it is "anti-alcohol."

antagonist—a drug that inhibits or counteracts the action of naturally produced substances on a receptor. Examples: *adrenergic antagonist, beta antagonist.* Cf. *agonist.*

antecolic—in front of the colon, e.g., antecolic anastomosis and antecolic gastrojejunostomy.

antecubital fossa—correct term for anterior cubital fossa, even if the latter is dictated. *Not* anticubital.

antegonial angle or notch—just in front of the gonion (the most inferior, posterior, and lateral point of the external angle of the mandible). An anatomical landmark in oral and plastic surgery.

antegrade continence enema (ACE) —an enema administered through a continent cutaneous appendicocecostomy created by the Malone procedure. It is used to improve bowel control in patients with fecal incontinence, severe constipation, or both due to neurologic disorders such as spina bifida and myelomeningocele. Enema fluid enters the proximal colon and flows in an antegrade direction, that is, in the direction of normal intestinal peristalsis, flushing impacted stool from above.

antegrade continence enema (ACE), **in situ appendix**—a procedure done for refractory constipation and overflow fecal incontinence due to neurogenic bowel. Also called *antegrade colonic enema* or *Malone antegrade colonic enema* (MACE).

antegrade scrotal sclerotherapy—treatment for varicocele consisting of puncture of dilated vein of the pampiniform plexus by scrotal access and injection of a sclerosing agent under fluoroscopy after control of venous drainage. This is an alternative to the traditional methods of choice, which include high vasal ligation and retrograde sclerotherapy, and the newer methods of microsurgical and laparoscopic ligation.

anterior apical aneurysm (AAA). Cf. *abdominal aortic aneurysm* (AAA).

anterior chamber acrylic implants (Oph).

anterior chamber maintainer (ACM)—an instrument used in intracapsular cataract extraction when the lens is subluxated.

anterior cruciate ligament (ACL).

anterior inferior communicating artery (AICA).

anterior lumbar interbody fusion (ALIF)

anterior mandibular positioning (AMP) **dental device**—a device designed to increase airway caliber and decrease airway resistance by moving the mandible forward during sleep, and used in treatment of obstructive sleep apnea.

anterior pelvic exenteration—a surgical procedure consisting of resection of the bladder, uterus, ovaries, and upper vagina en bloc.

anterograde Wenckebach cycle length (WBCL)—a term used in discussing the pacing of the heart or in electrophysiology testing.

anterolisthesis—spondylolisthesis with anterior displacement of a vertebral body on the one below it.

anthelix, antihelix—of the ear.

anthracenediones—a class of chemotherapy drugs, e.g., *mitoxantrone.*

Anthron heparinized antithrombogenic catheter—used in angiography.

anthropometry—measurement of the human body in order to assess general nutritional status of an individual or population group.

Antia-Buch chondrocutaneous advancement flap—a plastic surgery procedure in which a flap is used to repair moderate-sized defects on the helical rim of the ear. The skin of the helix and the underlying cartilage are either unilaterally or bilaterally advanced. Two variations of the flap exist: (1) The flap can be full thickness and detached on both the anterior and posterior surfaces of the helix. This construction allows for maximal extension of the flap, although the flap pedicle is relatively narrow. (2) The flap can also be designed with the posterior skin intact, leaving a broader flap base as Antia and Buch originally describe. The entire posterior skin is undermined to elevate the flap. Then, the flap is advanced with a dog ear that is removed posteriorly. The helix must be meticulously realigned.

Antia-Buch helical rim advancement flap—see *Antia-Buch chondrocutaneous advancement flap*.

anti-aliasing techniques (MRI)—mathematical methods for eliminating wrap-around and zebra artifacts. The artifacts appear because of the nature of the processing of the raw data that produce the image (two-dimensional Fourier transform, 2DFT). Doubling the size of the field of view (FOV), called oversampling, can be helpful, and newer imaging protocols include a "no phase wrap" function to eliminate aliasing artifacts.

antibacterial personal catheter—designed for intermittent self-catheterization in patients with incontinence and other voiding dysfunction, as well as for surgical and sampling procedures.

antibody—an immunoglobulin molecule, formed by a competent immune system in response to challenge by a foreign substance (antigen), which it neutralizes or destroys after binding to it chemically in lock-and-key fashion. See the following antibodies:

acetylcholine receptor (AChRab)
Acusyst Xcell monoclonal
ANA (antinuclear antibody)
anticardiolipin (ACL, ACA)
CCP
anti-CD11a humanized monoclonal
anti-CD18 humanized
anticentromere (ACA)
anticytoplasmic (ACPA)
anti-D (WinRho)
anti-EA
anti-EGF-receptor antibody for cancer
antiendomysial
antifibrin
anti-HA
anti-HAV
anti-IgE humanized monoclonal
anti-IL-8
anti-La
antimitochondrial
antineutrophilic cytoplasmic (ANCA)
antiphospholipid
anti-Ro
anti-Sm
anti-VEGF
AxSYM (to hepatitis C virus)

antibody *(cont.)*
Bexxar radiolabeled monoclonal
BR96-doxorubicin monoclonal
C100-3 hepatitis C virus (anti-HIV)
CC49 monoclonal
CD5+
CD18
cryptosporidiosis
dacliximab monoclonal
Diffistat-G polyclonal
Duffy blood antibody type
E5 monoclonal
Ha-1A monoclonal
HB_cAb
HB_eAb
HB_sAb
humanized anti-TAC (T-cell activated antigen) monoclonal
I-131 radiolabeled
IgM-RF (rheumatoid factor)
ImmuRAIT-LL2 (IgG 2A monoclonal)
islet cell (ICA)
Kell blood antibody type
Kidd blood antibody type
LDP-02 humanized monoclonal
LeuTech radiolabeled
Lewis blood antibody type
LymphoCide
MAb-170 monoclonal
MabThera (rituximab) monoclonal
monoclonal
Oncolym radiolabeled monoclonal
opsonizing
panel reactive (PRA)
PM 81 monoclonal
ProstaScint (CYT-356 radiolabeled with 111 indium chloride) monoclonal
ReoPro (abciximab) monoclonal
rhuFab
Rituxan (rituximab) monoclonal
7E3 monoclonal antiplatelet
thyroperoxidase
TI-23 cytomegalovirus monoclonal

antibody *(cont.)*
2C3 anti-VEGF (vascular endothelial growth factor)
WinRho SD (anti-D)
XMMEN-OE5 monoclonal

antibody molecules (immune globulins)—have heavy and light chains. There are five classes of heavy chains (G, A, M, D, and E), IgG, IgA, IgM, etc., and two classes of light chains (kappa and lambda).

Antia-Buch chondrocutaneous flap—for repair of full-thickness upper pole auricular (ear) defects. This technique achieves a natural auricular shape in three dimensions with minimal disruption of anatomic landmarks and avoids conspicuous scars.

anticardiolipin antibody (ACL, ACA).

anti-CCP antibody—a marker for rheumatoid arthritis and a predictor of the course of the disease.

anti-CD11a humanized monoclonal antibody—drug designed to specifically block the T-cells that are overactive in psoriasis. See *Xanelim.*

anti-CD18 humanized antibody—drug used for the prevention or alleviation of reperfusion injuries and mortality following treatment of shock.

anticentromere antibody (ACA)—appears in the majority of patients with CREST syndrome. See *CREST syndrome.*

anticipation (Genetics)—the progressively earlier appearance or increased severity of a familial disease in successive generations.

anticonvulsant hypersensitivity syndrome—a potentially fatal drug reaction with cutaneous and systemic reactions. The hallmark features of fever, rash, and lymphadenopathy

anticonvulsant *(cont.)*
are accompanied by multiorgan system abnormalities.

anticytoplasmic antibody (ACPA) **test** —detects autoantibodies to components of neutrophilic cytoplasm by immunofluorescence. Useful in diagnosing Wegener granulomatosis and gauging its extent and severity.

anti-D antibody (WinRho SD)—used in intermittent doses for treatment of childhood idiopathic thrombocytopenic purpura (also referred to as immunothrombocytopenic purpura).

anti-EA antibody—*EA* stands for *early antigen* of Epstein-Barr virus. Patients with chronic mononucleosis syndrome are thought to test positive to the antibody.

anti-EGF-receptor antibody—used in cancer treatment.

antiendomysial antibody test—blood test to detect celiac disease, a condition in which the gluten in wheat, oats, barley, and rye damages the small intestine.

antiestrogen drug—a drug that counteracts the effects of estrogen.

antifibrin antibody imaging—a method to diagnose deep vein thrombosis; it is thought to be a safer, faster, and more accurate way to detect blood clots than venography. In the procedure, a radiolabeled antifibrin antibody is injected into the patient. It then attaches itself to the fibrin in the clot; within an hour, imaging reveals the clot.

antigen—a molecule that can elicit antibody formation. See the following antigens.
bladder tumor (BTA)
bladder tumor-associated (BTA)
BPAG1 (BP antigen1, 230 kD BP
BPAG2 (BP antigen2, 180 kD BP

antigen *(cont.)*
Bu
CA1-18 tumor marker
CA 15-3
CA 19-9
CA 72-4
CEA (carcinoembryonic)
common acute lymphoblastic leukemia (CALLA)
ENA (extractable nuclear)
epithelial membrane (EMA)
Goa (Gonzales blood)
HbAg (or HBAg) (hepatitis B)
HB_eAg (hepatitis B *e*)
HB_sAg (hepatitis B surface)
Histoplasma capsulatum (HPA)
HLA (human lymphocyte)
inhalant
Jo-1
PHA (phytohemagglutinin)
PLA-I (platelet)
PSA (prostate-specific)
PSA-ACT
PSMA (prostate-specific membrane)
Rh (Rhesus) factor
SD
Sm
vWF (von Willebrand factor)

antigen enzyme immunoassay—a laboratory test for histoplasmosis.

antigenuria—the presence of one or more antigens in the urine.

Anti-Gliadin IgG, Anti-Gliadin IgA — ELISA autoimmune tests trademarked by Great Smokies.

anti-HA, anti-HAV (antibody to hepatitis A virus).

antihelix, anthelix—of the ear.

anti-IgE humanized monoclonal antibody—drug used to block or interfere with the process that leads to allergy symptoms in allergic rhinitis.

anti-IL-8 antibody for inflammation.

anti-La antibody—an unusual antibody found in patients with Sjögren disease. Cf. *anti-Ro*.

antimesenteric border of ileum—a surgical landmark; the side of the small bowel opposite the insertion of the mesentery.

antimicrobial catheter cuff—placed subcutaneously where a central venous catheter exits from the skin. It slowly releases silver ions which prevent infection from microorganisms along the catheter exit site.

antimitochondrial antibody.

Anti-MPO (p-ANCA) **ELISA autoimmune test**—used as a complement to the Anti-Pr-3 (c-ANCA) test. The two tests are used to differentiate between various forms of vasculitis.

antineutrophilic cytoplasmic antibody (ANCA)—indicative of an acute necrotizing vasculitis.

antinuclear antibody (ANA).

antiphospholipid antibody (aPLA)—found in the serum of women who experience recurrent spontaneous abortions. These antibodies inhibit the normal formation of syncytiotrophoblasts in the placenta and jeopardize the pregnancy.

antiphospholipid syndrome (APS)—a syndrome consisting of recurrent thromboses, spontaneous abortions, livedo reticularis, thrombocytopenia, neurologic disease, and antiphospholipid antibody (aPLA). See *antiphospholipid antibodies*.

anti-protrusio devices—used to bridge across the ischium to the ilium to compensate for poor or absent bone.

antipsychotic drug side effects—akathisia, extrapyramidal and pyramidal signs, and tardive dyskinesia.

antireflux flap valve—a valve constructed primarily of mucosa for urinary incontinence.

anti-RHO-D titer (Lab).

anti-Ro antibody—an unusual antibody found in patients with Sjögren disease. Cf. *anti-La*.

antisense (Genetics)—referring to the strand of a double-stranded nucleic acid that is complementary to the sense strand, which serves as a template for its formation.

antisense drugs—anticancer drugs consisting of small chemically modified stretches of single-stranded DNA, designed to prevent the production of certain cancer-causing proteins.

antisense oligodeoxynucleotides (also known as ODNs)—proposed as a new therapy for patients with cancer, including malignant brain tumors. Antisense ODNs have been used successfully to block glioblastoma gene expression in vitro and expression of multiple genes with the central nervous system of experimental animals.

Anti-Sept bactericidal scrub solution.

anti-Sm antibody—found in lupus erythematosus. The *Sm* is for *Smith*.

antistreptolysin titer (AST).

anti-Tamm-Horsfall protein—found in interstitial cystitis.

anti-teichoic acid titer (Lab).

antithrombin III (ATnativ)—drug used to inhibit blood coagulation in patients with an antithrombin III deficiency. It is given intravenously prior to surgery or obstetrical procedures to prevent the formation of thrombi and emboli. Note the unique spelling of *ATnativ*, with two initial capital letters.

antithymocyte globulin (ATG).

anti-TNF drugs (antitumor necrosis factor)—Procysteine, and pentoxifylline (Trental). Tumor necrosis factor has been linked to wasting syndrome and HIV activation in AIDS.

antitussives—a class of drugs used as cough suppressants.

anti-VEGF antibody—an inhibitor of angiogenesis (blood-vessel growth) that may hinder the growth of cancer tumors by starving their blood supply.

Antopol-Goldman lesion—subepithelial hematoma of the renal pelvis.

AnuloFlex—a flexible anuloplasty ring for mitral valve repair.

AnuloFlo—anuloplasty ring system.

anulus—the correct spelling, with one *n*. *Annulus* (with two *n*'s) is a deviant spelling of ancient vintage.

anulus of Zinn. *Not* annulus.

anuresis—inability of the kidneys to produce or excrete urine. Cf. *enuresis*.

anxiolytics—antianxiety drugs; minor tranquilizers.

AoBP (aortic blood pressure).

AO (American Optical) **indirect ophthalmoscope**.

AOIVM (angiographically occult intracranial vascular malformation).

A-OK ShortCut knife—an ophthalmic knife with a unique rounded tip and short length for intraocular incisions. Also called *ShortCut knife*.

A1cNow monitor—for use at home without a prescription by diabetes patients to obtain immediate glycated hemoglobin (HbA1c) or A1C results from a small drop of blood.

aortic connector system—for performance of sutureless anastomoses during coronary artery bypass graft procedures.

aortic root (*not* route)—Usage: "The patient underwent an aortic root reconstruction procedure with aortic valve replacement."

aortobifemoral reconstruction.

aortofemoral bypass graft (AFBG).

aortoiliac obstructive (or occlusive) **disease** (AIOD).

aortomyoplasty—a surgical treatment for heart failure in which the latissimus dorsi muscle is wrapped around the aorta and stimulated to contract during diastole to provide diastolic counterpulsation. In one technique, the latissimus dorsi muscle (LDM) is wrapped en bloc around the aorta and secured to itself (circumferential wrap). In a second technique (helical wrap), a 4-cm to 5-cm wide strip of the lateral portion of LDM is isolated and wrapped as a helical coil around the descending thoracic aorta. A newer third technique is called a wringer wrap, in which the oblique transverse portion of the LDM is wrapped clockwise around the superior portion of the descending thoracic aorta, coupled to the lateral portion of LDM, which is wrapped in a counterclockwise direction distal to the oblique transverse portion.

AOVM (angiographically occult vascular malformations).

APA (aldosterone-producing adenoma).

APAAP (alkaline phosphatase antialkaline phosphatase).

APACHE CV risk predictor—Internet-based product that can help physicians anywhere predict a patient's risk of death or serious complications before the patient elects to undergo an invasive heart procedure.

APACHE III (acute physiology and chronic health evaluation) **score**—originally designed as a predictor of death on admission to the ICU. It is now used to predict length of stay for long-term hospitalizations.

apallic syndrome—parasomniac conscious state.

A-pattern strabismus.

APC—see *argon plasma coagulation.*

APC (adenopolyposis coli) **gene**—implicated in the development of colorectal carcinoma.

APDDS—slang abbreviation for antibiotic prophylaxis before dental work (in patients at risk of bacterial endocarditis).

Apex irrigation system (ENT).

Apex Plus excimer laser—used in the treatment of myopia, hyperopia, and astigmatism. It combines an erodible mask with an Axicon prismatic lens system for ablation of hyperopia.

Apex universal drive (ENT).

Apgar score (named for Dr. Virginia Apgar, an anesthesiologist)—rating of the condition of the newborn infant, performed at one and five minutes after birth. The criteria are color, heart rate, respiration, reflex response to nose catheter, and muscle tone. "The infant's Apgars were 8 and 9 at one and five minutes."

1. Color: If the infant is pale or blue, the score for color is 0; if the body is pink and the extremities are blue, the score is 1; if the body and extremities are pink, the score is 2.

2. Heart rate: If the heart rate cannot be elicited, the score for heart rate is 0; if it is less than 100, the score is 1; if more than 100, the score is 2.

3. Respiration: If respirations can not be elicited, the score for respiration is 0; if irregular or slow, the score is 1; if respirations are good, crying, the score for this is 2.

4. Reflex response: If there is no reflex response to the nose catheter, the score is 0; if the infant grimaces, the score is 1; if the infant sneezes or coughs, the score is 2.

5. Muscle tone: If the infant is limp, the score for muscle tone is 0; if there is some flexion of the extremities, the score is 1; if the infant is active, the score is 2. All the subscore totals are added together for the total score on a scale of 1 to 10 at one and five minutes.

APGAR—in Family APGAR Questionnaire, the acronym formed from the initial letters of adaptability, partnership, growth, affection, and resolve. Sometimes abbreviated FAPGAR. See *Apgar score.*

apheresis (from Greek *aphairesis*, taking away)—removal of a component of the blood from the intravascular circulation. This process is used now as apheresis of plasma, erythrocytes, leukocyte fractions, platelets, and cold precipitable serum proteins in blood banking. It is used in treating babies who are Rh incompatible and is likely to be used in the future for selective apheresis of autoantibodies in the treatment of rheumatoid arthritis, systemic lupus erythematosus, and other autoimmune diseases. See *lymphapheresis, plasmapheresis.* Cf. *electrophoresis.*

A_1-PI (alpha$_1$-proteinase inhibitor)—see Zemaira.

aphtha (pl., aphthae), aphthous, adj., ("af-thus")—the small ulcers of the oral mucosa known colloquially as "canker sores." Cf. *abscess.*

apical impulse—a thrust noted over the apex of the heart. May be referred to as *PMI, point of maximal impulse.*

apico-abdominal bypass—a temporary bypass established between the left ventricle (cardiac apex) and the descending (abdominal) aorta.

APL (abductor pollicis longus).
APL (acute promyelocytic leukemia).
aPLA (antiphospholipid antibody).
APLD (automated percutaneous lumbar diskectomy).
Apley sign.
Apligraf (Graftskin)—living skin product that looks and feels like human skin, indicated for treatment of lower extremity venous ulcers. It has two primary layers, including an outer epidermal layer made of living human keratinocytes and a dermal layer consisting of human fibroblasts. The keratinocytes and fibroblasts are derived from donor tissue that is thoroughly screened for a wide range of infectious pathogens.
APML (acute promyelocytic leukemia).
apnea—see *obstructive sleep apnea* (OSA).
apnea/hypopnea index (AHI).
apocrine metaplasia—a change in the cells lining a breast duct so they appear similar to a lactating breast, often associated with mammary dysplasia.
Apo E-4 (apolipoprotein E-4)—thought to increase the risk for Alzheimer disease. It also appears to be associated with poor recovery from traumatic brain injury.
apolipoprotein E—the E4 allele of this gene may become a predictor of coronary heart disease mortality.
Apollo hip prosthesis.
Apollo knee prosthesis.
Apollo triple lumen papillotome.
apophysis—a projecting part of a bone; a bony outgrowth, such as a tubercle, process, or tuberosity, not separated from the main portion of the bone. Cf. *epiphysis, hypophysis*.
apoptosis ("AP-op-toe-sis")—programmed death of certain cells, such as erythrocytes and epithelial cells in the adult and cells of transitional organs in the fetus; may also occur in cells damaged by environmental factors or viral infection. Cells in cultures, other than stem cells and tumor cells, undergo apoptosis after about 50 cell divisions.
Apo-Zidovudine (Retrovir)—drug used to treat AIDS.
apparent—visible, obvious, evident. Cf. *aberrant*.
apparent life-threatening event (ALTE).
appendectomy, **inversion-ligation.**
appendicocecostomy—continent appendicocutaneous fistula, created surgically by the Malone technique, to provide access to the proximal colon for administration of antegrade enemas in patients with fecal incontinence, severe constipation, or both, due to neurologic disease. Also, *Mitrofanoff procedure*.
appendicular ataxia—muscular incoordination of the extremities.
appendicular bone mass measurement—see *amorphous silicon filmless digital x-ray detection arm artery*, *LIMA (left internal mammary artery)*.
appendogram—a contrast fluoroscopic exam to assess the size and shape of the left atrial appendage.
applanated condition—a wordy way of saying *applanation* (abnormal flattening of the cornea or lens).
applanation—flattening of the cornea by pressure.
applanation tonometry—measures intraocular pressure. See *Schiötz tonometry*.

applanometer—an instrument used to determine the intraocular pressure in testing for glaucoma. See *tonometry.*

Applebaum prosthesis and procedure—incudostapedial joint prosthesis for incus replacement surgery.

apple peel syndrome—jejunal atresia, caused by the distal small bowel coming straight off the cecum and twisting around the marginal artery like an apple peel.

apposition—the placing or bringing together of two adjacent parts, e.g., drawing together the cut edges of an incision on closure of a wound. Usage: "The wound edges were placed in apposition and sutured in place." Cf. *opposition.*

Appraise—diabetes monitoring system that allows patients to collect their own specimens for hemoglobin $A1_c$ and microalbumin.

apprehension test—refers to the apprehensive appearance of a patient in testing for a subluxed or dislocated shoulder. The arm is held abducted and extended while it is in external rotation, and the test is considered to be positive if the patient appears to be apprehensive. Usage: "There is a positive mild to moderate apprehension test."

approach—see *operation.*

APPT (Adolescent and Pediatric Pain Tool)—a scale used to measure pain in Ilizarov limb-lengthening procedures. It is a measurement of current pain, including a visual analog scale, a listing of 42 words that describe the qualitative aspects of pain, and two body diagrams. Cf. *HSC Scale.*

"aprenavir"—misspelling for *amprenavir.*

apron—excessive subcutaneous fat that hangs from the abdominal wall like an apron; also called *hanging panniculus.*

apropulsive gait—in which the patient has a weak push-off when walking.

aprosody (Psych)—lack of variation in voice features like pitch, loudness, tempo, and intonation, such as encountered in Parkinson disease.

APR total hip system—porous, coated cement fixation.

APS (antiphospholipid antibody syndrome).

APSAC (anisoylated plasminogen streptokinase activator complex). See *anistreplase.*

APSGN (acute poststreptococcal glomerulonephritis).

Apt-Downey alkali denaturation test—performed to rule out maternal source of bleeding in newborn.

Aptima Combo 2 and Aptima CT—assays for the detection of *Chlamydia trachomatis* and *Neisseria gonorrhoeae* from the widest variety of sample types: clinician-collected endocervical, vaginal and urethral swab specimens; patient-collected vaginal swab specimens; and female and male urine specimens.

A, P, T, M (aortic, pulmonic, tricuspid, and mitral valves)—listening areas for auscultation of heart murmurs.

APTT (activated partial thromboplastin time).

APUD (amine precursor uptake and decarboxylation).

apudoma—tumor composed of APUD cells; potentially malignant or overtly malignant gastrin-secreting tumor; the most frequent cause of the Zollinger-Ellison syndrome. See *APUD, Zollinger-Ellison syndrome.*

Aquacel Ag—a primary antimicrobial wound dressing made from sodium carboxymethylcellulose (NaCMC)

Aquacel *(cont.)* containing 1.2% silver in an ionic form.

Aquacel Ag Hydrofiber wound packing and dressing.

aquacise—a coined word denoting buoyant exercise in water.

Aqua-Flow collagen glaucoma drainage device—permanently implanted under the sclera (without entering the interior of the eye) for immediate reduction of eye pressure associated with open-angle glaucoma.

Aqua Glycolic—over-the-counter skin care line that contains glycolic acid.

Aquaphor gauze—non-adhering dressing.

aquaporin-1—protein identified as enabling the kidneys to form concentrated urine, a process that is critical for preventing severe dehydration during times of water deprivation. The discovery of this protein has potential implications for treatment of diseases associated with fluid retention or refractory edema, including congestive heart failure and cirrhosis.

AquariusNET—a streaming 2-D/3-D medical imaging server.

AquaShield—reusable, one-piece, completely waterproof orthopedic cast cover.

Aquasil Smart Wetting dental impression material.

Aquasorb transparent hydrogel dressing—a conformable gel dressing that promotes healing by maintaining a moist environment. Healing can be monitored because the dressing is transparent. Cf. *Curasorb, ClearSite,* and *Ventex.*

Aquaspirillum itersonii—a gram-negative organism.

aqueous flare (Oph)—scattering of slit-lamp light beam when the light is directed into the anterior chamber. This is found with increased protein in the aqueous and is an indication of iritis. See *cell and flare.*

arachidonic acid—an unsaturated fatty acid that occurs in certain fats and in animal phosphatides.

arachnoid (Greek *arachne*, spider)—the membrane between dura and pia mater; the weblike strands between it and the pia give rise to the name.

arachnophlebectomy—a procedure to eliminate spider veins. See *arachnophlebectomy surgical device*.

Arachnophlebectomy Needle—used with the arachnophlebectomy surgical device.

arachnophlebectomy surgical device—used to eliminate spider veins. The device consists of a needle with a fork-like head that captures the targeted vessel. The device is then rotated 360°, transecting the vessel. The procedure is repeated every 1 to 2 cm along the vessel, causing the vein to blanch. The body absorbs the destroyed tissue.

arbovirus (arthropod-borne virus)—any one of a group of viruses carried by mosquitoes and ticks. Arboviruses are the cause of some febrile diseases, such as yellow fever, and of types of viral meningitis. See *togavirus*.

ARC (AIDS-related complex).

arcade of Frohse—see *Frohse.*

Arcanobacterium haemolyticum—a bacterial throat infection seen in adolescents and young adults, and may mimic a viral exanthem, toxic erythema, or drug eruption.

ARCD (age-related cognitive decline).

arch bar—a wire or bar support, shaped to fit the arch of the teeth, used to splint a fractured jaw or loosened teeth. See *Winters arch bar.*

arch study—arterial imaging study, usually of the aortic arch.

ARDs (acid-related disorders).

ARDS (adult respiratory distress syndrome).

Arenberg-Denver implant—a pressure-sensitive unidirectional inner-ear valve implant. For use in patients with Mondini dysplasia, and to control endolymphatic hypertension and hydrops in Ménière disease, congenital hydrops, and large vestibular aqueduct syndrome.

AREx inhaler—a noninvasive device that delivers a drug through an inhaler rather than intravenously, thus allowing more flexibility for outpatients.

AREZ (anterior root exit zone).

ARF (acute renal failure)—a critical condition characterized by oliguria and rapid deterioration in renal function.

ARF (acute respiratory failure).

ArF excimer laser—used for tissue ablation.

argentaffin carcinoma.

arginine tolerance test (ATT)—for growth hormone.

Arglaes antimicrobial barrier film dressing—uses ionic silver in a controlled-release polymer film that forms an effective antimicrobial barrier. Also available in an island dressing. See *island wound dressing*.

Arglaes powder—a controlled-release ionic silver that protects against bacteria and fungi, but remains non-destructive to cells, designed to be used in a variety of settings, including pressure ulcers, postoperative wounds, minor burns, and line sites.

argon beam coagulator (ABC)—used for hemostasis in minimally invasive surgery instead of electrocautery, and for treating highly vascular pleural malignancies.

argon/krypton laser—a vitreoretinal laser used for iridotomies and trabeculoplasties, for management of glaucoma, and in macular procedures. May be used for other kinds of surgery.

argon laser—is used for photocoagulation in diabetic retinopathy and detached retina. May be used for other kinds of surgery. Cf. *laser*, CO_2 *laser*, *Nd:YAG laser*.

argon laser coagulation (ALC).

argon laser trabeculoplasty (ALT)—a procedure used in treating glaucoma and ocular hypertension which do not respond to medical management, before resorting to filtering surgery.

argon plasma coagulation (APC)—high-frequency energy is transmitted to tissue by ionized gas, thus reducing contact with the tissue to a minimum. This technique is being used during a number of gastrointestinal procedures.

Argosy Cameo CIC (completely-in-the-canal) **hearing aid** with digital magnetic sensing and remote adjustment of volume for various listening situations.

Argyle CPAP nasal cannula.

Argyle Turkel safety thoracentesis system.

Aria—coronary artery bypass graft which incorporates the proprietary biomaterial Thoralon in patients with few or no suitable native vessels.

Arias-Stella phenomenon.

ariboflavinosis—a vitamin deficiency state, indicated by flattening of the papillae of the tongue.

ARIES I, II—randomized, double-blind, placebo-controlled clinical trials of ambrisentan in patients with pulmonary artery hypertension.

Aries-Pitanguy correction of mammary ptosis.

aripiprazole—see *Abilify*.

ARM (age-related maculopathy).

arm and **lesser saphenous veins** (ALSVs)—an alternative for infrapopliteal arterial bypass grafts when the greater saphenous vein (GSV) is not available.

Armanni-Ebstein nephropathy—glycogen vacuolation of loops of Henle in diabetic patients, directly related to hyperglycemia and glycosuria.

arm board or **armboard**.

ARMD (age-related macular degeneration). See *dry age-related macular degeneration*; *wet age-related macular degeneration*.

Arndt-Gottron syndrome—scleromyxedema with corneal deposits.

Arneth grouping of polymorphonuclear neutrophils—according to the number of lobes in their nuclei, e.g., one lobe, class I; two lobes, class II; three lobes, class III, etc.

Arnett-TMP (trimandibular plate) **system** (Plas Surg)—a fixation device for orthognathic, craniofacial, midface, and mandibular applications.

Arnold nerve—the auricular branch of the vagus nerve.

Aromapatch nasal inhaler—OTC single-use patch indicated for aroma inhalation of essential oils.

AromaScan—aroma analysis device developed for use in beverage, food, and perfume industries, now being used to check breath samples for evidence of infection, producing a kind of "fingerprint" of the air. If the device produces a suspicion for lung infection, physicians can prescribe antibiotics while they await lab results.

Arouse-All—a combination of herbs focusing on maximum sexual performance.

Arrequi laparoscopic knot pusher ligator.

arrested heart surgery—surgery performed on a heart whose action has been arrested by injection of a cardioplegic drug, while all respiratory and circulatory functions are taken over by mechanical devices. Cf. *beating heart surgery*.

arrest of labor—stopping of progress in labor (*not* "a rest of labor").

arrhythmia mapping system—catheter-based system to aid in the diagnosis of complex ventricular tachyarrhythmias.

arrhythmogenic pulmonary vein—a pulmonary vein (extending from the ostium to its tributaries) that gives rise to single or multiple spontaneous discharges, with or without conduction to the left atrium.

arrow flap—a local skin fat flap shaped like an arrow for the reconstruction of the nipple. The arrow shape allows the scar to be broken on closure, minimizing postoperative wound contracture. Within the flap, a rib cartilage graft is used, and this provides additional support and projection for the skin and soft tissue envelope.

ArrowGard Blue Line catheter—a central venous catheter that contains chlorhexidine and silver sulfadiazine antiseptics bonded onto the outer surface to reduce the risk of catheter-induced bacteremia.

ArrowGard Blue Plus catheter.

Arrow-Howes multilumen catheter—provides multiple apertures with the use of only one venipuncture site, thus permitting hyperalimentation, central venous pressure monitoring, intravenous administration of medications, and blood sampling without the necessity of multiple needle punctures.

Arrow LionHeart—a heart-assist device implanted as long-term therapy for patients with end-stage heart failure who are not candidates for heart transplantation; some patients whose health improves markedly with this device may become eligible for transplant.

Arrow PICC—a radiology device for insertion of central venous lines.

Arrow pneumothorax kit—for nonsurgical treatment of pneumothorax, using percutaneous catheter-over-needle technique.

Arrowsmith corneal marker (Oph).

Arrow Twin Cath—multilumen peripheral catheter.

ARS (acute repetitive seizure) **disorder**.

ARS (alcohol-related seizures).

ArtAssist—compression dressing or wrap.

Artecoll (homogeneous polymethylmethacrylate [PMMA] microspheres)—a permanent wrinkle treatment consisting of collagen-coated microscopic plastic beads injected under the skin; the microspheres are evenly suspended in a solution of partly denatured 3.5% collagen.

arterial—referring to an artery. Cf. *arteriole*.

arterial blood gases (ABGs).

arterial line (A-line).

arterial obstruction, signs and symptoms of (also known as the classic five P's): pain, pallor, pulselessness, paresthesia, and paralysis.

arterial oxygen saturation (SaO_2).

arterial switch procedure—for correcting transposition of the great vessels.

arteriole—a tiny arterial branch. Cf. *arterial*.

arteriovenous oxygen difference (AVD O_2, AV DO_2, AVDO_2).

arteritis—inflammation of an artery or arteries. Examples: giant cell arteritis; Takayasu arteritis. Cf. *arthritis*.

artery of Adamkiewicz--the great anterior radicular artery.

Arthro-BST—arthroscopic probe for diagnosis of arthritis. Provides objective diagnosis of cartilage disease and evaluation of cartilage repair after therapy.

Arthopor acetabular cup (*not* Arthropor, although it is often pronounced that way). The acetabular component attached to the femoral stem constitutes the prosthesis used in hip arthroplasty. These sintered (calcareous) porous-coated hemispherical cups are made with holes in various shapes and sizes on the top to accommodate screws and locking pins. They come in three depths: low profile, deep profile, and extra deep profile. The cups are designated Arthopor I, II, and III.

arthritides ("ar-thrit-ih-dees")—plural form of *arthritis*.

arthritis—inflammation of a joint. Cf. *arteritis*.

ArthroCare Coblation-based cosmetic surgery system--used for skin resurfacing for treatment of wrinkles.

ArthroCare system—for rapid tissue removal, resection, and hemostasis in the knee and shoulder as well as

ArthroCare *(cont.)* for soft tissue sculpting of meniscus and articular cartilage, using Coblation technology. Also, *ArthroCare wand* and *ArthroWand.*

ArthroCare wand CoVac 70—a coagulation device.

ArthroCare wand TurboVac 90—a coagulation device.

Arthro-Flo system—provides powered irrigation for arthroscopy.

Arthro-Lok system—Beaver blades for arthroscopic surgery and all types of meniscal tears. Blades include banana, rosette, retrograde.

ArthroProbe laser system—a laser system for arthroscopic surgery, which provides both resection and hemostasis. Used through an arthroscopic cannula.

arthroscopic autologous chondrocyte transplantation—arthroscopic surgical technique for tissue-engineered cartilage grafting.

Arthro 7—an OTC arthritis drug available at health food stores.

Arthrosew—arthroscopic suturing device.

ArthroWand—used to apply radiofrequency in procedures using Coblation technology. See *CAPS ArthroWand.*

Arthus reaction—immune complex deposition in dermal walls; it can cause gangrene at the site of injection of an allergen. Named for a French bacteriologist (d. 1945).

artifact (Radiol)—a finding which mimics but is not a disease process, e.g., a nipple shadow resembling a lesion seen on a chest x-ray, a wrinkled film, or movement. Misleading images in radiology may be due to a variety of sources, such as patient movement, software or hardware failure, or human error. Examples:

artifact *(cont.)*
aliasing (wrap-around ghosting)
analog-to-digital (ADC) conversion quantization error
barium
beam hardening
black comets
braces
broadband noise detection error
calibration failure
chemical shift phenomena
coin
construction
corduroy
crescent
crinkle
cross-talk effect
crown
data-clipping detection error
data spike detection error
DC (direct current) offset
developer
distortion of limitations of image reconstruction algorithm
double exposure drift
eddy current
edge ringing
equipment
faulty RF (radiofrequency) shielding in MRI scanner room permitting coherent RF noise which distorts image
flow effect (MRI)
fog
foreign material (within the patient, within the MRI scanner room, within the MRI magnet bore)
geophagia
Gibbs phenomenon
glass eye
half-moon
image post-processing errors
imbalance of phase or gain
intensifying screen
kink

artifact *(cont.)*
kissing-type
large clothing
lettering
magic angle
magnetic susceptibility
main magnetic field inhomogeneity
mercury
misregistration
mitral regurgitation
moiré
movement
paramagnetic
patient motion
pellet
pica
pseudofracture
quadrature phase detector (QPD)
radiofrequency (RF) spatial distribution problem reconstruction
reticulation
screen craze
skin fold (skin crease)
skin lesion
slice profile
stimulated echo
subcutaneous injection of contrast
summation shadow
superimposition
swamp-static
temporal instability
traction
tree
truncation band
wheelchair
wrap-around ghost (aliasing)
wrinkle
zebra

artificial anterior chamber—a device used for modifying the donor button in endothelial lamellar keratoplasty. It is not used on the patient but in a sterile work area outside the operative field.

artificial blood
Fluosol plasma expander
Hemolink
Hextend blood plasma volume expander
pyridoxylated stroma-free hemoglobin (SFHb)
recombinant hemoglobin (rHb1.1)

artificial burr—Velcro analog used in staged closures of the abdomen, so named because reminiscent of burrs that appear on some plants.

artificial heart
CardioWest total (TAH)
Symbion J-7-70-mL-ventricle
University of Akron

artificial insemination–donor (AID).

artificial insemination–husband (AIH).

artificial lung—see *IVOX* (intravascular oxygenator).

artificial neural networks (ANNs)—the task-oriented computer algorithms modeled on the human brain. This is a diagnostic tool to predict the presence of pulmonary embolism by using findings from ventilation-perfusion lung scans and from clinical examination.

artificial nose—see *heat-moisture exchanger.*

artificial skin—see *Integra.*

artificial urinary sphincter (AUS)—for use in urologic reconstruction.

Artisan—a plastic intraocular lens (IOL) implanted in front of the natural lens in healthy eyes to correct nearsightedness in people with stable vision.

ARTMA (advanced real time motion analysis) **virtual patient technology**—used in endoscopic navigation system and telesurgery.

ASA triad—consisting of aspirin sensitivity, asthma, and nasal polyps. Also known as *Samter triad* and *triad asthma.*

ASO (Amplatzer septal occluder).

ARUM pin—for fixation of Colles fractures as an alternative to the usual intrafocal pinning procedure. It consists of a pin and a special nut. The pin is cut close to the nut, and the nut is designed so that it slides between the tendons very precisely.

ARV (AIDS-related virus)—the term given to the AIDS virus by the group of scientists working at U.C. San Francisco under Dr. Jay Levy. The virus is now officially known as *HIV*. See *HIV*.

aryepiglottic fold (AE fold).

arylcyclohexylamines—a category of drugs including phencyclidine (PCP), a street drug of abuse.

A.S. (*auris sinistra*)—left ear.

ASAP solution—mineral supplement solution that acts as a broad-spectrum antimicrobial agent.

A-scan—an ultrasound device used to differentiate abnormal from normal tissues in the eye.

Ascent guiding catheter—directs balloon catheters rapidly into coronary arteries or other sites where obstructions are treated.

ASC-H (atypical squamous cells, cannot exclude high-grade squamous intraepithelial lesion).

Aschoff-Tawara node—atrioventricular node.

ascitic—characterized by ascites or an accumulation of fluid in the peritoneal cavity. Cf. *acidic*.

ascribe—to attribute. Usage: "The patient ascribes occasional shortness of breath to the fact that she has put on a great deal of weight in the past four months, although she still smokes more than a pack a day." Cf. *describe*.

ASC-US (atypical squamous cells of undetermined significance).

AS-800—artificial sphincter for surgically treating urinary incontinence in women.

aseptic loosening—seen in some cemented custom-made prosthetic replacements for bone tumors of the limbs.

ASF (anterior spine fusion).

ASH (asymmetric septal hypertrophy) —the newer term for what was formerly called *IHSS* (idiopathic hypertrophic subaortic stenosis).

ash leaf spots in the eye—seen in cases of tuberous sclerosis.

ASI (active specific immunotherapy)—using the patient's own tumor to elicit an immune response.

ASIA impairment scale—classification of spinal cord injury established by the American Spinal Injury Association.

A—No motor or sensory function preserved in sacral segments.

B—Sensory but not motor function preserved in at least sacral segments.

C—Motor function preserved below the neurologic level; majority of key muscles have motor score <3.

D—Motor function preserved below the neurologic level; majority of key muscles have motor score of 3 or >.

E—Motor and sensory function normal.

Asian bird flu—see *avian flu*. Also known as "bird flu."

ASIF plates. (ASIF, Association for the Study of Internal Fixation.)

ASIS (anterior superior iliac spine).

A68 (Path)—a protein found in the brains of patients with Alzheimer disease. Cf. *ALZ-50*.

Aslera (prasterone)—drug for treatment of lupus erythematosus.

Asnis 2 guided screw system—for treatment of hip fractures.

ASO (Amplatzer septal occluder).

aspartate transaminase (AST) (formerly *SGOT*)—a liver function test.

Aspen electrocautery—used in arthroscopic procedures.

Aspen laparoscopy electrode—electrosurgical device used in laparoscopic surgical procedures.

Aspen ultrasound system—a maneuverable digital ultrasound system that utilizes high-frequency transducers, and enables the imaging of small body parts, such as breast, testicle, and thyroid.

Aspergillus—the fungus causing aspergillosis, which is seen in disseminated form in AIDS. See *Penicillium*.

aspheric—refers to the reflecting surface of a lens.

aspiration biopsy cytology (ABC).

aspiration-tulip device—used for in vitro percutaneous removal of rigid clots, such as a platelet-rich arterial plug.

aspartate aminotransferase (AST) (formerly called *SGOT*)—see *AST*.

aspheric custom ablation—laser procedure designed to produce a prolate cornea that more accurately mirrors the eye's natural curved shape.

ASPS (alveolar soft-part sarcoma)—soft tissue tumors as opposed to bone tumors.

assay—see *test*.

ASSI—bipolar coagulating forceps and disposable cranio blades (no hyphen and no period after *cranio*) and wire pass drills for use in neurosurgery and other surgical specialties. (ASSI, Accurate Surgical and Scientific Instruments Corporation.)

Assistant Free calibrated femoral-tibial spreader (Ortho).

Assistant Free self-retaining soft tissue retractor—used for soft tissue retraction in shoulder and hip surgery.

assisted same-day microsurgical arthroscopic lateral-approach laser-assisted (SMALL) **fluoroscopic diskectomy**.

association (Genetics)—the occurrence together in a population of two or more genetic characteristics more often than would be expected.

AST (acute stroke team).

AST (antistreptolysin titer).

AST (aspartate transaminase) (newer name for *SGOT*)—an enzyme whose level in the serum is elevated in myocardial infarction, liver disease, and other conditions.

astasia-abasia—inability to stand or to walk, although the legs are otherwise under control.

asthenic—lacking in strength and energy, or pertaining to an individual with an ectomorphic body build. Cf. *aesthetic*.

asthenopia—eye discomfort that feels like eyestrain and may also be accompanied by headache.

asthenospermic—poor motility of sperm.

asthma—synonym for reversible obstructive airway disease.

astigmatic keratotomy—surgical incision of the cornea to correct astigmatism.

astigmatism—an eye condition in which there is unequal curvature of one of the refractive surfaces of the eye, causing lack of sharpness in focus of a ray of light on the retina.

astigmatism with the rule—has the greater curvature along the vertical meridian of the eye. *Astigmatism against the rule* has the greater curvature in the horizontal meridian.

Astler-Coller modification of Dukes' C classification of carcinoma—provides a subscript for the C (C_1, C_2).

Aston cartilage reduction system—includes cartilage rasps and nasal scissors for nasal reconstruction.

Astra profiles (Lab)—blood chemistry analyzers.

Astringedent topical hemostatic solution—used by dentists. Does not contain epinephrine and can be infused with a Dento-Infuser. Also, *Astringedent X.*

ASTY colorimetric microdilution panel—a laboratory test to assess sensitivity of fungi to antifungal agents.

asymmetric septal hypertrophy (ASH) —newer term for *IHSS* (idiopathic hypertrophic subaortic stenosis).

asymmetric tonic neck reflex (ATNR) —alternative name for tonic neck reflex. Usage: "The ATNR and Moro reflexes are integrated."

asymptomatic left ventricular dysfunction (ALVD).

asyneresis—a localized reduction in ventricular wall motion.

Atavi atraumatic spine fusion system —for endoscopic posterolateral fusion procedure.

ataxia
appendicular
equilibratory
Marie
telangiectasia

atazanavir—a protease inhibitor used as an antiviral drug in treatment of HIV and AIDS.

ATFL (anterior talofibular ligament).

ATG (antithymocyte globulin)—drug used to prevent rejection of transplanted kidney.

atherectomy—the removal of atherosclerotic plaque from an artery by means of a rotary cutter introduced into the artery through a special catheter under radiographic guidance. Atherectomy methods include directional, extraction, and rotational.

atherectomy catheter—a catheter (such as AtheroCath and Simpson) used to retrieve cholesterol plaque from diseased arteries. See *Simpson atherectomy catheter*.

AtheroCath Bantam coronary atherectomy catheter—for performance of nonsurgical directional coronary atherectomy, a procedure for shaving obstructing plaque from coronary vessels.

atheroma—see *protruding atheromas*.

Athlete coronary guidewire—said to have optimal steering characteristics and unique stiffness, kink resistance, and pushability of the 3 cm radiopaque tip segment because of improved jointless spring technology (one-piece core wire). Used for recanalization of total coronary occlusion when conventional wires fail to cross.

Atkinson endoprosthesis—a silicone rubber tube with a preformed distal shoulder. Also, *Atkinson tube*.

Atkinson tube stent—used over Nottingham introducer.

Atkinson-type lid block—local eye anesthesia.

Atlantis SR—intravascular ultrasound imaging catheter.

Atlas HF ICD (implantable cardioverter-defibrillator)—cardiac resynchronization therapy debrillator.

Atlas shoulder prosthesis—for shoulder arthroplasty.

AtLast blood glucose monitoring system—enables diabetic patients to test their blood without painful fingersticks.

ATL duplex scanner—uses B-mode imaging and pulsed Doppler ultrasound in noninvasive evaluation of the extracranial carotid artery system.

ATL real-time Neurosector scanner—used in ultrasonography. (ATL, Advanced Technology Laboratories.)

ATL (acute tumor lysis) **syndrome**.

ATLS (advanced trauma life support) **examination**.

ATM (acute transverse myelitis).

ATN (acute tubular necrosis).

ATnativ (antithrombin III).

ATNR—see *asymmetric tonic neck reflex*.

ATO (arsenic trioxide)—drug used in treatment of multiple myeloma.

atomic force microscopy (AFM)—used by dental researchers to test strength and stiffness of dentin by pushing the atoms and molecules apart to observe how they respond. The goal is to create a tighter, more permanent bond between teeth and plastic-based fillings now used to repair most cavities.

ATP III—see *Adult Treatment Panel III*.

ATRA (all-trans retinoic acid).

Atraloc needle—double-pointed needle used for blood vessel anastomoses; the double point allows the needle to be passed in either direction without reversing it on the needle holder, thus saving time.

Atrauclip hemostatic clip.

atresia, **bilateral congenital aural**—see *stereolithography*.

atrial natriuretic peptide (ANP).

Atrial Fibrillation Follow-up Investigation of Rhythm Management (AFFIRM) **study**.

Atrial View Ventak AV implantable cardioverter-defibrillator.

Atridox (doxycycline hyclate 10%)—administered using the Atrigel drug delivery system. It is used for treatment of periodontal disease and is said to be faster, less painful, and less costly than scaling and root planing. Atridox is applied to the infected periodontal pocket as a fluid, where it molds to the shape of the problem area and quickly solidifies, releasing doxycycline for a period of seven days as it is bioabsorbed.

Atrigel—drug delivery system to administer (1) Atridox for periodontal disease and (2) leuprolide acetate over a 120-day period to treat patients with advanced prostate cancer.

atrio-His (pronounced "hiss") **tract or pathway in the heart**, as in *bundle of His*.

atrioventricular nodal reentry tachycardia (AVNRT).

Atrisorb FreeFlow—guided tissue regeneration barrier with doxycycline. Guided tissue regeneration barriers are used in conjunction with periodontal surgery to help regenerate bone and other tissues destroyed by periodontal disease.

Atrovent (ipratropium bromide)—inhalation solution drug for relief of bronchospasm in COPD.

Atrioverter—a very small implantable defibrillator device, specifically used to treat patients who do not respond to medical control of atrial fibrillation.

Atrium Vascular Products—a manufacturer of a variety of vascular surgical products, including Advanta VS, Advanta VXT, Advanta SuperSoft, Advanta SST PTFE vascular grafts, Advanta V12 stent graft system, Slider GDS (graft deployment system), and Ultramax coated knit-

Atrium *(cont.)*
ted velour vascular graft. Not to be confused with atrium of the heart.

ATS Open Pivot bileaflet heart valve.

ATT (arginine tolerance test)—a test for growth hormone.

attention-deficit disorder (ADD) (newer name for *minimal brain dysfunction* in children)—a group of developmentally inappropriate symptoms in children, such as moderate to severe distractibility, short attention span, hyperactivity, emotional lability, and impulsivity. Also called *hyperkinetic child syndrome, minimal brain damage, minimal cerebral dysfunction, minor cerebral dysfunction.*

attic defect plate—prosthetic implant for reconstruction of natural or surgically created defects of the bony attic of the middle ear.

at U—slang for *at the level of the umbilicus*.

atypical glandular cells (AGC)—a Bethesda System Terminology classification replacing the former term, AGUS or AGCUS (atypical glandular cells of undetermined significance), to avoid confusion with ASCUS. Attempts to identify whether the origin of the cells is endometrial, endocervical, or unqualified are also made. "Endocervical adenocarcinoma in situ" and "AGC, favor neoplastic" are included as separate AGC categories. AGC is an infrequent finding on an abnormal Pap smear. Cf. ASC-US.

atypical mole syndrome.

atypical squamous cells of undetermined significance (ASC-US)—in the 2001 Bethesda System Terminology, a new category of "atypical squamous cells" (ASC), replacing the category of "atypical squamous cells of undetermined significance" (ASCUS) and divided into qualifiers of (1) ASC of "undetermined significance" (ASC-US) and (2) "cannot exclude high-grade squamous intraepithelial lesion (HSIL or HGSIL), or (ASC-H). Cf. AGC.

AUA Symptom Index (Urol)—a seven-item patient questionnaire about benign prostatic hypertrophy, developed by the American Urological Association. Each item is rated on a scale of 1 to 5 and then totaled for the AUA Symptom Score.

AUB (abnormal uterine bleeding).

AuBMT (autologous bone marrow transplantation).

Auchincloss modified radical mastectomy.

AudioScope, Welch Allyn—an instrument for screening hearing loss in children; it is combined with an otoscope in a single device.

auditory brain stem response (ABR).

Auer body; rod—found only in myelogenous and monocytic leukemia.

Aufrecht sign of tracheal stenosis—faint breath sounds heard about the jugular notch.

augmentative communication device (also known as *alternative communication device*)—used by individuals with speech disorders such as cerebral palsy and autism as an alternative or adjunct to verbalizations. This can range from a simple picture board to a computerized system using a wireless connection to a computer.

Augustine guide and **scope**—for oral blind intubation of the trachea of patients presenting with difficult airways.

Aura desktop laser—for ENT surgery.

aural—pertaining to the ear, or to the sense of hearing, as aural acuity or aural surgery. Cf. *oral.*

Aura laser system—used in outpatient surgical and dermatologic procedures.

auramine-rhodamine stain (Path).

auramine-stained buffy coat smear—a rapid diagnostic test for mycobacteremia, with moderate sensitivity and high specificity.

auricular acupuncture—performed on the ear for treatment of various parts and organs of the body. The ear has many acupuncture points that correspond to parts and organs of the body.

auricular perichondritis—occurs as a result of ear piercing so high that it perforates the auricular cartilage, implanting infecting organisms, usually either *Pseudomonas aeruginosa* or *Staphylococcus*, and resulting in complications such as the need for incision and drainage, antibiotic irrigation, placement of drains, necrosis, liquefying chondritis, and cosmetic deformity.

auris dextra (A.D., AD)—right ear.

auris sinistra (A.S., AS)—left ear.

Aurora diode-based dental laser system—used for gingival surgery as well as recontouring, dental implant, and the removal of diseased soft tissue.

Aurora MR breast imaging system—a dedicated MRI system to detect lesions in patients with dense breasts for whom x-ray mammography may be unrevealing.

AUS—see *artificial urinary sphincter.*

Ausculscope—detects carotid bruits.

Austin Flint murmur of relative mitral stenosis—differs from the murmur of true mitral stenosis by having no audible opening snap.

Austin Moore hip prosthesis—named for Dr. Thomas Austin Moore. (No hyphen.)

Auth atherectomy catheter.

AUTI (asymptomatic urinary tract infection) (pronounced "ah-dee").

Autima II dual chamber cardiac pacemaker.

autoaugmentation (Urol)—a means of establishing a low-pressure, adequate capacity bladder. A large wide-mouthed mucosal diverticulum is fashioned to augment bladder storage capacity. See *urothelial augmentation.*

AutoCat, AutoCAT—automatic intra-aortic balloon pump.

Autoclix—fingerstick device for blood glucose testing.

autoclot—a preformed clot of the patient's blood, reinjected to stop bleeding.

autocrine motility factor (AMF)—a protein secreted by cancerous cells which can be detected in the urine. The test for AMF aids in early detection of bladder cancer.

Autoflex II—continuous passive motion (CPM) unit.

autogenous—a synonym for *autologous*, which is most often used to refer to blood transfusions of the patient's own blood (see *autologous transfusion*). *Autogenous* usually refers to a patient's own bone or bone marrow used for graft material (autograft).

Autolet—a fingerstick device for blood glucose testing.

AuTolo cure process—for treatment of chronic nonhealing wounds.

autoLog autotransfusion system—a device that provides autologous blood during surgical procedures by

autoLog *(cont.)* processing blood collected from a surgical site to produce washed red blood cells for return to the patient at a later time.

autologous augmentation of breasts—a surgical procedure primarily for mastectomy patients that originally used a transverse rectus abdominis musculocutaneous (TRAM) flap, advanced to a microvascular free TRAM flap approach, and now has been extended by the development of the deep inferior epigastric perforator (DIEP) flap in which the skin and subcutaneous tissue island are transferred based only on the perforating branches of the deep inferior epigastric vessels.

autologous bone marrow transplant (AuBMT).

autologous clot—used for control of hemorrhage. Some of the patient's blood is mixed with epsilon aminocaproic acid, and clot forms. This is then cut in small fragments. Gelatin sponge is then soaked in 50% diatrizoate sodium, and the clot alternated with strips of the gelatin sponge is injected into the bleeding vessels until hemorrhage stops.

autologous fat graft—use of the patient's own fat (to fill a cavity, such as that left by removal of a tumor or cyst).

autologous fibrin glue—used in surgery for acoustic neuromas, with blood for the glue taken at the time of routine blood draw. Used routinely to seal the ear and internal auditory canal in order to reduce the incidence of cerebrospinal fluid leak.

autologous fibrin tissue adhesive (AFTA)—uses a combination of ethanol and freezing to precipitate fibrinogen.

autologous growth factors (AGF)—properties in a patient's own blood that enable the orthopedic surgeon to speed healing and growth process of human bone.

autologous leukapheresis, processing, and storage (ALPS).

autologous osteochondral transplantation—joint surgery treatment.

autologous ovarian transplantation—procedure in which a strip of a woman's own cortical ovarian tissue is transplanted under her subcutaneous tissue—in the forearm, for example—to preserve ovarian function when undergoing sterilizing radiotherapy, chemotherapy, or oophorectomy.

autologous transfusion—transfusion of one's own blood or blood components, thereby eliminating risks (e.g., hepatitis and alloimmunization) associated with homologous blood transfusion. Also called *autogenous*.

autologous transplantation—the transplantation of cells, tissues, or organs in which donor and recipient are the same individual.

autolymphocyte-based treatment for renal cell carcinoma (ALT-RCC)—used in the treatment of stage IV metastatic renal cell carcinoma.

autolytic debridement—the process the body undertakes to remove dead tissue. During this process, enzymes present in the wound liquefy hard eschar and slough. Moist wound dressings that include hydrocolloids, transparent films, and hydrogels may be used to promote autolytic debridement.

automated cardiac flow measurement technology—see *ACM*.

automated cellular imaging system (ACIS)—HER2 protein expression system for the guidance of breast cancer therapy. (About 30% of breast cancer patients have a particularly aggressive cancer identified by the elevated expression of the HER2 protein. This protein is important for normal cell division; however, if patients overexpress this protein, their cancer can spread very rapidly.)

automated external defibrillator (AED)—used to provide a quick response and early defibrillation to victims of sudden cardiac arrest. This device is used by fire departments, corporations, and businesses that train employees in its use.

automated lamellar therapeutic keratoplasty system (ALTK)—keratoplasty system that uses extraocular techniques, unlike penetrating keratoplasty systems.

automated percutaneous lumbar diskectomy (APLD)—technique for treating a herniated lumbar disk. The procedure is performed under local anesthesia, and the herniated disk is extracted through a cannula inserted into the disk by using either pituitary forceps or a Nucleotome aspiration probe. The Nucleotome uses suction to aspirate nucleus pulposus into a side port and then a sleeve is pneumatically pushed across the portal opening, making a clean cut through the disk material.

Automator—a computerized device that attaches to the telescopic rods used in the Ilizarov leg lengthening procedure. Programmed to automatically adjust the hardware four times per day to increase bone distraction. Before this development, the adjustment was done manually by the patient.

autonopathy—jargon abridgement of autonomic neuropathy.

auto-obliteration—see *osteoneogenesis.*

AutoPap—automated screening device to analyze Pap smear slides for signs of cervical cancer prior to examination by trained personnel.

AutoPap 300 QC automatic Pap screener—a system used in labs to recheck Pap smear slides initially classified as normal.

Autoplex—Factor VIII inhibitor bypass drug (anti-anti Factor VIII) (yes, anti-anti).

autos—slang for *autograft transplant patients.*

Auto Segmentation—trademarked, sophisticated software tool that enables the neurosurgeon to quickly isolate and color-code critical structures, such as tumors and blood vessels, using a scan of a patient's brain.

autosomal dominant (Genetics)—a pattern of inheritance in which only one copy of an autosomal gene is required for expression; that is, expression occurs in heterozygotes as well as in homozygotes.

autosomal-dominant cerebellar ataxia (ADCA) **type II**. See *ADCA*.

autosomal-dominant retinitis pigmentosa (adRP).

autosomal recessive (Genetics)—a pattern of inheritance in which two copies of an autosomal gene (one on each chromosome of a pair) must be present for expression; that is, expression occurs in homozygotes but not in heterozygotes.

autosome (Genetics)—any chromosome other than a sex chromosome (hence neither X nor Y).

Auto Suture Multifire Endo GIA 30 stapler—for laparoscopic use in

Auto Suture *(cont.)* appendectomy, bowel resection, blebectomies, and wedge resections.

Auto Suture Premium CEEA stapler—used for circular anastomosis requiring double and triple stapling technique in intestinal procedures.

autotransfusion system—see *Cell Saver Haemolite.*

auxiliary transplant—a procedure in which the donor organ (or part of an organ, such as the liver) is placed alongside the patient's own damaged organ, sharing the same blood supply. Then it's a case of "survival of the fittest," and the stronger of the two organs takes over. The liver is the only organ that can regenerate, so only a portion of a liver can function until it grows to be normal size.

AV (atrioventricular) **bundle in heart**—a term used in electrophysiologic studies of supraventricular tachycardia. See *Kent bundle*.

Avandamet—see *rosiglitazone*.

Avanta metacarpophalangeal and proximal interphalangeal joint soft skeletal implants, made of Silflex II, a silicone elastomer (Hand Surg).

Avastin (bevacizumab)—combined with fluorouracil and leucovorin acetate with or without irinotecan, for metastatic colorectal cancer. Also used for kidney cancer, bevacizumab works by interfering with angiogenesis.

AVA 3Xi—advanced venous access device that is flexible enough for routine cardiac care and surgery, designed specifically for high-risk cardiovascular, trauma, and organ transplant surgeries.

aversion therapy (Psych)—a type of therapy used to change behavior patterns by associating them with unpleasant stimuli.

Avesta procedure kit—a laparoscopic surgical procedure kit that can be used to shorten and strengthen the uterosacral ligaments to support the vagina in posthysterectomy patients.

Aviane-28 (levonorgestrel and ethinyl estradiol)—oral contraceptive pill.

avian flu—a term used to describe the influenza viruses that infect birds, including wild birds such as ducks, and domestic birds such as chickens. Many forms of avian flu virus cause only mild symptoms in the birds or no symptoms at all. However, some of the viruses produce a highly contagious and rapidly fatal disease, leading to severe epidemics. These virulent viruses are known as "highly pathogenic avian influenza," and it is these viruses that cause particular concern. Until 1997 avian flu was believed to infect only birds; however, in 1997 it was discovered that the virus can occasionally infect people who have been in close contact with live birds in markets or farms. It is possible that a highly pathogenic avian flu virus could merge with a human flu virus and create a new virus that could be easily passed between humans.

avian influenza A (H5N1) **virus**—isolated in human patients in Hong Kong in 1997. Previously known to infect only birds.

Avitene—microfibrillar collagen hemostatic material; used like Gelfoam; applied topically for hemostasis in localized oozing, in areas inaccessible for suturing, and in procedures involving friable organs or vessels.

Avitene Ultrafoam collagen hemostat—collagen sponge used to obtain hemostasis in surgical procedures.

Avlimil (salvia rubus)—a natural supplement for female sexual dysfunction.

AVM (arteriovenous malformation).

AVM (atrioventricular malformation).

AV nodal Wenckebach cycle length (AVNW-CL)—a term used in discussing the pacing of the heart or in electrophysiology testing.

AVNRT (atrioventricular nodal reentry tachycardia).

AVNW-CL (AV nodal Wenckebach cycle length).

AvocetPT—a rapid prothrombin time (PT) meter.

AvWD (acquired von Willebrand disease).

Aware AccuMeter rapid HIV test.

Aware breast self-examination pad—consists of two 10-inch polyurethane circles with silicone lubricant sealed between them. Provides increased sensitivity on palpation that may help detect an abnormality.

Axcis—a proprietary Holmium:YAG laser device from CardioGenesis, used for percutaneous myocardial revascularization.

axial acetabular index (AAI)—hip dysplasia measurement in children with cerebral palsy.

axial images—MRI term.

axial proton-density-weighted image (MRI). Also, *axial T2-weighted image.*

axillobilateral breast approach (ABBA)—used in endoscopic thyroid surgery. This modification also improves cosmetic results by eliminating the parasternal incision, which results in hypertrophic scarring in a significant number of cases treated with breast approach.

axillofemoral bypass—used only in high risk patients.

axis—a real or imaginary straight line going through a structure, around which it revolves, or would revolve if it could. See *HPA* (hypothalamic-pituitary-adrenal) axis; transepicondylar (TEA). Cf. *access, excess.*

Axius Vacuum 2 stabilizer—used in beating-heart surgery to stabilize the area where the vessel is blocked.

Axostim nerve stimulator.

AxSYM antibody to hepatitis C virus test—a lab test used to help diagnose patients that may be infected with the hepatitis C virus. The test detects antibodies associated with hepatitis C virus.

AxSYM Free PSA test—combined with the total PSA test and a digital rectal exam to distinguish between cancerous and noncancerous prostate conditions.

AxyaWeld bone anchor system—uses suture material and bone anchors to secure soft tissue structures in surgical procedures, utilizing ultrasonic energy to weld polymeric materials, thereby eliminating knot-tying by the surgeon.

ayw1, ayw2, ayw3, ayw4, ayr—these are hepatitis B surface antigen (HB_sAg) subdeterminants.

azalides—a class of antibiotic drugs. The first drug in this group is azithromycin, which is similar to erythromycin.

Azo menopause tablets—a natural supplement for relief of hot flashes.

AZOOR (acute zonal occult outer retinopathy).

Azo urinary pain relief tablets—a natural supplement.

AZT (azidothymidine)—a drug name changed to zidovudine; dictators, however, often stick with the more easily pronounced abbreviation for the old name. When "AZT" is dictated, it may be transcribed *zidovudine (AZT)*.

azygos lobe, **azygos vein**—unpaired. (*Not* azygous or azygus.)

B, b

Baastrup syndrome—intervertebral disk collapse after severe lordosis, leading to "kissing spines."

babesiosis—infection with the tick-borne parasite *Babesia.*

Babinski sign—upward deviation of the great toe on stroking the sole of the foot, an indication of brain stem injury. A positive Babinski is an extensor plantar response: "The toes are upgoing." A negative Babinski is a flexor plantar response: "The toes are downgoing."

BA (bioactive) **bone cement**—consisting of Bis-GMA resin and bioactive-lasting fixation of implants to bone under weightbearing conditions.

BABYbird respirator (BABY, all caps)—a time-cycled infant ventilator. Also, *Bird respirator.*

BabyFace—3-D surface rendering accessory for diagnostic ultrasound systems that makes it possible for a physician to view a fetus in three full dimensions.

Babytherm IC—a thermostatically controlled gel mattress for warming newborns.

Bachmann anterior internodal tract in the heart.

bacillary angiomatosis (BA)—a condition in which nodular tumors made up of densely proliferating blood vessels appear in the skin, bone, brain, spleen, and other tissues. Caused by *Bartonella henselae* and detected by a serum immunofluorescent antibody test.

bacillus—see *pathogen.*

bacillus Calmette-Guérin (BCG)—an attenuated strain of tubercle bacillus, once used as a vaccine and still used in parts of the Third World, so it may turn up in past histories, especially now with drug-resistant TB becoming a problem. Variations include cell-free fractions, Glaxo, Montreal, Pasteur, Phipps, and Tice.

Bacillus circulans—a pathogen causing endophthalmitis, a complication of cataract extraction.

Bacillus coagulans (Lab).

BackBiter—grooved orthopedic instrument which cuts from the rear to allow easier access to the anterior horn of the meniscus.

BackTracker—assesses on-the-job low-back stress in flexion/extension, lateral flexion, and rotation.

backward failure—a phenomenon that occurs when all the blood returned to the heart cannot be pumped out. Venous pressure rises and the lungs and viscera congest.

Bacon-Babcock—operation for correction of rectovaginal fistula.

BacT/Alert—an automated blood culture system.

BACTEC—an automated blood culture system.

bacteria—see *pathogen.*

bacterial endophthalmitis—a serious postoperative complication of intraocular or cataract surgery.

bactericidal—see *cidal.*

bacteriophage—a virus that infects bacteria.

Bacteroides corrodens—a genus of anaerobic gram-negative rods, found normally in the oropharynx. Has been isolated from infected tonsils, in pharyngitis, pneumonia, and postoperative wound infections. Also called *Eikenella corrodens.*

Bactigras—wound dressing for the prevention of infection in minor skin loss injuries and ulcerative wounds.

baculovirus—an insect virus which is being used in research to develop an AIDS vaccine.

Baculovirus Expression Vector system (BEVS)—a process in which genetically engineered baculoviruses are injected into bioreactors containing proprietary insect cells. The engineered baculoviruses infect the cells and "program" them to manufacture a desired protein. After being supplied with nutrients and oxygen, the cells are harvested and the protein extracted.

BAEP (brain stem auditory evoked potential).

BAER (brain stem auditory evoked response) (pronounced "bear").

Baerveldt glaucoma implant—implantable intraocular device for treatment of glaucoma.

bagassosis—extrinsic allergic alveolitis caused by exposure to moldy sugar cane.

BagEasy—disposable manual respirator.

BAGF (brachioaxillary bridge graft fistula).

bagged—ventilated by hand using an Ambu bag. Usage: "The patient was being bagged via endotracheal tube in the emergency room."

Baggish hysteroscope—an operative sheath used in both Nd:YAG laser and conventional surgery in the uterine cavity as well as aspiration from the uterine cavity. Also, *Baggish contact panoramic hysteroscope.*

Bagolini lens—used in testing and assessing retinal correspondence in eye deviations.

bagpipe sign—a continuous wheeze at the end of expiration.

"bah-fawn"—phonetic for *bas-fond.*

Baim-Turi cardiac device.

Bair Hugger—brand of warming units and blankets.

Bair Paws—a warming gown and warming unit in one system.

Bakamjian flap (ENT)—a deltopectoral flap turned in a radical neck dissection.

Bakelite—strong, lightweight material used to make cystoscopy sheaths.

Bakes dilator (no apostrophe)—a common duct dilator.

BAK interbody fusion system—a system of spinal implants, surgical instruments, and procedures that aid

BAK *(cont.)* minimally invasive surgical placement of implants between the vertebrae to stabilize the spine and facilitate fusion. Also, *BAK/C* (cervical) and *BAK/T* (thoracic).

BAK surgical procedure—uses the BAK interbody fusion system to stabilize and fuse spinal vertebrae in patients with chronic back pain as a result of degenerative disk disease.

BAK Vista interbody fusion system—a radiolucent spine-stabilizing device implanted to treat lower back pain and leg pain stemming from degenerative disk disease.

BAL (bronchoalveolar lavage).

BAL Cath—a catheter used for bronchoalveolar lavage.

Baladi Inverter—a medical device that provides better access to the aorta in cardiac procedures than other clamps. The Inverter preserves the cylindrical shape of the aorta in beating-heart and still-heart procedures and thus provides less traumatic access than with a side-biting clamp.

balanced electrolyte solution (BES).

balanced salt solution (BSS) (Oph).

bald gastric fundus (Radiol)—absence of rugal folds when the gastric fundus is distended by gas or by the presence of barium from an (immediately previous) upper GI study.

Baldwin perineum needle.

Baldwin tube—ventilation tube for myringotomy surgery.

Baldy-Webster operation—for correction of uterine retrodisplacement.

Balke protocol—for cardiac exercise stress testing.

Ballard gestational assessment—a simplified score for assessment of fetal maturation of newly born infants and extremely premature infants. It includes a neuromuscular maturity exam which tests posture, square window, arm recoil, popliteal angle, scarf sign, heel to ear, and evaluates physical maturity to produce a maturity rating.

Ballard score—see *Ballard gestational assessment*.

Baller-Gerold syndrome—craniosynostosis.

ballism—intense and violent flailing movements. Also, *ballismus, hemiballism, hemiballismus*.

balloon brachytherapy—radiation treatment that delivers radiation from the inside out. The procedure involves the insertion of a balloon device, called the MammoSite catheter, through the skin incision and into the area where the cancer is removed. The small balloon is then inflated and radioactive material is used to provide radiation to the area twice a day for five days. After treatment is completed, the balloon is deflated and the device is removed.

balloon catheterization—used to stop bleeding following childbirth in order to avoid emergency hysterectomy postpartum. An interventional radiologist performs the dual procedure of embolization of the bleeding blood vessel and balloon catheterization to stop bleeding.

balloon dissector—used as an alternative to blunt dissection. The dissector is inserted with the balloon uninflated through a small incision and between the tissue layers. The balloon is then filled with air or saline to cause the desired dissection of the tissue planes.

Balloon-on-a-Wire—cardiac device.

balloon photodynamic therapy—a treatment for Barrett esophagus. The

balloon *(cont.)*
photosensitizing drug Photofrin is injected into a vein and concentrates in diseased tissue. When exposed to argon laser light, a chemical reaction occurs which kills the abnormal cells. The specially designed windowed centering balloon manipulates the treatment surface and improves the application of light.

balloon tuboplasty—opens blocked fallopian tubes without surgery. Technique is similar to that used in the Grüntzig balloon catheter angioplasty. In the tuboplasty, a guidewire is passed up through the uterus and eased through the fallopian tube to the point of blockage, which is then perforated. The balloon catheter is inserted and inflated to further enlarge the opening.

balloon wedge-pressure catheter.

Ball operation—for treatment of pruritus ani.

ball therapy—see *Swiss ball therapy*.

Baltic myoclonus—the benign form of Unverricht-Lundborg syndrome, a progressive myoclonus epilepsy associated with progressive dementia. See *Unverricht-Lundborg syndrome.*

banal-appearing nevomelanocytes—birth defects.

banana bag—a detox "cocktail" given IV to alcoholics. The solution contains thiamine, dextrose, and vitamins, the latter of which give it a yellow banana-like tint.

banana blade—a Beaver blade used in arthroscopic surgery.

banana sign—shape of the fetal cerebellum secondary to small size of the posterior fossa, seen in spina bifida.

bandage (see also *dressing)*
- Ace
- butterfly

bandage *(cont.)*
- Champ elastic
- Comperm tubular elastic
- E Cotton
- Elastic Foam
- Elastomull
- Esmarch
- Flexilite conforming elastic
- Fractura Flex
- Hydron Burn Bandage
- Kerlix
- Liquiderm liquid healing
- POP (plaster of Paris)
- Profore four-layer
- spica
- Tricodur Epi (elbow) compression support
- Tricodur Omos (shoulder) compression support
- Tricodur Talus (ankle) compression support
- Velpeau

bandage contact lens (BCL, bCL)—a contact lens placed over the cornea to protect it during healing following surgery or trauma.

bandeau (Plas Surg)—a narrow band or fillet; bandlike. A type of defect.

banding (Genetics)—a technique of staining chromosomes to reveal normal or abnormal distribution of genetic material.

banding of Molina—a dual-mesh gastroplasty banding technique.

band-ligator device—used to obtain large particle biopsies in the GI tract. It was originally designed for esophageal variceal ligation.

bands—immature neutrophils. More than 10% band cells indicates inflammation or infection.

band-snare technique (GI)—provides a large sample of mucosa and submucosa and can be used for either large particle biopsy or for endoscopic mucosal resection.

Banff score—of kidney transplant pathology.

Bang horseshoe-crab blood test—see *LAL test.*

banjo-string adhesion.

Bankart procedure—operation on the shoulder girdle to treat recurrent shoulder dislocation.

banner transposition flap—an ear reconstruction technique used to repair defects on the superior aspect of the helix. It was originally described with use of a flap of postauricular skin, but the loose preauricular skin can also serve as the donor site.

BAPS (biomechanical ankle platform system) **board**—a device used in physical therapy to treat gait disorders and improve range of motion and balance. Routines may be performed from level 1 to level 5.

BAR (biofragmentable anastomotic ring). Example: *Valtrac BAR*.

Bara-Med—a monoplace hyperbaric chamber, used for burn victims and patients with wounds.

Bárány symptom (ENT)—see *caloric testing*.

barbed sutures—sutures used in facial rejuvenation and other plastic surgery repairs. They are a bit like barbed wire that have little cuts in the side of the suture, allowing the barb to catch when it is passed through tissue. The catch allows the plastic surgeon to pull on the suture once it is in place and tighten the tissue. The sutures themselves are minimally invasive, require almost no downtime, and are low risk. See also *Quill self-anchoring suture*, *thread lift*, *feather lift*.

barbotage ("bar-bow-tahzh")—alternate injection and withdrawal of fluid. Usage: "Vancomycin 5 mg was then barbotaged into the Rickham reservoir."

Barcat technique, modified—treats distal hypospadias utilizing apposing, fully mobilized, meatal-based skin flaps.

Bardach modification (Plas Surg)—Obwegeser mandibular osteotomy.

Bard Biopty gun—see *Biopty gun*.

Bard BTA test—used for the detection of recurrent bladder cancer. Cf. *BTA stat test*.

Bard cardiopulmonary support system—a portable heart-lung machine that does not require opening the patient's chest. The patient's blood is shunted to an external machine via a narrow catheter inserted into the femoral vein up to the heart. The blood is oxygenated, warmed, and pumped back into the body via a second catheter threaded through the femoral artery.

Bard Clamshell Septal Umbrella—a device for closure of atrial and ventricular septal defects, similar to the Bard PDA Umbrella.

Bard Composix mesh graft material.

Bard EndoCinch endoscopic suturing system—used in endoscopic and endoluminal gastroplication procedures.

Bardenheuer bifurcation procedure, modified—a procedure for correction of radial ray defect, or club hand. See *pouce flottant*.

Bard Genie button tube—a G-tube for enteral nutrition.

Bard Memotherm—colorectal stent used for treatment of malignant obstructions arising from colon cancer.

Bard PDA (patent ductus arteriosus) **Umbrella**—device used to close patent ductus arteriosus defects in infants. The device is inserted via a

Bard *(cont.)*
catheter, positioning a balloon on each side of the orifice. When the balloons are expanded, slight pulling causes the arms or ribs of the umbrella to expand further and come flush to the orifice. Slight pushing then causes the arms of the other balloon to expand and come flush on the opposite side of the orifice, thus closing the patent ductus.

Bard Safety Excalibur—peripherally inserted central catheter introducer.

Bard sign—on cardiac palpation, a prominent and broad thrust sustained throughout ventricular systole in left ventricular hypertrophy.

Bard Sperma-Tex preshaped mesh.

Bard Stinger S ablation catheter—for the treatment of cardiac arrhythmias.

Bard TransAct intra-aortic balloon pump—a device to assist the heart before and after open heart surgery and complex balloon angioplasty procedures.

Bard Visilex mesh—graft material for laparoscopic hernia repair.

Bard XT coronary stent—a one-piece Y-shaped stent implanted in a patient. It is described as a modular zigzag design or a true bifurcated stent with a dedicated "trouser" balloon delivery system.

bare lymphocyte syndrome—a condition in which the lymphocytes do not express MHC class I and/or II antigens on their surface, resulting in severe combined immunodeficiency disease.

Bariatric Analysis and Reporting Outcome System (BAROS)—a proposed method for evaluating quality of life, metabolic indices, and other factors in patients who have undergone bariatric surgery for obesity.

barium artifact (Radiol)—overlooked dried barium on table tops, intensifying screens, or on patient gowns appearing to be within the patient and misleading the radiologist.

Barlow test—for dysplasia of the hip.

BAROS (Bariatric Analysis and Reporting Outcome System).

barotrauma—tissue injury caused by abnormally high or low atmospheric pressure, e.g., in flying, scuba diving; also, from high respirator pressures.

Barouk button space—used with conventional Keller arthroplasty technique for reconstruction of hallux valgus deformities.

Barouk microscrew—used with a shortening osteotomy for correction of hallux valgus.

Barouk microstaple—used with a closing wedge osteotomy for solid fixation using only a single implant.

Barraquer forceps and scissors—used in ophthalmology procedures.

Barr body—see *buccal smear; sex chromatin.*

barrel-stave osteotomies—the creation of barrel stave-shaped incisions in the skull of an infant with craniosynostosis, performed during cranioplasty procedure to allow for growth of the brain. Also, barrel stave-like osteotomies.

Barrett esophagus (BE)—one or more zones of metaplasia (cell transformation) in the distal esophagus, by which the normal squamous epithelium is replaced by columnar epithelium resembling that of the gastric mucosa. This change occurs chiefly in persons with hiatal hernia or gastroesophageal reflux disease, in whom the distal esophagus is repeatedly exposed to acid gastric juice.

Barrett *(cont.)*
The condition is associated with an increased risk of esophageal carcinoma. Various procedures may reduce the risk of malignant change. After an IV injection of a photosensitizing agent, which concentrates in zones of abnormal tissue, argon dye laser treatment of the lower esophagus selectively destroys sensitized metaplastic cells.

barrier—see *tissue regeneration barrier.*

barrier dressings.

Barron disposable trephine (Oph).

Barron donor corneal punch—steel blade with vacuum base to immobilize the cornea for cutting the button for transplantation.

Barron pump—four-speed pump used to control delivery of chemotherapeutic agents through an arterial line.

Barron radial vacuum trephine—corneal trephine made of solid steel.

Bartonella bacilliformis—a bacterial pathogen causing Carrión disease, a tropical infection.

Bartonella elizabethae—a bacterial pathogen isolated from a patient with endocarditis involving an artificial aortic valve.

Bartonella henselae—a bacterial pathogen causing bacillary angiomatosis and associated with cat-scratch disease. *B. henselae* is transmitted among cats by the cat flea and from cats to humans by means of a cat scratch.

Bartonella quintana—bacterial pathogen causing bacillary angiomatosis-peliosis. It was formerly called *Rochalimaea quintana* or *Rickettsia quintana* and was the cause of trench fever in World War I. *B. quintana* infection is transmitted by the human body louse.

Bartter syndrome—hypokalemic alkalosis, hyperaldosteronism secondary to adrenal cortical hyperplasia, hypertrophy and hyperplasia of the juxtaglomerular apparatus of the kidneys, and normal blood pressures associated with subnormal reactivity of blood pressures to angiotensin II.

basal calcitonin (bCT).

basal ganglia—gray masses in the cerebrum involved in motor coordination.

baseball stitch—Usage: "A baseball stitch of 00 chromic was used to complete the uterine repair."

base excess—one of the measurements on a blood gas study related to bicarbonate. Usage: "The arterial blood gases showed pH 7.35, PO_2 110, PCO_2 40 with a base excess of -3 and saturation of 95%."

base pair (bp)—a pair of complementary bases in a double-stranded nucleic acid. Adenine always pairs with thymine in DNA and with uracil in RNA; guanine always pairs with cytosine in both DNA and RNA. This pattern of pairing is the basis of DNA replication and RNA transcription.

bas-fond ("bah-fawn")—bladder fundus.

basic conditioning factors (BCF)—internal and external factors (sex, age, health, social factors) that contribute to individual diversity and affect self-care.

basicervical—more commonly used than *basocervical*. Usage: "basicervical femoral neck fracture."

basic fibroblast growth factor (bFGF)—one of several compounds the body uses to stimulate growth of blood vessels.

basic metabolic panel (BMP).

basidiobolomycosis—fungal disease caused by *Basidiobolus ranarum*, most often found in tropical regions of Africa. The fungus, usually limited to the skin, has also been found to invade the gastrointestinal and urinary tracts of some patients, producing nonspecific peptic ulcer-like symptoms such as fever, nausea, vomiting, anorexia, weight loss, and gastrointestinal bleeding.

Basidiomycetes—class of smut and rust fungi causing problems in allergic individuals who work around wheat and granaries.

basis pontis—the ventral portion of the pons; part of the brain stem.

BASMI (Bath Ankylosing Spondylitis Metrology Index).

Bassen-Kornzweig abetalipoproteinemia.

BAT (B-mode acquisition and targeting).

Batchelor technique—a modified procedure to correct hindfoot valgus deformity, achieving immediate stability.

Bateman UPF II bipolar endoprosthesis (Universal proximal femur)—hip replacement system made by Kirschner.

Bates-Jensen pressure ulcer status tool.

Bath Ankylosing Spondylitis Metrology Index (BASMI).

bathing trunks nevus (*not* bathing trunk nevus).

Batista procedure (left ventriculectomy)—radical surgical procedure for treatment of end-stage heart failure by removing a piece of the left ventricle, surgically reducing the size of the chamber, ultimately allowing the heart to beat more efficiently, as a possible alternative to heart transplantation.

Batista procedure—left ventricular reduction surgery.

Baton laser pointer—device used in minimally invasive surgery, allowing a surgeon to point out anatomical details on a video screen without having to physically point or use verbal descriptions. It is mounted on a lightweight headset and is activated by a small mouthpiece switch.

Batten disease—a form of cerebral macular degeneration.

batten graft—see *spreader graft*.

Battey-avium complex—see *MAC infection*.

Battle sign—discoloration (ecchymosis) over the mastoid process, a sign of basilar skull fracture.

batwing arms—see *brachioplasty*.

Bauhin, valve of—ileocecal valve.

Baumann, angle of.

Bayley Scales of Infant Development—from manual by Nancy Bayley.

Baylor bleeding score—identifies patients at increased risk for rebleeding following endoscopy.

bayonet bipolar forceps.

bayonet-type incision—a rectilinear incision with a jog near the middle, giving it a configuration like that of a rifle with a bayonet attached.

Bayou virus—a hantavirus pulmonary syndrome identified in the blood of patients from Louisiana and eastern Texas. The carrier is believed to be the rice rat (*Oryzomys palustris*).

Bazex syndrome—palmoplantar keratoderma with features similar to psoriasis on the hands, associated with carcinoma of the upper respiratory tract; this is a cutaneous marker to an internal malignancy.

B-bevel needle.

BB shot—small, 0.46 cm in diameter round pellet used in air rifles or BB guns. Usage: "There was a small BB-sized cystic lesion on the lateral thigh."

BCA (bichloroacetic acid).

B-cell (also called *B-lymphocyte*)—part of the immune system; some mature B-cells become plasma cells, which secrete antibodies, but not without help from T-cells, one variety of which is attacked by the AIDS virus. See *T-4 cell, helper cell.*

BCF (basic conditioning factors).

BCI (brain-computer interfaces).

BCL, bCL (bandage contact lens).

Bcl-2—see *BRCA*.

bcr/abl protein test—an indicator of an abnormality called the Philadelphia chromosome, which is present in 95% of patients with chronic myelogenous leukemia.

bCT (basal calcitonin).

BCT (breast-conserving therapy).

BCX-34—used to treat cutaneous T-cell lymphoma.

BDD (body dysmorphic disorder)—obsession and distress with physical appearance.

Bdellovibrio ("del′-o-vib′-re-o")—a genus of parasitic gram-negative organisms that live on certain other gram-negative bacteria.

BD Insyte Autoguard shielded intravenous catheter.

BDNF (brain-derived neurotrophic factor)—used to treat ALS (amyotrophic lateral sclerosis).

BDProbeTec ET system—for direct qualitative detection of *Chlamydia trachomatis* and *Neisseria gonorrhoeae.*

B-D (Becton-Dickinson) **spinal needle**.

BE (Barrett esophagus).

Beacon minimally invasive incontinence surgical line from UroMed.

Bead Block—use of polyvinyl alcohol (PVA) embolic microspheres for the treatment of hypervascular tumors and arteriovenous malformations. PVA beads are also being used to treat uterine fibroids.

beads of methylmethacrylate—see *methylmethacrylate, beads of.*

BEAM (brain electrical activity map, or mapping)—a computerized EEG that maps different areas of the brain.

Beamer injection stent system—a Percuflex stent that provides for contrast injection during ureteral stent placement. Can convert to drainage stent.

beam-hardening artifact (on CT scans)—streaks seen when the beam passes through tissues of vastly different densities (e.g., in petrous bone next to the brain, the parenchyma will be streaked).

beam splitter—used with an operating microscope to permit use of attachments that will enable a second person to look through the microscope with the surgeon; makes it possible to take photographs and videotape what is seen through the microscope.

beanbag shotgun rounds—refers to penetration of the chest by less-than-lethal shotgun rounds that look like beanbag pellets on chest radiographs.

"bear"—phonetic for *BAER*.

bear claw ulceration—large linear mucosal ulcerations in Crohn colitis.

Beare-Stevenson cutis gyrata syndrome—evident in newborns. Characterized by craniofacial anomalies, particularly craniosynostosis, ear defects, cutis gyrata, acanthosis nigricans, anogenital anomalies, skin

Beare-Stevenson *(cont.)*
tags, and prominent umbilical stump.

"bear hugger"—see *Bair Hugger.*

bear tracks (Oph)—a pattern of pigmentation at the back of the retina that has the appearance of footprints made by a bear. It is due to the clumping of pigment in the layer of cells behind the retina (retinal pigment epithelium). It is present from birth and has no significance in itself.

beaten silver appearance—increase in convolutional markings on x-rays of the skull.

beating heart surgery—any cardiac surgical procedure during which the heart continues to beat and maintain circulation. Various types of procedures can be performed on the beating heart, including keyhole heart surgery, minimally invasive direct coronary artery bypass (MIDCAB), off-pump coronary artery bypass (OPCAB), and robot-assisted coronary artery bypass (RACAB). All these surgeries are minimally invasive and are useful for bypassing critically blocked arteries on the front of the heart. These procedures are less difficult and risky than conventional open-heart surgery (coronary artery bypass grafting [CABG]), which requires stopping the flow of blood to and from the heart and placing the patient on heart-lung bypass. Cf. *arrested heart surgery.*

beat-knee syndrome—alternative term for prepatellar bursitis, carpet layer's knee, coal miner's knee, housemaid's knee.

Beau line—a transverse groove in the nail seen in fingernails. Can result from severe emotional or physical shock. Cf. *Mees line.*

Beaver blade (see also *blade*)
arachnoid shape
banana
cataract knife
discission knife
keratome
retrograde
rosette
sickle-shape

Beaver DeBakey blades—for hip surgery.

beaver fever—the hikers' and canoeists' "affectionate" term for giardiasis.

Bebax shoe (Peds).

Bechert lens-holding forceps.

Beck Depression Inventory (Psych).

Becker accelerator cannula—a liposuction cannula.

Becker nevus of the thigh with lipoatrophy.

Becker tissue expander/breast prosthesis—an inflatable tissue expander used to reconstruct the breast following mastectomy. Also serves as a permanent breast implant. Only the access port and tubing have to be removed in a brief outpatient procedure under local anesthesia with intravenous sedation.

Beckwith-Wiedemann syndrome—a congenital syndrome characterized by the presence of macroglossia, omphalocele, gigantism, and sometimes other associated anomalies.

becquerel (Bq)—the unit of measurement in the International System of Measurement (SI) that is the absorbed dose equivalent in radioactivity. See *International System.*

BED (binge eating disorder).

bedewing ("bee-doing") **of cornea**—swelling and superficial clouding of

bedewing *(cont.)*
the cornea, caused by increased intraocular pressure for an extended period of time. The surface of the cornea becomes "grainy" in appearance, thus interfering with the transmission of light rays. May also be referred to as *Sattler veil.*

Bedge antireflux mattress—egg-crate foam wedge used to elevate the upper body to prevent gastroesophageal reflux.

Bedwetting Store—a real store that carries bedwetting supplies.

beefy—having the appearance or texture of raw lean meat.

beer drinker's hyponatremia—a syndrome of hyponatremia in patients who consume excessive amounts of beer and have a poor dietary intake. Also called *beer potomania.*

"beetle" or "bee-toll"—phonetic for *BTL* (bilateral tubal ligation). Usage: "G3, P3, status post VBAC and beetle," or "'beetle' for contraception." Expand to *bilateral tubal ligation (BTL).*

behavioral mapping (Rehab).

Behavioral Pathology in Alzheimer Disease Rating Scale—rates behavioral symptoms in seven categories: delusional ideation, hallucinations, activity disturbance, sleep disturbance, depressive symptoms, anxiety, and aggressive behavior.

Behçet ("bay-shet") **syndrome**—severe uveitis and retinal vasculitis, optic atrophy.

bell-clapper deformity—an anatomic deformity that allows the spermatic cord to twist, which can result in occlusion of testicular blood flow. The tunica vaginalis completely surrounds the testis, which leads to inadequate posterior fixation of the testis and epididymis to the scrotal wall.

Bellini duct carcinoma—a rare variant of renal cell carcinoma.

Bell phenomenon—the eye rolls upward and outward on attempting to close the eye.

Bellucci scissors (ENT).

belly of muscle—the center of the muscle where its area of greatest mass lies. The site where an intramuscular injection may be given in certain large muscles in the arms, legs, and buttocks.

Belos compression pin.

Belzer solution—a solution that preserves organs until transplantation. Contains lactobionate and raffinose (to prevent cellular swelling) and some other ingredients (glutathione and allopurinol) that prevent oxidative damage, and still other ingredients that will help to restore adenosine triphosphate levels to normal after re-perfusion.

BEMA (bioerodible mucoadhesive)—pre-formed film designed for both systemic and local drug delivery across oral mucosal membranes.

Benchekroun valve—intussuscepted ileohydraulic valve for continent vesicostomy in the absence of an appendix.

bench method—refers to manual performance of a laboratory test (at a workbench, hence the name) rather than automated machinery. Usage: "Calcium determinations were 10.3 and 9.7 on the SMA, and 9.7 by bench method."

Bender Gestalt test (Neuro)—mental status examination.

Benecol margarine—contains a plant-derived substance (stanol esters), shown to help lower cholesterol. It is

Benecol *(cont.)*
sold as a nonprescription medical food product.

Benedikt ipsilateral oculomotor paralysis (Neuro).

BeneJoint—a topical drug for temporary relief of arthritis pain.

Benelli mastopexy (also, pursestring mastopexy; modified Benelli round block mastopexy)—a procedure used for true ptosis of breasts or tubular breast deformity.

Beneprotein instant protein powder—a concentrated source of high-quality protein designed to mix instantly into a wide variety of foods and beverages without compromising taste or texture. For use by patients who require additional protein to bolster their regular diet, to help promote skin health, wound healing, immune response and muscle strength. Easily mixes without clumping for easy tube feeding flushes and better acceptance when taken orally.

benign—normal, not showing evidence of disease or abnormality; a benign tumor is one that is not malignant.

benign intracranial hypertension (BIH).

benign necrotizing otitis externa (BNOE).

benign neglect—a program of doing essentially nothing when a disease is either beyond hope of cure by even the most radical methods, or is expected to resolve without any specific treatment. Also called *masterly inactivity.*

benign paroxysmal positional vertigo (BPPV)—a common form of vertigo that is precipitated by certain specific movements, such as bending over, looking upward, or even rolling over in bed.

benign prostatic hypertrophy or **hyperplasia** (BPH)—treated by a variety of surgical procedures and medications which are increasingly replacing the traditional treatment, TURP (transurethral resection of the prostate). Surgical procedures include laser resection, microwave thermotherapy, intraurethral coils and springs, balloon dilatation, cryotherapy, and focused extracorporeal ultrasound. Medical treatments include 5-alpha reductase inhibitors, alpha-adrenergic blockade, and antiandrogens.

Benik glove.

Benik joint support wraps.

Benirschke approach—surgical technique for treating calcaneal fractures. Named for Dr. Stephen K. Benirschke.

Benjamin binocular slimline laryngoscope (ENT).

Benjamin-Havas fiberoptic light clip—used as light source in laryngoscopes.

Benjamin pediatric laryngoscope.

Benjamin proverbs (Psych).

Bennett bone retractor.

Bennett fracture—alternative name for carpometacarpal thumb ray fracture, thumb fracture-dislocation, stave of thumb.

Bennett PR-2 ventilator—time-cycled ventilator, used mainly in treating children.

Bennett quadriceps plastic procedure—for traction contractures of the knee.

Bennett self-retaining retractor blade.

Bentley Duraflo II—extracorporeal perfusion circuit with universal biocompatibility protection to prevent blood reactions.

bent malleable retractor.

bentonite flocculation test—to diagnose trichinosis.

Bentson guidewire (Radiol).

benzalkonium chloride patch test—for allergies.

benzodiazepines—a class of drugs that includes antianxiety agents and sedatives.

BER (benign early repolarization).

Berens 3-character test—eye test used in small children who do not know the letters of the alphabet.

Berger disease—appears to be a variant of Henoch-Schönlein nephritis, but without the rash. Cf. *Buerger disease.*

Beriplast P—fibrin tissue glue.

Berkeley-Bonney retractor—a self-retaining three-blade abdominal retractor. See *Goligher modification.*

Berkeley optic zone marker.

Berkow formula—a method of assessing the percentage of body surface that has been burned. This is an adaptation of the Rule of Nines, but makes allowance for the age of the patient. In a one-year-old child, for example, the head is larger in proportion to body size; therefore, the head is rated at 19, while the head of an adult would be rated at 7. See *Rule of Nines.*

Berkson-Gage calculation—for determining breast cancer survival rates.

Berman locator—a magnetic device used in locating intraocular foreign bodies.

Bernese periacetabular osteotomy (PAO)—a joint-preserving technique that allows extensive corrections to be done without disturbing the abductor muscles. The surgeon can simultaneously do an arthrotomy and repair labral tears, without disturbing the blood supply to the acetabulum. Named for Berne, Switzerland, where the technique was developed.

berry aneurysm—abnormal berry-like dilatation of an artery.

Berryhill testing for functional capacity—an evaluation method used in occupational therapy and workers compensation cases.

Bertel position—used to visualize the floor of the orbits and the orbital fissures on x-rays.

Berwick dye (Gyn).

BES (balanced electrolyte solution).

Bessey-Lowry units—measure alkaline phosphatase. See also *Bodansky unit, King-Armstrong unit.*

Best right-angle colon clamp.

BeStent—a balloon-expandable stent for use in arteries measuring 2.5 mm to 5.5 mm in diameter.

BeStent2—Medtronic laser-cut stent for use after coronary arteries have been opened with balloon catheters in PTCA.

best spectacle-corrected visual acuity (BSCVA)—a term ophthalmologists use in referring to vision correction.

beta antagonist—see *antagonist*. Also known as *beta blocker.*

Beta-Cath system—an intracoronary catheter for use with beta irradiation, to prevent recurrence of stenosis after vascularization procedure.

Betadine Surgi-Prep (povidone-iodine) **Sponge Brush**.

beta-endorphin—an opiate-like peptide that acts on the central nervous system; it is of anterior pituitary origin. See *endorphins.*

beta interferon—see *interferon beta.*

beta isoform, 14-3-3—a variant of the 14-3-3 antigen, a marker for Creutzfeldt-Jakob syndrome detected by cerebrospinal fluid immunoassay.

beta-lactamase—an enzyme produced by certain bacteria which is able to split the beta-lactam chemical ring structure of penicillins and cephalosporins. Beta-lactamase-positive bacteria are resistant to the antibiotic effect of penicillins and cephalosporins.

betamethasone mousse—used topically for treatment of scalp psoriasis and other scalp dermatoses.

Betaseron needle-free delivery system—for use by multiple sclerosis patients to self-administer Betaseron (interferon beta-lb) for subcutaneous injection. It uses a burst of carbon dioxide to propel a stream of medication through the skin.

Bethesda rating scale—assigns a category for Pap smears in which the cells have abnormal features that quantitatively or qualitatively fall short of dysplasia, termed ASCUS (atypical squamous cells of uncertain significance).

Betz cells—large pyramidal cells forming layer of the gray matter of the brain. Vladimir Betz, Russian anatomist.

bevacizumab—see *Avastin*.

Bevan incision—vertical elliptical skin incision in the abdomen.

Bevel Wand—an ablation instrument used when cutting angles in meniscal repair procedures, for shoulder procedures, ACL stump removal, anterior meniscectomy, and removing soft tissue in elbow procedures.

BEVS (Baculovirus Expression Vector system).

BFE (blood flow enhancement).

bFGF (basic fibroblast growth factor).

BFNC (benign familial neonatal convulsions).

BFU-E (burst-forming unit—erythroid).

bG (blood glucose).

BHT (breath hydrogen test).

Biad SPECT imaging system.

Biafine RE (radiodermatitis emulsion)—used for protection against skin reactions induced by radiation therapy.

Biafine WDE (wound dressing emulsion)—used to manage dermal wounds, ulcers, and burns.

biannual—twice a year. See *biennial*.

bibasally—at the bases of both lungs (on chest x-ray).

Bible printer's lung—extrinsic allergic alveolitis caused by exposure to moldy paper.

biceps jerk (BJ) (Neuro).

bichloroacetic acid (BCA).

Bickel leg holder.

BiDil—a combination of hydralazine and isosorbide dinitrate, two older drugs that have been used in the past to treat various heart conditions, and are now being used in a new combination to treat advanced heart failure. In the clinical study, there was a significant decrease in mortality among African Americans. The results were so favorable that investigators halted the multi-center trial so that all the study participants suffering from advanced heart failure, including those on a placebo, could be given the combined drug treatment.

Bielschowsky head tilt—a test of oblique ocular muscle paralysis.

biennial—occurring every two years. Not to be confused with "biannual" (occurring twice a year).

Bier ("beer") **block anesthesia**—used in surgery of the extremities.

Bierman needle—used for bone marrow biopsy and aspiration.

BIFC (benign infantile familial convulsions).

biferious pulse (or bisferious)—see *bisferious pulse* (pulsus bisferiens, or biferiens).

bifidity—used to describe an iatrogenic deformity following rhinoplasty in which a retrograde cartilage-splitting or intracartilaginous incision was inappropriately performed in a patient with thick cartilages, resulting in a wide interdomal distance.

bifoil balloon catheter—see *percutaneous transvenous mitral commissurotomy.*

Bigliani/Flatow shoulder prosthesis—for shoulder arthroplasty.

BIH (benign intracranial hypertension).

Bihrle dorsal clamp and T-C needle holder—for fixation and suturing of the dorsal vein complex in urologic surgery.

BiLAP—bipolar cautery unit with cutting and coagulation functions.

bilateral juxtafoveal telangiectasis (BJT)—characterized by leaking parafoveal retinal capillaries resulting in retinal edema. It affects middle-aged and elderly patients and is treated with laser photocoagulation for macular edema.

bilateral PC-IOL (posterior chamber intraocular lens) **implantation**—used to correct pediatric aphakia.

bilateral ureteral obstruction (BUO).

bi-level positive airway pressure (BiPAP).

bilharziasis—another name for schistosomiasis. Infection with flukes of the genus *Schistosoma.*

biliary decompression (internal biliary drainage)—promotes Kupffer cell recovery in obstructive jaundice.

biliary reconstruction—a procedure using side-to-side anastomosis choledochocholedochostomy in liver transplant patients.

BiliBed—phototherapy system in which the infant, placed inside a special garment on a plastic film support, lies over the light source. The baby is exposed to light via a special section in the rear of the garment, eliminating the need for eye shielding.

BiliBlanket phototherapy system—an alternative to phototherapy light used to treat jaundice in newborn babies. This device consists of a small jacket that gives off high-intensity fiberoptic light.

BiliBottoms—light-permeable disposable phototherapy diaper for newborns with jaundice.

BiliCheck—handheld battery-powered system that measures bilirubin levels without needing a blood sample.

bili lights—slang for the fluorescent lights (bilirubin lights) used as phototherapy for infants with hyperbilirubinemia.

Bili mask—an eye shield used on infants undergoing phototherapy for bilirubinemia.

biliopancreatic diversion with duodenal switch—bariatric hybrid surgical procedure for weight loss and permanent weight control.

bilirubinometer—see *Colormate TLc BiliTest System.*

Billroth gastroenterostomy. Billroth I is a partial resection of the stomach (65-75%), and anastomosis of the end of the stomach to the duodenum. (The stomach is first tapered to the size, or caliber, of the duodenum.) The Billroth II is used for duodenal ulcer; a gastrojejunostomy is performed, bringing the jejunal loop up to the remnant of the stomach posteriorly through a hole in the transverse mesocolon, or anterior to the transverse colon. The antecolic anastomosis is used more frequently because it is a simpler procedure.

biloma—encapsulated collection of bile due to biliary tract injury.

Binet classification of chronic lymphocytic leukemia (CLL)—classifies CLL according to the number of lymphoid tissues that are involved, as well as the presence of anemia and thrombocytopenia.

Stage A patients have fewer than three areas of enlarged lymphoid tissue. Enlarged lymph nodes of the neck, underarms, and groin, as well as the spleen, are each considered "one group," whether unilateral (one-sided) or bilateral (on both sides).

Stage B patients have more than three areas of enlarged lymphoid tissue.

Stage C patients have anemia plus thrombocytopenia.

Bing auditory acuity test. A vibrating tuning fork is placed at the mastoid process and the acoustic meatus is closed off and opened. If the patient hears a decrease and increase in sound (a positive Bing), hearing is normal or the hearing loss is sensorineural. If the patient does not notice any difference in sound (a negative Bing), there is a deficit in conductive hearing.

binge, bingeing—overindulging in excessive amounts of food (as in bulimia) or alcohol.

binge eating disorder (BED).

binocular infrared oculographic (BIRO) **system**—allows binocular recordings with simultaneous measurements of horizontal and vertical eye movements.

bioabsorbable closure device—bovine collagen plug and anchor used after angioplasty to stop bleeding.

bioabsorbable polymeric material (BPM).

bioactive (BA) **bone cement**.

bioactive glass—developed to promote intimate contact between bone and any foreign material or implant forming a bone/implant interface to produce a layer of what is known as biologically active apatite, which chemically bridges the host tissue and the implant material.

bioartificial kidney—a device for patients in renal failure. The bioartificial kidney includes a cartridge that filters the blood as in traditional kidney dialysis. That cartridge is connected to a renal tubule assist device, which is made of hollow fibers lined with a type of kidney cell called renal proximal tubule cells. These cells are intended to reclaim vital electrolytes, salt, glucose and water, as well as control production of immune system molecules called cytokines, which the body needs to fight infection.

Biobrane adhesive—a biosynthetic skin substitute. The adhesive is used to protect clean superficial abrasions and burns. It maintains a clean wound until healing takes place, or is removed when autografting is necessary and possible. See *Biobrane glove, Biobrane/HF.*

Biobrane glove—a glove-like wrapping made of a biosynthetic skin substitute. It is used to protect clean excised burn wounds of the hand until healing occurs, or is removed when autografting is possible.

Biobrane/HF—experimental skin substitute made from human neonatal fibroblasts cultured in a mesh of Biobrane, which is a dressing made of a thin layer of silicone bonded to nylon mesh. Researchers believe this

Biobrane/HF *(cont.)* graft could replace cadaveric allograft skin for temporary wound closure after burn wound excision.

BioBypass—gene-based angiogenic therapy designed to stimulate new blood vessel formation in the heart and other tissues affected by inadequate blood flow.

biocavity laser—a semiconductor laser scalpel with a blood analysis system built into the handle to give a surgeon immediate feedback on whether cells being removed are cancerous.

Biocell RTV implant—saline-filled breast implant used as an alternative to, or replacement of, gel-filled or silicone implants.

Bioceram two-stage series II, or **type S**—endosteal dental implants.

Bio-Chromatic hand prosthesis.

Bioclot protein S assay—a test for the anticoagulant protein S, which is considered an important naturally occurring anticoagulant in human blood. Measuring deficiency in protein S can identify patients at risk for clotting disorders such as deep venous thrombosis and pulmonary embolism.

Bioclusive transparent dressing—a clear, waterproof sterile dressing that protects the wound, permits continuous wound monitoring, is vapor permeable (thus preventing skin maceration), and prevents dehydration of the wound.

BioComFold foldable intraocular lens (IOL)—intraocular lens which allows greater optical shifts along the anteroposterior axis during accommodation.

Biocoral (Neuro)—processed madreporic coral. See *madreporic coral.*

Biocor porcine stented aortic and mitral valves and **stentless porcine aortic valve**.

Biocor 200—a high performance oxygenator device that replaces the function of the lungs during open-heart surgery.

biocrime—the threat or use of biological agents for individual objectives, such as revenge or financial gain.

BioCuff—bioresorbable screw and spiked washer implant, used for reattachment of torn rotator cuff tissue to bone.

Biodel—biodegradable polymer formed into wafers or beads impregnated with a chemotherapy drug or antibiotic. Used to treat osteomyelitis and malignant gliomas.

Biodex system—for multijoint testing and rehabilitation.

BiodivYsio—phosphorylcholine-coated coronary stent.

bioerodible mucoadhesive (BEMA).

Bio-eye—hydroxyapatite ocular implant that allows motility and fibrovascular ingrowth. It can be coupled directly to an artificial eye.

biofeedback therapy—used in occupational therapy: *electromyographic feedback*—used to increase or decrease muscle function; *goniometric biofeedback*—used to study range of motion; and *thermal biofeedback*—used to treat vascular problems like Raynaud syndrome and reflex sympathetic dystrophy.

Biofilter hemoconcentrator—used in open heart surgery to prevent fluid overload.

BioFIT Herbgels—a line of "natural" remedies, nutrients, and food products.

Biofix system—bioabsorbable fixation rod made of Dexon sutures.

biofragmentable anastomotic ring (BAR).

Biofreeze with Ilex—topical analgesic drug that may be used to enhance benefits of ultrasound, electrical stimulation, and massage therapy.

BioGlue—surgical adhesive used for repair of aortic dissections.

bio-interference screw (Ortho).

Bio-Intrafix system—a soft tissue tibial fixation system for anterior cruciate ligament repair, an alternative to the widely used bone-patellar tendon-bone graft repair.

Biojector 2000—jet injection systems for needle-free drug delivery.

biologically-active apatite—see *bioactive glass.*

Biologically Quiet screw—trade name for a screw used in anterior cruciate ligament reconstruction. The biodegradable screw does not have to be removed. About six weeks postoperatively it begins to metabolize, and by six months the space that had been occupied by the screw has been replaced by new cancellous bone marrow.

Biologically Quiet suture anchor—a mini-screw implant for soft tissue repair in the shoulder.

BioLogic-DT system—a blood detoxification system used for treating acute hepatic coma.

BioLogic-HT system—used for whole-body extracorporeal hyperthermia treatment for AIDS patients.

Biolox ball head—ceramic head for total hip replacement and hemi-arthroplasty.

Biomatrix ocular implant—an implant made of hydroxyapatite and used in patients who have had enucleation or evisceration of an eye. About six to eight weeks after surgery, the blood vessels and tissues have grown into the implant, and the artificial eye is then attached to the implant. This lets the artificial eye move naturally with the other eye, for very good cosmetic effect. See *enucleation, evisceration, hydroxyapatite.*

BioMend—type 1 collagen membrane made from bovine Achilles tendon and utilized in dental implants.

biomicroscope—a microscope used to visualize living tissue in the body. Used synonymously with slit lamp in ophthalmology. It permits study of the structures of the eye, with the intense beam of light permitting visualization through the tissues of these structures. See *slit-lamp biomicroscopy.*

Bionicare 1000—a stimulator system used to reduce pain and symptoms of osteoarthritis of the knee.

Bionx SmartNail bioresorbable implant—used to maintain fixation and accurate alignment of small bone fractures, osteochondral fragments, or osteochondritis dissecans lesions.

BIO-OSS (all caps)—a bone filler used in oral and maxillofacial surgery. This is a bovine-derived natural bone matrix with all protein removed. Once implanted, it will be invaded by lamellar bone and is osteoconductive, which means it becomes vascularized just as normal bone.

Biopatch—foam wound dressing.

Bioplus dispersive electrode (Cardio).

BioPolyMeric graft for femoropopliteal bypass.

BioPort collection and transport system—a sterile, self-contained device to preserve the viability of aerobic microbial specimens.

biopsy—see *operation*.

Biopty (*not* biopsy) **cut needle**—a needle used in breast biopsy and prostate biopsy.

Biopty (*not* biopsy) **gun**; **Bard Biopty gun**—a device used in needle core breast biopsy and prostate biopsy.

BioRCI screw—orthopedic screw used for fixation of bone-tendon-bone or soft-tissue grafts during anterior cruciate ligament and/or posterior cruciate ligament reconstruction.

bioresorbable implants—experimental implants for repair of facial fractures and osteotomies. Most common polymers used are polyglycolic acid (PGA), polylactic acid (PLA), and levo-PLA.

Biosafe PSA4—can measure prostate-specific antigen on even a small blood sample collected by the patient.

BioScrew bio-absorbable interference screws—used in knee arthroscopy.

BioSorb resorbable urology stent products.

BioStar strep A OIA (optical immunoassay) **Max test**—accurate, rapid strep test which can be used to assist in selection of appropriate antibiotic treatment.

Biostent—an agent to prevent restenosis following balloon angioplasty.

BioStinger—low-profile fixation device developed for the performance of BioStinger meniscal fixation surgical technique.

biosurgery—a rapidly growing field in which surgeons use solutions or gels to enhance or replace traditional invasive surgery. Used in areas such as wound care, burn care, cosmetic augmentation, orthopedics, and reduction of tissue adhesions in surgery.

Biosyn suture—synthetic monofilament suture with similar features to a braided suture, without promotion of bacterial growth.

Biot breathing—an irregular breathing commonly found in meningitis.

Bio-Tense—a relaxation tool that looks much like the sunglasses given to patients following cataract surgery. It combines specific audio frequencies delivered through stereo headphones with continuous flashing *flicker phenomena* to relax patients with hypertension, depression, insomnia, chronic pain, headaches, and arthritis.

Biotrack coagulation monitor—with only one drop of blood, can calculate the APTT value to assess heparin levels while a cardiac catheterization is being performed.

Bio-Tract—proprietary strain of *Lactobacillus salivarius* which inhibits *Helicobacter pylori* bacteria in vitro.

Bio-Vascular Probe—a medical instrument used in vascular surgery procedures.

BioZ system—a digital noninvasive cardiac function monitoring system used as an alternative to the invasive right heart catheter for monitoring critically ill patients.

BiPAP (bi-level positive airway pressure).

biphasic helical CT scan—computed tomographic study in which an imaging agent is injected, scans are taken (the arterial phase), and delayed scans (the delayed phase) are additionally performed.

biplane sector probe—used with Bard Biopty gun to perform transrectal prostatic ultrasonographic biopsy.

bipolar affective illness (also *manic-depressive*; *bipolar disorder*)—alternating attacks of mania and depression.

bipolar coagulation—electrosurgery using a pair of electrodes. Tissue be-

bipolar *(cont.)*
tween them is coagulated by flow of current from one to the other. Also, *bipolar forceps*.

bipolar disorder—see *bipolar affective illness*.

bipolar esophageal recording.

bipolar urological loop—a device used in endoscopic surgical procedures such as resection of prostate tissue and nonmalignant tumors of the bladder wall. It is said to offer the benefit of tissue resection in a saline environment physiologically compatible with the human body.

BIPP (bismuth-iodoform-paraffin paste)—ribbon gauze used to pack the ear canal after surgery.

BI-RADS—breast imaging and reporting data system of the American College of Radiology. Mammographic findings may be characterized by the term *BI-RAD* followed by an arabic numeral, e.g., BI-RAD 3.

Category 0: Need additional imaging evidence
Category 1: Negative
Category 2: Benign finding
Category 3: Probably benign finding
Category 4: Suspicious abnormality
Category 5: Highly suspicious for malignancy

Birbeck granule—identification of this part of a Langerhans cell is diagnostic of histiocytosis X. Also called *X-body*.

birdcage splint—descriptive term for a splint used on a digit with a crush injury. Usage: "The wound was dressed and a birdcage splint was applied to the index finger."

Bird cup (Ob-Gyn)—attached to a vacuum source to facilitate vacuum-assisted vaginal deliveries. Also, *Bird OP cup*, for posterior presentations.

bird flu—see *avian flu*. Also known as *Asian bird flu*.

birdlike facies (Neuro)—refers to a "pinched" facial expression in which eyes are squinting and lips are slightly pursed.

bird's nest filter (BNF)—temporarily placed caval filter to treat a patient for phlegmasia cerulea dolens and limb-threatening ischemia due to sudden complete occlusion of thigh and iliac veins. Suitable and effective for short-term use during caval thrombolysis. See *Gianturco-Roehm bird's nest vena cava filter*.

Bird respirator—see also *BABYbird respirator*.

birdshot chorioretinopathy—autoimmune ophthalmologic disease of unknown cause, diagnosed by positive HLA-A29 titer. Also, *birdshot retinochoroidopathy*.

Birkhauser eye testing chart.

birth defect—see *congenital melanocytic nevi* (CMN); *encephalocraniocutaneous lipomatosis* (ECCL).

birthing ball—a physical therapy ball that can support up to 300 pounds. A woman in labor sits on the ball in a natural, comfortable, squatting-type position, which opens the pelvic outlet, supports pressure points, and helps gravity work with the woman's body to speed labor.

bisferious pulse (or biferious) (pulsus bisferiens, or biferiens)—a pulse with two beats, sometimes palpable in combined aortic stenosis and aortic regurgitation.

Bishop-Koop ileostomy—a procedure to decompress an intestinal graft, such as might be performed during complete intestinal transplantation.

bishop's nod—rhythmic nodding of the head, synchronous with the pulse, in aortic regurgitation. Cf. *de Musset sign.*

Bishop score of cervical ripening (Ob-Gyn)—a score for estimating the prospects for induction of labor in a primigravida. A score of less than or equal to 4 would be considered an unfavorable cervix. See *dinoprostone*.

Bismuth classification, types I-IV—a typing system for cholangiocarcinoma. Also *Bismuth-Corlette classification.*

BIS (Bispectral Index) **Sensor**—a one-piece sensor used to acquire the signals necessary to produce the Bispectral Index. Noninvasive, direct, quantitative measurement of the effects of anesthetics on the brain.

bite line—a horizontal line of whitened, thickened buccal mucosa caused by habitual biting or chewing of the surface.

bite sign—x-ray evidence of avascular necrosis. Gouged-out areas of bony destruction look similar to small animal bites, hence the name.

biventricular pacing—a therapy in which wires are implanted in both of the two lower chambers of the heart so that both sides of the heart are paced at the same time. This therapy is being evaluated for its use in the treatment of congestive heart failure. It affects more than 3 million people in the U.S.

Bivona TTS (tight-to-shaft) **tracheostomy tube**.

BJ (biceps jerk) (Neuro).

Bjerrum scotoma—further development of Seidel scotoma.

BJT (bilateral juxtafoveal telangiectasis).

BKS-1000 refractive set (Barraquer-Krumeich-Swinger)—used to section and reshape the cornea.

black cohosh—herbal remedy shown to be effective for menopausal symptoms, especially hot flashes.

black comets (Radiol)—artifacts on radiographs. Characteristic streaks resulting from dirty automatic film processor.

Black Creek Canal virus—identified in a single case of hantavirus pulmonary syndrome in southern Florida. The carrier is believed to be the cotton rat (*Sigmodon hispidus*).

Blackfan-Diamond syndrome—a rare hypoplastic anemia seen in infants and young children; caused by defective erythropoiesis and lack of adequate nucleated erythrocytes in the bone marrow, but with normal platelet and leukocyte counts. Also known as *Josephs-Diamond-Blackfan syndrome*.

black hairy tongue—discoloration and alteration of the surface texture of the tongue by fungal infection.

blackout—loss of consciousness; syncope.

black-patch delirium—hallucinations caused in some patients with both eyes patched.

Black spanner strut—a modular ossiculoplasty prosthesis, named for Dr. Bruce Black.

bladder blade—a protective surgical device used to isolate the bladder and protect it from injury during surgery in that region.

bladder cancer-specific nuclear matrix protein (BLCA-4).

bladder carcinoma classification—see *Jewett classification*.

bladder neck closure (BNC)—a salvage procedure sometimes performed in conjunction with continent urinary diversion procedures, when attempts at achieving outlet competence have repeatedly failed.

bladder neck support prosthesis—for control of urinary incontinence. The device is an elastic vaginal pessary with two prongs on one side of the ring that elevate the bladder neck against the pubic bone and facilitate pressure transmission around the bladder neck.

BladderScan—uses noninvasive ultrasound technology to rapidly reveal the amount of urine in a patient's bladder. The instrument's use in long-term care facilities may translate into fewer catheterizations and resulting infections for residents.

BladderScan BVI 2500—a portable transabdominal bladder ultrasound scanner.

Bladder Tumor assay—a method of monitoring urinary specimens. The test is said to be more sensitive than cytology in detecting low-grade carcinomas that may have insufficient cellular activity for cytologic identification.

blade or **knife**
- Acra-Cut Spiral craniotome
- Alcon crescent
- Alcon pocket
- arachnoid-shape
- ASSI disposable cranio blade
- banana
- Bard-Parker
- Beaver cataract knife
- Beaver DeBakey
- Beaver discission knife
- Beaver keratome
- Bennett self-retaining retractor

blade *(cont.)*
- bladder
- Curdy
- Dyonics disposable arthroscope
- Eschmann
- 5-prong rake
- Franceschetti-type freeblade
- Hebra
- K-Blade
- LaserSonics EndoBlade
- LaserSonics Nd-YAG Laserblade scalpels
- Merlin bendable
- MVR
- Paufique
- RAD40 sinus
- sickle-shape
- Superblade
- Swann-Morton surgical
- 3-prong rake
- Typhoon microdebrider

blade of grass sign (Radiol)—a V- or wedge-shaped radiolucent area, clearly demarcated from the adjacent bone, seen when involvement of the lytic phase of diaphyseal Paget disease is present in a long bone. Paget disease has three distinct phases visible radiographically: a lytic phase, a sclerotic phase, and a mixed lytic-sclerotic phase.

Blaivas classification of urinary incontinence.

Blake drains—flat, round, and hubless silicone nonclogging wound drains.

Blakeley classification—for classifying the degrees of muscular incoordination.

Blakemore-Sengstaken tube—a triple-lumen tube. It is useful in stopping hemorrhage from gastric and esophageal varices, to suction gastric contents, and in differentiating between bleeding from esophageal varices and other causes of upper gastrointestinal

Blakemore-Sengstaken *(cont.)* bleeding. This tube has a gastric balloon (always inflated), an esophageal balloon, and a gastric tip that permits suction.

Blalock-Taussig procedure (Cardio)—for blue baby syndrome.

Bland-Garland-White syndrome—see *ALCAPA syndrome.*

blastocoel (also spelled blastocoele)—the cavity in the blastula of the developing embryo.

blastocyst—a very early (preimplantation) embryo, consisting of 50-200 cells, produced by repeated cleavage of a zygote (fertilized oocyte). It is a roughly spherical structure consisting of an outer cell layer (the trophectoderm), which will develop into the fetal membranes and placenta; a fluid-filled cavity (the blastocoel); and a cluster of pluripotent cells (the inner cell mass), which will develop into the body of the fetus.

blastomere—a pluripotent cell of the inner cell mass of a blastocyst.

Blazer II XP cardiac ablation catheter—an ablation catheter to treat atrial flutter and tachycardia. Wires running inside a tube connect to an electrical system that allows a physician to view the heart's action on a viewing screen. This ablation catheter is also connected to a generator that delivers radiofrequency (RF) energy to the tip of the catheter in the heart. The RF energy generates heat that destroys abnormal heart tissue responsible for causing tachycardia. Also referred to as the *EPT-1000 XP cardiac ablation catheter*.

BLCA-4 (bladder cancer-specific nuclear matrix protein).

bleb, filtering (Oph).

Bledsoe brace—for knee and lower extremity fractures.

bleed (noun)—a hemorrhage, usually gastrointestinal. Intracranial bleeds are common in very premature infants. See *sentinel bleed.*

bleeding time—see *Duke; Ivy.*

blend current 2—a setting on an electrocoagulator.

blepharitis—inflammation of the eyelid margin.

Blessed Information Memory Concentration (IMC) **test**—a cognitive screening test used to evaluate patients with dementia and Alzheimer disease. Scores are given as the number of errors out of a possible 34. Also called *Blessed IMC test.*

blind esophageal brushing (BEB)—a method of diagnosing infectious esophageal disease in patients with AIDS. This technique protects the endoscopist from exposure to HIV better than the standard procedure of esophagogastroduodenoscopy.

blind headache—the old lay name for any headache preceded by ocular phenomena. May still appear in past histories, in the patient's words.

Blinkeze external lid weights—a treatment for lagophthalmos; the weights, made of tantalum, have adhesive backs and are placed on the upper lids.

BlisterFilm—transparent dressing.

Bloch, clear cells of.

Bloch equation—MRI term.

Block cardiac device.

Blom-Singer indwelling low pressure voice prosthesis—a prosthetic device used to improve esophageal speech in patients after laryngectomy. See also *Panje voice button.*

blood, artificial—see *artificial blood.*

bloodborne—referring to infections transmitted by blood transfusion, contaminated surgical or dental instruments, needles shared by intravenous drug abusers, or other means whereby blood is transferred from one person to another.

blood-brain barrier—barrier by which many substances that pass easily through vessel walls in other parts of the body are chemically prevented from passing through blood vessel walls into central nervous system tissue.

blood coagulation factors—see *coagulation factors, blood.*

blood flow enhancement (BFE) **device**—a compact wearable device for the localized enhancement of blood flow to the extremities. Electrical signals induce a directional wavelike contraction of the underlying muscle tissue that significantly improves the supply of blood to the extremities.

blood flow
high shear
superior mesenteric artery

Bloodgood syndrome—see *fibrocystic breast syndrome.*

blood glucose (bG).

blood oxygenation level-dependent (BOLD) **response**—a change in the MRI signal of the brain that reflects variations in the oxygen saturation of cerebral capillary and venous blood. An increased signal indicates a rise of saturated (oxygenated) hemoglobin, paralleling increased neural activity. A reduction in signal indicates a rise in reduced (deoxygenated) hemoglobin. Such a change may result from either a relative increase in cerebral metabolism or a relative decrease in cerebral blood flow, and is thought to reflect inhibition or suppression of neuronal firing patterns. These effects are detected with a T2-weighted imaging protocol.

blood patch—a method of stopping postspinal tap headaches. The patient's own blood is injected into the epidural space and seals the hole in the dura made by the spinal tap needle. This prevents leakage of cerebrospinal fluid, the cause of the headache pain, also called *postspinal headache.*

blood perfusion monitor (BPM)—incorporates laser and fiberoptic technology to provide continuous tissue perfusion data. See *Laserflo.*

blood pool—the circulating blood, into which radionuclides are injected for various types of circulatory scans.

blood pressure—see *zero diastolic blood pressure.*

Blood Shield—a device that attaches easily to the tip of a conventional suction catheter to limit the degree of splash which occurs during vascular graft flushing, and to increase the efficiency of a standard suction tip in collecting shed blood for autotransfusion.

blood-type diet—controversial food plan based on a person's blood type. It postulates that an individual's digestive and immune systems are influenced by blood type (A, B, AB, O), and that optimal nutrition and weight control can be achieved by selecting foods that have been categorized as beneficial for a particular blood type.

blooming artifacts—occurs in ultrasonography when a bolus injection of contrast agent is used.

Bloom syndrome—a genetically transmitted syndrome whose manifesta-

Bloom *(cont.)*
tions are short stature, sun-sensitive facial erythematous lesions, and susceptibility to diarrhea and respiratory infections with a compromised immune system. Individuals with this condition have a striking predisposition to develop various neoplasms at an early age.

blot test—see *Western blot electrotransfer test.*

blow-by oxygen—a tube with humidified flowing oxygen is positioned near the patient's nose and allowed to blow by. FiO_2 (forced inspiratory oxygen) is not precise.

blow-in fracture.

blown pupil—slang for a dilated pupil unresponsive to light in a brain-damaged patient.

blow-out fracture—a result of blunt impact to the orbit. It usually involves the floor of the orbit.

Blue Angel syndrome—a pathological infatuation in which partners in a relationship sacrifice themselves and their own best interests.

blue bloater—a patient with severe respiratory failure, showing dyspnea, cyanosis, and peripheral edema due to right ventricular failure. Cf. *pink puffer.*

blue diaper syndrome—tryptophan malabsorption.

blue-dot sign—when, in testicular torsion, the infarcted appendix epididymidis can be seen through the scrotal skin.

Blue FlexTip catheter—a cardiac catheter with a special blue flexible tip to decrease the risk of vessel perforation.

Bluemax BM500—see *ALS Bluemax BM500.*

Bluemyst aerosol spray—device used for pulmonary delivery of drugs.

blue rubber-bleb nevus syndrome.

blue toe syndrome—multiple emboli of atheromatous material in small arteries, causing cyanosis and pain in the toes.

blue velvet syndrome—feelings of euphoria, excitement, or depression, following repeated intravenous injections of strong analgesics with talcum filler. Signs include apical thrust, tachycardia, systolic murmur, pulmonary rales, hepatomegaly, ankle edema.

blue "whale tail" of the Octopus stabilizer—a term used in beating heart surgery in which the Octopus tissue stabilizer is slowly tightened and the heart allowed to beat for approximately four cardiac cycles prior to the final tightening of the blue "whale tail" to eliminate any compression and then lock the arm/stabilizer in place.

Blumberg sign—rebound tenderness over the site of a suspected abdominal lesion, a sign of possible peritonitis.

Blumenthal irrigating cystitome—used during cataract surgery.

Blumer shelf—in anorectum.

Blumgart technique—for hepaticojejunostomy.

blunt dissection (also, *blunt finger dissection* and *finger dissection*)—separating tissues with the fingers or a sponge.

blunted costophrenic angle—on chest x-ray, a costophrenic angle that is flattened or distorted by scarring or pleural fluid.

Bluntport disposable trocar—used in minimally invasive surgeries, such as laparoscopy.

BLU-U—blue light photodynamic therapy (PDT) illuminator used in the Levulan PDT System for treatment of nonhyperkeratotic actinic keratoses of the face or scalp.

B-lymphocyte—see *B-cell.*

Blythe uvulopalatoplasty—performed with standard electrocautery.

BM (bone marrow).

BMD (bone mineral density).

BMI (body mass index).

B-mode—see *B-scan.*

B-mode acquisition and targeting (BAT, BMAT)—radiation therapy technique that uses sonar to identify the exact location of treatment. Used to treat prostate cancer.

BMP (basic metabolic panel)—a group of 8 tests that usually includes glucose, calcium, sodium, potassium, carbon dioxide (CO_2, bicarbonate), chloride, BUN, and creatinine. *Not* BNP (brain natriuretic peptide).

BMP (bone morphogenic protein).

BMP cable system—used for trochanteric reattachment, fracture fixation, and cerclage cabling.

BMT (bone marrow transplantation).

BMX mouthwash—Benadryl, Maalox, Xylocaine.

BNC (bladder neck closure).

BNCT (boron neutron capture therapy).

BNF (bird's nest filter).

BNMSE (Brief Neuropsychological Mental Status Examination).

BNOE (benign necrotizing otitis externa).

BNP (brain natriuretic peptide). *Not* BMP (basic metabolic panel).

Boas sign (also **point, test**)—tender area to the left of the twelfth thoracic vertebra. May be mentioned in workups for gallbladder disease and is indicative not of cholecystitis or cholelithiasis but gastric ulcer. Do not confuse with *psoas.*

boat hook—a combination of a Sinskey hook and an iris hook. The boat hook is used to manipulate an intraocular lens. It is so named because it is similar in shape (a C curve going in one direction with a straight short tip going in the opposite direction) to boating hooks used by sailors.

bobby pin-like configuration—complication of retrograde balloon cautery endopyelotomy in which the electrocautery wire breaks inside the body after firing. To effect atraumatic removal of the wire, the catheter is twisted and the wire is wrapped around the tip.

Bochdalek hernia—congenital hernia through a hiatus in the posterolateral part of the diaphragm because of the persistence of the pleuroperitoneal canal in an infant.

Bodansky unit—unit of measurement of alkaline phosphatase. Very high levels (over 100 Bodansky units) are seen in primary biliary cirrhosis. Alcoholic liver disease, cholestatic hepatitis, and drug-induced cholestasis also produce high alkaline phosphatase levels. Also, *King-Armstrong* and *Bessey-Lowry* measurements of alkaline phosphatase.

body
Auer
Barr
Councilman
creola
cytomegalic inclusion
cytoplasmic inclusion
Gamna-Gandy
Heinz
Hirano
inclusion
Lafora inclusion
Lewy inclusion
lyssa inclusion

body *(cont.)*
Negri inclusion
Pick inclusion
psammoma
vitreous
X-body

body box—an airtight chamber with clear doors where one sits to have lung volumes measured. Breathing is accomplished through a mouthpiece.

body dysmorphic disorder (BDD).

body floss technique—a method of straightening a tortuous iliac artery during an intravascular procedure. A guidewire is placed in the aorta with one end emerging from a brachial artery access incision and the other from a femoral artery incision. Gripping one end of the wire with each hand, the operator uses a series of push-pull maneuvers (similar to those used in flossing teeth) to provide a straight channel for catheter manipulation.

Body Glue—an autologous gluelike gel used in plastic surgery. A small amount of the patient's blood is drawn and processed to release human growth factors, resulting in a glue-like substance that is applied to the surgical area. This reportedly promotes faster, more efficient healing.

body mass index (BMI)—a ratio between weight and height (weight divided by height x 705). The BMI is considered a more objective assessment of relative fitness and in determining obesity:

18.5 - 24.9	acceptable range
25 - 29.9	overweight
30 - 34.9	obese
35 - 39.9	severe obesity
40 - 49.9	morbid obesity
50 and above	supermorbid obesity

body of Luys (subthalamic nucleus)—an important "way-station" in the extrapyramidal system. Also called *corpus Luysii* and *nucleus of Luys.*

body surface area (BSA)—calculations by various methods from height and weight for infants, small children, and adults. The BSA is preferred over simple weight to compute the ideal dosages of certain drugs, as well as for determining fluid, electrolyte, and caloric needs of infants and small children. The West nomogram is widely used to calculate BSA.

body surface Laplacian mapping (BSLM)—noninvasive way to map out the heart's electrical activity in patients with arrhythmias. This technique utilizes Laplacian electrodes to translate the three-dimensional heart into a two-dimensional picture.

Boehler angle (or Böhler)—radiologic view of the two superior surfaces of the calcaneus.

Boerema hernia repair—used to repair type 2 paraesophageal hernia, often followed by gastropexy to prevent volvulus following the repair.

Boerhaave syndrome—a spontaneous rupture of the esophagus.

boggy uterus—undesirable soft, spongy uterus felt on abdominal palpation following delivery, rather than firm uterus which is needed to stop hemorrhaging.

Böhler angle—see *Boehler angle.*

Bohlman triple-wire technique—posterior cervical fusion for stabilization of cervical spine fracture.

BOLD (blood-oxygenation level-dependent) **response**—term in MR imaging of the kidney. See *blood oxygenation level-dependent response*. Also *BOLD effect, BOLD signal, BOLD contrast enhancement*.

Boltzmann distribution—MRI term.

bolus—a single dose of a drug given intravenously over a few minutes, usually by the I.V. push method. A bolus produces immediate therapeutic levels of the drug and is used in emergency situations. See also *chase bolus; I.V. push.*

bolus chase—see *chase bolus.*

bolus-chase technique—used in angiography and MRI scan.

bombé—curved or swelling outward.

bombesin—a polypeptide found in mammalian and amphibian tissues. High levels occur in human brain and intestine; elevation of serum levels is noted in certain pulmonary and thyroid malignancies. Persistent elevation after radiotherapy for small-cell lung cancer is an unfavorable prognostic sign.

Bonaccolto utility and splinter forceps—for ophthalmology use.

Bondek absorbable sutures.

bone age according to Greulich and Pyle (Radiol).

bone and limb growth velocity ratios (Ortho, Ped).

bone bruise sign—diagnostic of anterior cruciate ligament tear on magnetic resonance imaging.

Bone Bullet suture anchor—used to attach soft tissue to bone in hallux valgus repair, midfoot reconstruction, scapholunate ligament reconstruction, ulnar or radial collateral ligament reconstruction, PIP joint ligament reconstruction, and profundus tendon reattachment.

bone cement—see *adhesive.*

bone conduction (ENT)—refers to the transmission of sound through the bones of the skull to the cochlea and auditory nerve. Bone conduction is tested by holding an activated tuning fork against the mastoid bone. Normally the sound is heard twice as long by air conduction as by bone conduction. See *Weber test, air conduction, Rinne test.*

bone-cutting forceps.

bone density measurements—a study performed with amorphous silicon filmless x-ray technology.

bone in bone sign—abnormal finding on lumbar spine x-rays, in which a vertebra appears to enfold a small replica of itself. This is a characteristic finding seen in osteopetrosis.

Bone-Lok—device for the surgical reconstruction and fixation of small bones.

bone marrow edema pattern on MR imaging—seen in an epiphysis and may indicate posttraumatic or stress fractures, osteonecrosis, transient osteoporosis, reactive changes underlying degenerative articular disease, and a self-resolving condition referred to as *transient bone marrow edema syndrome.*

bone marrow stromal cell—any stem cell found in bone marrow that is not involved in hematopoiesis (blood cell formation). These are mesenchymal stem cells, some of which can differentiate into specialized connective tissue cells such as bone, cartilage, and fat.

bone marrow transplantation (BMT).

bone mineral density (BMD)—new application as a predictor of breast cancer in older women. Ironically, the higher the bone mineral density and the smaller the risk for osteoporosis, the greater the risk of advanced breast cancer. BMD itself is not the cause of breast cancer but a marker for hormone levels. Women are advised not to discontinue their

bone *(cont.)* efforts to maintain bone mass through diet or medication.

bone morphogenetic protein—a protein involved in the formation of bone and cartilage. Bone morphogenetic protein 2 (BMP2) belongs to a superfamily called transforming growth factor beta (TGF-beta). BMP2 is an indication of osteoporosis risk.

bone paste (skeletal repair system)—injectable biomaterial that may soon replace the painful pins and screws and casts used to hold fractures in place while healing. The material hardens in 15 minutes. As the fracture heals, the hardened biomaterial is replaced by living bone.

bone-patellar tendon-bone (BPTB) **graft**.

BonePlast—bone void filler; biocompatible plaster-of-paris-based material that resorbs and is replaced with bone during the healing process.

bone replacement material—see *graft*.

bone scan—see *TSPP rectilinear bone scan*.

bone surface lesions—may be endosteal, intracortical, paracortical, parosteal (juxtacortical), periosteal, or subperiosteal.

bone wax—a sticky material prepared from beeswax and used to control bleeding on bony surfaces.

bone window—CT setting which optimizes the visualization of osseous structures. See *brain window, pulmonary parenchymal window, soft tissue window, subdural window.*

Bonney test—used for diagnosis of stress incontinence. It produces continence by restoring the anterior vaginal wall hammock. See *Miyazaki-Bonney test*.

bony island (Radiol)—benign developmental abnormality consisting of a localized zone of increased density in a long bone.

Bookler swivel-ball laparoscopic instrument holder—features a clamp tip for holding instruments such as trocars and graspers.

Bookwalter retractor system—a metal circular frame on a post to which many retractors are clamped to expose the surgical field from all directions. Used in colorectal, vaginal, and small-incision surgery. Note on spelling: There is no *Buckwalter* or *Buchwalter retractor*.

BOOP (bronchiolitis obliterans with organizing pneumonia).

Boorman gastric cancer typing system (types 1-4):
1 polypoid carcinoma
2 ulcerocancer
3 ulcerating and infiltrating carcinoma
4 diffusely infiltrating carcinoma

boots—see *Zzooties*.

Booth wire osteotomy.

Bordetella—genus of small gram-negative coccobacilli, or rods, of the family *Brucellaceae,* formerly *Haemophilus*. The organism causing whooping cough is *B. pertussis* (formerly *Haemophilus pertussis)*.

Bores radial marker—used in refractive eye surgery.

Bornholm disease (also called "devil's grip")—caused by coxsackievirus.

boron neutron capture therapy (BNCT)—for treatment of brain tumors. Patients are injected with a nontoxic boron compound that accumulates in the brain. A beam of low-energy neutrons is then fired at the tumor area, reacting with the compound to produce cancer-killing

boron *(cont.)*
nuclear particles. It is reportedly far less traumatic than current treatments and has fewer side effects. Currently the treatment is only available at nuclear reactor sites, where the beams can be safely generated.

Borrelia burgdorferi—tick-borne spirochete that causes Lyme disease.

bortezomid—see *Velcade*.

Bosker TMI system—a transmandibular implant (TMI) for cosmetic reconstruction of the mandible or to treat fractures caused by accident or radiation therapy. Mandibular fixation device using an osseointegrated rigid box-frame structure which can induce bone growth in the mandible.

Bosker transmandibular reconstructive surgical system—a procedure (named for a reconstructive maxillofacial surgeon) utilizing a transmandibular approach.

boss (noun), **bosselated** (adj.)—a rounded eminence, as on the surface of a bone or tumor; for example, bosselated surface.

Boston Scleral Lens—a contact lens that covers the entire sclera, restoring sight to the blind and visually impaired due to certain corneal or ocular surface diseases.

Bosworth procedure—repair of acromioclavicular separation, using screw fixation of the clavicle to the coracoid.

bother score—see *International Prostate Symptom Score.*

bouche de tapir ("boosh duh tahpeer") (Fr., tapir's mouth)—elongation of the face, so that it resembles that of a tapir, caused by extreme weakness of the muscles about the mouth.

Bouin solution—a fixative for gastrointestinal biopsy specimens (and other tissue specimens).

bounce home sign (or **test**)—to differentiate between meniscal tear and joint effusion. The patient assumes the supine position and relaxes the muscles around the knee. The examiner places one or both hands on the heel of the patient's foot and passively flexes the knee to about 15°. While ensuring that the musculature is still relaxed, the knee is passively extended (the bounce home) while examiner palpates the end-feel. A rubbery end-feel indicates meniscal tear; a mushy end-feel indicates joint effusion.

Bourns-Bear ventilator—volume-cycled ventilator that delivers a pre-set volume of air.

Boutin thoracoscope.

boutonnière deformity of the finger.

bovied (lowercase)—verb form denoting the use of the Bovie electrocautery.

Bovie ultrasound aspirator.

bovine heterograft—see *graft.*

bovine lavage extract surfactant—see *surfactant, heterologous.*

bovine pericardium strips—used to seal air leaks during surgical stapling of emphysematous lung tissue in lung volume reduction surgery. See *Peri-Strips.*

bovine spongiform encephalopathy (BSE)—also known as "mad cow disease." This malady causes progressive degeneration of brain tissue and produces symptoms of agitation, clumsiness, and eventual death in cows. It is believed that this disease can be spread to humans by ingesting meat from infected animals. BSE causes symptoms strikingly similar to the human brain infection called Creutzfeldt-Jakob disease.

Bowen Hutterite syndrome—a very rare disorder inherited as an auto-

Bowen *(cont.)*
somal recessive genetic trait. Major symptoms may include low birth weight, microcephaly, a prominent nose, an underdeveloped jaw, rockerbottom feet, and failure to thrive.

Bowen wire tightener—tightens stainless steel wires and breaks them at precisely the proper length. Also, Bowen wire cutters and wire holders.

Bowman layer of the cornea (Oph).

bow tie procedure—see *Alfieri mitral valve procedure.*

bow-tie repair—another name for *Alfieri-plasty*.

bow-tie sign—an abnormality seen on x-ray which is associated with a cervical facet fracture. The body and facet of the cervical vertebra rotate and overlap, causing a shadow in the shape of a bow tie to appear.

boxcarring (Oph)—segmentation of blood in retinal vessels; a sign of death.

boxer's fracture—caused by striking close-fisted hand on hard object, as in boxing. Usage: "Preliminary interpretation of x-rays of the left hand is of a boxer's-type fracture of the distal aspect of the second metacarpal."

boxer's knuckle—injury of the extensor hood with extensor tendon subluxation.

boxer's nose—a nasal deformity (usually from a fracture) that looks like that which boxers often acquire in their occupation.

Boyle uterine elevator—used to retract the uterus during hysterectomy. Replaces standard self-retaining retractors and bowel packing. Consists of a long rod with a cervical cup on one end. Advantages are that a small abdominal incision can be used, and less manipulation of abdominal contents helps to avoid postoperative catheterization and decreases total hospital length of stay.

Boynton needle holder.

bp (base pair).

BPA (burst-promoting activity).

BPAG1 (BP antigen 1, the 230 kD BP antigen) and **BPAG2** (BP antigen 2, the 180 kD BP antigen)—protein markers for bullous pemphigoid.

BPD (biparietal diameter) (Ob-Gyn).

BPD (bronchopulmonary dysplasia).

BPI (bactericidal/permeability-increasing) **protein**—a human host-defense protein that kills bacteria, neutralizes endotoxins, and inhibits neovascularization. Used to develop new antifungal agents.

BPM (bioabsorbable polymeric material)—a new embolic agent incorporated into Guglielmi detachable coils, used in treating aneurysms.

BPM (blood perfusion monitor).

BPPV (benign paroxysmal positional vertigo).

BPTB (bone-patellar tendon-bone) graft—a technique used in anterior cruciate ligament reconstruction.

BPTI (brachial plexus traction injury) **syndrome**.

BPTT (brachial plexus tension test).

Bq (becquerel).

BRACAnalysis—comprehensive gene test used to detect hereditary breast and ovarian cancer. The BRCA1 and BRCA2 gene mutations are believed to be responsible for 90 percent of early-onset hereditary breast and ovarian cancers.

brace (see also *braces for children* and *orthosis)*
Aircast Swivel-Strap

brace *(cont.)*
Bledsoe
Breg
Cast Boot hip abduction
chair-back
clamshell
CRS (counter rotation system)
Cruiser hip abduction
C.Ti.2
dial-in, block-lock knee
DonJoy GoldPoint knee
DonJoy IROM
49er knee
Friedman Splint
gait lock splint (GLS)
Galveston metacarpal
Jewett
Ilfeld-type abduction
Kallassy ankle
Kicker Pavlik harness
Liberty CMC thumb
KS 5 ACL
Kydex
Lenox Hill
LSU reciprocation-gait orthosis
Moon Boot
Newport MC hip orthosis
Nextep knee
OS-5/Plus 2 knee
Palumbo knee
PMT halo system
postoperative flexor tendon traction
Rhino Triangle
Rolyan tibial fracture
Seton hip
SmartBrace
SmartWrap elbow
Swede-O-Universal
Swivel-Strap
TLSO (thoracolumbosacral)
Townsend knee
UBC (Univ. of British Columbia)
Ultrabrace
Wheaton Pavlik harness

braces artifact (Radiol)—orthodontic hardware degrading image quality on CT and MRI studies of the neck and posterior fossa structures.

braces for children—polypropylene hip abduction brace for treating hip dysplasia in toddlers up to 2 1/2 years of age. The following are trademarks:
Cast Boot
Cruiser hip abduction
Friedman Splint
Kicker Pavlik harness
Rhino Triangle

brachial—refers to the arm, as in brachial plexus, a network of nerves located partly in the neck and partly in the axilla. Cf. *branchial, bronchial.*

brachial neuritis—a condition characterized by acute onset of severe pain in the shoulder followed by muscle weakness and gradual recovery. Diagnosed by electromyography. Also known as *Parsonage-Turner syndrome.*

brachial plexus tension test (BPTT)—aids in differentiating between local arm conditions causing pain, and cervical/brachial plexus conditions with pain referral into the arm.

brachioaxillary bridge graft fistula (BAGF)—used for patients on chronic hemodialysis when sites for direct arteriovenous anastomosis are no longer usable.

brachioplasty—surgical procedure for patients with batwing arms. The hanging skin of the upper inner arm is excised, but the procedure is effective only for patients with extra skin, not extra fat.

brachioradialis transfer—Ober-Barr procedure for weakness of the triceps muscle.

brachiosubclavian bridge graft fistula (BSGF)—used for patients on chronic hemodialysis when sites for direct arteriovenous anastomosis are no longer usable.

BrachySeed—iodine ^{125}I drug for treatment of prostate cancer.

BrachySeed Pd-103—a palladium-103 brachytherapy implant for the treatment of prostate cancer and other selected localized tumors of the head, neck, lung, pancreas, breast, and uterus.

brachytherapy—interstitial implantation of radioactive isotopes, permitting the localized delivery of high doses of radiation to a tumor mass.
afterloading brachytherapy
balloon
BrachySeed Pd-103
Checkmate intravascular
episcleral plaque
high-dose-rate (HDR)
intraluminal
intravascular
IOHDR (intraoperative high-dose-rate)
I-Plant brachytherapy seeds
low-dose radiation (LDR) seed
Novoste Beta-Cath system
permanent
remote afterloading (RAB)
Syed template interstitial gynecologic
Symmetra I-125 brachytherapy seeds
Ultraseed
vascular

Brackmann facial nerve monitor.

Brackmann II EMG system—used in complex cranial motor nerve monitoring.

Braden score—measures potential for alteration of skin integrity in bedridden patients.

bradyarrhythmia—a disturbance in the heart rhythm, resulting in a slow, irregular heartbeat.

bradykinin—endogenous peptide that causes vasodilation, induces contraction of smooth muscle, and induces hypotension.

bradyphemic (Neuro)—afflicted with slow speech.

bradyrhythm—incorrect dictation for *bradyrhythmia*.

Bragg peak (Radiol, Neuro)—photon beam therapy.

Brailler—see *Perkins Brailler*.

brain attack—a concept developed to educate the public on the warning signs of stroke, transient ischemic attacks, and amaurosis fugax.

brain-computer interfaces (BCI)—a technology that may allow people completely paralyzed by neurodegenerative diseases to regain some movement or ability to communicate with those around them.

brain-controlled devices—devices that may enable paraplegics to use their limbs and enhance amputees' control of prostheses.

brain death—irreversible coma.

brain death syndrome—state in which brain function, including autonomic control, is totally and permanently absent. See *Harvard Criteria for Brain Death*.

brain-derived neurotrophic factor (BDNF).

brain electrical activity map (BEAM).

brain or **intraventricular temperature monitoring**—difficult to monitor as there are no commercially available devices yet for measuring brain temperature.

brain natriuretic peptide (BNP)—a test used to determine if dyspnea is due to heart failure or from pul-

brain *(cont.)*
monary disease. BNP rises when heart failure is present or gets worse and drops when heart failure is successfully treated. Also *B-type brain natriuretic peptide. Not* BMP (basic metabolic panel).

brain plasticity—the phenomenon that allows remodeling of detailed connections in the brain during learning and underlies the progressive development of behavioral skills and abilities. Researchers are investigating the use of electrical stimulation of the nucleus basalis to magnify and accelerate plasticity changes involved in stroke recovery.

brain sand—see *sand, brain.*

brain stem—two words traditionally, both as a noun and an adjective, but it is frequently found in the literature as one word.

brain stem auditory evoked potential (BAEP).

brain stem auditory evoked response (BAER).

brain tests, noninvasive
- BAEP—brain stem auditory evoked potential
- BAER—brain stem auditory evoked response
- EP—evoked potential
- ER—evoked response
- MEP—multimodality evoked potential (a combination of visual, somatosensory, and brain stem auditory evoked potential)
- SEP—somatosensory evoked potential
- SER—somatosensory evoked response
- VEP—visual evoked potential
- VER—visual evoked response

brain window—CT setting which optimizes radiologic visualization of intracranial anatomy. See *bone window, pulmonary parenchymal window, soft tissue window, subdural window.*

branched calculus (Radiol)—staghorn calculus.

branched chain DNA assay—uses a series of DNA probes to capture, target, and amplify viral RNA in a specimen. Cf. *polymerase chain reaction.*

branchial arches, cleft—pertaining to gill-like structures in embryo that become modified into structures in the ear and neck. Cf. *brachial, bronchial.*

branchio-oto-renal (BOR) **syndrome**—rare, autosomal dominant genetic disorder involving branchial cleft and renal anomalies, hearing loss, and other otologic manifestations.

branch point plaque—an atherosclerotic plaque that develops at the juncture between a major coronary artery and a smaller branch vessel.

branch retinal vein occlusion—said to be second only to diabetic retinopathy as the most common form of retinal vascular disease.

Brandt cytology balloon—used for esophageal brushing to diagnose fungal esophagitis and esophageal cytomegalovirus in AIDS patients.

Brandt-Daroff exercises—a method of treating benign paroxysmal positional vertigo.

Branemark endosteal implants (ENT).

Branham sign—compression over an arteriovenous fistula causing slowing of the pulse, which gives a positive sign. Also called *Nicoladoni-Branham sign.*

Branhamella catarrhalis (new genus—formerly *Neisseria).*

Brantigan interbody fusion cage.

brash—burning sensation in the stomach. Cf. *water brash.*

BRAT diet—for children who, after having been on intravenous fluids, are started on *bananas, rice cereal, applesauce*, and *toast*.

Braun enteroenterostomy. Also *Braun anastomosis.*

Brava breast enhancement device—a nonsurgical breast enhancing and shaping system that uses tension-induced tissue growth to enlarge breasts.

Bravo pH monitoring system—a device used to measure esophageal pH to aid in the diagnosis of gastroesophageal reflux disease (GERD).

brawny edema—a chronic swelling in which deposition of connective tissue fibers in edema fluid has caused induration. Also called *tough edema* or *brawny induration.*

Braxton Hicks contractions—sometimes called *false labor*. Light, irregular contractions, usually painless; may become more intense, frequent, and regular later in pregnancy.

BRCA1, BRCA2 (breast cancer one and two)—oncogenes thought to act as a tumor suppressor in breast cancer. An estimated 85% of women who inherit a defective copy of BRCA2 will develop breast cancer during their lifetime, as compared to 10% of women in the general population.

BreakAway absorptive wound dressing.

breakthrough syndrome, normal perfusion pressure (in giant arteriovenous malformations).

BreastAlert—differential temperature sensor (DTS) screening device for early detection of breast disease.

breast bolster—device that helps to increase tissue depth of the breast during fine needle biopsy. It is most effective in moderately large breasts that are flaccid and easily compress to a thin tissue depth.

Breast Cancer System 2100—a system that uses thermal imaging to help differentiate between benign and malignant breast lesions.

BreastCheck—a handheld electronic device for breast self-examination. It uses miniature pressure sensors which are glided over the breast, gently "palpating" in a manner similar to the human hand.

breast-conserving therapy (BCT)—breast cancer treatment limited to lumpectomy, axillary dissection, and radiation therapy.

BreastExam—used by physicians for breast cancer detection. See *Breast-Check.*

breast fibrocystic disease, stages of:
- mazoplasia—in patients in late teens and early 20s
- adenosis—early 30s and 40s
- cystic disease—late 30s through 40s and early 50s

breast imaging and reporting data system of the American College of Radiology (BI-RADS).

breast imaging technique—see *digital tomosynthesis.*

breast reconstruction donor sites for autogenous tissue—transverse rectus abdominis myocutaneous flap, latissimus dorsi, gluteal free flap, lateral transverse thigh flap or "saddle bags," and Rubens flap, a modification of the deep circumflex iliac artery iliac crest flap. See *Rubens flap.*

breast reconstruction pattern—see *fleur de lis pattern.*

breast reduction technique—a short-scar procedure that uses the inferior pedicle (tissue situated on the bottom part of the breast) to give consistent, controllable results over breast shape. By retaining fat and parenchyma (the main tissue of the breast) centrally beneath the nipple and areola, direct contouring of the breast with consistent control over shape becomes possible. Very little reliance is placed on postoperative settling, with essentially no bottoming out.

Breathe-Easy nasal splint—postoperative nasal splint to aid in septal stabilization.

Breathe Right nasal strips—temporary treatment for nasal congestion, including a version with Vicks mentholated vapors.

breath excretion test
breath hydrogen excretion
breath pentane
^{14}C-cholylglycine breath excretion
^{14}C-urea breath excretion
Helicobacter pylori breath excretion

breath-hold MR cholangiography in adults and children vs. **non-breath-hold** studies in infants.

breath hydrogen excretion test—serves two functions: (1) a screening test in premature infants to detect necrotizing enterocolitis; (2) a reliable indicator of lactose intolerance at high levels of concentration; not reliable at lower concentration levels. See also *breath excretion test* entries.

breath pentane—an indicator of heart transplant rejection. Measurement of breath pentane via gas chromatography is considered a marker for cardiac transplant (allograft) rejection. Previously found to correlate closely with the severity of an inflammatory process, breath pentane may replace expensive and hazardous fluoroscopic or echocardiograph-guided bioptome biopsies of the transplanted heart. See also *breath excretion test* entries.

Brecher and Cronkite technique—for platelet counting.

Breg bracing products—for postoperative orthopedic conditions.

Breisky-Navratil retractor (Ob-Gyn) —used in sacrospinous ligament fixation. Also, Navratil retractor.

Bremer AirFlo Vest—for thoracic stabilization. Can be used in CT and MRI scanning, where movement causes artifact.

Bremer Halo Crown system—for cervical traction and stabilization. Can be used in CT and MRI scanning.

bremsstrahlung photon—one of the numerous ways electrons interact with matter.

Brent pressure earring—used for treating earlobe keloids.

Brescia-Cimino AV fistula—arteriovenous fistula, used as hemodialysis access.

Breslow classification system—pathologic classification of melanoma.

Bretschneider-HTK cardioplegic solution.

Brett syndrome (also *Janus syndrome*) —used to indicate an occasional radiologic finding of a clear lung on one side and opaque shadow on the other side. This aspect is observed in Fallot tetralogy with atresia of a branch of pulmonary artery or in truncus arteriosus with solitary pulmonary artery.

Breuerton view—a special x-ray view of the hand, to permit visualization of early changes of the joints from rheumatoid arthritis.

Brevibacterium linens.

Brevi-Kath epidural catheter—spring-guide catheter used for the administration of local anesthetics into the epidural space for pain management.

Brewster retractor—used in gynecologic surgery.

Bricker ureteroileostomy.

Bridge Assurant—a biliary stent delivery system.

Bridge extra support over-the-wire renal stent system—a metal mesh tube (stent) and a delivery system, used to hold open the renal artery when it is blocked by an atherosclerotic plaque. The delivery system is a guidewire and thin flexible tube (catheter) with a deflated balloon on the end. Using the delivery system, the physician inserts the stent through a small incision in a leg artery and threads it up to the narrowed or blocked renal artery. The expanded stent opens the artery so blood can flow more freely to the kidney. The stent is permanent and the artery lining will grow over it in about 8 weeks. The increased flow of blood to the kidney reduces the risk of kidney failure, high blood pressure, stroke and heart attack in patients who have narrowed or blocked renal arteries.

bridging osteophytes—osteophytes on adjacent vertebrae that meet and fuse, forming a "bridge" across the joint space.

bridle suture (*not* bridal)—used in eye surgery.

Brief Neuropsychological Mental Status Examination (BNMSE).

Brief Pain Inventory (BPI)—a self-report questionnaire that measures the impact of pain on mood, ability to work, interactions with people, sleep, and enjoyment of life.

bright signal—MRI term.

brim sign (Radiol)—in Paget disease, a thickened pelvic brim.

bris—the Jewish circumcision rite, from the Hebrew *berith*. Also, *briss*.

Bristow coracoid process transfer—for recurrent anterior dislocation of the shoulder. The procedure stabilizes the shoulder.

BriteSmile—teeth-whitening laser device.

brittle bone disease (osteogenesis imperfecta)—marked by a china-blue discoloration of the sclerae.

broach—an elongated, tapered, and serrated cutting tool for shaping and enlarging holes.

broad beta disease—hyperlipoproteinemia type 3, one of a group of inherited disorders of fat metabolism.

Broca motor speech area of the brain (Neuro).

Brockenbrough-Braunwald sign—spike-and-dome configuration of pressure gradient at cardiac catheterization in which the pulse pressure is unchanged or actually reduced following an extrasystolic beat. It is believed to reflect worsening of obstruction of the left ventricular outflow tract during the potentiated beat, with diminished stroke volume and aortic pulse pressure.

Brockenbrough cardiac device.

Brockenbrough needle—used in diagnostic cardiovascular procedures, such as with a Mullins sheath in transseptal catheterization.

Broders index (devised by A. C. Broders, an American pathologist)—a classification of the malignancy of tumors, based on the degree of differentiation, and therefore the aggressiveness, of the tumor; graded from 1 to 4, grade 1 representing the

Broders *(cont.)*
most differentiation and the best prognosis, and grade 4 the least differentiation and the poorest prognosis.

Brodie abscess—centrally placed radiographic lucency in the metaphysis adjacent to the growth plate, usually in adolescents and associated with subacute or chronic hematogenous osteomyelitis. Named for Benjamin Brodie in 1832.

Brolin antiobstruction stitch—a stitch used in stapled Roux-en-Y enteroenterostomy.

bromocriptine-dopamine agonist—drug that has been found to help stave off craving for alcohol in men who inherited the minor allele (A1) of the gene for the D2 dopamine receptor (DRD2). While no studies have included women, researchers believe this drug may help the 69% of alcoholics who have the A1 allele. More studies and easier identification tests are needed before widespread clinical use, but physicians may give alcoholics a trial of the drug without determining whether the patient has the inherited gene. Its effectiveness (or lack thereof) would be considered diagnostic.

bronchial solution (from the Brompton Hospital in London)—drug used for analgesia in terminal cancer patients. Contains cocaine, morphine sulfate, Compazine, ethyl alcohol, and syrup. Also, *Brompton mixture*.

bronchial—refers to the bronchi and bronchial tubes. Cf. *bronchiole, brachial, branchial.*

bronchial artery embolization—for treatment of bronchial bleeding and life-threatening hemoptysis.

bronchial dehiscence—disruption of the anastomosis secondary to airway ischemia in the watershed area in lung transplantation. These areas may heal spontaneously, require stenting or dilatation, or go on to bronchial stricture or rejection. See *watershed region.*

bronchial sleeve resection—procedure to treat centrally located lung cancer, while sparing distal parenchyma. It requires full mobilization of the hilum and dissection of the bronchi and vessels. Successful reconstruction involves frozen section analysis of regional lymph nodes and confirmation of free margins prior to bronchial anastomosis.

bronchial washings cytology.

bronchiole—one of the smaller branches into which the segmental bronchi divide. Cf. *bronchial.*

bronchiolitis obliterans—a term for signs of chronic rejection of a transplanted lung. Also called *progressive parenchymal restriction*. As the process continues, the radiologist sees the lungs decrease in size, the vascular markings decrease, and the interstitial markings increase.

bronchiolitis obliterans with organizing pneumonia (BOOP)—cryptogenic organizing pneumonia or proliferative bronchiolitis. Forms of this disease may be referred to as *idiopathic BOOP* and *BOOP reactions*. Cf. *obliterative bronchiolitis*.

bronchiolocentric—used in radiologic reports, as in "abnormalities are bronchiolocentric."

Bronchitrac L catheter—a flexible suction catheter designed specifically to reach the left lobe of the lung without having to twist the catheter or reposition the patient.

bronchoalveolar lavage (BAL).

Broncho-Cath—a double-lumen endobronchial tube.

bronchogram, tantalum—using powdered tantalum.

bronchopleuromediastinal fistulectomy—the excision of a fistula extending from a bronchus across the pleural cavity to the mediastinum.

bronchoprovocation testing—administration of an agent known to induce or aggravate bronchoconstriction.

bronchovisceral fistulectomy—the excision of a fistula between a bronchus and a nearby viscus, e.g., liver, pancreas, stomach.

bronze diabetes—diabetes with accompanying pancreatic damage. Also called *iron storage disease*.

bronze disease—Addison disease; called *bronze* because one of the symptoms of this hypofunction of the adrenal glands is a bronze or brownish color of the skin.

Brooke Army Hospital splint—used in tendon repair.

Brooke ileostomy.

Brooker classification—a system of classifying periarticular heterotopic ossification following total hip arthroplasty. It consists of grades 1 through 4, with grade 1 showing islands of bone in the periarticular soft tissues and grade 4 showing osseous ankylosis (complete bony fusion) of the hip.

Broselow tape or **chart**—used to determine a child's weight. It is part of trauma cart equipment.

Broström procedure—repair of ankle ligament injuries using direct suturing to reconstruct a ligament with available tissue and reimplant into the bone.

browlift—cosmetic surgery employing tiny incisions without hair removal and using laser-digital camera science.

Browlift BoneBridge system—an instrument allowing browlift suture fixation without implant.

Brown-Adson tissue forceps.

Brown-Brenn stain—a method of tissue staining for gram-positive organisms.

Brown dermatome—oscillating blade-type dermatome.

Browne—see *Denis Browne clubfoot splint*.

Brown-Hopps stain—a method of tissue staining for gram-negative organisms.

Brown-McHardy pneumatic dilator—used in treatment of dysphagia associated with achalasia. The unit of measure used in procedures with this dilator is p.s.i. ("sigh"), pounds per square inch.

Brown-Roberts-Wells (BRW) **stereotactic system**—consisting of an arc system, frame, stereotactic adapter used in performing stereotactic procedures on the brain.

brown sugar, or sugar, packing for wound. Usage: "The chest was then packed with brown sugar, a perforated interface drape was placed over the brown sugar, and a customized wound VAC sponge was inserted."

Brown tendon sheath syndrome—the superior oblique tendon is short, causing strabismus.

Brown two-portal technique—for endoscopic carpal tunnel release.

Bruce protocol—staging on cardiac treadmill test. Scored in mets—1 met equals 3.5 ml O_2/kg/min. There are six stages, I through VI.

Bruch membrane—glassy-appearing membrane of the choroid of the eye. (K.W.L. Bruch, Swiss anatomist.) Usage: "Vascularization was found of the inner part of Bruch membrane in the enucleated eye."

Brudzinski sign—a positive sign in meningitis. Bending a patient's neck (pressing the chin toward the sternum) produces flexion of the knees and hips.

Brueghel syndrome—see *Meige syndrome.*

Bruel-Kjaer transvaginal ultrasound probe.

Bruel-Kjaer ultrasound scanner—used in intracavitary prostate ultrasonography. Usage: "Incremental multiplane scanning of the prostate and seminal vesicles in real-time mode was performed using the Bruel-Kjaer ultrasound scanner, type 1846, and a 7 MHz 112° rectal multiplane transducer, type 8551."

Bruening syringe—for Teflon insertion into vocal cords.

Brugada syndrome—the occurrence of sudden cardiac death in the setting of the following electrocardiographic findings: right bundle branch block pattern with ST-segment elevation in the right precordial leads. The right bundle branch block may be incomplete while the ST-segment elevation is minimal. The ECG findings are not constant.

Bruhat maneuver—CO_2 laser surgery neosalpingostomy.

Bruininks-Oseretsky test of motor proficiency (Phys Ther).

bruit ("broo'ee") (pl., bruits)—a sound or murmur heard on vascular auscultation, especially an abnormal one. See *aneurysmal bruit*; *interscapulovertebral arterial bruit*.

brunescent—dark brown, as in brunescent cataract.

Bruno-Helfand physical therapy—combines whirlpool, electrical stimulation, foot and toe exercises, to improve circulation.

Bruns bone curette.

Bruser skin incision—in knee surgery.

Brushfield spots—frequently found on the iris of patients with Down syndrome.

brush marks (Oph)—lid margin vascular dilation.

brux, bruxism—to grind the teeth spasmodically. Usage: "She complained of a weak chin and malocclusion, and desired a normal bite and profile. She bruxes and clenches, but denied any TMJ (temporomandibular joint) pain or dysfunction."

BRW (Brown-Roberts-Wells) **CT stereotaxic guide**—may also be used with MRI and PET scan techniques.

Bryant traction—used on small children for the correction of congenital hip dislocation, or for stabilization of femur fractures. Overhead suspension is used, so that the hips are flexed to 90°.

BSA (body surface area)

B-scan (also called *B-mode)*—an ultrasound technique which permits visualization of structures by delineating echoes from these structures in various shades of gray. It can differentiate between the lumen of an artery and the arterial wall, to determine the thickness of the wall.

BSCVA (best spectacle-corrected visual acuity).

BSD-2000—uses hyperthermia to treat tumors deep in the body and precisely heat surface tumors by directing radiofrequency/microwave energy.

BSE—see *bovine spongiform encephalopathy.*

BSGF (brachiosubclavian bridge graft fistula).

BSS (balanced salt solution) (Oph).

BSS Plus—balanced salt solution with added bicarbonate, dextrose, and glutathione, used as a sterile intraocular irrigating solution. It is better than plain BSS in preserving the integrity of the corneal epithelium following surgery.

B strep—refers to group B streptococcus, a significant cause of meningitis.

B symptoms—fever, night sweats, weight loss, etc.; criteria for inclusion of the letter B in the staging of Hodgkin disease.

BTA (bladder tumor antigen, bladder tumor-associated antigen).

BTA stat test—rapid, single-step immunoassay of the urine to detect recurrent bladder cancer. The disposable test device contains two monoclonal antibodies that detect the presence of a newly identified human complement factor H-related protein (hCFHrp). The BTA stat test is said to be simpler and faster than urine cytology and is simpler than the original Bard BTA test.

BTA Trak assay—urine test for bladder tumor-associated antigen (BTA), a marker for transitional cell carcinoma of the bladder.

BTX-A (botulinum toxin, type A).

B-type brain natriuretic peptide (BNP)—see *brain natriuretic peptide.*

Bu antigen—a recently discovered antigen at the HLA-B locus.

bubble boy disease—see *pegademase bovine.*

bubble study (contrast echocardiography)—a technique where a substance containing "microbubbles" is rapidly injected into a peripheral vein or selectively into the heart. The passage of these microbubbles into the ultrasound beam generates many tiny echoes that temporarily opacify the blood pool being imaged. The microbubbles look like bright sparkles which move with the blood flow. Agitated saline solution, a mixture of saline and the patient's blood, indocyanine green dye and other substances can be used as echo-contrast material. Injection into a peripheral vein will opacify the right heart chambers and aid in detecting an intracardiac right-to-left shunt. These microbubbles do not pass through the lungs; therefore, visualization of intracardiac left-to-right shunts or mitral regurgitation requires echo contrast injection via selective left heart catheterization.

bubble ventriculography—used in diagnosing hydrocephalus.

buccal—pertaining to the cheek, as in "no buccal or posterior pharyngeal lesions." Cf. *buckle.*

buccal mucosa (*not* buckle)—the mucosa lining the inside of the cheek.

buccal smear—test used in X-chromosome determinations; made from cells scraped from the buccal mucosa, placed on a slide, and stained; demonstrates the Barr bodies (sex chromatin) seen in normal females.

"Buchwalter" or "Buckwalter"—misspellings for *Bookwalter retractor.*

bucket-handle pattern of fracture—seen in a metaphyseal lesion of the distal femur in abused infants.

bucket-handle tear of the knee meniscus.

Buck-Gramcko retractor.

buckle (Oph)—a surgical procedure for repair of retinal tears, as in scleral buckle. Cf. *buccal*.

Buck restrictor (Ortho).

Buck traction—used on the leg and in knee injuries. Also used as a temporary measure to help reduce muscle spasm, while the patient is awaiting surgical repair for fracture of the hip.

Budd-Chiari syndrome—acute parenchymatous jaundice. Related terms:
Budd disease
Budd jaundice
Chiari disease
Rokitansky disease
von Rokitansky disease

Budde halo retractor system (Neuro).

buddy splint—used in dislocation of fingers or toes; the dislocated digit is taped to an adjacent digit (its buddy), which acts as a splint.

Budin toe splint—treats overlapping toes and hammertoes.

Buechel-Pappas total ankle prosthesis—a 3-piece titanium and ultra-high-molecular-weight polyethylene prosthesis that can be used to restore a functioning ankle joint even in a patient with previous fusion.

Buerger Allen exercise (Phys Ther)—used to increase circulation.

Buerger disease—an inflammatory disease of the blood vessels which can lead to ischemia and gangrene. Cf. *Berger disease.*

buffalo hump—a zone of focal edema over the upper mid back, seen especially in Cushing syndrome and in prolonged adrenal steroid therapy.

buffy coat—layer of white blood cells found on centrifugation of anticoagulated blood between the plasma and the red cells. You may hear of a test being "buffy coat positive." See *buffy coat smear.*

buffy coat smear—used in diagnosis of lupus erythematosus, in determining the presence of certain protozoa and fungi in the peripheral blood, and for some bone marrow exams.

Buford complex—a normal anatomic variant distinguished by a cordlike middle glenohumeral ligament that originates directly from the superior labrum at the base of the biceps tendon and crosses the subscapularis tendon to insert on the humerus. This unusual-appearing anatomical variation may lead the surgeon to confuse this complex with a sublabral hole or a pathologic labral detachment.

Bugbee electrode.

bulbosity—the condition of being bulbous; used in describing a nasal tip in plastic surgery procedures.

bulimia nervosa—binge eating followed by self-induced vomiting or purging.

bulimorexia—an eating disorder including features of both *anorexia nervosa* (severe caloric restriction due to distortion of body image, with dangerous nutritional deficiency) and *bulimia nervosa* (binge eating followed by self-induced vomiting or purging).

Bullard intubating laryngoscope.

bull's eye lesion—a skin lesion consisting of concentric rings of erythema.

bunching suture.

bundle-nailing method of treating bone shaft fractures—a two-step method. It lacks the stability of Küntscher method but has the advantage that no bone-damaging boring of the medullary canal is needed.

bunionectomy
Joplin
Keller
Kreuscher
scarf osteotomy
tricorrectional
Wu

bunion last—used in management of hyperkeratotic lesions of the foot. See *last*.

bunionplasty—coined term for bunionectomy.

Bunnell
active hand and finger splints
finger extension splint
knuckle bender
tendon transfer

Bunny boot—orthopedic brace.

BUO (bilateral ureteral obstruction).

Burch colposuspension—for stress incontinence.

Burch iliopectineal ligament urethrovesical suspension.

burden (Genetics)—the total impact of a genetic disorder.

Burhenne steerable catheter with basket inserted.

buried bumper syndrome—a complication of gastrostomy tube placement whereby the tube migrates anteriorly to lie partially or completely outside the gastric wall, where it becomes embedded in the abdominal wall as the gastric site heals and reepithelializes behind it. The internal "bumper" of the gastrostomy tube burrows into the gastric mucosa and becomes permanently embedded. It must be freed surgically and a new gastrostomy tube inserted.

buried penis—an infrequent congenital penile deformity in which the penile shaft is buried below the surface of the prepubic skin because of an abnormally prominent suprapubic fat pad and dense fascial bands retracting and tethering the penis.

buried vaginal island—see *vaginal wall sling procedure.*

Bürker chamber for macrophage counting.

Burkitt lymphoma—one of the cancers to which AIDS patients are particularly susceptible.

burn diagram—see *Lund Browder.*

burning mouth syndrome (BMS)—characterized by chronic orofacial pain usually unaccompanied by mucosal lesions or other clinical signs. Several oral sites are usually affected (lips, palate, tongue). Symptoms include oral burning, dry mouth, thirst, dysgeusia, change in eating habits, irritability, and depression. Most commonly seen in postmenopausal women of Asian-American or American Indian heritage, and most often found in the western United States.

burning vulvar syndrome—see *vulvar vestibulitis syndrome.*

burns classification

first degree—erythema, involving only epidermis. Only superficial destruction of tissue and no blistering.

second degree—entire epidermis and some of the dermis involved. There are blisters, mottling of the surface, and pain. In deeper burns, hair follicles and sebaceous glands may be destroyed.

third degree—full thickness of skin injury.

fourth degree—extends to subcutaneous tissue, muscle, or bone. There may be charring.

Burow solution (*not* Burrow, but pronounced the same).

burst-forming unit-erythroid (BFU-E).

burst fracture—a type of spiral column injury, commonly caused by motorcycle or automobile accidents or falls from great heights, causing the vertebral body to explode or burst.

burst-promoting activity (BPA).

burst-suppression activity—a finding on an EEG.

BUS (Bartholin, urethral, Skene) **glands**.

Buselmeier shunt—a vascular access shunt, used in performing dialysis.

butoconazole nitrate—see *Gynazole-1*.

butterfly bandage.

butterfly diagram—a method of analyzing gait style.

butterfly drain—a soft tissue drain consisting of a butterfly needle connected to a Vacutainer; used after surgery.

butterfly effect—irregularities in the radiation cloud surrounding each (brachytherapy) seed.

butterfly flap—technique used in hand surgery for treatment of incomplete syndactyly.

butterfly needle—a fine-gauge needle with color-coded plastic tabs on each side (like wings of a butterfly) for gripping while inserting. Useful for drawing blood from a hand vein or used for scalp vein I.V. in premature infants.

butterfly rash—a rash that has a shape roughly like that of a butterfly; it is seen over the malar area and bridge of the nose in systemic lupus erythematosus.

butterfly shadow—on x-ray.

Button and **Button-One Step gastrostomy devices**—skin-level, nonrefluxing feeding devices available in sizes for both children and adults.

button cecostomy—creation of a cecal fistula for management of fecal incontinence.

buttonpexy fixation—internal fixation procedure for stomal prolapse in pediatric patients.

button sequestrum—a round lucent defect with a bony density, or sequestrum, in its center. It is a radiographic manifestation of eosinophilic granuloma.

butyrylcholinesterase inhibitors—a class of drugs for treatment of Alzheimer disease.

B-VAT (Baylor Visual Acuity Test). Mentor BVAT is a computer screen chart used in testing visual acuity.

BVM device (bag-valve-mask)—a resuscitating device consisting of a ventilating bag with a valve, attached to a mask.

Bx Sonic stent.

Bx Velocity—a sirolimus-coated coronary stent.

bypass circuit (Cardio).

bypass tract—see *nodo-Hisian* (or *nodohisian*.

C, c

CA (cardiac-apnea)—see *CA monitor.*

CA—slang for *carcinoma.*

CAB (combined androgen blockade)—significantly increases survival in patients with advanced prostate cancer.

CABG ("cab-bage")—coronary artery bypass graft. Usage: "The patient underwent a CABG," or "The patient was given a CABG."

CAD (computer-aided diagnosis).

CAD (coronary artery disease).

CADD-Prizm pain control system (PCS)—drug delivery system that provides measured therapy for management of pain.

CADD pump—computerized ambulatory drug delivery device.

Cadence AICD (automatic implantable cardioverter-defibrillator).

Cadet cardioverter-defibrillator.

CADstream—dedicated image processing system for breast MRI.

Caesar grasping forceps—used for foreign body retrieval.

café au lait macules (CALMs)—may be treated with the frequency-doubled Q-switched neodymium:YAG laser and the Q-switched ruby laser.

Caffinière prosthesis—cemented prosthesis used in replacement of the trapeziometacarpal joint.

CA15-3 RIA—a radioimmunoassay for monitoring breast cancer, based on two monoclonal antibodies which react with circulating antigen expressed by human breast carcinoma cells. This monitors a breast cancer patient's response to therapy. Used in the manner of carcinoembryonic antigen.

CAGE (cutting, annoyance, guilt, eye-opener)—an acronym for questions about cutting down on drinking, annoyance at others' concern about drinking, feeling guilty about drinking, and using alcohol as an eye-opener in the morning. Referred to as the CAGE test or CAGE screening tool for alcoholism, its brevity gives it an advantage in a busy medical office.

CAGEIN (catheter-guided endoscopic intubation)—used at the start of endoscopy as a method to intubate the esophagus in patients who have constricted anatomy, such as from Zenker diverticulum.

caisson disease—decompression sickness (called "the bends"), seen in workers and divers who work for long periods of time under water, breathing air at higher than atmospheric pressure, and then come up too quickly. The name is from the watertight structures in which underwater construction is performed, as in building bridges or tunnels.

cake mix kit—for hematopoietic progenitor assay.

Calahist Clear—topical cream for skin itching.

calamus scriptorius—the lowest portion of the floor of the fourth ventricle, shaped like a writing pen (hence its name). Used in surgical correction of syringomyelia.

Calandruccio triangular compression fixation device—used for fixation of the distal tibia.

calcarine fissure—sulcus on medial surface of the occipital lobe; the visual cortex is around this fissure.

calcar reamer (Ortho).

Calcibon—used for filling and reconstruction of bone defects.

calciphylaxis—an untreatable, rare, generally fatal, necrotizing cutaneous syndrome.

Calcitek drill system—for use in oral and maxillofacial surgery.

Calcitek spline dental implant system.

Calcitite—alloplastic material used as bone replacement. It is a solid hydroxyapatite, similar to cortical bone. See *hydroxyapatite*.

calcium-free and magnesium-free Hanks balanced salt solution (CMF-HBSS)—used in a laboratory for cell culture.

calcium channel blockers—a class of drugs commonly used to treat angina, hypertension, and arrhythmias, and now a part of some chemotherapy protocols. Certain types of cancer are resistant to the effects of chemotherapy agents, but this resistance can be overcome with the use of calcium channel blockers such as nifedipine and verapamil. See also *P-glycoprotein*.

calcium entry blockers—alternative name for calcium channel blockers.

calcium pyrophosphate deposition (CPPD) **of the spine**—a relatively uncommon arthropathy characterized by clinical features of pseudogout, radiographic manifestations of chondrocalcinosis, and the pathological deposition of calcium pyrophosphate crystals in hyaline and fibrocartilage. It is sometimes the cause of mechanical low back pain or nerve root compression syndrome. Also called *CPPD disease*.

calculi—see *cat's-eye calculi*.

Calcutript—a lithotripter used for stone disintegration in the ureter.

Caldwell view—occipitofrontal view for x-raying the ethmoid and frontal sinuses.

caliber—the internal diameter of a needle; also known as the *bore*. Cf. *caliper*.

calibration failure—MRI term.

Calibri forceps (Oph).

Caligamed—an ankle orthosis that can be worn in a shoe to offer full immobilization of the ankle joint. It is used to treat chronic ankle instability, immediate post-injury immobilization, protection postoperatively after ligament restructuring, or as a conservative treatment for torn ligaments.

caliper (often plural)—instrument with two curved legs used to measure a width or thickness indirectly—for

caliper *(cont.)* example, the thickness of a skin fold. Examples: Jameson, Lange skin-fold, Machemer, Osher, Stahl, Tenzel, Vernier. Cf. *caliber.*

CALLA (common acute lymphoblastic leukemia antigen).

Callaway formula—used to calculate a person's optimal daily calorie intake: Multiply your weight by 4.3 and your height in inches by 4.7. Add these results together plus 655 calories. From this resulting number subtract your age multiplied by 4.7. That number represents the number of calories you burn at rest. Multiply that by 1.3 and you get the number of calories you burn with moderate activity. If you keep within that calorie count, you will lose weight; if you go below the lower number, your metabolism will slow down.

Calleja exercises (Ortho).

callotasis distraction (Ortho)—bone lengthening by gradual mechanical distraction using an external fixation device. Also called *distraction osteogenesis.*

callous (adjective)—hard, as "There is a callous area on the heel of the left foot." Cf. *callus.*

callus (noun)—localized growth of a hard, horny epidermal material, as "There is a callus on the palm of the hand, near the ring he is wearing on his ring finger." Cf. *callous.*

callus distraction—a technique that corrects limb shortening by callus formation and induces bony union of nonunited fractures.

Cal Mag Fizz—an over-the-counter effervescent blend of calcium and magnesium for better absorption.

Calmette-Guérin—see *bacillus Calmette-Guérin.*

CALMs (café au lait macules).

Calnan-Nicolle synthetic joint prosthesis—used to lengthen a shortened metatarsal.

caloric testing of vestibular function—stimulates the labyrinth by instilling fluid into the ear (either above or below body temperature). Resulting nystagmus lasting more than two minutes indicates hyperirritability of the labyrinth. Absence of response indicates eighth nerve damage. Also called *cold water calorics.* See *Bárány symptom.*

calorimeter—a device to measure an individual's caloric burn.

Caluso PEG tube—a percutaneous endoscopic gastrostomy tube.

calusterone—an androgen used experimentally in treatment of carcinoma.

calvarium—frequently dictated but incorrect term for *calvaria.*

Calypso Rely catheter—rapid-exchange PTCA balloon angioplasty catheter.

CAM (complementary and alternative medicine).

CAM (cystic adenomatoid malformation).

Cambridge Biotech HIV-1 urine Western blot test—a supplemental, more specific test for urine samples found to be reactive for antibody to HIV-1.

cameral fistula—a very rare condition of the coronary arteries, with an arteriovenous fistula between the artery and one of the cardiac chambers. Also called *coronary artery cameral fistula.*

Camey ileocystoplasty—see *LeDuc-Camey ileocystoplasty.*

Camey reservoir—a continent supravesical bowel urinary diversion, performed for bladder reconstruction to treat invasive bladder cancer. Also, *Camey ileocystoplasty.*

Camino intracranial catheter—inserted into the lateral ventricle, subarachnoid space, or subdural space, this catheter uses a transducer to monitor intracranial pressure.

Camino microventricular bolt—a catheter with a transducer on the end. Used to monitor intracranial pressure and facilitate draining of cerebrospinal fluid through a ventriculostomy.

CAMIS (computer-assisted minimally invasive surgery).

Camitz palmaris longus abductorplasty—for severe thenar atrophy secondary to carpal tunnel syndrome.

CA (cardiac-apnea) **monitor**—for newborns.

cAMP (cyclic adenosine monophosphate)—a second-messenger neurotransmitter.

Campbell de Morgan spots—see *cherry angioma*.

Campral (acamprosate calcium)—a medication for the treatment of alcoholism.

Camptosar (irinotecan)—antineoplastic drug for metastatic cervical, colon, and rectal carcinoma.

Campylobacter fetus—a gram-negative organism causing enteritis in AIDS patients.

Campylobacter jejuni—enteric pathogen in humans, probably transmitted by infected animals, or from consumption of contaminated water or foods of animal origin.

CAM tent (Peds).

Cam (controlled ankle motion) **walker**—an air-filled ankle-support device, looking something like a padded boot with a rocker foot. (Note: Only the initial letter in *Cam* is capitalized.)

Canal Finder System—for use in endodontic applications, and specialized biomaterials for dentistry and other medical specialties.

canaliculus—a small canal; generally refers to the one that leads from the lacrimal punctum to the lacrimal sac of the eye. Cf. *colliculus*.

canalith repositioning maneuver—used to resolve or decrease intensity of symptoms in patients with disorders of the vestibular system with a component of benign postural vertigo.

canals (or canaliculi) **of Sondermann**—blind outpouchings from the canal of Schlemm.

Canavan disease—a devastating inherited neurological disorder most commonly affecting children of Jewish ancestry.

c-ANCA (cytoplasmic antineutrophil cytoplasmic antibody)—a marker for Wegener granulomatosis. It is sometimes paired in laboratory tests with p-ANCA. Cf. *ANCA*, *p-ANCA*.

Cancell—a biologic drug especially popular in the Midwest and Florida. Proponents claim it returns cancer cells to a primitive state from which they can be digested and rendered inert. The FDA has found no basis for the claims.

cancellous (adj.)—descriptive term for a reticular, spongy, or lattice-like structure, mainly of bony tissue.

cancellus (noun)—any structure arranged like a lattice.

cancer—a term for malignant neoplasm often used interchangeably with *carcinoma*. The word *cancer* is derived from the Latin word for 'crab' and first used for malignant ulcerations by the Roman medical writer Celsus (1st century AD).

cancer *(cont.)*
Much earlier, Greek writers including Hippocrates used the Greek word *karkinos*, also meaning 'crab', and its derivative *karkinoma,* for malignant disease. The association between malignancy and crabs has been variously explained: (1) malignant tumors were thought to gnaw or erode tissue like the claws of a crab, and (2) the dilated veins on the surface of a cancerous breast seemed to suggest the outline of a crab with outstretched claws. Cf. *carcinoma* and *sarcoma*.

cancer classifications—see *classification and staging*.

cancerization—malignant degeneration.

cancer marker—see *tumor marker*.

Candela 405-nm pulsed dye laser.

Candida albicans—a fungus which can disseminate in AIDS, but is also an exceedingly common cause of dermatitis, vaginitis, and thrush in persons with intact immune systems. Also, esophageal candidiasis is seen in AIDS patients.

Candida glabrata—a pathogen causing vaginitis.

C&S, C and S—culture and sensitivity. Do not confuse with *CNS* (central nervous system).

CA 19-9—tumor marker which is a sialylated Lewis A antigen expressed by many adenocarcinomas of the digestive tract.

candy-cane stirrups—stirrups used to elevate the patient's feet while maintaining flexion and abduction of the thighs during therapeutic or surgical procedures performed in the lithotomy position. Each foot is supported by a sling consisting of two straps, one passing behind the ankle and the other under the ball of the foot. Each sling hangs from the tip of a cane-shaped metal support that is mounted on the operating table. Usage: "Her legs were then placed in the candy-cane stirrups in the dorsal lithotomy position."

canker sore—see *aphtha*.

Cannon catheter—a 15-French polyurethane dual-lumen catheter with nonfused arterial and venous ends containing side holes. The catheter has an attachable hub assembly for retrograde tunneling, allowing for precise tip and cuff positioning. It is used for vascular access for hemodialysis.

cannon waves—a phenomenon in which the two chambers of the heart may contract at the same time, when the heart loses coordination of the atria and ventricles. Blood then flows upward across the mitral and tricuspid valves, and a venous wave is seen in the neck.

Cannulated Plus screw system.

can-opener capsulotomy (Oph)—a method of entering the anterior lens capsule in preparation for cataract extraction in which many small tears are joined together to create a continuous circular incision, much as a kitchen can-opener chews its way around the lid of a can. Usage: "A capsulorrhexis was then made for 270.° At the 12 o'clock position, the tear extended radially, and the remaining 3 clock hours of the capsulorrhexis were finished using a can-opener capsulotomy."

canstatin—a collagen fragment that inhibits angiogenesis. It has a variety of anticancer applications.

Cantlie line—the plane separating the right and middle hepatic vein territories, not marked by any anatomical feature but usually running along or

Cantlie *(cont.)*
to the right of the line joining the gallbladder fossa with the inferior vena cava.

Cantor tube—see *mercury artifact*.

CA1-18 tumor marker—a tumor-associated antigen used in diagnosis and management of GI and lung cancer patients.

CAPD (continuous ambulatory peritoneal dialysis).

Capetown aortic prosthetic valve.

capillary blood sugar (CBS).

capillary leak syndrome—extravasation of plasma fluid and proteins into the extravascular space, sometimes resulting in fatal hypotension and reduced organ perfusion; an adverse effect of aldesleukin (interleukin-2) therapy.

Capio CL transvaginal suture-capturing device—for suturing a sling to Cooper ligament through a transvaginal approach without the need for an abdominal incision.

Capio suture capturing device.

Capiox SX—gas and heat exchange oxygenation system.

capnograph (*capno-* pertains to carbon dioxide)—a graph displaying the results from an infrared spectrometer. The capnograph shows the results as CO_2 wave forms, and as numbers denoting value for $ETCO_2$ (end-tidal carbon dioxide concentration).

capnography—used in anesthesiology to record measurement of end-tidal carbon dioxide.

CaPPi (calcium pyrophosphate)—one of the salts of which bone is composed.

capravirine—an antiretroviral agent for HIV-infected patients.

Caprosyn suture—a rapidly-absorbed monofilament synthetic suture, indicated for use in general soft tissue approximation and/or ligation.

CAPS ArthroWand—collagen shrinkage wand used in arthroscopic surgery.

Capset (calcium sulfate) **bone graft barrier**—applied following bone graft procedure to keep grafted bone or bone substitute from migrating and to prevent unwanted tissue formation before the grafted material has had time to integrate and heal.

CAPS-free diet:
C caffeine
A alcohol
P pepper
S spicy foods

capsule endoscopy—a technique using a disposable video capsule swallowed by the patient that allows visualization of much of the small bowel not within reach of standard upper and lower endoscopy. It allows more access to the small bowel for patients with an obscure source of gastrointestinal bleeding. Other potential uses for the capsule are under investigation. This technology may be particularly helpful in discovering the cause of bowel bleeding when standard upper endoscopy and colonoscopy are negative. See *PillCam video capsule*.

capsulorrhexis (also capsulorhexis)—circular anterior capsulotomy; rupture of a structure enveloping an organ, vessel, or joint. See *continuous circular capsulorrhexis technique, posterior capsulorrhexis with optic capture,* and *two-stage capsulorrhexis for endocapsular phacoemulsification*.

CAPSure ArthroWand—applies radiofrequency to achieve capsular shrinkage.

CapSure steroid-eluting electrode.

CAPS X Wand—thermal ArthroWand for performing capsular shrinkage.

CAPS *(cont.)*
It can access all joint capsule areas and provides access to both anterior and posterior compartments. It is used in conjunction with an arthroscopic Bankart repair.

caput—the head; also used in reference to the expanded part of an organ or muscle. Cf. *caput medusae*.

caput medusae—dilated veins around the umbilicus. So named because of the resemblance to the snakes which formed the hair of Medusa in Greek mythology. Seen in patients with cirrhosis of the liver, and in some newborns. Cf. *caput*.

Carabello sign—a rise in arterial blood pressure during left heart catheter pull-back in patients with severe aortic stenosis.

carbacephems—a class of antibiotics similar to cephalosporins. Example: Lorabid (loracarbef).

CarboFlex—a five-layer odor-control wound dressing.

carbolfuchsin stain—Tilden method, to study mouth organisms.

Carbomedics prosthetic heart valve (CPHV).

carbonaceous material—smoke inhalation debris deposited in the nose and upper respiratory tract.

carbonate-apatite (Lab).

carbon dioxide laser—see *laser*.

carbon fiber—synthetic ligament material.

carbon-14—see *^{14}C-urea breath excretion test*.

Carbo-Seal—zero-porosity cardiovascular composite graft.

carboxyhemoglobin—levels measured in patients exposed to fires and in attempted suicides using automobile exhaust. Carbon monoxide binds competitively with hemoglobin molecules, excluding oxygen.

carcinoembryonic antigen (CEA)—present in many cases of carcinoma, particularly of the lung, digestive tract, and pancreas. It is valuable in testing treated cancer patients for recurrence of metastases.

carcinoma—a term for malignant neoplasm often used interchangeably with *cancer*. It is derived from the Greek word *karkinos* meaning 'crab' and its derivative *karkinoma,* for malignant disease. Carcinoma develops from epithelium, either glandular (adenocarcinoma) or squamous (squamous carcinoma). Cf. *cancer* and *sarcoma*.

carcinoma ex pleomorphic adenoma—a type of malignant pleomorphic adenoma (appearing as two or more distinct forms of tumor) that usually occurs in the salivary glands of older adults. An epithelial malignancy arises in a preexisting mixed tumor, with metastasis only of the malignant epithelial component. Also called *malignant mixed tumor.*

carcinoma in situ (CIS).

carcinoma of bladder classification—see *Jewett classification*.

cardiac allograft vascular disease (CAVD)—cardiac disease occurring after heart transplantation.

Cardiac Assist intra-aortic balloon catheter—a device to assist the heart before and after open-heart surgery and complex balloon angioplasty procedures.

cardiac device—see *device* and specific categories, such as *catheter.*

cardiac hybrid revascularization procedure—in which minimally invasive surgery is first used to treat the principal coronary artery, while interventional therapies such as balloon angioplasty and coronary

cardiac *(cont.)*
stenting are then used to treat other blocked vessels.

Cardiac Protect—combines noninvasive electron beam computed tomography to detect plaque in coronary arteries, with patented methodology to determine which of 16 subclasses of cholesterol is causing plaque build-up.

cardiac resynchronization therapy defibrillator (CRT-D).

cardiac retraction clip—used to retract the fatty layer over the heart during coronary artery anastomosis.

cardiac risk factors—elevated blood lipids, obesity, habitual dietary excesses, lack of exercise, hypertension, cigarette smoking, and stress.

cardiac shock wave therapy (CSWT).

cardiac sling—used to support the heart and expose the circumflex branch of the coronary artery during surgery.

Cardiac STATus—rapid assay to rule out myocardial infarction.

Cardiac T rapid assay—a rapid bedside assay to diagnose myocardial infarction. Uses cardiac troponin T, which is found inside the cardiac muscle and released into the blood only when cells are damaged.

cardiac troponin T—used to test for myocardial infarction. The protein troponin T is elevated in myocardial infarction and is cardiac-specific, unlike CK-MB which may indicate other muscle injury. Also, the diagnostic window for troponin T is from one hour (before CK-MB shows up) to 14 days (long after CK-MB has returned to normal).

Cardia Salt Alternative—a salt substitute used by hypertensive patients.

Cardima Pathfinder—microcatheter for diagnosis of cardiac tachyarrhythmia.

CardioBeeper CB-12L—cardiac monitoring device that allows for transmission of a complete 12-lead ECG, utilizing prefitted reusable electrodes, over a standard telephone line.

Cardioblate BP—a surgical ablation tool.

Cardioblate XL—a surgical ablation pen.

Cardioblate saline-irrigated cooled-tip radiofrequency ablation pen.

Cardiocap 5—a patient monitor designed for use in the operating room, ambulatory surgery unit, induction area, or PACU.

CardioCard—stores digital electrocardiogram records on an optical memory card.

CardioCoil coronary stent—a self-expanding stent used for prevention of re-stenosis following PTCA.

CardioFix Pericardium—a patch for intracardiac repair and pericardial closure.

CardioFlow—a patented extract from the tomato which has been shown in human trials to have a powerful effect on blood platelets, thereby reducing the propensity to excessive blood clotting.

Cardiofreezer cryosurgical system.

cardiogenic shock—inability of the heart to maintain adequate blood flow for vital functions.

cardiokymography (CKG)—for measuring interference in pacemaker function. Cardiokymography is used clinically at some institutions for detecting segmental wall motion abnormalities of the heart. It may interfere with cardiac pacemaker function and can cause the pacemaker to operate at its upper rate limit.

Cardiolite scan—a cardiac scan showing areas of myocardial infarction, using the radioactive imaging agent ^{99m}Tc sestamibi (Cardiolite).

Cardiomed Bodysoft epidural catheter—thermosensitive material of catheter softens when warmed to body temperature, minimizing patient trauma.

Cardiomed endotracheal ventilation catheter.

Cardiomed thermodilution catheter.

cardiomyoplasty—a surgical treatment for weakened heart muscle leading to congestive heart failure. In cardiomyoplasty, the latissimus dorsi muscle is surgically excised except for a pedicle that contains its blood and nerve supply. It is then inserted into the chest cavity through an opening created by excision of the second rib on the anterior chest. Two pacing electrode leads are placed in the muscle flap, and two sensing leads are placed on the heart itself. These leads are connected to a programmable pulse pacemaker which is placed surgically beneath the rectus abdominis muscle. The pacemaker synchronizes the contraction of the muscle flap to the R wave of the heart's own electrical rhythm. The number of bursts from the pacemaker is gradually increased after surgery until, after a few months, the skeletal muscle contracts with every heartbeat or every other heartbeat. After exposure to burst stimulation from the pacemaker, the skeletal muscle gradually changes its muscle fibers at the cellular level until they resemble those of heart muscle, which can contract repeatedly without fatigue.

CardioPass—a layered small-bore vascular graft.

cardioplege (verb)—a coined term meaning to administer cardioplegia. Usage: "I therefore elected to cross-clamp the aorta again, go back on full bypass, cardioplege the patient, and harvest a vein from the right thigh."

cardioplegic solution—an iced solution injected into the coronary arteries during open-heart surgery to produce cardiac arrest. Composed of calcium, magnesium, potassium, chloride, and sodium bicarbonate in solution, it produces cardiac standstill, and protects the myocardium from damage due to intracellular ion imbalance and acidosis.

Cardiopoint—cardiac surgery needles.

cardiopulmonary support system (CPS).

cardiorrhexis—rupture of a ventricle.

CardioSEAL septal occluder—a cardiac implant used in a minimally invasive, catheter-based procedure to close heart defects.

Cardiosol—a patented human organ preservation solution designed for use during heart transplantation and open-heart surgery. Also, *HK-Cardiosol* and *CP-Cardiosol.*

Cardio Tactilaze peripheral angioplasty laser catheter—contains an Nd:YAG laser to vaporize atheromatous plaques.

CardioTec scan—a cardiac scan showing areas of myocardial infarction, using the radioactive imaging agent ^{99m}Tc teboroxime (CardioTec). Used for emergency scans, it clears rapidly from the blood to allow subsequent scans, if necessary.

cardiothoracic ratio (CTR).

cardiotocography—method of fetal monitoring.

CardioWest total artificial heart (TAH)—a device used in transplant-eligible critically ill patients suffering from irreversible failure of both sides of the heart. Formerly known as the Jarvik heart.

Cardizem Monovial—advanced infusion delivery system for the injectable form of Cardizem, prescribed for certain heartbeat irregularities.

CareLink monitor—allows patients to collect data by holding a small antenna over their implanted GEM II DR/VR implantable cardioverter-defibrillator, allowing physicians to obtain the data via the Internet.

CARES (Cancer Rehabilitation Evaluation System)—cancer-specific health-related quality-of-life assessment.

CARF (Commission on Accreditation of Rehabilitation Facilities).

Caring Behavior Assessment (CBA) **tool**—used to assess the caring behaviors of primary healthcare providers.

Carlesta—an over-the-counter topical preparation for the prevention and treatment of skin irritation associated with adult incontinence.

Carmeda—heparin biocompatible surfaces on cannulas used in arrested heart surgery.

Carmeda BioActive Surface—extracorporeal circuit whose surface reduces thrombogenesis and preserves platelet function.

C-arm fluoroscopy—image intensifier, portable x-ray unit used in the operating room.

carmine dye (also called *cochineal extract*)—color additive extracted from dried female cochineal insects and commonly used in fruit drinks, candy, yogurt, and other foods. It can cause anaphylactic shock in some people.

carmustine wafer—biodegradable wafer impregnated with carmustine, inserted into the cavity after surgical removal of recurrent glioblastoma multiforme, delivering medication directly to brain tumor site.

carneous degeneration—tissue change producing a fleshy texture. Also, carnification.

Carney complex—a multiple neoplasia syndrome with cardiac, endocrine, cutaneous, and neural tumors together with spotty pigmentation of the skin, particularly on the face, lips, and trunk, and of mucous membranes. It may simultaneously involve multiple endocrine glands such as the pituitary, adrenals, and testes. It includes the LAMB syndrome and the NAME syndrome.

Caroli disease—congenital dilatation of the intrahepatic biliary ducts.

Carolina rocker—a wheelchair on a rocker platform, used in physical therapy for patients with stroke, and also for tardive dyskinesia.

carotene—the yellow or red coloring found in egg yolk, carrots, and sweet potatoes. Cf. *creatine, creatinine, keratin*.

carotid angioplasty with stenting—noninvasive alternative to carotid endarterectomy. A balloon catheter is threaded from groin to neck and pushed into the clogged section under fluoroscopic guidance. After flattening of plaque and removal of the balloon, another catheter deposits the metal stent to keep the artery open.

CarotidCoil stent—designed to resist compression after placement in the

CarotidCoil *(cont.)* neck arteries to maintain blood flow to the brain.

carotid intima-media thickness (c-IMT)—a marker for future cardiovascular and cerebrovascular events.

carotid sinus massage—used as the provocative test for the detection of sinus node disease, which is the most common indication for pacemaker implantation.

carpal compression test—performed by applying direct pressure on the carpal tunnel, and considered by many to be more sensitive and specific than the Tinel or Phalen tests.

Carpal Lock cock-up splint (Phys Ther).

carpal tunnel syndrome (CTS)—caused by repetitive hand motions, such as prolonged keyboard use, or hammering, filing, or writing, resulting in compression of the soft median nerve against the volar carpal ligament by the nine comparatively harder tendons that are in the tunnel with it. Depending on the degree of pressure, symptoms range from aching and numbness over the median nerve distribution (but sparing the little finger), to constant hypesthesia and paralysis of the abductor pollicis brevis. Also, *repetitive strain injury.*

Carpentier-Edwards Perimount RSR pericardial bioprosthesis—a tissue heart valve designed for patients with small heart valves. It is implanted in a position that improves blood flow and decreases the need for anticoagulant drugs.

Carpentier-Edwards Physio anuloplasty ring.

carperitide study—a recombinant human atrial natriuretic polypeptide in phase 2 clinical trials for acute respiratory distress syndrome.

carphology—purposeless plucking at clothing or bedclothes; sometimes seen in dementia or terminal illness.

"car-pon-tee-aye"—phonetic for *Carpentier.*

CarraFilm—transparent film dressings used as wound coverings for wounds with light exudate.

CarraSmart foam—a self-adhesive foam dressing with water-attracting properties used for skin ulcers, pressure sores, burns, abrasions, and lacerations. This smart foam manages the moisture balance of a wound with its absorption and evaporative properties.

Carra Sorb H—a calcium alginate wound dressing used in the management of heavily exuding wounds.

Carra Sorb M—a freeze-dried gel with aloe vera gel extract, containing acemannan, used for the medium exudating wound.

Carrasyn hydrogel—wound dressing.

carrier (Genetics)—an individual who is heterozygous for an abnormal gene, carrying a copy of it on one chromosome of a pair but a normal gene on the other chromosome.

Carrión disease—a tropical infection caused by *Bartonella bacilliformis.*

Carroll-Girard screw (Orthodontia)—not *Carrel-Girard.*

Carr-Purcell-Meiboom-Gill sequence—MRI term.

Carr-Purcell sequence—MRI term.

Carswell grapes—clusters of tubercles around the smaller bronchioles, looking like a bunch of grapes; seen in pulmonary tuberculosis.

Carter pillow—a foam cushion which immobilizes and elevates simultaneously; often used in replantation procedures.

Carter-Thomason suture passer—for ligation of bleeding vessels in the abdominal wall as well as other laparoscopic surgical applications.

Carticel autologous cultured chondrocytes—a tissue repair product used to grow a patient's own cartilage cells to repair knee damage.

Cartilade—shark cartilage that presently has a use patent as a drug for inhibition of angiogenesis.

CAS (contralateral acoustic stimulation).

CAS (coronary artery scan).

Casale vesicostomy—a technique similar to the "full Monti" using a single piece of bowel to gain additional length for continent urinary diversion. Do not confuse with *Casola cecostomy.*

caseation—necrosed tissue resembling cheesy material.

CA 72-4—a cancer antigen serum tumor marker to monitor metastatic gastric cancer.

CASH (classic abdominal Semm hysterectomy).

Casola cecostomy—percutaneous placement of a cecostomy catheter for colonic decompression in adults. Do not confuse with *Casale vesicostomy.*

cast—a laboratory term referring to an elongated mass formed by inspissation of semisolid material in a tubular structure. Found in the urine or sputum in certain abnormal conditions.

CAST (Cardiac Arrhythmic Suppression Trial)—a cardiac protocol. May be followed by a roman numeral.

casting material
- Cotton Loader position
- Fractura Flex
- Gypsona
- Hexcelite
- hip spica
- MaxCast
- Minerva-type
- Risser localizer
- Sarmiento
- spica

Castanares face-lift scissors.

Castaneda anastomosis clamp.

Castaneda bottle—used in the culture of certain organisms from blood.

Cast Boot—polypropylene hip abduction brace for treating hip dysplasia in toddlers up to 2 1/2 years of age.

Castleman disease—a rare B-cell lymphoproliferation disorder that occurs in two forms. The more common localized Castleman disease often presents as an asymptomatic mediastinal mass and usually is cured by surgical removal of the mediastinal mass. The rarer form, multicentric Castleman disease, often presents as multisystem illness with widespread lymphadenopathy. It has a poor prognosis but may respond to prednisone, chemotherapy or surgical removal of affected nodes and spleen.

Castroviejo-Colibri forceps.

cast syndrome—a rare but sometimes fatal condition in which a body cast occludes the blood supply to the duodenum.

CAT ("cat") (computerized, or computed, axial tomography). Also called *ACAT, CT,* and *CAT scan*. See *computed tomography scan*.

cataract—opacity of the lens of the eye, or its capsule, or both. Types include *brunescent, mature, posterior subcapsular*, *senile,* and *traumatic.*

Catarex—surgical device for cataract removal through a 1 to 2 mm hole created in the lens capsule. It uses a mechanical energy source, with the procedure taking less than 10 minutes.

catastrophizing—an exaggerated negative mental set brought to bear during painful experiences. It is believed that the tendency to catastrophize during painful stimulation contributes to more intense pain experience and increased emotional distress.

catch—term for a sharp, localized pain, usually in the chest, and provoked or aggravated by drawing a breath (inspiration).

CATCH 22—acronym for the major features of microdeletion of chromosome 22q11:
C cardiac defect
A abnormal face
T thymic hypoplasia
C cleft palate
H hypocalcemia

cat cry syndrome—a chromosome abnormality including multiple heart and eye abnormalities, mental retardation, microcephaly, and a mewing cry, thus its name. Also called *cri du chat syndrome*.

cat's eye calculi (Radiol)—gallstones in the common bile duct resulting from metallic surgical clips from previous surgical procedure, so-called because of radiographic appearance of stones.

cat's eye pupil (also, *cat's eye reflex*) —unusual appearance of the pupil resembling that of a light shining into a cat's eye. It is seen in retinoblastoma.

cat's eye reflex—sign of retinoblastoma.

catgut—see *surgical gut*.

cathepsin D—lysozomal enzyme used to label fibroblasts, macrophages, sweat ducts and glands, smooth muscle, and stratum granulosum in normal tissue, and now being used as a prognostic marker in breast tumors.

catheter
ablation
Abscession fluid drainage
AccuSet introducer
Accu-Vu sizing
Achiever balloon dilatation
ACS Concorde
ACS Endura coronary dilation
ACS OTW (over-the-wire) Lifestream coronary dilatation
ACS OTW (over-the-wire) Photon
ACS RX Comet coronary dilatation
ACS Tourguide II guiding
AcuNav ultrasound
Ahn thrombectomy
Alert
Alzate
Amazr
Angiocath PRN
AngiOptic microcatheter
Anthron heparinized
antibacterial personal
arrhythmia mapping system
ArrowGard Blue Line
ArrowGard Blue Line Plus
Arrow-Howes multilumen
Arrow Twin Cath
Ascent guiding
atherectomy
AtheroCath
AtheroCath Bantam coronary atherectomy
Atlantis SR
Auth atherectomy
BAL
balloon biliary
balloon wedge-pressure
Bard Safety Excalibur

catheter *(cont.)*
Bard Stinger S ablation
BD Insyte Autoguard shielded intravenous
Beta-Cath system
bifoil balloon
Blazer II XP cardiac ablation
Blue FlexTip
Brevi-Kath epidural
Bronchitrac L
Burhenne steerable
Calypso Rely
Camino intracranial
Camino microventricular bolt
Cannon
Cannon retrograde tunneling
Cardiac Assist intra-aortic balloon
Cardima Pathfinder microcatheter
Cardiomed Bodysoft epidural
Cardiomed endotracheal ventilation
Cardiomed thermodilution
Cardio Tactilaze peripheral angioplasty laser
Cath-Finder
CCOmbo
Celsius control endovascular
Celsius DS (dual sensor) diagnostic/ablation
central venous (CVC)
Cheetah angioplasty
Chemo-Port
Chilli cooled ablation
Cholangiocath
CliniCath peripherally inserted
Closure System by VNUS
Cohen
Comfort Cath I or II
Conceptus Soft Seal cervical
Conceptus Soft Torque uterine
Conceptus VS (variable softness)
Constellation mapping
Cook TPN
Cool Tip
Cordis Predator PTCA balloon
Cordis Trakstar PTCA balloon

catheter *(cont.)*
coudé
CrossSail coronary dilatation
CryoVasc
cuffed tunneled
cutdown
Cutting Balloon microsurgical dilatation
Dale Foley
Datascope
decompression
Dorros infusion/probing
Double J indwelling
Double J ureteral
Du Pen long-term epidural
DuraGlide3 stone balloon
EAC (expandable access catheter)
EchoMark
Edwards-Cohen
EndoCPB (endovascular cardio-pulmonary bypass)
Endosound endoscopic ultrasound
Endotak C lead
EnSite cardiac
EPT-Dx steerable diagnostic
EPT-1000 XP cardiac ablation
Erythroflex
e-TRAIN 110 AngioJet
Evert-O-Cath
eXamine cholangiography
Explorer 360° rotational diagnostic
Explorer ST fixed curve diagnostic
Express PTCA
FACT (Focal Angioplasty Catheter Technology)
Falcon coronary
Fast-Cath introducer
Fino vascular
Flexima ureteral
Flexguard Tip
Flexxicon Blue dialysis
Fogarty adherent clot
Fogarty balloon biliary
Fogarty graft thrombectomy
Force balloon dilatation

catheter *(cont.)*
Freeway PTCA
Freezor cryocatheter
Frontrunner XP CTO (chronic total occlusion)
FX miniRAIL RX PTCA
Gold Probe bipolar hemostasis
Grollman
Groshong
Grüntzig balloon (Gruentzig)
Hartzler ACX-II or RX-014 balloon
HealthShield mediastinal wound drainage
HemoGlide dialysis
HemoSplit long-term hemodialysis
Hickman
Hieshima coaxial
Hohn central venous
Hurwitz dialysis
Hydrolyser microcatheter
ICP (intracranial pressure)
Illumen-8 guiding
ILUS (intraluminal ultrasound)
Infiniti
Infuse-A-Cath
InfusaSleeve II
Insemi-Cath
Intracath
Intran disposable intrauterine pressure measurement
intravascular ultrasound (IVUS)
intrepid PTCA angioplasty
ITC balloon
IVUS (intravascular ultrasound)
Jackman orthogonal
Jelco intravenous
JL4 (Judkins left 4 cm curve)
JL5 (Judkins left 5 cm curve)
Jocath Maestro coronary balloon
Jography angiographic
Joguide coronary guiding
Judkins 4 diagnostic
Kaye tamponade balloon
KDF-2.3
Kifa

catheter *(cont.)*
Kinsey atherectomy
Kish urethral illuminated
KISS (kidney internal splint/stent)
Koala intrauterine pressure
Kontron
L-Cath peripherally inserted neonatal
Lifestream coronary dilatation
Livewire Duo-Decapolar
Livewire TC ablation
MammoSite RTS (radiation therapy system)
MapCath
Marathon guiding
Mark IV Moss decompression-feeding
Maverick Monorail balloon
Maverick over-the-wire balloon
Maverick2 Monorail
Max Force
Mercator atrial high-density array
Metricath
MicroMewi multiple sidehole infusion
Millar MPC-500
Millenia balloon
More-Flow
Moss decompression feeding
MS Classique balloon dilatation
multiflanged Portnoy (for hydrocephalus shunts)
Multipurpose-SM
Naviport deflectable tip guiding
NaviStar DS (dual sensor) diagnostic/ablation
Neo-Sert umbilical vessel
nephrostomy-type
NeuroVasx (Sub-Microinfusion)
Nexus 2 linear ablation
NoProfile balloon
NovaCath multi-lumen infusion
Nutricath
OmniCath atherectomy
Omni Flush shape

catheter *(cont.)*
On-Command (male and female)
OpenSail balloon
Opti-Plast XT balloon
Oracle Focus
Oracle Megasonics
Oracle Micro
Oracle Micro Plus
Oreopoulos-Zellerman
Outback re-entry
Pace bipolar pacing
P.A.S. Port
P.A.S. Port Fluoro-Free
Pathfinder
Percuflex APD all purpose catheter with Fader Tip
Periflow peripheral balloon
PermCath double-lumen ventricular access
Phantom V Plus
PIC (peripherally inserted)
PICC (peripherally inserted central)
Pico-ST II
pigtail
Pipelle endometrial suction
Polaris X steerable diagnostic
Polaris-Dx steerable diagnostic
PolyFlo
Polystan
Powerline
ProCross Rely over-the-wire balloon
Pro-Flo XT
Quantum Maverick
Quinton Mahurkar dual lumen
Ranfac cholangiographic
Reddick cystic duct cholangiogram
Reddick-Saye screw
Redifurl TaperSeal IAB
Reliance urinary control insert
remote access perfusion (RAP) cannula
Response CV
Response electrophysiology
Rigiflex TTS balloon

catheter *(cont.)*
Rivas vascular
R1 Rapid Exchange balloon
Racz epidural
Rebar microcatheters
Revelation microcatheters
Rhythm Catheter
RIC fluid exchange resuscitation
Robert G. Edwards
Rosch-Uchida transjugular liver access needle-catheter
Sable
Samuels Micro-Scler
SCA-EX ShortCutter
Schon hemodialysis
SCOOP 1; SCOOP 2
Seroma-Cath
SET three-lumen thrombectomy
Shaldon
Sherpa guiding
Simpson atherectomy
Simpson peripheral AtheroCath
Skinny dilatation
Slinky
SmartCath esophageal balloon
soaker
Soft Torque uterine
Soft-Vu Omni flush
Solo catheter with Pro/Pel coating
SoloPass
Sones woven Dacron
Speedicath intermittent
Speedy balloon
SPI-ARgent II peritoneal dialysis
SpineCATH
split sheath
Spyglass angiography
Stamey-Malecot
StatLock dialysis
Steerocath-A ablation
Steerocath-Dx octapolar and valve mapping
Steerocath-T ablation
Stinger ablation
St. Jude 4F Supreme electrophysiology

catheter *(cont.)*
Stormer balloon
Sub-Microinfusion
Suction Buster
Supreme electrophysiology
SureCuff
surgically implanted hemodialysis (SIHC)
Swan-Ganz
swan-neck
Swartz SL Series Fast-Cath introducer
Syntel latex-free embolectomy
Tactilaze angioplasty laser
Targis microwave catheter-based system
Taut cystic duct
Tenckhoff peritoneal dialysis
Tennis Racquet
thermodilution
Tis-u-trap endometrial suction
Torcon NB selective angiographic
torque tube
Tourguide guiding
Tracker-18 Soft Stream
transluminal extraction (TEC)
transtracheal oxygen
Trellis infusion
T-TAC (transcervical tubal access)
TTS (through the scope)
TUN-L-KATH epidural
twist drill
Uldall (*not* Udall) subclavian hemodialysis
Ultra 8 balloon
UltraLite flow-directed microcatheter
umbilical artery (UAC)
Ureflex
UroMax II
vanSonnenberg-Wittich
Vas-Cath
Vector and VectorX large-lumen guiding
Venaport guiding

catheter *(cont.)*
Ventra
Ventrix
Ventureyra ventricular
Verbatim balloon
Veripath peripheral guiding
vessel-sizing
Visa II PTCA
Vision PTCA
Vitesse Cos laser
Vitesse E-II
VNUS Restore
Vueport balloon-occlusion guiding
Was-Cath
whistle-tip ureteral
Witzel enterostomy
Workhorse percutaneous transluminal angioplasty balloon
Wurd
XL-11
Xpeedior 60
Xpeedior 100
X-trode electrode
Z-Med
Zuma guiding

catheter balloon valvuloplasty—performed for severe calcific aortic stenosis.

catheter-directed thrombolysis and endovascular stent placement—treatment for SVC (superior vena cava) syndrome.

catheter vitrector—Verbatim balloon probe.

Cath-Finder—catheter tracking system, part of the P.A.S. Port system that tracks the catheter tip during placement, without fluoroscopy.

CathLink implantable vascular access device.

CathScanner ultrasound imaging system—a device using an intravascular catheter for ultrasound imaging of the blood vessels.

Cath-Secure—a hypoallergenic tape with an attached fastener to hold a triple-lumen central catheter in place.

Cath-Shield—a surgically implantable cover for attachment of a catheter to an implantable drug delivery system.

CathTrack catheter locator system—handheld device used to determine catheter tip placement.

cat-scratch disease (CSD)—a *Bartonella henselae* infection acquired through the bite or scratch of a cat.

Cattell Infant Intelligence Scale.

cauda—tail, or structure resembling a tail. See *tail*.

caudate, adj., having a tail, as in "caudate lobe." Cf. *chordate, cordate*.

cauliflower ear—slang term for an external ear deformed by repeated or severe trauma, as in boxers and wrestlers.

cautery (electrocautery)
- BiLAP bipolar
- bipolar
- Concept handheld
- Mira
- NeoKnife
- Op-Temp
- Scheie ophthalmic
- wet field

CAVD (cardiac allograft vascular disease).

CaverMap—a nerve stimulator device used intraoperatively during rectal surgery to stimulate the cavernous nerve while monitoring penile tumescence. Assists in sparing vital nerves typically damaged during prostate cancer surgery.

Cavernotome—device used to prepare the corpora cavernosa for implantation of a penile prosthesis.

cavernous hemangioma—one of the most common benign intraorbital tumors, found typically within the cone of the extraocular muscles. Removal of cavernomas located in the basal, inferomedial, and lateral aspect of the orbit may be done by a microneurosurgical transconjunctival approach. Other surgical approaches include transcranial and direct orbital.

Caves-Schultz-Stanford bioptome—an instrument for obtaining a biopsy of the myocardium via a transvenous catheter.

Cavilon barrier ointment—forms an occlusive barrier to block transepidermal water loss.

Cavitron ultrasonic surgical aspirator (CUSA)—used in the resection of lung tumors. It can fragment and aspirate tissue at a selected margin from a tumor, leaving airways and vessels intact to be ligated. This operation can be performed in a bloodless fashion with direct visualization of adequate margins. It can also be used to resect large masses of residual germ cell tumor following chemotherapy by insertion directly through the tumor pseudocapsule, fragmenting the giant mass and collapsing the pseudocapsule, facilitating exposure of mediastinal vessels and nerves. The collapsed pseudocapsule can then be excised, allowing the underlying lung to expand normally.

cavum conchal cartilage graft—a graft harvested from the lower cavernous portion of the concha of the auricle, used in rhinoplasty. See also *cymba conchal cartilage graft*.

cavum velum interpositum (CVI)—an anatomical structure in the brain that may appear as a cyst in the pineal region on neonatal sonograms. Usually it has a characteristic inverted

cavum *(cont.)* helmet shape and is situated beneath the fornices and above the internal cerebral veins.

C-bar web-spacer—a device used to prevent burn contractures. It is a plastic appliance that fits around the wrist and has a protrusion that supports the thumb and stretches the web space so that the configuration of the thumb and the rest of the fingers is much like a letter *C*.

CBF (cochlear blood flow) (ENT).

CBFV (cerebral blood flow velocity).

C-bloc—continuous nerve block system for management of postoperative pain. A portable infusion pump creates a continuous pain blockade by infusing local anesthetic through a catheter placed alongside a nerve.

CBP (chronic bacterial prostatitis)—may be treated with the antibiotic Maxaquin.

CBS (capillary blood sugar)—a test for hypoglycemia. It enables a patient to take a blood sugar reading by a fingerstick.

CBT—see *cognitive behavior therapy*.

CBV (cerebral blood volume).

CBWO (closing base wedge osteotomy).

cc (cubic centimeter)—the SI unit used for volume of tissue or other solid objects, whereas mL (milliliter) is used to measure liquids. The dictated "Estimated blood loss was 200 cc" should be corrected to "200 mL."

C Cap (compliance cap)—a device on containers of medications for glaucoma, to help patients track medication compliance.

C-CAP (custom contoured ablation pattern) **method**—treatment system used to remove microscopic amounts of tissue from the cornea in order to correct off-center ablation. The treatment restores the cornea's normal shape.

CCB (calcium channel blocker).

CCD (central collodiaphyseal angle) in the shaft and neck of long bones.

CCE (clubbing, cyanosis, and edema).

CCE (counterflow centrifugation elutriation).

CCH (C-cell hyperplasia).

CCH (circumscribed choroidal hemangioma).

^{14}C-cholylglycine breath excretion test—highly sensitive test indicating bacterial overgrowth in small intestine or ileal disease. See *^{14}C-urea breath test*.

CCK-HIDA—see *HIDA-CCK scintigraphy*.

CCO (continuous cardiac output).

CCOmbo catheter—measures pressures inside the heart with continuous cardiac output (CCO).

CCPD (continuous cyclical peritoneal dialysis)—method of maintenance dialysis in patients with end-stage renal disease.

CCS (Certified Coding Specialist).

CCS-P (Certified Coding Specialist-Physician-based).

CCRT (continuous renal replacement therapy).

CCUP (colpocystourethropexy).

CD (color Doppler).

CDA (chenodeoxycholic acid)—drug used to dissolve gallstones in patients at higher surgical risk, who are slender, who have noncalcium gallstones, and who tend to have higher serum cholesterol levels. Cf. *2-CdA*.

CDAD (*Clostridium difficile*-associated diarrhea).

CDC—the Centers (*not* Center) for Disease Control and Prevention in

CDC *(cont.)* Atlanta, Georgia, federal clearinghouse for information on epidemic diseases. In addition to being a pool of information for researchers and practicing physicians, the CDC sometimes has investigational drugs available.

CDC/IDSA/ASBMT Guidelines for the Prevention of Opportunistic Infections in Hematopoietic Stem Cell Transplant Recipients. CDC (Centers for Disease Control). IDSA (Infectious Diseases Society of America). ASBMT (American Society of Blood and Marrow Transplantation).

CDCR (conjunctivodacryocystorhinostomy).

CD4-IgG—a drug used to treat HIV-positive mothers and babies.

CD5+ monoclonal antibody—used in treating graft-versus-host disease.

CD8 AIS CELLector—a device used in treatment for Kaposi sarcoma, a rare form of skin cancer that affects HIV-positive patients. The CD8 AIS CELLector isolates the patient's CD8 cells, which serve to separate and multiply the patient's own cancer-killing cells. Additional applications include the processing of stem cells for transfusion or bone marrow transplantation, and the treatment of cancer and AIDS.

CD18 antibodies—may, in the future, help reduce some kinds of heart damage after a heart attack. In research trials, the antibodies prevent the attachment to the artery walls of polymorphonuclear leukocytes which form as a result of heart injury, usually attaching first to arterial walls and then squeezing through them into the heart tissue. With CD18 antibodies, the PMNs continue to circulate harmlessly through the body.

CD26—a protease. This HIV co-receptor acts as a door for cell penetration. Scientists hope to use this new target to develop a vaccine for all HIV strains.

CDH (congenital dysplasia of the hip). Also, dislocation.

CD Horizon Eclipse spinal system.

CD Horizon M8 multiaxial screws for lumbar fixation.

CD Horizon Sextant spinal system—used in minimally invasive spinal fusion.

CDI (Cotrel-Dubousset instrumentation).

CDI 2000 blood gas monitoring system—bedside (point of care) monitoring system that measures arterial pH, PCO_2, and PO_2. The system decreases therapeutic decision time and is advantageous for patients needing frequent blood gas monitoring. Lack of blood loss and reduced infection risk to patient and operator are major advantages.

cDNA (complementary DNA).

CDP (computerized dynamic posturography).

CDR (computed dental radiography).

Cd-texaphyrin—photosensitizing drug used in laser surgery.

CE (capillary electrophoresis)—a technique for rapid separation and analysis of peptides and proteins.

CE (center edge) **angle**—see *Wiberg center edge angle*.

CEA (carcinoembryonic antigen).

CEA (carotid endarterectomy).

CEAker—an anti-CEA monoclonal antibody labeled with indium 111; used to detect recurrent colorectal carcinoma.

CEAP classification—used in diagnosis of chronic venous disease of the lower extremities: assesses **c**linical manifestations, **e**tiologic factors, **a**natomic involvement, and **patho**physiologic features.

CEA-Scan—diagnostic imaging product for screening of colorectal cancer. The technique uses radiolabeled antibodies in conjunction with technetium Tc 99m to detect tumors within hours, using conventional gamma cameras. The use of a small fragment of antibody will reduce immune reactions by patients to the foreign protein.

ceased to breathe (CTB).

CEA-Tc 99m—carcinoembryonic antigen (a monoclonal antibody) plus ^{99m}Tc (a technetium isotope) imaging agent. See *RAID, ImmuRAID*.

Cebotome—orthopedic tool by Zimmer. Also, *Neurairtome, Surgairtome.*

CECT (contrast enhancement of computed tomographic) head and body imaging.

Cedell fracture—fracture of posterior process of the talus which may result in tarsal tunnel syndrome.

CeeOn heparinized intraocular lens.

cefazolin and dextrose—used for treatment of respiratory tract infections.

Celestin latex rubber tube—used in dilation of the esophagus in treatment for peptic stricture.

celiac dimple—the anatomic area of slight depression in the abdomen.

celiacography—used to diagnose hemangiomata.

cell
- adult stem
- Betz
- Bloch
- bone marrow stromal
- clue

cell *(cont.)*
- Deiters
- diploid human
- eating (phagocyte)
- embryonic germ
- embryonic stem
- eukaryotic
- foam
- gelbe
- germ
- glitter
- ground-glass
- HeLa
- helle
- helper
- hematopoietic stem
- heterokaryon
- hybrid
- hybridoma
- inducer
- islet
- koilocytotic
- Kulchitsky
- Kupffer
- LAK (lymphokine-activated killer)
- Leydig
- LUCs (large undifferentiated cells)
- macrophage colon-forming (M-CFC)
- mast
- multinucleated giant
- multipotent adult progenitor cells (MAPC)
- NK (natural killer)
- null
- oligopotent progenitor
- oxyphil
- peripheral blood progenitor (PBPC)
- Pelger-Huët
- phagocyte
- primordial germ
- progenitor
- Sézary
- somatic
- stem
- suppressor

cell *(cont.)*
T&B (T and B)
Tart
T-cell (thymus)
T-8 suppressor
T-4
theca
thymus dependent
TRC
umbrella
universal donor
zymogen

cell and flare (*not* flair) (Oph)—an accumulation of white blood cells and an increase of protein in the aqueous which can be seen on slit-lamp examination of the anterior chamber of the eye. A sign of iritis or ciliary body inflammation.

Cellano phenotype (Kell blood group) —see *McLeod blood phenotype*.

cell assay test—see *Raji cell assay test*.

cell-based therapy—a form of treatment in which stem cells are induced to differentiate into specific cells of the type required to repair damaged or depleted adult cell populations or tissues.

cell culture—growth of cells in vitro on an artificial medium.

cell division—a process by which a single cell divides to form two daughter cells, with nothing left over; preceded by division and reapportionment of genetic material in the nucleus (mitosis in somatic cells, meiosis in gametes).

Cellect graft preparation device—a bone marrow aspiration technique for iliac crest cell harvest, used to obtain osteogenic graft material that is rich in cells that can be prepared by surgeons without subjecting the patient to an iliac crest graft harvesting procedure. The Selective Retention process can be quickly performed intraoperatively and delivered to the patient at a reasonable cost.

cell line—a self-perpetuating or self-renewing colony of cells grown in culture and having an indefinite life span.

Cellegesic (nitroglycerin ointment)—a medication for the treatment of chronic anal fissures, with the potential for broader use in hemorrhoids and dyspareunia.

cell-mediated immunity (CMI).

cell nuclear replacement (CNR)—a procedure that involves removing the nucleus of a human donor egg, replacing it with the genetic material from the nucleus of an easily obtainable cell, such as skin, heart, or nerve from the patient, and then stimulating this cell to divide. Once a group of cells has been formed, stem cells can be extracted a few days later.

Cellolite—a form of patty material (see *cottonoid patty*) produced as an alternative to cottonoid; made of polyvinyl alcohol foam cross-linked with formaldehyde, and impregnated with particles of barium sulfate.

cellophane crackles—sounds resembling crunching of cellophane present on auscultation of the lungs in patients with diffuse interstitial pulmonary fibrosis.

Cellpatch—an investigational drug delivery system that enables both the formation of a standardized small epidermal bleb and exposure of the circular base of the bleb to drug. The epidermis is split off by suctioning without bleeding or discomfort in a layer superficial to dermal capillaries and nociceptor nerves. Transdermal invasion is thus avoided.

cell ratio—see *helper-suppressor*.

cell recovery system (CRS)—an automated medical device used to brush and retrieve cells from surfaces of internal organs, such as the bladder. The endoscopic procedure is minimally invasive and can be performed in a physician's office.

Cell Saver Haemolite—a washed red cell autotransfusion system for use in low-volume blood loss procedures. Can be used intraoperatively and postoperatively.

cell seeding (of vascular grafts)—the seeding of a vascular graft with the patient's own cells by various methods. Also, graft seeding technique.

CellSpray—a product that is sprayed on skin to treat patients with severe burns.

celltrifuge—a coined word for a device to remove white blood cells from blood of patients with leukemia.

Cellugel ophthalmic viscosurgical device (OVD)—viscoelastic solution for use in the anterior segment of the eye. It is used to create and maintain space, to protect the corneal endothelium and other intraocular tissues, and to manipulate tissues during surgery.

cellular xenograft rejection—rejection reaction involving the transplantation of cells or tissue of animal origin, thought to be T-cell mediated as in an allograft rejection response.

cellular xenotransplantation—transplantation of tissue or cells of animal origin, more successful than solid organ xenotransplantation.

Celsior—an organ preservation solution used to preserve the heart prior to cardiac transplantation and to promote graft function in the initial 48 hours after cardiac transplant.

Celsius control endovascular catheter—used in procedures employing hypothermia.

Celsius DS (dual sensor) diagnostic/ablation catheter—used in treatment of atrial flutter.

cement—see *adhesive*.

cementless jumbo cup—used in revision hip arthroplasty.

Cementless Spotorno (CLS) **hip arthroplasty stem**.

cementless surface replacement arthroplasty (CSRA)—technique that replaces damaged joint-bearing surfaces and restores normal anatomy, with minimal bone resection and insertion of cementless prosthesis.

cementophyte—an excrescence of cement (such as methylmethacrylate), the result of a previous arthrotomy, in contrast to osteophyte, which is a bony excrescence or osseous outgrowth.

Cemex system (Ortho)—an integrated system that contains, prepares, and extrudes bone cement.

Cenflex central monitoring system.

Centauri Er:YAG laser system—for tooth procedures, including decay removal, cavity preparation for restorations, and related applications. It works by vaporizing the bacteria along with the decay to provide a virtually sterile area for restoration. Reportedly eliminates the need for traditional dental anesthesia and the drill.

center-edge (CE) **angle of Wiberg**.

Center for Epidemiological Studies–Depression (CES-D) **scale**.

Centers for Disease Control and Prevention (CDC).

centigray (cGy)—an SI unit of absorbed radiation dose equal to 1 rad. See *gray*.

centimeter (cm) (often pronounced "sona-meter")—type the abbreviation "cm" in a report when dictated with a numeral. The measurement is written out only when dictated without a numeral (e.g., "visibility was limited to a very few centimeters beyond the junction").

centimorgan (cM) (Genetics)—in genetic linkage studies, a unit that represents 1% recombination. Synonym: map unit.

centistoke—a unit of measurement of plasma viscosity and serum viscosity.

central venous catheter (CVC)—an intravenous catheter inserted into the subclavian vein (occasionally into the internal jugular vein) and advanced so that the tip is just above the right atrium. Used to administer fluids, drugs, or total parenteral nutrition on a long-term basis.

Centralign Precoat Hip prosthesis—precoat cemented hip replacement components by Zimmer.

centric relation-centric occlusion (CR/CO).

centriole—either of two organelles that migrate to opposite poles of a cell in preparation for cell division and form the points of focus of the chromosomal spindle during mitosis.

centromere—the central region of a chromosome at which the long and short arms are attached.

cEOEs (click-evoked otoacoustic emissions)—see *Echocheck*.

cephalopelvic disproportion (CPD)—a condition in which the head of the fetus is too large to enter the pelvic outlet; used in ultrasound and x-ray pelvimetry reports.

cephalosporins—a group of antibiotic drugs with a broad spectrum of antibacterial activity, divided into first-, second-, and third-generation cephalosporins. This designation has nothing to do with when these antibiotics were discovered or first marketed, but instead divides them by their therapeutic antibiotic properties. First generation, such as Ancef (cefazolin) and Keflex (cephalexin), are generally inactivated by bacteria that produce penicillinase. Third generation, such as Suprax (cefixime) and Fortaz, Tazidime (ceftazidime), show the greatest activity against gram-negative bacteria and resistant strains of bacteria.

CeQUAL protocol—Cedars Quantitative Analysis, a cardiac rehabilitation therapy protocol. Type the acronym; do not expand.

c-erbB-2 oncogene levels (Lab)—determined in breast cancer patients before therapy as an important biomarker to assess the extent of disease spread in the lymph nodes. Also, serum c-erbB-2 levels are elevated in patients with advanced-stage colorectal cancer and liver metastasis.

cerclage—encircling, hooping, banding. Also *cervical cerclage*, used for incompetent cervix in pregnancy. See *Dall-Miles cable grip*.

cerebellopontile angle tumor—a brain tumor located between the cerebellum and the pons. It involves cranial nerves V through VIII. Spasms of eyelid muscles, oscillating eye movements, loss of corneal sensation, and impaired hearing are characteristic symptoms.

cerebral blood flow velocity (CBFV).

cerebral blood volume (CBV).

cerebral perfusion pressure (CPP).

cerebral salt-wasting (CSW) **syndrome** —a condition characterized by ex-

cerebral *(cont.)*
cessive natriuresis and subsequent hyponatremic dehydration in patients with intracranial disease. It must be differentiated from the syndrome of inappropriate [secretion of] antidiuretic hormone (SIADH).

cerebrospinal fluid rhinorrhea—leakage of cerebrospinal fluid from one or both nostrils due to an abnormal communication between the subdural space and the nasal cavity. Causes include head trauma, surgery on the nose, sinuses, or anterior cranial fossa, and intracranial infection. Invasion of the subdural space by pathogenic microorganisms from the upper respiratory tract can lead to life-threatening meningitis. The condition is treated endoscopically by the intranasal approach.

cerebrovascular accident (CVA)—a stroke.

Ceretec—technetium 99m (Tc-99m) contrast imaging agent commonly used with SPECT imaging to detect cerebrovascular accidents. It may also be used to help diagnose Alzheimer disease.

ceroid-like histiocytic granuloma—see *xanthogranulomatous cholecystitis*.

cerotinic acid—a saturated fatty acid.

Cerrobend radiation cutouts—electronic imaging ports (radiotherapy).

Certified Coding Specialist (CCS).

Certified Coding Specialist–Physician-based (CCS-P).

Certified Medical Transcriptionist (CMT)—an individual who has satisfied the requirements for voluntary certification through the American Association for Medical Transcription (AAMT).

Certified Nurse Midwife (CNM).

Cervex-Brush—used to simultaneously obtain ectocervical and endocervical cells for cytologic exam.

cervical aortic arch—an anomaly in which the aortic arch retains a cervical position. (The heart and aortic arches begin as cervical structures and migrate to the thorax during fetal development.) It is of no clinical significance in terms of symptomatology, but important in the differential diagnosis of pulsatile masses in the neck.

cervical collar or **support**
AOA halo traction
Bremer Halo Crown
Georgiade visor
Houston Halo traction
Miami Acute Collar
Miami J collar
Philadelphia collar
Plastizote
PMT halo system

cervical intraepithelial neoplasia (CIN)—a designation to describe preinvasive lesions of the cervix. The degree of abnormal cytology is expressed in grades 1-3. CIN-2 is severe dysplasia.

cervical rib—a congenital anomaly in which an extra rib arises from a cervical vertebra. There is controversy over whether this is a normal variant or a condition requiring surgery.

cervicography, cervigram (Ob-Gyn)—a noninvasive technique for photographing the cervix. It is similar to colposcopy but less expensive. Colposcopy requires extensive expertise to perform and to read, but cervicography, in combination with a Pap smear, appears more reliable in detecting malignant and premalignant lesions than either procedure alone.

cervicouterine junction—the junction between the cervix and the body of the uterus (corpus uteri). The term is not official anatomic terminology but is frequently dictated in gynecology and radiology imaging reports.

CES (cranial electrical stimulation).

CES-D (Center for Epidemiological Studies–Depression) scale.

Cetus trial—a trial of tumor necrosis factor in conjunction with interleukin-2 in the treatment of cancers that have been unresponsive to other therapy. Cetus is the corporation that manufactures tumor necrosis factor. See *tumor necrosis factor*.

cf. (L., *confer*, compare).

CF (counting fingers) (Oph).

CFA digital camera—produces high-resolution pictures for ophthalmologic detection of retinal problems, which can then be stored on a computer.

C_3F_8 gas (perfluoropropane)—used in pneumatic retinopexy, for correcting detached retina.

C-fiber—small unmyelinated nerve fiber.

CFIDS (chronic fatigue immune dysfunction syndrome).

CFL (calcaneofibular ligament).

CF-200Z Olympus colonoscope—enables high-power magnified observation of the surface of colorectal neoplasms.

CFU (colony-forming unit).

CFU-E (colony-forming unit—erythroid).

CFU-GM (colony-forming unit—granulocyte, monocyte).

CFU-meg or **CFU-MK** (colony-forming unit—megakaryocyte).

CF-UM3 echocolonoscope.

CG Future anuloplasty system—a mitral valve repair technique involving a low-profile band designed to remodel the anulus so as to maintain apposition of the anterior and posterior leaflets. Developed by valve-repair surgeons Colvin and Galloway.

CGL (chronic granulocytic leukemia).

cGy (centigray).

Chadwick sign—purplish or bluish discoloration of the cervix and vaginal mucosa, a normal finding in pregnancy early in gestation. Also, *Jacquemier sign*.

CHAG (coralline hydroxyapatite Goniopora)—a bone graft substitute material made by conversion of the calcium carbonate structure of reef-building sea corals into pure hydroxyapatite.

chair—see *wheelchairs* for list of chairs used in Rehabilitation reports.

chair-back brace (Ortho).

Chait percutaneous cecostomy—an antegrade colonic enema technique involving the percutaneous insertion of a tube into the cecum. Patients with fecal incontinence, or their caregivers, can use the cecostomy to administer a small-volume phosphate enema followed by a saline enema to quickly and completely evacuate and cleanse the large intestine, emptying through the anal opening.

chalazion—chronic inflammatory granulomatous process of a meibomian gland. See *meibomian cyst, tarsal cyst*.

ChAM (charcoal alveolar macrophage) **index**.

chamfer reamer (lowercase *c*).

Champ cardiac device.

Champion Trauma Score (CTS)—a scoring system used to evaluate multiple trauma injuries.

Chan wrist rest—a device used by ophthalmic surgeons to stabilize their hands, particularly when performing vitrectomies.

Chance fracture—a fracture of the lumbar vertebrae caused by extreme forward flexion of the spine above and below a seat belt during an automobile accident. Dr. C. Q. Chance first described this type of traumatic spinal fracture in 1948. Also known as a *seat belt fracture* and a *fulcrum fracture* because the seat belt acts as the point of a fulcrum which separates the upper and lower segments of the spinal column.

chandelier sign—extreme tenderness of the uterine adnexa, elicited on pelvic examination. (The term fancifully implies that the pain causes the patient to leap into the air and cling to the chandelier.)

channel opener

K

$K_{(ATP)}$

potassium

channel osteotomy—exposure osteotomy that provides improved access to posterior talar dome lesions, especially for the use of osteochondral autograft.

charcoal—see *activated charcoal.*

charcoal alveolar macrophage (ChAM) index—a laboratory test performed on bronchoalveolar lavage fluid that has been permeated with charcoal, used in the diagnosis of aspiration pneumonia.

Charcot-Bouchard aneurysm—aneurysmal formation in small arteries within the neural parenchyma.

Charcot-Leyden crystals—found in sputa of patients with bronchial asthma. Also, in aspiration of visceral larva migrans lesions. See *visceral larva migrans.*

Charite artificial disk for the spine—designed to treat severe low back pain by replacing a damaged or worn-out spinal disk with an artificial one. The new disk, made of two metal endplates and a plastic core, offers an alternative to the traditional surgery that fuses two bones in the lower spine.

Charles Bonnet syndrome—condition wherein elderly patients see strange figures or objects during hallucinations.

Charles flute needle (Oph).

charley horse—a painful spasm in a lower extremity, generally due to injury or strain.

Charnley Howorth Exflow system—a sterile air system for operating rooms to reduce infection rate, particularly used during arthroplasties.

Charnley reamer—used in hip replacement.

Charnley wire tightener—used in total hip arthroplasty.

CHART (continuous hyperfractionated accelerated radiotherapy).

chase bolus—an imaging technique in which a bolus of dye is injected, and the bolus is "chased" by a digital imaging camera. Also, *bolus chase.*

Chattanooga Balance System—a computer system attached to two foot pads. Used to document postural sway and instability in patients with strokes, head injuries, and neuromuscular disorders.

Cheatle slit—for takedown of colostomy.

Cheatle syndrome—see *fibrocystic breast syndrome.*

checkerboard mosaic pattern—appearance of unilateral nevus achromicus and congenital agminated Spitz nevi.

Check-Flo introducer—used to introduce balloon, electrode, closed-end, and other catheters; the seal on this prevents blood reflux and air aspiration.

checking—fine control of voluntary movement; the act of stopping a motion when its goal or purpose has been attained.

Checkmate intravascular brachytherapy system—used for recurrent blockage of coronary arteries in patients previously treated with coronary artery stents.

cheese worker's lung disease—extrinsic allergic alveolitis caused by exposure to moldy cheese.

Cheetah angioplasty catheter.

cheilectomy ("ky-LEK-to-me")—(1) excision of a lip; (2) an operative procedure in which bone edges that impede joint motion are removed, e.g., in hallux rigidus.

chelation therapy—oral or intravenous administration of medications such as ethylenediaminetetraacetic acid (EDTA) to remove metals such as lead, iron, and calcium from the body. It is used in alternative medicine, although its efficacy as a treatment for atherosclerosis has not yet been established in mainstream medicine.

chemical shift imaging (CSI) (Radiol).

chemical shift phenomena (MRI term) —spatially mismapped signals occurring at the interface of tissues with different chemical shifts. Fat suppression technique is helpful.

chemoembolization—the use of DSM (degradable starch microspheres) administered simultaneously with a chemotherapy drug. These microspheres temporarily block the blood flow at the capillary level. The chemotherapy drug is then concentrated in the region of the cancer and achieves high tissue uptake. See *DSM*.

Chemo-Port catheter—for administration of chemotherapeutic agents or for the delivery of nutritional fluids.

chemoprevention—administration of a natural or man-made agent to retard or prevent development or progression of cancer.

chemosis—edema of the conjunctiva of the eye.

chemotherapy code for evaluating progress:
- -2 definitely worse
- -1 probably worse
- 0 no change since last scan
- +1 probably better
- +2 definitely better

chemotherapy drugs—see *medication*.

chemotherapy-induced nausea and vomiting (CINV).

chemotherapy protocol—see individual main entries alphabetically throughout the book. Also listed under *medication*.

Chemstrip bG—a plastic strip used in checking blood glucose. Cf. *Dextrostix*, used in a similar manner. The blood spot on the treated strip is wiped off and rinsed with water, and then the resulting color is compared with a color chart, which gives the blood glucose value.

Chemstrip MatchMaker blood glucose meter—for self-testing by diabetics.

ChemTrak AccuMeter—screens for *H. pylori* bacteria commonly associated with stomach ulcers.

ChemTrak *Helicobacter pylori* test—a one-step test that can detect the presence of *H. pylori* within minutes during an office visit.

Cheng-Ferkel grading system—grading system used during arthroscopy to determine the extent of osteochondral lesions (uses letters A through F).

Cherf leg holder—supports lower extremity during knee and hip surgery.

Cherney incision—lower transverse abdominal incision.

cherry angioma—benign hemangioma that is a round, cherry-red, dome-shaped papule; usually seen in the elderly. Called *Campbell de Morgan spots,* or *De Morgan spots.*

Cherry-Crandall test—of serum lipase.

cherry-red endobronchial lesions of Kaposi sarcoma—a finding on bronchoscopy.

Chester-Erdheim disease—a rare lipid storage disorder characterized by hardening of the growth areas of the long bones of the body. Lipid cell deposits (histiocytes) are found in various vital organs of the body such as heart, lungs, peritoneum, kidneys, and other tissues. Severity of the disease differs with each patient, but the outcome is generally fatal.

chest
flail
funnel

chest PT—the use of positioning (postural drainage) and clapping with a cupped hand over the patient's chest and back (frappage) to loosen pulmonary secretions. The patient may cough up the secretions, or they may be suctioned out. Also, *percussion.*

chest shell—used for noninvasive extrathoracic ventilation (NEV) during transport.

chevron incision—the name derives from the V shape of the incision.

C'H_{50}—total hemolytic complement.

CHF (congestive heart failure).

Chiari I malformation (Peds).

Chiba tip on Skinny needle—used in percutaneous transhepatic cholangiography.

Chick CLT—operating table and frame for orthopedic surgery.

Chilaiditi ("ky-la-dee-tee") **syndrome**—interposition of the colon (sometimes the small intestine) between the liver and the diaphragm. This is a result of a congenital anomaly of the diaphragm or the falciform ligament, which is a fold of peritoneum from the diaphragm to the surface of the liver.

chilblain—local cutaneous inflammation caused by exposure to cold and damp.

Child class (A, B, and C)—a classification system for esophageal varices.

Child classification of hepatic risk criteria—class A, class B, and class C. Relates to operative risk.

Child-Pugh class A, B, or **C**—used in hepatic disease.

Child Pugh scale—a scale for grading bleeding esophageal varices, grades A-C.

Child-Turcotte classification—used in hepatic surgery.

Child-Turcotte-Pugh classification—used to assess the severity of cirrhosis; degrees of cirrhosis classified as class A, B, or C. Also called *Child class.*

Chilli cooled ablation catheters—incorporating real-time position management (RPM) navigation technology.

chimera ("ki-mé-ra," named for a monster of Greek myth)—an organism composed of cells derived from at least two genetically different zygotes, from the same or different species; it can occur naturally, but the term usually refers to the laboratory

chimera *(cont.)* creation of an artificial zygote by replacement of the nucleus of a cell with a cell nucleus taken from another individual.

Chinese fingertrap—a tube formed of flat strips of flexible material obliquely interwoven in such a way that, once a finger is firmly inserted in the tube, efforts to withdraw it tighten the tube by reducing its circumference. Originally a toy, it is used in orthopedics to apply traction to a finger during surgery or fracture healing.

chink—a small diamond-shaped (or triangular-shaped) opening between the posterior ends of the vocal cords in vocal cord dysfunction. A "chink" is opposed to complete closure of the space between the vocal cords. See *vocal cord dysfunction*.

chin-to-jugulum distance—a term used in assessing ankylosing spondylitis.

Chlamydia pneumoniae **bodies**—detected in atherosclerotic lesions. Seropositivity for *C. pneumoniae* is associated with an increased intima-media thickness in the common carotid artery but not plaque status in hypertensive men at high risk for cardiovascular disease.

Chlamydia trachomatis—a gram-negative organism.

chloracetate esterase (Leder stain).

chocolate agar—a culture medium.

chocolatization—brown discoloration of a blood culture medium by metabolic products of certain organisms, including *Streptococcus pneumoniae*, growing on the medium.

Cho/Dyonics two-portal endoscopic system (Hand Surg).

choked disk—edema and hyperemia of the optic disk, usually associated with increased intracranial pressure. Also called *papilledema*.

Cholangiocath—used in GI surgery.

cholecystectomy—see *operation*.

cholecystitis—see *xanthogranulomatous cholecystitis*.

cholecystocholedocholithiasis—gallstones in gallbladder and common duct.

cholecystokinin (CCK)—thought to be one of the important hormones regulating gallbladder contraction. See *noncholecystokinin substance*.

choledochofiberscope—Olympus URF-P2 translaparoscopic.

cholescintigraphy—radionuclide test; ^{99m}Tc PIPIDA is injected intravenously, giving prompt visualization of the liver, bile ducts, and gallbladder. Absence of dye in the gastrointestinal tract indicates obstruction of the common duct. If the gallbladder is not visualized, this is an indication of acute cholecystitis or of obstruction of the cystic duct or hepatic duct. See *PIPIDA*.

Cholestech LDX system with the TC (total cholesterol) and **glucose panel**—used to measure cholesterol and glucose levels at the same time from a single drop of blood and receive the results within five minutes. The system consists of a portable blood analyzer and disposable test cassettes and measures total cholesterol, HDL cholesterol, triglycerides, and glucose levels, and provides a calculated LDL cholesterol.

Cholesterol Manager—home cholesterol management kit. It consists of two parts: CholesTrak, a device to determine cholesterol levels, and Total-Lo, a chewable plant-derived tablet taken with each meal to block absorption of cholesterol in the intestines.

Cholesterol 1,2,3—a test for cholesterol via the skin using the palm of the hand. Note: No spaces between comma and number.

CholesTrak home cholesterol test—used by patients with high cholesterol who are trying to achieve better cholesterol levels through diet and exercise. See also *Cholesterol Manager*.

Choletec (technetium ^{99m}Tc mebrofenin)—hepatobiliary imaging agent.

chondrocutaneous advancement flap—used in reconstruction of full-thickness marginal defects of the ear.

chondromalacia patellae (*not* patella, even though only one knee is involved); *patellae* is (Latin) genitive case, meaning *of the patella*.

Chonstruct chondral repair system—used for repair of chondral defects of the articular cartilage. A paste consisting of a mixture of the patient's cancellous bone and articular cartilage is used as an anatomic patch for repair of the defect with a supportive matrix to promote new cartilage formation.

Chopart ankle dislocation of navicula and cuboid across talus and calcaneus.

chordate—having a notochord (primitive backbone). See *caudate, cordate*.

chordae—plural of *chorda*; e.g., chordae tympani. Do not confuse with *chordee*.

chordee—a congenital defect that involves stricture of the fibrous tissue of the penis and that causes the penis to bow. This condition is often associated with a hypospadias. Do not confuse with *chordae*.

chordoma (*not* cordoma)—a malignant tumor arising from the embryonic remains of the notochord (primitive backbone).

chordotomy—see *cordotomy*.

chorionic villi biopsy (CVB).

chorionic villous sampling (CVS)—a biopsy of placental (chorionic) villi performed in early pregnancy to detect genetic defects in the fetus. Under ultrasonic guidance, tissue is aspirated from the villous area of the chorion either by a catheter inserted through the cervix or by needle puncture of the abdominal wall. The risk of miscarriage after chorionic villus biopsy is 2-4%.

chorioretinopathy, birdshot (Oph).

choristoma—a benign tumor containing tissues foreign to the tissue in which the tumor is found, e.g., bone found in muscle tissue.

choroidal hemangioma—benign vascular hamartoma.

choroidal neovascularization (CNV).

choroidal neovascular membrane.

Chow technique—a modified technique for performance of endoscopic carpal ligament release through an open slotted cannula, performed under local anesthesia without a tourniquet; developed by Dr. James Chow.

Chrisman and Snook procedure—modification of the Elmslie procedure using half of the peroneus brevis tendon to correct lateral ankle instability.

Christmas disease—factor IX deficiency (hemophilia B). See *hemophilia A*. Named for the child in whom it was first identified.

Christmas tree appearance of pancreas (Radiol).

Christmas tree pattern—seen in the skin eruption of pityriasis rosea.

Christoudias fascial closure device—for closing wounds.

chromatid—either of the two parallel strands into which a chromosome divides during mitosis; each will become a chromosome of a daughter cell.

chromatin—older, general term for the nucleoprotein fibers of which a chromosome is composed.

chromatography
affinity
gas

ChromaVision digital analyzer—an automated intelligent microscopy system used for prenatal screening for Down syndrome and for HIV and cancer detection.

chromomere—a densely coiled region of chromatin on a chromosome; chromomeres are responsible for the beaded appearance of chromosomes.

chromopertubation—a test used in the evaluation of infertility. Dye is injected into the cervix through the vagina; a laparoscopic incision permits visualization of where the dye goes, to determine if the fallopian tubes are patent. Also called *chromohydrotubation*.

chromosomal aberration (Genetics)—any abnormality in the structure of one or more chromosomes or in their number.

chromosomally mediated-resistant *Neisseria gonorrhoeae*—a penicillin-resistant gonococcus.

chromosomal satellite (Genetics)—a small mass of chromatin seen at the distal extremity of the short arm of each of the two chromatids derived from an acrocentric chromosome.

chromosome—any of a group of paired structures in the cell nucleus (23 pairs in human cells), consisting chiefly of long coiled strands of DNA, that determine the genetic makeup of an organism. One of each pair is contributed by each parent. Chromosomes are made up of subunits called genes, each of which codes for a specific trait.

chromosome 14q—a tumor marker for patients with nonpapillary renal cell carcinoma (RCC). Patients with 14q deletion are found to have higher stages and grades of nonpapillary RCC.

chronic—persistent or prolonged, as in chronic bronchitis, chronic steroid therapy.

chronic bacterial prostatitis (CBP).

chronic fatigue immune dysfunction syndrome (CFIDS)—newer name by the Centers for Disease Control for what is usually called *chronic fatigue syndrome*.

chronic fatigue syndrome (CFS) (also known as *chronic fatigue immune dysfunction syndrome, myalgic encephalomyelitis, postviral fatigue syndrome,* and *yuppie flu*)—characterized by fatigue, irritability, sleep loss, forgetfulness, and muscle pain. Many of the patients are also depressed, and whether this is one of the symptoms of the disease or relates to the isolation, exhaustion, pain, and the fact that many physicians do not recognize this as a disease entity is not known. Symptoms last for months or even years, and seem to affect more women than men. See also *chronic fatigue immune dysfunction syndrome.*

chronic idiopathic urticaria (CIU)—relapsing hives of unknown cause.

Chronic Pain Coping Inventory (CPCI)—used as a predictor of depression in patients suffering chronic pain.

chronic intestinal pseudo-obstruction—syndrome manifested by signs and symptoms of obstruction but without true mechanical obstruction. See *familial visceral neuropathy*.

Chronicle implantable hemodynamic monitor.

chronic lunger—a pejorative term not used in the patient's presence. Usage: "The patient is a chronic lunger who no longer smokes." It refers to a patient who has had chronic long-term lung disease, particularly tuberculosis or chronic obstructive pulmonary disease.

chronic myeloid leukemia (CML).

chronic myelomonocytic leukemia (CMML).

chronic otitis media with effusion status post bilateral myringotomy with tympanostomy tube (COME s/p BMTT).

chronic pulmonary emphysema (CPE).

chronic regional pain syndrome—see *complex regional pain syndrome (CRPS)*.

chronotherapy—a technique for administering chemotherapy drugs that follows the body's biorhythms; it shows increased effectiveness in shrinking tumor size when compared to standard administration schedules.

Chrysalin—synthetic peptide used to accelerate healing of chronic wounds.

CHRYS CO_2 laser—a portable carbon dioxide laser as small as a desktop computer. Intended for use in physician offices and outpatient surgery centers.

chrysiasis—a rare blue-gray skin discoloration that occurs in sun-exposed sites of some patients who receive gold salts for treatment of psoriatic arthritis.

CHST6 (carbohydrate sulfotransferase-6) **gene assay**—a laboratory test to diagnose macular corneal dystrophy. CHST6 is a causative gene for macular corneal dystrophy.

CHUK (conserved helix-loop-helix ubiquitous kinase)—protein that is believed to play a key role in inflammatory response. Identification of this protein may help treat a number of inflammatory diseases, including rheumatoid arthritis, inflammatory bowel disease, septic shock, and asthma.

Churg-Strauss syndrome—allergic granulomatosis.

chymonucleolysis—use of chymopapain to break down nucleus pulposus of herniated disk. Rarely used but will continue to appear in dictation as patients return with continued back problems.

Ciaglia percutaneous tracheostomy introducer—allows for bedside placement of tracheal tube for fewer complications than traditional open surgical technique.

Cibis ski needle—a flat needle used as an aid in placing an encircling band in retinal surgery.

C-IBS (constipation-predominant irritable bowel syndrome).

Cica-Care topical gel sheeting—adhesive topical gel sheeting used for the management of hypertrophic and keloid scars and to lessen the overall effect of scarring following surgery.

CIC (clean intermittent catheterization).

CIC (completely-in-the-[ear] canal) **hearing aid**. See *Argosy Cameo* and *Unitron Esteem*.

ciclesonide—inhaled corticosteroid for asthma. See *Alvesco*.

cidal level (serum cidal; bactericidal): the amount of an antibiotic needed in the blood to kill an organism.

CIE (countercurrent immunoelectrophoresis)—test for amebic antigen.

CIF-4 needle (Oph).

cilantro—kills harmful salmonella bacteria and shows promise as a safe, natural food additive that could help prevent foodborne illness.

Cilco Slant lens—a single-piece intraocular lens with a design that incorporates slanted haptics and a low profile for easy insertion through the longer scleral tunnel and more acute angle of entry now used in intraocular lens surgery. *Slant* is a trade name. Also called *Slant lens*.

Cilostazol for Restenosis (CREST) **study**.

CIN (cervical intraepithelial neoplasia).

CINA (Clinical Institute Narcotic Assessment) **scale**—a scale for withdrawal symptoms.

cinacalcet HCl—see *Sensipar*.

cinchonism ("sin-koh-nism") (from cinchona, the plant from which quinine is obtained)—the manifestations of quinine toxicity: tinnitus, blurred vision, nausea, headache, and possibly thrombocytopenia.

cinctured—encircled. Verb/adjective form coined from noun *cincture*.

cineangiography—studies of the cardiac vasculature performed by teams including cardiologists and radiologists. The cine (motion picture) films can be studied later by many physicians.

cine CT (computed tomography) **scanner**—provides a movie of the contractions of the heart wall and the blood flow in the brain. It can evaluate coronary artery bypass graft function, detect regional thickening of the myocardium or abnormalities in wall motion, and estimate cardiac output. Also, *ultrafast CT*.

cine view in MUGA (cinematograph in multiple gated acquisition) **scan**—a moving picture of the cardiac cycle, constructed from individual frames, of which each is a composite image of one point in the cardiac cycle obtained by cardiac gating.

cingulate gyrus ("sing-gyu-late")—an elevation of the brain surface, just above the corpus callosum.

CINV (chemotherapy-induced nausea and vomiting).

CIP (chronic intestinal pseudo-obstruction).

CIPA—see *congenital insensitivity to pain and anhidrosis*.

Cipro XR (ciprofloxacin)—extended-release formulation of the drug.

circinate ("sur-sin-ate")—ringlike or circular.

circinate-pattern interstitial keratopathy—occurs in soft contact lens wearers.

circinate retinopathy—a condition marked by white spots encircling the macular area, which results in complete foveal blindness.

circle of death—attributed to an aberrant obturator artery that can bleed from both sides of an injury because of existing anastomosis. In laparoscopic herniorrhaphies, there is the danger of not identifying the aberrant artery because of the limited visibility of abdominal and pelvic anatomy. If inadvertently cut, it may bleed profusely, resulting in the death of the patient. It is, therefore, important that physicians performing laparoscopic procedures be able to identify internal anatomy "with

circle *(cont.)*
their eyes closed," so to speak, and that they anticipate such anomalies.

Circon video camera—used for arthroscopy. The camera is connected to the arthroscope and provides color reproduction reported to be almost identical to that perceived by the human eye. Also, *Saticon and Newvicon*, *Vidicon vacuum chamber pickup tube for camera*.

Circon videohydrothoracoscope—an instrument that allows for viewing and irrigation through the same port during thoracoscopy, a minimally invasive surgical procedure.

Circon-ACMI electrohydraulic lithotriptor probe (Urol).

CircPlus—compression dressing or wrap.

circulation—see *extracorporeal circulation*.

circularplasty—see *endoventricular circular patchplasty*.

circulator boot therapy—an external compression device attached to the lower extremity and timed to the cardiac cycle. As the heart pumps and the pressure head of the blood reaches the extremity, the boot gives the blood an extra push to force it through diseased vessels. The device also helps stimulate alternative blood vessels to bring oxygenated blood to diseased parts of the extremity.

Circulon dressing or wrap.

circumduction ("sur-kum-duk-shun") —the rotational movement, active or passive, of an eye, or of an extremity. Cf. *sursumduction*.

circumduction-adduction shoulder maneuver—see *Clancy test*.

circumferential fracture—extends completely around the skull, leaving the skull essentially in two pieces.

circumferential wrap—see *aortomyoplasty*.

circumscribed choroidal hemangioma (CCH).

circus-movement tachycardia (CMT).

circus senilis (often used interchangeably with *arcus senilis)*—a hazy gray ring around the periphery of the cornea, composed of lipid droplets.

CIRF (cocaine-induced respiratory failure).

CirKuit-Guard—device for cardiovascular and vascular surgery.

cirsodesis ("sur-sod-ee-sis")—ligation of varicose veins.

CIS (carcinoma in situ).

cisplatin (cis-platinum—an antineoplastic drug. When cisplatin first appeared, it was called *cis-platinum*, although this term is rarely used today. *Cisplatin* (lowercase *c*) is the current approved name in all nomenclature systems. If a doctor dictates cis-platinum, it would be better to type the internationally recognized name, cisplatin.

cisternography—see *oxygen cisternography*.

cite—to bring forward, as for illustration; to quote, as proof or by way of authority; to summon to appear. Usage: "It may be necessary to cite an example." Cf. *site*.

Citrobacter amalonaticus (formerly *C. freundii*)—associated with enteritis, septicemia, urinary tract infections, pneumonia, and burn and wound infections.

Citrobacter braakii—a newly formed specific genomospecies 6 of the *Citrobacter freundii* complex.

Citrobacter koseri.

Citscope—a disposable arthroscope.

citta ("sit'-ah")—the craving for unusual foods during pregnancy (strawberries, pickles, etc.).

CIU—see *chronic idiopathic urticaria.*

CIWA (Clinical Institute Withdrawal Assessment) **detox protocol**—guidelines for assessing and treating withdrawal symptoms from a variety of toxic substances including drugs and alcohol. Also, *CIWA-A scale.*

CK (creatine kinase).

CK (conductive keratoplasty).

CK_1, CK_2, CK_3—isoenzymes of creatine kinase.

CK/AST (creatine kinase/aspartate aminotransferase) **ratio**.

CKC (cold knife cone) **biopsy**.

CKPT (combined kidney and pancreas transplant).

CLA (conjugated linoleic acid).

Cladosporium—an inhalant antigen.

Clagett-Barrett esophagogastrostomy.

clamp or **clip**
- Absolok extra absorbable ligating clip
- Acland microvascular clamp
- Atrauclip hemostatic clip
- Benjamin-Havas fiberoptic light clip
- Best right-angle colon clamp
- Bihrle dorsal clamp
- cardiac retraction clip
- Castaneda anastomosis clamp
- Cope crushing clamp
- Cope modification of Martel intestinal clamp
- Cunningham clamp
- Dardik clamp
- DuVal lung-grasping clamp
- Filshie female sterilization clip
- Fukushima C-clamp
- Glassman clamp
- Goldstein Microspike approximator
- Gregory clamp
- Gusberg hysterectomy clamp
- Hemoclip
- Hem-o-lok
- Jahnke anastomosis clamp
- Klintmalm clamp

clamp *(cont.)*
- Lane bone-holding clamp
- Ligaclip
- Locke clamp
- Masters intestinal
- Mayfield three-pin skull clamp
- mosquito clamp
- Multiclip
- Neuromeet nerve approximator
- Olsen cholangiogram clamp
- Omed bulldog vascular clamp
- Parker-Kerr intestinal clamp
- Perneczky aneurysm clamp
- Raney clip
- Right Clip
- Sarot bronchus clamp
- Secu clip
- Selverstone clamp
- side-biting clamp
- Sugita right angle aneurysm clip
- Verbrugge bone clamp
- Wertheim clamp
- Zinnanti Z-clamp
- Z-clamp

clamshell brace (Ortho).

clamshell incision—same as transverse anterior thoracotomy incision.

Clancy test—also called the circumduction-adduction shoulder maneuver. It is said to be 95% sensitive and specific for diagnosing rotator cuff tendinopathy, including partial tears.

Clanton and DeLee classification—grading system for osteochondritis dissecans (uses Arabic numerals).

Clarion cochlear implant—a hearing implant for pediatric patients. It bypasses ear damage, sending electric signals directly to the auditory nerve. These signals are then interpreted by the brain as sounds.

Clarion HiFocus electrode—the component of the Clarion cochlear implant that is implanted into the inner ear. This electrode has been

Clarion *(cont.)*
approved for treatment of hearing impairment in children as young as 18 months of age.

Clarion multi-strategy cochlear implant (ENT)—for use in post-lingually deafened adults.

Clark classification of malignant melanoma, levels I-IV. Named for the pathologist who devised it, Wallace H. Clark, Jr., M.D.

Clark-Elder classification—a classification of malignant melanoma. See also *Clark* and *Elder*.

Clarke-Reich micro knot pusher—for use with suture sizes 6-0 and smaller.

Clarke sign (or **test**)—to help diagnose chondromalacia patellae. The patient lies relaxed with the knee extended. While the examiner presses down gently on the upper pole of the patella, the patient is asked to contract the quadriceps muscle. If this causes retropatellar pain and the patient cannot hold a quadriceps contraction, the test is considered positive.

Clark perineorrhaphy (Gyn).

Clarus spinescope—a percutaneous spinal endoscope used for treatment of chronic spinal pain by interventional anesthesiologists.

classic abdominal Semm hysterectomy (CASH)—transabdominal hysterectomy done via laparoscopy, pioneered by German surgeon Kurt Semm. It leaves the extrafascial, highly vascularized vascular stem, the corresponding nerves, and the topography of the ureter untouched during extracervical enucleation (removal of part or all of a mass in its entirety) of the fascia of the uterine body, removing the uterus. Because the cardinal ligaments are preserved as well as the nerve supply of the cervical fascia, transvaginal sexual sensations are not impaired. Suspension of the cervical fascia at the supporting ligaments of the uterus can be performed in this procedure.

classic triad of Rigler—see *triad of Rigler.*

classification, **grade,** or **stage**
- Altmann congenital aural atresia
- Astler-Coller modification of Dukes classification
- Baylor bleeding score
- Behavioral Pathology in Alzheimer Disease Rating Scale
- Bethesda rating scale for Pap smears
- Binet classification of chronic lymphocytic leukemia
- Bismuth classification, types I-IV
- Bismuth-Corlette classification
- Blaivas urinary incontinence
- Blakeley
- Breslow classification for malignant melanoma
- Broders tumor index
- Brooker periarticular heterotopic ossification (PHO)
- burns classification
- CEAP
- chemotherapy code
- Child esophageal varices
- Child hepatic risk criteria
- Child-Pugh A, B, C classification
- Child-Turcotte classification
- Child-Turcotte-Pugh classification
- CIN (cervical intraepithelial neoplasia)
- Clanton and DeLee
- Clark-Elder malignant melanoma
- Clark malignant melanoma
- cleaved cell non-Hodgkin lymphoma

classification *(cont.)*
Coleman congenital aural atresia
concussion grades
Couinaud
de la Cruz classification of congenital aural atresia
Delbet fracture classification
DeSmet criteria
diabetes mellitus classification
diastasis of ankle sprain classification
Dukes-Astler-Coller adenocarcinoma
Dukes carcinoma
Edmondson-Steiner grading of hepatocellular carcinoma
Elder malignant melanoma
Erlanger and Gasser peripheral nerve classification
FAB (French/American/British)
FIGO classification
Floyd peripheral nerve
Forrest classification of gastroduodenal ulcer
Framingham criteria for heart failure
Fredrickson lipid disorders
Frykman classification of hand fractures
Glasgow classification of choledocholithiasis
Greenwich grading system
Gurd criteria
Gustilo fracture
Harvard Criteria for Brain Death
Healey classification
Highet and Sander criteria of Mackinnon and Dellon, modified
Highet and Sander criteria of Zachary and Holmes, modified
HIV children classification
Hoehn and Yahr Parkinson staging
House-Brackmann facial weakness scale

classification *(cont.)*
Hunt and Hess neurological
Hyams grading system for esthesioneuroblastoma
hypertension standard
ICD-9, ICD-10 (International Classification of Diseases) (coding)
IMIG (International Mesothelioma Interest Group) classification
International Society for Heart and Lung Transplantation
Jewett classification of bladder carcinoma
Judet epiphyseal fracture classification
Karnofsky performance rating
Karnofsky status classification
Kazangia and Converse fracture
Keith-Wagener classification of retinopathy
Keith-Wagener-Barker stages of hypertensive retinopathy
Kiel classification of non-Hodgkin lymphoma
Killip heart failure
Klatskin tumor classification
Lauge-Hansen classification of ligamentous ankle fractures
Lenke classification of adolescent idiopathic scoliosis
leukemia classification
Lichtman radiographic classification of Kienböck disease
Lukes-Collins classification of non-Hodgkin lymphoma
lymph node location system of neck
lymphoplasmacytic lymphoma
Mackinnon and Dellon criteria
Mallampati airway assessment
Marx classification of microtia
Masaoka staging system, modified
Mayo Clinic criteria to determine patient survival

classification *(cont.)*
Mayo Clinic system for primary biliary cirrhosis
Meurmann congenital aural atresia
Modic disk abnormality classification
modified Masaoka staging system
modified Stahl classification of Kienböck disease
MSTS (Musculoskeletal Tumor Society) staging system
murmur grades
Neer (shoulder fractures I, II, III)
NYHA (New York Heart Association) classification of congestive heart failure
Olerud and Molander fracture
osteoarthritis grading
Pauwels femoral neck fracture
Pulec and Freedman congenital aural atresia
Rai classification of chronic lymphocytic leukemia
Reese-Ellsworth classification of retinoblastoma
Rye histopathologic classification of Hodgkin disease
Samsoon modification of Mallampati airway classes I through IV
Schuknecht congenital aural atresia
Singh-Vaughn-Williams arrhythmia
Stahl classification of Kienböck disease
Stanford Dependency Index
TNM malignant tumor
tuberculosis
Universal Spine Classification
Van Herick grading system
van Heuven anatomic classification of diabetic retinopathy
Visick grading system for post-gastrectomy carcinoma recurrence
White and Panjabi criteria

classification *(cont.)*
WHO (World Health Organization) classification of papillary urothelial neoplasms of the bladder
WHO/ISUP (International Society of Urological Pathology) classification of papillary urothelial neoplasms of the bladder
Wiberg classification of patellar types
WNM system

Clauss modified method of plasma fibrinogen measurement.

claustrum—thin layer of gray matter lateral to the external capsule of the brain. Cf. *colostrum, clostridium*.

claviculotomy, claviculectomy technique—used for tumors that transgress the neck, thoracic inlet, and axilla, offering maximal exposure for excision, vascular control, and preservation of vital structures.

clavus (pl., clavi)—a corn on the foot or toe.

clean-catch urine specimen—an uncontaminated urine specimen obtained by first thoroughly washing the genitalia. The urine stream is started and then, midstream, the specimen is caught without the urine stream or container touching the genitalia or perineum.

cleansers, wound
Dey-Wash skin wound cleanser
DiaB Klenz wound cleanser
MicroKlenz wound cleanser
Optipore wound-cleaning sponge
Puri-Clens wound cleanser
Sea-Clens wound cleanser
Shur-Clens wound cleanser
UltraKlenz wound cleanser

ClearCut 2—an electrosurgical handpiece by Medtronic used in tissue cutting and coagulation.

Clearglide optical vessel dissector—for use in the creation and dissection of operative cavities in extraperitoneal spaces.

ClearLight—a high-intensity light-based treatment for acne.

ClearSite borderless dressing—gauze scrim and a 1 cm printed top film in an open-weave design that allows monitoring of wound healing and complete visualization of the wound site even after extended use. Cf. *Aquasorb, Curasorb, and Ventex.*

ClearSite Hydro Gauze dressing—dressing with a thin layer of ClearSite gel that maintains a moist environment for healing.

clear to auscultation and percussion (CTAP).

ClearView Blower/Mister device—a device used to facilitate coronary artery grafting procedures performed on a beating heart. A tube with a tip that can be bent by the surgeon to the desired configuration delivers a mist of air and saline to clear the arteriotomy site of retrograde blood flow.

ClearView CO_2 laser—includes a device to continually evacuate smoke generated by laser use.

cleaved cell non-Hodgkin lymphoma—cellular classification of one type of non-Hodgkin lymphoma.

Cleland ligament—in the hand; keeps the skin sleeve from twisting around the bone of the digit. It may be referred to in operative procedures for Dupuytren contracture. See also *Grayson ligament*; they are not synonymous.

click-evoked otoacoustic emissions (cEOEs).

Climara Pro (estradiol and levonorgestrel)—estrogen replacement patch.

clindamycin and benzoyl peroxide—see *Duac*.

Clinical Global Impression of Change (CGIC)—measures Alzheimer patient's clinical change relative to baseline.

Clinical Institute Narcotic Assessment (CINA).

Clinical Institute Withdrawal Assessment-Alcohol (CIWA-A) **scale**—psychological/physiological scale used to assess the degree of alcohol withdrawal that a patient is experiencing. For a score above 10, the patient is given a drug such as Librium (chlordiazepoxide) or Valium (diazepam) to produce sedation and prevent seizures.

Clinical Triage Instrument—used in emergency departments to aid in devising treatment program for HIV-infected patients.

CliniCath peripherally inserted catheter.

clip—see *clamp*.

Clirans T-series—hollow-fiber-type dialyzer for urea clearance.

clitoridectomy—(also referred to as "excision")—female genital mutilation consisting of removal of entire clitoris, both prepuce and glans, with removal of adjacent labia. See also *infibulation* and *Sunna circumcision*.

CLL (chronic lymphocytic leukemia)—seen primarily in late adulthood, usually after age 50.

CLO (congenital lobar overinflation).

Clobetasol E cream (clobetasol propionate emollient cream 0.05%)—topical drug for the topical treatment of inflammatory and pruritic corticosteroid-responsive dermatoses of the scalp.

clock drawing test—an easy to score and administer, cultural and educa-

clock *(cont.)*
tional bias-free test in which the patient is given a circle, asked to draw a clock, and then put the hands on the clock to make it read 2:45.

Clolar (clofarabine)—drug for the treatment of children with refractory or relapsed acute lymphoblastic leukemia.

clone—any aggregation of cells, ranging up to a complete organism, derived asexually from a single ancestral diploid cell.

cloning, human—generation of an embryo by somatic cell nuclear transfer. See *reproductive cloning, research cloning, therapeutic cloning*.

clonogenic assay—single cell suspensions of tumor cells are cultured in soft agar and then exposed to various chemotherapy agents. The soft agar permits the selective growth of tumor cells. Sensitivity and resistance are estimated by a count of surviving clones of cells.

Clonorchis sinensis—liver fluke.

clonus—see *drawn ankle clonus*.

C-loop of duodenum (Radiol).

cloretazine—a medication for relapsed or refractory acute myelogenous leukemia (AML).

closed fracture—one in which there is no break in the skin. Formerly called *simple fracture*.

closed intramedullary pinning (CIMP) —a closed technique for correcting displaced fractures of the epiphysis of the neck of the radius. An incision is made in the shaft of the radius to gain access to the epiphysis. A Kirschner wire is inserted through a drill hole and gently hammered through the medullary canal to the epiphysis. The tip of the K wire secures the fracture fragment. To correct lateral displacement of the fragment, the wire may be rotated 180° on its long axis, creating torque which slides the fragment back in its place. The K wire is then cut at the other end where it exits from the shaft, and the skin incision is closed.

Closer, The—provides minimally invasive closure of an arterial access site in the femoral artery following a diagnostic procedure such as coronary angiography.

CloseSure procedure kit—used in full-thickness suturing of trocar wounds.

closing base wedge osteotomy (CBWO).

clostridial bacteremia—in cancer patients, most frequently associated with *Clostridium perfringens* and *C. septicum*.

clostridial collagenase—derived from *Clostridium histolyticum* and used for enzymatic wound debridement in preparation for skin grafting.

Clostridium difficile—organism isolated from meconium and feces of infants, from wounds, and from the urogenital tract of asymptomatic people.

***Clostridium difficile*-associated diarrhea** (CDAC).

closure system by VNUS—catheters used for endovascular coagulation of blood vessels in patients with superficial vein reflux.

Clo-Sur P.A.D.—a pressure-applied hemostatic dressing used after cardiac catheterization.

CLOtest (*Campylobacter*-like organism)—a trademark term for the test for *H. pylori*. *Campylobacter* is the former name of *Helicobacter*.

Clot Stop drain—a drain with an antithrombogenic covering, used in cosmetic surgery.

clotrimazole/betamethasone dipropionate—see *Lotrisone.*

clotting factors—see *coagulating factors.*

clove hitch—a sailor's knot; also used in surgery.

cloverleaf skull (Ger., Kleeblattschädel).

CLSE (calf lung surfactant extract)—see *surfactant, heterologous.*

CLS (Cementless Spotorno) **stem insertion.**

clubbing, cyanosis, and edema.

clubbing of the fingers and toes—thickening and bulbous enlargement of the tissue at the base of the nail; often seen in patients with cystic fibrosis, ulcerative colitis, cirrhosis of the liver, and cardiopulmonary disease.

clubfoot splint—see *Denis Browne.*

club sandwich tympanoplasty technique—in which multiple layers of EpiFilm disks are placed at several locations to minimize the formation of adhesions, enhance epithelial cell formation, and minimize chronic inflammation of the graft.

clue cells—a term used in reference to a Pap smear. They are so-called because their presence is a clue to possible infection with *Gardnerella vaginalis* (formerly *Haemophilus vaginalis*).

cm (centimeter).

cM (centimorgan).

CME (cystoid macular edema) (Oph).

CMF-HBSS (calcium-free and magnesium-free Hanks balanced salt solution).

CMI (cell-mediated immunity).

CMI/O'Neil cup (Ob-Gyn)—attached to a vacuum source to facilitate vacuum-assisted vaginal deliveries. Available in both anterior and posterior presentations.

CMJ (corticomedullary junction) phase imaging on CT scan.

CML (chronic myelocytic leukemia)—mostly in adults age 20 to 50.

CML (chronic myeloid leukemia).

CMML (chronic myelomonocytic leukemia).

CMN (congenital melanocytic nevi).

CMRNG (chromosomally mediated-resistant *Neisseria gonorrhoeae*)—a penicillin-resistant gonococcus.

CMT (Certified Medical Transcriptionist).

CMT (circus-movement tachycardia).

CMV (cytomegalovirus).

CNM (Certified Nurse Midwife).

CNP (C-type natriuretic peptide)—a peptide found in endothelial cells, a possible factor in endotoxin shock and atherosclerosis.

CNR (cell nuclear replacement).

C/N ratio (contrast-to-noise)—a term used in MRI scans.

CNRB (cervical nerve root block)—used in treatment of patients with cervical radicular pain.

CNS (central nervous system). Not to be confused with *C&S* (culture and sensitivity). See *C&S.*

CNV (choroidal neovascularization).

CNVM (choroidal neovascular membrane) (Oph).

coags—slang for coagulation studies.

CoaguChek—self-testing device that measures blood coagulation levels (prothrombin time).

coagulation factors (blood)

- I fibrinogen
- II prothrombin
- III thromboplastin
- IV calcium ions
- V proaccelerin (accelerator globulin, AcG)

coagulation *(cont.)*
VI factor VI (which is rapidly destroyed by thrombin; hence, it cannot be identified by its activity in the serum) is assumed to be the active form
VII proconvertin (or serum prothrombin conversion accelerator, SPCA)
VIII antihemophilic factor (or von Willebrand factor)
IX plasma thromboplastin component (Christmas factor)
X Stuart factor (or Stuart-Prower factor)
XI plasma thromboplastin antecedent
XII Hageman factor
XIII fibrin stabilizing factor

Coagulin-B—adeno-associated virus-based gene therapy drug for the treatment of hemophilia B.

Coaguloop resection electrode (new use)—an instrument used for resection, ablation, and fulguration in the bladder.

coagulum pyelolithotomy—procedure for removal of kidney stones. Coagulum is introduced through two Intracaths, and cryoprecipitate and calcium chloride mixture are instilled simultaneously. After 7 minutes an incision is made in the pelvis of the kidney, and the stones, now surrounded by the gel that has formed, are easily scooped out without rough edges traumatizing the renal tissues.

coal tar, crude—*not* cold tar.

coal tar shampoo.

Coat-A-Count PSA IRMA and **Coat-A-Count Free PSA IRMA**—tests for the detection of prostate cancer.

Coats disease (Oph)—unilateral, congenital (but not familial) vascular anomalies of the retina. It is sometimes confused with retinoblastoma, but fluorescein angiography and ultrasound help differentiate between the two entities. Coats disease is frequently seen in young boys.

coaxial sheath cut-biopsy needle—see *PercuCut cut-biopsy needles*.

Cobactin E—a proprietary strain of *Lactobacillus acidophilus* that inhibits *E. coli* 0157:H7.

cobalamin C methylmalonic acidemia—a nutritional deficiency thought to be responsible for certain skin diseases.

Coban dressing, wrapping—an elastic dressing.

COBAS Amplicor HBV monitor test—laboratory test that uses polymerase chain reaction technique to detect hepatitis B virus DNA.

COBAS Amplicor HCV assay (or **test**).

Cobb angle—measurement in kyphoscoliosis. Usage: "Seven patients had a thoracic curve with a mean preoperative Cobb angle of 69° (range 47 to 112°)." "Instrumentation begins with a convex compression force to shorten not only the posterior column but also the convexity of the scoliotic deformity while reducing the Cobb angle."

Cobb-Ragde needle—a double-prong ligature carrier for bladder neck suspension.

Cobb syndrome—characterized by the presence of spinal and vertebral angiomas.

cobblestone appearance of mucosa—a radiographic finding in advanced Crohn disease on small bowel follow-through exam. The cobblestone appearance is caused by submucosal edema and deep transverse and

cobblestone *(cont.)*
longitudinal ulcers in the distal ileum.

cobblestone degeneration (Oph)—atrophic condition in which sharply outlined rounded lesions appear in the peripheral retina. Also called *paving stone degeneration.*

cobblestoning—coarsely lumpy appearance of a mucosal surface, such as the tongue, nasal mucosa, or conjunctiva, caused by inflammation.

Cobe gun—a staple gun.

Cobe Optima—a hollow-fiber membrane oxygenator for use in ECMO (extracorporeal membrane oxygenation) systems.

COBE Spectra Apheresis System—an instrument for bone marrow cell processing.

COBE 2991 Cell Processor—an instrument for bone marrow cell processing.

Coblation (trademark coined from "cool ablation")—a patented process that uses radiofrequency (RF) energy applied to a conductive medium, like saline, to remove target tissue in a relatively cool process without damage to surrounding tissue as might occur with heat-driven electrosurgical techniques. Used in orthopedics, plastic surgery, and ears, nose, and throat procedures, and investigationally in cardiovascular procedures.

Coblation Channeling—a minimally invasive procedure for volumetric reduction of tissue, used primarily for treating a variety of upper airway disorders, including snoring, but also in knee and spinal surgery.

Coblation tonsillectomy—a nonheat-driven process that causes a low temperature molecular disintegration of tonsillar tissue, resulting in minimal tissue damage to surrounding areas. See *Coblation.*

cobra head plate (Ortho).

Cobra malleable multielectrode surgical ablation system with fluid-cooled and bipolar options.

Coburn equiconvex lens—an intraocular lens with an equal curvature from anterior to posterior.

cocaine-induced respiratory failure (CIRF)—the sudden onset of dyspnea, pulmonary edema, and respiratory failure caused by cocaine.

coccygodynia—pain in the coccyx and neighboring region.

cochineal extract—see *carmine dye.*

Cochlea Dynamics sound processing technology—digitally programmable products for persons with hearing loss.

cochlear blood flow (CBF).

cochlear implant—electronic device that provides direct electrical stimulation to the auditory fibers in the inner ear. See *Clarion*; *Contigen Bard.*

cochleosacculotomy—see *Schuknecht.*

cockade image—a well-defined lytic lesion with a central calcification resembling a cockade. A cockade is a badge in the form of a rosette or knot, worn on a hat. It is a classic finding for intraosseous lipoma of the calcaneus.

Cockcroft-Gault equation or **formula** —used to quickly calculate renal function by estimating creatinine clearance from serum creatinine. This equation takes into account the patient's age, weight, and sex. It is used to adjust the dosage of certain drugs which are excreted by the kidneys. It is of particular value in elderly patients whose kidney func-

Cockcroft *(cont.)*
tion may be compromised but whose therapy cannot be postponed until a 24-hour urine collection for creatinine clearance is completed.

cocktail—used in *banana bag, detox cocktail, GI cocktail, green lizard, immunosuppressant cocktail.*

Co-Cr-Mo pin—named after the chemical symbols of its components (cobalt, chromium, molybdenum).

code black—emergency department jargon for a patient who has expired.

Codere orbital floor implant.

Codman exercises—to increase range of motion in a stiff shoulder. The patient bends over at a 90° angle at the waist and, with a weight held in each hand, moves the arms in arcs.

Codman triangle—an abrupt cutoff of periosteal new bone at the edge of a lesion, representing a mass elevating the periosteum, and often associated with malignancy.

codon—a triplet of three nucleotide bases in a DNA or RNA molecule, specifying a particular amino acid.

Cody tack operation—for treatment of progressive endolymphatic hydrops (Ménière disease). Similar to the Fick sacculotomy.

Coe-pak—hard- and fast-set periodontal paste.

coffee-grounds material, vomitus, emesis—indicative of blood in the gastric contents. Usage: "She has vomited twice. This was productive of stomach contents and bile, no hemoptysis, hematemesis, or coffee-grounds material." The appearance of the vomitus is similar to that of the grounds left over after roasting coffee. Note: Coffee grounds, *not* coffee ground.

Coffey ureterointestinal anastomosis.

Coffin-Lowry syndrome—mental retardation and congenital deformities.

Cofield total shoulder system.

CO_2Guard (typed as one word)—filters gas in laparoscopy and hysteroscopy.

cognitive behavior therapy (CBT).

cogwheel breathing—jerkiness or intermittency of breath sounds on inspiration, due to sudden expansion of previously collapsed air sacs.

cogwheel gait—muscle jerkiness due to spasticity in patients with Parkinson disease.

cogwheel phenomenon (sign)—jerky movement about a joint caused by alternating spastic resistance and relaxation during passive range of motion examination; a hallmark of Parkinson disease.

cogwheel rigidity—a type of muscle rigidity seen in Parkinson disease.

Cohen catheter—a catheter used to introduce an embryo fertilized in vitro into the uterine cavity.

Cohen reimplantation—a procedure to prevent vesicoureteral reflux in patients having undergone continent cystostomies.

Coherent CO_2 (carbon dioxide) **surgical laser**—Series 2000 Ultima or Novus photocoagulators used in eye surgery.

Coherent UltraPulse 5000C laser—used for aesthetic facial resurfacing and treatment of acne scars, superficial skin cancers, moles, and warts.

Coherent VersaPulse device.

Cohn cardiac stabilizer—for retraction and stabilization of the heart during minimally invasive beating-heart surgical procedures.

coin test—for pneumothorax. One coin is pressed against the anterior chest and tapped with another, while the

coin *(cont.)*
posterior chest is auscultated. A characteristic sound is diagnostic of pneumothorax.

CO_2ject system—allows for routine use of carbon dioxide gas as a replacement for the more expensive iodinated contrast media currently used in angiographic procedures.

Colapinto needle—transjugular liver biopsy needle used in interventional radiology.

Colaris test—predictive medicine test that assesses an individual's risk for colon cancer based on the presence of a mutation of either of two genes. These same mutations, when found in women, are also said to substantially increase their risk of endometrial cancer.

CO_2 laser (carbon dioxide laser). See *argon laser, laser, Nd:YAG laser*.

colchicine poisoning—drug intoxication resulting from toxic doses of colchicine used primarily in the treatment of gout.

cold cup biopsy—a method of obtaining tissue for histologic examination. Cold cup biopsies of the lower urinary tract require rigid endoscopic access and the use of biopsy forceps and Bugbee electrodes.

cold-dissection technique—where a scalpel, knife, or other sharp instrument is used to resect tissue without the use of cautery or other hot instrument source.

cold knife cone (CKC) **biopsy**.

cold water calorics—a test for vertigo, nystagmus, and vestibular function, with cold water gently injected by syringe into the ear canal. Also, *ice water calorics test*.

Coleman classification of congenital aural atresia.

CollaCote—collagen wound dressing.

collagen hemostatic material for wounds—initially acts as a hemostatic agent when applied to a wound. Continued application seems to aid and hasten the body's own repair mechanisms. The most abundant collagen is type 1, extracted from bovine hide. Other sources include porcine, chicken, and bovine tendon. See also *cleansers*; *dressing*
Avitene
bucrylate
Collastat
Contigen glutaraldehyde
cross-linked
CosmoDerm
CosmoPlast human-based implant
cryoprecipitate
Endo-Avitene
Hemaflex sheath
Helitene
Hemopad
Hemotene
Instat
Surgical Nu-Knit hemostatic material
Surgicel
Unilab Surgibone
Zyderm I or II
Zyplast

collagen absorbable suture—made of beef tendon.

collagenous colitis—see *microscopic colitis*.

colitis
collagenous
lymphocytic
microscopic
pseudomembranous (PMC)
single-stripe (SSC)
toxic

collagen injection, **periurethral**—given to women for stress urinary incontinence.

collagen injection, transurethral—given for stress incontinence after radical prostatectomy, although not in men with severe bladder neck dysfunction or scarring.

collagen meniscus implant (CMI)—tissue-engineered biological meniscus implant designed to regenerate damaged meniscal tissue.

Collagraft bone graft matrix—non-osteoconductive bone-void filler that provides healing and fusion rates equivalent to an autograft without the risks of viral transmission and donor-site morbidity problems.

Collamer—foldable intraocular lens for use in cataract surgery. It varies in length to accommodate the natural shape of the human eye.

CollaPlug (Oral Surg)—wound dressing.

collar—see *cervical collar.*

collar-button abscess of the palm.

collar-button appearance in colon (Radiol).

Collastat—collagen hemostatic sponge with proposed advantages over Avitene. It is said not to shred or pull apart after absorbing tissue fluids, and it costs less.

CollaTape—tape used with wound dressing.

collateralization—formation of collateral vessels.

collateral vessels—vascular channels that are newly formed from existing ones to maintain the circulation of a tissue or organ whose normal blood supply has been impaired by disease or injury. Cf. *collateralization*.

CollectFirst system—used for intraoperative and postoperative autotransfusion.

collecting system (Radiol)—on an intravenous pyelogram (IVP), the nonexcretory portions of the kidney, which collect newly formed urine and conduct it to the ureter; the minor and major calices and the renal pelvis.

collicular fracture of the medial malleolus.

colliculus—a small protuberance. Cf. *canaliculus*.

Collier sign—when the upper lid is elevated, showing more sclera above the iris than is usually seen, producing the so-called thyroid stare; a sign of thyroid disease. Cf. *Dalrymple sign*.

collimation (Radiol)—in scanning.

Collin-Beard procedure—resection of the levator muscle, with advancement onto the tarsal plate.

Collins solution—used for preservation of a liver which is to be transplanted; the liver may be kept in this solution for about six hours before implantation. Ringer solution may be used for this purpose if the liver is to be kept for a shorter period.

Collis-Nissen fundoplication—used in association with transthoracic parietal cell vagotomy for advanced gastroesophageal reflux with peptic stricture and Barrett metaplasia.

Collis-Nissen gastroplasty—a procedure for gastroesophageal reflux.

collodion—a topical protectant used to keep a surgical wound dry.

colloidal bismuth subcitrate—drug used for reduction of *H. pylori* in the mouth.

colloid oncotic pressure (COP)—measurement of brain edema after cryogenic (vasogenic) brain injury.

colloids—used as blood replacement, including dextrose, hetastarch, plasma protein fraction, and serum albumin. See *crystalloids*.

colloid shift on liver-spleen scan.

ColoCARE—a noninvasive home test to detect early warning signs of colorectal disease.

colocolic intussusception—a term that may be confusing because *colocolic* might be misunderstood as *colonic* or simply stuttering. *Intussusception* is the prolapse of one part of the intestine into an adjoining part. In colocolic intussusception, the colon prolapses into itself rather than the intestine prolapsing into the colon.

colocolponeopoiesis—technique used to create a new vagina in females with congenital vaginal aplasia or in males having a sex change operation. A portion of the sigmoid colon is resected, carefully preserving its blood supply. Using sutures or a stapler, the colonic segment is formed into a conduit for use as a vagina. Also called *modified Kun colocolpopoiesis*.

colony-forming unit (CFU).

colony-forming unit-granulocyte, monocyte (CFU-GM).

colony-forming unit-megakaryocyte (CFU-meg or CFU-MK).

Colorado microdissection needle (Neuro).

color Doppler—a computer used with sonography of blood vessels computes the speed of the blood flow and demonstrates it in different colors to the radiologist.

colorectal cancer (CRC).

colorectal cancer screening—includes fecal occult blood testing, flexible sigmoidoscopy, barium enema, and colonoscopy.

Colorgene DNA hybridization test— a DNA probe test to detect herpes simplex virus in two hours rather than waiting days for culture results.

Colormate TLc BiliTest system—transcutaneous bilirubinometer for monitoring newborn jaundice.

colostomy shift en masse—a novel technique in which the colostomy is shifted along with a rim of skin and abdominal wall tissue. This provides additional length of distal bowel if needed during pull-through anastomosis.

colostrum (Ob-Gyn)—a thin, milky fluid which is secreted by the mammary glands around the time of parturition. It contains antibodies which provide the baby with passive immunization. Cf. *claustrum*.

colpocystourethropexy (CCUP).

colpoperineopexy—see *abdominal-sacral colpoperineopexy.*

colposuspension—see *vaginal-psoas colposuspension*.

columnization of contrast medium—an abnormal finding on x-ray. For example, the entire ureter is not usually visualized on a single film except when an obstruction is present, such as from a stone. In that case the contrast appears lined up, as in a column. Usage: "Columnization of contrast was noted in the left ureter on intravenous pyelogram."

CombiDerm absorbent cover dressing.

combined androgen blockade (CAB).

Combitube—a relatively new device used for blind insertion emergency intubation.

comb sign—vascular jejunization of the ileum (alteration of the mucosal pattern so that it resembles that of the jejunum) as seen on CT scan in a Crohn disease patient.

Comed—a line of post-traumatic and postsurgical footgear.

COME s/p BMTT (chronic otitis media with effusion, status post bilateral myringotomy with tympanostomy tube).

Comfeel Ulcus—a synthetic (hydrocolloid) occlusive dressing for lower extremity ulcers.

Comfort Cast, Comfort Cast Stirrup—foot and ankle casting system with four adjustable parts, reducing the need for crutches.

Comfort Cath I or II—male external catheter.

ComfortFlex—see *Hanger ComfortFlex.*

comitant—accompanying, following, or related to deviation of the eye. Here is the definition supplied by an ophthalmologist: *Comitant* refers to the eye's deviation in the same amount in all positions of gaze. Let's say it's an in-turning eye and it deviates 10 diopters of inward deviation, and that deviation is the same in upgaze, downgaze, right gaze, and left gaze; we call that *comitant deviation* or *comitant esotropia*. If the deviation varies in different gaze positions, we call it *noncomitant*; it is more likely to be paralytic. Cf. *concomitant*.

Commander PTCA wire line.

Command instrument system—cutting instruments used in the femoral canal for joint replacement.

Command PS pacemaker.

Commission on Accreditation of Rehabilitation Facilities (CARF).

commissure of Gudden—located within the optic chiasm.

Commit lozenge—over-the-counter nicotine-containing lozenge for smoking cessation.

Companion 314—a nasal CPAP system designed for in-home use to treat adults with obstructive sleep apnea.

Companion 2 self blood glucose monitoring device. See *SBGM*.

compartment syndrome of the hand or anterior compartment of leg—a condition characterized by raised pressure within a closed space with a potential to cause irreversible damage to the contents of the closed compartment.

Compass hinge—used to prevent joint contractures following elbow or finger trauma or surgery. This external device measures the degree of passive and active range of motion exercises. The numbered calibrations for degrees of motion at the outside of the edge of this circular device resemble those on a compass.

compensated—corrected or mitigated; said of a defect or disability, as in compensated congestive heart failure; compensated hearing loss, hearing loss improved with a hearing aid; edentulous and compensated, toothless but fitted with dentures.

compensated dysphagia for solid foods—the patient's attempt to deal with the effects of congenital esophageal stenosis. Stenosis may be treated by endoscopic bougienage or balloon dilatation.

Comperm tubular elastic bandage—provides 360° compression and support for sports injuries, postcast support, postburn scarring, sprains, and strains.

complementary and alternative medicine (CAM)—a broad range of healing philosophies that include acupuncture, chiropractic, homeopathy, herbs and supplements, massage, and body and mind therapies.

complementary DNA (copy DNA, cDNA)—DNA transcribed from a complementary strand of RNA by the action of reverse transcriptase.

complement-dependent cytotoxicity (CDC) **assay**—method of detection for serum anti-HLA antibodies. Also, *PRA assay*.

complement fixation—a type of serologic test in which the consumption of a serum protein, called complement, is taken as evidence that the expected antigen-antibody reaction has occurred. Cf. *compliment*.

completely in the [ear] **canal** (CIC)—hearing aids, referring to the ear canal, particularly suited to patients with presbycusis.

complex
AIDS-related (ARC)
anisoylated plasminogen streptokinase activator (APSAC)
Battey-avium
Buford
Carney multiple neoplasia syndrome
Eisenmenger
Ghon
Golgi
K
MAC (*Mycobacterium avium* complex)
MAI (*Mycobacterium avium-intracellulare*) complex
nipple-areola (NAC)
ostiomeatal
Pierre Robin
Ranke
sling ring
triangular fibrocartilage (TFCC)

complex regional pain syndrome (CRPS)—a perplexing condition that can occur following injury, usually to an extremity. Patients with this syndrome experience burning pain along with autonomic and tissue changes in the region of the injury. This group of symptoms has also been referred to as *reflex sympathetic dystrophy* (CRPS type I) or, in the case of a known nerve injury, *causalgia* (CRPS type II). This condition is also known as *chronic regional pain syndrome*.

complex tone test—a diagnostic auditory procedure to identify hemispheric dysfunction. It is used in psychology and psychiatry to evaluate psychoacoustic aspects of the hearing process.

compliance—a patient's following of physician's directions and advice regarding diet or medicinal treatment. *Noncompliance*, when the patient is not cooperative.

Compliant pre-stress system—a prosthetic bone implant device that helps native bone grow into implant and heal.

compliment—an expression of admiration or praise. Cf. *complement*.

Composite Cultured Skin—treatment for severe burns.

composite dressings—products which combine physically distinct components into a single dressing. See *dressing*.

Composix E/X mesh—two-layer mesh with a tissue-impervious ePTFE layer that goes next to viscera and minimizes adhesions. The upper layer is a polypropylene that allows tissue ingrowth and reduces or eliminates the need for transfixation sutures.

compromise—impairment or damage to a normal structure or function, as in neural compromise, circulatory compromise, and compromise of the immune system.

CompuCAM—digital intraoral camera.

Compuscan Hittman computerized electrocardioscanner—used in studies of ventricular septal defect, pulmonary stenosis, and Ebstein

Compuscan *(cont.)* anomaly of the atrioventricular valve. Usage: "Tapes were analyzed with a Compuscan Hittman computerized electrocardioscanner and graded according to the method of Lown and Woolf."

computed dental radiography (CDR)—computerized imaging system that utilizes an electronic sensor where dentists would normally use x-ray film. Images appear almost instantly on a computer monitor.

computed tomography angiographic portography (CTAP).

computed tomography angiography (CTA).

computed tomography laser mammography (CTLM)—breast imaging device that creates contiguous cross-sectional slice images of the breast, without compression of the breast or x-rays.

computed tomography (CT) **scan** (also called *computerized axial tomography*, or *CAT scan*)—an application of computer technology to diagnostic radiology. Instead of exposing a film after passing through the patient, x-rays are detected and recorded by a scintillation counter. The x-ray tube moves around the patient on a frame called a *gantry*, rotating through an arc and "cutting" across one plane of the patient. A series of scintillation counters are so placed that each detects the rays passing through the patient at a different angle. (Alternatively, a single counter may rotate in perfect alignment with the x-ray source.) Data on the amount of x-ray that penetrates the patient at each angle are collected from the counters, digitized, stored, and analyzed by a minicomputer programmed to generate a cross-sectional image of the patient corresponding to the plane cut by the moving x-ray beam. Contrast medium may be injected into the circulation immediately before CT scanning. Intravenous contrast enhances the sensitivity of CT scanning of certain structures and body regions and improves the visibility of some tumors.

computer-aided diagnosis (CAD).

computer-assisted arthritis detection—see *amorphous silicon filmless digital x-ray detection technology.*

computer-assisted minimally invasive surgery (CAMIS).

computerized dynamic posturography (CDP)—used to evaluate the presence of vestibular and balance disorders.

computerized phonoenterography—a system using computerized analysis of bowel sounds to aid in diagnosis of intestinal obstruction and paralytic ileus.

computerized texture analysis of lung nodules and lung parenchyma—a viable alternative to a histologic examination in patients with focal or diffuse lung diseases.

computerized tomographic hepatic angiography (CTHA).

COMT (catechol-O-methyltransferase)—inhibitors that work to enhance the effectiveness of levodopa by blocking one of the main enzymes responsible for breaking down levodopa in the bloodstream before it reaches the brain.

concealed straight leg raising test—a method for the physician to determine the extent of the patient's disability. If it appears that the patient is not cooperating in the straight leg raising test or is malingering, the

concealed *(cont.)* examining physician will pretend to examine the patient's feet but actually will be noting how high up the patient's feet will go with the legs extended. Usage: "There is negative concealed straight leg raising at 90° bilaterally."

Conceive Fertility Planner—a software program that uses the natural fertility signs of a woman's body to assist couples who are trying to conceive.

concentric plaques in carotid arteries.

Concentric retriever system (CRS)—a small metal wire with a loop at the end that removes clots from arteries and thereby restores blood flow to the brain.

Concept bipolar coagulator—an electronic coagulator for hemostasis of tiny bleeders; effective in a wet field (under irrigation or in a bloody field).

Conceptus Robust guidewire—used for fallopian tube catheterization.

Conceptus Soft Seal cervical catheter—designed for atraumatic transcervical access to the uterus.

Conceptus Soft Torque uterine catheter—designed to allow easy, accurate placement at tubal ostium.

Conceptus VS (variable softness) **catheter**—used for fallopian tube catheterization.

Concise cementing sculps—a series of disposable spoon and trowel-shaped instruments that are used to remove excess cement while it is still soft, without scratching the prosthesis.

Concise compression hip screw system.

concomitant—together, along with, accompanying, associated with. Cf. *comitant*.

concordant (Genetics)—said of twins who both exhibit a certain trait.

concussion grades

grade 1—no loss of consciousness, but symptoms may include some transient confusion, inability to maintain a thought process, dizziness, headache, nausea, vomiting, and blurred vision; may resolve within 15 minutes.

grade 2—no loss of consciousness, but symptoms may include transient confusion, amnesia, dizziness, headache, and general disorientation; may persist for 15 minutes or more.

grade 3—a brief or prolonged loss of consciousness, but symptoms of confusion, amnesia, and general disorientation may persist from a few minutes to 24 hours.

condition—see *disease* or *syndrome*.

conditioned insomnia—a form of chronic insomnia, caused by negative association between the characteristics of the customary sleep environment and sleeping.

conductive keratoplasty (CK)—a surgical device to treat farsightedness that uses radiofrequency waves, instead of a laser, to reshape the cornea. Heat-causing radiofrequency waves pass through a tiny probe as thin as a human hair that is guided in a circle around the edge of the cornea. It is less invasive than laser surgery.

conduit—see *ileal conduit*.

condylomatous atypia—a form of low-grade squamous intraepithelial lesion (LGSIL) noted on cervical Pap smear that is characteristic of human papillomavirus infection.

coned-down view—a study limited to a small area by the use of a cone that narrows and focuses the x-ray beam.

C100-3—hepatitis C virus antibody (anti-HIV), diagnostic of hepatitis C.

C1q ("C-one-q") **assay**—one of a series of complement components or inhibitor proteins, numbered C1 to C9 (not a subscript), related to antibody-antigen reactions. The test is used to detect immune complexes in rheumatoid arthritis.

condom—see *device.*

conductive keratoplasty (CK)—nonlaser treatment for presbyopia. It uses radio waves to reshape the cornea and bring near vision back into focus. The procedure is typically performed only on one eye, helping the patient to maintain distance vision. Minimally invasive and painless, CK is performed in less than three minutes in the doctor's office under topical anesthesia.

coned-down view—a radiographic study limited to a small area by the use of a cone that narrows and "focuses" the x-ray beam.

cone of extraocular muscles—an anatomical structure referred to in MRI reports on cavernous hemangioma and other orbital pathology.

confabulation—invention of stories about one's past, often bizarre and complex, to fill in gaps left by amnesia; a typical feature of Korsakoff syndrome in chronic alcoholics.

Confide HIV test kit—a home collection HIV testing kit. A kit is sent confidentially to a home address, the recipient takes a blood sample, returns the specimen by mail, and phones for results.

confocal microscope (Oph).

Conformant contact-layer wound dressing.

conformer—that part of an eye prosthesis which covers the surface of an artificial eye sphere.

congenital—present at birth, but not necessarily genetic.

congenital dysplasia (or dislocation) **of hip** (CDH)—see *developmental dysplasia of the hip* (DDH).

congenital esophageal stenosis—considered a diagnosis of exclusion. It is suggested on the basis of barium studies when a long, smooth, concentric area of esophageal narrowing is seen radiographically in patients with a life-long history of dysphagia for solids (often associated with recurrent food impactions) and with no other risk factors for the development of esophageal strictures. Symptoms are usually relieved by endoscopic bougienage or balloon dilatation.

congenital glenoid dysplasia (Ortho).

congenital insensitivity to pain and anhidrosis (CIPA)—a rare inherited disease characterized by a lack of pain sensation and thermoregulation. Although lacking pain sensation, some patients do have tactile hyperesthesia; thus, anesthetics are a necessity during surgery, and temperature management must be maintained. Also referred to as *hereditary sensory and autonomic neuropathy type IV (HSAN-IV).*

congenital lobar overinflation (CLO).

congenital melanocytic nevi (CMN) —birth defect.

congenital sensory neuropathy with anhidrosis (CSNA).

Congo red—a dye used in the laboratory to stain amyloids. Has been found to prevent the formation of

Congo *(cont.)*
memory-robbing plaques in Alzheimer disease and may stop the cell-killing that leads to adult-onset diabetes mellitus. The discovery of Congo red's effect may also provide fundamental information about the aging process.

congruous acetabulum, egg-shaped.

conical cecum—cone-shaped appearance of the cecum on radiography, indicative of Crohn disease or colonic tuberculosis.

conjugated estrogens (CE)—given to renal transplant patients to decrease bleeding complications secondary to uremic coagulopathy. Favored over fresh frozen plasma.

conjugated linoleic acid (CLA)—natural supplement that has been shown to reduce body fat in people who are obese. See *Tonalin*.

conjunctivodacryocystorhinostomy (CDCR).

connective tissue disease (CTD).

consanguinity—relationship by descent from a common ancestor.

consensual light reflex—constriction of the pupil of one eye in response to stimulation by light of the retina of the other eye. See *direct light reflex*.

consensus (*not* concensus and *not* consensus of opinion). Consensus means general opinion, or conclusion after discussion with a number of people, so the word *opinion* is redundant.

conserved helix-loop-helix ubiquitous kinase—see *CHUK*.

"consil"—phonetic for Konsyl, a bulk laxative.

consolidative process (Radiol)—abnormal process that increases the density of a tissue or region.

Constellation—an advanced mapping catheter for electrical mapping of complex right atrial tachycardias.

constipation-dominant irritable bowel syndrome (C-IBS).

contact dissolution—also known as *direct solvent dissolution or litholysis* and *transhepatic gallbladder litholysis* for the treatment of gallstones. Products used for contact dissolution include MTBE, ethyl propionate, and isopropyl acetate.

construction artifact (Radiol)—also called *superimposition artifact*. See *summation shadow artifact*.

consultand—a patient or client who is referred for counseling.

consumption coagulopathy—a disorder, such as disseminated intravascular coagulation (DIC), characterized by the abnormally regulated activation of procoagulant pathways resulting in decreased levels of hemostatic components. *Not* conception coagulopathy.

contact-layer wound dressings—thin, nonadherent sheets placed directly on an open wound bed to protect the wound tissue from direct contact with other agents or dressings applied to the wound. They are porous to allow wound fluid to pass through for absorption by an overlying dressing. See *dressing*.

Contegra pulmonary valved conduit—a bioprosthetic heart valve made from a segment of cow (bovine) jugular vein.

contig (Genetics)—a continuous sequence of DNA that has been assembled from overlapping cloned DNA fragments.

Contigen Bard collagen implant.

Contigen glutaraldehyde cross-linked collagen—used for urethral injection for urinary incontinence.

Contigen implant—an alternative to surgical procedures or wearing external pads for urinary incontinence.

Contigen *(cont.)*
Via periurethral or transurethral cystoscopy, this liquid collagen implant is injected submucosally on either side of the urethra near the bladder neck until the urethral lumen is just occluded and offers normal resistance to the flow of urine from the bladder.

contiguous images (in computed tomography scan)—a series of scans without intervals of unexamined tissue between them.

continent catheterizable appendicovesicostomy using the Mitrofanoff principle—a procedure done for continent urinary diversion. See *Mitrofanoff principle.*

continent ileovesicostomy—*see Monti procedure.*

continent supravesical bowel urinary diversion—for bladder reconstruction to treat invasive bladder cancer. Examples: Camey reservoir, continent urinary diversion, Kock pouch, Mainz pouch, Rowland pouch, and sigmoid colon reservoir.

continent vesicostomy—a technique that involves a segment of tubularized bladder with an antireflux flap valve constructed primarily of mucosa for urinary incontinence.

continuous arteriovenous hemofiltration (CAVH)—a procedure that filters toxins from the blood of patients in renal failure. It has a lower risk of side effects than hemodialysis because the equipment is simpler and blood is removed from the patient's body at a much slower rate.

continuous circular capsulorrhexis technique (Oph).

continuous cyclical peritoneal dialysis (CCPD).

continuous passive motion (CPM).

continuous positive airway pressure (CPAP).

continuous renal replacement therapy (CCRT)—continuous administration of hemofiltration or hemodialysis.

continuous subcutaneous insulin infusion (CSII)

continuous venovenous hemodialysis (CVVHD).

continuous wave Doppler examination.

Continuum MR-compatible infusion system—enables patients to receive intravenous medications safely and continuously during the course of a scanning procedure.

Contour closed end stent.

contoured tilting compression mammography—uses a paddle-shaped rather than flat compression component in the mammography unit. This technique is said to provide more comfort for the patient, since the paddles conform more to the individual's breast shape.

Contour MD implantable single-lead cardioverter-defibrillator.

Contour Profile—anatomically shaped silicone breast implant for breast reconstruction or augmentation.

Contour stent with HydroPlus coating.

Contour V-145D and **LTV-135D**—implantable cardioverter-defibrillator devices.

Contour VL Percuflex stent—variable length stent.

contraction fasciculations—rhythmic, brief twitching of a muscle during weak voluntary or postural contractions. Seen in some elderly patients and those with neurogenic muscle atrophy.

contractions—see *Braxton Hicks contractions*.

contracture—see *Volkmann contracture*.

contralateral acoustic stimulation (CAS)—used in studies of comparative hearing.

contrast echocardiography—ultrasound technique used to diagnose blood flow abnormalities in heart muscle. It uses Optison contrast agent.

contrast material-enhanced scan—MRI term.

contrast medium—see *medication*.

contrast-to-noise (C/N) **ratio**—MRI term.

contrecoup injury—referring to an injury, as to the brain, occurring at a site opposite the point of contact.

Contreet—hydrocolloid nonadhesive foam, and adhesive foam antimicrobial dressing.

controlled spontaneous vaginal delivery (CSVD).

Control-Release pop-off needle.

conus medullaris—cone-shaped lower end of spinal cord.

conventional spin-echo MR imaging vs. breath-hold fast spin-echo or multishot spin-echo echo-planar imaging—MRI term.

convergence test (Oph)—locates breaking point of fusion at near vision.

Convergent color Doppler—a more powerful color imaging capability that is reportedly easier to use, and a more sensitive way to image blood flow dynamics.

conversion disorder—a psychiatric diagnosis in which the loss of function on presentation mimics organic disease. Although rare, it is most common in adolescents and young adults. A patient with conversion disorder may present with progressive bilateral lower-extremity weakness and impaired gait.

convertible slip knot—a knot that converts between a locking and slipping configuration, useful in microsurgical, endoscopic, and laparoscopic applications. See *Aberdeen knot*.

convex linear array—term used in B-scan, Doppler, and color Doppler imaging. See *B-scan*.

convolutions of Gratiolet ("grah-tee-olay")—small convolutions that are buried beneath the lateral surface of the occipital lobe of the brain.

convulsions
benign familial neonatal (BFNC)
benign infantile familial (BIFC)

Cook endoscopic curved needle driver—allows endoscopic suturing using standard curved needle sutures so that tissue approximation, anatomical reconstruction, and hemostasis can be performed endoscopically.

Cook needle—an aspiration biopsy needle.

Cook TPN (total parenteral nutrition) **catheters** (single and double lumen).

cookie—see *Gelfoam cookie*.

cookie cutter—see *Freeman*.

Cool Comfort—a D-ring thumb and wrist splint.

CoolGlide—aesthetic laser system for permanent hair reduction.

CoolSpot—skin-cooling device that provides surface cooling to upper layers of skin during dermatological laser treatments.

Cool Tip catheter—used in catheter ablation treatment of atrial arrhythmias.

Coomassie-blue stain.

Cooperman event probability—a clinical scoring system used to predict cardiac morbidity.

Cooper syndrome—see *fibrocystic breast syndrome.*

Coopervision irrigation/aspiration handpiece (Oph). Usage: "The residual cortex was aspirated with the Coopervision irrigation/aspiration handpiece."

COP (colloid oncotic pressure).

Copalis—acronym for **co**upled **pa**rticle **li**ght scattering, trademarked by Sienna Biotech, Inc. See *Copalis ToRC.*

Copalis ToRC—completely automated total antibody assay that detects *Toxoplasma gondii*, rubella, and cytomegalovirus in human serum.

Copalis treponemal antigen total antibody assay. See *Copalis*.

COPD Lung Profiler—a free Internet-based lung health support tool for patients suffering from COPD (chronic obstructive pulmonary disease).

Cope crushing clamp—used in bowel resection.

Cope modification of a Martel intestinal clamp—used in GI surgery.

copper-binding protein (CBP) **test**.

copper-vapor pulsed laser.

copper wire effect, copper-wiring—narrowing of arterioles in the retina; seen in some patients with arteriosclerosis in the funduscopic examination.

cor (noun)—the heart. Cf. *core, corps*.

coracoacromial—pertaining to coracoid and acromial processes.

coralline hydroxyapatite Goniopora (CHAG).

cordate—heart-shaped. Cf. *caudate, chordate*.

cord blood—blood in the umbilical cord and placenta, particularly in the context of childbirth and the immediate postpartum period.

Cordguard II—a device used by an obstetrician to clamp and cut the umbilical cord and obtain an uncontaminated neonatal blood sample immediately after birth.

Cordis Bioptome sheath.

Cordis-Hakim shunt—used in the Kasai procedure for biliary atresia. See *Kasai procedure*.

Cordis Predator PTCA balloon catheter—used in interventional cardiac treatment.

Cordis Trakstar PTCA balloon catheter—used in interventional cardiac treatment.

cordotomy, chordotomy—words used interchangeably by many dictionaries and journals, although *cordotomy* seems to be the preferred spelling. See *Rosamoff cordotomy*.

corduroy artifact (Radiol)—results from grid synchronization problems.

cord, vocal (*not* chord) (ENT).

core (noun)—the central part of something; (verb)—to take out the core of something. Cf. *cor, corps*.

Core aspiration/injection needle—for laparoscopic surgery.

Core-Assure—bone and vertebral body biopsy kit.

Core CO_2 insufflation needle for laparoscopic surgery.

CORE status—emergency notification of a cardiac or respiratory emergency within a healthcare facility.

Core trocar and cannula systems for laparoscopic surgery.

Cor-Flex wire guides—used with Cook Micropuncture catheter system.

Corflo—a brand name for enteral feeding tubes, percutaneous access catheters for use in enteral procedures, and medical pumps used for enteral feeding.

Corin hip system—total hip arthroplasty and hemiarthroplasty cemented system.

CorLink device—a device for gaining access through the skin to the pericardial space or the peripheral vascular system.

Cormet hip resurfacing system.

CorlS interference screw—machined from allograft cortical bone and designed for reattaching soft tissue grafts to bone in the knee.

Cormed ambulatory infusion pump—permits outpatient therapy in patients receiving chemotherapy, heparin, hyperalimentation, or other ambulatory infusion treatment.

corneae, limbus—see *limbus corneae*.

cornea guttata—degenerative condition of the cornea caused by dystrophy of the endothelial cells.

corneal exhaustion syndrome—a result of long-time wear of contact lens.

corneal forward shift—a progressive forward shift of the cornea for up to 6 months after performance of photorefractive keratectomy (PRK); this shift may not represent true corneal ectasia.

corneal impression test (CIT)—allows cells from the cornea to be tested for signs of rabies before blood, skin, or saliva tests can pick up the disease.

corneal reflex—closure of the eyes on stimulating the cornea.

Corneal Ring (Oph)—a product designed to correct myopia by reshaping the curvature of the cornea.

CorneaSparing LTK (laser thermal keratoplasty) **system**—a noncontact simultaneous laser application for correction of hyperopia, presbyopia, and overcorrection resulting from laser treatments for myopia.

corner fracture—metaphyseal lesion commonly found in abused infants.

corner mouth lift—a plastic surgery procedure in which a triangle is excised just above the commissure, with the suture line following the upper lip vermilion border and extending slightly beyond the corner. It may or may not be performed as an adjunct to lip lift. See *lip lift*.

corn picker's pupil—unilateral mydriasis afflicting workers exposed to belladonna or jimsonweed.

Corometrics maternal/fetal monitor.

coronal CT scan of sinuses—used to diagnose sinusitis. A limited four-slice coronal CT scan of the sinuses provides more information than plain films and has a much-reduced radiation dose and cost than a full CT scan.

coronal orientation—MRI term.

coronal SPIR image (MRI). See *SPIR*.

coronal T1-weighted MR image (spin echo).

coronary anastomotic shunt—used in cardiopulmonary bypass surgery to keep the operating field clear of blood while protecting the heart through distal perfusion.

coronary artery scan (CAS) by Ultrafast CT—a simple, low-cost, and noninvasive diagnostic scan that identifies patients at risk for atherosclerosis and coronary disease episodes by detecting and quantifying calcium in the coronary arteries.

coronary artery scoring—controversial but widely used method of determining calcium plaquing in the coronary arteries using imaging techniques.

coronary atherectomy—an alternative to balloon angioplasty. It works on the Roto-Rooter principle, with suc-

coronary *(cont.)*
tion apparatus utilized to remove the excised plaque.

coronary devices for treatment of ischemic heart disease include *stents* (Palmaz-Schatz and Gianturco-Roubin), *atherectomy* (directional, rotational, and extraction), and *excimer laser angioplasty*.

coronary radiation therapy (CRT).

coronary remodeling—focal enlargement or shrinkage of the lumina of atherosclerotic arteries during plaque formation. Shrinkage has also been demonstrated as a mechanism of arterial remodeling in vessels that have undergone balloon angioplasty and directional atherectomy.

coronary-subclavian steal syndrome—a rarely occurring retrograde blood flow seen postoperatively in patients who have had a coronary artery bypass graft (CABG).

corps ("core") (noun)—corpus; also, a group or body of individuals organized and under common direction (e.g., the medical corps). Cf. *cor, core, corpse*.

corpse—a dead body. Cf. *corps*.

corpus callosum—mass of white matter in the depths of the longitudinal fissure connecting the two cerebral hemispheres.

corpus cavernosum penile electromyography—predicts cavernous smooth muscle function.

corpuscles—see *malpighian corpuscles*.

corpus Luysii—see *body of Luys*.

CorRestore System (Cardio).

corset platysmaplasty—cosmetic surgery for the aging neck. The platysma is used to contour the neck like a corset, producing fewer contour irregularities.

Corti—see *organ of Corti*.

cortical mapping (of the brain).

cortical ring sign—caused by abnormal orientation of the scaphoid on x-ray (rotary subluxation). Also known as the *signet-ring sign*.

cortical spoking.

cortical thumb—a condition in which the thumb lies flat on the palm, with the fingers over it; this is suggestive of a corticospinal lesion.

corticomedullary junction (CMJ) phase imaging on CT scan.

corticotropin-releasing factor (CRF)—a human peptide used for the reduction of edema and inflammation in patients with brain cancer, asthma, and rheumatoid arthritis.

corticotropin-releasing factor (CRF) **receptor antagonist**—a new class of antidepressant drugs. CRF, a neurotransmitter that promotes release of ACTH (adrenocorticotropic hormone) from the pituitary gland, is intimately involved in the body's stress response. There is evidence that excessive production or activity of CRF may play a role in the development of abnormal emotional states such as major depression and post-traumatic stress disorder. By blocking the action of CRF at its receptor sites in the pituitary gland, CRF receptor antagonists may modulate the stress response and relieve the symptoms of these and other mood disorders.

cor triatriatum—a cardiac anomaly in which there are three atria. Also, *triatrial heart*.

cor triatriatum dexter—rare congenital anomaly in which an obstructive membrane is located in the right atrium.

Corynebacterium—gram-positive organism that causes infection in immu-

Corynebacterium (cont.) nosuppressed patients, particularly pneumonia in AIDS patients.

Cosamine DS—combination of glucosamine and chondroitin sulfate.

CoSeal—resorbable synthetic sealant for use in sealing vascular grafts.

Cosgrove-Edwards anuloplasty system.

Cosman ICP Tele-Sensor—implantable telemetric pressure sensor used in hydrocephalus shunts to measure intracranial pressure and to diagnose shunt blockage and function. Also, *Cosman Tele-Monitor System*.

CosmoDerm (1 and 2) **human-based collagen implant**—sterile injectable liquid made of highly purified human collagen, a natural protein that supports the skin. It is injected into the skin to correct soft tissue defects such as wrinkles and acne scars. Also contains lidocaine, which numbs the skin at the site of injection. Used for minor skin defects. Cf. *CosmoPlast*.

CosmoPlast human-based collagen implant—sterile injectable liquid made of highly purified human collagen, a natural protein that supports the skin. It is injected into the skin to correct soft tissue defects such as wrinkles and acne scars. Also contains lidocaine, which numbs the skin at the site of injection. Used for more serious defects. Cf. *CosmoDerm*.

Cosmos II pacemaker—a dual chamber or DDD pacemaker.

CoStasis—postsurgical paranasal sinus packing containing collagen and thrombin.

Costello protocol—laser ablation of prostate in benign prostatic hypertrophy.

costolateral areas—an area of body including the ribs and the sides.

costophrenic angle (CPA)—the acute angle formed by the ribs (chest wall) and the periphery of the diaphragm, particularly as seen on a standard PA chest film.

costosternal angle.

cot—see *finger cot*.

cotinine test—assay of a nicotine degradation product in urine, useful in measuring the subject's level of tobacco use.

Cotrel-Dubousset instrumentation (CDI)—used for posterior spine stabilization and fusion (with bone graft). See *Kaneda device*. Kaneda and Cotrel-Dubousset procedures may be performed at the same time or separately.

Cotrel traction—treatment for adult scoliosis. Uses a leather head halter, pelvic girdle, and a system of pulleys. Also, *Cotrel-Dubousset*.

Cottle elevator (Neuro).

Cotton-Berg syndrome—proximal end tibia fracture; fender fracture.

Cotton-Loader position cast (Ortho).

cottonoid patty (pattie)—used to stem hemorrhage and to protect the exposed brain in surgery. Cf. *Cellolite*.

Cotton procedure—a cartilage graft to the cricopharyngeal area; for subglottic stenosis.

cotton-wool exudates of retina—microinfarcts of nerve fiber layer that resemble tufts of cotton.

cotton-wool sign—radiographic sign of Paget disease of the cranium. Do not confuse with cotton-wool spots of the retina.

cotyledon—subdivision of the uterine surface of a discoidal placenta.

coudé catheter—bent (or elbowed).

cough CPR—a technique used in cardiac catheterization and emergency medicine in which the patient force-

cough *(cont.)* fully and repeatedly coughs. Coughing converts ventricular arrhythmias to a normal sinus rhythm.

Couinaud classification—a grading system for liver disease, using roman numerals that correspond to the segment of liver involved. Usage: "The hepatectomy consisted of a segmentectomy VIII (according to Couinaud classification)." This means that segment VIII of the liver was involved in the procedure.

Coulter counter—for platelet count.

Coulter HIV-1 p24 antigen assay—an antigen test kit for screening of blood donors for HIV-1 during the initial period when donors may actually be infected but still have negative antibody tests with current testing.

coumarin pulsed-dye laser (Pulsolith)—used in lithotripsy.

Councilman bodies—seen in hepatocytes in viral hepatitis.

Councilman chisel—an autopsy instrument used for splitting bone.

countercurrent immunoelectrophoresis test (CIE).

counterflow centrifugal elutriation—a technique which removes some lymphocytes from patients who had allogenic bone marrow transplant to decrease the incidence of graft-versus-host disease.

counterstaining technique—a procedure used in intraoperative ultrasonography of the liver with injected contrast medium. Dye injected into branches of the portal vein adjacent to a liver segment that has been embolized arterially with tumor cells outlines the zone of tissue that must be resected.

counting fingers (or *count fingers*) (CF)—a term used in eye examinations. Usage: "Visual acuity was limited to counting fingers in the right eye, and hand movements in the left eye."

counts, kick—see *kick counts*.

coup de sabre ("coo-da-sob") (Fr., stroke of a sword)—linear scleroderma usually found over the scalp or forehead.

coupled suturing—technique for microvascular anastomosis which is an adaptation of a type of continuous stitch used in the garment industry, generally using 9-0 and 10-0 nylon.

COUP-TF—thyroid hormone receptor auxiliary protein.

Cournand cardiac device.

Courvoisier sign—a sign of malignancy. A palpable and nontender gallbladder with severe jaundice usually suggests malignancy rather than cholelithiasis.

CoVac 50 and **CoVac 70**—suction ArthroWand.

CoVac Wand—used in arthroscopy to treat meniscal tears and facilitate soft tissue removal. It ablates tissue and evacuates the wispy free-floating remnants. Using suction, it prevents clogging and improves visibility by eliminating bubbles.

Covaderm composite wound dressing.

Coverlet adhesive dressing.

Cover-Roll adhesive gauze.

Cover-Strip wound closure strips—uses a hypoallergenic adhesive. In some wounds these may be an alternative to sutures. They have a porous gauze strip that permits air to enter and exudate to pass through.

CoverTip safety syringe—designed to protect against accidental needle sticks.

cover-uncover test (Oph)—assesses eye muscle deviation.

Cowboy Collar—brachial plexus injury control.

COWS (cold to the opposite, warm to the same)—a mnemonic device to help remember the Hallpike caloric stimulation response. Usage: "Caloric testing produced COWS." See *caloric testing*.

coxarthrosis—see *end-stage coxarthrosis* (Ortho).

coxibs—cyclooxygenase-2 inhibitors. The generic names of these drugs end in *coxib* (without hyphen)—e.g., celecoxib.

Coxiella burnetii—rickettsia that causes Q fever. See *Q fever*.

Cox maze III procedure—see *maze procedure; maze cut-and-sew protocol*.

COX (cyclo-oxygenase) **pathway**—a prostaglandin.

coxsackievirus, A and B—a virus that causes meningitis and paralytic disease.

COX-2 inhibitors—a class of nonsteroidal anti-inflammatory drugs for osteoarthritis, rheumatoid arthritis, acute pain, and primary dysmenorrhea. They work by inhibiting cyclooxygenase-2 (COX-2), responsible for producing pain and inflammation, without affecting COX-1, which protects the stomach lining. Inhibition of COX-1 is thought to be the cause of serious GI side effects in NSAIDs.

CP (costophrenic) **angle**.

CPAP (continuous positive airway pressure) ("see-pap")—provides positive pressure in lungs even when the patient exhales fully, to prevent lungs from collapsing.

CPB (cardiopulmonary bypass).

CP-Cardiosol—used in cardiopulmonary bypass.

CPCI (Chronic Pain Coping Inventory).

CPD (cephalopelvic disproportion).

CPD (chorioretinopathy and pituitary dysfunction) **syndrome**—characterized by severe, early-onset chorioretinopathy, trichosis, and evidence of pituitary dysfunction.

CPE (chronic pulmonary emphysema).

CPHV OptiForm mitral valve—used in patients requiring mitral valve replacement. The OptiForm mitral valve has a flexible sewing cuff that can be sculpted to fit mitral annular anatomy, thus ensuring tissue compliance with the valve. *CPHV* is an acronym for *Carbomedics prosthetic heart valve*.

CPI (conventional planar imaging).

CPK (creatine phosphokinase)—serum enzyme that can be chemically distinguished into three isoenzymes or fractions: the MB isoenzyme, elevated in myocardial infarction; the MM isoenzyme, elevated in cerebral infarction; and the BB isoenzyme, sometimes elevated in uremia and other conditions. When separated in the laboratory by electrophoresis, these isoenzymes appear as distinct bands in a visual display. Hence the expression "*MB band* is roughly synonymous with *MB isoenzyme*." Do not confuse *creatine* with *creatinine*.

CPM (continuous passive motion) **devices**—see *Autoflex II*.

CPP (cerebral perfusion pressure).

CPPD (calcium pyrophosphate deposition; disease).

CPS (cardiopulmonary support) **system**—heart-lung machine.

CPT (Current Procedural Terminology) (coding).

CPT hip system.

CPVG (cryopreserved vein graft).

crack—street name for rock cocaine, a concentrated, smokable form of the drug which is highly addicting. Cf. *crank*.

cracked pot sound—(1) a percussion sound like that heard when striking a cracked pot and indicates a pulmonary cavity; (2) a sound on percussion caused by the separation of cranial sutures in children with increased cranial pressure, e.g., as seen in hydrocephalus. Also called *Macewen sign*.

cracker test—for the presence of Sjögren disease. Usage: "She has a negative cracker test in the sense that if we were to give her a soda cracker, she would easily be able to swallow without drinking water."

cradle cap—seborrheic dermatitis manifested as thick yellowish scales, often seen on the scalp of infants.

Crafoord-Senning heart-lung machine.

Cragg endoluminal graft—see *Cragg Endopro System 1*.

Cragg Endopro System I—a covered stent design, used in Cragg endoluminal graft procedure as adjunct to balloon angioplasty of long complex iliac stenosis. The stent is covered with woven fabric graft and is a flexible, self-expanding endoprosthesis of nitinol wire.

Cragg thrombolytic brush—a mechanical thrombolysis system to dissolve clots in hemodialysis access grafts.

cranial electrical stimulation (CES)—introduced by Saul Liss for relief of pain and anxiety, there being a noted correlation between depression and chronic pain. The Liss CES device is used for chronic headache pain and is similar to TENS application.

cranial nerves, twelve—written with roman numerals, I to XII.

I olfactory
II optic
III oculomotor
IV trochlear
V trigeminal
VI abducens
VII facial
VIII vestibulocochlear (acoustic)
IX glossopharyngeal
X vagal
XI accessory
XII hypoglossal

CranioCap—custom-made cranial orthosis for treatment of deformational plagiocephaly.

cranioplastic powder—used for repair of cranial defects.

craniosacral therapy (CST)—a hands-on light-touch method of assisting in the natural flow of cerebrospinal fluid within the system. The CST method of evaluating and enhancing the function of the physiological body system called the craniosacral system was developed by John E. Upledger, an osteopathic physician, and is referred to as *Upledger CST*.

craniosynostosis (craniostosis)—premature closure of the sagittal suture in newborns, resulting in scaphocephaly and other associated compensatory deformational changes. When treated early (less than 2-3 months of age), a simple suturectomy or resection of the synostotic suture provides correction. By 6 months of age, patients require major craniofacial reconstructive procedures. See also *endoscopic strip craniectomy, helmet-molding therapy,* and *scaphocephaly.*

crank—slang term for the street drug methamphetamine ("speed"), which is snorted or injected. Cf. *crack*.

Crawford graft inclusion technique (Cardio)—with direct branch vessel reattachment.

CRC (colorectal cancer).

CR/CO (centric relation-centric occlusion)—used in maxillofacial surgery when discussing bite patterns.

CRE (cAMP response element)—a DNA sequence that acts as a binding site for proteins.

C-reactive protein (CRP)—an acute-phase reactant that is elevated in many inflammatory conditions, such as cardiovascular disease. The protein is high when there is an inflammatory response and returns to undetectable as the response clears. Elevation of CRP probably doesn't occur unless arteriosclerosis (increasingly recognized as an inflammatory rather than a degenerative process) is already present. Thus, CRP is considered a good marker of arteriosclerotic disease.

creatine—a nitrogenous substance that is found in muscles, brain, and blood of vertebrates. Cf. *carotene, creatinine, keratin.*

creatine phosphokinase—see *CPK.*

creatinine clearance, 24-hour—a measure of kidney function, calculated from the serum creatinine level and the amount of creatinine excreted in the urine in 24 hours. Cf. *creatine, creatinine.*

creatinine, serum—a waste product of protein metabolism, elevated in kidney disease. Cf. *creatine.*

CREB (cAMP response element binding) **protein**—regulates genes for neurotransmitter synthetic enzymes.

Credé ("kre-day") **maneuver**—massaging the lower abdomen over the bladder to promote complete emptying in patients with neurological damage. Usage: "Bladder Credé was ordered." Cf. *Credé method.*

Credé method—expressing the placenta from the uterus by pushing the uterus down into the pelvis and squeezing it. Cf. *Credé maneuver.*

crenated—having a shriveled or pitted surface.

creola bodies (lowercase *c*)—balls of desquamated epithelium. Often found in the sputa of asthmatics.

crepitance—a possible mispronunciation of the noun *crepitus* (a crackling sound), influenced by the sound of the adjective *crepitant*. *Crepitance* is probably here to stay, and if clearly dictated, it should be transcribed, even though this non-word has yet to be recorded in dictionaries. The spelling *crepitants* is wholly erroneous an unacceptable in this setting.

crepitant rales—fine crackling or bubbling sounds heard on auscultation of the breath sounds.

creps—slang for *crepitus* (crackling sounds in lungs).

crescendo-decrescendo murmur—increases from quiet to louder and then decreases again. May be diagnostic of aortic stenosis when heard as a systolic murmur. In aortic insufficiency it is heard as a diastolic murmur. Also, *diamond-shaped murmur.*

crescent artifact—see *kink artifact.*

crescent sign (Radiol)—a crescentic lucent zone that separates the fragment from the remainder of the femur, in a fracture in the subchondral bone in avascular necrosis. The crescent sign is seen in a radiograph of the hip joint, which reveals a thin, curvilinear lucent line parallel to the cortical margin of the femoral head. Interruption of the blood supply to

crescent *(cont.)*
the femoral head leads to ischemic necrosis of the marrow and bone that it supplies. Eventually the bone infarcts and insufficiency fractures may ensue.

crescentic base wedge osteotomy—a rotational osteotomy whose axis is near the first metatarsal base. Used for correction of hallux valgus and similar to an opening base wedge osteotomy.

CREST (Cilostazol for Restenosis) **study**.

CREST syndrome (see also *CRST*)
C calcinosis cutis
R Raynaud phenomenon
E esophageal dysmotility
S sclerodactyly
T telangiectasia

cribogram—a special mattress wired with sensing devices. An infant who is suspected of hearing loss is placed on it and a computer compares the baby's movements with the stimulation.

cribriform—perforated like a sieve.

crick—painful spasm, usually in the neck.

Cricket—small, light pulse oximeter.

cri du chat (cat's cry)—an indication of a chromosomal irregularity causing mental retardation; the name derives from the catlike cry emitted by these children.

Crigler-Najjar syndrome—one of the reasons for liver transplant in children.

Crikelair otoplasty (ENT).

crinkle artifact—see *kink artifact*.

crisis—see *Dietl crisis*.

crisscross heart—a heart with crossing of the atrioventricular valves.

"crit"—slang for hematocrit. It should always be expanded in medical reports.

criteria (pl.)—standards or means by which conclusions are arrived at. Usage: "On EKG there were voltage criteria for left ventricular hypertrophy." See *DeSmet criteria*; *Jones criteria, revised*; Ranson criteria; *Rome I and Rome II criteria*.

Crit-Line III—a blood monitoring system that is noninvasive and standalone. It enables real-time measurement of hematocrit, blood volume, and oxygen saturation. Also, *Crit-Scan*.

crochetage—notch or notching, a finding on electrocardiogram.

crock—pejorative slang for difficult patient.

Crohn disease—regional enteritis; a chronic granulomatous inflammatory disease.

Cröhnlein procedure (Oph).

cromolyn sodium—see *Steri-Neb*.

Cronin S dermal-fat flap, modified—used in nipple-areola reconstruction in autologous breast reconstruction.

cross-chest adduction test—also referred to as horizontal adduction test. It is used for diagnosing rotator cuff tendinitis.

cross clamp (noun); **cross-clamp, cross-clamped** (adj., verb).

cross-cover test—measures degree of eye deviation.

crossed coil—MRI term.

crossed reflex—in which stimulus applied to one side produces a response on the contralateral side.

crossed-swords technique (Oph)—Usage: "The inferior oblique muscle was reattached using the crossed-swords technique."

crossfire radiation therapy—a procedure for treating brain tumors. Doctors attach a metal frame to the

crossfire *(cont.)* skull with screws to hold the head still and help aim the beams. The beams are fired from hundreds of points, following paths that intersect only at the tumor. Working together, they kill the tumor while sparing other tissue.

CrossFlex LC coronary stent—for improving luminal diameter and maintaining patency in ischemic coronary arteries secondary to discrete de novo stenosis or restenosis of native coronary arteries. It is an over-the-wire product that is placed via a balloon catheter during PTCA procedures.

crosshatch pattern (Oph)—see *fishbone pattern*.

crosslinking nucleotides—see *XLnt*.

crossover (crossing over) (Genetics)—exchange of genetic material between members of a chromosome pair.

CrossSail—coronary dilatation catheter.

cross-talk effect—MRI term.

cross-tunneling incision—used in performance of lipectomy. Usage: "A cross-tunneling incision was made and a 1.8 and a 2.4 mm triple-hole cannula used."

crowded carpal sign—in which frontal radiographs of the wrist reveal overlap of the distal carpal row with the proximal carpal row. This overriding gives rise to the "crowded carpal" appearance and is diagnostic of volar perilunate dislocation.

crowncork tympanoplasty (ENT)—a total reconstruction of the tympanic membrane. A composite graft of tragal cartilage and perichondrium is fashioned. It looks like a crown on top of a bottle cork. It is used in correcting subtotal or total defects of the tympanic membrane, found in surgery for middle ear malformation.

CRP (canalith repositioning procedure)—measures vertigo. A vibrational device is held against the mastoid process of the ear that is affected with benign paroxysmal positional vertigo.

CRP (C-reactive protein).

CRPS—see *complex regional pain syndrome*.

CRRT (continuous renal replacement therapy).

CRS (cell recovery system).

CRS (Concentric retriever system).

CRS (counter rotation system)—type of brace used to correct internal and external tibial torsion in children. Consists of a hinged device with rods that attach to footplates glued onto both shoes. It allows kicking and crawling, and children can sleep in it comfortably.

CRST syndrome (see also *CREST*)

C calcinosis cutis
R Raynaud phenomenon
S sclerodactyly
T telangiectasia

CRT (coronary radiation therapy).

CRTD (cardiac resynchronization therapy defibrillation) **system**.

cruciate incision—cross-shaped.

crude coal tar (*not* cold tar)—used in treatment of psoriasis.

Cruiser hip abduction brace—polypropylene hip abduction brace for treating hip dysplasia in toddlers up to 2½ years of age.

crush technique—in balloon angioplasty, a technique for the treatment of atherosclerotic plaque that develops at the juncture between a major coronary artery and a smaller branch vessel (branch point plaque).

crush *(cont.)*
The procedure involves the placement of a drug-eluting stent in the side branch, with 4-5 mm extending into the main artery. An angioplasty balloon is inflated in the main artery to crush, or fold over, the end of the stent, and a second drug-eluting stent is placed in the main vessel. An angioplasty balloon is then threaded through all three stent layers into the side branch, another balloon is threaded into the main artery, and the side-by-side, or "kissing," balloons are inflated at the same time so that both stents expand in a tubular shape. The crush technique ensures that there are no gaps between the two stents, thereby minimizing the risk of arterial tearing (dissection) and, it is hoped, long-term renarrowing.

crust—a hard, friable, irregular layer of dried blood, serum, pus, tissue debris, or any combination of these adherent to the surface of injured or inflamed skin. Also, scab.

crutched-stick-type endoprosthesis—a descriptive term used for a biliary duct stent.

Crutchfield skeletal traction tongs.

Cryer criterion—pelvic fracture classification based on potential for hemorrhage and associated injuries, useful in helping anesthesiologist evaluate a surgical patient.

CryoCor—cardiac cryoablation system, used to convert atrial flutter to normal sinus rhythm.

cryoablation for prostate cancer—a minimally invasive procedure performed under general or local anesthesia. It involves freezing and destroying cancerous tumors inside the body, using advanced ultrasound technology to locate the tumor and a cryoprobe to freeze tissue. The body absorbs the dead tissue over time.

CRYOcare system—used in endometrial cryoablation as treatment for dysfunctional uterine bleeding.

cryocrit—the percentage of red and white blood cells re-added to arrive at this value. Cf. *cytocrit*.

Cryo/Cuff ankle dressing—reduces swelling and pain by applying cryotherapy and compression.

Cryo/Cuff boot—boot filled with ice and water, covering foot and ankle. Exerts pressure up to 40 mmHg.

cryogens—supercooled gases such as helium or nitrogen, used to cool the magnet at the heart of a magnetic resonance scanner.

CryoHit—allows surgeons to ablate localized tumors by freezing diseased cells during a minimally invasive procedure using ultrathin probes. The system is compatible with interventional MRI (I-MRI), which provides real-time video images of the tissue during surgery.

CryoLife-O'Brien valve—a stentless porcine heart valve.

cryomagnet—an MRI magnet in which a cryogen is used to bring the wires of the magnet coil into a superconducting state.

cryophake (Oph)—an instrument using extremely cold temperatures to remove a cataract. Example: *Keeler cryophake*.

cryoprecipitate—drug used to control bleeding in patients with uremia and prolonged bleeding time. Contains fibrinogen, factor VIII, fibronectin, and factor XIII. It is used as a last resort in life-threatening bleeding because of the risk of viral transmission. See *DDAVP*.

cryopreserved embryo—an embryo, usually one produced by in vitro fertilization, that has been stored in the frozen state because it exceeded the needs of the moment.

cryopreserved vein graft (CVG).

cryoprobe—instrument used to apply extreme cold to tissues, as in cryosurgery.

cryostat—a device containing a microtome for sectioning frozen tissue.

cryosurgery—a treatment that kills some types of cancer cells by freezing them with liquid nitrogen. It is used in prostate cancer if there has been no spread to other tissue. Cryosurgery is performed under spinal or general anesthesia, with the aid of an ultrasound probe that is inserted into the rectum. The ultrasound converts sound waves into images on a TV monitor; this functions as a guide for inserting the probes, through which the liquid nitrogen is administered. The ice ball that is formed within the prostatic tissue and tumor can be seen on the screen. And the neat thing (in the housekeeping sense) is that the dead cells are absorbed by the body. This is a form of therapy that can be repeated, if the cancer should recur.

CryoValve-SG—human allograft heart valve processing method. It depopulates the native cells of a donor heart valve, leaving a collagen matrix with the same functionality as other cryopreserved heart valves.

CryoVasc catheter—a catheter for the treatment of chronic cardiac ischemia.

"crypto"—slang term for cryptococcosis, infection with *Cryptococcus neoformans*, or cryptosporidiosis, which is seen in AIDS patients. As with all slang, when in doubt, ask the dictator for clarification.

cryptochrome—a newly discovered light-sensitive pigment in the eye that has been found to mediate the circadian rhythm, the biological timer regulating many body functions.

Cryptococcus neoformans—rare cause of lytic bone lesions; an AIDS infection.

cryptogenic (idiopathic) **epilepsy**—a condition of recurring seizures for which no cause can be assigned.

cryptosporidiosis antibody—immunostimulant for AIDS patients, obtained from cow's milk.

Cryptosporidium—a protozoan parasite. Sometimes referred to as the slang term "crypto."

crystalloids—a substance in solution that can pass through a semipermeable membrane. Usage: "Fluids: 1600 cc of crystalloids." Normal saline solution and lactated Ringer solution are crystalloids used as blood replacement.

cry, uterine (Ob-Gyn). Usage: "Curettage was done, with good uterine cry." *Uterine cry* refers to the sound of the uterus as it is being scraped clean of debris, during the curettage. The uterus is a smooth and firm muscle, and once all the lining and debris are removed by sharp curettage, the smooth muscle emits a "cry" when it is clean and smooth once again. Note: Some physicians pronounce "cree" (probably from French *cri*, as in *cri du chat*), others "cry" (long *i*).

CSD (cat-scratch disease).

CSDH (chronic subdural hematoma).

CSF (cerebrospinal fluid).

CSF (colony-stimulating factor).

CS-5 cryosurgical system—used for cryoablation of prostatic tissue and liver metastases and other gynecological, urological, and general surgical applications.

C-shaped curves.

C sign—a C-shaped line formed by the medial outline of the talar dome and the inferior outline of the sustentaculum tali. This is a sign of subtalar coalition on x-ray of the foot.

Cs131 (Cesium-131) **Seed**—a new isotope for low-dose-radiation (LDR) seed brachytherapy for the treatment of prostate cancer and other malignancies. When placed inside or near a tumor, Cs131 Seeds deliver radiation directly to cancer cells while reducing or eliminating damage to surrounding tissue. This new isotope represents the first major advancement in LDR seed brachytherapy in more than 18 years.

CSII (continuous subcutaneous insulin infusion).

CSQI (continuous subcutaneous infusion)—pain-control method utilizing a butterfly needle inserted subcutaneously and connected to an intravenous line. It is used for patients who will receive narcotic medication for more than 48 hours and who cannot receive intravenous medication due to poor veins or other problems. The system can be coupled with a patient-controlled analgesia pump which allows the patient to select the time when the medication is most needed for pain control and administer it. *Sub-Q-Set* is the trade name for one continuous subcutaneous infusion device.

CSRA (cementless surface replacement arthroplasty).

CSVD (controlled spontaneous vaginal delivery).

CSVT (central splanchnic venous thrombosis).

CSW (cerebral salt-wasting) **syndrome**.

CSWT (cardiac shock wave therapy).

CT (computed tomography).

CTA (computed tomographic angiography).

CTAP (clear to auscultation and percussion). The abbreviation should be expanded in medical transcripts.

CTAP (CT angiographic portography).

CTB—slang abbreviation for *ceased to breathe.*

CTCL (cutaneous T-cell lymphoma)—also called *mycosis fungoides*.

CT colonography—computed tomographic imaging study of the colon.

CTD (connective tissue disease).

CTDx electrostimulation system—helps decrease symptoms associated with repetitive stress injury of the wrist while providing wrist support.

C-Tek anterior cervical plate system—available in both fixed- and slotted-hole versions to accommodate the physician's surgical technique.

C-terminal assay for PTH (parathormone; parathyroid hormone).

CTE:YAG (CrTmEr:YAG) **laser**.

CTFC (corrected TIMI frame count)—a quantitative method of assessing coronary artery flow during angiography.

CT gantry—the bridgelike frame on a CT scanner on which the traveling crane of the scanner moves.

CTHA (computerized tomographic hepatic angiography).

C.Ti.2 Brace—a six-point knee support especially for ACL (anterior cruciate ligament) deficient knees.

CT laser mammography (CTLM)—a "painless mammogram" that requires no breast compression, uses no x-rays, and produces detailed cross-sectional images of the tissue.

CTLC (contact transscleral laser cytophotocoagulation).

CTLM (computed tomography laser mammography).

CTMP (contrast threshold for motion perception).

CTNS—a gene associated with cystinosis. Neuropathic cystinosis is characterized by an accumulation of the amino acid cystine in cells, leading to severe organ damage, primarily in the kidneys. Most patients develop the disease within their first year of life, and many die of kidney disease before the age of 10.

CT PE (computed tomography pulmonary embolus) **protocol**.

CT PEG (CT-guided percutaneous endoscopic gastrostomy)—for placement of a gastric feeding tube without open surgery.

CTR (cardiothoracic ratio).

C-TRAK handheld gamma detector—measures the accumulated radioactivity in a nodule after radionuclide injection.

CTS (carpal tunnel syndrome).

CT scanner—see *scanner.*

CT/SPECT fusion—digitally fused CT and radiolabeled monoclonal antibody SPECT images. Used to detect tumors.

CT with slip-ring technology.

C225—monoclonal antibody antineoplastic.

C-type acupuncture needle—used with a guiding tube to assure straight entry into the skin. B-type needles are used without guiding tubes.

C-type natriuretic peptide—see *CNP.*

cubic centimeter (cc).

cubital tunnel syndrome—caused by compression of the ulnar nerve at the elbow. Cf. *carpal tunnel syndrome*.

Cueva cranial nerve electrode monitoring device.

cuffed tunneled catheter—a catheter used in vascular access for hemodialysis.

cuirass ("kwe-ras´")—a covering for the chest. Also, *cuirass respirator*.

CUI (Cox-Uphoff International) **tissue expander**.

cul-de-sac—a blind pouch; a saclike cavity or tube open at only one end, e.g., the rectouterine pouch, or pouch of Douglas.

culdolaparoscopy—surgical technique that combines culdoscopy with laparoscopy and microlaparoscopy.

culdoplasty, modified McCall posterior—performed at the time of abdominal hysterectomy to decrease the incidence of posthysterectomy vaginal vault prolapse and enterocele formation.

Cullen sign—a bluish discoloration around the umbilicus, indicative of a ruptured ectopic pregnancy or acute hemorrhagic pancreatitis.

culture and sensitivity (C&S)—a lab test in which an organism is grown on a nutrient medium containing several antibiotic-laden disks. A lack of growth around a disk shows that the organism is sensitive to that antibiotic. Do not confuse *C&S* with *CNS* (central nervous system).

cultured autologous melanocytes—applied to superficially dermabraded skin for treatment of vitiligo.

cultured epithelial autografting—a technique to cover a burn wound in patients with massive burns, who do

cultured *(cont.)* not have enough skin of their own for grafting. Small pieces of their remaining skin are cultured into new skin.

culture medium—a nutrient and protective fluid or semisolid material in which a culture is grown in vitro.

Cun-Meter—a mathematical search square which is a point-search aid used to assess position of acupuncture points. Measurements are registered in Cun, which is the width of the thumb joint. With these measuring instruments, width is first measured, after which readings can be taken at any time from a scale of 0.5 to 2.5 Cun.

Cunningham clamp—for male urinary incontinence.

cup-cage acetabular device—used in revision hip arthroplasty.

Cupid's bow contour or **sign**—curvature of the endplate of the fourth and fifth lumbar vertebrae, which mimics the curvature of Cupid's bow (aimed cephalad) on x-ray. It is considered a normal variant.

cupping—method of stimulating acupuncture points by applying suction through a metal, wood, or glass jar in which a partial vacuum has been created. This technique produces blood congestion at the site and therefore stimulates it. Used for low backache, sprains, soft-tissue injuries, and helping remove fluid from lungs in chronic bronchitis.

cup-to-disk ratio (Oph).

Curaderm hydrocolloid dressing material.

Curafil hydrogel dressing.

Curafoam foam wound dressing.

Curagel hydrogel dressing—absorbs excess exudate while it cools and cushions a wound. It has a top layer of polyurethane designed to help control evaporation and leave no residue to irritate the wound when removed.

Curasorb calcium alginate dressing—reacts with sodium ions in wound exudate to form a nonadherent gel that provides a moist healing environment, reducing possible maceration of healthy skin surrounding a wound. It can be trimmed and customized for a variety of wound shapes and sizes and can be used for packing deep wounds. Cf. *Aquasorb, Ventex.*

Curdy blade (Oph).

^{14}C-urea breath excretion test—highly sensitive test diagnostic for *Helicobacter pylori,* using urea labeled with the radionuclide carbon-14. Patients are given a dose of ^{14}C-urea and "cold" urea, with breath samples taken at 30- and 60-minute intervals, and ^{14}C-urea measured in exhaled CO_2. See also *breath pentane test, ^{14}C-cholylglycine breath test, ^{14}C-urinary excretion, Helicobacter pylori breath test.*

^{14}C-urinary excretion—measurement of ^{14}C-urea in urine after oral dose, correlates with ^{14}C-urea breath test for diagnosis of *H. pylori*. See also *^{14}C-urea breath test.*

Curling ulcer—gastric or duodenal ulcers seen in patients who have suffered severe burns over large areas of the body.

Curlin 2000 Plus—a portable infusion pump.

Current Procedural Terminology (CPT) (coding).

Curschmann spirals—formed elements that have been found in the sputa of asthmatic patients.

curve of Spee—a curved line extending along the summits of the buccal cusps from the first premolar to the third molar. Named for a German embryologist, Ferdinand von Spee.

curvilinear incision (*not* curvalinear)—a curved incision.

CUSA (Cavitron ultrasonic aspirator).

Cu-Safe 300—IUD specifically designed to decrease unwanted side effects, such as bleeding, pain, and expulsion, while providing simplicity of insertion, ease of removal, and fair contraceptive protection.

CUSALap—ultrasonic accessory that provides simultaneous fragmentation, irrigation, and aspiration.

Cushieri maneuver, two-hand—a maneuver used in laparoscopic cholecystectomies.

cushingoid (*not* cushinoid)—having the appearance or symptoms of Cushing disease, as in "cushingoid facies."

Cushing response—a neurologic indication of intracranial pressure. As intracranial pressure increases, the systolic blood pressure increases noticeably, while the diastolic pressure changes little, if at all. The increased difference between the two blood pressures is significant as an indication of the onset of late-stage intracranial pressure. Cf. *Cushing triad.*

Cushing syndrome—a symptom complex including moon facies, buffalo hump, abdominal distention, hypertension, amenorrhea (in women), impotence (in men), muscle wasting and weakness, fat pad formation, skin darkening, and skin thinning. More common in women than men. Caused by taking large amounts of steroids for long periods of time or by the excess production of cortisol. Cf. *Cushing response.*

Cushing triad—rising blood pressure, bradycardia, and widening pulse pressure are indicative of cerebral hemorrhage and cerebral edema. See *Cushing response*.

custom contoured ablation pattern (C-CAP) **method**.

CustomCornea Wavefront system—see *wavefront measurement*.

cut—a CT (computed tomography) section or image; a scan. See *tangential cut*.

cutaneous T-cell lymphoma (CTCL).

cut-biopsy needle—see *PercuCut*.

cut, clamp, and tie—the basic operating program: first, make or extend an incision or dissection; second, clamp with hemostats any vessels severed in the process ("bleeders"); third, tie ligatures around the ends of the severed vessels and remove the hemostats. Alternatively, bleeding vessels may be coagulated with electric current or sealed with metal clips.

cutdown catheter—inserted in the cutdown to a vein when no veins are accessible to a needle in an emergency situation.

Cutinova Cavity wound filling material.

Cutinova Hydro—hydrocolloid transparent and flexible dressing that does not leave a residue on the wound.

Cutler-Beard bridge flap procedure—for reconstructing large defects of the upper eyelid, with flaps from the lower lid and the median forehead. Similar to the modified Hughes procedure of the lower eyelid.

Cutting Balloon—microsurgical dilatation catheter system for treatment of

Cutting *(cont.)*
coronary artery disease. It uses microsurgical blades mounted longitudinally on an angioplasty balloon to open narrowed arteries.

cutting loops—used with resectoscopes.

CVA (cerebrovascular accident, called *stroke* or *brain attack*)—the result of a severe cerebrovascular occlusion in which symptoms do not resolve within 24 hours, and in which there is a long-term residual deficit. See *TIA*.

CVB (chorionic villi biopsy)—used in prenatal diagnosis of many birth defects. It can be performed at 8 to 11 weeks, rather than the 17 to 20 weeks needed for amniocentesis.

CVC—see *central venous catheter*.

CVEMC—a chemotherapy protocol consisting of cisplatin, vincristine, etoposide, mesna, and cyclophosphamide.

C-VEST system—ambulatory radionuclide monitoring system.

CVI (cavum velum interpositum).

CV Peri-Guard patch—a glutaraldehyde cross-linked bovine pericardium for cardiac repair.

CVProfilor DO-2020—cardiovascular profiling device.

CVS (chorionic villous sampling).

CVT-124—a highly selective adenosine A_1 receptor antagonist used in the treatment of edema associated with congestive heart failure.

CVVHD (continuous venovenous hemodialysis).

C-wire Serter (C-wire fitting into C-serter system)—a handheld, battery-driven device for inserting C-wires into place in bones in hand and foot surgery.

cyanoacrylate (Superglue)—a tissue adhesive.

CyberKnife Express—a combination of software and hardware that significantly speeds up radiosurgery treatments using the CyberKnife.

CyberKnife radiosurgery—used to treat locally advanced pancreatic cancer as well as lesions anywhere in the body when radiation treatment is indicated. CyberKnife radiosurgery administers a high dose of radiation in a single or small number of treatments, with minimal toxicity to surrounding tissues and organs.

CyberKnife stereotactic radiosurgery/radiotherapy system—uses a linear accelerator, robotic arm, and image-guided technology to provide non-invasive treatment of tumors and other conditions affecting the brain, head, neck, and cervicothoracic spine.

Cybex test—apparatus used in testing and measuring the strength of a muscle as it is involved by a joint going through range-of-motion testing, as in shoulder girdle muscles or hip and thigh muscles.

cyclic adenosine monophosphate (cAMP).

cyclic vomiting syndrome—digestive disorder that for the most part affects children, characterized by chronic nausea, vomiting, extreme fatigue, motion sickness, abdominal pain and, in some cases, vertigo that may last for hours to days. The exact cause of cyclic vomiting syndrome is not known.

cyclomania—a mild form of bipolar disorder which includes hypomania and depression.

cycloplegia—pathologic or induced paralysis of the ciliary muscle of the eye; paralysis of accommodation.

cyclops lesion—localized anterior fibrosis of the knee, often occurring after anterior cruciate ligament reconstruction and leading to loss of knee extension.

Cyclops procedure—technique used to cover a large soft tissue defect after excision of a breast, chest wall muscles, and clavicle or ribs. The opposite breast, which must be large, is rotated intact across the chest wall to completely cover the surgical defect.

cyesis ("si-e'-sis")—pregnancy. Usage: "Her symptoms of acute nausea and vomiting are probably secondary to cyesis."

CYFRA 21-1—a tumor marker detected in the serum of patients with non-small cell lung cancer. May also be useful as a tumor marker for breast carcinoma and gynecology neoplasm.

Cyma line—a term used in foot x-ray reports.

cymba conchal cartilage graft—a graft harvested from the upper part of the concha of the auricle, used in rhinoplasty. See also *cavum conchal cartilage graft*.

Cymetra—brand name for LifeCell micronized AlloDerm, a nonsurgical soft tissue replacement material used in facial plastic surgery.

Cypher sirolimus-eluting coronary stent—a combination drug device intended to help reduce restenosis (reblockage) of a treated coronary artery. The stent's treatment process is controlled by a polymer coating that gradually releases the drug sirolimus into the vessel lining to prevent scar tissue growth.

CYP3A4—naturally occurring enzyme present in the small intestine that can interfere with drug metabolism. Grapefruit juice has been found to decrease levels of CYP3A4 and improve drug efficacy.

CYP2D6 (cytochrome P450 2D6)—drug-metabolizing enzyme that is estimated to act upon 25% of all prescription drugs, notably Prozac, Paxil, Zoloft, Effexor, hydrocodone, Risperdal, and Allegra.

CYP2D6 test—drug screen for the CYP2D6 drug-metabolizing enzyme. It determines whether a person will metabolize certain drugs at a slow, intermediate, fast, or superfast rate.

Cyriax physiotherapy—for treatment of tennis elbow, consisting of deep transverse friction over the extensor origin and manipulations.

cystic adenomatoid malformation.

cysticercosis—infestation with a larval form of tapeworm.

cystitome (Oph)—an instrument used to open the capsule of the lens of the eye. Cf. *cystotome*.

cystocolpoproctography—fluoroscopic imaging for the detection and measurement of prolapse of pelvic organs.

cystoid macular edema (CME).

cystometrogram (CMG).

cystotome (Urol)—an instrument used for incising the bladder. Cf. *cystitome*.

cytoblast—the cell nucleus. Cf. *cytoplast*.

cytocidal—cell-killing or destroying. Usage: "The cytocidal properties of this drug could be useful if those we are trying should prove less than effective." See *cidal*.

cytocrit—the sum of the percentage of white blood cells and the percentage of red blood cells. Cf. *cryocrit*.

cytogenetics—the branch of biomedicine that studies the relationship of the microscopic appearance and configuration of chromosomes and their behavior during cell division to the genotype and phenotype of the individual.

cytokeratins—proteins that form the intermediate filaments of the cytoskeleton.

cytokines—proteins produced by the body in response to HIV infection and other stressors. Their action is not yet well understood. Tumor necrosis factor (TNF) and interleukins 1 and 6 are cytokines.

cytomegalic inclusion body.

cytomegalovirus (CMV)—herpesvirus that causes several diseases in AIDS patients, including intestinal disease, retinitis that can lead to blindness, and other problems.

cytomegalovirus encephalitis—an opportunistic infection of the brain by cytomegalovirus, seen in patients with immunodeficiency. Variable symptoms include seizures, clouding of consciousness, and other symptoms similar to those of the HIV dementia complex.

cytomegalovirus hepatitis.

cytomegalovirus retinitis—an infection of the retina caused by one of a group of herpesviruses. This is one of a number of opportunistic infections seen in AIDS.

cytometry

EPIC-C or EPICS Profile flow
FACScan (fluorescence-activated cell sorter) flow
flocculation flow
flow
laser scanning (LSC)
multiple sort flow
Urocyte diagnostic

cytoplasm—all components of a cell exclusive of the cell membrane and the nucleus; it consists of a fluid medium containing water, electrolytes, nutrients, wastes, proteins, enzymes, and organelles (ribosomes, mitochondria, Golgi apparatus).

cytoplasmic autoantibody against neutrophils (cANCA)

cytoplasmic inclusion body.

cytoplasmic inheritance—transfer of genetic material by genes present in cytoplasm.

cytoplast—a cell whose nucleus has been removed, but which remains viable for a period of time. Cf. *cytoblast*.

CytoPorter—drug delivery system that transports drugs across lipid barriers (e.g., skin, cellular membranes) into the interior of cells for optimal therapeutic effect.

cytoreductive surgery—surgical removal of malignant tissue, also called *debulking*.

CytoRich preservative—fixative and preservative used in cell pathology.

cytosine—a pyrimidine (symbol C), one of the four nucleotide bases found in DNA and RNA; in the formation of a double-stranded nucleic acid, it always pairs with the pyrimidine thymine (T) in DNA and with the pyrimidine uracil (U) in RNA.

cytoskeleton—the cells that comprise the bony skeleton.

cytostatic—bringing to a halt; stopping or suppressing the growth of cells and their reproduction; also, an agent that accomplishes this.

cytotoxic cells—"killer" T-cell lymphocytes, also called *T-8 cells*. T-4 cells are the lymphocytes affected by the virus, but they are needed to activate the cytotoxic cells. As AIDS re-

cytotoxic *(cont.)*
search has shown, loss of one piece of the immune system makes it ineffective, as the interactions are multiple and complex.

Czaja-McCaffrey rigid stent introducer/endoscope—used for insertion of tracheal stents.

D, d

DAD (diffuse alveolar disease).

Dacogen (decitabine)—an anticancer compound.

Dacomed snap gauge—used in testing impotence; will break if an erection occurs during sleep, thus indicating that the impotence is not organic in nature. See *snap gauge band*.

Dacron synthetic ligament material.

dacryocystorhinostomy (DCR).

Dafilon suture—nonabsorbable polyamide surgical suture for skin closure. Used in plastic, ophthalmic, and microsurgery procedures.

dagger sign—a single central radiodense line on frontal x-ray of the lumbar spine that is related to ossification of supraspinous and interspinous ligaments. It is diagnostic of ankylosing spondylitis.

Dagrofil suture—nonabsorbable polyester braided suture for use on muscles and in orthopedic procedures.

Dale Foley catheter holder.

Dalkon shield—intrauterine device.

Dall-Miles cable grip system—cerclage application for bone grafting and fracture fixation.

Dalrymple sign ("dal-rimpl")—the widened eyelid opening typical of the "stare" in hyperthyroidism. Cf. *Collier sign*.

DALM (dysplasia-associated lesion or mass).

dalton—unit of measurement of the molecular weight of proteins (measured in kilodaltons), which constitute aeroallergens.

Damato Campimeter—used to measure visual fields.

Damus-Kaye-Stansel operation—for repair of congenital heart defect.

DANA (designed after natural anatomy) **shoulder prosthesis**.

dance medicine—holistic multidisciplinary approach to on-site treatment of injured dancers beyond traditional orthopedic care, often using a staff of orthopedic surgeons, physical therapists, massage therapists, a psychologist, a nutritionist, a podiatrist, a naturopathic physician who performs acupuncture, a family medicine practitioner, and a chiropractor.

Dance sign—a slight retraction of the tissue in the right iliac region in some cases of intussusception.

Dandy-Walker syndrome—congenital hydrocephalus caused by blockage of the foramina of Magendie and Luschka. Can be diagnosed on fetal ultrasound.

DAP/TMP (dapsone plus trimethoprim)—drug used in therapy for *Pneumocystis carinii* pneumonia.

dapsone plus trimethoprim (DAP/TMP).

Darco shoe—brand name for postoperative podiatric shoe.

Dardik Biograft—modified human umbilical vein graft; used as a substitute for saphenous vein graft in revascularization procedures on the lower extremities.

Dardik clamp—used in liver transplantation surgery.

dark-field microscopy—a microscopic technique using special lighting that makes it easier to identify *Treponema pallidum*, the organism that causes syphilis.

Darkschewitsch, nucleus of—also, depending on which dictionary you consult, spelled *Darkshevich, Darkschevich.*

Darrach procedure—extensor carpi ulnaris tenodesis, or surgery on distal radioulnar joint.

darusentan—an endothelin A-selective endothelin receptor antagonist treatment for patients with uncontrolled hypertension.

darwinian medicine (also evolutionary medicine)—subscribes to the theory that the most enduring widespread illnesses, such as heart disease, cancer, and mental illness, are due to pathogens rather than lifestyle or genes.

DASH (dietary approaches to stop hypertension) **diet**—established by the National Institutes of Health as a way to lower blood pressure and cholesterol levels. It may have health benefits that go beyond its stated purpose of lowering people's risk of heart disease. In addition to consumption of fruits, vegetables, and whole grains, the DASH diet advises people to consume low-fat and fat-free dairy foods and lean meat, poultry, and fish.

dashboard knee—a knee injury in a motor vehicle accident.

Dash pacemaker—a single-chamber rate-adaptive pacemaker.

data clipping detection error—MRI term.

Datascope catheter—used to position an intra-aortic balloon pump.

data spike detection error—MRI term.

Daumas-Duport glioma pathology grading scale.

Dautery osteotome.

DAVA (desacetyl vinblastine amide)—see *vindesine sulfate.*

DAVF (dural arteriovenous fistula) (Neuro).

David Letterman sign—in which the scapholunate dissociation distance is wider than 2 mm on x-ray. Also known as Terry-Thomas sign (for actor Terry-Thomas).

Davies repair—Z-plasty technique for unilateral cleft lip.

da Vinci robot—computer-guided robotic device that allows surgeons to operate remotely using minimally invasive surgical techniques.

Davol drain—see *Relia-Vac.*

Davydov vagina construction (Ob-Gyn) —a technique used to create a new vagina in patients with congenital vaginal aplasia, or males having a sex-change operation. See also *colocolponeopoiesis*, *Frank and McIndoe*, *Abbe-McIndoe procedures*.

dawn phenomenon—hyperglycemia occurring before dawn in both type 1 (insulin dependent) and type 2 (non-insulin dependent) diabetics; an early morning hyperglycemia.

daxial—see *paxial*.

DayTimer carpal tunnel support—prevents wrist flexion while allowing useful range of motion.

D blood typing and antibody screening—formerly Rh blood typing. Related terminology includes D incompatibility (when a D negative woman is pregnant with a D positive fetus); D hemolytic disease; D antibody; administration of D immunoglobulin or Rho(D) immune globulin; weak D; and D isoimmunization.

DBM (demineralized bone matrix).

DC (direct current) **offset**—MRI term.

DCA (directional coronary atherectomy) —treatment for coronary artery disease.

DCA (directional coronary angioplasty) (also, atherectomy).

DCC (deleted in colorectal carcinoma) **gene**—implicated in the development of colorectal carcinoma.

DCFS (Department of Children and Family Services)—a government agency that investigates charges of child abuse.

DCH (diffuse choroidal hemangioma).

D-chiro-inositol—a drug that is found naturally in fruits and vegetables. It helps the body use insulin and may be effective in promoting ovulation in patients with polycystic ovary syndrome, thus reducing the risk for diabetes and heart attacks due to high levels of insulin, blood pressure, and triglycerides.

DCIA (deep circumflex iliac artery).

DCIS (ductal carcinoma in situ).

D_{CO}—pulmonary diffusion capacity.

DCP (dynamic compression plate).

DCR (dacryocystorhinostomy)—a laser endonasal procedure.

DCS (decompression sickness).

DCS (dorsal column stimulator, or stimulation)—implanted for relief of pain.

DCS (D-cycloserine)—a medication approved for the treatment of tuberculosis, used off-label in concert with psychotherapy, as an effective treatment for some anxiety-related disorders.

D-cycloserine (DCS).

DDCT (decubitus digital communication treatment)—a device that stimulates a normal wound healing response in patients with chronic wounds by creating an electric induction field around the sore, especially indicated for pressure ulcers (bed sores).

DDD pacemaker (Cardio).

DDH (developmental dysplasia of the hip)—newer term for *congenital dysplasia of the hip*.

D-dimer—an indirect marker of thrombin and plasmin generation. Cf. *t-dimer*.

DDT ([fluorescein] **dye disappearance test)**.

DEATH—mnemonic for Dressing, Eating, Ambulating (walking), Toileting, and Hygiene such as bladder control (basic ADLs). Cf. *SHAFT*.

DeBakey woven Dacron.

debris ("duh-bree")—amorphous and necrotic material.

debulking—a process in which the inner "core" (or bulk) of a tumor is removed. This permits the outer portion to, in effect, "cave in" a bit, thereby permitting easier removal of the whole tumor. If the "outer wall"

debulking *(cont.)*
portion of the tumor does not readily separate from the attached tissue, at least the total volume of the tumor is somewhat reduced and hence does not exert as much pressure on the adjacent structures as it did before.

deceleration—slowing, as in "deceleration of contractions." Slang, *decels*.

decerebrate rigidity—seen in metabolic disorders that affect upper brain stem function, evidenced by clenched teeth, and arms and legs stiffly extended. Cf. *decorticate rigidity.*

decidua—that part of the endometrium of the pregnant uterus that is shed at parturition.

decision—the settling of a controversy; a conclusion arrived at or a choice made. Cf. *discission.*

decitabine—see *Dacogen*.

de Clérambault syndrome—erotomanic delusions; a psychosis in which a person is under the delusion that another person, often famous or celebrated, is engaged in erotic communication with the subject and that the object of the delusion was the first to fall in love and the first to make advances. The amorous delusion is always directed toward the same individual throughout the episode, and the subject rationalizes the object's paradoxical behavior (such as failing to respond to phone calls or letters). Celebrities are frequently victims of persons with de Clérambault syndrome.

decompression catheter—utilizes thermal energy at the site of the pathology, used to treat herniated disks. See *electrothermal procedure*.

decompression sickness (DCS)—see *caisson disease*.

decorticate rigidity—seen in lesions which damage the internal capsule of the brain and nearby structures, evidenced by flexion of the fingers, wrist, and arm, plantar flexion, and internal rotation of the leg. Cf. *decerebrate rigidity.*

decrepit rotator cuff—indicative of an irreparable rotator cuff tear.

decubitus digital communication treatment (DDCT).

decubitus ulcer—bed sore, pressure sore, trophic ulcer. Decubitus means "lying down" and these synonymous terms refer to the ulcerated areas of ischemic necrosis on the tissues that overlie bony prominences (sacrum, hips, greater trochanters, lateral malleoli, heels, and other areas where there may be pressure and friction). They are usually seen in patients who have been bedridden for long periods of time, who are emaciated or paralyzed, or in whom pain sensation is absent.

deep brain stimulation—works by using electrical impulses to block abnormal nerve signals that cause tremors and other symptoms of Parkinson disease.

deep inferior epigastric (artery) **perforator** (DEIP) **flap**—used in autologous bilateral breast reconstruction.

deep lamellar endothelial keratoplasty (DLEK)—a surgical procedure that replaces the endothelium without corneal surface incisions or sutures. Also, *deep lamellar keratoplasty* (DLK). Compare *endothelial lamellar keratoplasty (ELK)*.

deep lateral femoral notch sign—imaging term used to describe a secondary sign of anterior cruciate ligament tear in the knee. Also *lateral femoral notch sign*.

deep posterior talotibial ligament (DPTTL).
deep-seated—so far below the surface that it is unsusceptible to superficial examination, study or treatment, as in a deep-seated infection. *Not* deep-seeded.
deep tendon reflexes:
- 4+ brisk, hyperactive, clonus
- 3+ is more brisk than normal, but does not necessarily indicate a pathologic process
- 2+ normal
- 1+ is low normal, with slight diminution in response
- 0 no response

deep venous insufficiency (DVI).
deep venous thrombosis (DVT).
defensins—naturally occurring peptides with antimicrobial activity. Investigators have for the first time found defensins in tissues of the eye and in tears, suggesting that purified defensins may be useful in treating eye infections.
deferiprone—see *Ferriprox.*
defervesce—to experience reduction of fever. The word is a back-formation from *defervescence*.
defibrillator
- Alert
- Alert Companion II
- Angstrom MD
- Atlas HF ICD (implantable cardioverter-defibrillator)
- Atrial View Ventak AV implantable cardioverter-defibrillator
- automated external (AED)
- Cadence AICD (automatic implantable cardioverter-defibrillator)
- Cadet cardioverter-defibrillator
- cardiac resynchronization therapy (CRT-D)
- Contour MD implantable single-lead cardioverter-defibrillator

defibrillator *(cont.)*
- Contour V-145D and LTV-135D implantable cardioverter-defibrillator
- Endotak C lead
- Endotak DSP
- Epic HF ICD (implantable cardioverter-defibrillator)
- FirstSave automated external (AED)
- ForeRunner automatic external
- Gem DR implantable
- GEM II DR/VR implantable cardioverter-defibrillator
- GEM III AT dual chamber ICD (implantable cardioverter-defibrillator)
- GEM III AT implantable cardioverter-defibrillator
- Guidant Ventak Prizm
- HeartStart home
- Heartstream ForeRunner automatic external
- ICD (implantable cardioverter-defibrillator)
- Jewel AF implantable
- LifeVest wearable cardiac
- Medtronic Gem automatic implantable
- Medtronic InSync implantable cardioverter
- Medtronic Micro Jewel II
- Medtronic Sprint lead for cardioverter-defibrillator
- Micron Res-Q implantable cardioverter-defibrillator
- PCD Transvene implantable cardioverter-defibrillator
- Photon DR dual-chamber implantable cardioverter-defibrillator
- Phylax AV cardioverter-defibrillator
- Porta Pulse 3
- Powerheart automatic external cardioverter-defibrillator

defibrillator *(cont.)*
Res-Q ACD (arrhythmia control device) implantable cardioverter-defibrillator
Res-Q Micron implantable cardioverter-defibrillator
Sentinel implantable cardioverter-defibrillator
smart
St. Jude Pacesetter Atlas DR ICD (implantable cardioverter-defibrillator)
tiered-therapy programmable cardioverter-defibrillator (PCD)
Ventak AV III DR implantable cardioverter-defibrillator
Ventak Mini III implantable
Ventak Prizm
WCD 2000 system wearable
Zoll

defibrillation threshold (DFT).

deficient vs. deficit—terms sometimes confused in neuropsychiatric dictation. Usage: "Nonetheless he is still intellectually deficient" (*not* deficit).

Definition PM (Pre-Mantle) **femoral component**—used in orthopedic surgery.

Deflux injectable gel—drug for treatment of vesicoureteral reflux in children. The substance is injected into the wall of the bladder near the opening of one or both ureters, creating a bulge in the tissue and making it harder for the urine to reflux.

deformity (see also *disease*)
bell-clapper
boutonnière finger
buried penis
flexion contracture
gibbous
Haglund
Hill-Sachs lesion

deformity *(cont.)*
hallux abductovalgus
hallux extensus
inverted Napoleon hat sign
lemon sign
Michel
mucolipidosis III (pseudo-Hurler)
polly-beak nasal
pseudo-Hurler
sabre shin
supratip nasal tip
uni-tip

deglutition mechanism (Radiol)—the coordinated sequence of muscular contractions in the mouth, pharynx, and esophagus involved in normal swallowing, as demonstrated in a barium swallow or upper GI series.

degradable starch microspheres (DSM)—injected into an artery at the same time as a chemotherapy drug to temporarily block the blood flow at the capillary level (chemo-embolization). The chemotherapy drug is then concentrated in the region of the cancer, and high tissue uptake is achieved. DSM has a short half-life and does not occlude the local circulation long enough to produce ischemia, and in conjunction with a chemotherapy drug can be administered repeatedly.

DEHP (di[2-ethylhexyl]phthalate)—chemical used to soften plastics in IV tubing, nasogastric and feeding tubes, and the bags that hold blood or IV solutions. The FDA has determined that the substance is harmful to humans and has advised the medical community to use alternative products when possible; however, the FDA has not banned the product.

DEI (diffraction-enhanced imaging).

Deiters cells (ENT)—in the organ of Corti.

déjà vu (Fr., already seen)—the incorrect feeling that one has seen or experienced something before, a feeling which frequently precedes seizures. Cf. *jamais vu*.

Dejerine onion peel sensory loss—sensory loss starting from mouth and nose and extending concentrically outward in an "onion peel" distribution.

De Juan forceps.

Deklene—blue monofilament polypropylene suture used in cardiovascular surgery and in neurosurgery.

Deknatel (Shur-Strip)—a sterile wound closure tape.

de la Cruz classification—congenital aural atresia.

delta-shaped anastomosis—shaped like a *V* or Greek capital delta (Δ), used in gastrointestinal anastomoses.

delayed pulmonary toxicity syndrome (DPTS)—a lung disorder seen in breast cancer patients in the weeks following treatment with a combination of chemotherapy and bone marrow transplantation. If the inflammation is detected early and the body's inflammatory response modified through steroids, lung toxicity can be prevented or significantly minimized.

delayed xenograft rejection (DXR)—delayed rejection reaction in response to transplantation of cells, tissue, or solid organ of animal origin.

Delbet fracture classification, types I-IV—the most widely accepted system of classification of femoral head and neck fractures in children.

Delbet splint—used for heel fractures.

De Lee retractor (Ob-Gyn).

deletion (Genetics)—a chromosomal aberration in which part of a chromosome is completely lost.

"dello-vibrio"—a phonetic spelling of *Bdellovibrio*, a genus of parasitic gram-negative organisms that live on certain other gram-negative bacteria. Although this is not a word you will often hear, who would think to look under the *B*'s?

DeLorme boot—see *quadriceps boot*.

Delrin joint replacement biomaterial.

delta—When a dictator gives a lab value such as "delta of 35," the reference is to the anion gap.

delta OD_{450}—in amniocentesis, testing for bilirubinemia in erythroblastosis fetalis.

Delta 32 TACT (tuned aperture computed tomography)—a breast imaging device.

De Mayo two-point discrimination device.

dementia
- frontotemporal (FTD)
- Lewy body
- multi-infarct (MID)
- non-Alzheimer
- subcortical
- subcortical ischemic vascular (SIVD)

DEMENTIA—a mnemonic for the reversible causes of dementia:
- **d**rugs
- **e**motional disorders
- **m**etabolic and endocrine disorders
- **e**yes, ears
- **n**utritional disorders, normal pressure hydrocephalus
- **t**umors, trauma
- **i**nfection
- **a**therosclerosis (and strokes)

Dementia Rating Scale (DRS)—used in detecting patients with dementia of the Alzheimer type.

demineralization—reduction in the amount of calcium present in bone, due to disease or immobilization, as seen on x-ray.

demineralized bone matrix (DBM).

de Morsier syndrome—agenesis of the olfactory lobes, hypoplasia of the thalamus, dystrophy of the cerebral hemispheres, and absence of development of the gonads at puberty. Also, *de Morsier-Gauthier syndrome.*

de Musset sign—rhythmic shaking of the head caused by carotid artery pulsations; a sign of aortic insufficiency. Cf. *bishop's nod.*

denaturation—the conversion of DNA from the double-stranded to the single-stranded state.

denatured homograft (Surg).

dendritic lesion—having a branched appearance.

dengue hemorrhagic fever (DHF)—a disease on the increase in the U.S. and Latin America. The recent introduction of the *Aedes albopictus* mosquito to the U.S. will increase the probability of more severe disease, according to the CDC.

Denis Browne clubfoot splint—talipes hobble splint. Named for Dr. Denis (pronounced "Denny") Browne, Hospital for Sick Children, London, England.

Dennis-Brown pouch (Urol).

Dennis-Varco pancreaticoduodenostomy.

Dennyson-Fulford extra-articular subtalar arthrodesis—for correction of supple hindfoot valgus deformities in children.

densitometer, densitometry
accuDEXA bone
DEXAscan bone
dynamic spiral CT lung
Norland bone

densitometer *(cont.)*
Prodigy bone
QDR-1500 or QDR-2000 bone
Sahara
video (VD)

de novo inflammatory growth—beginning, recurring, or new inflammatory growth. Usage: "De novo tissue was generated from mesenchymal precursors."

densitometry—determination of variations in density (for example, bone density) by comparison with that of another material or with a certain standard. See *dual photon densitometry.*

dens view of cervical spine (Radiol)—a view of the odontoid process of the second cervical vertebra on x-ray. The word *dens* is not an eponym.

dental bonding materials
Cerestore
Dicor
Empress
Fortress
Hi-Ceram
In-Ceram Zirconia
Optec

dental implant—see *implant*.

DentaScan—a program for multiplanar reformation that processes axial CT scan information to obtain true cross-sectional images and panoramic views of the mandible and maxilla; this optimizes the ability to detect tumor involvement in the mandible and maxilla.

DentCAM—a virtual reality articulator used in dentistry, orthodontics, and jaw surgery.

DentiPatch lidocaine transoral delivery system—dental anesthetic patch for the prevention of pain from oral injections and soft tissue dental procedures.

Dento-Infuser—an instrument used by dentists to infuse Astringedent, a topical hemostatic solution.

DENT-X—intraoral dental x-ray unit.

denuded—uncovered, deprived of a normal surface.

Denver Developmental Screening Test—rating scale for development of fine motor skills, gross motor skills, language, and personal/social skills in infants and preschool children.

Denver nasal splint—a quickly applied adhesive nasal splint.

Denver PAK (percutaneous access kit) includes a Denver ascites shunt designed for subclavian vein placement.

Denver pleuroperitoneal shunt—for control of chronic pleural effusions.

Denys-Drash syndrome—an inherited renal disease.

deodorized opium tincture (DOT).

Deon hip prosthesis—made of a titanium alloy which can be implanted with or without cement.

deoxyribonucleic acid—see *DNA*.

DePalma staple procedure—a technique that fixes the gracilis tendon to the ischial tuberosity. Also called *stimulated graciloplasty*.

Department of Children and Family Services (DCFS).

Department of Transportation (DOT) **physical**.

depth—the deepest portion of a surgically excised specimen, as in "The margins and depths of the specimen are free of malignant cells."

depth-resolved NIRS—permits the noninvasive assessment and quantification of certain characteristics of specific blood and tissue that is deep in the body and surrounded, or behind, other more superficial blood and tissue (e.g., in the brain and behind the scalp and skull). See *NIRS*.

DePuy Global Advantage shoulder eccentric humeral head.

DePuy Global shoulder glenoid component with a fin.

DePuy total hip system with porous coating. Also, Profile.

de Quervain disease—inflammation of the long abductor and short extensor tendons of the thumb, with accompanying tenderness and swelling. Also called *Quervain disease*.

Dercum disease—see *adiposis dolorosa*.

Dermablend—a cover cream used to cover vitiligo, birthmarks, etc.

Dermabond—a topical skin adhesive (2-octyl cyanoacrylate) which is an alternative to sutures or staples. Used to close incisions made to repair facial deformities such as cleft lip and palate.

dermabrasion—an abrasion procedure for acne scars, performed after anesthetizing and freezing the skin with Freon; scars are abraded with fine sandpaper, diamond fraises, or abrasive brushes. See *diamond fraise*.

Dermacea—wound and skin care product line.

Derma-Gel hydrogel sheet.

Dermagraft-TC—a human fibroblast-derived temporary skin substitute, used as a short-term wound covering for severe burns. Also used for diabetic foot ulcers.

Dermagran ointments and dressings—used to treat decubitus ulcers.

Derma K laser (Surg)—uses both pulsed Er:YAG and CO_2 laser energy to perform skin rejuvenation.

DermaLase laser system (Surg)—used in surgical procedures that involve incision, excision, ablation, vaporization, and/or coagulation of soft tissue.

Dermalene—linear polyethylene monofilament suture material.

Dermalon—monofilament nylon suture material.

Dermal Regeneration Template—used in conjunction with Integra artificial skin.

DermaMend foam wound dressing.

DermaMend hydrogel dressing.

Dermanet contact-layer wound dressing.

Dermapor glove—allows the escape of water and heat from hand perspiration but keeps out water and external irritants, resulting in drier and less irritated hands.

Dermapulse—pressure control zone therapy for pressure sores.

DermaScan—used with skin rejuvenation devices.

DermaSeptic—small electronic device that delivers broad-spectrum antimicrobial ions directly into the skin in a process known as iontophoresis, providing highly effective treatment for conditions such as cold sores, pimples, and warts, where infection lies on or beneath the skin surface.

Dermasof—semiocclusive reinforced gel sheeting for treatment of hypertrophic and keloid scar tissue.

DermAssist hydrocolloid dressing material.

DermAssist wound filling material.

Dermatell hydrocolloid dressing material.

Dermatology Index of Disease Severity (DIDS)—a severity-of-illness index for inflammatory skin diseases.

dermatographism or **dermographism**—the property of abnormally sensitive skin by which strokes or writing with a pointed object are reproduced on the skin surface as raised red lines. Also called *skin writing*.

Dermatophagoides farinae—a mite; it may be one of the principal sources of antigen in house dust in some areas. Cf. *Dermatophagoides pteronyssinus.*

Dermatophagoides pteronyssinus—a mite that may be one of the principal sources of antigen in house dust in some areas. Cf. *Dermatophagoides farinae.*

dermatophyton control—used as a control with PPD testing.

dermatoscope—handheld microscope that allows magnification of the skin x 10 and replaces previously used inflexible and expensive stereomicroscopes which were cumbersome and time-consuming. Important in the diagnosis of malignant melanoma for which an oil or disinfectant solution is applied to the skin and a halogen light at an angle of 20° is used to make the horny layer of the skin more translucent.

dermatoscopy—see *dermoscopy*.

Derma 20 laser system (Surg)—pulsed Er:Yag laser intended for general dermatological applications, including skin surfacing.

DermMaster—macroabrasion system that does not use aluminum oxide. Used for skin resurfacing and other aesthetic/dermatology applications. Also, *DermMaster Salt-A-Peel, DermMaster II, DermMaster II Plus.*

dermographism—see *dermatographism.*

dermoscopy (dermatoscopy) using epiluminescent microscopy—the fastest and simplest procedure to differentiate tinea nigra from a melanocytic lesion.

desats, desatting—slang for *desaturating.*

Descemet membrane—between the endothelial layer of the cornea and the substantia propria.

descemetocele—herniation of Descemet membrane.

Deschamps ligature carrier.

describe—to explain or characterize in words. Cf. *ascribe.*

DES (diethylstilbestrol) **daughter**—a female exposed in utero to diethylstilbestrol, formerly prescribed for bleeding and other complications of pregnancy and now known to affect fetal development of the genital tract.

DES (drug-eluting stent).

desiccated (*not* dessicated)—dried.

Desilets-Hoffman introducer—used to introduce balloon, electrode, and other catheters.

DeSmet criteria—for grading osteochondral fragment stability.

desmoplastic small round-cell tumor (DSRCT)—a histologic entity that is uniform in appearance and is characterized by the presence of poorly differentiated small round cells, but also abundant fibrous stroma and a specific multidirectional immunohistochemical profile.

DeSouza exercises—to encourage position change of fetus.

desquamative interstitial pneumonitis (DIP)—an early stage of idiopathic pulmonary fibrosis.

desulfatohirudin—naturally occurring anticoagulant or thrombin inhibitor drug derived from leeches. Brief form is *hirudin*.

detergent worker's lung—extrinsic allergic alveolitis caused by exposure to detergent powder.

detemir—see *insulin detemir*.

Detour bar—a brand name for a protein bar used by body builders and athletes.

Detsky modified risk index score—a clinical scoring system used to predict cardiac morbidity.

detubularization principle—the use of ileum, ileocecum, or the sigmoid colon for conduit material in a continent urinary diversion procedure when the appendix is absent or must be preserved intact.

De Vega tricuspid anuloplasty—performed on children.

developer artifact (Radiol)—flawed images with areas resembling lesions resulting from darkroom problems.

developmental dysplasia of the hip (DDH).

developmental causes of limb-length discrepancy—avascular necrosis of hip, hip dislocation, idiopathic, Klippel-Trenaunay-Weber syndrome, linear scleroderma, local tumor, melorheostosis, neuromusculature, osteomyelitis, slipped capital femoral epiphysis, talectomy, trauma.

developmental dysplasia of the hip (DDH)—newer term for *congenital dysplasia of the hip*.

developmental milestones—the mastery of activities or skills expected at a certain age for normal child development.

Devers dissector, straight or curved—used in keratoplasty procedures.

Devex cage—see *Devex mesh* (referred to by either name).

Devex mesh—a spinal intervertebral body fixation orthosis.

Devic disease—neuromyelitis optica, a form of acute multiple sclerosis.

device—a quick-reference list of medical devices and systems found in medical and surgical dictation.

Common devices such as *catheter, endoscope, pacemaker, stent, tube,* and many others appear as main entries throughout the book.
ABI Vest airway clearance system (the "Vest")
Ablatherm HIFU (high-intensity focused ultrasound)
Absolok endoscopic clip applicator
Acapella chest physical therapy
Ac'cents permanent lash liner
accelerometer
Accellon Combi biosampler
Accel stopcock
Accu-Line knee instrumentation
AccuProbe
AccuSharp instrument
AccuSpan tissue expander
Accutome low-speed diamond saw
ACD (active compression-decompression) resuscitator
ACG knee instrumentation
ACL (anterior cruciate ligament) drill guide
Acland-Banis arteriotomy set
ACM (automated cardiac flow measurement) technology
AcroFlex-100 artificial disk
Acryl-X-II bone cement removal system
ACS Anchor Exchange
ACTID (analgesic cell therapy implantable device)
Actis venous flow controller (VFC)
active compression-decompression (ACD) resuscitator
actocardiotocograph
Acufex arthroscopic instruments
Acufex bioabsorbable suture anchor
AcuFix anterior cervical plate (also SC-AcuFix)
AcuPressor myotherapy tool
AcuTrainer electronic bladder retraining

device *(cont.)*
adaptive focusing technology (AFT)
adjustable leg and ankle repositioning mechanism (ALARM)
Adkins strut
Adolescent and Pediatric Pain Tool
ADTRA composite external fixator ring
advanced cardiac life support (ACLS)
AdvanTeq II TENS unit
Aerochamber
AeroTech II nebulizer
AERx electronic inhaler
Aescula left ventricular (LV) lead
Aesop 2000 surgical robot
Aestiva/5 MRI anesthesia machine
Agris-Dingman submammary dissector
air entrainment
Air-Limb
Air Supply
air trousers
Akros extended care mattress
Alert Companion II defibrillator
Alexa 1000 breast lesion diagnostic
AlloDerm
Allon ThermoWrap
Aloka SSD ultrasound system and probes
Alphastar operating room table
Alphatec small fragment system (SFS)
ALS Bluemax BM500 light source
Alta reconstruction rod
ALVAD (abdominal left ventricular assist device)
Amadeus microkeratome
Ambu bag
Ambulator shoe
AME bone growth stimulators
Ameflow
AME PinSite Shields
A.M.E. tongue retaining

device *(cont.)*
- Amicus separator
- Amis 2000 respiratory mass spectrometer
- amorphous silicon filmless digital x-ray detection technology
- Amplatz ventricular septal defect
- Amsler grid
- AMS Sphincter 800 urinary prosthesis
- anal EMG PerryMeter sensor
- anatomic graduated components (AGC)
- Anchorlok soft-tissue anchor
- Ancure endovascular repair
- Andrews spinal frame/table
- AneuRx stent-graft
- AngeFlex leads
- Angio-Seal hemostatic puncture closure
- ankle air stirrup
- AnkleCiser exerciser
- Anspach surgery instruments
- anterior chamber maintainer (ACM)
- A1cNow monitor
- APACHE CV Risk Predictor Internet-based product
- Apex universal drive
- AbioCor implantable replacement heart
- Accolade
- acetabular cage
- Acorn cardiac support
- Actifier high-tech pacifier
- air entrainment
- Alert defibrillator
- AliMed positioner
- Ambulette paratransit van
- AMP (anterior mandibular positioning) dental
- Amplatzer ductal occluder
- Andorscope i-Stethos stethoscope
- Androflo monitor
- Androgram
- Androscope Stethos stethoscope

device *(cont.)*
- Androsonix biological sound monitor
- anti-protrusio
- Apollo triple lumen papillotome
- applanometer
- Aqua-Flow collagen glaucoma drainage
- AquariusNET
- AquaShield
- arachnophlebectomy surgical
- arch bar
- AREx inhaler
- argon beam coagulator (ABC)
- Argyle CPAP nasal cannula
- Arnett-TMP (trimandibular plate) system
- Aromapatch nasal inhaler
- AromaScan
- Arrequi laparoscopic knot pusher ligator
- Arrow LionHeart heart assist
- Arrow PICC system
- Arrow pneumothorax kit
- Arrowsmith corneal marker
- Arthro-BST arthroscopic probe
- ArthroCare Coblation-based cosmetic surgery
- ArthroCare wand
- ArthroCare wand CoVac 70
- ArthroCare wand TurboVac 90
- Arthopor acetabular cup
- Arthrosew arthroscopic suturing
- ArthroWand
- artificial anterior chamber
- ARTMA virtual patient technology
- ARUM pin
- AS-800 artificial sphincter
- Aspen electrocautery
- Aspen laparoscopy electrode
- Aspen ultrasound system
- aspiration-tulip
- Assistant Free calibrated femoral tibial spreader
- ASSI wire pass drill

device *(cont.)*
Atlas HF ICD (implantable cardioverter-defibrillator)
Atrigel drug delivery
Atrioverter
augmentative communication
AutoCat (AutoCAT) automatic intra-aortic balloon pump
Autoclix fingerstick
Autoflex II CPM unit
Autolet fingerstick
Automator
AutoPap 300 QC automatic Pap screener
Auto Segmentation software tool
AVA (advanced venous access) 3Xi
Avesta procedure kit
Avitene Ultrafoam collagen hemostat
AvocetPT (prothrombin time) meter
Aware breast self-examination pad
Axcis Holmium:YAG laser
Axius Vacuum 2 stabilizer
Axostim nerve stimulator
AxyaWeld bone anchor
BabyFace 3-D surface rendering accessory
Babytherm IC gel mattress
BackBiter orthopedic instrument
BackTracker
Baim-Turi cardiac
Bair Hugger warming body cover
Bair Paws warming gown and unit
Bakelite material
Bakes dilator
Baladi Inverter
balloon dissector
Balloon-on-a-Wire cardiac
band-ligator
BAPS (biomechanical ankle platform system) board
Bara-Med
Bard Biopty gun
Bard Clamshell Septal Umbrella
Bard Composix mesh
Bard EndoCinch

device *(cont.)*
Bard PDA (patent ductus arteriosus) Umbrella
Bard Safety Excalibur catheter introducer
Bard TransAct intra-aortic balloon pump
Barouk button space
Barouk microscrew
Barouk microstaple
Barron disposable trephine
Barron donor corneal punch
Barron pump
Barron radial vacuum trephine
Baton laser pointer
BDProbeTec ET
Beacon incontinence surgical line
beam splitter
Bedge antireflux mattress
Bellucci scissors
Belos compression pin
Bentley Duraflo II perfusion circuit
Berkeley optic zone marker
Berman locator
Beta-Cath radiation therapy
Betadine Surgi-Prep (povidone-iodine Sponge Brush
Bevel Wand ablation instrument
BFE (blood flow enhancement)
Bickel leg holder
BiliBottoms phototherapy diaper
Bili mask
bilirubinometer
bioabsorbable closure
bioartificial kidney
Biobrane glove
BioBypass
Biocor 200 oxygenator
Biofilter hemoconcentrator
biofragmentable anastomotic ring
bio-interference screw
Biologically Quiet screw
Biologically Quiet suture anchor
Biolox ball head
Bionicare 1000 stimulator

device *(cont.)*
Bioplus dispersive electrode
BioRCI orthopedic screw
BioScrew bio-absorbable interference screw
Bio-Tense relaxation tool
Bio-Vascular Probe
biplane sector probe
bipolar urological loop
Bird cup
Bird Nest filter (BNF)
birthing ball
BIS (Bispectral Index) Sensor
bladder blade protective surgical
BladderScan
Blood Shield
Bluemax BM500
Bluemyst aerosol spray
Blumenthal irrigating cystitome
Bluntport disposable trocar
BLU-U (blue light photodynamic therapy) illuminator
BM500
BMP cable
boat hook
body box
Bone Bullet suture anchor
Bone-Lok
Bookler swivel-ball laparoscopic instrument holder
Bores radial marker
Bovie ultrasound aspirator
bovine pericardium strips
Bowen wire tightener
Boyle uterine elevator
Boynton needle holder
brain-controlled
Brandt cytology balloon
Brava breast enhancement
Bravo pH monitoring
BreastAlert differential temperature sensor (DTS) screening
breast bolster
BreastCheck handheld electronic device for breast self-exam

device *(cont.)*
BreastExam breast exam
Breathe Right nasal strips
Bremer AirFlo Vest
Brent pressure earring
Brockenbrough cardiac
Browlift BoneBridge
Brown dermatome
Brown-McHardy pneumatic dilator
Bruel-Kjaer transvaginal ultrasound probe
Bruening syringe
Bruns bone curette
BRW (Brown-Roberts-Wells) CT stereotaxic guide
BSD-2000
Button and Button-One Step gastrostomy
BVM (bag-valve-mask)
bypass circuit
CADD pump
Calandruccio triangular compression fixation
calcar reamer
Calcitek spline dental implant
calipers
calorimeter
Cam (controlled ankle motion) walker
CAM tent
candy-cane stirrups
Cannulated Plus screw system
Capio CL transvaginal suture-capturing
Capio suture capturing
CAPS ArthroWand
CAPSure ArthroWand
CapSure steroid-eluting electrode
CAPS X Wand
cardiac sling
CardioBeeper CB-12L
Cardioblate BP surgical ablation tool
Cardioblate XL surgical ablation pen

device *(cont.)*
CardioCard
CardioSEAL septal occluder
C-arm fluoroscopy portable x-ray unit
Carolina rocker wheelchair
Carpentier-Edwards Physio anuloplasty ring
Carroll-Girard screw
Carter pillow
Carter-Thomason suture passer
Castanares face-lift scissors
Castaneda bottle
Catarex surgical
catheter vitrector
Cath-Finder
CathLink
CathScanner ultrasound imaging system
Cath-Shield
CaverMap nerve stimulator
CaverMap surgical
Cavernotome
Caves-Schultz-Stanford bioptome
Cavitron ultrasonic surgical aspirator (CUSA)
C-bar web-spacer
C Cap (compliance cap)
CD8 AIS CELLector
CD Horizon M8 multiaxial screws for lumbar fixation
Cellect graft preparation
Cellpatch drug delivery
Cellugel ophthalmic viscosurgical (OVD)
cementless jumbo cup
CFA digital camera
Charite artificial disc for the spine
ChemTrak AccuMeter
chest shell
Cholesterol 1,2,3 testing
Christoudias fascial closure
ChromaVision digital analyzer
Cica-Care topical gel sheeting
Clarion HiFocus electrode

device *(cont.)*
Clarke-Reich micro knot pusher
ClearCut 2
Clearglide optical vessel dissector
ClearLight
ClearView Blower/Mister
CoaguChek
Coaguloop resection electrode
Coblation technology
Cochlea Dynamics sound processing technology
Cohn cardiac stabilizer
Colormate TLc BiliTest bilirubinometer
Combitube
ComfortFlex
Command cutting instrument
Commander PTCA wire line
Compliant
CompuCAM digital intraoral camera
Conceive Fertility Planner
Conceptus Robust guidewire
confocal microscope
Contigen Bard collagen implant
Convergent color Doppler imaging technology
CoolSpot skin-cooling
COPD Lung Profiler
Core trocar and cannula
CorLink
CorlS interference screw
Cotrel-Dubousset instrumentation (CDI)
Cottle elevator
Councilman chisel
Cournand cardiac
CoVac 50
CoVac 70
CoVac Wand
CoverTip safety syringe
Cowboy Collar
CPM (continuous passive motion)
CPS (cardiopulmonary support) heart-lung machine

device *(cont.)*
Crafoord-Senning heart-lung machine
Cragg thrombolytic brush
cribogram
Cricket oximeter
Crutchfield skeletal traction tongs
CRYOcare endometrial cryoablation
Cryo/Cuff boot
CryoHit
cryophake
cryoprobe
cryostat
CT with slip-ring technology
C-TRAK handheld gamma detector
CUI (Cox-Uphoff International) tissue expander
Cun-Meter
cup-cage acetabular
Curlin 2000 Plus infusion pump
Cu-Safe 300
CUSALap
Cutting Balloon microsurgical dilatation catheter
CV Profilor DO-2020
C-wire Serter (C-wire C-Serter)
CyberKnife Express
CyberKnife stereotactic radiosurgery/radiotherapy
cystitome
cystotome
CytoPorter drug delivery
Dacomed snap gauge
Dalkon shield
Damato Campimeter
Darco shoe
Dautery osteotome
da Vinci robot
DayTimer carpal tunnel support
DDCT (decubitus digital communication treatment)
defibrillator
Definition PM (pre-mantle) femoral component
DeLorme quadriceps boot

device *(cont.)*
De Mayo two-point discrimination
dental anti-snoring
Delta 32 TACT (tuned aperture computed tomography)
DentCAM
DentCAM articulator
Dento-Infuser
DENT-X intraoral dental x-ray unit
Dermapor glove
DermaSeptic
DermMaster macroabrasion
Deschamps ligature carrier
Desilets-Hoffman introducer
Devers dissector
Dexterity PneumoSleeve
DHS (dynamic hip screw)
Dialock implantable access port
diamond bur
Diamond-Flex instruments
diamond fraise
Diamond-Lite
Diamond pocket maker
DiaPhine corneal trephination
Diasensor 1000 for blood glucose
DICOM (digital imaging and communications in medicine)
Digikit pneumatic tourniquet
DigiMatch
Digirad 2020 TC Imager
DigiSound
digital Add-On Bucky image acquisition
digital fundus imager
digital IC-Green (indocyanine green) fluorescein dye videoangiography
Digital OsteoView 2000
digital signal processing (DSP)
DIGIT-grip
Digitrapper MKIII esophageal sphincter pressure assessment
Digitron digital subtraction imaging
Dilamezinsert (DMI)

device *(cont.)*
DIMAQ integrated ultrasound workstation
DirectFlow arterial cannula
DirectRay direct-to-digital technology
Disetronic Insulin Pen
Disk-Criminator
disposable aortic rotating punch
Dissectron
Diva laparoscopic morcellator
Doc-U-Dose dosimeter
Dome Wand
domino connectors
donor-recipient plug exchange
Dormia noose
dorsal column stimulator (DCS)
double umbrella
Douvas roto-extractor
DPAP Stealth
D-Prevent
Draeger high vacuum erysiphake
Draeger tonometer
Dr. B's mouthpiece
Drionic electrical iontophoresis
DSP Micro Diamond-Point
Dualine digital hearing instrument
Dubecq-Princeteau angulating needle holder
Ducor tip
Duette instruments
Duet vascular sealing
Dura-Kold ice wrap
Durasul large diameter head
Durathane cardiac
Duval disposable dermatome
dynamic compression plate
Dynamic Cooling Device (DCD)
Dynasplint knee extension unit
DynaVox 2 communication
DynaWell spinal compression
DyoVac suction punch
Eagle II survey spirometer
Eagle Vision-Freeman punctum plug

device *(cont.)*
EarCheck Pro reflectometer
ear oximeter
EBI SPF-2 implantable bone stimulator
E.CAM photon emission camera
EchoFlow blood velocity meter (BVM-1)
Eclipse ST cyclotron
Eclipse TENS unit
ECTA (enzyme-catalyzed therapeutic activation) technology
EDA (extravasation detection accessory)
Elasto-Gel shoulder therapy wrap
elastomeric sleep appliance
Electro-Acuscope
Electro-Mate cutting and coagulating
electron-beam CT technology
electronic portal imaging
electro-oculogram apparatus
Electroscope disposable scissors
El Gamal cardiac
Eliminator ArthroWand
Eliminator dilatation balloon
Ellik kidney stone basket, evacuator, elevator
Elmor tissue morcellator
EMA (elastic mandibular advancement)
EMA-T (elastic mandibular advancement-titration)
Embol-X arterial cannula and filter
Embosphere microspheres
Embrace heart stabilizer
Emerge DualMesh biomaterials
emergency infusion (EID)
EMI scanner
Enclose anastomosis assist
end-effectors
Ender nail
Endius endoscopic access
Endius TriFix thoracolumbar pedicle screw

device *(cont.)*
endoanal coil
EndoAnchor
Endo Babcock surgical grasper
Endo Clip applier
endocut cautery
Endodissect instrument
endoesophageal MRI coil
Endofix absorbable interference screw
Endoflex
Endo-Gauge tissue thickness measurement
Endoloop suture instrument
EndoLumina invasive light delivery catheter
EndoMate Grab Bag
Endopath bladeless trocar
Endopath ES endoscopic stapler
Endopath laparoscopic trocar
Endopath Linear Cutter
Endopath Optiview optical surgical obturator
Endopath TriStar trocar
Endopearl
Endo-P-Probe
endorectal coil
endoscopic suction cap
Endo Shears
Endo Stitch endoscopic suturing
EndoStitch instrument
Endotak Reliance
Endotrac endoscopic instruments
endovaginal coil
endovaginal ultrasound (EVUS)
EndoWrist
Enduron acetabular liner
Enfant pediatric vision testing system
Ensemble contrast imaging (ECI)
ENTec Coblator Plasma Surgery
ENTec Plasma Wand
Entera-Flo
Enteryx

device *(cont.)*
Entree thoracoscopy trocar and cannula
EPIC-C or EPICS Profile flow cytometer
EpiE-ZPen auto injector
Epi-Grip
Epistat double balloon
Epitrain elbow support
equalizer airway
Equinox occlusion balloon
Eros-CTD (clitoral therapy device)
Esclim estradiol transdermal
E-Scope electronic stethoscope
Escort balloon stone extractor
esophageal pill electrode
estrogen/progesterone transdermal delivery
ESU (electrosurgical unit) dispersive (grounding) pad
e-Touch technology
ETS Flex 45-3.5 endoscopic stapler
EU-M30S
Euro-Collins multiorgan perfusion kit
EVac wand
Evershears
Evolve Cardiac Continuum
ExAblate 2000 system
ExacTech blood glucose meter
Exact-Fit ATH hip replacement
Excelart MRI
eXcel-DR (disposable/reusable) instruments
Expandacell sinus pack
Extractor three-lumen retrieval balloon
eXtract specimen bag
extravasation detection accessory (EDA)
Extra View balloon
ExtreSafe needles, lancets, phlebotomy devices, catheters, syringes
E-Z Flex jaw therapy

device *(cont.)*

E-Z Tac soft-tissue reattachment
eZY WRAP orthopedic products
face-lift scissors
FACScan (fluorescence-activated cell sorter) flow cytometer
FACSVantage cell sorter
FasT-Fix
Faulkner folder
FeatherTouch automated rasp
Felig insulin pump
Female Condom, The
FemCap contraceptive
femoral canal restrictor
FemoStop femoral artery compression arch
FemSoft insert continent
fenestrated Drake clip
fiducial box
Filcard temporary removable vena cava filter
filiforms and followers
FilterWire embolization
FilterWire EX embolization
Finesse cardiac
Finger Blocking Tree
finger cot
fingerstick blood glucose testing
Firm D-Ring wrist support (Rolyan)
Fisch drill
FISH, The
fixation
Fixion intramedullary humeral nail
FlashPoint optical localizer
Fletcher-Suit applicator
Fletcher-Suit-Delclos (FSD) mini colpostat tandem and ovoids
Flexicath silicone subclavian cannula
Flexiflo Lap G laparoscopic gastrostomy kit
Flexiflo Lap J
Flextend
F. L. Fischer microsurgical neurectomy bayonet scissors

device *(cont.)*

Flimm Fighter percussor machine
Flo-Rester
FlossBrite
Flow-Guard introducer
FlowGun
FloWire ultrasound
Flu-Glow fluorescein-impregnated paper strip
fluorescence-activated cell sorter (FACS)
Fluor-i-Strip
FluoroCatcher
FluoroPlus Angiography
FluoroPlus Cardiac digital imaging
FluoroPlus Roadmapper
FluoroScan
Fluoro Tip cannula
Flutter chest percussion therapy
FocalSeal, FocalSeal-S
Forma water-jacketed incubator
Fox shield
Freedom arthritis support
FreeDop
Freeman cookie cutter areola marker
Freeman femoral component with a Rotalok cup
Freeman Punctum Plug
Freestyle aortic root bioprosthesis
Freezor cryocatheter
Freezor Xtra surgical cardiac cryoablation
fria pelvic continent aid
Friedländer marker
Frigitronics probe
Frontier 3 x 2
Fukushima cranial retraction
Fukushima-Giannotta instruments
Gaffney joint
GAIT (great toe arthroplasty implant technique) spacer
Galileo intravascular radiotherapy
gamma counter probe

device *(cont.)*
Gamma Knife radiosurgical instrument
Gamma locking nail
Gammex RMI DAP meter
Gardner chair
Garrett dilator
GasBGon filter seat cushion
Gatch bed
GDx
GDx Access
Geenan cytology brush
gelatin compression boot
Gelfoam cookie
Gellhorn pessary
gel pads
GelPort
Gemini paired helical wire basket
GEM-Premier analyzer
Generation 6 integrated radiotherapy
GenesisXP
Gen-Probe hybridization kit
Gensini cardiac
GenStent biologic gene-based therapeutic
GentlePeel skin exfoliation
Gentle Touch appliance
Genutrain P3
Georgiade visor
GE Senographe 2000D digital mammography
Geo-Mattress
GEO Structure spinal implant
GE Tesla Double-Doughnut Magnet MRI machine
Ghajar guide
Gherini-Kauffman Endo-Otoprobe
Gianturco-Roehm bird's nest vena cava filter
Gianturco wool-tufted wire coil
Gingrass and Messer pins
Girard Fragmatome
Glassman stone extractor
GliaSite radiation therapy
glide

device *(cont.)*
GlideCath instruments
Glidewire
Gluck rib shears
GlucoWatch
Goldenberg footplate shoe
Goldman-McNeill blepharostat
Goldmann applanation tonometer
Goldmann campimeter
Goodale-Lubin cardiac
GoodKnight 418A, 418G, 418P CPAP
Goodwin sound
Gore cast liner
Gore 1.5T Torso Array
Gore Smoother Crucial Tool
gouge
Gould electromagnetic flowmeter
Gould polygraph
GraNee needle (Riza-Ribe grasper needle)
Greenfield IVC filter
Greenwald cutting loop
Greenwald flexible endoscopic electrodes
Grieshaber manipulator
Grignolo-Tagliasco-Zingirian projection campimeter
Grinfeld cannula
G-suit
Guardsman femoral screw
GuardWire Plus angioplasty
Guglielmi Detachable Coil
Guidant Ventak Prizm defibrillator
Guidant Vigor-DR pulse generator
Gullstrand slit lamp
gurney
Gyroscan ACS NT MRI scanner
Gyrus endourology
HAART (highly active antiretroviral therapy)
Haemonetics Cell Saver
Hakim-Cordis pump
Hall dermatome
Hall valvulotome

device *(cont.)*
Hammer mini-tubular external fixation valve
Hancock II tissue valve
H&M anti-snoring
Hanger ComfortFlex knee prosthesis
HappySkin Acne Light
Hardy-Sella punch
Harmonic Scalpel
Harmony breast pump
Harpoon suture anchor
Harrington rod
Harris-Galante porous-coated femoral component
Harrison-Nicolle polypropylene pegs
Harvard 2 dual syringe pump
Harvard pump
Hasson blunt-end cannula
Hasson graspers
Hasson open laparoscopy cannula
Hasson SAC (stable access cannula)
Hasson trocar
Hastings frame
HBS (headless bone screw)
Healey revision acetabular component
hearing aid
HeartSaver VAD artificial heart
HeartStart home defibrillator
HearTwave EP (electrophysiology)
heat-moisture exchanger (HME)
HeatProbe
Hedrocel
Heel Float gel insert
Heffington lumbar seat spinal surgery frame
heliX knot pusher
Hellberg-Kupka scissors
Helmholtz coil
Hemaflex PTCA sheath with obturator
Hemaquet PTCA sheath with obturator

device *(cont.)*
Hemasurer/LS red blood cell filtration
Hemi Sling
Hemoccult Sensa
HemoCue photometer
hemodialyzer
HemoDoppler
Hemopad
Hemopump
hemostatic eraser
Hemotherapies liver dialysis unit
Henning instruments
Hepcon
Hep-Lock infusion
Herbert bone screw
Herbert-Whipple bone screw
HercepTest HER2 protein expression
Hewlett-Packard ear oximeter
Hexcelite
Hex-Fix
Heyer-Schulte tissue expander
high-resolution multileaf collimator
Hilger facial nerve stimulator
Hi-Per cardiac
HipNav process
HipSaver
HiSonic ultrasonic bone conduction hearing
Hi Speed Pulse Lavage
Histofreezer cryosurgical wart treatment
Hoffmann external fixation
Hoffmann mini-lengthening fixation
Holladay-Godwin cornea gauge
HomeChoice Pro with PD Link
HomeTrak Plus compact cardiac event recorder
Honan balloon
Honan manometer
hookah
Hopkins 70° rigid telescope for laryngoscopy
Horn Endo-Otoprobe

device *(cont.)*
Hot/Ice Cold Therapy Cooler
Hot Sampler
Hotsy Cautery
Houston Halo
Howmedica Universal compression screw
Hoyer lift transfer
HPCD (hemostatic puncture closure device)
Hp Chek
HRL (Hardy-Rand-Littler) screening plates
H-TRON insulin pump
Hubbard hydrotherapy tank
Hulka tenaculum
Humalog Mix 75/25 Pen (insulin lispro protamine suspension, insulin lispro injection)
HumatroPen
HumidAire heated humidifier
HUMI uterine manipulator/injector
Hummer microdebrider
Hummingbird wand
Humulin 70/30, Humulin R, and Humalog Pens
Hunter-Sessions balloon
HydroBlade keratome
HydroBrader irrigating/aspirating dermabrader
HydroBrush keratome
Hydrocollator
hydrogel sheets
Hydromer coagulation probe
HydroSurg laparoscopic irrigator
Hydro ThermAblator
Hyfrecator coagulator
Hylashield, Hylashield Nite
Hypafix nonwoven tape
hyperbaric chambers
iBOT 3000 stair-climbing and balancing wheelchair
IceSeeds
ICLH (Imperial College, London Hospital) orthopedic apparatus

device *(cont.)*
Ideal cardiac
I-Flow nerve block infusion kit
Ile-Sorb absorbent gel
IMED infusion
Imount instruments
IMP-Capello arm support
implantable gastric stimulator (IGS)
Import vascular access port with BioGlide
Import vascular access port with dual lumen
Impress Softpatch
incentive spirometer
Incert
In Charge diabetes control
Incise Pouch
In-Exsufflator cough machine
Infamyst aerosol spray
inferior turbinate
InFix interbody fusion
Infuse-a-Port
Infuse bone graft
Injex
InnerVasc sheath
InnovaTome microkeratome
InPath
INRO surgical nails
Inspirator implantable
inspiratory muscle trainer (IMT)
Inspiron
InstaTrak
Insuflon
InSurg laparoscopic stone baskets
InSync cardiac stimulator
Intacs
Integrated Wound Manager
Integris 3-D RA (rotational angiography)
Integrity AFx AutoCapture pacemaker
intense pulsed light source (IPLS)
Intercept Esophageal Internal MR Coil

device *(cont.)*
Intercept Vascular 0.030-inch Internal MR Coil
Intercept Vascular guidewire
interferential stimulator
Inter Fix RP (reduced profile) threaded spinal fusion cage
Inter Fix spinal fusion cage
InterStim neurostimulation
Intrabeam intraoperative radiotherapy (IORT)
Intracell
intracoronary Doppler flow wire
IntraDop
Intra–Op autotransfusion
Invisalign
INVOS 3100 (and 3100A) cerebral oximeter
Ioban antimicrobial incise drape
iodophor-impregnated adhesive drape
Iowa trumpet
I-Plant brachytherapy seeds
iris hook
Irrijet DS
Ishihara plates
ISI laparoscopic instruments
IsoMed implantable drug pump
i-STAT
Itrel 3 spinal cord stimulation
IVAC electronic thermometer
IVAC volumetric infusion pump
iWALKfree crutch
JACE W550
Jackson spinal surgery and imaging table
Jaeger eye chart
Jaeger lid plate
Jamar dynamometer
Jameson calipers
Jarit Rotator
Jeter lag screws or position screws
Jet-X internal fixator
JJ Aligner grid
Jobst jaw bra

device *(cont.)*
Joe's hoe
Joystick
J-wire
Kambin and Gellman instrumentation
KAM Super Sucker
Kanavel brain-exploring cannula
Karl Storz Calcutript
Katena spoon and spatula
Kaycel towels
Kaye tamponade balloon
K-Caps
KCD (kinestatic charge detector)
K-Centrum anterior spinal fixation
keel bone
Kellan hydrodissection cannula
Kempf internal screw fixation
Kendall AV Impulse
Ken nail
Kennedy pack or splint
KeraVision Intacs intracorneal ring
Key-Med dilator
Kid-Kart
Killip wire
Kim-Ray Greenfield caval filter
kinestatic charge detector (KCD)
Kinetec hip CPM machine
King cardiac
Kirklin fence
Kirschenbaum foot positioner
Kirschner Medical Dimension
Kish urethral illuminated catheter set
Kitano knot
Kiwi vacuum extraction cup
Klearway
Klein pump
KLS centre-drive screws
K9 Scooter
Knodt rod
Koch phaco manipulator/splitter
KOH colpotomizer system
Kold Kap
Köper Knit

device *(cont.)*
Kostuik internal spine fixation system
Kraff nucleus splitter
K-Sponge
Kuhn-Bolger seeker
Kuhn frontal sinus curette
Kusch'kin wheelchair
Kuske breast template
Küttner blunt dissector
LADARVision
Laerdal resuscitator
laminaria applicator
Landolt pituitary speculum
Landolt ring
Lange skin-fold calipers
LaparoLith
LaparoSAC single-use obturator and cannula
laparoscopic Doppler probe
LaparoSonic coagulating shears
Lap-Band adjustable gastric banding (LAGB)
Lap Sac
lap tape
LapTie
Lapwall
laser
Lawrence Add-A-Cath trocar and sheath
leading bar
Lea Shield contraceptive
Legacy Phaco-Emulsifier
Legasus Sport CPM
Lehman cardiac
Leibinger miniplate
Leksell stereotaxic frame
LeMaitre Glow 'N Tell tape
Leonard Arm
Leslie Parachute stone retrieval
LeukoNet Filter
lever arm
Levulan Kerastick
Lexer gouge

device *(cont.)*
LHE (light- and heat-based electrical) apparatus
Lido Lift
LifeShirt
LifeSite hemodialysis access
LifeVest
LiftMate patient transfer
Ligaclip
LigaSure hemostasis tool
Light Talker
Lilliput neonatal oxygenator
LIMA-Lift
LIMA-Loop
Lindorf lag screws or position screws
Lindstrom arcuate incision marker
linear cutter stapler
Link Lubinus SP II hip replacement
Linvatec cannulated interference screw
Linvatec microdebrider
LINX-EZ cardiac
LionHeart left ventricular assist (LVAD)
lion jaw tenaculum
liposhaver
Liquid Ice
Liss CES (cranial electrical stimulation)
Listerine PocketPaks
LithoCatch immobilization
lithotrite
Littleford-Spector introducer
Lloyd-Davies scissors
LMA-Unique
LNOP Neo adhesive sensor
long-edge medullary nail
Long45 endocutter
long Gamm locking nail
long taper/stiff shaft Glidewire
LoPro ArthroWand
low-resistance rolling seal spirometer
L-shaped trocar

device *(cont.)*
LT-CAGE lumbar tapered fusion
Lunderquist-Ring torque guide
Luque rods and sublaminar wires
Lusk instruments
Lutrin photosensitizer
LVAS (left ventricular assist system) implantable pump
lymphatic mapping
Lymphedema Alert Bracelet
Lyo-Ject syringe
MAC (Miami Acute Care) collar
Mackay-Marg tonometer
Mackinnon-Dellon Disc-Criminator
Macroplastique continent implant
Maddacrawler
MagnaPod pain relief magnets
Magnes 2500 WH (whole head) imager
Mainstay urologic soft tissue anchor
Makler insemination
Malis CMC-II bipolar coagulator
malleus nipper
Malmstrom cup
Maloney Endo-Otoprobe
Mammomat Novation digital mammography
Mammotome handheld breast biopsy
Mandibular Excursiometer
mandibular repositioning oral appliance
Man facelift expander
Mark II Kodros radiolucent awl
Mark II Sorrells
Mark VII cooling vest
Marlow Primus instrument collection
Marsupial pouch-like belt
Maryland dissector
Masimo SET (signal extraction technology)
Master Flow Pumpette
Matritech NMP22 test kit
Matroc femoral head
Maxima Forté blood oxygenator

device *(cont.)*
Maxima II TENS unit
May anatomical bone plates
Mayfield-Kees headholder
Mayo-Gibbon heart-lung machine
McGaw volumetric pump
McGee platinum/stainless steel piston
McGovern nipple
McKinley EpM pump
McNeill-Goldman blepharostat
Mectra Tissue Sample Retainer
Medela breast pump
Medelec DMG 50 Teflon-coated monopolar electrode
Medfusion 2001 syringe infusion pump (also, Medfusion 2010)
medical holography
Medicon surgical instruments
Medigraphics 2000 analyzer
Medi-Jector Choice
MediPort
MedJet microkeratome
Medoff sliding fracture plate
Medrad automated power injector
Medrad MRInnervu endorectal colon probe
Medstone STS shock wave generator
Medtronic Activa tremor control therapy
Medtronic distal perfusion kit
Medtronic Pisces Quad Plus
Medtronic Hemopump
Medtronic Inspire
Medtronic Jewel AF implantable
Medtronic Micro Jewel II
Medtronic Octopus
Medtronic SynchroMed pump
Medtronic tremor control therapy
MedX physical therapy
MegaDyne all-in-one hand control
MegaDyne E-Z clean laparoscopic electrodes
membrane delamination wedge

device *(cont.)*
MemoryTrace AT cardiac
Mentor BVAT computer screen chart
Mercedes tip cannula
Merci Retriever
Merocel sponge
Merry Walker ambulation
Messerklinger sinus endoscopy set
Metricath catheter/transducer
Miami J collar
MIC disposable cytology brush
Microblator
microdebrider
Micro Diamond-Point microsurgery instruments
microendoscopic diskectomy (MED) instrumentation
MicroFrance BackBiter
MicroFrance minimally invasive surgical instruments
MicroFrance pediatric BackBiter
MicroFrance Selesnick lateral skull base instrument
Micro-Imager
MicroMed DeBakey ventricular assist
Microny II SR+ pulse generator
Microplaner blade
Microplaner soft tissue shaver
Micropuncture Peel-Away introducer
microSelectron-HDR (high-dose-rate) brachytherapy source
MicroSmooth probe
Microtaze
MicroTeq portable belt
microtome
MicroVas vascular treatment system
Microvit cutter
Micro-Z stimulator
Midas Rex pneumatic instruments
Mighty Bite Zimmon lateral biopsy cup
Mijnhard electrical cycloergometer

device *(cont.)*
Miltex surgical instruments
MIMCOM (multimode imaging confocal optical microscope)
Minerva neurosurgical robot
Mini-Acutrak
Mini-Med Continuous Glucose Sensor
Mirena intrauterine (IUD)
Miser tube
mist stick
Mitek anchor system
Mitek BioKnotless anchor
Mitek side effect electrode
Miya hook ligament carrier
MMS-10 Tympanic Displacement Analyzer
Mobin-Uddin umbrella filter
Modulap probe
Modulock posterior spinal fixation
Moe instrumentation
Molnar disk
Monolyth oxygenator
Monoscopy locking trocar with Woodford spike
monster rongeur
Morscher titanium cervical plate
Morse taper stem
Moss T-anchor needle introducer gun
MOST Options modular instruments
M2A Swallowable Imaging Capsule
Mullins cardiac
Multibite biopsy forceps
Multifire Endohernia clip applier
Multileaf Collimator (MLC)
Multilok hand operating table
Multi Podus (boot)
MultiVac ArthroWand
MUSTPAC
Myosplint
Myotherm XP cardioplegia delivery system
Myself female incontinence

device *(cont.)*
Nagahara phaco chopper and phaco chop technique
Nakao snare I and II
NanoWalker
NAPA (nocturnal airway patency appliance)
Nathanson liver retractor
Nashold TC electrode
Natural-Knee system
Navarre interventional radiology
NBIH cardiac
NB200 vascular access
Nellcor Symphony
Neocontrol magnet technology
Neo-EpCAM cancer detection kit
NeoNaze
Neoprobe 1000 detector
Neoprobe 1500 portable radioisotope detector
Neoprobe detector
nerve block infusion kit
NervePace
NeuroCybernetic Prosthesis
NeuroLink II
NeuroMate robotic technology
Neuromed Octrode implantable
Neuromeet nerve approximator
Neuroperfusion pump
Neuroprobe
Neuroshield cerebral protection
Neuro-Trace
New England Baptist acetabular cup
NexGen complete knee replacement
Nezhat-Dorsey Trumpet Valve hydrodissector
Nibbler
Nibblit laparoscopic
Nidek MK-2000 keratome
NightOwl pocket polygraph
NIM-Spine system neural integrity monitor
ninety-ninety (90/90) intraosseous wiring
NIRS (near infrared spectroscopy)

device *(cont.)*
nitinol mesh-covered frame
NonSpil drug delivery
NordiPen human growth hormone injection
Nottingham introducer
Novacor left ventricular assist system (LVAS) implantable pump
NovolinPen
Novus Verdi diode-pumped green photocoagulator
Nucleotome
Nucleotome Flex II
NuTech Plexipulse
Nu-Tip disposable scissor tip
Nycore cardiac
Nylok self-locking nail
Oasis thrombectomy
obturator
Obwegeser-Dalpont internal screw fixation
Oculaid capsular tension ring
ocutome
Ogden anchor
Ojemann cortical stimulator
olive ring
olive wire
Olympia VACPAC support
Olympus EU-M30S endoscopic ultrasonography receiver
Olympus UM-1W endoscopic probe
Omega splinting material
OmniFilter
Omni-Flexor
one-shot anastomotic instrument
One Touch blood glucose meter
Onyx finger pulse oximeter
Opal Photoactivator
OpenAnchor
optical coherence reflectometry (OCR)
optical pachometer
Opti-Gard patient eye protector

device *(cont.)*
Optistat power contrast injector
Orbasone noninvasive therapeutic
Orfizip wrist cast
Origin balloon, tacker, trocar
Orion anterior cervical plate
OR1 electronic
Ortho Dx
Orthofix Cervical-Stim
Orthofix intramedullary nail
Orthofix ISKD (intramedullary skeletal kinetic distractor)
OrthoGuard AB bone pin sleeve
Ortho-Ice Multipaks
Ortholav equipment
OrthoNail
OrthoPak II bone growth stimulator
Orthoplast jacket
OrthoSorb absorbable pin
OSCAR bone cement removal
Osciflator balloon inflation syringe
oscillating saw
OSI arthroscopic leg holder
OSI well leg holder
OssaTron
Osteonics Omnifit-HA hip stem
Osteonics Trident PSL acetabular shell
Osteopatch
OsteoStim implantable bone growth stimulator
OsteoView 2000
Ousley insertion spatula
OutBound
outflow cannula
Ovès cervical cap
Ovès fertility cap
OV-1 surgical keratometer
oximeter
Oxylator EM-100 resuscitation
OxiMax pulse oximetry
Oxymizer
Oxymizer Pendant
Oxytrak pulse oximeter

device *(cont.)*
Pacesetter APS pacemaker programmer
Pacesetter Trilogy DR+
pachometer
Pach-Pen
PACS (Picture Archiving and Communications Systems)
Padgett baseline pinch gauge
Padgett hydraulic hand dynamometer
Padogram vascular diagnostic
palisade screen
pallidal brain stimulation
Panje voice button
Papercuff
Paradigm insulin pump
ParaGard intrauterine (IUD)
Paramax cruciate guide
Parasmillie double-bladed graft-harvesting knife
Paratrend 7 and 7+
Parietex composite mesh
Pari LC Plus reusable nebulizer
Pari LC Star reusable nebulizer
P.A.S. Port Fluoro-Free
Passager introducing sheath
Pavlik harness
PC Polygraf HR
PD Access with Peel-Away needle introducer
Peakometer
Pearce nucleus hydrodissector
PEG-Intron Redipen injection syringe
Pennig dynamic wrist fixator
Pennig minifixator
People-Finder
Perclose A-T
Perclose closure
PercuGuide
PercuPump disposable syringe and injector
percutaneous gastroenterostomy
PerDUCER pericardial access

device *(cont.)*
- PerFixation screws
- PerFix Marlex mesh plug
- Peri-Strips Dry
- Perkins Brailler
- Perkins tonometer
- Perl-Rad sleep disorder aid
- PERM (Electropneumatic Platform for Motor Rehabilitation)
- Peyman vitrector
- Phantom nasal mask
- PharmaSeed (palladium Pd 103 seeds
- Philips ultrasound machines
- PhotoDerm PL
- PhotoDerm VL
- Photon cataract removal
- photonic stimulator
- Photopic Imaging ultrasound
- Physios CTM 01
- Physio Partner support mechanism
- Picasso phone
- Picker Magnascanner
- piezo electrical stimulator
- Pigg-O-Stat
- PillCam ESO video capsule
- Pilot audiometer
- PINC polymer
- Pinn.ACL guide
- Pinpoint stereotactic arm
- Pittman IMA retractor
- Pixsys FlashPoint
- Plasma Scalpel
- Plastizote collar
- platinum coil
- platysma Kaye face-lift
- PLC-55 stapling
- Pleatman sac
- PlegiaGuard
- Plexus mattress
- PM positioner, also adjustable PM positioner
- PMT AccuSpan tissue expander
- Pneumo Sleeve
- Pocket Pachymeter

device *(cont.)*
- point-search acupuncture instruments
- Polaris cage
- Poly-Dial insert
- polylactide absorbable screw
- Polyrox
- Polystan cannula
- Poppen Ridge Sensitometer
- portable blood irradiator
- Port-A-Cath
- Portex
- Positrol cardiac
- Posture S'port
- potential acuity meter (PAM)
- Potts scissors
- Powerheart
- PowerSculpt cosmetic surgery
- Precision Osteolock
- Precision QID
- Premium Plus CEEA disposable stapler
- preperitoneal distention balloon (PDB)
- PREP Pap smear
- Presto cardiac
- Prime ECG (electrocardiographic) mapping
- Probe cardiac
- Prodigy lens inserter
- Profore four-layer bandaging
- ProForma double-lumen papillotome
- ProLease
- PROloop electrosurgical
- Propel cannulated interference screws
- ProPoint
- Prosorba column pheresis
- Prostar, Prostar Plus, and Prostar XL percutaneous closure
- ProstaLund CoreTherm system
- Prostatron
- ProstaSeed ^{125}I radiation treatment
- prosthetic disk nucleus (PDN)

device *(cont.)*

ProtectaCap, Protect Cap+ Plus
Protectaid contraceptive sponge
Protect-a-Pass suture passer
ProteinChip
Protocult
Protouch
Pro-Trac
Protractor
public access defibrillation (PAD)
Pulmicort Turbuhaler
Pulmios inhaler
PulmoSphere
pulsatile catheter (PUCA) pump
PulseDose technology
pulse oximetry
PulseSpray
PumpMate system
punctum plug
Pursuer CBD Helical or Mini-Helical stone basket
PVCM (paradoxical vocal cord motion)
Pylon intramedullary nail
pyogenic liver abscess (PLA)
PZT (plumbeous zirconate titanate) tip
QuantX color quantification tools
Quest medical tape and hard pledget
Questus Leading Edge arthroscopic grasper-cutter
Questus Leading Edge sheathed arthroscopy knife
QuickDraw venous cannula
QuickSeal arterial closure system
QuickVue UrinChek 10+ urine test strips
Quikheel lancet
RAD55 self-irrigating suction bur
radioimmunoluminography (RILG)
radiolucent spine frame
RadiStop radial compression
Radstat
rake

device *(cont.)*

RAMP Reader
Rancho cube
Rand microballoon
RAP (remote access perfusion) cannula
RapidFlap cranial fixation
Rashkind cardiac
Rashkind double umbrella
Raulerson syringe
Ray-Tec sponge
Ray threaded fusion cage (TFC)
Razi cannula introducer
RazorVac ArthroWand
RDX coronary radiation catheter delivery
ReAct NMES
real-time color flow Doppler
real-time position management (REAL) tracking
Rebif in a thin-needle pre-filled syringe
reciprocating saw
Reddick-Saye screw
Reese dermatome
Reese stimulator
Refinity Coblation
reflectant spectral photometer
ReFlex Wand
Regency SR+
Regent aortic heart valve
Reitan CatheterPump
Relia-Flow
Reliance CM femoral component
Reliance urinary control insert
ReliefBand NST (nerve stimulation therapy)
Relton-Hall spine frame
renal tubule assist (RAD)
Repela surgical glove
Repose surgical
RESPeRATE apparatus
Res-Q ACD (arrhythmia control device)
Res-Q Micron

device *(cont.)*
resipump
Resolve Quickanchor
Respiradyne
Respironics CPAP (continuous positive airway pressure) machine
Respironics nasal mask
Respitrace machine
Response GM
Resuscitaire radiant warmer
RetCam 120 digital camera
Retisert
Retrox fractal active fixation lead
Reveal Plus implantable loop recorder
Reveal Plus insertable loop recorder
Revo retrievable cancellous screw
Revo rotator cuff repair
rhBMP-2/ACS (recombinant human bone morphogenetic protein-2/absorbable collagen sponge)
Rheolog
RhinoBur rhinoplasty bur
rhinoplasty
Rhino Rocket
rhytidectomy
Richards Solcotrans Plus
Riechert-Mundinger stereotactic
Riester otoscope
ring stand
Rigiflex TTS balloon
RigiScan
RinoFlow
Risser localizer cast
Risser table
R-Med Plug
Robicsek Vascular Probe (RVP)
Robodoc
ROC and ROC XS suture fasteners
Rochester bone trephine
rod-sleeve instrumentation
Roeder loop
roentgen knife

device *(cont.)*
Roho air-filled mattress
Rolyan Firm D-Ring wrist support
Rossiter stretching program
Rotablator
RotaLink rotational atherectomy
Rotalok cup
Roth Grip-Tip suture guide
Rothman Gilbard corneal punch
Roth retrieval net
roticulating endograsper
Roto-Rest bed
Roy-Camille plates
Ruiz-Cohen round expander
Ruiz microkeratome
RUMI uterine manipulator and injector
Russel (one *L*) gastrostomy kit
Russell-Taylor (R-T) nail
Rutzen ileostomy bag
Saber Bisector ArthroWand
SACH (solid-ankle, cushioned heel) heels
sacral nerve stimulation (SNS) implantable
Sadowsky hook wire
SAF-T shield
Sahara Clinical Bone Sonometer
Salz nuclear splitter
Sand process
SANS (Stoller afferent nerve stimulation)
SAPHFinder surgical balloon dissector
SAPHtrak balloon dissector
Sarns aortic arch cannula
SatinCrescent tunneler
SatinShortcut
SatinSlit keratome
SAVANT
Savary dilator
scalp electrode
Scanmaster DX x-ray film digitizer
Scanning-Beam Digital X-ray (SBDX)

device *(cont.)*
SCD (sequential compression device)
Schanz screw
Schiek back support
Scholten endomyocardial bioptome and biopsy forceps
SciTojet needle-free injector
scleral expansion band (SEB)
Scopettes, Scopettes Jr.
Scorpio total knee
Scully Hip S'port
SEA (side entry access) port
Secur-Fit HA (hydroxyapatite) hip
SeedNet cryotherapy
segmentally demineralized bone technology
Segura CBD (common bile duct) basket
Seidel humeral locking nail
Seidel intramedullary fixation
semidisposable monocrystant antimony pH electrodes
sequential compression (SCD)
Semmes-Weinstein nylon monofilaments
Senning intra-atrial baffle
Senographe 2000D digital mammography imaging
Sensability lubricated plastic sheet
SensiCath optical sensor
Sepacell RZ–2000
Seprafilm
Servo pump
sewing capsule
SharpShooter
Shaw I and Shaw II scalpel
Sheffield pedobarograph
Shepherd internal screw fixation
Shuffors internal screw fixation
SI (sacroiliac) belt
side-cutting Swanson bur
Side-Fire reflecting dish
SieScape imaging technology

device *(cont.)*
signal-averaged electrocardiogram (SAECG)
Silencer
Silent Nightshirt sleep kit
Silent Nite, Silent Nite Soft oral appliance
silicone flexor rod
Silipos Distal Dip
SI-LOC
Silon tent
Silverstein stimulator probe
Simal cervical stabilization
Simplicity spirometer
SimpliCT
Single-Day Baxter infuser
Sinskey hook
SiPAP
SJM-Seguin anuloplasty ring
Skil saw
Skimmer RRP laryngeal shaver
Skin Skribe
Skylight gamma camera
slip-ring CT technology
SmartFlow
SmartMist
Smart Scalpel
SmokEvac electrosurgical probe
SNOAR (sleep nocturnal obstruction airway repositioner) Open Airway Appliance
Snore Aid Plus
Snore-Cure
Snore-Ezzer
Snoremaster snore remedy
Snore-No-More
Snore Peace
Snore Tec
Snorex
Snore-X mouth guard
snoring control
Soehendra dilator
Soehendra stent retriever
Sofamor spinal instrumentation

device *(cont.)*
SofPulse
SoftLight
Soft N Dry Merocel sponge
Soft Palate Lifter, Adjustable
Soft Shield collagen corneal shield
soft tissue shaving cannula (liposhaver)
Soft Touch cup
SolarGen 2100s laser
SoLight
Soluset
SomaSensor
SOMATOM Volume Zoom CT
Sonablate 200
sonicator
SonoCT real-time compound imaging
SonoHeart handheld digital echocardiography
SONOLINE Sierra ultrasound imaging
Sonolith Praktis
SonoSite 180 hand-carried ultrasound
Sonotron
Sophy programmable pressure valve
Sorbie Questor elbow
Spacemaker balloon dissector
Space-Saver volumetric pump
Spectraprobe-Max probe
Spectrum tissue repair
Speculite
SpF Spinal Fusion Stimulator
Sphygmocorder
Spiessel lag screws, position screws, internal screw fixation
SpinaLogic 1000 bone growth stimulator
SpineAssist robot
SpineWand
Spira-Valve implantable
Splintrex
spondylophyte impaction set
sponge dissector

device *(cont.)*
SprayGel adhesion barrier
spring-loaded silo
spud dissector
Squirt wound irrigation
S-ROM femoral stem prosthesis
SRT (smoke removal tube) vaginal speculum
S.S.T. small bone locking nail
Statak
Statham electromagnetic flow meter
StatLock Universal Plus
Stat 2 Pumpette
Steeper powered Gripper
Steffee plates and screws
Steinhauser lag screws, position screws, or internal screw fixation
Steinmann pin
StereoGuide
stereotactic vacuum-assisted biopsy (SVAB)
Steri-Drape
steroid-eluting electrode
Stim Plus
St. Jude Medical Port-Access
St. Jude Pacesetter Atlas DR ICD (implantable cardioverter-defibrillator)
Staccato drug delivery
Stammberger circular punch
Starfish NS (non-sternotomy) heart positioner
Step trocar
Stimuplex Dig RC (remote control) peripheral nerve stimulator
Stomeasure
Stone Cone nitinol stone retrieval
STOO Series Ten Thousand Ocutome
STOP (selective tubal occlusion procedure) contraceptive
Storz Calcutript
Storz cholangiograsper
Storz radial incision marker
StraightShot arterial cannula

device *(cont.)*
StraightShot Magnum handpiece
Strata hip system
Stratasis TF (tension free) urethral sling
STRETCH cardiac
Stryker leg exerciser
Stryker microdebrider
Stulberg hip positioner
Stylet esophageal MRI coil
Summit LoDose collimator
Super-9 guiding cardiac
Super Pinky
SuperQuad assistive
supradescemetic keratoprosthesis
Supramesh
SureCell Chlamydia test kit
SureCell herpes (SC-HSV) test kit
Sure-Closure
SureSight
Suretac
Suretac IXC
surgical isolation bubble (SIBS)
Surgical No Bounce Mallet
Surgicel Fibrillar absorbable hemostat
Surgidyne
SurgiLav Plus machine
Surg-I-Loop
Surgiport
SurgiScope robotic microscope
Surgisis IHM (inguinal hernia matrix)
Surgitron
Surgi-Vision Intercept urethral coil
SutureGroove gold eye weights
Suture/VesiBand organizer
SVAB (stereotactic vacuum-assisted biopsy)
Sweet Tip pacing lead
Swenson papillotome
SwingAlong walker caddy
Symbion J-7-70-mL-ventricle total artificial heart
Symmetra I-125 brachytherapy seeds

device *(cont.)*
Symmetry endobipolar generator
Synergy neurostimulation
Synthes CerviFix
Synthes compression hip screw
Synthes dorsal distal radius plate
Synthes drill
Synthes mini L-plate
Synthes transbuccal trocar
Syringe Avitene
Szabo-Berci needle drivers
Tagarno 3SD cine projector
Take-apart scissors and forceps
Talent LPS endoluminal stent-graft
TandemHeart percutaneous ventricular assist
tangent screen
Tanne corneal punch
Tanner mesher
Tanner-Vandeput mesh dermatome
tantalum mesh, plate, ring, wire
TAPET (tumor amplified protein expression therapy)
Tardy MicroBur
targeted cryoablation
Targis microwave catheter-based
Taylor pinwheel
TCu380A IUD (intrauterine device)
Tebbetts rhinoplasty set
Techstar and Techstar XL
Techstar percutaneous closure
Teflon paste injection for incontinence
Telangitron
TeleCaption decoder
Telescopic Plate Spacer (TPS)
telesensor
Teller acuity card (TAC)
Tender Touch Ultra cup
Tendril DX
Tendril SDX
Tennant nuclear ball rotator
Tenzel calipers
Terry keratometer

device *(cont.)*
Test of Incremental Respiratory Endurance (TIRE)
ThAIRapy Vest
Therabite jaw motion rehabilitation system
TheraGym exercise balls
TheraSnore, also Adjustable TheraSnore
Thermal Angel
thermistor
Thermoflex
Thermophore
Thermoscan Pro-1-Instant thermometer
Thermoskin arthritic knee wrap
Thermo-STAT
TherOx 0.014 infusion guidewire
The Viewing Wand surgical digitizer
ThinLine EZ pacing lead
Thora-Port
Thoraseal
Thoratec VAD (ventricular assist device)
Thornton adjustable positioner (TAP)
Thornton double corneal ruler
Thornton 360° arcuate marker
threaded interbody fusion cage
threadwire saw
TiMesh
TissueLink Monopolar Floating Ball
tissue morcellator
TMZF femoral component, Accolade
TOA (Thornton oral appliance)
Todd-Wells guide
tongue display unit (TDU)
tongue stabilizer
Tono-Pen tonometer
Toomey syringe kit
TQA (transcutaneous access flow)
TracerCAD

device *(cont.)*
Tracer hybrid wire guide
trache "go bag"
Trachlight
Trak Back
Transcend implantable gastric stimulator)
Transvac transdermal patch
transvaginal suturing (TVS) system
TraumaJet needle
Travenol infuser
TriActiv system
Triangle gelatin-sealed sling material
Trident ceramic acetabular insert
TriFix spinal instrumentation
triflange acetabular cup
TriGen FAN nail
TriGen intramedullary nail system
Trilogy acetabular cup
Triosyn T-1000 respirator
Trippi-Wells tongs
Trocan disposable CO_2 trocar and cannula
trochanteric Gamma locking nail
Tru-Area Determination wound-measuring
Trufill n-BCA (N-butyl cyano-acrylate)
TruJect
Trumpet Valve hydrodissector
TruWave pressure transducer
T-Span tissue expander
tube harvester
Tubex injector
tulip probe
tulip tip
Tum-E-Vac
Turbo Whisker
turnbuckle functional position splint
Turvy internal screw fixation
Tutofix cervical pin
2010 Plus Holter
TwinFix
Twisk needle holder, forceps, scissors combination instrument

device *(cont.)*
Two-Photon Excitation (TPE)
UC strip catheter tubing fastener
UHMWPe (ultra-high molecular weight polyethylene) ball liner
Ultima C femoral component
Ultra-Drive bone cement removal system
Ultraject
Ultraseed ultrasound brachytherapy
Ultrasonic Biomicroscope (UBM)
ultrasonic dissection coagulator
Ultratome
Uniflex femoral nail
Uniflex intramedullary nail
UniPuls electro-stimulation instrument
UniShaper keratome
Universal fixation screws
University of Akron artificial heart
unreamed femoral nail (UFN)
Urologic Targis
Uroloop
UroVive balloon
USCI cannula
USCI Goetz bipolar electrodes
USCI NBIH bipolar electrodes
U-Titer
Vabra aspirator
V.A.C. (vacuum-assisted closure)
Vac-Lok cushion
Vac-Pak Pad
Vacurette
Vacutainer
Vairox high compression vascular stocking
Valchev uterine manipulator
Validyne manometer
V-Amour female condom
Vancenase Pockethaler
Vannas capsulotomy scissors
VaporTrode electrode
Variflex cardiac
VariLift spinal cage
VasoSeal VHD (vascular hemostatic)

device *(cont.)*
VasoView Uniport
VCS vascular clip applier
vectis lever
Vector intertrochanteric nail
VED (vacuum erection device)
vein contrast enhancer (VCE)
Veley headrest
VenaFlow compression
Vena Tech LGM filter
ventilation-exchange bougie
Ventritex Angstrom MD
ventricular containment
ventricular geometry change
ventroposterolateral thalamic electrode
venturi mask
Vernier calipers
Versadopp 10 probe
Versa-Fx femoral fixation
Versalab ultrasonic medical
vertebral body impactor
Vesica bladder neck stabilization kit
V5M Multiplane transducer
V510B Biplane TEE transducers
VHS variable-angle hip fixation
Vibracare percussor machine
Vibram-soled rockerbottom shoe
Vibrant Soundbridge
videoendoscopic surgical equipment
Viewing Wand
Viringe vascular access flush
Visijet Hydrokeratome
Visilex mesh
Visuflo blood flow
VitaCuff antimicrobial cuff
VitaCuff attachable cuff
Vitalograph spirometer
Vitatron catheter electrode
Vitrax viscoelastic
vitrector probe
vitreous cutter
V-MAX
VNUS Closure catheter/radiofrequency generator

device *(cont.)*
Vocare bladder
Volutrol
Von Lackum surcingle
Voptix corneal
Vortex router
Vortex stabilization
Voxgram
Voyager aortic
Vozzle Vacu-Irrigator
VPL (ventroposterolateral) thalamic electrode
WACH (wedge adjustable cushioned heel) shoe
Wagner distraction
walkaway
Wallace Flexihub central venous pressure cannula
Wallace pipette
Wallach pencil
Wallstent with Unistep
Warm 'n Form lumbosacral corset
Wartenberg pinwheel
Wartner wart removal system
Water-Pik irrigator
Watzke Silicone sleeve
wavefront measurement
weapon otologic instrument
wearable cardioverter-defibrillator (WCD)
Wedeen wire passers
Wedge electrosurgical resection

Wehbe arm holder
WEST-foot
whale tail of Octopus tissue stabilizer
Whittlestone Physiological Breast-milker, The
Wholey wire
Williams cardiac
Wilson-Cook (modified) wire-guided sphincterotome
Wiltse pedicle screw
Wiltse rods

device *(cont.)*
Wissinger rod
Wixson hip positioner
Wizard cardiac
Wizard microdebrider
wobble board
Wolvek sternal approximation fixation instrument
Wound Stick measuring
Wrightlock posterior fixation
Wristaleve
Xillix LIFE endoscopic system
Xillix LIFE-Lung system
XKnife software
Xomed dacryocystorhinostomy (DCR) drill
X-PRESS vascular closure system
XPS Sculpture system
XPS StraightShot
XT cardiac
X-10 Crosslink plates
Yang-Monti ileovesicostomy
Yankauer curette (curet)
Yasargil bayonet scissors
Yellow IRIS workstation
Yperwatch gamma control watch
Zebra exchange guidewire
Zeiss ophthalmology instruments
Zenith AAA (abdominal aortic aneurysm) endovascular graft
ZEUSS robot
Zielke instrumentation
Zipper Medical neck band
Ziramic femoral head
Zirconia orthopedic prosthetic heads
Zone Specific II meniscal repair
ZTT I and ZTT II acetabular cups
Zucker and Myler cardiac
ZUMI uterine manipulator
Zyoptix
Zywave aberrometer

devil's grip—see *Bornholm disease.*

devil's pinches—factitious purpura; psychogenic purpura. Recurrent painful bruising, consciously or unconsciously self-inflicted.

dewlap—redundant skin hanging below the chin.

DeWrap—a three-layer compression system is designed to deliver sustained, graduated compression for management of lower extremity edema and ulcerations associated with venous insufficiency.

Dexamet stent.

DEXA (dual energy x-ray absorptiometry) **scan**—for bone density determination.

Dexon mesh—a synthetic (polyglycolic acid filaments) and stretchable fabric used in surgery on soft-tissue organs, e.g., liver, spleen, that do not hold sutures well. The idea is to salvage the organ by enclosing it within the mesh, suturing the mesh to the organ at 1/2 to 1/4 inch intervals. The mesh is absorbed by the body tissues in four to six weeks, by which time healing should have taken place.

Dexon Plus suture—a coated synthetic absorbable suture with a timed coating that lasts for 7 hours.

Dexon II suture—an improved Dexon suture which, according to the manufacturer, ties more securely and has better overall strength.

Dextrostix—trade name of plastic strip with reagent areas that change color in the presence of glucose in a drop of capillary blood (usually obtained from the ear lobe or finger stick). Used in monitoring and control of diabetes. Cf. *Chemstrip bG.*

Dexterity PneumoSleeve device—used in hand-assisted laparoscopic surgery.

Dey-Wash skin wound cleanser—saline solution in an aerosol can which sprays under pressure to gently debride and cleanse wounds.

DFA test (direct fluorescent antibody)—for *Legionella pneumophila*. See also *IFA*.

D5/normal saline—incorrect dictation for D5 in half-normal saline (a mixture of dextrose and saline).

DFT (defibrillation threshold).

DGHAL (Doppler-guided hemorrhoidal artery ligation).

DG (Davis & Geck) **Softgut suture**—surgical chromic suture.

DHS—a registered trademark for a dynamic hip screw, an implantable prosthetic device used to achieve a stable repair of femoral neck fracture. Sometimes dictated: *DHS dynamic hip screw* or *DHS plate with 95-mm DHS screw,* with *DHS* used as a modifier to refer to the system or appliance used, and plate and screw to give the dimensions of each component.

Diabetes A1c Initiative—a national awareness campaign to educate diabetics as to the importance of keeping hemoglobin A1c levels below 7%.

diabetes, bronze—see *bronze diabetes.*

diabetes mellitus classifications—from the American Diabetes Association to replace the terms *juvenile onset* and *adult onset*, as follows:

type 1 diabetes mellitus—results from the body's failure to produce insulin, the hormone that "unlocks" the cells of the body, allowing glucose to enter and fuel them. It is estimated that 5-10% of Americans who are diagnosed with diabetes have type 1 diabetes.

type 2 diabetes mellitus—results from insulin resistance, a condition in which the body fails to properly use insulin, combined with relative insulin deficiency. Most Americans

diabetes *(cont.)*
who are diagnosed with diabetes have type 2 diabetes.

prediabetes—a condition that occurs when a person's blood glucose levels are higher than normal but not high enough for a diagnosis of type 2 diabetes. There are 41 million Americans who have pre-diabetes, in addition to the 18.2 million with diabetes.

gestational diabetes—a condition that occurs when a pregnant woman who does not have diabetes develops a resistance to insulin because of the hormones of pregnancy. It affects about 4% of all pregnant women. Gestational diabetes is further divided into two major classes: class A_1 is non-insulin dependent (NIDDM); class A_2 is insulin dependent (IDDM). Class A_2 is further divided into subgroups:

• preexisting diabetes—women who already have insulin-dependent diabetes and become pregnant.

• class B—diabetes developed after age 20 but present less than 10 years, with no vascular complications.

• class C—diabetes developed between age 10 and 19 or present for 10-19 years, with no vascular complications.

• class D—diabetes developed before age 10 or present more than 20 years; vascular complications are present.

• class F—diabetic women with kidney disease called nephropathy.

• class H—diabetic women with coronary artery or other heart disease.

• class R—diabetic women with retinopathy (retinal damage).

• class T—diabetic women who have undergone kidney transplant.

Diabetes Plus—a nutritional supplement (in cans).

diabetic ketoacidosis (DKA).

diabetic macular edema (DME).

diabetic-neuropathic osteoarthropathy (DNOAP).

diabetic triopathy—a triad of diabetic complications consisting of nephropathy, retinopathy, neuropathy.

DiabetiSweet sugar substitute—an artificial sweetener.

DiaB Gel hydrogel dressing.

DiaB Klenz wound cleanser.

Diacyte DNA ploidy analysis—a way to identify aneuploid tumor of the prostate which may require aggressive treatment, such as tumors with intermediate Gleason scores.

Diagnex Blue test—lab test for gastric acid. (Diagnex Blue is a trademark.)

DIAGNOdent—laser device that assists in early diagnosis of tooth decay.

Diagnostic and Statistics Manual, Fourth Edition Text Revision (mental health).

Diagnostic Relative Groups (DRGs).

dial a haptic (Oph).

dial-in, block-lock knee braces—above-the-knee braces that can be set so that the ankle is at an angle of 90 degrees.

Dialock—implantable access port for patients undergoing hemodialysis therapy.

dialyze, dialyzes, dialyzed—to undergo or having undergone dialysis. Usage: "The patient dialyzes from a PermCath in the right internal jugular."

diamagnetic—MRI term.

diamond bur—instrument used to abrade or smooth; for example, to resect an osteophyte.

Diamond-Flex instruments—a variety of flexible endoscopic instruments that can be formed into desired shapes.

diamond fraise—an instrument used in dermabrasion.

Diamond-Lite—titanium cardiovascular surgical instruments.

Diamond pocket maker—used in preparing the pocket for the corneal donor button in deep lamellar endothelial keratoplasty (DLEK).

diamond-shaped murmur—a systolic heart murmur that first grows louder and then softer, the same as a crescendo-decrescendo murmur. Named for diamond-shaped tracing on phonocardiogram.

diamond-shaped posterior chink—a characteristic shape (dashed circle) of the vocal cords during paradoxical narrowing of the vocal cords during inspiration in a patient with vocal cord dysfunction.

Dianon prostate profile and diagraph—an oncology trend report showing results over time of PSA, PAP, and LASA-P in patients with prostate cancer.

diaphanography—transillumination of the breast, with photography of the transilluminated light on infrared-sensitive film.

diaphanoscope—instrument for transilluminating a body cavity.

diaphanous—see-through, transparent. See *diaphanoscope.*

DiaPhine corneal trephination device—uses a diamond dissection blade.

diaphragmatic hump—a finding on radiography, due to distortion of the diaphragm by enlarged liver or liver tumor.

diaphysis—the shaft of a long bone between the ends (the epiphyses). *Cf. diastasis, diathesis.*

DIAPPERS—an acronym for causes of transient urinary incontinence:

D delirium
I infection
A atrophic urethritis, vaginitis
P pharmaceuticals
P psychological (especially severe depression)
E excess urine output
R restricted mobility
S stool impaction

diarrhea-predominant vs. constipation-predominant irritable bowel syndrome.

Diascan—a glucose monitoring system.

Diasensor 1000—a sensor that measures the blood glucose level using near-infrared technology, without the need of a finger prick for a blood sample.

diastasis—separation (or dislocation) of two bones that are normally attached without the presence of a true joint; sometimes refers to the separation of muscles, as in diastasis recti abdominis. Cf. *diaphysis, diathesis.*

diastasis of ankle sprain—latent or frank classifications of traumatic syndesmotic sprain of the ankle. Latent diastasis is seen on stress radiographs only, and frank diastasis is obvious on plain radiographs.

diastatic fracture—involves separation of the bones at the suture line of the skull, or marked separation of the bone fragments.

Diastat vascular access graft—used for dialysis access.

Diatest—breath test kit that enables physicians to diagnose the early stages of insulin resistance and type 2 diabetes.

diathermy—see *ultrasound diathermy.*

diathesis—constitution of the body that predisposes one to certain diseases or conditions. Usage: "The patient

diathesis *(cont.)*
appeared to have a hemorrhagic diathesis, although there was no family history of hemophilia." Cf. *diaphysis, diastasis.*

Dibbell unilateral cleft lip nasal reconstruction.

dibenzodiazepines—a class of antipsychotic drugs. See *clozapine.*

DIC (disseminated intravascular coagulation).

DIC (drip infusion cholangiography)

DIC (differential interference contrast) **microscopy.**

dicentric (Genetics)—referring to an abnormal chromosome that has two centromeres.

DICOM (digital imaging and communications in medicine) (teleradiology) —the industry standard for transfer of radiologic images and other medical information between computers.

DID (delayed ischemic deficit).

didelphys—see *uterus didelphys.*

"didge"—phonetic for *dig*, slang for *digitalis, digoxin,* or *digitoxin*, hence ambiguous. Do not expand *dig* unless the exact sense is clear from other data.

Dieckmann intraosseous (IO) **needle**—used to deliver drugs and fluids through the bone marrow. Because children's veins are so small, administering drugs intravenously is very difficult and slow, but, in an emergency, using this needle, the physician can get to the bone marrow within 30 seconds. The easiest point to access the marrow (which is said to be much like a noncollapsible vein) is just below the knee.

diener ("dee-ner")—an assistant in a laboratory or morgue.

DIEP (deep inferior epigastric [artery] perforator) flap.

dietary and natural supplements *(see also medications)*
AlitraQ
Avlimil (salvia rubus)
Azo menopause tablets
Azo urinary pain relief tablets
cilantro
BioFIT Herbgels
conjugated linoleic acid (CLA)
D-chiro-inositol
Enzogenol
epoxyeicosatrienoic acids
Essiac
EstroLogic
Femaprin
femoré intimacy cream
Gerson dietary
Hoodia (*Hoodia gordonii*)
hydrazine sulfate
Iscar
Kangaroo Kids NutraPops
L-Camipure (L-carnitine tartrate)
Limitrol-DM
MigraHealth
MigraSpray
Migre Lief
NutriMan TNT (*Tribulus terrestris* extract)
Nu-Trim
Nuzyme dietary
Oralife mouth rinse
Osteo Bi-Flex
Perative
phytochemicals
phytostanol
phytosterol
Polyphenon E
Prelief (calcium glycerophosphate)
Promensil
Quintessence nutritional supplement
Salonpas
Satietrol Complete
seabuckthorn seed oil
ShanStar Cranberry
Skinny Pill

dietary *(cont.)*
Skinny Pill for Kids
Spirulina Pacifica nutritional supplement
Stacker 2 diet supplement
Stacker 3 with Chitosan
StriVectin-SD
Tonalin (conjugated linoleic acid)
Trinovin
Vitacor Plus
Wobenzym
Zeavision (zeaxanthin)

Dietl crisis—when a kidney twists on its pedicle, cutting off blood flow.

Dieulafoy gastric lesion—a congenital defect in a submucosal artery lining the stomach. It can burst and cause massive hemorrhage. Also referred to as a *cirsoid aneurysm*, *caliber-persistent artery*, *submucosal arterial malformation*, or *vascular malformation*.

DIF (digital image fusion) **procedure**.

"diff"—medical slang for WBC differential. See *differential*.

differential interference contrast microscopy (DIC).

differential in white blood cell count:
eosinophils—range 5-6%
basophils—range 0-1%
lymphocytes—range 20-40%
monocytes—range 0-7%
polymorphonuclear neutrophils (PMNs or polys)—range 50-70% of total white blood cells

differential renal function (DRF) **on MR urography**.

differentiation—a developmental process characterized by an increase in the organization or complexity of a cell or tissue, accompanied by specialization of function.

Diffistat-G—uses a polyclonal antibody in a test for *C. difficile* diarrhea.

Diff-Quik stain—a stain for diagnosing *Helicobacter pylori*.

diffraction-enhanced imaging (DEI)—imaging method using a single-energy x-ray source to detect breast tumors. The method produces sharply defined pictures by reducing scattering and helping visualize low-contrast areas not visible with traditional mammography.

diffuse alveolar disease (DAD)—term for idiopathic pulmonary fibrosis.

diffuse toxic goiter (DTG).

diffusion tensor magnetic resonance imaging (DT-MRI)—can make detailed three-dimensional maps of nerve pathways in the brain, heart muscle fibers, and other soft tissues.

diffusion-weighted imaging—ultrafast MRI technique that shows exactly which brain tissue is dead following a stroke and helps to determine whether the patient has had a transient ischemic attack (TIA). Victims of TIA usually recover fully but run a high risk of major strokes at a later time. It is also useful in diagnosing Alzheimer disease. See *perfusion-weighted imaging*.

dig ("didge," "dij")—slang for *digitalis, digoxin, or digitoxin,* hence ambiguous. Do not expand *dig* unless the exact sense is clear from other data.

Digene HIV RNA test.

DiGeorge anomaly (DGA). Also, *DiGeorge syndrome*.

DiGeorge syndrome—thymic hypoplasia. Congenital aplasia of the thymus and parathyroid glands; pure T-cell deficiency, but with B-cell function intact. Cf. *Nezelof syndrome*.

digestive-respiratory fistula (DRF)—a coated Wallstent used for palliative treatment.

Digikit—finger and toe pneumatic tourniquet that prevents nerve trauma that could occur with the use of a Penrose drain as a tourniquet.

DigiMatch—pinless total hip arthroplasty.

Digirad 2020 TC Imager—solid-state gamma camera for use in nuclear medicine.

Digiscope—automated camera used to identify diabetics with diabetic retinopathy before they sustain permanent damage and lose vision.

DigiSound—two-channel digital signal processing hearing instrument.

digital Add-On Bucky—x-ray image acquisition system that produces filmless, digitized images.

digital fundus imager—digital camera and recording system for color and/or fluorescein angiography by ophthalmologists and optometrists.

digital holography system—uses data collected by computed tomography and magnetic resonance scanners to produce a three-dimensional image called a Voxgram. These images help clinicians diagnose craniofacial problems, create the surgical treatment plan and templates, and intraoperatively measure and reconstruct deformities.

digital image fusion (DIF) **procedure**—for diagnostic mapping and treatment of complex cardiac arrhythmias.

digital IC-Green (indocyanine green) fluorescein dye) **videoangiography**—provides enhanced imaging of subretinal diseases.

digital movement analysis (DMA)—a new instrumental approach to assessing oral tardive dyskinesia by means of digital image processing of a video signal, which tracks five paper dots placed around the patient's mouth and detects perioral tremor as a sign of parkinsonism.

Digital OsteoView 2000—amorphous silicon flat panel x-ray detection system, capable of detecting both osteoporosis and arthritis.

digital parabola (Radiol)—term related to toe lengths in x-ray reports.

digital radiography—low-dose, reduced-dose digital technique for follow-up radiographs in pediatric orthopedic patients.

digital signal processing (DSP)—technology for hearing aids.

digital storage—a term used in cineangiography. Usage: "High resolution images from magnetic tape were transmitted to digital storage to serve as guiding or map views for subsequent angioplasty."

digital subtraction angiography (DSA)—an interventional radiological procedure which allows visualization of the small vessels. Iodinated contrast material is injected via venous catheter, and a computer subtracts out all the tissues until only the vessels visualized by contrast material are left; any vessels blocked by occlusion or stenosis are then readily apparent.

digital subtraction macrodacryocystography (Oph).

digital-to-analog converter—MRI term.

digital tomosynthesis—a 3-D picture of the breast using x-rays, available now only for research purposes. Digital tomosynthesis of the breast is different from a standard mammogram in the same way a CT scan of the chest is different from a standard chest x-ray. Digital tomosynthesis takes multi-

digital *(cont.)*
ple x-ray pictures of each breast from many angles. The breast is positioned the same way it is in a conventional mammogram, but only a little pressure is applied—just enough to keep the breast in a stable position during the procedure. The x-ray tube moves in an arc around the breast while 11 images are taken during a seven-second examination. Then the information is sent to a computer, where it is assembled to produce clear, highly focused 3-dimensional images throughout the breast.

Digitek—an antiarrhythmic medication.

DIGIT-grip—a computer-based device used by physical therapists to rehabilitate patients with hand injuries. It displays a digital readout of either total grip strength or the strength of the middle/index fingers or ring/little fingers.

Digitrapper MKIII—device for ambulatory assessment of lower esophageal sphincter (LES) pressures and esophageal motility disorders.

Digitron—a digital subtraction imaging system.

Dilamezinsert (DMI)—urologic instrument consisting of a dilator and inserter to aid in penile prosthesis implantation.

Dilapan—synthetic laminaria for cervical dilatation. See *Laminaria*.

DILE (drug-induced lupus erythematosus).

dilute Russell viper venom—see *Russell viper venom*.

dilutional hematocrit—when too much water or crystalloid dilutes the blood, lowering the hematocrit. *Not* delusional.

DIMAQ integrated ultrasound workstation.

Dimension Free Prostate-Specific Antigen (FPSA) **Flex reagent cartridge**—used in FPSA test to help diagnose prostate cancer and distinguish between cancerous conditions and benign conditions.

DIMOAD syndrome—diabetes insipidus, diabetes mellitus, optic atrophy, and deafness.

Dinamap blood pressure monitor and Oxytrak pulse oximeter—to measure oxygen saturation.

Dingman-Denhardt mouth gag.

Dingman mouth gag.

diode laser.

DioPexy probe—for treatment of retinal detachment, an alternative treatment to cryopexy. The procedure employs transscleral retinal photocoagulation.

DIP (desquamative interstitial pneumonitis).

diploid ('double')—referring to the full complement of chromosomes in a somatic cell, 23 pairs in human beings.

diploid human cell—a cell having 46 chromosomes.

dipslide—see *Uricult dipslide*.

dipstick technique—topical application of liquid nitrogen to skin warts. Although it can cause intense pain, the cure rate is said to be 93 to 97%.

dipyramidole (Canadian spelling). In the U.S., the correct drug name is dipyridamole (Persantine).

dipyridamole echocardiography test—may demonstrate exercise-induced myocardial ischemia, which might be "EKG-silent," by providing evidence of the ischemic event. Also an agent to reduce blood viscosity.

dipyridamole thallium stress test—a chemical equivalent of the treadmill stress test, used when patients cannot take the standard treadmill test.

dipyridamole *(cont.)*
Dipyridamole (Persantine), given orally or intravenously, dilates the coronary arteries and increases the blood flow to the heart, reproducing the effects of exercise. A radioisotope, thallium, is then injected into a vein. A scanning device will record the passage of the thallium and demonstrate the areas that receive adequate amounts of blood and which are occluded. See *thallium stress test.*

directed differentiation—modification of a stem cell culture, for example by the addition of growth factors, so as to induce differentiation into a specific cell type.

DirectFlow arterial cannula—introduced through a thoracic trocar or incision and used to deliver oxygenated blood during cardiopulmonary bypass surgery. Also used to introduce and remove the Heartport Endoclamp aortic catheter.

direct fluorescent antibody test (DFA).

Directigen latex agglutination test—identifies pathogens by detecting specific antigens in cerebrospinal fluid and urine.

directional coronary angioplasty (DCA)—method of treating stenosis of a saphenous vein free-graft coronary artery bypass graft. Alternative treatment to percutaneous transluminal coronary balloon angioplasty.

directional coronary atherectomy (DCA)—cardiac catheterization procedure in which a catheter with a small mechanically driven cutter is inserted into the plaque-containing artery. A rotating blade shaves off the plaque, which is pushed into a storage chamber in the catheter and removed with the catheter. Also, *rotational coronary atherectomy.*

direct light reflex—light reflex in which the response occurs in the eye that was stimulated. See *consensual light reflex.*

direct myocardial revascularization (DMR).

DirectRay—uses direct-to-digital technology to capture and convert x-ray energy into digital images using a full-field (14" x 17") digital image-detector array.

direct solvent dissolution or litholysis—for the treatment of gallstones. See also *contact dissolution or litholysis* and *transhepatic gallbladder litholysis.*

DirectView CR 900—imaging system device.

direct vision internal urethrotomy (DVIU).

dis-, see *dys-*.

DISA S-Flex coronary stent—laser-sculpted implant used to open and maintain blood flow in the coronary arteries.

disc—alternate spelling of *disk.* See *disk.*

discission—the incision, or cutting into, as of a capsule of a cataract, or of the cervix uteri. Cf. *decision.*

disconjugate gaze—when the eyes do not work in unison. Alternate spelling, *dysconjugate.* Apparently either spelling is acceptable.

discordant (Genetics)—referring to twins of which one shows an inherited trait and the other does not.

discordant cellular xenograft—transplantation of tissue from a distantly related species, such as the pig.

discordant organ xenograft—transplantation of a solid organ from a distantly related species, such as the pig.

Discovery bone densitometers—a line of bone densitometers, including the Discovery QDR. It combines 10-second bone density measurements with 10-second assessment of vertebral fracture status.

Discovery LS—imaging system that combines CT and PET scanning technology to provide very detailed images. The resolution is so fine that it can identify early stages of cancer or cancer recurrence. It takes about 30 minutes and is considered to be a cost-effective means of diagnosis and treatment.

Discovery QDR—see *Discovery bone densitometer.*

discreet—circumspect, prudent, using or showing good judgment in conduct and in speech. Usage: "I hope you will be most discreet in using this information." Cf. *discrete.*

discrete—separate, composed of distinct parts or discontinuous elements. Usage: "There were large, discrete nodules noted in the neck." (A mnemonic device to help remember this spelling: *discrete* means separate; note that the *t* separates the two *e*'s.) Cf. *discreet.*

disease, disorder, or **condition** (see also *lesion*)
ACAD (atherosclerotic carotid artery disease)
acanthosis
ACD (allergic contact dermatitis)
achondroplastic dwarfism
acrodysostosis
acromesomelic dysplasia
acute inflammatory demyelinating polyradicular (AIDP) neuropathy
acute promyelocytic leukemia (APML)
acute repetitive seizure (ARS) disorder

disease *(cont.)*
acute zonal occult outer retinopathy (AZOOR)
adenocarcinoma in situ (AIS) of the cervix
adenomatous hyperplasia (AH)
adiposis dolorosa
adolescent idiopathic scoliosis (AIS)
adRP (autosomal-dominant retinitis pigmentosa)
adult chronic immune thrombocytopenic purpura (ITP)
age-associated memory impairment (AAMI)
age-related macular degeneration (AMD)
aggressive angiomyxoma
AILD (angioimmunoblastic lymphadenopathy with dysproteinemia)
AIOD (aortoiliac obstructive)
AIP (acute intermittent porphyria)
air-space
Alder-Reilly morphological abnormality
aldosterone-producing adenoma (APA)
allergic bronchopulmonary aspergillosis (ABPA)
Alström
alveolar soft-part sarcoma (ASPS)
AML (acute myeloblastic leukemia)
AML (angiomyolipoma)
AMMOL (acute myelomonoblastic leukemia)
AMOL (acute monoblastic leukemia)
AMPPE (acute multifocal placoid pigment epitheliopathy)
anterolisthesis
Antopol-Goldman lesion
AOIVM (angiographically occult intracranial vascular malformation)
aortoiliac obstructive (or occlusive) (AIOD)

disease *(cont.)*
aphtha
apical impulse
apocrine metaplasia
appendicular ataxia
applanated condition
APSGN (acute poststreptococcal glomerulonephritis)
argentaffin carcinoma
Armanni-Ebstein nephropathy
ARS (acute repetitive seizure) disorder
Arthus reaction
ash leaf spots in the eye
astasia–abasia
asthenopia
asymmetric septal hypertrophy (ASH)
auricular perichondritis
babesiosis
bacillary angiomatosis (BA)
bacterial endophthalmitis
basidiobolomycosis
Bassen-Kornzweig abetalipo-proteinemia
Batten
beaver fever
Becker nevus of the thigh with lipoatrophy
Bellini duct carcinoma
benign intracranial hypertension (BIH)
benign necrotizing otitis externa (BNOE)
benign paroxysmal positional vertigo
benign prostatic hypertrophy or hyperplasia (BPH)
Berger
bipolar affective illness
birdshot chorioretinopathy
black patch delirium
body dysmorphic disorder (BDD)
bone surface lesion
Bornholm (devil's grip)

disease *(cont.)*
bovine spongiform encephalopathy (BSE)
brittle bone disease (osteogenesis imperfecta)
broad beta
bronchiolitis obliterans with organizing pneumonia (BOOP)
bronze (Addison)
bubble boy
Buerger
bull's eye lesion
buried penis
Burkitt lymphoma
C. difficile-associated diarrhea (CDAD)
caisson
calcium pyrophosphate deposition (CPPD)
cameral fistula
Campbell de Morgan spots
Canavan
carcinoma ex pleomorphic adenoma
carcinoma in situ (CIS)
cardiac allograft vascular (CAVD)
cardiogenic shock
carneous degeneration
Caroli
Carrión
Castleman
CATCH 22 (microdeletion of chromosome 22q11)
cat-scratch (CSD)
central splanchnic venous thrombosis (CSVT)
cerebrospinal fluid rhinorrhea
Chester-Erdheim
chronic bacterial prostatitis (CBP)
chronic subdural hematoma (CSDH)
circinate-pattern interstitial keratopathy
cobalamin C methylmalonic acidemia
cobblestone degeneration
columnization of contrast media

disease *(cont.)*
combined hernia
common acute lymphoblastic leukemia antigen (CALLA)
compound volvulus
congenital esophageal stenosis
congenital insensitivity to pain and anhidrosis (CIPA)
connective tissue (CTD)
consumption coagulopathy
cradle cap
craniosynostosis (craniostosis)
cryptogenic (idiopathic) epilepsy
Curling ulcer
cutaneous T-cell lymphoma
cyclomania
cyclops lesion
cystic adenomatoid malformation (CAM)
cytomegalovirus retinitis
de Quervain
Dercum
desmoplastic small round-cell tumor (DSRCT)
detergent worker's lung
Devic
devil's grip
devil's pinches
diabetic triopathy
diabetic-neuropathic osteoarthropathy (DNOAP)
Dieulafoy gastric lesion
diffuse alveolar (DAD)
diffuse toxic goiter (DTG)
DIP (desquamative interstitial pneumonitis)
dry age-related macular degeneration (ARMD)
dumbbell tumor
duodenal ulcer perforation (DUP)
dysfibrinogenemia
dyskaryosis
dyskeratosis
dysphagia lusoria
dysthymia

disease *(cont.)*
Eales
egg-shaped congruous acetabulum
elastosis perforans serpiginosa
ELD (episodic laryngeal dyskinesia)
endoscopy-negative reflux (ENRD)
ENL (erythema nodosum leprosum)
eosinophilic pustular folliculitis
ependymitis granularis
epidermodysplasia verruciformis
epidermolysis bullosa acquisita
equilibratory ataxia
Erb palsy
Erdheim-Chester
ER/PR-negative infiltrating ductal carcinoma of the breast
erythema migrans (EM)
erythematous vulvitis en plaque
erythroplasia of Queyrat
esophageal achalasia
Ewing sarcoma
extrahepatic cholangiocarcinoma
Fabry lipid storage
facioscapulohumeral dystrophy (FSHD)
familial adenomatous polyposis (FAP)
farmer's lung
female sexual arousal disorder (FSAD)
fibrodysplasia ossificans progressiva (FOP)
fingerprint dystrophy
fish meal lung
fish tank granuloma
Fleischner
flock worker's lung
foamy esophagus
forme fruste
Fournier gangrene
fragmentation phase of Legg-Calvé-Perthes (LCP)
Freiberg
Fuchs phenomenon
furrier's lung

disease *(cont.)*
gas-forming liver abscess
GAVE (gastric antral vascular ectasia)
germ cell tumor (GCT)
gestational trophoblastic (GTD)
giant anorectal condyloma acuminatum
giant cell arteritis (GCA)
glioblastoma multiforme
glomus tumor
glucose-6-phosphate dehydrogenase (G-6-PD) deficiency
graft versus host
granulomatous mastitis
Grover skin
GTD (gestational trophoblastic)
Gudden atrophy
gumma
Haglund deformity
hairy-cell leukemia
hardware (traumatic pericarditis)
hemangiolymphangioma
hemangiopericytic meningioma
hemangiopericytoma
hepatic venous web
hepatitis A (infectious hepatitis)
hepatitis B (serum hepatitis)
hepatitis C (chronic hepatitis)
hepatitis D
hepatitis E
hepatitis F
hereditary nonpolyposis colorectal cancer (HNPCC)
hereditary sensory and autonomic neuropathy type IV (HSAN-IV)
herpes whitlow infection
herpes encephalitis
herpesvirus
HGD (high-grade dysplasia)
HIB (*Haemophilus influenzae* type B)
Hill-Sachs lesion or deformity
HIV-associated thrombocytopenia
Hollenhorst plaques

disease *(cont.)*
Holt-Oram atriodigital dysplasia
homocystinuria
hordeolum
hour-glass constriction of hip capsule
human granulocytic ehrlichiosis (HGE)
Hunner interstitial cystitis
Hunner ulcer
hypertrophic obstructive cardiomyopathy (HOCM)
hypertrophied nasal turbinate
hypothenar hammer syndrome
ICE (immunoglobulin-complexed enzyme) disorders
idiopathic CD4+ lymphocytopenia (ICL)
idiopathic (cryptogenic) epilepsy
idiosyncratic asthma
ileosigmoid knot
inborn error of metabolism
inflammatory bowel (IBD)
interstitial cystitis (IC)
intracranial aneurysm (ICA)
intraepidermal blistering (pemphigus)
intramural duodenal hematoma after blunt abdominal trauma
intraosseous pneumatocyst, cervical spine
iron storage
ischemic penile gangrene
Jadassohn-Dössekker
Janeway lesions
Kandahar sore
kaposiform hemangioendothelioma
Kawasaki
Kienböck lunatomalacia
Kimmelstiel-Wilson
Kniest dysplasia
König
Kousseff syndrome
kraurosis vulvae
Krukenberg tumor

disease *(cont.)*
Kugelberg-Welander
Kussmaul respiration
lactobezoar
Lafora body
laryngospasm
Lassa fever
late luteal phase dysphoric disorder (LLPDD)
lateral hypopharyngeal pouches (LHPs)
leather-bottle stomach gastric carcinoma
Leber
legionnaires'
Letterer-Siwe
Lewis upper limb cardiovascular
Lhermitte-Duclos
lichen planus
ligamentization
lipid storage
Listeria meningitis
Little League elbow
littoral cell angioma
locked-in syndrome
longitudinal melanonychia
low-grade dysplasia (LGD)
low-grade squamous intraepithelial lesion (LSIL)
lupus pernio
Lyme
Lyme lymphocytic meningo-radiculitis
lymphangioleiomyomatosis (LAM)
lymphocytic interstitial pneumonitis (LIP)
lymphogranuloma venereum (LGV)
lymphomatoid papulosis (LyP)
Lynch and Crues Type 2 lesion
lytic (or osteolytic) lesion
MAC (*Mycobacterium avium* complex) infection
macrometastasis
macro-orchidism
macular degeneration

disease *(cont.)*
mad cow disease (bovine spongiform encephalopathy) (BSE)
Madura foot
MAI (*Mycobacterium avium*-intracellulare) infection
malacoplakia of kidney
Malassezia furfur pustulosis
malignant mixed mullerian tumor (MMMT)
MALToma
maple bark stripper's
maple-syrup urine (MSUD)
Marburg hemorrhagic fever
Marchiafava-Bignami
Martorell hypertensive ulcer
Masson tumor
MC (multifocal choroiditis)
meat wrapper's asthma
Mediterranean lymphoma
Meige disease or syndrome
melorheostosis
membranous croup
MEN (multiple endocrine neoplasia)
meningococcal supraglottitis
meralgia paresthetica
Merkel cell carcinoma (MCC)
metaphyseal lesion of the distal femur
methylmalonic acidemia
microchimerism
micro-dots
micrometastasis
Miescher cheilitis granulomatosa
milk leg
Milroy
minimal change
moccasin-type tinea pedis
Mondini dysplasia
Mondor
mucormycosis
multifocal chorioretinitis
multigenic carcinogenesis
multiple endocrine neoplasia (MEN), type 2b

disease *(cont.)*
mummification
mushroom worker's lung
Mycobacterium abscessus
mycosis fungoides palmaris et plantaris
mycotic aneurysm
myocardial remodeling
myositis ossificans (MO)
NANB (non-A/non-B) hepatitis
nasal T-cell/natural killer cell lymphoma
necrotizing enterocolitis (NEC)
necrotizing fasciitis
neonatal acne
nesidiodysplasia
neural tube defects (NTD)
neuro-Behçet
neuroimmune dysfunction
new variant Creutzfeldt-Jakob (nvCJD)
NHL (non-Hodgkin lymphoma) tumors
Niemann-Pick
nil disease (lipoid nephrosis)
nonalcoholic fatty liver (NAFLD)
nonalcoholic steatohepatitis (NASH)
nonerosive reflux (NERD)
non-nasal CD56+T/NK (natural killer) cell lymphoma
non-small cell lung carcinoma (or cancer) (NSCLC)
nonseminomatous germ cell tumor
nonspecific esophageal motility disorder (NEMD)
nonspecific urethritis (NSU)
non-ST segment elevation myocardial infarction (non-STEMI)
nonvalvular AF (atrial fibrillation)
nosocomial
no-view cataract
NTG (normal-tension glaucoma)
obliterative bronchiolitis
obsessive-compulsive disorder (OCD)

disease *(cont.)*
ocular rosacea
onychopachydermoperiostitis
ophthalmic pneumocystosis, AIDS-associated
optic neuritis
Ormond
osteomesopyknosis
otospondylomegaepiphyseal dysplasia (OSMED)
painter's encephalopathy
pantaloon hernia
paroxysmal nocturnal hemoglobinuria (PNH)
Patella
paving stone degeneration
PCNSL (primary central nervous system lymphoma)
pediatric autoimmune neuropsychiatric disorders associated with streptococcus (PANDAS)
peliosis hepatis
Pelizaeus-Merzbacher
penile gangrene and penile necrosis
peptic ulcer (PUD)
perforating folliculitis
perforating verruciform collagenoma
periarticular heterotopic ossification (PHO)
periorbital infantile myofibromatosis
peritoneal melanosis
pernio, perniosis
pes anserine bursitis
PID (primary immune deficiency)
pilomatrix carcinoma
pizza lung
plus
PMDD (premenstrual dysphoric disorder)
Pneumocystis carinii pneumonia (PCP)
Pneumocystis choroidopathy
pneumoparotitis
polly-beak nasal deformity

disease *(cont.)*
polymorphous light eruption
Pompe glycogen storage disease, type II
portal hypertensive gastropathy (PHG)
postprandial lipemia
poststernotomy mediastinitis (PSM)
post-transplantation lymphoproliferative disorders (PTLD)
post-transplant diabetes mellitus (PTDM)
Pott puffy tumor
preinvasive urothelial neoplasia
premenstrual dysphoric disorder (PMDD)
primary biliary cirrhosis (PBC)
primary immune deficiency (PID)
primary pure teratoma
primary sclerosing cholangitis (PSC)
primary trimethylaminuria (fish-odor syndrome)
progressive multifocal leukoencephalopathy (PML)
progressive osseous heteroplasia
progressive parenchymal restriction
prolapsing redundant arytenoids
proud flesh
pseudodermachalasis
pseudo-Hurler deformity
pseudolaminar necrosis
pseudomembranous colitis (PMC)
pseudomyotonia
psoriatic onychopachydermoperiostitis
pulmonary alveolar proteinosis (PAP)
pulmonary sequestration
pyogenic granuloma
Q fever
quadriceps tendon rupture
Quervain
raccoon eyes
rachitic rosary

disease *(cont.)*
radiation-related optic neuropathy (RON)
reactive airways (RAD)
reactive perforating collagenosis (RPC)
rectal linitis plastica (RLP)
Rector-Gordon-Healey-Mendoza-Spitzer type IV renal tubular acidosis
recurrent respiratory papillomatosis (RRP)
Reese retinal telangiectasia
reflex sympathetic dystrophy (RSD)
Regnauld-type degeneration
Reis-Bückler corneal dystrophy
renal cell carcinoma (RCC)
repetitive strain injury (RSI)
retrobulbar neuritis
reversible obstructive airway (ROAD)
rhabdomyolysis
rhagades
rhinocerebral aspergillosis (RA)
Richter hernia
Riedel struma
rippling muscle
Roger
Rosai Dorfman
Roth-Bernhardt
rugger-jersey spine
sabre shin deformity
sacrococcygeal pilonidal sinus
sagging brain
salmon-patch hemorrhages
salon sink radiculopathy
sarcoglycanopathy
satellite lesion
scaphocephaly (sagittal synostosis)
Scheuermann
schizencephaly
schneiderian papilloma, inverted
Schönlein-Henoch purpura
scleroderma
scleroderma sine scleroderma

disease *(cont.)*
sclerosing encapsulating peritonitis
sebaceous miliaria
sedentary death syndrome (SeDS)
segmental mediolytic arteriopathy
sentinel bleed
sentinel clot
severe childhood autosomal recessive muscular dystrophy (SCARMD)
sexually transmitted (STD)
short-limb dwarfism
short-segment Barrett esophagus (SSBE)
silent
silent prostatism
Sinding Larsen–Johannson
single-stripe colitis (SSC)
sink-trap malformation
skier's tear
skip metastasis
Sly
small cell lung carcinoma (or cancer) (SCLC)
solar keratosis
spinal epidural hematoma
spondylodiskitis
spontaneous nipple discharge (SND)
squamous cell carcinoma (SCC)
Staphylococcus aureus septicemia
Stargardt dystrophy
Still
streptococcus A infection
stress-related mucosal (SRMD)
string phlebitis
subcortical atherosclerotic encephalopathy (SAE)
subcortical dementia
subependymal heterotopia
subepithelial hematoma of the renal pelvis
suberosis
syringolymphoid hyperplasia with alopecia and anhidrosis (SLHA)

disease *(cont.)*
systemic lupus erythematosus
talcosis
Takayasu arteritis
terrible triad of the shoulder
Terrien degeneration
thoracic splenosis
thromboembolic (TED)
thyrotoxicosis factitia
thyrotoxicosis medicamentosa
Tis
Tornwaldt bursitis
toxic colitis
transient aplastic crisis (TAC)
transitional cell carcinoma of the bladder (TCCB)
transient neonatal diabetes mellitus (TNDM)
trichinosis
trichosis
tularemia
tumoral calcinosis
typhlitis
upper airway dysfunction (UAD)
Van Bogaert
vascular Parkinson
vasomotor rhinitis
veno-occlusive (VOD)
vestibular adenitis
vestibulodynia
VHL (von Hippel-Lindau)
Vincent infection
vipoma endocrine tumor
vitreoretinopathy
Voerner
Vogt-Koyanagi-Harada
von Hippel-Lindau (VHL)
von Recklinghausen
wandering spleen
Warthin tumor
watermelon stomach
Wegener granulomatosis
Werdnig-Hoffmann
Wernicke
wet age-related macular degeneration (ARMD)

disease *(cont.)*
Wharton tumor
wheat weevil
Whipple
wood pulp worker's lung
Woringer-Kolopp
wreath pattern corneal infiltrates
xanthelasma
xanthogranulomatous cholecystitis
X-linked familial spastic paraparesis
X-linked severe combined immunodeficiency (X-SCID)

Disetronic Insulin Pen—does not use a prefilled cartridge but allows a diabetic patient to fill the insulin reservoir with economical vial insulin.

DISH (diffuse idiopathic skeletal hyperostosis).

disk, disc (Gr., diskos, L., discus)—a circular or rounded flat plate. Note: *Disk* appears to be the preferred spelling, although *disc* is also used, especially in names of anatomic structures.

Disk-Criminator—used to check localization of stimuli.

disk diameter (dd or DD)—1.5 mm (the diameter of the optic nerve head); used in measuring the size of a fundal lesion or in describing its location. Also, *disc diameter.*

diskectomy
APLD (automated percutaneous lumbar)
SMALL (same-day microsurgical arthroscopic lateral-approach laser-assisted) fluoroscopic

diskectomy with Cloward fusion.

disorder—see *disease*.

disposable aortic rotating punch—used in cardiovascular bypass surgery. It has a patented rotating blade and is said to have unique cutting action.

disproportion—see *cephalopelvic.*

dissecans—see *osteochondritis.*

dissection, dissector (see also *device*)
blunt
Cavitron
Clearglide optical vessel
Creed
Desmarres corneal
Devers
Dingman breast
Falcao suction
finger
Kitner
Küttner blunt
Neivert
Nezhat-Dorsey Trumpet Valve hydrodissector
Pearce nucleus hydrodissector
Rhoton
sharp and blunt
spontaneous coronary artery (SCAD)
spud
Trumpet Valve

Dissectron—ultrasonic neurosurgical aspirator console and a broad line of related hand pieces.

disseminated intravascular coagulation (DIC)—results from imbalance between the mechanisms of coagulation and of fibrinolysis. Can be induced by infection (meningococcal meningitis, Rocky Mountain spotted fever, septicemia), trauma, shock, complications of pregnancy and parturition, and myelocytic leukemia. Clinical manifestations range from widespread bleeding to widespread intravascular thrombosis, and both of these may occur together.

disseminated lupus erythematosus *(not* erythematosis)—see *systemic lupus erythematosus.*

dissociated vertical divergence (DVD).

Distaflo bypass graft—used an alternative to vein cuffs and patches when

Distaflo *(cont.)* adequate autologous saphenous vein is not available.

distal articular set angle (DASA).

distal tibial osteotomy—pediatric and adult foot and ankle surgery.

distention—the state of being expanded, stretched. Also, *distension.*

distortion product otoacoustic emission (DPOAE)—used in studies of comparative hearing.

distraction laminoplasty—decompression of the lumbar spinal canal with maximal bone preservation. The technique involves the application of a distraction force in conjunction with an undercutting laminoplasty technique.

distraction osteogenesis surgery—performed on children with facial deformities caused by congenital problems such as hemifacial microsomia. Suitable patients are identified after evaluation of breathing, bone structure, and soft tissues of the face. Also, bone-lengthening technique such as the Ilizarov procedure. See *callotasis distraction.*

Diva laparoscopic morcellator—used in SMART (surgical myomectomy as reproductive therapy) procedures to remove uterine fibroids.

divergence (Genetics)—a variation between DNA sequences in two related genes, or in the resulting amino acid sequences in coded proteins, due to mutation.

diverticulum of Kommerell, normal variant—a diverticulum of the aorta, named for Dr. Burckhard Kommerell.

Dix-Hallpike position (ENT)—for Epley canalith repositioning.

Dix-Hallpike test—for paroxysmal positional nystagmus.

dizygotic twins—fraternal twins, produced by two oocytes, each of which is fertilized by a distinct sperm.

DJD (degenerative joint disease).

DJJ (duodenojejunal junction).

DKA (diabetes ketoacidosis).

DLCO (diffusing capacity of the lung for CO) (carbon monoxide).

DLEK—see *deep lamellar endothelial keratoplasty.*

DLK—see *deep lamellar keratoplasty.*

DLP elongated one-piece arterial cannulae (EOPA).

DLT (double lung transplant) **recipient**.

DMA (digital movement analysis).

DMARDs (disease-modifying antirheumatic drugs)—thought to slow down the basic destructive rheumatoid arthritis process, e.g., oral or injectable gold, methotrexate, azathioprine, Cytoxan (cyclophosphamide), Plaquenil (hydroxychloroquine).

DMAST (Dyna Med anti-shock trousers)—an antishock garment that is noninflatable, has no tubes or valves, and has no risk of puncture. Used by NASA, the military, and paramedics. See also *MAST.*

DME (diabetic macular edema).

DME (drug metabolizing enzyme).

DMI (Dilamezinsert).

DMR (direct myocardial revascularization)—a minimally invasive cardiac catheterization procedure using laser technology to revascularize ischemic heart muscle.

DMVA (direct mechanical ventricular actuation)—ventricular assist device that can begin biventricular support in as little as three minutes, because insertion is technically easy. There is no need for systemic anticoagulation as it has no cannulas in any blood vessels. It is said to decrease the need for drug support for a failing

DMVA *(cont.)* heart, provide prolonged circulatory support without cardiac trauma, and increase cardiac output. Currently DMVA is used as a temporary measure to sustain patients whose hearts fail while they wait for a suitable donor heart for heart transplantation.

DNA (deoxyribonucleic acid)—the genetic material of all cellular organisms, contained chiefly in the nucleus and forming the chromosomes. It is a polymer (long chain of repeating units) in which molecules of deoxyribose (a five-carbon sugar) are linked by phosphate bonds and carry side-chains of adenine, guanine, cytosine, and thymine. These four substances (the first two purines and the second two pyrimidines) carry the genetic blueprint for the synthesis and arrangement of all the substances and structures in the body.

DNA histogram—in which individual cell nuclei are visualized in the context of their relationship and position. It can reveal tumor types and patterns that may be useful in cancer diagnosis and treatment.

DNA ploidy analysis—a test on biopsy tissue of the prostate that correlates well with the Gleason score for severity of cancer. The test may help physicians and patients make more informed decisions about whether radical prostatectomy should be performed.

DNA polymerase-alpha—a tumor marker. When found in frozen tissue sections of patients who have had an exploratory thoracotomy for early non-small cell lung carcinoma, the presence of this marker can be used to indicate those patients who will most likely suffer an early relapse of the disease and a poorer prognosis.

DNA sequencing—method of genetic testing that identifies mutations not found by other methods.

DNOAP (diabetic-neuropathic osteoarthropathy).

DNS (dysplastic nevus syndrome)—can lead to malignant melanoma.

Dobbhoff gastrectomy feeding tube.

DOBI (dynamic optical breast imaging system)—uses dynamic functional imaging to detect angiogenesis associated with growth of malignant lesions and is designed to offer a noninvasive and pain-free method to distinguish between malignant and benign breast lesions.

dobutamine stress echocardiography (DSE).

Docke murmur—diastolic murmur associated with stenosis of left anterior descending artery of the coronary distribution.

Doc-U-Dose—multidose packaging and prescription management system.

Döderlein bacillus—a strain of lactobacillus normally seen in the vagina. It is considered a benign bacterium and maintains the normal acid pH of the vagina. Also, Doederlein.

Döderlein laparoscopic hysterectomy—vaginal hysterectomy combined with laparoscopic technique to dissect uterus and adnexa and develop bladder flap. Can be used for patients with adhesions or previous cesarean sections, who might not otherwise be candidates for vaginal hysterectomy. Also, Doederlein.

Dodick laser photolysis system—uses an Nd:YAG laser for cataract removal.

dog-boning—a surgical complication caused when an angioplasty balloon

dog-boning *(cont.)* becomes excessively expanded at either end of a stent (similar in appearance to a dog bone).

dog-ear, dog-eared (noun, adj.)—a deformity that occurs in closing a wound or incision, as dictated in plastic surgery reports. Usage: "The patient had a rather irregular closure with dog-ears on both sides and poor contour of the abdominal flaps."

Dohlman endoscopic repair of Zenker diverticulum—procedure in which the diverticulum is exposed with a bivalved endoscope with one blade in the pouch and the other blade in the cervical esophagus. Under direct visualization, the common wall between the pouch and the esophagus is ablated, usually with a CO_2 laser.

Dohlman plug—used to treat perforated corneal ulcers.

dolichocephalic—long head.

DoLi S—extracorporeal shock wave lithotriptor by Dornier.

doll's eye sign—dissociation between movements of the eyes and those of the head. A positive sign indicates damage to cranial nerves III, IV, and VI.

domain—(1) a region of the amino acid sequence of a protein, or the corresponding segment of a gene, that can be equated with a particular function; (2) an English word meaning territory, used in a medical context as follows: "The abdominal domain accommodated the small and large bowel."

Dome Wand—provides increased contact with curved tissues. Also used for front and side ablations, for anterior cruciate ligament notchplasty, and in certain cases of shoulder surgery to resect Bankart lesions.

dominant (Genetics)—said of a gene whose expression is the same in heterozygotes (individuals with only one copy of the gene) as in homozygotes (individuals with two copies of the gene).

domino connectors—descriptive term for connectors on a spinal instrumentation device used to correct scoliosis.

DonJoy GoldPoint knee brace.

DonJoy IROM brace.

DonJoy knee splint. Usage: "A dry sterile dressing was then applied, followed by a DonJoy splint holding the knee out in extension."

donor island harvesting—a method of obtaining micro- and minigrafts from a hairbearing strip.

donor-recipient plug exchange—switching osteochondral plugs from damaged and healthy condyles; that is, the plug from the healthy condyle (usually the posterior) is placed in a hole created by removing a plug from the damaged condyle, that plug being placed in the hole left by removing the donor plug.

donor-specific transfusion (DST).

"doops"—phonetic for *dupes*, slang for *duplicates*.

DOOR syndrome—inherited disorder characterized by hearing impairment, malformations of the nails and certain bones, mental retardation, and other abnormalities. DOOR is an acronym for the characteristic abnormalities associated with the disorder: **d**eafness, **o**nychodystrophy, **o**steodystrophy, and mild to severe mental **r**etardation.

Doppler echocardiography—useful for assessment of left ventricular dias-

Doppler *(cont.)*
tolic function in ischemic heart disease.

Doppler-guided hemorrhoidal artery ligation (DGHAL).

Doppler instruments
blood flow detector
fetal heart monitor
IntraDop intraoperative
intraoperative
ultrasonic blood flow detector
ultrasonic fetal heart monitor

Doppler perfusion index (DPI)—the ratio of hepatic artery to total liver blood flow. May be a prognostic indicator of early death in colorectal cancer patients who have undergone supposedly curative surgery.

Doppler sonography of the SMA (superior mesenteric artery)—noninvasive method to detect inflammatory disease of the small bowel.

Doppler tissue imaging (DTI) (Cardio)—used for transesophageal echocardiography (TEE) imaging on the V5M Multiplane and V510B Biplane TEE transducers. TEE imaging with DTI shows tissue motion with high resolution, which may enable cardiologists to differentiate normal versus ischemic or infarcted tissue; visualization and timing of contractile impulse; qualitative measurement of myocardial wall velocity; quantification in M-mode for high temporal resolution and reduced subjectivity of wall motion analysis.

Doppler waveform analysis (Radiol)—noninvasive study of blood vessels. See *duplex ultrasound* and *ultrasound*.

Dopplette—a small Doppler monitor.

Doptone monitoring—of fetal heart tones.

Dorc surgical instruments.

Dorello canal—an opening in the temporal bone which is the point of entry of the sixth cranial nerve into the cavernous sinus.

Dorendorf sign—of aortic arch aneurysm, evidenced by fullness of supraclavicular groove.

doripenem—a medication for the treatment of urinary tract infections.

Dormia noose—a surgical device used for grasping. Usage: "The ligamentum teres hepatis was grasped with a Dormia noose and pulled up through the gastric tube to close the perforated ulcer." The Dormia noose can be left in place, secured with Kocher forceps for several days until closure is certain.

Dornier compact lithotriptor—a much smaller, less expensive, mobile, and user-friendly lithotriptor. Effective for treatment of kidney stones, with a low incidence of complications and adverse effects.

Dornier Epos Ultra—extracorporeal shock wave therapy for the treatment of plantar fasciitis.

Dor procedure—see *endoventricular circular patchplasty*.

Dorros—infusion and probing catheter.

dorsal (adj.)—referring to the back or to any posterior part or surface, e.g., the dorsal surface of the hand is the back of the hand. See *dorsum*.

dorsal column stimulator (DCS) (also *spinal cord stimulation*)—a controversial and risk-prone procedure for pain relief. It is said by some to be a procedure of last resort. One of the pioneers in percutaneous and transcutaneous electrical nerve stimulation no longer uses it, but other surgeons and anesthesiologists do.

dorsal lithotomy position *(not* dorsolithotomy).

dorsal penile nerve block (DPNB)—a technique to reduce behavioral stress and modify the adrenocortical stress response in neonates undergoing circumcision.

dorsum (noun)—back; posterior aspect. See *dorsal.*

dosimeter—a device worn continuously by a person whose occupation involves exposure to x-rays or other radiation, to monitor cumulative exposure. Also called a *film badge*.

Dos Santos needle—for aortography.

DOT (deodorized opium tincture)—a medication prescribed for pain.

DOT physical—Department of Transportation physical.

Dott-Dingman self-retaining cleft palate gag.

Dott mouth gag.

Dotter-Judkins PTA (percutaneous transluminal angioplasty)—involves dilatation of the lumen of a stenotic femoral artery in patients who are not good risks for femoral-popliteal bypass surgery. A special catheter is directed to the site of the atheromatous lesion under fluoroscopy, and then progressively larger catheters are introduced over a guidewire. See *PTA*.

double anterior horn sign—knee meniscal displacement. Can be seen with either medial or lateral bucket-handle tears or in association with double posterior cruciate ligament or fragment-in-notch signs.

double-armed suture—a suture with a needle at each end. See *suture.*

double-blind study—a study in which neither the patient nor the physician knows if the drug administered is a test medication or a placebo.

double bubble flushing reservoir—in patients with hydrocephalus.

double bubble sign—seen in infants with choledochal cysts and obstructive jaundice. Usage: "Plain films show the double bubble sign, with a large air bubble that represents the stomach; the second bubble represents air dilating the duodenum that is proximal to the point of blockage." Also, ultrasound appearance of a fetus with fluid-filled stomach and duodenum which, along with polyhydramnios, indicates duodenal atresia.

double contrast arthrography—used for evaluation of ligamentous injuries of the knee, but thought to be not as accurate as single-contrast arthrography or the newer arthroscopic techniques. With the double contrast technique, more time is available for air to enter the joint, causing misleading findings.

double contrast barium enema (Radiol)—a modification of the barium enema procedure. After the standard barium enema examination has been completed, the patient expels most of the barium, and the colon is then inflated with air. The coating of barium remaining on the surface may outline masses or defects not seen during the standard examination.

double dip—an upper and lower endoscopy performed together.

double dose delay (DDD)—contrast studies.

double helix—two DNA strands wound around each other and united by their base pairs (adenine with guanine, cytosine with thymine).

doubled semitendinosus and gracilis autograft (DST&G).

double exposure artifact (Radiol)—a darkroom error.

double exposure drift—MRI term.

double freeze-thaw sequence—term used to describe technique in percutaneous or laparoscopic cryotherapy for tumor ablation.

double halo sign—seen on CT scan of ulcerative colitis. It is characterized by an inner soft tissue density ring comprising the mucosa, lamina propria, and muscularis mucosae; a central low-density ring comprising the submucosa; and an outer soft tissue density ring comprising the muscularis propria and serosa. Also called *target sign*.

double helix acquisition—used in CT scanning.

Double J indwelling catheter stent—trademark, from Surgitek (Urol).

Double J ureteral stent (Urol).

double lung transplant (DLT) **recipient**.

double-orifice repair—a reliable and safe surgical correction of mitral regurgitation in Barlow disease. Another name for *Alfieri-plasty*.

double PCL (posterior cruciate ligament) **sign**—a low-signal-intensity band that is parallel and anteroinferior to the PCL on sagittal MR images and is a highly specific indicator of a bucket-handle meniscal tear.

double plate Molteno implant (Oph).

DoubleStent biliary endoprosthesis.

double stripe sign—see *parallel track sign*.

double-T pouch urinary diversion—a bladder augmentation technique for continent urinary diversion in adult patients. It is used when the appendix is unavailable.

double-twist knot (DTK) **technique**—an easy-to-tie sliding knot for arthroscopic repair of rotator cuff tears and glenoid labrum lesions. It is a modified lark's head knot that can be tied only on a double suture.

double umbrella device—used in closure of a patent ductus arteriosus.

double-wall sign (Radiol)—detection of free intraperitoneal air.

double whammy syndrome (Oph)—voluntary eye propulsion; the ability to voluntarily propel and retract one or both eyes.

Douek-MED Bioglass middle ear device—enables surgeons to reconstruct the ossicular chain, using a biocompatible, nonporous material that forms a physiochemical bond with soft tissue and bone.

douglasectomy—laparoscopic procedure for treatment of painful uterine retroversion which involves resection of the cul-de-sac of Douglas.

doula—an individual contracted to provide either labor or postpartum support for a pregnant woman. Doulas often work under the supervision of midwives but do not perform nursing jobs or deliveries.

Douvas roto-extractor (Oph).

dowager's hump—kyphosis due to osteoporosis of the spine.

Downey texture discrimination test.

downgoing toes—in a normal response to the Babinski test, the great toe curls downward when the sole of the foot is stroked; thus, a negative Babinski is a flexor plantar response: "The toes are downgoing." Cf. *upgoing*.

doxorubicin (epi-Adriamycin, epi-ADR, EPI)—a chemotherapy drug.

Doyle Shark nasal splint—maintains a patent nasal airway and prevents synechiae and postsurgical adhesions.

DPA (Designated Power of Attorney) for Health Care.

DPAP Stealth—a real-time interactive positive airway pressure device used for treatment of sleep apnea. It uses a flow-sensing and measurement device to monitor all air moving through the breathing circuit. It responds with a rapid increase in air pressure when a critical reduction is detected, as in sleep apnea. The device intermittently assists the breathing process and restores patency before oxyhemoglobin desaturation and/or arousal from sleep occurs.

DPI (Doppler perfusion index).

DPN (diabetic peripheral neuropathy).

DPOAE (distortion product otoacoustic emission).

DPPC (dipalmitoyl phosphatidylcholine) **test**—an accurate predictor of respiratory distress syndrome and fetal lung maturity. DPPC is the major surface-active component of the mature fetal lung surfactant.

D-Prevent—an electrical device for improving circulation and preventing DVT, pulmonary embolism, or other circulatory ailments.

DPTS (delayed pulmonary toxicity syndrome).

DPTTL—see *deep posterior talotibial ligament.*

Draeger high vacuum erysiphake (Oph).

Draeger tonometer—a handheld applanation tonometer; used to measure intraocular pressure.

drain
- Blair silicone
- Blake wound
- butterfly
- Chaffin-Pratt
- Clot Stop
- Davol
- endoscopic retrograde biliary (ERBD)

drain *(cont.)*
- J-Vac closed wound
- Molteno implant
- Nélaton rubber tube
- Penrose
- Quad-Lumen
- Relia-Vac
- Shirley wound
- Solcotrans closed vacuum-drainage
- Stryker
- Thora-Drain III three-bottle chest
- Thora-Klex chest

Drake clip—used in clipping intracranial aneurysms.

Drake-Willock automatic delivery system—used in peritoneal dialysis with Tenckhoff catheter.

DRAM (de-epithelialized rectus abdominis muscle) **graft**—a free flap that can be used in reconstruction in patients with cranial-dural defects.

Draw-a-Bicycle test—a mental status examination. Also, *DAB test.*

Draw-a-Flower test—a mental status examination. Also, *DAF test.*

Draw-a-House test—a mental status examination. Also, *DAH test.*

Draw-a-Person test—a mental status examination. Also, *DAP test.*

drawer sign—in testing for ligamentous instability or for rupture of the cruciate ligaments of the knee.

drawn ankle clonus.

DRC (dynamic range control) **algorithm**—see *dynamic range control algorithm.*

DRD (dopa-responsive dystonia).

DRE (digital rectal examination).

DRESS—see *drug reaction with eosinophilia and systemic symptoms.*

dressing (see also *adhesive; bandage)*
- AcryDerm border island
- AcryDerm Strands absorbent wound
- Acticoat silver-based burn

dressing *(cont.)*

Actisorb silver
Acu-Derm I.V./TPN
AlgiDERM alginate wound
Algidex wound
alginate wound
AlgiSite alginate wound
Algosteril alginate wound
Allevyn
Aquacel Ag Hydrofiber wound packing
Aquacel Ag wound
Aquaphor gauze
Aquasorb transparent hydrogel
Arglaes antimicrobial barrier film
Arglaes powder
ArtAssist
artificial burr (Velcro analog)
Bactigras
barrier
Biafine WDE (wound dressing emulsion)
Biobrane adhesive
Bioclusive transparent
Biopatch foam wound
BreakAway absorptive wound
BlisterFilm transparent
brown sugar, or sugar, wound packing
CarboFlex wound
Carra Film adhesive film
CarraSmart foam
Carra Sorb H
Carra Sorb M
Carrasyn hydrogel wound
Chinese fingertrap
CircPlus compression
ClearSite Hydro Gauze
ClearSite transparent wound
Clo-Sur P.A.D.
Coban
CollaCote
collagen hemostatic material
CollaPlug
CollaTape

dressing *(cont.)*

collodion
CombiDerm absorbent cover
CombiDerm hydrocolloid
Comfeel Ulcus
composite
Conformant contact-layer wound
contact-layer wound
Contreet
Covaderm composite wound
Coverlet adhesive surgical
Cover-Roll adhesive gauze
Cover-Strip wound closure strips
Cryo/Cuff ankle
Curaderm
Curafil
Curafoam
Curagel hydrogel
Curasol
Curasorb calcium alginate
Cutinova Cavity
Cutinova Hydro
Deknatel (Shur-Strip)
Dermacea alginate wound
Derma-Gel hydrogel sheet
Dermagraft-TC
Dermagran hydrogel
DermaMend hydrogel
Dermanet contact-layer wound
DermAssist glycerin hydrogel
DermAssist hydrocolloid
Dermatell hydrocolloid
DeWrap three-layer compression
DiaB Gel hydrogel
DiaB Klenz wound cleaners
DuoDerm compression
DuoDerm hydroactive gel for wound hydration
Dyna-Flex compression
Elastikon elastic tape
Elasto-Gel hydrogel
Elastomull
elta (trademarked) dermal hydrogel
EpiFilm otologic lamina
Epi-Lock polyurethane foam wound

dressing *(cont.)*
ExuDerm hydrocolloid
Exu-Dry absorptive
Fibracol collagen-alginate
Fibracol collagen hemostatic wound
Flexderm hydrogel sheet
Flexzan foam wound
foam
Fuller shield
FyBron alginate wound
Gelocast Unna boot compression
Gentell alginate wound
Gentell foam wound
Glasscock
GraftCyte gauze wound
Graftskin
Handages
Humatrix Microclysmic Gel
hyCURE collagen hemostatic wound
hyCURE G hydrogel
Hydrasorb foam wound
Hydrasorb Plus
Hydrocol hydrocolloid
hydrocolloid
Hydrofiber
hydrogel gel
hydrophilic semipermeable absorbent polyurethane foam
Hypergel
Iamin Gel wound
Iamin hydrogel
Inerpan
Intelligent Dressing
IntraSite gel
Iodoflex absorptive
Iodosorb absorptive
IPM Wound Gel
Isovis wound protector
island wound
jaw bra compressive
Kalginate alginate wound
Kaltostat wound packing
Kling adhesive
Kling fluff rolls and sponges

dressing *(cont.)*
Kollagen
Lakeside cotton
Lapwall
Liquiderm liquid healing bandage
Lyofoam C
Lyofoam tracheostomy
marshmallows
Maxorb alginate wound
Medifil collagen hemostatic wound
Medipore Dress-it
Mepitel contact-layer wound
Mepore absorptive
MeroGel nasal
Mesalt
Mesalt impregnated absorbent
Mitraflex foam wound
Mitraflex multilayer wound
MPM hydrogel
Multidex wound filling material
MultiPad absorptive
Normigel hydrogel
N-Terface contact-layer wound
Nu-Derm hydrocolloid
Nu Gauze
Nu-Gel hydrogel
Oasis wound dressing
O'Donoghue
Omiderm transparent adhesive film
OpSite Flexigrid transparent adhesive film
OrCel bilayered cellular matrix
OsmoCyte pillow
Oxiplex
PanoGauze hydrogel-impregnated gauze
PanoPlex hydrogel
Polyderm foam wound
PolyMem foam wound
Polyskin II
PolyWic wound filling
Primapore absorptive wound
Primer compression
Pro-Clude transparent adhesive film
ProCyte transparent adhesive film

dressing *(cont.)*
Profore four-layer bandage system
Promogran (oxidized regenerated cellulose and collagen)
PuraPly wound
Quinaband
RepliCare hydrocolloid
Repliderm
Reston foam wound
Restore alginate wound
SAF-Gel hydrogel
SeaSorb alginate wound
Seprafilm tissue barrier
Shur-Strip (Deknatel)
SignaDress hydrocolloid
Silon wound
Silverlon wound packing strips
SiteGuard MVP transparent adhesive film
SkinTegrity hydrogel
Sofsorb absorptive
SoftCloth absorptive
Soft N Dry Merocel
Sof-Wick
SoloSite hydrogel
SoloSite wound gel
Soothies
SorbaView composite wound
Sorbsan topical wound
SpyroDerm
Stratasorb composite wound
Sure-Closure
SurePress compression
Suresite transparent adhesive film
Suture Strip Plus
Synthaderm
TAB (tumescent absorbent bandage)
Tegaderm transparent
Tegagel hydrogel
Tegagen HG alginate wound
Tegagen HI alginate wound
Tegapore contact-layer wound
Tegasorb
Thera-Boot compression

dressing *(cont.)*
THINSite with Biofilm
3M Clean Seals
Tielle absorptive
Transeal transparent adhesive film
TransiGel hydrogel-impregnated gauze
Transorbent
transparent adhesive film
TubeLok tracheotomy
tumescent absorbent bandage (TAB)
Ultec hydrocolloid
Uniflex polyurethane adhesive surgical
Unna-Flex compression
Unna-Pak compression
Vari/moist
Veingard
Velpeau
Ventex
Viasorb
Vigilon
wet-to-dry
Woun'Dres hydrogel
WoundSpan Bridge II
Xeroform
Zipzoc stocking compression

DREZ (dorsal root entry zone) **lesion** (Neuro).

DREZ-otomy—a surgical procedure to treat spasticity and pain in the lower limbs.

DRF (differential renal function)—on MR urography.

DRF (digestive-respiratory fistula).

DRGs (Diagnostic Relative Groups) (hospital coding).

Drionic electrical iontophoresis device—for hyperhidrosis.

drip infusion cholangiography (DIC)—not to be confused with diffuse intravascular coagulopathy.

Dripps-American Surgical Association score—a clinical scoring system to predict cardiac morbidity.

drip test and suction test—used during laparoscopic procedures. In lieu of absorbent sponges or packs to absorb or remove blood from the surgical field, the laparoscopic surgeon depends on a flow of heparinized saline. Introduced into the surgical field, this flushes away blood and prevents clotting in nooks and crannies and on instruments. The saline is continuously removed from the site by the suction apparatus. Although the saline infusion is commonly referred to as a "drip," the equipment involved is much more sophisticated than an IV drip. The saline is heated and delivered under pressure (hence more of a squirt), and the flow may be pulsed to dislodge clots. The "drip" equipment as well as the suction apparatus must be checked for proper function before surgery.

driveline infection—can occur in patients on left ventricular assist device for extended period of time.

drooping shoulder sign—x-ray finding diagnostic of inferior subluxation of the shoulder. It occurs following fracture of the surgical neck and may be secondary to hemarthrosis or musculoligamentous injury.

drop attacks—episodes of dropping objects but remaining conscious; a form of petit mal epilepsy. Also may be experienced by narcoleptics who have sudden brief periods of unconsciousness.

droplet spread—transmission of respiratory and other infections by fine mists of respiratory secretions expelled into the air by coughing or sneezing.

DRS (Dementia Rating Scale).

DR-70 tumor marker test—for detecting lung cancer tumors and quantifying levels of tumor marker in patients. The DR-70 is a noninvasive procedure compared to other cancer detection methods such as biopsies. It is a biochemical probe that has shown early indications of being one of the most sensitive tumor marker tests in current use. The test is based on the detection of submicroscopic ring-shaped particles (RSP) that appear to be shed in detectable quantities by malignant cells, both in the lab and in the human body.

drug categories or classifications
- ACE (angiotensin-converting enzyme) inhibitors
- agonists
- allylamines
- alpha$_1$-proteinase inhibitor
- aminobiphosphonates
- aminoglycosides
- aminosterols
- anabolic steroids
- antagonists
- anthracenediones
- antiestrogen
- anti-TNF (tumor necrosis factor)
- antitussives
- anxiolytics
- arylcyclohexylamines
- bacteriostatics
- benzodiazepines
- beta antagonist
- beta blocker
- butyrylcholinesterase inhibitors
- calcium channel blockers
- carbacephems
- cephalosporins
- COX-2 inhibitors
- dibenzodiazepines
- DMARDs (disease-modifying antirheumatic drugs)
- fusion inhibitors

drug *(cont.)*
H_2 blockers
hERG blocker
HIS fusion inhibitors
imidazotetrazines
immunoliposomes
matrix metalloprotease inhibitor (MMPI)
MSTRs (multiple signal transduction regulators)
oligozymes
oxazolidinones
PDE4 (phosphodiesterase 4) inhibitor
prokinetic agent
pyranocarboxylic acid
SAANDs (selective apoptotic antineoplastic drugs)
SAARD (slow-acting antirheumatic drug)
selective estrogen receptor modulator (SERM)
SERM (selective estrogen receptor modulator)
serotonin type-3 receptor antagonists
slow-channel blocking drugs
statin drugs
superparamagnetic iron oxide (SPIO) class of imaging agents
TAT (thrombin-antithrombin III complex) inhibitor
thiazolidinediones (TZDs)
USPIO (ultrasmall superparamagnetic iron oxide)

drug-eluting stent (DES)—a vascular stent used in the treatment of occlusive vascular disease (atherosclerosis). The stent is coated with a time-release drug intended to slow down restenosis and allow the vessel to heal.

drug-induced lupus erythematosus (DILE).

drug metabolizing enzyme (DME)—human enzyme that helps to metabolize drugs within the body. Individual responses to drugs are affected by genes, and some people may have a hidden genetic "glitch" in which a drug dose deemed safe in most people is metabolized so slowly as to be fatal.

drug reaction with eosinophilia and systemic symptoms (DRESS)—also known as *hypersensitivity syndrome*. It has a mortality rate of about 10%.

DRUJ (distal radioulnar joint) **prosthesis**—for painful radioulnar joint instability after failure of Kapandji-Sauve or Moore-Darrach procedure.

drusen—small hyaline globular pathological growths formed on Bruch membrane.

dry age-related macular degeneration (Oph)—breakdown or thinning of retinal pigment epithelial cells, leading to atrophy of these light-sensitive, photoreceptor cells.

dry eye—keratoconjunctivitis sicca. See *Schirmer test*.

dry heaves—gagging or retching without emesis.

Dryvax (smallpox vaccine, dried, calf lymph type).

DS (duplex sonography).

DSA (digital subtraction angiography).

DSE (dobutamine stress echocardiography).

DSM (degradable starch microspheres).

DSM-IV-TR—Diagnostic and Statistics Manual, Fourth Edition, Text Revision (mental health).

DSP (digital signal processing).

DSP Micro Diamond-Point microsurgery instruments.

DSRCT (desmoplastic small round-cell tumor).

DST (donor-specific transfusion)—used before kidney transplantation, to

DST *(cont.)*
identify any possible incompatibility between donor and recipient and thus possibly prevent rejection of a transplant.

DST&G (doubled semitendinosus and gracilis) **autograft**—a technique for anterior cruciate ligament (ACL) reconstruction in which the ACL autograft consists of the semitendinosus and gracilis tendons. Both tendons are dissected, placed side by side, sutured together, and then folded, using a weaving Krackow-type stitch of Tycron. One end of the doubled tendons is attached to a screw in the femur, the other end to a screw in the tibia.

D-Tach removable needle—separates from the suture with a slight pull, but does resist inadvertent removal of the needle, which makes for faster interrupted suturing. See *pop-off needle*.

DTAFA (descending thoracic aorta-to-femoral artery) **bypass graft**—used for treatment of aortoiliac disease when opening the abdomen is contraindicated or ill advised.

DTG (diffuse toxic goiter).

DTI (Doppler tissue imaging).

DTICH (delayed traumatic intracerebral hematoma)—a frequent complication following closed head trauma. The patient is relatively asymptomatic after the head injury for several hours to several days, but then suddenly presents with a neurological deficit. A CT scan is diagnostic, revealing either the presence of a new intracranial hematoma or enlargement of an existing one. Proposed causes of DTICH include poor clotting as shown by the prolonged PT and PTT noted in head-injury patients or local cerebral ischemia which leads to necrosis and blood vessel rupture.

D-stix—slang for Dextrostix.

DTK (double-twist knot).

DT-MRI (diffusion tensor magnetic resonance imaging).

DTU-one Ultrasure—see *UltraSure DTU-one imaging system*.

DU (duplex ultrasound).

Dua antireflux stent—named for Dr. Dua.

Duac (clindamycin and benzoyl peroxide)—a topical drug used for the treatment of inflammatory acne vulgaris.

dual chamber Medtronic.Kappa 400 pacemaker (yes, a period between Medtronic and Kappa).

dual chamber pacemaker (Cardio).

dual energy x-ray absorptiometry (DEXA).

Dualer Plus—system for documenting range of motion and completing AMA impairment ratings for spine and extremities.

Dualine digital hearing instrument—uses digital signal processing (DSP) and a digital loudness control.

DualMesh—a biomaterial by Gore-Tex, used for repair of hernias and soft tissue deficiencies to permit a secure closure.

dual mesh gastroplasty banding technique—see *banding of Molina*.

dual photon densitometry—test recommended for diagnosis of osteoporosis through comparative height measurements. Loss of height means the patient is losing trabecular bone and should undergo further testing for osteoporosis.

dual switch valve (DSV)—a valve for shunting hydrocephalus that avoids overdrainage-related problems such

dual *(cont.)*
as subdural hygromas/hematomas or slit-like ventricles with the high risk of proximal catheter obstruction.

Duane retraction syndrome—a congenital, usually unilateral, disorder of eye movement, affecting females more often than males. The affected eye usually has complete absence of abduction, and partial absence of adduction (sometimes the reverse). The involved eye retracts into the orbit on adduction, and demonstrates pseudoptosis. There is also paresis or failure of convergence. Also known as *Stilling-Türk-Duane syndrome.*

Dubecq-Princeteau angulating needle holder—a 5 mm needle holder indicated for use in laparoscopic procedures.

Dubin and Amelar varicocele.

Dubowitz scale for infant maturity—a 24-hour test to correlate the neurological function with fetal gestational age. Usage: "The infant was 38 weeks' gestational age by Dubowitz."

duck—hospital slang for male urinal.

duck waddle—a test of the integrity of the knee joints and menisci, in which the patient is required to "walk" in a squatting position.

Ducor tip—a blend of two polyurethane materials, used as a catheter tip in coronary arteriography. It is said to be softer than the "standard" multipurpose catheter tip.

Ducrey bacillus—see *Haemophilus ducreyi.*

ductal carcinoma in situ (DCIS).

duct ectasia—an inflammatory lesion that possibly accounts for 1% of all operative breast lesions. Also called *plasma cell mastitis*. See also *granulomatous mastitis.*

ductions—monocular rotations (with the other eye covered):
abduction—outward rotation
adduction—inward rotation
infraduction—downward movement
supraduction—upward movement

ductions and versions (Oph).

Duecollement maneuver—in hemicolectomy.

Duette—collective trade name for catheters, probes, and baskets used in endoscopic retrograde cholangiopancreatography. Each instrument has a double lumen (hence the name) to facilitate multiple procedures: insertion of guidewires and other instruments as well as injections of drugs.

Duet vascular sealing device—used to seal the arterial access site following catheterization procedures such as angiography, angioplasty, and stenting.

Duffy blood antibody type—factor in agglutination. See also *Kell, Kidd, Lewis, Lutheran.*

Duhamel pull-through procedure—for correction of Hirschsprung disease. It involves excision of the aganglionic segment of the proximal colon and anastomosis between the normal remaining bowel and the posterior wall of the healthy segment of the rectum. Also, Duhamel laparoscopic pull-through anastomosis. Cf. *Lester Martin modification of Duhamel procedure.*

Duke bleeding time—the number of minutes it takes for a small incision in the skin (by puncture of the earlobe), made with a lancet, to stop bleeding.

Duke pouch—for continent urinary diversion. A resected segment of colon is used to form the pouch.

Dukes-Astler-Coller adenocarcinoma classification—uses letters and arabic numbers (A1, B1, etc.). See *Dukes classification*.

Dukes classification of carcinoma, named for Cuthbert E. Dukes, a British pathologist. Classes:
A invading mucosa and submucosa
B invading muscularis
C spread to regional lymph nodes; distant metastasis

Duke treadmill exercise score—of prognostic value in patients with suspected coronary artery disease.

Dulaney intraocular implant lens.

dullness—see *shifting dullness.*

dumbbell-shaped shadow (Radiol).

dumbbell tumor—a tumor that penetrates two nearby anatomic structures with a narrow bridge in between.

Dumon tracheobronchial stent.

dumping syndrome—symptoms of palpitations, sweating, and weakness, sometimes seen after gastrectomy and gastric bypass, and caused by rapid emptying of gastric contents into the small intestine (hence "dumping").

dunk, dunked—medical jargon for the inversion of the appendiceal stump before tying the pursestring suture. Usage: "A 2-0 silk pursestring suture was then placed around the stump of the appendix, and the appendiceal stump was dunked."

Dunlop synoptophore test—for eye vergence.

duodenal bulb (Radiol)—onion-shaped dilatation of the duodenum immediately below its origin at the pylorus.

duodenal C-loop (Radiol)—C-shaped loop of the duodenum as it courses around the head of the pancreas.

duodenal seromyectomy—a partial denudation procedure to clear the duodenum of metastatic tumor. "Right hemicolectomy and seromyectomy of the duodenum at the site of adhesion was performed in this patient with Dukes class C primary adenocarcinoma of the ascending colon adherent to the duodenum."

duodenal sweep (Radiol)—the normal course of the duodenum, from the pylorus and around the head of the pancreas to the ligament of Treitz, as visualized with contrast medium in an upper GI series.

duodenal switch—a procedure for pancreaticobiliary diversion that eliminates the need for the antrectomy and vagotomy that is done with a Roux-en-Y gastrojejunostomy.

duodenal ulcer perforation (DUP).

duodenojejunal junction (DJJ).

duodenum deformed by scarring.

DuoDerm dressing—a wound dressing used in treatment of leg ulcers, pressure sores, and superficial wounds. Also, *DuoDerm CGF* (control gel formula) *dressing*.

DuoDerm hydroactive gel for wound hydration.

Duodopa (levodopa/carbidopa)—liquid drug for intraduodenal infusion. It is used for the treatment of patients with late-stage Parkinson disease when treatment with conventional oral levodopa is difficult.

DUP (duodenal ulcer perforation).

dupe(s)—slang for *duplicate(s)*.

DUPEL—iontophoretic drug delivery system allowing for simultaneous treatment at two sites, thus cutting treatment time in half.

Du Pen long-term epidural catheter—used for long-term access to the epidural space for the delivery of preservative-free morphine sulfate to relieve intractable pain in cancer patients.

duplex pulsed-Doppler sonography.

duplex ultrasound—simultaneous high resolution real-time sonography and Doppler color spectral analysis. Used to diagnose a variety of conditions, including deep venous thrombosis. Shows areas of blood flow in color contrast on a video screen to demonstrate movement of blood. Since sonography does not require use of contrast media, it is less painful, less expensive, and quicker than contrast studies such as venograms. Individuals allergic to certain contrast media are thus spared allergic reactions. See also *Doppler* and *ultrasound*.

duplication (Genetics)—the formation or presence of two identical segments of a chromosome.

Dupont distal humeral plate.

Duracon total knee system.

DuraGen—an absorbable dural graft matrix used as a dura substitute for repair of the dura mater in spinal and cranial surgical procedures. It is used for the closure of the dural membrane that covers the brain and spinal cord.

DuraGen dural graft matrix—a collagen matrix for dural closure or dural onlay patch graft. Do not confuse with the possibly spurious or foreign estradiol brand Duragen-20.

DuraGlide3 stone balloon—single-use triple-lumen balloon catheter for removal of biliary stones from the common bile duct.

Dura-Guard patch—processed sterile animal tissues for use as surgical implants.

Dura-Kold wrap—reusable ice wrap for postoperative and rehabilitation cold therapy.

dural arteriovenous fistula (DAVF).

dural tail sign (Radiol)—seen on contrast-enhanced T1 weighted MR images as a thickening of the dura mater that resembles a tail extending from a mass; a sign of meningioma.

Duran AnCore anuloplasty system—for mitral and tricuspid repair.

Duraphase prosthesis—inflatable penile prosthesis.

Durapatite graft.

Durapore—easy to tear but strong surgical tape.

DuraPrep surgical solution—an iodophor scrub.

DuraScreen—a waterproof, long-lasting sunscreen.

Durasphere—an injectable bulking agent for the treatment of stress urinary incontinence due to intrinsic sphincter deficiency. It is injected under the mucosal lining of the bladder neck and urethra, expands, and then closes the bladder neck.

Durasul—highly wear-resistant polyethylene material used in Sulzer Natural-Knee implants.

Durasul large diameter head system—for orthopedic hip implant applications.

Durathane cardiac device.

Dura-II positional penile prosthesis.

DuraView OL-1 flexible nasopharyngoscope—for endoscopic visualization in nasopharyngeal procedures.

Duret hemorrhage—blood effusion in the brain stem due to herniation.

Durie and Salmon—classification of multiple myeloma in three stages.

Durkan CTS (carpal tunnel syndrome) **gauge**—a positive screening test for carpal tunnel syndrome.

dusky, duskiness—a bluish skin color from cyanosis.

Duval disposable dermatome.

Duval distal (caudal) **pancreaticojejunostomy**—a drainage technique that was used more in the past than at present. The term may be encountered in a patient's past history.

Duval lung-grasping clamp.

DuVries hammer toe repair.

DVA (dynamic visual acuity).

DVD (dissociated vertical divergence) —when the eyes do not move together and the deviating eye tends to move up and out.

DVI (deep venous insufficiency)—see *Hunter tendon rod*.

DVI (digital vascular imaging).

DVIU (direct vision internal urethrotomy).

DVP (draining vein pressure).

DVT (deep venous thrombosis).

dwell time—in radiology, the amount of time that the imaging device is focused on one area.

Dwyer correction of scoliosis—a procedure using an internal device of clips, screws, and a cable to straighten the spinal column. A clip is applied to each vertebra involved; a screw with a screw head that has a hole in it is screwed through a hole in the clip and into the bone. A braided titanium cable is run through the holes protruding from the screw heads and tightened (after grafts of cancellous iliac bone or pieces of rib bone have been placed between the vertebrae). Tension is then applied to the cable.

Dwyer osteotomy—calcaneal osteotomy as seen in ankle surgery.

DXR (delayed xenograft rejection).

dye exclusion test—measures bone marrow viability.

dye laser—a type of laser used to remove birthmarks such as port wine stains by pinpointing and vaporizing the abnormal blood vessels which cause these marks. No anesthesia is necessary, as the procedure is essentially painless. The yellow-orange dye inside the laser is sensitive to the color red, therefore zeroing-in on the blood vessels with light energy that turns into heat, thus vaporizing the vessels or skin tumors consisting of blood vessels. It cannot be used for correction of varicose veins.

Dyna-Flex compression dressing or wrap.

Dynaflex penile prosthesis—for male impotence.

Dynalink—self-expanding biliary stent system.

Dyna-Lok system—a plating system incorporating the advantages of both the rigid and semirigid system for spinal instrumentation.

Dyna Med anti-shock trousers (DMAST)—see *DMAST*.

dynamic compression plate (DCP) (Ortho). Usage: "When the reduction was considered satisfactory, DCPs were bent to conform with the patient's anatomy and secured in place with an assortment of cortical and cancellous screws."

dynamic computerized tomography—rapid sequential CT scanning after an intravenous bolus injection of contrast medium for detection of microadenomas that are isodense with surrounding tissues on conventional (delayed) CT scans.

dynamic conformal therapy—an irradiation technique focusing radiation precisely on malignancies, no matter how irregular the shape. This technique allows physicians to deliver more effective treatments with fewer side effects and minimizes radiation effects on healthy tissue

dynamic *(cont.)*
surrounding the tumors under treatment.

Dynamic Cooling Device (DCD)—reduces pain and trauma to patients during laser therapy by delivering a short burst of the cooling agent to the target area immediately prior to the laser treatment.

Dynamic Flotation—pressure control zone therapy for pressure sores.

dynamic graciloplasty—a technique for correcting fecal incontinence in which the gracilis muscle is wrapped around the anus to create a new sphincter. Several weeks later, a standard cardiac pacemaker is implanted in the lower abdomen and electrodes placed on the gracilis muscle. Continued stimulation of the muscle by the pacemaker actually changes the type of muscle fibers to ones which resist fatigue and can maintain a sustained contraction around the anus. When the patient needs to defecate, the pacemaker is temporarily turned off with an external magnet.

dynamic nasopharyngoscopy—diagnostic procedure for evaluation of obstructive sleep apnea.

dynamic optical breast imaging system (DOBI).

dynamic range control (DRC) **algorithm**—used in digital radiography. It has been shown to improve image quality and contrast in poorly penetrated regions of digital chest images.

dynamic spiral CT lung densitometry—used to differentiate air trapping from compensatory hyperinflation in children.

DynaPulse 5000A—ambulatory blood pressure monitor.

Dynasplint knee extension unit—a device that provides ongoing dynamic stress while patients are asleep or at rest.

Dynasplint shoulder system—applied for treatment of adhesive capsulitis (frozen shoulder).

DynaVox 2—an augmentative communication device that uses a wireless computer connection and software designed to aid nonverbal communication.

DynaWell—medical compression device used with MRI or CT to provide a more accurate diagnosis of spinal conditions by providing the weight and load of upright posture.

Dyonics disposable arthroscope blade.

Dyovac suction punch for arthroscopy.

dysconjugate gaze—see *disconjugate.*

dysfibrinogenemia—a condition in which there is abnormality of fibrinogen, an essential clotting factor.

dysfunctional *(not* dis-)—abnormality of function of an organ.

dysgeusia—persistent alteration in taste perception.

dyskaryosis—aberrant nuclear arrangement or structure; may be seen in malignancy or cell death. Cf. *dyskeratosis.*

dyskeratosis—aberrant keratin production and/or deposition. Cf. *dyskaryosis.*

dysmorphism—any developmental error resulting in an abnormal appearance or configuration.

dysphagia—difficulty in swallowing due to mechanical problems with the GI tract, esophageal infection or ulcers, or strokes. Cf. *dysphasia.*

dysphagia lusoria (from *lusus naturae,* freak of nature)—esophageal compression by anomalous right subcla-

dysphagia *(cont.)*
vian artery. An aberrant right subclavian artery is the most common aortic arch anomaly in adults.

dysphasia—impairment or loss of the power to use or understand speech; caused by disease of, or injury to, the brain. Cf. *dysphagia.*

dysplasia
acetabular
acromesomelic
Barlow hip
bronchopulmonary
cervical intraepithelial neoplasia (CIN)
congenital dysplasia of hip (CDH)
congenital glenoid
DALM (dysplasia-associated lesion or mass)
developmental dysplasia of hip (DDH)
fibromuscular (FMD)
high-grade (HGD)

dysplasia *(cont.)*
Holt-Oram atriodigital
hypohidrotic ectodermal (HED)
Kniest
low-grade (LGD)
Mondini
multilineage
refractory cytopenia with multilineage (RCMD)

dysplasia-associated lesion or mass (DALM)—detected by colonoscopy in patients with long-standing ulcerative colitis. A DALM is an indication for colectomy in a patient with high-grade dysplasia and malignancy.

dysprosody—change in the rhythm of speech due to neurologic or psychiatric disease. Cf. *hyperprosody.*

dysthymia—mood disorder. Usage: "Secondary to her disabling organic illness, she has developed a chronic dysthymia."

E, e

EAAT2 protein—a gene deficiency present in ALS (amyotrophic lateral sclerosis) (Lou Gehrig disease), due to aberrant ribonucleic acid which halts the production of this protein. A new test is being developed to detect this aberrant ribonucleic acid in the hopes of early detection of ALS.

EAC (expandable access catheter)—facilitates embolectomy and angioplasty procedures. In its collapsed state, the EAC is inserted into either the iliac, femoral, or popliteal artery. In its expanded state, the EAC lumen is wide enough so that an angioscope with either a Fogarty embolectomy catheter or an angioplasty balloon can be placed inside it.

Eagle-Barrett syndrome (prune-belly syndrome)—congenital absence of one or more layers of the abdominal wall musculature, often accompanied by other congenital anomalies.

Eagle equation—a scoring system used to predict cardiac morbidity.

Eagle straight-ahead arthroscope.

Eagle II survey spirometer.

Eagle Vision-Freeman punctum plug (Oph)—see *Freeman punctum plug*.

Eales disease—characterized by neovascularization and recurrent hemorrhage of retinal vessels. Seen principally in young men.

ear—may easily be confused with "air" when the dictator says "air-bone gap" in audiology (*never* "ear bone gap" or "airborne gap"). Cf. *ear oximeter*.

EarCheck Pro—an instrument that can detect the presence of middle ear effusion through acoustic reflectometry (sonar-like technology). It is reported to be comparable in accuracy to a tympanometer but does not require an airtight seal or pressurization of the ear canal.

Earle sign—a boggy swelling in the prostate; with urethral disruption following a pelvic injury, it could be associated with a pelvic fracture.

ear lobe crease (ELC)—diagonal ear lobe creases are associated, in a graded fashion, with higher rates of cardiac events in patients admitted to the hospital with suspected coronary disease.

EarlyBird study—a noninterventional prospective cohort study seeking to determine which children develop insulin resistance and why.

ear oximeter (*not* air)—a photoelectric device that is attached to the ear and measures oxygen saturation of the blood that passes through the ear. See *Hewlett-Packard ear oximeter*.

earring, Brent pressure—used to treat earlobe keloids.

Easi-Lav—a system for gastric lavage. Used in patients with upper GI bleeding, it delivers a greater volume of lavage in less time than standard methods.

"eastem"—see *e-stim*.

Eastern Cooperative Oncology Group (ECOG)—performance status in cancer patients.

EAST test (Vasc Surg)—an acronym for external rotation, abduction, stress test. With the hands/arms held straight up (as in a holdup), the hands are opened and closed. In a positive EAST test, the patient reproduces the symptoms for which medical care was sought.

eating cell (phagocyte).

EATL (enteropathy-associated T-cell lymphoma).

Eaton agent (*Mycoplasma pneumoniae*) —used thus in dictation: "primary atypical pneumonia, possibly due to the Eaton agent."

EBI bone healing system—noninvasive system for treating nonunion and failed arthrodesis with electromagnetic fields. (EBI, Electro Biology, Inc.).

EBIORT (electron beam intraoperative radiotherapy) **procedure**—bypasses the radiosensitive skin and the superficial structures, thus allowing radiation to be administered to the surgically exposed tumor.

EBI SPF-2 implantable bone stimulator.

EBL (endoscopic band ligation)—a procedure for treating bleeding esophageal varices, said to have fewer side effects than sclerotherapy. Also, *endoscopic variceal ligation* (EVL).

EBL (estimated blood loss)—estimated by measuring blood in the suction bottle and weighing the sponges that have soaked up blood.

EBNA (Epstein-Barr nuclear antigen) **test**.

Ebola virus—acute hemorrhagic febrile disease, highly fatal, endemic to areas of Africa at this time. See also *Marburg fever*.

EBRT (external beam radiation therapy).

EB (Euler-Byrne) **score**.

Ebstein cardiac anomaly (*not* Epstein, as in Epstein-Barr virus).

EBT (electron beam tomography).

eburnated bone; eburnation.

EBV (Epstein-Barr virus).

E-CABG (endarterectomy and coronary artery bypass grafting).

E-CABG (endoscopic coronary artery bypass graft).

E.CAM—photon emission camera used for whole-body emission tomography and general imaging procedures with variable angle techniques. Also referred to as *E.CAM positron emission tomography* (PET) *imaging system*.

ECC (emergency cardiac care).

ECCE (extracapsular cataract extraction).

Eccentric Y retractor—adjustable finger retractor for use in laparoscopic procedures.

ECCL—see *encephalocraniocutaneous lipomatosis.*

Eccocee—a mid-range compact ultrasound diagnostic system.

Eccovision acoustic rhinometry system—used to obtain quantitative measurements of the nasal cavity.

ECE (esophageal capsule endoscopy) —see *PillCam video capsule.*

E-CFC (erythroid colony-forming cells).

echocardiographic automated border detection—a technique that allows continuous measuring of left ventricular cavity area (and thus volume) by differentiating the acoustic backscatter characteristics of blood from myocardial tissue within a defined area of the heart, replacing more invasive techniques such as catheter insertion.

echocardiography—a noninvasive cardiac diagnostic procedure. From the sonographic pattern are determined the dimensions, position, and movements of the chamber walls and valve leaflets, and any possible deformities. See *dobutamine stress echocardiography*, *M-mode, sector scan, transesophageal echocardiogram*, and *two-dimensional echocardiography*.

echo characteristics (ultrasonography) —the frequency, intensity, and distribution of echoes produced by a structure or region.

Echocheck—a hearing screening device for infants and children that works by recording click-evoked otoacoustic emissions (cEOEs).

Echo-Coat ultrasound biopsy needles.

echocolonoscope—endoscopic sonographic transducer in combination with a colonoscope.

EchoEye—3-D ultrasound imaging system that is placed in front of a catheter or probe to provide tissue imaging during surgery.

EchoFlow blood velocity meter system (BVM-1)—enables physicians to evaluate and quantify blood flow in vessels using ultrasound technology.

echogastroscope—used for endoscopic ultrasonography.

Echols retractor (Neuro).

EchoMark catheter—an angiographic catheter that contains a wire and transducer sensitive to ultrasound signals. As the catheter is advanced, ultrasound (rather than x-rays) is used to correctly position the catheter in the vessel.

echo planar imaging (EPI)—MRI term.

echo sign (Neuro)—repetition of the last word of a sentence or phrase, indicating brain pathology.

echo time (TE)—given in milliseconds (msec)—MRI term.

ECI (Ensemble contrast imaging).

EC-IC (extracranial-intracranial) **bypass** —for complete carotid occlusions or intracranial carotid stenosis not treatable by endarterectomy.

Eckhout vertical gastroplasty (named for Clifford V. Eckhout, MD).

ECLIA—see *electrochemiluminescence immunoassay.*

Eclipse ST cyclotron—used with PET scan imagers.

Eclipse TENS unit—see *TENS.*

Eclipse TMR laser—a holmium laser device used in transmyocardial revascularization (TMR) to create pathways within the heart muscle.

ECLS (extracorporeal life support)—the term currently preferred to ECMO (extracorporeal membrane oxygenation). ECLS provides circulatory and/or respiratory support using a basic extracorporeal perfusion system over a period of days or

ECLS *(cont.)*
a few weeks until the native heart or lungs recover after open heart surgery.

ECM (extracellular matrix).

ECMO (extracorporeal membrane oxygenation) ("ek-mo")—a technique used in infants with serious lung problems at birth with poor prognosis for survival. The baby's blood is circulated through a machine that removes carbon dioxide and adds oxygen, thereby functioning for the lungs while they mature or heal.

ECochG (electrocochleography)—test to estimate hearing loss.

ECOG (Eastern Cooperative Oncology Group) **performance status scale**—a rating system prognostic for cancer survival and quality of life, by which eligibility for some forms of chemotherapy is determined. The scale ranges from 0 to 5, 5 being dead. Patients in the upper ranges are unlikely to respond to chemotherapy.

E. coli **0157:H7**—a strain of *Escherichia coli,* causing outbreaks of severe diarrheal disease in the U.S. Transmission occurs through contaminated food and water and directly from person to person. It is particularly dangerous for children and the elderly.

E. coli **L-asparaginase**—a chemotherapy drug for acute lymphoblastic leukemia. *E. coli* is a gram-negative bacterium which provides the enzyme L-asparaginase aminohydrolase contained in this version of L-asparaginase. Some people who are allergic to the *E. coli*-derived version of the drug can be given *Erwinia* L-asparaginase, from the gram-negative bacterium *Erwinia*.

ECOM (endotracheal cardiac output monitoring).

EcoNail—a nail lacquer that contains the antifungal drug econazole and a drug-absorption-enhancement compound. It is used to treat fungal infections of the fingernails and toenails.

economy class syndrome—condition where a blood clot in the leg is related to long-haul air flights in cramped space that limits ambulation.

ECP (extracorporeal photochemotherapy).

ECRB (extensor carpi radialis brevis).

ECRL (extensor carpi radialis longus).

ectasia—expansion or dilatation of a duct or vessel.

ecstatic—exhibiting great elation or enthusiasm. Cf. *ectatic*.

ECT (electroconvulsive therapy).

ECTA (enzyme-catalyzed therapeutic activation) **technology**—focuses on treatment of drug resistance in cancer.

ectatic—stretched or distended. Cf. *ecstatic*.

ectoderm—the outermost of the three germ layers of the early embryo, all of which are derived from the inner cell mass of the blastocyst. As fetal development progresses it gives rise to the skin, the nervous system, dental enamel, and the ocular lenses.

ectodermal groove—embryonic feature that lies between the maxillary and mandibular facial prominences. Incomplete fusion is thought to cause facial aplasia cutis (failure of development of skin).

Ectra system—for endoscopic release of the transverse carpal ligament in carpal tunnel syndrome.

ECU (environmental control unit)—enables severely disabled individuals to perform everyday functions with use of computer commands activated by blow tubes or mouth sticks. Each system is designed to meet the needs of the individual.

ECV (external cephalic version).

EDA (extravasation detection accessory).

EDAS (encephaloduroarteriosynangiosis).

EDC (extensor digitorum communis).

eddy currents; eddies—MRI terms.

edema
brawny
cystoid macular edema (CME)
flash pulmonary
1+ to 2+ pitting
tough

EdgeAhead phaco slit knife—used in cataract surgery. Note: *EdgeAhead* is one word.

edge detection (ED)—a term used in MRI scans.

edge ringing artifact (Gibbs phenomenon, truncation band)—an MRI artifact caused by limitation of the image reconstruction algorithm.

edible vaccines—created from a genetically engineered food product (e.g., potato) containing a toxin produced by *E. coli*. Volunteers who ate portions of the potato in separate doses over a 21-day period showed an increase in antibodies in the blood, and some had increase in antibodies in the lining of the digestive tract. The director of the government agency funding the study stated, "Edible vaccines offer exciting possibilities for significantly reducing the burden of diseases like hepatitis and diarrhea . . . in the developing world where storing and administering vaccines are often major problems."

Edinburgh Postnatal Depression Scale (EPDS)—a self-rated measure specifically designed for use in primary care settings. Its main feature is the exclusion of items which might reflect physical discomfort and thus confuse depression with the somatic effects of childbirth.

Edinger-Westphal nucleus—the parasympathetic nucleus from which arises the oculomotor nerve (cranial nerve III), for constriction of the pupil and accommodation of the lens for near vision.

Edmondson grading system—in small hepatocellular carcinoma.

Edmondson-Steiner histologic grading of hepatocellular carcinoma (grades I, II, II, IVa).

EDR (extreme drug resistance) **assay**—a test performed prior to chemotherapy.

EDRT (endothelium-derived relaxant factor).

Edwards-Cohen catheter—a device used for the introduction of an embryo into the uterine cavity after fertilization in vitro.

Edwards woven Teflon aortic bifurcation graft.

Edwin Shaw Hospital for Rehabilitation.

EEA stapler (end-to-end anastomosis).

EECP (enhanced external counterpulsation).

EEC (ectrodactyly-ectodermal dysplasia-clefting) **syndrome**—including hypertelorism, cleft lip or palate, or both, and possibly seizures.

"ee-DAY-feeks"—phonetic for *idée fixe*.

EEL (external elastic lamina).

EEPLND (extraperitoneal endoscopic pelvic lymph node dissection).

EES (expandable esophageal stent).

efface—used in plastic and reconstructive surgery to describe obliteration of a deformity by covering it with a graft. Usage: "A flat onlay graft was inserted through an intercartilaginous incision into a precise pocket to efface the deformity."

effacement—abnormal flattening of the contour of a structure.

effect (noun)—an immediate result produced by an agent or cause. Usage: "The surgical procedure produced a good cosmetic effect." Examples: proarrhythmic effect, Somogyi effect, Tyndall effect.

effect (verb)—to execute, accomplish, bring to pass. Usage: "This therapy should effect a cure" or, in surgery, "closure was effected." *Effect* is most often used as a noun. Cf. *affect*.

efferent—moving away from the center. Cf. *afferent*.

Efficacy Sources Inventory—a 3-part survey to measure a patient's performance in daily activities, vicarious experience of exercise, and verbal encouragement to exercise received from others.

effusion—escape of a fluid into a part. Examples: pericardial and pleural. Cf. *infusion*.

EFM (electronic fetal monitoring)—uses telephone transmission of data and remote sensory devices for patient monitoring.

Egan mammography—a set of procedures for mammographic examination developed by Robert L. Egan, M.D., the author of a standard textbook and many articles on mammography.

EG/BUS (external genitalia/Bartholin glands, urethra, and Skene glands).

EGCg, EGCG (epigallocatechin gallate)—a compound in green tea that inhibits activity of an enzyme required for cancer cell growth. A purified caffeine is separated from green tea.

EGD (esophagogastroduodenoscopy).

EGF (epidermal growth factor).

EGF-R (endothelial growth factor receptor) **small molecule inhibitors**—used in the treatment of psoriasis.

egg-shaped congruous acetabulum—a favorable finding in Legg-Calvé-Perthes disease.

egg shelling procedure—kyphosis correction surgery.

eggshell procedure—pedicle subtraction osteotomy.

egoisme à deux—a phenomenon sometimes seen when both members of a couple deny they have a problem, such as one individual's dementia.

EGTA (esophageal gastric tube airways).

EHL (electrohydraulic lithotripsy).

Ehlers-Danlos syndrome—increased laxity and elasticity in the supporting structures of the joints; can also follow neurosyphilis or severe rheumatoid arthritis.

EIA (enzyme-linked immunoassay)—used in the detection of AIDS-associated retroviruses.

EIA-2 (enzyme-linked immunoassay)—detects the presence of the hepatitis C virus in blood.

EIB (exercise-induced bronchospasm).

EIC (extensive intraductal carcinoma).

eicosapentaenoic acid (EPA)—a marine fatty acid, analogue of arachidonic acid that is found in fish, some other marine oils, and also possibly in seaweeds. Some researchers think that a diet rich in EPA may be protection against

eicosapentaenoic *(cont.)* thrombosis in patients with high serum cholesterol and triglyceride levels.

EID (emergency infusion device)—percutaneous central venous large-bore catheter.

EIFT (embryo intrafallopian transfer).

800 Series Blood Gas and Critical Analyte System—provides diagnostic measurements of blood gas, electrolytes, metabolites, and CO-oximetry from a single blood sample in a compact and user-friendly format.

EIP (extensor indicis proprius).

Eisenmenger complex—congenital heart anomaly.

EIT (endoscopic injection therapy).

EIWA (Escala Inteligencia Wechsler Para Adultos)—the Wechsler Adult Intelligence Scale for administration to adults who speak only Spanish.

EKG (electrocardiograph) **leads**
augmented leads: aVF, aVL, aVR
cardiac leads: I, II, III, V1 to V6

EKG-silent—see *dipyridamole*.

EKP—see *endokeratoplasty*.

"ek-SIGH-trin"—see *Xcytrin*.

ELA (euglobulin lysis activity).

Elastalloy Ultraflex Strecker nitinol stent.

ELAS (endoluminal laser ablation of the greater saphenous vein) **procedure**.

elastic fibers stain (Weigert)—a special tissue stain to reveal the presence of elastin (a fibrous microscopic cell protein) found in skin and vessels.

Elastikon elastic tape—for pressure dressings.

Elasto-Gel hydrogel sheet.

Elasto-Gel shoulder therapy wrap—used for giving heat treatments for shoulder injuries.

Elastomull—an elastic gauze bandage, a double-woven stretch dressing.

elastosis perforans serpiginosa—skin disease in which abnormal elastic tissue fibers, other connective tissue elements, and cellular debris are expelled from the papillary dermis through the epidermis.

elbow fat pad sign (Radiol)—seen in a plain lateral radiograph of the elbow. Intra-articular hemorrhage due to skeletal injury (usually fracture of the radial head in an adult) causes distension of the synovium and forces the fat out of the fossa, producing triangular radiolucent shadows anterior and posterior to the distal end of the humerus.

Elbowlift suspension pad.

ELBW (extremely low-birth-weight) infants.

ELC (ear lobe crease).

ELCA (excimer laser coronary angioplasty).

ELD (episodic laryngeal dyskinesias).

Elder classification—a classification of tumor-infiltrating lymphocytes in malignant melanoma. Named for pathologist D. E. Elder, M.D.

EleCare—a nutritionally complete amino acid-based medical food and infant formula with iron.

Elecsys Anti-HBs immunoassay and **Elecsys PreciControl Anti-HBs**—for the qualitative determination of total antibodies to the hepatitis B surface antigen in human serum and plasma.

Elecsys proBNP immunoassay—automated laboratory blood test used in the diagnosis of congestive heart failure. The test can detect a protein molecule (N-terminal pro-B-type-natriuretic peptide or NT-proBNP) in the blood that is secreted almost

Elecsys *(cont.)* exclusively by the heart. A high amount of NT-proBNP in the blood suggests congestive heart failure and provides information about its severity. The higher the blood level of NT-proBNP, the more serious is the condition. Also, *NT-proBNP immunoassay.*

elective lymph node dissection (ELND).

electrically generated pain management techniques—see *pain management techniques.*

electrical stimulation—see *"e-stim."*

electric zone—see *triangle of pain.*

Electro-Acuscope—microcurrent electrical nerve stimulator that generates complex waveforms that automatically adjust to meet the needs of injured tissue. Used in treating carpal tunnel syndrome. Also, *Electro-Myopulse.*

electrocardiogram—see *signal-averaged electrocardiogram* (SAECG).

electrocardiographic gating with electron-beam CT technology.

electrocautery—see *cautery.*

electrochemiluminescence immunoassay (ECLIA)—a highly specific method of detecting antibodies.

electrochemotherapy—a therapy in which a split-second electrical impulse is applied to the skin in combination with topical chemotherapy. It opens up skin pores, allowing the chemotherapeutic agent to seep in and more effectively target cancerous cells. It is relatively painless and involves no cutting or stitching, so there is none of the disfigurement that might be associated with surgery.

electroconvulsive therapy (ECT).

electrocorticography—procedure performed to clarify the origin of tumor-related seizures.

electrode data—When a neurosurgeon dictates: "The electrode was connected with zero two zero negative polarity," it should be written *0-2/0 negative.*

electroejaculation—an infertility procedure on anejaculatory males under anesthesia. A probe inserted into the rectum administers an electric shock, causing ejaculation.

electrogalvanic stimulation—used in treatment of fractures. See *pulsing current.*

electrohydraulic lithotripsy (EHL)—has the merit of being less costly than laser lithotripsy, but it requires a dual endoscope arrangement to target the stones precisely and avoid bile duct injury.

Electro-Mate cutting and coagulating device—an instrument used in laparoscopic procedures.

electromechanical dissociation (EMD) **of the heart**.

electromyography of penile corpus cavernosum muscles—a diagnostic tool to evaluate cavernous smooth muscle and its autonomic innervation.

electron-beam angiography of coronary arteries—minimally invasive procedure performed on the electron-beam tomography scanner.

electron-beam computed tomography (CT)—method of examining the cardiovascular system.

electronic fetal monitoring (EFM).

Electronic HouseCall system—allows full 2-way audio and video communication between a patient and a physician 24 hours per day, collecting vital signs and automatically

Electronic *(cont.)*
recording them in a central database so that caregivers have real clinical information about the patient's condition.

electronic portal imaging device (EPID)—a device used for online treatment verification in complex radiation therapy treatments.

electro-oculogram apparatus (Oph)—used in determining saccadic velocity.

electrophoresis—a process in which charged particles (such as ions), suspended in liquid, are moved under the influence of an applied electrical field. Note the different root words in electrophoresis (*phoresis*, carrying, transmission) and plasmapheresis (*apheresis*, separation).

electrophysiologic study (EPS).

electroporation therapy—application of high electric field pulses of short duration to create temporary pores (holes) in membranes of cells for easier and more efficient entrance of potential tumor-killing drugs.

electroretinogram, -graphy (ERG).

Electroscope—disposable scissors used in laparoscopic procedures.

electrostimulation—see *pulsing current*.

electrothermally assisted capsulorrhaphy (ETAC)—surgical method for treating glenohumeral instability of the shoulder. Thermal energy (laser or radiofrequency) is applied at a temperature of 65°C arthroscopically to "loosen" capsuloligamentous tissues, which causes shrinkage of the collagen fibers.

electrothermal procedure—utilizes decompression catheter to dissolve herniated disks. See *decompression catheter*.

electrotransfer test—see *Western blot electrotransfer test*.

elemental diet—for burn patients, a high-nitrogen liquid diet that requires almost no digestion and produces little residue.

Elestat (epinastine HCl)—a medication for the prevention of itching associated with allergic conjunctivitis.

elevator
Boyle uterine
Cottle
Ellik
Endotrac
Freer
Gimmick
Hough ("huff") hoe
McGlamry
Molt periosteal
OSI extremity
Somer uterine
Toriumi sharp and dull suction

El Gamal cardiac device.

elicit—to draw out. Usage: "We could elicit little information as to the patient's past medical history." Cf. *illicit*.

ELIFA (enzyme-linked immunofluorescent assay).

Eligoy metal alloy—used in joint replacement.

Eliminator ArthroWand—ablation instrument used in rapid volumetric tissue removal in subacromial decompression and anterior cruciate ligament reconstruction and for very heavy synovial incisions. The wand passes easily through most cannulas.

Eliminator dilatation balloon.

ELISA (enzyme-linked immunosorbent assay)—the first "AIDS test" used by blood banks to diminish the chance of HIV infection through a blood transfusion. ELISA can also be used as a screening test for hepatitis C.

Elite dual chamber rate-responsive pacemaker—marketed by Medtronic, weighing only $1^1/2$ oz., and using CapSure SP leads.

Elite Farley retractor—adjustable retractor for all types of spinal surgery.

ELK—see *endothelial lamellar keratoplasty*.

Ellestad protocol—treadmill stress test.

Ellik kidney stone basket, evacuator, elevator.

Ellis fracture (Oph/Plastic)—a fracture of the zygomaticomaxillary complex (ZMC), grades 1 through 3.

ELM (epiluminescence light microscopy).

Elmor tissue morcellator—a tissue morcellator powered by radiofrequency energy that is used to isolate, contain, and remove large tissue masses during laparoscopic surgery.

Elmslie triple arthrodesis—used for podiatric surgical correction of post polio pes calcaneovalgus deformity.

ELND (elective lymph node dissection).

eloquent areas of the brain—seizures starting from a focus in these areas will produce an aura.

"el-tack"—phonetic for *LTAC* (long term acute care [facility]).

elta (trademarked lowercase) **dermal hydrogel dressing**.

EL2-LS2 flexible video laparoscope.

EL2-TF410 laparoscope—a flexible laparoscope.

elusion—an adroit or clever escape; escape notice of. Usage: "Elusion of a fourth parathyroid gland indicated its possible congenital absence." Cf. *allusion, illusion*.

ELVT (endolaser venous therapy).

EMA (epithelial membrane antigen).

embolism vs. embolus—terms sometimes confused. Embolism is the process whereby a vessel becomes obstructed by material carried in the circulation; an embolus is that material, usually a clot but sometimes fat (from the marrow of a broken bone), amnionic fluid, injected materials, or air.

embolotherapy—embolization of hypervascularized tumors and arteriovenous malformations, cutting off blood supply.

Embol-78—a liquid embolic material used for vein embolization.

embolus—see *embolism*.

Embosphere microspheres—device for occluding the blood supply to uterine fibroids during uterine artery embolization. The device is also used to treat hypervascularized tumors and arteriovenous malformations with embolization, or embolotherapy.

Embol-X arterial cannula and filter system—protects against the risk of stroke and other neurologic deficits during cardiovascular procedures by capturing emboli (including aortic plaque) that may be released into systemic circulation.

EMBP (estramustine binding protein) (Neuro).

Embrace heart stabilizer—stabilizes desired areas of the heart, which, in turn, creates a relatively stationary coronary artery during beating heart or off-pump coronary bypass surgery. The device uses stabilization "feet" to hold the epicardium in place parallel to the coronary artery, allowing the surgeon to bypass the blocked artery without resorting to the traditional method of stopping the heart and employing the heart-lung machine.

embryo—an organism in the earliest stages of development; for human beings, the embryonic stage extends

embryo *(cont.)* from fertilization until the end of the eighth week of gestation.

embryo biopsy—a procedure performed when an in vitro fertilized embryo has reached the 8-cell stage, in which a laser is used to make a hole in the envelope surrounding the embryo and a single cell is removed using a pair of tiny pipettes for the purpose of genetic diagnosis. The 7-celled embryo that remains is just as viable as the 8-celled one and remains in the petri dish while the biopsied cell is being studied genetically.

embryoid body—a spheroidal clump or colony of partially differentiated cells that develops spontaneously in a culture of embryonic stem cells. Cells isolated from embryoid bodies may be used to start lines of multipotent stem cells.

embryonic germ cell—a pluripotent stem cell derived from the gonadal ridge of a 5-week to 8-week embryo. With continued normal development these cells differentiate into gametes (oocytes or sperm). Their properties and developmental potential are similar but not identical to those of embryonic stem cells.

embryonic stem cell—a primitive, undifferentiated, pluripotent stem cell derived from the inner cell mass of an embryo in the blastocyst stage.

embryo intrafallopian transfer (EIFT).

embryo provider—a person who has custody of an embryo and the authority to make decisions regarding its disposition; not necessarily either biological parent of the embryo.

embryoscopy—the use of a fiberoptic endoscope to visualize a fetus in the first trimester. This technique allows greater access to very tiny fetuses than ultrasonographically guided prenatal diagnostic testing.

EMD (electromechanical dissociation). Usage: "He was defibrillated into asystole and treated with atropine, but he went into an EMD and we were unable, despite continued and adequate CPR, to resuscitate him."

EMERALD (Enhanced Myocardial Efficacy and Recovery by Aspiration of Liberalized Debris) study.

Emerge—part of the DualMesh line of biomaterials. It is designed for rapid deployment in laparoscopic repair of incisional and ventral hernias.

emergency infusion device (EID).

emergency medical services (EMS).

emergency medical technician defibrillation (EMT-D).

Emergency Medical Treatment and Labor Act (EMTALA)—designed to prevent the dumping of underinsured patients from private emergency rooms to public emergency rooms for financial reasons. You may hear this referred to in emergency department or psychiatric dictation.

emergency orders of detention (EOD).

EMF (endomyocardial fibrosis).

EMG (electromyography)—electrical nerve study. Do not confuse with ENG (electronystagmogram).

eminence—a bony projection. Cf. *imminent*.

EMI ("emmy") **scanner**—the original CT scanner. (EMI, Electrical Musical Instruments.)

EMIT (enzyme-multiplication immunoassay technique)—used in toxicology screens on urine samples.

EMLA (eutectic mixture of local anesthetics [lidocaine and prilocaine]) **anesthesia**.

EMLA cream (lidocaine and prilocaine)—applied to the skin topically and covered with a dressing for 60 minutes. It provides a level of anesthesia complete enough for dermal procedures that an additional injection of lidocaine is often not needed.

empiric risk (Genetics)—an estimate of the probability that a genetic trait will recur in a family based on past experience rather than on knowledge of the causative mechanism.

empty can sign—a test for supraspinatus tendinitis. The deltoid muscle is responsible for most of the range of the arm's abduction (20° to 90°) and is assisted by the trapezius, rhomboid, and supraspinatus muscles. Resistance to abduction, with the arm at 90° and the thumb pointed down, isolates the supraspinatus muscle and is used to detect weakness or pain. Such a response is known as the empty can sign and is commonly seen in rotator cuff impingement. Also, *empty beer can sign*.

empty nest syndrome—restlessness and depression in parents whose children have grown up and left home.

empty nose syndrome (ENS)—a side effect of surgical removal of diseased turbinates in order to provide adequate airflow for breathing. Enhancement of nasal air flow can create a subjective sense of inadequate pulmonary ventilation. Also known as *secondary atrophic rhinitis*.

empty sella syndrome—diagnosed in a patient with an enlarged sella turcica, where there is no tumor present and the sella fills with air on CT or MRI scan.

EMR (endoscopic mucosal resection).

EMS (emergency medical services).

EMS (encephalomyosynangiosis).

EMS (endolymphatic mastoid shunt).

EMS (eosinophilia-myalgia syndrome).

EMTALA ("em-tall-uh")—see *Emergency Medical Treatment and Labor Act*.

EMT-D—see *emergency medical technician defibrillation*.

EMV grading, Glasgow Coma Scale—E = eyes; M = motor; V = voice. Written as $E_2M_4V_2$. The Glasgow Coma Scale goes to 8. See *Glasgow Coma Scale*.

ENA (extractable nuclear antigen).

EnAbl system—a thermal ablation system used to treat excessive uterine bleeding.

ENANB hepatitis—enterically transmitted non-A, non-B hepatitis.

ENBA (Epstein-Barr virus nuclear antigen).

en bloc dissection of bladder, reproductive organs, perineum, rectum, and pelvic lymph nodes.

en bloc laminectomy (Neuro, Ortho).

en bloc transplantation of small pediatric kidneys into adult recipients, using an interposition technique—averts the complication of vascular thrombosis and provides adequate mass to achieve a normal level of renal function. The successful technique places the allografts using vascular anastomoses in continuity.

en bloc vein resection—performed in the treatment of pancreatic adenocarcinoma adherent to the superior mesenteric-portal vein.

encapsulated liposomes—see *liposomes*.

encephalocraniocutaneous lipomatosis (ECCL)—birth defects appearing as skin nevi on head, neck, and trunk of infants.

encephaloduroarteriosynangiosis (abbreviated EDAS)—surgical treatment for moyamoya disease, in which a scalp artery is dissected over the course of several inches, then a small temporary opening in the skull directly beneath the artery is made. The artery is then sutured to the surface of the brain and the bone replaced. Cf. *encephalomyosynangiosis*.

encephalomyosynangiosis (abbreviated EMS)—surgical treatment for moyamoya disease. The temporalis muscle of the forehead region is dissected, and through an opening in the skull it is placed onto the surface of the brain. Cf. *encephaloduroarteriosynangiosis)*.

Enclose anastomosis assist device—designed to eliminate the need for partial clamping of the aorta during off-pump or beating-heart coronary artery bypass grafting procedures.

Encompass cardiac network—system that connects to all major cardiac x-ray and ultrasound systems using the industry-standard DICOM communications protocol, creating a central repository of digital images from multiple modalities together with the associated physician findings reports.

endarterectomy and coronary artery bypass grafting (E-CABG).

end-biting forceps.

end-effectors—the working ends of robotic instruments (graspers, scissors, etc.).

Ender nail, or rod, fixation—used for fixation of long bone fractures.

End-Flo laparoscopic irrigating system.

Endius endoscopic access system—for noninstrumental posterolateral spinal fusion.

Endius TriFix—thoracolumbar pedicle screw system. Uses the Dome screw design and Diamond connectors.

endoanal coil—used in MRI studies to image the lower colon.

EndoAnchor—for securing mesh in laparoscopic hernia repair.

Endo-Avitene—a microfibrillar collagen hemostatic material, used in an endoscopic delivery system.

Endo Babcock—surgical grasping device.

Endobag—laparoscopic specimen retrieval system.

endobronchial needle aspiration—to diagnose endobronchial small cell carcinoma.

Endocare renal cryoablation—freezes and destroys diseased tissue in place, eliminating the necessity for nephrectomy in patients with renal carcinoma.

EndoCinch suturing system—used for treatment of gastroesophageal reflux disease. See also *Bard EndoCinch*.

Endo Clip applier—laparoscopic clip applier.

EndoCoil biliary stent—for malignant obstruction of the bile duct due to pancreatic cancer.

EndoCoil esophageal stent to treat a stenosis.

EndoCPB (endovascular cardiopulmonary bypass) **catheter**.

endocut cautery device.

endoderm—the innermost of the three germ layers of the early embryo, all of which are derived from the inner

endoderm *(cont.)* cell mass of the blastocyst. As fetal development progresses it gives rise to the respiratory and digestive systems, including the liver and the pancreas.

Endodissect—reticulating (or roticulating) dissecting instrument.

endoesophageal MRI coil—tiny probe that is inserted through the mouth and nestles in the esophagus, giving an image of the aorta that is nine times sharper than the standard MRI provides.

end-of-dose deterioration—a loss of symptom control in patients, such as those on L-Dopa for Parkinson disease.

EndoFit aortic endovascular grafts—see also *AccuSet introducer catheter.*

Endofix absorbable interference screw (Ortho)—bioabsorbable device made of a polyglyconate polymer. Used in bone-tendon-bone fixation in anterior cruciate ligament surgery.

Endoflex—minimally invasive endoscopic lumbar diskectomy scope and instrument system.

Endo-Gauge—device used to measure the thickness of tissue in laparoscopic wedge biopsy of the liver.

endogenous morphine (endorphins).

Endo-GIA suture stapler.

Endo Grasp device—used in minimally invasive lung surgery.

Endo Hernia stapler—used in laparoscopic hernia repairs.

endokeratoplasty (EKP)—alternative to full penetrating keratoplasty, performed with the automated lamellar therapeutic keratoplasty. See *endothelial lamellar keratoplasty (ELK).*

Endoknot suture—used in minimally invasive surgeries such as laparoscopy.

endolaser venous therapy (ELVT)—minimally invasive laser closure of varicose veins. A special laser-tipped fiber is passed through a small catheter inserted into the greater saphenous vein. As the laser is activated, the resulting heat at the tip causes a reaction in the walls of the vein, causing them to stick together. The varicosities associated with this vein then disappear as blood from the lower leg reroutes through the deeper circulation.

endoleak—flow of blood from arterial lumen into the aneurysm sac, a phenomenon consisting of persistent blood flow outside of an endograft into the aneurysm sac after endovascular aneurysm repair. There are five types identified as follows:

type 1—endoleak originating proximally or distally at the intended site of attachment.

type II—endoleak originating from retrograde branch vessels.

type III—arising from a defect in the fabric of the graft or at junction zones between members of modular grafts.

type IV—occurring as a result of diffuse leakage through the interstices of the graft.

type V—when the aneurysm sac remains pressurized and enlarged in the absence of a demonstrable leak on imaging studies.

Endoloop—disposable chromic ligature suture instrument.

EndoLumina invasive light delivery catheter—illuminated bougie for transillumination of esophagus, using a silicone-sheathed fiberoptic bundle bonded to a soft, clear, flexible tip. Also for general, colorectal, and gynecological laparoscopic surgery.

endoluminal gastroplication procedure—see *Bard EndoCinch endoscopic suturing system.*

endolymphatic hypertension.

endolymphatic mastoid shunt (EMS)—a surgical procedure that establishes communication between the endolymphatic sac and the cerebrospinal fluid space, for treatment of vertigo in patients with Ménière disease.

EndoMate Grab Bag—an endoscopic specimen retrieval bag.

Endomed LSS—total laparoscopic system.

endometrial ablation—used as a treatment for dysfunctional uterine bleeding. Ablation of the uterine lining with hysteroscopy is less invasive than hysterectomy.

Endo-Model rotating knee joint prosthesis—permits flexion of the joint up to 165°.

endomyocardial fibrosis (EMF)—a severe and progressively restrictive form of cardiomyopathy.

endonuclease—an enzyme that cleaves bonds in a strand of DNA or RNA.

Endopath bladeless trocar—creates a smaller fascial defect, thus causing less trauma and improving cannula retention.

Endopath EMS hernia stapler.

Endopath ES—reusable endoscopic stapler.

Endopath laparoscopic trocar—used for laparoscopic surgery, as in inguinal hernia repair.

Endopath Linear Cutter—a surgical stapler, used in minimally invasive surgery.

Endopath Optiview optical surgical obturator—allows visually guided trocar entry for laparoscopic surgery.

Endopath TriStar trocar—used in minimally invasive surgery. Allows use of the fingertip technique of placing the trocar precisely and with much less force than conventional trocars.

Endopath Ultra Veress needle—used for insufflation during obstetric and gynecologic laparoscopic procedures.

Endopearl—bioabsorbable device that provides enhanced fixation of soft tissue grafts within the femoral socket during ACL reconstruction of the knee.

endophthalmitis—inflammation of the internal structures of the eye or the adjacent tissues.

Endo-P-Probe—used in combination with standard ultrasound machines for endorectal ultrasonography.

endoprosthesis—crutched-stick type biliary duct stent. See *prosthesis*.

endopyelotomy procedure—minimally invasive procedure for primary ureteropelvic junction obstruction. It has no major negative impact on eventual open pyeloplasty if that should become necessary.

endorectal coil—MRI term.

EndoRetract—a retractor used in minimally invasive surgery.

endorphin (endogenous morphine)—natural morphine-like compound produced by the brain.

EndoSaph vein harvest system—used in minimally invasive harvesting of the saphenous vein for CABG procedures.

endoscope

AO (American Optical) indirect ophthalmoscope
AudioScope
Augustine guide and scope
Ausculscope

endoscope *(cont.)*
Baggish hysteroscope
Benjamin binocular slimline laryngoscope (ENT)
Benjamin pediatric laryngoscope
Boutin thoracoscope
Bullard laryngoscope
CF-200Z Olympus colonoscope
CF-UM3 echocolonoscope
choledochofiberscope
Circon videohydrothoracoscope
Citscope disposable arthroscope
Clarus spinescope
Czaja-McCaffrey endoscope
dermatoscope
diaphanoscope
Digiscope
DuraView OL-1 flexible nasopharyngoscope
Dyonics disposable arthroscope
Eagle arthroscope
echocolonoscope
echogastroscope
EL2-LS2 flexible video laparoscope
EL2-TF410 laparoscope
Electro-Acuscope
endometrial resection and ablation (ERA) resectoscope sheath
EVIS 140 endoscope reprocessing system
falloposcope
FG-36UX linear scanning echoendoscope
Flexiblade laryngoscope
flexible steerable nasolaryngopharyngoscope
Futura resectoscope sheath
Gautier ureteroscope
gonioscope
Gynecare Versascope hysteroscope
Holinger anterior commissure laryngoscope
Iglesias fiberoptic resectoscope
Imagyn microlaparoscope
indirect laser ophthalmoscope

endoscope *(cont.)*
InjecTx cystoscope
Kantor-Berci video laryngoscope
Karl Storz flexible ureteropyeloscope
Killian-Lynch laryngoscope
Kleinsasser anterior commissure laryngoscope
Landry vein light Venoscope
Lewy suspension laryngoscope
Lindholm operating laryngoscope
lingoscope
Mascot indirect ophthalmoscope endoscope
Microprobe laser microendoscope
MicroSpan microhysteroscope
MiniSite laparoscope
Morganstern continuous-flow operating cystoscope
mother and baby endoscope
Navigator flexible endoscope
OLM (ophthalmic laser microendoscope)
Olympus CF-1T100L video colonoscope
Olympus CF-200Z colonoscope
Olympus CYF-3 OES cystofiberscope
Olympus ENF-P2 laryngoscope
Olympus EVIS 140 endoscope
Olympus EVIS Q-200V videoendoscope
Olympus GF-UM3 and CF-UM20 ultrasonic endoscope
Olympus GIF-EUM2 echoendoscope
Olympus GIF-1T10 and GIF20 echoendoscope
Olympus JF1T10 fiberoptic duodenoscope
Olympus JF-UM20 echoendoscope
Olympus OSF sigmoidoscope
Olympus SIF10 enteroscope
Olympus TJF-100 endoscope

endoscope *(cont.)*
Olympus URF-P2 translaparoscopic choledochofiberscope
Olympus VU-M2 and XIF-UM3 echoendoscope
Olympus XQ230 gastroscope
OPERA STAR SL
orascope microfiberoptic
Ossoff-Karlan laryngoscope
Panoramic 200 nonmydriatic ophthalmoscope
Pentax EUP-EC124 ultrasound gastroscope
Pentax FG-36UX echoendoscope
Pentax-Hitachi FG32UA endosonographic system
percutaneous discoscope
Pixie minilaparoscope
Primbs-Circon indirect video ophthalmoscope
Riester otoscope
Shapshay/Healy laryngoscope
SIF10 Olympus enteroscope
Sine-U-View nasal endoscope
sinuscope
Sonde enteroscope
STAR (specialized tissue aspirating resectoscope)
Storz infant bronchoscope
SurgiScope
Surgiview laparoscope
3-Dscope laparoscope
TJF-100 Olympus endoscope
URF-P2 choledochoscope
Valle hysteroscope
van Loenen operating keratoscope
variable stiffness endoscope
VerreScope
video Hydrolaparoscope
videolaseroscopy
Visicath
visuscope
Weerda laryngoscope
Welch Allyn AudioScope
WuScope laryngoscope

endoscope *(cont.)*
XQ230 Olympus gastroscope
Zeiss EndoLive endoscope

endoscopic aspiration mucosectomy.

endoscopic band ligation—see *EBL.*

endoscopic biliary endoprosthesis—a relatively safe and effective palliative procedure for patients with unresectable carcinoma of the gallbladder. The prosthetic stent is placed endoscopically beyond the stricture with the goal of producing free flow of bile, a 30% fall in the patient's bilirubin, and relief of pruritus.

endoscopic brow lift—minimally invasive procedure in which the eyebrows are "lifted" to smooth wrinkles and remove excess fat and skin.

endoscopic coronary artery bypass graft (E-CABG).

endoscopic cryotherapy—method of treating various gastrointestinal conditions with cryotherapy through the endoscope.

endoscopic division of incompetent perforating veins—a minimally invasive procedure for the treatment of venous ulceration of the lower leg. It is said to be as effective as open surgical exploration but leads to fewer wound healing complications with its endoscopic exploration of the subfascial area through a small incision.

endoscopic injection therapy (EIT).

endoscopic laser cholecystectomy—see *laparoscopic laser cholecystectomy.*

endoscopic laser dacryocystorhinostomy.

endoscopic ligation—a surgical treatment for bleeding esophageal varices.

endoscopic mucosal resection (EMR) —surgical therapeutic method based

endoscopic *(cont.)*
on principles of strip biopsy for resection of flat lesions of the gastrointestinal tract. Researchers believe applying EMR to esophageal dysplasia, a precancerous condition, would decrease incidence of esophageal cancer.

endoscopic mucosectomy—a procedure for treatment of early gastric carcinoma.

endoscopic optical coherence tomography (EOCT)—uses light instead of sound to produce images with a 10-fold greater resolution.

endoscopic papillectomy (EP).

endoscopic plantar fasciotomy (EPF).

endoscopic posterolateral fusion (PLF)—lumbar fusion procedure performed endoscopically to treat degenerative disk disease through one access port.

endoscopic procedure
capsule endoscopy
double dip endoscopy
double dip upper and lower endoscopy
ECE (esophageal capsule endoscopy)
endoscopic thoracic sympathectomy (ETS)
Enteryx
"fetoscopy"
flexible transgastric peritoneoscopy (FTP)
functional endoscopic sinus surgery
gasless anterior neck skin lifting method
lasertripsy
off-pump coronary revascularization with endoscopic saphenous vein harvesting (OPCRES)
PillCam video capsule
tattooing of colonic neoplasms
trimodal spectroscopy

endoscopic *(cont.)*
VFSS (videofluoroscopy swallowing study)
video-stroboscopic laryngoscopy

endoscopic retrograde cholangiography (ERC).

endoscopic retrograde cholangiopancreatogram (ERCP).

endoscopic sewing machine technique—to place sutures in the region of the lower esophageal sphincter and gastric cardia. The sewing machine involves suction and a needle device to carry a suture through the muscularis propria.

endoscopic sphincterotomy (ES).

endoscopic, staple-assisted esophagodiverticulostomy—see *esophagodiverticulostomy*.

endoscopic strip craniectomy—precedes helmet-molding therapy in infants (less than 3 months of age) to correct sagittal craniosynostosis. Endoscopic technique for early correction of sagittal synostosis is said to be safer, decreases blood loss, operative time, hospital costs, and provides early surgical results. See *craniostosis*, *helmet-molding therapy*, and *scaphocephaly*.

endoscopic suction cap—device used to facilitate endoscopic mucosal resection.

endoscopic thoracic sympathectomy (ETS)—minimally invasive procedure to treat excessive sweating (hyperhidrosis). Two needle holes are made in the axillary area. Then, using endoscopic equipment that includes a small camera, specific nerves are identified and divided. This essentially blocks the signal from the sympathetic nervous system to the sweat glands. The outpatient procedure takes about an hour,

endoscopic *(cont.)*
and the results are reportedly immediate.

endoscopic transpapillary catheterization of the gallbladder (ETCG)—a procedure to dissolve gallstones. The gallbladder is catheterized using an ERCP catheter. The catheter with a hydrophilic guidewire is passed through the nose and advanced via a retrograde approach through the common bile duct. The ERCP catheter is then exchanged for a radiopaque Teflon biliary dilating catheter that allows the guidewire to be inserted into the cystic duct and gallbladder. The next day the patient undergoes both extracorporeal shock wave lithotripsy and infusion of solvent through the catheter to dissolve gallstones.

endoscopic ultrasound-guided fine needle aspiration (EUS-FNA)—provides visualization of peripancreatic tumors and their relationship to the surrounding structures as well as enabling cytologic diagnosis of the tumor and adjacent lymphadenopathy. It is a tool for the imaging and staging of peripancreatic tumors.

endoscopic ultrasonography (EUS)—examination of the esophagus and stomach with ultrasound using an echogastroscope. It can measure the thickness of the gastric folds and determine the depth to which carcinoma has invaded the stomach wall in order to stage esophageal and gastric carcinomas.

endoscopic ultrasound-assisted band ligation—technique for resection of submucosal tumors.

endoscopic variceal ligation (EVL)—see *EBL*.

endoscopic variceal sclerotherapy (EVS).

endoscopy-negative reflux disease (ENRD)—in which no findings are apparent on upper endoscopy in a patient who suffers from gastroesophageal reflux.

Endo Shears—used in minimally invasive surgery.

endosonography—insertion of sonographic transducers in upper or lower GI endoscopy.

Endosound endoscopic ultrasound catheter.

endostatin—drug used in cancer treatment and potentially other diseases that depend upon new blood vessel growth, such as in some forms of blindness and arthritis. Endostatin is a natural antiangiogenic protein that has been found to inhibit the growth of blood vessels, thereby “starving” cancerous tumors.

Endo Stitch—suturing device for endoscopic suturing.

Endotak lead defibrillator (Cardio)—provides increased electrode surface area and reduced system resistance in an implantable defibrillator. Also, *Endotak C lead* and *Endotak DSP*.

Endotak Picotip cardiac defibrillation lead.

Endotak Reliance—endocardial leads for implantable defibrillators.

endotension—term applied to the enlargement of an aneurysmal sac that remains pressurized after repair and continues to enlarge in the absence of a demonstrable endoleak.

endothelialize—the regeneration of a functional endothelium over the surfaces of the implanted devices, such as stents.

endothelial lamellar keratoplasty (ELK)—corneal transplant proce-

endothelial *(cont.)*
dure that makes use of a hinged, thick, large-diameter corneal flap. Also, *PLT, PLK, EKP*. Compare *deep lamellar endothelial keratoplasty*.

endothelium-derived relaxant factor (EDRT).

endotoxin activity assay—test to rule out gram-negative infection. Results are available in about an hour.

Endotrac cannula, elevator, obturator, probe, rasp, retractor—endoscopic instruments used in carpal tunnel procedures.

endotracheal cardiac output monitoring (ECOM)—monitoring devices incorporated into a standard endotracheal tube to allow for continuous cardiac output monitoring of patients undergoing surgery or on respiratory support.

endovaginal coil—MRI term.

endovaginal ultrasound (EVUS)—ultrasound probe is placed directly into the vagina to obtain a measurement of the uterine lining and detailed images of the uterus. This procedure has been found to identify 96% of uterine cancer and 92% of uterine disease in postmenopausal women who experience abnormal vaginal bleeding.

endovascular aortic repair (EVAR)—for treatment of high-risk patients with infrarenal aneurysms.

endovascular coil embolization procedure—an interventional neuroradiology technique also used to treat cerebral hemorrhage from a ruptured aneurysm.

endovascular stent-grafting—used for treatment of abdominal aortic aneurysm. A wire and fabric-covered stent are inserted into the body via the catheter system. The delivery catheter is advanced through the leg to the site of the aneurysm, and the self-expanding stent-graft is released. The graft lines the existing vessel and provides a new path for blood to flow past the aneurysm.

endoventricular circular patchplasty—the removal, following myocardial infarction, of the infarcted (dead) area of heart tissue or a resultant aneurysm. Infarct exclusion surgery allows the surgeon to return the left ventricle to a more normal shape and to improve function. Also known as *Dor procedure* or *modified endoventricular circularplasty.*

EndoWrist—instruments used with the da Vinci robot surgical system for endoscopic mitral valve repair.

end point—the point in an analysis at which the chemical reaction is complete, or at which the reading or interpretation of test results is feasible.

end-stage—referring to a progressively deteriorating condition that has reached the point of lethal (terminal) functional impairment of an organ or organ system (end-stage renal failure, end-stage lung disease).

end-stage coxarthrosis—treated by total hip arthroplasty.

end-stage liver disease (ESLD).

end-stage renal disease (ESRD).

end-tidal carbon dioxide ($ETCO_2$)—the partial pressure or maximal concentration of carbon dioxide (CO_2) at the end of an exhaled breath, expressed as a percentage of CO_2 or mmHg (normal values equal 5% to 6% CO_2 or 35-45 mmHg). A capnometer measures the partial pressure or maximal concentration of

end-tidal *(cont.)* CO_2 at the end of exhalation. During CPR, the amount of CO_2 excreted by the lungs is proportional to the amount of pulmonary blood flow; thus, measuring it is a noninvasive method of monitoring the efficacy of ongoing effort and the outcome of CPR.

Endur-acin (sustained-release nicotinic acid)—a medication for the treatment of hyperlipidemia.

Enduron acetabular liner—a ball liner made with UHMWPe (ultra-high molecular weight polyethylene) for extra strength to prevent cracking.

EnfaCare infant formula. *Not* Infacare.

en face ("ahn fahs") (Fr., in front, head on). Usage: "X-rays revealed left chest wall and diaphragmatic pleural plaques, the former seen both in profile and en face."

Enfamil ProSobee Lipil—infant formula containing DHA and ARA at the levels clinically shown to benefit mental and visual development.

Enfant pediatric vision testing system—a noninvasive, child-friendly medical device that tests for visual deficits using visual evoked potential technology. It records the brain's response to light and can detect vision problems such as amblyopia early in a child's life when these conditions are correctable. It reportedly has 97% sensitivity in detecting vision deficits in children as young as 6 months of age.

enfuvirtide—see *Fuzeon*.

ENG (electronystagmography)—evaluation of the acoustic nerve. Do not confuse with EMG (electromyography).

engaged, **engagement**—said of the fetal head as it enters and becomes lodged in the superior pelvic strait.

En Garde spring coil fixation system—a device that allows a surgeon to "suture" by delivering the fixation coil through a small-gauge needle.

Englert forceps (Plas Surg).

enhanced external counterpulsation (EECP)—a noninvasive outpatient procedure to relieve angina pectoris by improving perfusion to ischemic areas of the heart.

Enjuvia—a drug for treatment of menopausal symptoms.

ENL (erythema nodosum leprosum).

enlargement of Beck drill hole—a minimally invasive method of external frontal sinus surgery.

enoximone—see *Perfan I.V.*

ENP (extractable nucleoprotein).

ENRD—see *endoscopy-negative reflux disease.*

ENS (empty nose syndrome).

Ensemble contrast imaging (ECI)—used with Sonoline Elegra ultrasound platform to improve detection and characterization of organ tumors.

EnSite—cardiac catheter and cardiac mapping procedure.

EnSite 3000—imaging system that provides a 3-D graphical display of the heart's electrical activity.

Entamoeba histolytica—parasite which can be very virulent in AIDS.

ENTec Coblator Plasma Surgery System—provides precise, rapid incisions and channeling of submucosal tissue with minimal thermal injury to surrounding tissue, using Coblation technology. Used for physician-office tonsillotomy, to debulk the tonsil rather than remove it.

ENTec Plasma Wands—used to apply radiofrequency in Coblation-Channeling techniques.

Entera-Flo—enteral feeding pump for use with Entera closed tube feeding products that look like boxed drink containers.

enteral—pertaining to the small intestine or to administration of a drug or solution via the small intestine. Example: enteral feedings via tube. Cf. *parenteral*.

"Enteralflex"—phonetic for Enteroflex feeding tube.

Entereg (alvimopan)—a medication used for the treatment for postoperative ileus.

enterically transmitted non-A, non-B hepatitis (ENANB).

Enterobacter liquefaciens—now *Serratia liquefaciens*.

Enterobacter sakazakii—formerly *E. cloacae*.

enterocleisis—closure of a wound in the intestine. Also, occlusion of the lumen of the intestine. Cf. *enteroclysis*.

enteroclysis—the injection of a nutritional or medicinal liquid into the bowel. Cf. *enterocleisis*.

enterocystoplasty—a secondary bladder augmentation technique for urinary incontinence.

Enteroflex feeding tube. *Not* Entroflex or Enteralflex.

enterokinase—an enzyme of the small intestine.

enteropathy-associated T-cell lymphoma (EATL)—a highly aggressive neoplasm.

enteroscope vs. endoscope—soundalikes that can be confused in dictation; the former is used for the small intestine, the latter for upper or lower GI tract.

Entero-Test—a method for retrieving duodenal contents without intubation; the patient swallows a nylon line coiled inside a gelatin capsule.

enterotoxigenic *Escherichia coli* (ETEC).

Entero Vu (barium sulfate for suspension)—low-density contrast medium used in "see-through" radiographic studies of the small bowel.

Enterra—gastrointestinal "pacemaker" that stimulates nerves lining the stomach to control digestion. Useful in patients with severe gastroparesis that causes continual nausea, vomiting, and pain.

Enteryx—a permanently implanted device used to help patients with symptoms of gastroesophageal reflux disease. The device is a solution made up of a polymer and a solvent that is implanted by injection into the wall of the lower esophagus. After the injection, the solvent separates away, leaving the polymer to solidify into a spongy material that is intended to help prevent the reflux.

Enteryx endoscopic procedure—the endoscopic injection of a liquid polymer into the muscle of the lower esophageal sphincter, using a needle catheter, after which the polymer solidifies into a spongelike permanent implant. This permanent implant may help improve the barrier between the stomach and esophagus by supporting and improving the elasticity of the lower esophageal sphincter to reduce, and sometimes prevent, acid reflux into the esophagus.

Entity pacemaker.

Entree Plus and **Entree II trocar and cannula systems**—for laparoscopic

Entree *(cont.)* surgery. Also referred to as *Core trocars and cannulas.*

Entree—thoracoscopy trocar and cannula.

EntriStar PEG (percutaneous endoscopic gastrostomy) **tube**—polyethylene feeding gastrostomy (or jejunostomy) tube inserted using percutaneous endoscopy. It has a larger internal diameter than other tubes to avoid clogging. The catheter end closes for insertion and removal but opens into a flow-through, three-dimensional star shape in the stomach to maintain tube position and prevent tip obstruction.

Entristar skin-level gastrostomy tube—primary placement with radiologic guidance in patients with amyotrophic lateral sclerosis.

"Entroflex"—phonetic for Enteroflex feeding tube.

EntSol nasal wash system—therapy for nasal and sinus congestion.

enucleation—removal of the eyeball, without taking the eye muscles or the remaining orbital contents. Also, shelling out a tumor from its bed without rupturing it. See also *evisceration, exenteration, extirpation.*

enuresis—bedwetting. Enuresis differs from incontinence in that enuresis more commonly refers to involuntary discharge of urine during sleep. Cf. *anuresis.*

Envacor—a lab test of two HIV proteins.

Envision TD—intravitreal implants with fluocinolone acetonide, in the treatment of diabetic macular edema and posterior uveitis.

Envoy middle ear implantable system—uses a piezoelectric sensor to detect sound vibrations from the malleus bone, which is attached to the back of the eardrum. The system converts those vibrations into electrical signals that are amplified, filtered, and then transmitted as mechanical vibrations through another piezoelectric transducer to the stapes bone, resulting in significant restoration of hearing.

Enzogenol—antioxidant drug derived from the bark of the *Pinus radiata* tree in New Zealand.

enzymatic debriding agents—agents that are selective in removing necrotic tissue. They loosen necrotic debris so that surgical debridement may be avoided. Enzymatic agents act on materials such as collagen, protein, fibrin, elastin, and nucleoproteins. See *dressing.*

enzyme immunoassay technique—screens drugs in the urine that have been present for up to 7 days.

enzyme-linked immunoassay (EIA).

enzyme-linked immunofluorescent assay (ELIFA).

enzyme-linked immunosorbent assay (ELISA).

EOA (esophageal obturator airway).

EOCT (endoscopic optical coherence tomography).

EOD (emergency orders of detention). Usage: "Psychiatric consultation was ordered to evaluate the mental status and to make decisions for EOD."

EOG (electro-oculogram)—used in sleep studies. Usage: "EOG does show some rapid eye movement."

EOPA (elongated one-piece arterial).

EOPA CAP—facilitates peripheral or central arterial cannulation techniques. EOPA (elongated one-piece arterial) cannulae. CAP (central arterial pressure).

eosinophilia-myalgia syndrome (EMS)—multisystem disease with neuromuscular manifestations, the correct name for the group of symptoms resulting from the use of the amino acid L-tryptophan. The clinical picture of severe myalgia, fever, cramps, weakness, and arthralgias can be confused with myositis or trichinosis unless a history of L-tryptophan use is established.

eosinophilic pustular folliculitis—a pruritic skin condition with sterile follicular pustules on an expanding erythematous plaque. Biopsy of pustules at the advancing edge of the plaque shows an eosinophilic abscess within the follicle or sebaceous gland. Before its association with AIDS, this condition had been reported mostly in Japan and affected mostly males.

EP (endoscopic papillectomy).

EP (evoked potential).

EPA (eicosapentaenoic acid).

EPAP (expiratory positive airway pressure).

EPDS (Edinburgh Postnatal Depression Scale).

ependyma—cells lining the fluid-filled central cavity of the brain and spinal cord.

ependymitis granularis—granular inflammation of the lining membrane of the ventricles of the brain.

ependymoma—tumor originating from ependymal cells lining the ventricular system of the central nervous system.

EPF (endoscopic plantar fasciotomy).

"epi"—slang term for epinephrine (Adrenalin). Can also refer to epithelial cell seen in urinalysis.

EPI (echo planar imaging) (MRI term).

epi-ADR, epi-Adriamycin (doxorubicin).

EPIC-C or **EPICS Profile flow cytometer**.

Epicel autologous skin cells—a tissue repair product.

Epic HF ICD (implantable cardioverter-defibrillator)—cardiac resynchronization therapy debrillator.

Epic ophthalmic 3-in-1 laser system.

epicritic two-point sensation (Neuro).

EPID (electronic portal imaging device).

epidermal growth factor (EGF)—a protein involved in the maturation of the epidermis; in the newborn it hastens eyelid opening and tooth eruption. It is given to increase the rate of corneal healing after corneal transplant surgery and is used to accelerate wound healing in partial-thickness wounds and second-degree burns.

epidermodysplasia verruciformis—a rare lifelong disease that is a model of cutaneous genetic cancer induced by specific human papillomaviruses.

epidermolysis bullosa acquisita—a rare mechanobullous disease presenting as skin blistering and scarring at sites of trauma in inflammatory bowel disease.

epididymal sperm aspiration (ESA).

epididymovasostomy—see *microsurgical epididymovasostomy*.

epidural blood patch—injection of the patient's own blood into space around the spine. This is done to repair holes or tears in the spinal fluid sac; it leads to a temporary blood clot that allows time for the sac wall to repair itself.

epidural neuroplasty—pain-relieving procedure in which a catheter is inserted into the epidural space and an

epidural *(cont.)* anesthetic injected directly into the site of nerve injury or adhesion.

EpiE-ZPen (epinephrine 0.3 mg and 0.15 mg)—an autoinjector for use by patients in the emergency treatment of allergic reactions. The device resembles a fountain pen, with a pocket clip for easy carrying. It is disposable and contains a cartridge filled with epinephrine with push-button activation.

EpiFilm club sandwich technique for tympanoplasty—see *club sandwich technique.*

EpiFilm otologic lamina—a biological dressing used to enhance healing of exposed bone during otologic surgery.

Epi-Grip—a medical device used in cardiopulmonary bypass surgery to improve the presentation and isolation of the bypass site.

EpiLaser—laser-based hair removal system.

epileptic equivalent—as in migraine equivalent, some or all of the symptom complex without the convulsion. See *migraine equivalent*.

epileptogenic focus—the area in which tumor-related seizures originate.

Epi-Lock—polyurethane foam wound dressing.

epiluminescence light microscopy (ELM)—high-resolution microscopy used in detecting malignancies in pigmented skin lesions of reticulated black solar lentigo.

epinastine HCl—see *Elestat*.

epinephrine—drug used as an adjunct with local anesthetic to prolong the effectiveness of the anesthetic agent used and to constrict superficial blood vessels. Also, *racemic epinephrine.* Cf. *"epi."*

epiphysis—the end of a long bone, usually wider than the long portion of the bone. Cf. *apophysis, hypophysis, hypothesis*.

episcleral plaque brachytherapy—treatment of subretinal fluid caused by circumscribed choroidal hemangiomas. Cf. *lens-sparing external beam radiation therapy*.

episodic laryngeal dyskinesia (ELD)—another name for vocal cord dysfunction (VCD).

EpiStar Diode Laser System—for hair removal and treatment of vascular and pigmented skin lesions.

Epistat double balloon—used in treatment of uncontrolled epistaxis.

epistaxis—nasal bleeding.

epithelial ingrowth—a complication of endothelial lamellar keratoplasty.

epithelial membrane antigen (EMA)—pathologic finding in benign cystic mesothelioma.

epithelial turn-in flap—used for reconstruction of the internal lining in full-thickness nasal defects.

epitheliosis—the condition of being epithelialized. You will likely hear this term in pathology dictation.

EpiTouch—a laser used for hair removal and in the treatment of tattoos and pigmented lesions.

Epitrain (Ortho)—an elastic elbow support with contoured silicone inserts.

Epivir/Retrovir (lamivudine/zidovudine)—combination AIDS drug.

EPL (extracorporeal piezoelectric lithotriptor)—see *Piezolith-EPL*.

epoxyeicosatrienoic acids—compounds produced naturally in the body that trigger arteries to dilate and help prevent adhesion of monocytes to artery walls, thus lessening atherosclerotic plaque buildup.

EPS (electrophysiologic study)—used to assess ventricular arrhythmias.

Epstein-Barr virus (EBV)—the herpes-like virus known to cause mononucleosis, with evidence that it plays a part in susceptibility to Burkitt lymphoma, and possibly to AIDS.

EPT-Dx steerable diagnostic catheters.

ePTFE (expanded polytetrafluoroethylene)—used for facial implants in plastic and reconstructive surgery.

EPT-1000 XP cardiac ablation catheter—see *Blazer II XP*.

Epworth Sleepiness Scale—for evaluation of effects of obstructive sleep apnea.

Epzicom (abacavir sulfate 600 mg and lamivudine 300 mg)—a fixed-dose combination of antiretroviral drugs for the treatment of HIV infection.

Equate *Legionella* water test—an on-site detection of *Legionella* bacteria in water supplies.

equilibratory ataxia—the disturbance of equilibratory coordination, with abnormal gait and station. On testing gait and station, the physician is ruling in/out lesions of the vermis, labyrinthine-vestibular apparatus, and frontopontocerebellar pathways.

Equinox occlusion balloon system—for occluding and controlling distal blood flow during vascular procedures. The balloon is introduced via the SilverSpeed guidewire.

equipment artifact (Radiol)—produced by some equipment, such as surgical sponges or pillows used for patient positioning, that is not radiopaque as advertised.

equivalent—as in anginal equivalent, migraine equivalent, epilepsy equivalent. An atypical pain syndrome in which the location or character of the pain differs from that usually experienced. Usage: "It is not clear whether this left shoulder discomfort radiating down his arm is arthritic or may be an anginal equivalent."

ER (estrogen receptor).

ER (evoked response) (Neuro).

ERA (endometrial resection and ablation) **resectoscope sheath**—used for minimally invasive procedures such as endometrial resection and ablation, myomectomy, and polypectomy.

ERBD (endoscopic retrograde biliary drainage).

Erb-Duchenne paralysis—see *Erb palsy*.

erbium:YAG infrared laser (Er: YAG) —now approved for use directly on teeth. The laser has been shown to be as safe and effective as high-speed drills for removing dental decay.

Erb palsy—injury to the fifth and sixth cervical roots, causing flaccid paralysis of the entire arm, without involving the small muscles of the hand. Also called *Erb-Duchenne paralysis* and *Duchenne paralysis*.

ERC (endoscopic retrograde cholangiography).

ERCP (endoscopic retrograde cholangiopancreatogram)—study of the gallbladder, pancreas, and biliary system through an endoscope and a special cannula.

ErCr:YAG (erbium chromium: yttrium-aluminum-garnet) **laser**.

Erdheim-Chester disease—a rare lipid storage disorder characterized by hardening of the growth areas of the long bones of the body. Lipid cell deposits (histiocytes) are found in various vital organs of the body such as heart, lungs, peritoneum, kidneys,

Erdheim *(cont.)*
and other tissues. Severity of the disease differs with each patient, but the cause is unknown and the outcome is generally fatal.

ErecAid system—nonsurgical treatment for erectile impotence.

ERG (electroretinogram)—see *flicker electroretinogram.*

Ergos O_2 pacemaker—a dual chamber rate-responsive pacemaker.

Erich arch bar (Oral Surg).

Erlanger and Gasser—classification of peripheral nerves.

Ernest-McDonald soft IOL folding forceps—used for placement of thin, soft intraocular lenses.

Ernst, space of—pterygoid-superior constrictor space.

erogenous zones—areas of the body that produce feelings of sexual desire when stimulated. Cf. *aerogenous.*

Eros-CTD (clitoral therapy device)—treatment for female sexual dysfunction (FSD).

ER/PR (estrogen receptor/progesterone receptor).

ER/PR-negative infiltrating ductal carcinoma of the breast—estrogen receptor-negative and progesterone receptor-negative ductal carcinoma of the breast.

ERT (estrogen replacement therapy).

ERT patch—for treatment of vasomotor symptoms related to menopause.

erythema migrans (EM)—a rash that appears after a bite of the tick (*Ixodes dammini*) that transmits the organism (*Borrelia burgdorferi*) that causes Lyme disease. The rash is circular in form, target-like, may disappear and reappear, often in another site (hence migrans). It may be the first symptom of Lyme disease. See *target lesion.*

erythema nodosum leprosum (ENL)—a skin complication of leprosy.

erythematous vulvitis en plaque—see *vulvar vestibulitis syndrome.*

Erythroflex—a hydromer-coated central venous catheter that resists thrombus formation.

erythroplasia of Queyrat—an intraepidermal squamous cell carcinoma that presents as a well-demarcated moist red patch on the penis. Also referred to as *carcinoma in situ of the glans penis.*

ES (endoscopic sphincterotomy).

ESA (epididymal sperm aspiration).

ESAT-6 protein—may be effective in diagnosing *Mycobacterium tuberculosis.*

Escala Inteligencia Wechsler Para Adultos (EIWA).

escape pacemaker (Cardiol). Unless an escape pacemaker takes over pacing the ventricles, ventricular standstill occurs and there will be only P waves on the EKG tracing.

Eschmann blade (*not* Ashman)—used to debride wounds. Usage: "I also used the Eschmann blade to superficially debride the proximal forearm and remove necrotic subcutaneous tissue from that location."

Esclim—estradiol transdermal drug system for treatment of vasomotor symptoms of menopause, vulvar and vaginal atrophy, and abnormal vaginal bleeding.

escutcheon—the triangular-shaped area over the pubic bone.

E-Scope—electronic stethoscope that allows amplification of heart, breath, and Korotkoff sounds without accentuation of background noise. Can be used with hearing aid or second listener.

Escort balloon stone extractor—designed for easy cannulation and fluoroscopic visibility.

ESLD (end-stage liver disease).

Esmarch ("Ez-mark") **bandage**—used as a tourniquet.

esodeviation ("ee-so")—inward deviation of the eye; also, *esotropia, esophoria.*

EsophaCoil self-expanding esophageal stent—used to minimize dysphagia and help restore swallowing and nutritional intake for patients with malignant strictures.

esophageal achalasia—failure of the esophagogastric sphincter to relax in swallowing, resulting in dilation. It is treated with laparoscopic Heller myotomy and Toupet fundoplication.

esophageal dysmotility (Radiol)—seen on upper GI series; abnormality in the strength or coordination of peristaltic movements in the esophagus.

esophageal gastric tube airways (EGTA).

esophageal obturator airways (EOA).

esophageal pill electrode—a disposable EKG lead encased in a gelatin capsule which is swallowed by the patient. Two attached wires exit through the patient's mouth and are attached to an EKG machine. When the gelatin capsule dissolves, electrical activity from the heart can be detected. The esophageal electrode is thus better able to record the electrical activity of the atrial contraction which is obscured with standard EKG leads.

esophageal sling procedure—see *ligamentum teres cardiopexy*.

esophageal stenosis, congenital—see *congenital esophageal stenosis*.

esophageal stretching—a treatment for esophageal atresia. Four pledgeted sutures are attached to the esophagus proximally and distally, placed under traction, and tightened daily. The procedure allows the esophagus to lengthen by 5 to 10 cm in 6 to 19 days.

esophageal Z-Stent with Dua antireflux valve.

esophagodiverticulostomy, endoscopic, staple-assisted—surgical treatment for Zenker diverticulum. A bivalved endoscope is placed through the mouth to expose the cricopharyngeus. Similar to the Dohlman procedure, one blade is placed in the Zenker diverticulum and the other in the cervical esophagus. Under endoscopic visualization with a 0° Hopkins rod telescope, a GI stapler is used to resect the common wall.

esophagogastroduodenoscopy (EGD)—examination of the esophagus, stomach, and duodenum using an endoscope.

esotropia—turning inward of the eye; crossed-eye or cross-eyed.

ESP—automated blood culture system.

esprolol plus Viagra (sildenafil citrate)—drug regimen thought to protect men with heart disease who are also taking Viagra.

ESRD (end-stage renal disease).

Essex-Lopresti lesion—disruption of the distal radioulnar joint.

Essiac—one of the most popular herbal cancer drug alternatives in North America, comprised of four herbs—burdock, Turkey rhubarb, sorrel, and slippery elm. Although illegal in the U.S., it is nevertheless widely available. Researchers at the Memorial Sloan-Kettering Cancer Center claim it has no anticancer effect. The herbal formula was named by spelling backward the name of the developer, a nurse named Rene Caisse.

"ess-pep"—phonetic for *SPEP* (serum protein electrophoresis)

Essure sterilization system—a nonsurgical but permanent alternative to tubal ligation in women. The procedure takes about 10-20 minutes in a doctor's office using local anesthesia. During the implantation procedure, a doctor uses a special catheter to insert one of the devices into each of a woman's two fallopian tubes. The device works by causing scar tissue to form over the implant, blocking the fallopian tube and preventing fertilization of the egg by thc sperm. It is an irreversible procedure.

Estalis—combination estrogen/progesterone transdermal drug delivery system.

Esterman visual function score—used as the standard, adopted by the American Medical Association, for rating visual field disability (glaucoma). Obtained from the patient's responses to a disability questionnaire. Scores range from I-4-e to V-4-e. (Benjamin Esterman, M.D.)

esthetic(s)—relating to pleasing appearance, beautiful. While *aesthetic* is preferred in artistic contexts, *esthetic* is often seen in plastic, dental, and maxillofacial surgery journals.

e-stim—short form for *electrical stimulation*. It should be expanded in medical transcripts.

estramustine binding protein (EMBP).

Estring—an estradiol-loaded silicone vaginal ring for treatment of postmenopausal women with symptoms of urogenital aging.

estrogen—may prevent stress-induced constriction in the arteries, as estrogen opens arteries and allows blood to flow freely in conditions of cold-related stress. Angina and heart attacks occur more often in cold weather.

estrogen receptor (ER)—a cytoplasmic protein. Estrogen receptor tests of breast cancer tissue reflect the degree of hormone dependency of that particular breast cancer. If there is a high degree of hormone dependency, an oophorectomy may be performed to alter the course of the disease.

estrogen replacement therapy (ERT)—drug regimen used to treat symptoms of stress urinary incontinence. Estrogen (given orally, as a transdermal patch, or applied vaginally as a topical cream) has long been used to counteract the symptoms of vaginal dryness, hot flashes, and fatigue experienced by postmenopausal women. It is now known that decreased levels of estrogen have an adverse effect on the function of the urethra as well as the genitalia. The urethra has a concentration of estrogen receptors similar to that of the vagina. Decreased estrogen levels alter nerve conduction and elasticity of the urethral mucosa. Restoring estrogen levels to normal appears to decrease stress urinary incontinence in some women.

EstroLogic—a natural supplement for estrogen balance.

ESU (electrosurgical unit) **dispersive** (grounding) **pad**.

ESWL (extracorporeal shock wave lithotripsy). See *lithotriptor*.

ET (embryo transfer).

ETAC (electrothermally assisted capsulorrhaphy).

etafilcon A (Acuvue)—disposable contact lens.

ETCG (endoscopic transpapillary catheterization of the gallbladder).

$ETCO_2$ (end-tidal carbon dioxide).

ETEC (enterotoxigenic *Escherichia coli*).

Ethalloy TruTaper cardiovascular needle.

ethanol—alcohol, EtOH.

ethers—see *dihematoporphyrin ethers*.

Ethibond—polyester suture with prethreaded Teflon pledgets.

Ethicon—manufacturer of Teflon paste and numerous surgical products.

Ethiflex—a synthetic suture material. Ethibond, Ethiflex, and Ethilon sutures are all manufactured by Ethicon, but they have different coating materials.

Ethilon—a monofilament nylon suture with extremely low tissue reactions. It comes in black, green, and clear and is a nonabsorbable suture.

ethylene vinyl alcohol (EVAL).

E to A changes—egophony on auscultation of the chest. On chest examination the patient's "e" sounds like "a" through a stethoscope. The sound of "e" indicates normal lung, "a" indicates consolidated lung.

EtOH (lowercase "t")—ethanol, ethyl alcohol.

e-Touch technology—combines data from regular ultrasound with a force-feedback mechanism to produce a medical virtual reality (VR) experience without goggles or gloves. Example: Touch the image of a fetal cheek with a handheld stylus, and signals sent from the computer to mechanical motors in the stylus simulate the sensation of pressing against soft skin. Move the stylus across the fetus's face and feel the contours of its nose, lips, and ears.

e-TRAIN 110 AngioJet catheter.

ETS (endoscopic thoracic sympathectomy).

ETS Flex 45-3.5—45-mm endoscopic linear stapler.

ETT (exercise tolerance test)—see *MPHR and Bruce protocol*.

EUA (examination under anesthesia).

euboxic—said of a laboratory test whose result falls within the "normal" box on the automated report printout.

EUCAST—a laboratory test using spectrophotometric determination techniques to determine fungal susceptibility to antifungal agents.

Eucerin—proprietary name of wool fat-based cream.

eugenics—the theory or practice of preserving genetic traits that are considered positive or advantageous within a population while annihilating traits considered undesirable; methods range from manipulating the reproductive behavior or outcomes of a population to involuntary sterilization and genocide.

eugenic tourism—traveling to a country where cloning and inheritable genetic modification is legal in order to undergo a procedure which is illegal or ethically unacceptable in one's own country.

euglobulin lysis activity (ELA).

eukaryote—any organism whose cells have a true nucleus containing genetic information stored in chromosomes.

eukaryotic cells—cells with a true nucleus.

Eular (extended release oxymorphone) —an opioid drug for osteoarthritis pain.

Euler-Byrne (EB) **score**—a method of evaluating the severity of gastroesophageal reflux using the number of episodes in a specified period of time. Also *Euler-Byrne index, Euler-Byrne formula*.

EU-M30S—endoscopic ultrasonography receiver from Olympus.

Euro-Collins multiorgan perfusion kit—used for organ procurement and preservation.

EUS (endoscopic ultrasonography).

EUS-FNA (endoscopic ultrasound-guided fine needle aspiration).

eutectic mixture of local anesthetics (EMLA) (lidocaine and prilocaine) **anesthesia**.

euthymic—normal thymus gland function.

euthyroid—normal thyroid gland function.

EVac—wet field wand for tissue ablation, coagulation, and suction in tonsillotomy.

EVac CAT—minimally invasive procedure for the treatment of snoring, with the creation of channels in the soft palate.

evac'd, evaced, e-vac'd—brief forms for *evacuated*, meaning transported via air ambulance. *Evacuated* should be transcribed.

Evacet—liposome-encapsulated doxorubicin for treatment of metastatic breast cancer.

EVAL (ethylene vinyl alcohol)—used for liquid embolization of spinal angiomas (as in Cobb syndrome). EVAL (not a glue) is used in the same way as cyanoacrylate.

Evans-Burkhalter protocol—rehabilitation following tendon repair.

Evans tenodesis—reconstruction of the peroneus brevis tendon to treat chronic lateral ankle instability by reattaching the tendon to the muscle in a slightly overlapped fashion.

EVAR (endovascular aortic repair).

Eve procedure—the transfer of vascularized seventh rib, fascia, cartilage, and serratus muscle to other anatomic areas to reconstruct severe defects. The procedure is named for Eve, who in the Bible was said to be created from one of Adam's ribs.

Evershears—a surgical instrument that combines a curved scissors tip at the end of a bipolar electrocautery. Used in laparoscopic surgery.

Evershears II bipolar curved scissors—bipolar curved scissors with cutting and coagulating capability indicated for use in laparoscopic surgical procedures.

Evert-O-Cath—drug delivery catheter.

evisceration—(1) removal of the contents of the eyeball, but leaving the shell of sclera—see *enucleation*; (2) disemboweling; exenteration; extirpation; splitting open of a surgical wound and subsequent spillage of its contents.

EVIS 140 endoscope reprocessing system.

EVL (endoscopic variceal ligation).

EVOH (ethylene vinyl alcohol copolymer).

evoked potential (EP)—a noninvasive way to examine the functional integrity of the central nervous system. It demonstrates the response of the brain to electrical stimulation. EPs are used as indicators, both diagnostic and prognostic, in patients with head injuries. See *brain tests, noninvasive*.

evoked response (ER) (Neuro)—see *brain tests, noninvasive*; also *EP*.

evolutionary medicine—see *darwinian medicine.*

Evolution XP scanner—an ultrafast CT scanner.

Evolve Cardiac Continuum—designed to support physicians in a systematic approach from open-chest surgery to endoscopic beating-heart surgery,

Evolve *(cont.)*
integrating computer and robotic technology.

EVS (endoscopic variceal sclerotherapy)—to control variceal hemorrhage, particularly due to portal hypertension.

EVUS (endovaginal ultrasound).

Ewald tube—used in gastric lavage.

Ewart sign—pericardial effusion.

Ewing sarcoma—osteosarcoma.

ExAblate 2000 system—medical device that uses MRI-guided focused ultrasound to target and destroy benign uterine fibroids. The treatment requires repeated targeting and heating of fibroid tissue while the patient lies inside the MRI machine. The procedure can last as long as three hours. Fibroids close to sensitive organs such as the bowel or bladder and those outside the image area cannot be treated.

Exactech total knee system.

Exact-Fit ATH—hip replacement system.

ExacTech blood glucose meter—for self-testing by diabetics.

examination—see *test*.

eXamine cholangiography catheter.

excavatum, pectus—*not* excurvatum.

Excelart—short-bore MRI with wide opening, said to be very quiet.

eXcel-DR (disposable/reusable) **instruments**
a-fiX cannula seals
eXcel-DR pneumo needle
eXpose retractor
eXtract specimen bag
heliX knot pusher

Excel GE—electrochemical glucose monitoring test strip for use with Glucometer Elite R meters.

excess—the degree or state of surplus, or beyond the usual. Usage: "There was excess peritoneal fluid present." See *base excess*. Cf. *access, axis*.

excimer laser—*excimer,* a word coined from *excited dimer*. The laser uses ultraviolet light.

excimer laser coronary angioplasty (ELCA)—used in percutaneous revascularization for coronary artery disease.

excision—removal, as of an organ, by cutting. Cf. *incision*.

Excluder bifurcated endoprosthesis—a low-profile self-expanding cardiac stent.

exenterative surgery for pelvic cancer—removal of organs and adjacent structures of the pelvis. Usually performed to surgically ablate cancer involving urinary bladder, uterine cervix, and/or rectum.

Exercise Self-efficacy Scale—used to measure a patient's confidence in treadmill performance ability.

exercise tolerance test (ETT).

EX-FI-RE external fixation system—for reduction and fixation of long bones and for limb lengthening.

ex-fix—external fixator, external fixation.

EXIT (ex utero intrapartum treatment) **procedure**—surgical treatments of the fetus.

ex lap—slang; expand to *exploratory laparotomy.*

exodeviation—outward deviation of the eye; also, exotropia, exophoria.

Exogen SAFHS (sonic accelerated fracture healing system)—a low-intensity ultrasound therapy in an in-home, non-invasive, portable unit.

exon—a coding sequence of DNA in a gene, that is, a sequence that functions to direct the synthesis of a protein. Compare *intron*.

Exorcist—a respiratory compensation technique—MRI term.

expandable access catheter (EAC).

expandable esophageal stent (EES).

expandable metallic stent—used as an alternative to the plastic stent. It offers ease of insertion and lack of migration. Its risks include erosion of adjacent vital structures, difficulty in adjustment or removal, and overgrowth of malignant tissue.

Expandacell sinus pack—used to prevent lateralization of the middle turbinate after functional endoscopic sinus surgery, absorb postoperative fluids, and aid in maintaining antibiotic at the surgical site.

"expedior"—see *Xpeedior 100 catheter.*

Expedium MIS spine system—a spinal fixation system for the treatment of degenerative disk disease.

expiratory positive airway pressure (EPAP).

expire—to exhale, or to take one's last breath, i.e., to die.

explorer—see *Xplorer imaging.*

Explorer ST fixed curve diagnostic catheters.

Explorer 360° rotational diagnostic catheters.

Explorer X 70 intraoral radiography system.

eXpose (trademark) **retractor**—comes in three shapes: inflatable triangle, U, and wand shapes. (Note the initial lowercase *e* and capital *X*.)

exposure osteotomy—various types of osteotomies used especially for osteochondral or autologous chondrocyte grafts.

express—see *X-PRESS vascular closure system.*

expressivity (Genetics)—the extent to which a genetic trait or defect is expressed in individuals carrying the relevant gene; for some genes it may vary widely among individuals.

Express PTCA catheter (percutaneous transluminal coronary angioplasty).

Express2 coronary stent system—a laser-cut balloon-expanded stent. The Express2 stent (combined with Maverick balloon catheter technology, Bioslide hydrophilic coating designed to reduce friction, and proprietary Crimp 360 technology to secure the stent to the balloon) is said to offer greater flexibility and trackability. There is no space between the name and the numeral.

exquisite—said of extremely severe pain or tenderness, as exquisite tenderness of the breast.

exstrophy—congenital eversion of an organ, as of the bladder.

extended right hepatectomy—a surgical option in patients with hilar bile duct cancer.

extension (*not* extention).

extensive intraductal component (EIC) —risk factor leading to recurrence in young women with breast cancer.

external beam radiation therapy (EBRT)—using linear accelerator or cobalt machine, to irradiate internal structures from an external source.

external cephalic version (ECV) (Ob-Gyn)—repositioning of a fetus using I.V. terbutaline and vibroacoustic stimulation. It is performed to avoid vaginal breech delivery or cesarean section.

external elastic lamina (EEL).

extinction phenomenon—when the patient is touched in the same area on both sides of the body and perceives it on only one side. May be indicative of a lesion of the sensory cortex.

extirpation—see *evisceration.*

extra-articular harvest—occurs in bone graft harvesting from iliac crest and Gerdy tubercle that contributes to increased morbidity of the graft.

extracapsular cataract extraction (ECCE).

extracellular matrix (ECM).

extracorporeal circulation—using the heart-lung machine to provide circulation outside the body during heart surgery.

extracorporeal life support (ECE).

extracorporeal membrane oxygenation therapy (ECMO).

extracorporeal photochemotherapy (ECP)—see *Theralux*.

extracorporeal photoimmune therapy—involves use of ultraviolet or visible light and compounds that are activated by such light to alter function of blood cells or blood components. See also *photophoresis*.

extracorporeal piezoelectric lithotriptor (Piezolith-EPL)—device with a single-focus dish which directs all of the shock waves to the renal stone or gallstone, eliminating any unfocused shock waves that could cause the patient pain or discomfort (thus eliminating the need for anesthesia). The stone is reduced to fragments 2 mm or less in size which are then readily passed by the patient.

extracorporeal shock wave lithotripsy (ESWL)—see *lithotriptor*.

extract—see *XTRAC*.

extractor—an instrument to remove a metal implant from bone. See *Glassman stone extractor*.

Extractor three-lumen retrieval balloon.

eXtract specimen bag—an expandable bag for isolating organs or specimens retrieved during laparoscopic surgery, e.g., a gallbladder with stones, to prevent stone spillage in abdomen.

extradural clinoidectomy—a surgical approach to enter the anterior cavernous sinus, to expose aneurysms of the C4–C6 segments of the internal carotid artery, to resect the dural attachment and hyperostotic bone, and as part of a transcavernous approach to produce wider exposure of basilar artery aneurysms of the upper clival region.

extraperitoneal excision of lower one-third of ureter—a urologic procedure making a bladder cuff without an initial vesicotomy, without injury to the opposite ureteric orifice. It is used to treat urothelial tumors of the kidney and ureter. Advantages of this procedure are said to be minimal blood loss, a small vesicotomy, and easy suturing of the bladder.

extrapyramidal signs (or symptoms)—involuntary movements such as tics or tremors, or impairment of involuntary movement such as rigidity, secondary to antipsychotic drugs or chemical imbalances in the brain. See *tardive dyskinesia*. Cf. *pyramidal signs, akathisia*.

Extra Sport coronary guidewire—coronary guidewire marketed under the ACS Hi-Torque group of guidewires.

extravasation detection accessory (EDA)—for use during contrast-enhanced CT studies performed with a power injector. The EDA keeps contrast material from leaking into surrounding soft tissues by halting the infusion when extravasation is detected.

extravasation of contrast—leakage of contrast medium from the structure

extravasation *(cont.)* into which it is injected through a perforation or other abnormal orifice.

Extra View balloon—used in laparoscopic procedures to create extraperitoneal space.

extreme drug resistance (EDR) **assay.**

extremis, in—at the point of death.

ExtreSafe—needles, lancets, phlebotomy devices, catheters, syringes, and butterflies that minimize the risk of accidental needle sticks.

Exubera (inhaled insulin)—inhaled drug that is a dry powder formulation of insulin, developed for patients with type 1 and type 2 diabetes.

exudate, cotton-wool.

ExuDerm hydrocolloid dressing material.

Exu-Dry absorptive dressing.

ex utero intrapartum treatment (EXIT) **procedure**.

ex vivo (L., outside of the living body)—usually means about the same as *in vitro*. Usage: "He mentioned that in the near future there will be a commercial concern which is able to grow blood ex vivo and to have the cells then harvested for therapeutic transfusions."

ex vivo liver-directed gene therapy—used for the treatment of familial hypercholesterolemia. A liver segmentectomy is performed and the specimen delivered to the laboratory, where hepatocytes are isolated and exposed to a recombinant retrovirus. The hepatocytes are then harvested and infused back into the patient via the mesenteric vein.

Exxcel ePTFE soft vascular graft.

eye of the Scotty dog—the target point on oblique views of the spine for medial branch nerve block by spinal injection.

eye movement tracking techniques—electro-oculography, infrared scleral reflection technique, Purkinje image tracking, scleral search coil, and video pupil scanning. They are valuable for early detection and localization of central nervous system lesions.

Eysenck Personality Inventory—a 6-item inventory used to measure neuroticism; that is, a tendency to worry and be anxious, irrational, and shy as well as to suffer from feelings of guilt and low self-esteem.

EZ Detect—colorectal screening test kit.

ezetimibe—see *Zetia*.

E-Z Flap—a mini-plate system constructed from titanium, used in neurosurgical procedures.

E-Z Flex jaw therapy—patented mandibular rehabilitation exercise system designed to treat pain in jaws and the sides of the face.

EZ-Screen Profile—urine drug screening test for marijuana, cocaine, opiates, amphetamines, and PCP. The device was developed primarily for employers. The screening device is about the size of a credit card, no laboratory evaluation is required, and results are available in less than 10 minutes on site.

E-Z Tac soft-tissue reattachment system—cuts operative procedure time by securing soft tissues without sutures, without knot tying, and without the need for a guidewire.

eZY WRAP—orthopedic products including splints, abdominal binders, elbow supports, rib belts, and foam positioners.

F, f

F—Plasma F is plasma cortisol, or a dictator may speak of "free F in the urine."

FA (femoral anteversion)—hip dysplasia measurement in children with cerebral palsy.

Fab (fragment, antigen-binding)—acronym, as used in Fab fragment, Fab region, Fab segment. See *digoxin immune Fab (ovine) fragments.*

FAB (French/American/British)—morphologic classification of acute nonlymphoid leukemia, as used in the format, FAB T2N1M0 (no subscripts). See *TNM classification.*

M1 myeloblastic, with no differentiation
M2 myeloblastic, with differentiation
M3 promyelocytic
M4 myelomonocytic
M5 monocytic
M6 erythroleukemia

fabere sign—acronym for the maneuvers of Patrick test for hip-joint disease: **f**lexion, **ab**duction, **e**xternal **r**otation, **e**xtension.

Fabry lipid storage disease (Oph)—verticillate (whorl-shaped) keratopathy.

facet denervation—treatment for disabling spinal pain that fails to respond to conservative treatment. Also known as *percutaneous radiofrequency facet rhizotomy.*

facial—pertaining to the face. Cf. *falcial, fascial.*

facial resurfacing—used to describe laser and chemical peel ablation of facial blemishes.

facies (singular noun), as in "The facies is tense and anxious."

facilitated angioplasty—so-called when adjunctive angioplasty is performed immediately after atherectomy or excimer laser angioplasty.

facioscapulohumeral dystrophy (FSHD).

facioscapulohumeral (FSH) **muscular dystrophy**.

faciotomy, medial (*not* fasciotomy)—a term coined for a somewhat rare procedure, also referred to as four-walled osteotomy or facial bipartition, for the skeletal treatment of orbital hypertelorism.

FACS (fluorescence-activated cell sorter)—FACS-sorted cells.

FACScan (fluorescence-activated cell sorter) **flow cytometer**.

FACSVantage cell sorter.

Factive (gemifloxacin)—a potent quinolone antibiotic drug for the treatment of respiratory and urinary tract infections.

factor (see also *coagulation factors)*
autocrine motility (AMF)
basic fibroblast growth (bFGF)
blood coagulation
brain-derived neutrotrophic (BDNF)
cardiac risk
coagulation
corticotropin-releasing (CRF)
epidermal growth
fibroblast growth
human fibroblast growth factor-I (FGF-I)
IGF-1 (insulin-like growth factor 1)
IL4-PE (interleukin-4-*Pseudomonas* exotoxin fusion protein)
Leiden
leukemia inhibitory (LIF)
megakaryocyte growth and development (MGDF)
Michelangelo
nerve growth (NGF)
recombinant human insulin-like growth (rhIGF)
recombinant platelet-derived growth (rPDGF)
ReFacto antihemophilic (recombinant)
Repifermin (keratinocyte growth factor 2 [KGF-2])
Rh (Rhesus)
rheumatoid (RF)
Stuart
thymic humoral
tumor necrosis (TNF)
vascular endothelial growth (VEGF)
von Willebrand (vWF)

FACT (Focal Angioplasty Catheter Technology) coronary balloon angioplasty catheters.

FACT (Functional Assessment of Cancer Therapy)—a scale for assessing the functional capabilities of cancer patients while undergoing therapy.

factor V Leiden—inherited trait that causes clotting disorders (thrombophilia). You may also hear it referred to as *Leiden factor*.

Factor III multimer assay.

Faden retropexy—posterior fixation suture procedure used in strabismus surgery.

Fader Tip ureteral stent—a Percuflex stent with a tip that dissolves in one to two hours in the body, leaving a wide hole for maximum drainage.

fadir sign—acronym for maneuvers used to test the hip joint: **f**lexion, **ad**duction, **i**nternal **r**otation.

Fagan test—used to detect retardation in infants. A six-month-old is shown a picture for a certain period of time. Later, the infant is shown the same picture and a new picture. The amount of time the infant looks at the new picture correlates with overall intelligence.

failed back surgery syndrome (FBSS) —seen in patients who have persistent back pain following back surgery. Further testing often reveals a migrated disk fragment, another disk herniation at a different level, previously undetected lateral recess syndrome (stenosis), a tethered nerve root, an anomalous root, or tumor above the level of the previous surgery.

failure to thrive (FTT)—in infants or the severely debilitated, or a patient making no progress despite treatment.

Fajersztajn crossed sciatic sign.

falcial—see *falcine region*. Cf. *facial, fascial*.

Falcinelli OOKP—a two-stage surgical technique for osteo-odontokeratoprosthesis (OOKP).

falcine region—either the region of the falx cerebelli or the falx cerebri. Also *falcial*.

Falcon coronary catheter.

fallen fragment—diagnostic of unicameral bone cyst on radiography. A portion of the wall of the cyst undergoes a pathologic fracture and subsequently floats down (falls) via gravity into the dependent portion of the cyst.

falloposcope (flexible fallopian tube endoscope).

falloposcopy—an imaging method used in diagnosis and treatment of infertility by providing views of the interior of the fallopian tube. In this procedure, a flexible catheter is inserted into the fallopian tube, after which a flexible fallopian tube endoscope (falloposcope) with imaging fibers is inserted and slowly withdrawn while taking images of the lumen of the tube.

Fallot pentalogy—tetralogy of Fallot plus atrial septal defect. See *Fallot trilogy, tetralogy of Fallot*.

Fallot trilogy—congenital cyanotic heart disease that includes pulmonary stenosis and atrial septal defect, but does not have any ventricular septal defect. See *Fallot pentalogy, tetralogy of Fallot*.

Falope ring (Ob-Gyn).

false labor—see *Braxton Hicks contractions*.

false memory syndrome (Psych)—a controversial condition in which an adult patient "recalls" episodes of childhood sexual abuse and sometimes memories of satanic ritual and child sacrifice for which there is no documentation available. The psychiatric community is split over the issue, some believing the patient's memories are of actual events; others believe the memories to have been prompted by overzealous counselors and the patient's desire to please the counselor. The American Psychiatric Association has issued a position statement on the syndrome and guidelines for evaluating patients with restored memories of traumatic events from infancy and childhood.

false negative—a test result that is normal or negative despite the presence in the patient of a disease or condition that would be expected to produce an abnormal or positive test result.

false positive—an abnormal or positive test result in a patient who is healthy or free from the condition tested for.

falx cerebri—a sickle-shaped fold of tough connective tissue partially separating the two cerebral hemispheres.

familial—referring to a trait or defect that is more prevalent among the members of a given family than in the general population.

familial adenomatous polyposis (FAP)—an inherited autosomal dominant disease. Affected individuals develop polyps throughout the GI tract, most frequently in the colon. Surgical measures include total proctocolectomy and end ileostomy, total proctocolectomy with ileoanal pouch anastomosis (IPAA), and total abdominal colectomy with ileorectal anastomosis.

familial visceral neuropathy—an inherited disorder characterized by

familial *(cont.)* polyneuropathy, ophthalmoplegia, leukoencephalopathy, and intestinal pseudo-obstruction. The latter is caused by destruction of the gastrointestinal myenteric plexus resulting in dysmotility, early satiety, bloating, nausea and vomiting, abdominal distention, diarrhea, weight loss, and malnutrition. Neuronal destruction of other parts of the peripheral and central nervous system may be present as well. This syndrome can be fatal.

Family Assessment Measure III (FAM III)—a self-reporting measure of overall family functioning.

Family Inventory of Life Events and Changes (FILE)—a self-report instrument that records normative and non-normative changes, life events, and strains experienced by the family unit.

Family Medical Leave Act (FMLA).

FAMMM (familial atypical multiple mole melanoma) **syndrome**.

FAM III (Family Assessment Measure III).

FANA (fluorescent antinuclear antibody).

F&G (feeder and grower)—a term used to describe normal infants. Usage: "The infant was basically an F&G in the nursery."

FAPGAR—Family APGAR questionnaire. See *APGAR*.

FAP (familial adenomatous polyposis).

FAPs (fibrillating action potentials).

Faraday shield—MRI term.

faradic (electrical) **stimulation**—named for Michael Faraday, English physicist, 1791-1867.

farmer's lung disease—extrinsic allergic alveolitis caused by exposure to moldy hay.

farnesoid X receptor (FXR) **agonist**—an agent that may provide hepatoprotection in conditions of cholestasis by increasing the capacity for bile excretion from the hepatocyte and by decreasing bile acid biosynthesis.

Farr test—a specific test for anti-DNA antibodies in screening for systemic lupus erythematosus (SLE). High titers of anti-DNA antibodies would be diagnostic of SLE.

farsightedness—see *presbyopia*.

Fas—one of a family of cell-surface death receptors. One of the better known of this family is the smaller type 1 receptor for the cytokine tumor necrosis factor (TNF).

fascial—pertaining to the subcutaneous layer of fascia found throughout the body and encountered during surgery. Cf. *facial, falcial*.

fascia lata suburethral sling—used in treating recurrent urinary stress incontinence.

Fast-Cath introducer catheter.

Fastex—proprioceptive and agility test.

fast-Fourier transform (FFT)—MRI term.

fast low-angle shot (FLASH)—MRI term.

F.A.S.T. (First Access for Shock and Trauma) **1 System**—provides rapid, reliable access to a patient's blood stream to administer drugs and fluids for intraosseous infusion through a sternal insertion site.

fast spin-echo acquisition (MRI)—2-D or 3-D technique used in MR cholangiography.

FastTake electrochemical blood glucose monitoring system.

FASTak suture anchor system—used in arthroscopic surgery.

FasT-Fix—meniscal anchor and repair system.

fastidious organisms—microorganisms that are difficult or impossible to culture on standard laboratory media because they require special nutrients or grow only at a certain temperature, pH, or concentration of oxygen or carbon dioxide.

FastPack System—fully automated blood analyzer designed to perform quantitative immunoassay tests in physician offices and small labs.

fast track product—a designation by FDA that means the agency will facilitate the development and expedite the review of a drug if it is intended for the treatment of a serious or life-threatening condition and it demonstrates the potential to address unmet medical needs for such a condition.

fast-twitch fibers (Sports Med)—fast runners have relatively more of these in their skeletal muscles than the rest of the population.

FasTrac guidewire—hydrophilic-coated guidewire for smooth tracking.

fat- and water-suppressed T2-weighted images (MRI)—used in the diagnosis of optic neuritis.

fat-blood interface (FBI) **sign**—diagnostic of lipohemarthrosis on radiographs of the knee.

fat depot ("de-po")—area in the body of deposit of stored fat. Usage: "The face was very bony, showing loss of fat depots."

fat doctor—bariatrician; a specialist in treating obesity.

fat embolism syndrome (FES)—a type of adult respiratory distress syndrome. A complication of long-bone fracture or trauma to fatty tissues, FES occurs when an embolus of fat lodges in the lungs.

fat pad sign—distention and displacement of fat adjacent to a joint capsule, in elbow or knee, visible on x-ray with joint flexion. A sign of fracture within the joint. Usage: "X-rays of the right elbow show no acute bony injury or any posterior fat pad sign per the radiologist's interpretation."

FAT SAT—slang for fat saturation technique.

fat towels (or wound towels)—used in surgery to protect tissues, to keep them from losing moisture.

Faulkner folder—an instrument that holds an intraocular lens in a folded position for insertion in cataract surgery.

faulty RF (radiofrequency) **shielding in MRI scanner room**.

Favaloro-Morris retractor.

FAZ (foveal avascular zone) (Oph).

FBI (fat-blood interface) sign (Radiol) —a very suggestive sign of underlying fracture extending into the joint. Fat-fluid interface is seen on multiple lateral radiographs of the knee secondary to lipohemarthrosis.

FBI (food-borne illness).

FBSS (failed back surgery syndrome).

FCE—see *Functional Capacity Evaluation*.

FCIS (Flint Colon Injury Scale).

$F_E CO_2$ (fraction of expired carbon dioxide)—recorded numerically on a capnograph.

FCPA2 laser—ultrafast ultracompact laser, for use in medical diagnostics and therapy.

FCR 9501HQ—a high-resolution storage phosphor imaging agent.

FCT (foraminal compression test).

FCU (flexor carpi ulnaris).

FCXM (flow cytometry crossmatch).

FDG (18-fluorodeoxyglucose) **positron emission tomography**.

FDI (frequency domain imaging)—in ultrasound.

FDP (fibrin degradation products).

FDT (fluorescein disappearance test).

feather lift—see *thread lift*.

FeatherTouch automated rasp—part of the XPS 2000 Microresector system instrument set, used in rhinoplasty.

FeatherTouch CO_2 laser—used in skin resurfacing to treat deep lines, wrinkles, scars, and hair transplantation.

FEB (fluorinated ethylene propylene).

fecal occult blood test (FEOT)—blood present in stool in too small an amount to be detected by naked-eye observation, but detectable by chemical testing or microscopic examination. See *guaiac*; *Hemoccult Sensa*; *Hemoccult II*; *occult blood*.

fecalogram—slang term for an imaging study in an improperly prepared patient, showing stool in the colon.

fecal-oral route—the route by which some intestinal and other pathogens are transferred from person to person; contamination of food or water, or direct physical contact, where the infected person's feces leads to ingestion of the pathogen.

Fechtner syndrome—a form of hereditary thrombocytopenia associated with giant platelets, and characterized by interstitial nephritis, congenital cataracts, and neurosensory deafness associated with Alport syndrome.

Federici sign—a sign of gas in the abdomen, or peritonitis, when cardiac sounds are heard on abdominal auscultation.

feedback microwave thermotherapy—for clinical benign prostatic hyperplasia.

feeder and grower (F&G).

feeder layer—a layer of cells (usually mouse embryonic fibroblasts treated with gamma radiation to prevent them from proliferating) on which a stem cell culture is maintained.

feeding mean arterial pressure (FMAP).

feeding solution—see *medication*.

feeding tube—see *tube*.

FEF_{25-75} (forced midexpiratory flow).

Felig insulin pump—worn externally.

fellow—the holder of a fellowship for teaching or research, an academic appointment carrying a stipend and providing facilities for postdoctoral study or research. Teaching fellow, research fellow.

felon—an abscess of the fingertip. See *herpes whitlow*.

Female Condom, The—provides protection against pregnancy and the transmission of sexually transmitted diseases.

female genital mutilation—see *Sunna circumcision*, *clitoridectomy*, and *infibulation*.

female sexual dysfunction (FSD)—including symptoms such as lack of lubrication and lack of blood flow to the genital area.

Femaprin—over-the-counter natural menopause drug.

FemCap—a nonhormonal latex-free contraceptive device that can be worn for up to 48 hours at time and is made of non-allergenic material. It is available at a low cost (typically $2-3 per month) and reusable for up to two years. It is believed to be an effective mechanical barrier which covers the cervix completely and potentially protects the cervix from the invading sperm, bacteria, and viruses.

FemCard—short for FemExam TestCard, a line of point-of-care (POC) diagnostic tests to aid in the diagnosis and management of infectious vaginitis. Specimen: vaginal fluid (vaginal swab); results available in approximately 2 minutes. Marketed tests: pH and amines; *G. vaginalis* PIP (proline iminopeptidase) activity.

"femister"—phonetic for Phemister.

"fem-la"—phonetic for FMLA (Family Medical Leave Act).

femoral canal restrictor (Ortho).

femoré—over-the-counter women's intimacy cream that reportedly heightens sexual response. Trademarked without an initial capital letter.

FemoStop femoral artery compression arch.

fem-pop—femoral-popliteal.

FemSoft insert—small, single-use liquid and silicone device for the treatment of stress urinary incontinence in women. The self-inserted device slides into and conforms to the urethra and creates a seal at the bladder neck to prevent unintended leakage. Available by prescription only.

femtoliter (fL)—unit of measurement in mean corpuscular volume (MCV). One-quadrillionth of a liter.

femtosecond laser (Pulsion-FS) and **femtosecond-pulse intrastomal laser microkeratome** (20/10 Perfect Vision)—replaces microkeratomes, which use blades to create a corneal flap prior to laser vision correction procedures.

FEN (fluids, electrolytes and nutrition). Sometimes dictated as a heading.

fencing-in—placing of laparoscopic or thoracoscopic ports too close together, which interferes with maneuverability of the instruments. See also *sword-fighting*.

fenestra ovalis; **fenestra vestibuli**—see *vestibular window*.

fenestrated Drake clip—for clipping of intracranial aneurysm.

fenestrated drape—sterile surgical drape with round opening to expose just the operative site.

fenestrated tracheostomy tube—tracheostomy tube with an opening on its upper surface that permits the patient to talk while still keeping the airway open.

fenestrating—the making of openings. Cf. *festinating*.

fenestration—a window-like inclusion in a cell caused by large cellular spaces called *vacuoles*.

FEN-GI—pronounced as a word, dictated as a heading. Translates to "fluid, electrolytes, and nutrition and gastrointestinal."

fen-phen or **phen-fen diet**—weight loss program that consisted of the anorectic medications fenfluramine and phentermine, and a reduced-calorie ADA diet. Fenfluramine has since been taken off the market due to association with cardiac valvular dysfunction.

Feridex I.V. (ferumoxides injectable solution)—a contrast medium used in MRI scans to aid in detection of primary and metastatic liver cancer, imaging lesions as small as 3 mm.

fern test—used in obstetrics to determine the level of estrogen secretion; so-called because of the fernlike appearance of the cervical and uterine mucus when it dries on the glass slide.

Ferrans and Powers Quality of Life Index, Cardiac Version—measures subjective perception of quality of life.

Ferriprox (deferiprone)—a heavy iron chelating agent for the treatment of thalassemia.

Ferris chart—measures visual acuity.

Ferrlecit (sodium ferric gluconate)—drug used for iron supplementation in patients with iron-deficiency anemia.

ferromagnetic materials and MRI—a combination resulting in danger to patients having MRI scans. Ferromagnetic materials on or in a patient's body can result in burns and tissue tears during an MRI scan. Usually these are easy to detect, but shrapnel, prostheses, aneurysm clips, or pacemakers may be forgotten. At least one fatality has been reported because a stainless steel neurosurgical clip was actually ferromagnetic (there are several types of stainless steel). This shows once again the importance of accurate medical records, as operative reports should contain exact information about metallic implants.

fertilization—the process whereby male and female gametes (sperm and oocyte) unite to form a zygote.

FES (fat embolism syndrome).

$FeSO_4$—chemical symbol for iron sulfate.

FESS (functional endoscopic sinus surgery).

FES (functional endoscopic sinus) **surgery**.

Festalan (pancrelipase)—a medication that contains the enzymes needed to break down food into simpler substances that the intestines can absorb. Pancrelipase is used in people with pancreatic problems where the pancreas is producing little or no pancreatic enzymes.

festinating gait—the short, accelerating steps seen in patients with Parkinson disease. Cf. *fenestrating*.

fetal fibronectin (fFN) **test**—a diagnostic test using cervical mucus to detect the presence of the protein, fetal fibronectin, to aid in detecting symptoms in women that may cause premature delivery.

fetal hydantoin syndrome—disorder that is caused by exposure of a fetus to phenytoin (Dilantin), an anticonvulsant drug prescribed for epilepsy. Major symptoms may include abnormalities of the skull and facial features, growth deficiencies, underdeveloped nails of the fingers and toes, and/or developmental delays.

fetal magnetocardiography—imaging procedure that can detect fetal heart defects in utero.

fetal neuron allotransplantation—the implantation of fetal cells of human origin into adult brains; used successfully to treat patients with Parkinson disease.

fetal-pelvic index—a method of determining the presence of fetal-pelvic disproportion which is said to be more accurate than estimated fetal weights by ultrasonography, the use of the Mengert index, or x-ray pelvimetry. A positive fetal-pelvic index indicates fetal-pelvic disproportion and the need for a cesarean section. A false negative result can occur in the presence of a malpositioned fetus.

fetal pig cell transplantation—a procedure in which fetal pig cells are transplanted into the brains of Parkinson disease patients to restore dopamine to natural levels. (Parkinson disease patients cannot produce enough dopamine, causing the brain to lose communication with the rest of the body.)

fetal small parts—the extremities of a fetus as felt through the mother's abdominal wall.

fetal tissue transplant—used successfully to restore sight in patients with advanced retinitis pigmentosa and macular degeneration.

fetal ventral mesencephalic tissue transplantation—performed on parkinsonian patients in hopes of improving cognitive function.

FETENDO or **fetendo** (Ob-Gyn)—a coined word used to describe a fetoscopic approach, allowing the surgeon to work not only inside the uterus but also inside the fetus to view, endoscopically, the fetal trachea, esophagus, and bladder.

fetoscopy—an endoscopic technique for direct visualization of the fetus.

fetus—a developing organism from the end of the embryonic period (eight weeks of development in human beings) until birth.

FEV (forced expiratory volume). The subscript, as in FEV_1, indicates the number of seconds in which the forced expiratory volume is measured.

FFL (floral variant of follicular lymphoma).

FFP (fresh frozen plasma).

FFT (fast-Fourier transform)—MRI term. See *Fourier analysis*.

FGF (fibroblast growth factor).

FGF-I (human fibroblast growth factor-I).

FGFR2 (fibroblast growth factor receptor 2).

FG-36UX linear scanning echoendoscope.

Fiberlase—flexible and disposable beam delivery system for CO_2 surgical lasers developed for Surgilase unit.

fiberoptic bronchoscopy (FOB).

fiberoptic, **fiber optic**, **fibreoptic**—these three different spellings appear in different books and journals, with *fiberoptic* the most common. *Fibreoptic* is a British spelling. See *Luxtec fiberoptic system*.

fiberoptic intracranial pressure monitor—instrument under development to measure brain temperature.

FiberScan laser system.

Fiblast (trafermin)—basic fibroblast growth factor (bFGF) drug used for the treatment of strokes and coronary artery disease.

Fibracol collagen-alginate dressing—nonadherent dressing that maintains its integrity when wet. It is used for treatment of ulcers, burns, and donor sites.

Fibrel (injectable porcine derivative collagen)—a wrinkle treatment that purportedly stimulates the patient's own collagen production.

fibrillar Surgicel—see *Surgicel Fibrillar absorbable hemostat.*

fibrillating action potentials (FAPs).

Fibrillex (NC-503)—drug for the treatment of secondary amyloidosis.

fibrin degradation products (FDP)—important in coagulation process. Also, they show up on MRI scans, indicating that an earlier hemorrhage has occurred.

fibrin glue—a surgical adhesive. Usage: "I reconstituted the anterior wall of the sella with a piece of nasal septal cartilage, and then over this I applied fibrin glue in which I placed a piece of subcutaneous fat."

fibrin sealant—liquid biological tissue glue composed of thrombin and fibrinogen (blood products). It is used to stop air leaks and control bleeding in surgical and orthopedic procedures.

fibroblast growth factor (FGF).

fibrocystic breast syndrome—may be "a rose by any other name." A number of eponyms are used to identify this syndrome, including *Bloodgood syndrome*, *Cheatle syndrome*, *Cooper syndrome*, *Reclus I syndrome* or *disease*, *Schimmelbusch disease* or *syndrome*, and *Tillaux-Phocas* or *Phocas syndrome*. Cystic breast syndrome may also be called *blue dome syndrome*, *chronic cystic mastitis*, and *mastopathia chronica cystica*. Although there may be minute differences of meaning among these terms, they may also be used less discriminately. See also *breast fibrocystic disease stages*.

fibrodysplasia ossificans progressiva (FOP)—a rare hereditary disorder that manifests as ossification of skeletal muscle and connective tissue and congenital deformity of the bones. Occurs in childhood. No effective therapy is known.

fibrofatty infiltration of the pancreas.

fibroglandular tissue—a term used on mammogram reports, referring to the dense stroma of tissue made up of fibrous glandular tissue.

fibroid embolization—performed by an interventional radiologist, who makes a small incision in the groin (less than one-quarter inch), places a catheter into the femoral artery, and guides it to the uterine artery via x-ray imaging. Small particles are then injected into the uterine artery, cutting off the blood supply to the fibroid and dramatically shrinking it. A general anesthetic is not required.

fibroinflammatory pseudotumor of the middle and inner ear—characterized by total deafness in the affected ear and lack of response to caloric stimulation, destruction of inner ear structures, and atypical widening of parts of the labyrinth. A pseudotumor is a tumefactive fibroinflammatory lesion.

fibromuscular dysplasia (FMD).

fibrose—a verb meaning to form fibrous tissue. Cf. *fibrous*.

FibroSpect study—a noninvasive approach to detect liver fibrosis.

fibrous—an adjective describing something composed of fibers. Cf. *fibrose*.

fibroxanthogranulomatous—see *xanthogranulomatous cholecystitis*.

fibula free flap—fibula osteocutaneous free tissue reconstruction of midface.

Fick method—calculates cardiac output. The oxygen content of exhaled air is measured to determine oxygen consumption in a patient undergoing cardiac catheterization. This is then compared to the oxygen levels from an arterial blood sample and a venous blood sample. The differences in oxygenation are used to calculate the cardiac output.

Fick sacculotomy—procedure for treatment of progressive endolymphatic hydrops (Ménière disease). Picks are introduced through the footplate of the stapes to puncture the saccule, thus producing a permanent fistula in the saccular wall to drain endolymph into the perilymphatic space. See *Cody tack operation*.

FID (free induction decay)—MRI term.

fiducial box—a device used with Leksell base frame in Gamma Knife surgery.

field gradient; field lock—MRI terms.

field of view (FOV)—MRI term.

FiF (functional intact fibrinogen) **test**.

FIGO (Fédération Internationale de Gynécologie et Obstétrique)—used in staging adenocarcinoma of the endometrium, e.g., FIGO II.

figure-4 position—so-called because in this position the patient lies with the right side of the body up and brings the right ankle up to rest on the left knee, forming the figure *4*.

Filcard temporary removable vena cava filter—used in local thrombolytic therapy.

fil d'Arion silicone tube (Oph).

FILE (Family Inventory of Life Events and Changes).

filiform—threadlike.

filiforms and followers—used to dilate a urethral stricture.

filling defect—a zone within a tubular structure that is not filled by injected contrast medium (usually a tumor or abnormal mass).

filling factor—MRI term.

film badge—see *dosimeter*.

filmy adhesion.

Filshie female sterilization clip—comparable to the Hulka clip and to tubal rings.

Filtek A1 (Dentistry)—a restorative dental composite.

filtered-back projection (Radiol).

filtering bleb—a tiny, surgically coated vesicle, or blister, placed over a passageway into the eye to provide drainage in treatment of open-angle glaucoma.

filter replacement fluid (FRF)—given intravenously during CAVH (continuous arteriovenous hemofiltration) to maintain fluid balance.

FilterWire, FilterWire EX—an embolization prevention device with an off-center filter attached to a guidewire.

filum terminale—threadlike extension of the spinal cord from conus medullaris to the tip of the dural sac.

FIM (Functional Independence Measure).

fine-angled curet (*not* Fine) (Neuro).

Fine Lines—see *Restylane*.

fine-needle aspiration biopsy (FNAB). Also, *Skinny needle, Chiba needle*.

Finesse cardiac device.

Finesse Dacron patch angioplasty.

Fine-Thornton scleral fixation ring—ophthalmic instrument that provides fixation of globe without injury.

Finger Blocking Tree—a hand therapy product for use during finger or thumb blocking exercises.

finger cot—surgical glove material to fit just one finger.

finger fracture—blunt dissection performed with the surgeon's fingers.

finger friction—used to test hearing acuity. Usage: "She cannot hear finger friction in either ear." Rubbing thumb and index finger together makes an audible rubbing sound. It may not be heard by someone with hearing loss.

fingerprint dystrophy—a corneal dystrophy characterized by fine, wavy, concentric lines that may be associated with a map- or dot-like pattern.

fingerstick devices for blood glucose testing: Autoclix, Autolet, Monojector.

fingers-to-floor distance—term used in assessing spinal mobility in ankylosing spondylitis.

finger-to-nose test (F to N). The patient is asked to touch his nose with the index finger of one hand and then the other, with the eyes closed, alternating hands and increasing speed. In a variation of this test, the patient is asked to touch his nose and then the

finger *(cont.)* examiner's finger at a distance of 12 to 18 inches, with increasing speed. This test is used to evaluate the patient's coordination, and may be one of the neurologic tests administered in the physical examination.

finger-trap phenomenon (Ortho)—a rise in compartment pressure soon after fracture reduction and fixation.

Finkelstein sign; **test**—for synovitis of the abductor pollicis longus tendon.

Finney Doc-U-Dose—see *Doc-U-Dose.*

Finney Flexi-Rod penile prosthesis.

Finn hinged knee replacement prosthesis.

Fino vascular catheter—a thrombectomy catheter for treatment of deep vein thrombosis.

FIRDA (frontal irregular rhythmic delta activity)—in EEG. Usage: "Since the amplitude of the FIRDA was greatest over the left hemisphere, it may in this instance also suggest a possible left frontal structural lesion."

Firm D-Ring wrist support—a splint (manufactured by Rolyan) used to restrict wrist flexion and extension to help decrease pain and inflammation associated with severe tendinitis or ligament damage of the wrist.

First Check Ecstasy—an OTC test for the illegal drug Ecstasy.

"first-lipped"—phonetic for *pursed-lipped breathing*.

first pass effect—metabolic action of the liver on drugs. A drug that is taken orally first passes through the liver before reaching the general circulation to exert any systemic effect. For some drugs the first-pass effect is so extensive that almost all of the drug dose is immediately metabolized. Some drugs are not metabolized and are excreted unchanged through the kidneys. A decreased rate of drug metabolism occurs in patients with liver diseases and hepatitis, impaired liver function due to aging, or immature liver function in premature infants.

first pass view (in multiple gated acquisition scan, or MUGA)—an image or set of images obtained immediately after injection of radionuclide into the circulation, when its concentration in the blood pool is at its highest.

FirstSave—automated external defibrillator (AED).

first-toe Jones repair.

Fisch drill (ENT)—named for Professor Ugo Fisch of University of Zurich.

FISH—Glassman viscera retainer. It looks a bit like a flounder; it retains viscera and omentum during closure of the peritoneal cavity, then folds into a narrow roll for easy removal.

fishbone pattern—seen in sclerotic white retinal arterioles and venules in lattice degeneration of the retina. Also called *crosshatch pattern*.

Fischer sign—an obsolete sign: in tuberculosis of the mediastinal or peribronchial glands, after bending the patient's head as far back as possible, auscultation over the manubrium sterni will sometimes reveal a continuous loud murmur caused by the pressure of the enlarged glands on the large mediastinal vessels. See also *fissure sign*.

Fisher exact test.

fish meal lung disease—extrinsic allergic alveolitis caused by exposure to fish meal.

fishmouth-type reimplantation—used in urology surgery. Usage: "The ureter was bivalved and a fishmouth-type reimplantation performed."

fish-odor syndrome—primary trimethylaminuria, a rare condition that causes an individual to emit the odor of rotting fish. Caused by excessive bodily emission of trimethylamine (TMA), the problem may be a by-product of digestion of choline-rich foods such as saltwater fish, eggs, and liver.

FISH (fluorescence in situ hybridization) **protocol in bone marrow transplantation**—method to monitor engraftment in bone marrow transplantation patients.

fishtank granuloma—a skin infection caused by bacteria that live in aquatic environments. It is contracted by cleaning tanks without using gloves.

fish vertebrae—biconcave deformities of the vertebral bodies, characteristic of disorders in which there is diffuse weakening of the bone. The name is derived from the actual appearance of a fish vertebra, which normally has depressions in the superior and inferior surfaces of each vertebral body. This sign is typical for osteopenia.

fissula—a little groove. Cf. *fissura, fistula*.

fissura—fissure, a general reference to a groove or cleft, e.g., fissura cerebri lateralis (fissure of Sylvius). Cf. *fissula, fistula*.

fissure sign (Radiol)—the decreased uptake of radionuclide, in perfusion scintigraphy of the lungs, in the periphery of each lobe, making the fissures visible; caused by a variety of diseases and artifacts. Do not confuse with *Fischer sign*.

fistula (cf. *fissula, fissura*)—aberrant passage from one organ to another, or from an organ through to the outside surface of the body. Types:
AV (arteriovenous)
brachioaxillary bridge graft
brachiosubclavian bridge graft
Brescia-Cimino AV
cameral
colovesical
digestive-respiratory (DRF)
dural arteriovenous (DAVF)
nuisance
perilymphatic (PLF)
rectovaginal
ventriculocoronary arterial
vesicovaginal

fistula in ano—an abnormal tract or passage that arises within the anal canal and ends somewhere on the skin adjacent to the anus.

Fitz-Hugh and Curtis syndrome—gonococcal perihepatitis in women with a history of gonorrheal salpingitis.

5-HIAA (hydroxyindoleacetic acid)—a lab test of substance found in the urine of patients with carcinoid tumors of intestine.

5-HT1, 5-HT2 receptors—two types of serotonin receptors present in the central nervous system which are stimulated by certain drugs such as buspirone (BuSpar) to relieve anxiety. Serotonin is also known as *5-hydroxytryptamine (5-HT)*.

5-HT3 receptors—a serotonin receptor found in the chemoreceptor trigger zone of the brain and in the GI tract. The stimulation of these receptors is thought to trigger the vomiting reflex. The antiemetic drug ondansetron (Zofran) is the first drug in the class of 5-HT3 receptor blockers and is used to prevent vomiting in chemotherapy patients.

5-lobe infiltrate—on chest x-ray, a pulmonary infiltrate involving all lung lobes (3 right, 2 left).

5′nucleotidase (5′NT) ("five prime nucleotidase").

5-prong (or five-prong) **rake blade**—a self-retaining retractor blade.

five-view chest x-ray (*not* 5-U)—AP, PA, lateral, and both oblique views. Usage: "A five-view chest x-ray series was obtained."

fixation device—any appliance placed surgically in or on a bone to stabilize a fracture during healing. See *device, implant, prosthesis.*

fixation switch diplopia—may be experienced by adults with a history of strabismus since childhood, if a change in their refractive error or use of glasses encourages fixation with their nondominant eye. If correctly diagnosed, this seldom-recognized cause of acquired diplopia in adults may be successfully treated with the proper optical management.

fixative (Path)—see *glycol methacrylate, Hollande solution, Zenker.*

Fixion intramedullary humeral nail—an expandable nail that does not require interlocking screws for fracture fixation of humerus, tibia, and femur.

FK-565—a drug used to treat HIV-positive patients.

fL (femtoliter).

FLACC pain scale—an acronym for faces, legs, activity, cry, and consolability, a pain scale used as an assessment tool in preverbal pediatric patients. It measures changes in scores in response to analgesics.

Flack node—see *sinoatrial node*.

flail chest (*not* frail)—movement of the chest wall inconsistent with respirations; caused by rib fractures.

FLAIR (fluid-attenuated inversion recovery) (MRI term).

flanking sequence—a region of a gene that either precedes or follows a transcribed DNA sequence.

flap (see also *graft*)
abdominal
anterolateral thigh
Antia-Buch chondrocutaneous advancement
Antia-Buch helical rim advancement
arrow
axial
Bakamjian
banner transposition
bipedicle
butterfly
Chinese
chondrocutaneous advancement
Cronin S dermal-fat
cross-finger
Cutler-Beard bridge
deep inferior epigastric (artery) perforator (DIEP)
deltopectoral
distant pedicle
epithelial turn-in
E-Z titanium
fibula free
free
free flap transfer
free perforator
gluteus myocutaneous
gracilis myocutaneous
groin
Gunderson conjunctival
Iselin
island
Karapandzic lip
Kazanjian midline forehead
lateral island
lateral transverse thigh (LTTF)
latissimus dorsi myocutaneous
liver

flap *(cont.)*
lumbar artery perforator
maple leaf
Martius labial fat pad
Martius urethral repair
McCraw gracilis myocutaneous
medial thigh
Moberg advancement
modified Martius
neurovascular
neurovascular pudendal–thigh fasciocutaneous
O-to-T advancement
Palva
perineal artery fasciocutaneous
Pontén-type tubed pedicle
Randall-Tennison triangular
random transposition (rhomboid or Limberg)
rectus abdominis myocutaneous (RAM)
Rubens
Singapore fasciocutaneous
sliding plus pivoting
supercharged TRAM
superior gluteal artery perforator (SGAP)
superior inferior epigastric (artery) perforator (SIEP)
thenar
Thom
TRAM (transverse rectus abdominis myocutaneous)
transposition
transverse rectus abdominis myocutaneous
triangular island
tubularized cecal
tummy tuck
V-Y island
Wolfe
YV advancement

flap surgery—uses both pedicled and free-tissue transfer in reconstructive surgery to salvage severely traumatized limbs.

flap tracheostomy—may be useful in the management of pediatric patients who require long-term bypass of the upper airway.

flap (*not* flat) **valve**.

flap valve principle—a technique in which the appendix or an alternative conduit is placed in the urinary reservoir in an antireflux manner whereby pressure in the conduit is directed against the semirigid wall, compressing the lumen of the catheterizable tube. Variations of the Mitrofanoff principle have been used to achieve fecal continence. Also called *Mitrofanoff principle*.

flare—sudden exacerbation; a sudden outburst; a spreading out. Also a term used in ophthalmology, as in *aqueous flare, cell and flare, Tyndall effect*. (*Not* flair, which means an aptitude or bent, as in "She has a flair for writing.")

FLASH (fast low-angle shot)—an MRI term. Usage: "FLASH images were obtained with gradient echo technique."

flashlamp-pulsed Nd:YAG laser—used in lithotripsy by converting light into thermal energy.

flashlamp-pumped pulsed dye laser—used to treat uncomplicated and recalcitrant warts.

FlashPoint—image-guided surgical instruments that utilize CT and MRI data to provide surgeons with real-time visual localization of surgical instruments relative to a patient's anatomy during image-guided surgical procedures.

flash pulmonary edema—the appearance of acute or sudden pulmonary edema, often in the presence of marked systolic hypertension.

flash pulmonary edema with anuria—an atypical presentation of renovascular hypertension.

FlashTab—quick-dissolving oral tablet that requires no intake of liquid. This dosage form may be used in the future with a variety of medications and should be particularly useful for children or the elderly.

flat (or flattened) **affect**—diminished emotional response; apathy.

flat electroencephalogram—flat or isoelectric EEG recorded for at least 10 minutes in the absence of hypothermia or central nervous system depressants.

flatliner—patient whose EEG shows no cerebral activity.

Flatow/Bigliani shoulder prosthesis—for shoulder arthroplasty.

Flatt finger/thumb prosthesis.

flat tube pressure sensor—enables rotary ventricular assist devices (VADs) to autoregulate by directly and continuously measuring blood pressure. This in turn lets VADs adjust pumping rates in response to patient activity levels and perfusion needs, allowing better control of congestive heart failure.

flavonols—plant substances that appear to have protective properties. These can be found in a range of foods, including onions, chocolate, tomatoes, and red wine. Usage: "The patient was advised to reduce her fat intake and eat foods rich in flavonols."

flax seed oil—a nutritional supplement, a vegetable source of omega-3.

Fleischner disease—osteochondritis of the middle phalanges of the fingers.

Fleischner lines—coarse linear shadows on a chest radiograph, indicating bands of subsegmental atelectasis.

Fleischer ring—a deposit of iron, ring-shaped, in the cornea; seen with keratoconus. See *Kayser-Fleischer ring*.

Fleischner sign—(1) a prominent central pulmonary artery seen on chest x-ray in acute pulmonary embolism; (2) a wide gap between a thickened, patulous ileocecal valve and narrowed ulcerated terminal ileum.

"flem"—phonetic for phlegm (starts with *ph*, *g* is silent).

flesh-eating bacteria—see *streptococcus A infection*; *necrotizing fasciitis; and toxic shock syndrome.*

Fletcher-Suit applicator—an appliance used for the insertion of radiation sources for treatment of carcinoma of the endometrium. Also, *Fletcher applicator*.

Fletcher-Suit-Delclos (FSD)—a mini-colpostat tandem and ovoids system. It is used for insertion of radioactive seeds for therapy of cervical cancer.

fleur de lis pattern—a breast reconstruction pattern used for latissimus dorsi reconstruction. This technique provides enough skin and fat overlying the muscle to create sufficient volume without necessitating an implant.

Flex-A-Min (glucosamine chondroitin MSN) **tablets**.

FlexDerm hydrogel sheet.

Flexeril—a skeletal muscle relaxant drug. Often misspelled *Flexoril* because of its association with flexor muscles.

Flexguard tip catheter (Cardio).

Flexiblade laryngoscope—rigid laryngoscope with flexible blade for placement of tracheal tube and for examination and visualization of the upper airway.

flexible fallopian tube endoscope (falloposcope) (Gyn).

flexible steerable nasolaryngopharyngoscope.

flexible transgastric peritoneoscopy (FTP)—examination and surgery of abdominal organs (intestine, liver, pancreas, gallbladder, and uterus) performed by means of a flexible endoscope that is passed through the mouth into the stomach and from there through an incision into the peritoneal cavity; less invasive than laparoscopy.

Flexicath silicone subclavian cannula.

Flexiflo Lap G laparoscopic gastrostomy kit—believed to be an alternative to surgical gastrostomy and PEG. It uses a T-fastener that helps affix the stomach to the abdominal wall without tedious suturing and which can raise or lower the stomach for better visibility and retract it for stability during tube insertion. See *PEG*.

Flexiflo Lap J—a laparoscopic jejunostomy kit for direct jejunal feeding tube placement. This is fitted with a Brown/Mueller T-Fastener set.

Flexiflo Stomate low-profile gastrostomy tube—does not require endoscopy for removal.

Flexima ureteral catheter.

flexion contracture—a fixed or irreversible deformity or malpositioning at a joint in flexion. Usage: "There was a significant flexion contracture and varus contracture at the knee." *Flexion* and *varus* in the example indicate that the joint is fixed in partial flexion with a varus (bowleg) deformity.

Flexisplint—flexed arm board used as a restraint after brachial embolectomy or placement of an AV fistula in the forearm.

Flexlase 600—laser system for treatment of benign cutaneous vascular and pigmented lesions.

Flex microwave catheter ablation system.

flexor—a muscle that flexes a joint. Cf. *flexure*.

FlexPosure endoscopic retractor—used to facilitate exposure and allow simultaneous use of other instruments during endoscopic spinal surgery.

FlexSure HP test—noninvasive test for serum IgG antibodies to *Helicobacter pylori*.

Flextend—a pacing lead that delivers low pacing thresholds to the heart.

flexure—the bent part of an organ or structure. Cf. *flexor*.

Flexxicon and **Flexxicon Blue catheters**—dialysis catheters with flexible tips.

Flexzan foam wound dressing.

F. L. Fischer microsurgical neurectomy bayonet scissors—used in electrosurgery, craniofacial surgery, and skull base surgery.

flicker electroretinogram (ERG)—used in predicting outcome in central retinal vein occlusion (such as development of neovascularization of the iris). It is recorded at 5 Hz steps, at frequencies 5 to 30 Hz. Usage: "ERG recordings were made using a Ganzfeld sphere and a xenon strobe with a flash duration of 20 microseconds."

"flick-ten-yule"—see *phlyctenule*.

Flieringa scleral ring—applied to maintain the shape of the globe of the eye when vitreous is lost.

Flimm Fighter—percussor machine for patients with cystic fibrosis. Provides optimal postural drainage. See also *Vibracare*.

Flint Colon Injury Scale (FCIS)—a system of scoring abdominal trauma. A low FCIS correlates with less severe injuries. See also *PATI*.

flip angle—MRI term.

flipped meniscus sign—knee meniscal displacement identified on x-ray.

FLK—pejorative slang for funny-looking kid.

floaters—translucent specks of various sizes and shapes that float across the visual field; due to small bits of protein on cells floating in the vitreous.

Floating-Harbor syndrome—a disorder characterized by short stature, delayed language skills, and a triangular shaped face. A broad nose, deep-set eyes, and wide mouth with thin lips give the affected patient a distinctive appearance. The disorder was named after the hospitals at which the first two patients were seen: the Boston Floating Hospital and Harbor General Hospital in California. The cause of the disorder is not known.

flocculation—bentonite flocculation test for trichinosis.

flock worker's lung—lung disease caused by nylon fibers (previously thought to be inert), affecting workers in nylon flocking factories.

floppy—general term used to describe lack of muscle tone in extremities of newborns, due to hypoxia.

floppy guidewire—high-torque guidewire used in catheterization. See also *high-torque floppy guidewire*.

floral variant of follicular lymphoma (FFL)—normal lymph node structure altered in this type of lymphoma in such a way that, under the microscope, follicles are seen surrounded by atypical lymphocytes arranged in a scalloped pattern that resembles the petals of a flower.

Flo-Restors—devices for controlling backbleeding in microvascular anastomoses.

Florida pouch—a continent urinary reservoir using a detubularized right colonic segment as the urinary reservoir, thus allowing a large-capacity, low-pressure pouch.

FloSeal matrix hemostatic sealant—stops heavy bleeding during surgery.

FlossBrite—a patented plastic-molded toothbrush-shaped dental floss device.

Flo-Stat fluid management system—used in outpatient endometrial resection/ablation (OPERA) procedures.

Flo-Thru intraluminal shunt—a blood vessel occluder.

flow cytometry—a method to detect recurring bladder cancer by examining the DNA of urothelial cell sediment in urine specimens. It is thought to be more accurate than urine cytology.

flow cytometry crossmatch (FCXM)—method of detection for serum anti-HLA antibodies.

flow-dependent vascular remodeling—a compensatory mechanism whereby the diameter of an artery increases as a result of increased blood flow and decreases as a result of decreased flow. In the presence of atherosclerosis, two types of remodeling may be seen. Positive remodeling (the Glagov phenomenon) is a structural change in which the arterial wall bulges outward and the lumen remains uncompromised. With negative remodeling there is an increase in intima and media thickness (IMT) at the expense of inner

flow *(cont.)*
diameter, with little increase of external diameter. In hypertension, vascular remodeling also involves IMT, which normalizes wall stress. Recent studies in human coronary arteries showed that regions exposed to low shear stress were associated with increased IMT and outward remodeling (increased external elastic lamina, EEL).

flow effect artifact (MRI)—distortions caused by blood flow or cerebrospinal fluid (CSF) flow appearing as abnormal signal intensity within a vessel or CSF space, a band of noise across the image, or a spatially misregistered signal. Gating (timing of images) is helpful.

Flowers mandibular glove—a chin prosthesis developed by Dr. Robert Flowers.

Flow-Guard—introducer technology that features a longer body for easier access during conventional and minimally invasive cardiovascular procedures.

FlowGun—suction/irrigation for minimally invasive surgical procedures.

FloWire—a Doppler ultrasound medical device that measures blood flow impairment in blood vessels.

Flowtron DVT—a pump system used during and after surgery to prevent deep venous thrombosis.

flow volume loop—a term used in spirometry reports.

Floyd classification of peripheral nerves.

flu—see *Asian bird, avian flu, bird flu.*

fluasterone—a synthetic drug version of dehydroepiandrosterone (DHEA). Potential uses include prevention or treatment of cancer, lupus erythematosus, rheumatoid arthritis, multiple sclerosis, as well as management of obesity and type 2 diabetes mellitus.

fluctuance—when dictated, transcribe fluctuancy.

fluctuancy (adj. fluctuant)—refers to the tactile quality of confined fluid. The palpating fingers of the physician can displace this fluid and perhaps even set up waves in it, as in compressing a balloon filled with water. Palpation or manipulation of a cyst, mass, organ, or body cavity containing fluid causes a characteristic feeling to be transmitted to the fingers due to the wavelike shifting (fluctuation) of the fluid. Anything that displays the property of fluctuancy is said to be fluctuant.

fluences—pulse energy densities in laser surgery.

Flu-Glow—a fluorescein-impregnated paper strip used to diagnose corneal abrasion or the presence of a foreign body in the eye. The strip is moistened with a sterile solution and placed on the conjunctiva of the lower lid. Any break in the corneal epithelium will permit the fluorescein to be absorbed, and the defect will appear as a bright green fluorescence under appropriate lighting. No defect, no glow. Cf. *Fluor-i-Strip.*

fluid-attenuated inversion recovery (FLAIR).

fluid output, insensible. See *insensible fluid output.*

fluids, electrolytes, and nutrition (FEN).

fluids, electrolytes, and nutrition and gastrointestinal (FEN-GI).

FLU-OIA—rapid (15-minute) test for detection of influenza A and B.

fluorescein angiography—evaluates the anatomic and physiologic states

fluorescein *(cont.)* of blood vessels in the choroid and retina after intravenous injections of fluorescein dye.

fluorescein dye disappearance test (DDT)—evaluates patients with possible partial nasolacrimal outflow obstruction.

fluorescein uptake (Oph).

fluorescence-activated cell sorter (FACS)—an automated lab tool which separates individual cells in a sample by fluorescence and size.

fluorescence in-situ hybridization (FISH) **protocol**—a procedure in which a fluorescent microscope is used to visualize a section of tumor embedded in paraffin and stained to study the chromosome pattern.

fluorescence overlay antigen mapping (FOAM).

fluorescence spectroscopy—see *spectrofluorometry*.

fluorescent cytoprint assay—an in vitro chemosensitivity assay that dissociates malignant cells from stromal tissue to facilitate the selection of the most effective chemotherapy regimen.

fluorescent treponemal antibody absorption (FTA-ABS)—a test for syphilis.

Fluor-I-Strip—ophthalmic strips; corneal disclosing agent (fluorescein sodium).

FluoroCatcher digital last-image hold, designed to reduce patient and operator radiation exposure.

FluoroNav virtual fluoroscopy system—surgical imaging device that provides information in multiple views simultaneously without having to reposition the C-arm.

Fluoropassiv thin-wall carotid patch—thin-wall patch with reduced thrombogenicity for use in carotid artery repair.

FluoroPlus angiography—provides real-time subtraction images for immediate diagnosis; minimizes radiation exposure.

FluoroPlus Cardiac—real-time digital imaging for cardiac catheterization lab. Provides instant display of all injection cycles, allowing immediate decisions during interventional procedures.

FluoroPlus Roadmapper—provides instant display of high-quality diagnostic images, enabling filmless diagnosis and decisions during PTA and ERCP procedures.

FluoroScan (no space)—a mini C-arm imaging system with high resolution, used for intraoperative imaging. This type of imaging is often referred to in podiatric surgical procedures.

fluoroscopic cystocolpoproctography—see *cystocolpoproctography*.

fluoroscopic diskectomy (Ortho).

fluoroscopic road-mapping technique—used in radiologic invasive vascular procedures.

fluorosilicone oil—a type of substitute for vitreous humor, this drug is used to float and help facilitate the removal of a dislocated intraocular lens.

Fluoro Tip cannula—used in ERCP. Has a radiopaque distal tip for location on fluoroscopy.

FluoroTrak—fluoroscopy-based surgical navigation system.

flush—method of taking blood pressure in infants.

flush aortogram (Cardio).

Flutter device—hands-free chest percussion therapy device that provides positive expiratory pressure to

Flutter *(cont.)*
patients with mucus-producing respiratory conditions. It is a small, handheld, pipe-shaped device that allows patients to clear their own airways of accumulated mucus and is used by patients with respiratory diseases such as cystic fibrosis, bronchitis, and bronchiectasis.

flying spot excimer laser system—designed to correct low to moderate nearsightedness and astigmatism. The small-beam laser pulses 55 times a second and is directed by an active corneal tracking device that scans eye position 4000 times a second, rapidly hopping from one side of the cornea to the other to allow for thermal relaxation of tissue.

FMAP (feeding mean arterial pressure).

FMLA (Family Medical Leave Act). May be pronounced as a word, "femla."

fmoles/mg (femtomoles/mg)—a measurement used with estrogen and progesterone receptors to determine if a patient with breast cancer should be categorized as positive or negative. (Greater than 10 fmoles/mg is considered positive.)

fMRI (functional MRI).

FNAB (fine-needle aspiration biopsy).

FNA cytology (fine-needle aspiration).

FNH (focal nodular hyperplasia)—MRI term.

FO (foot orthosis).

FOAM (fluorescence overlay antigen mapping)—a technique to evaluate bullous skin disorders.

foam cell (foamy histiocyte)—a cell which has a ground-glass-appearing cytoplasm due to accumulation of fat, glycogen, or other material.

foam dressing—made from hydrophilic polyurethane foam, with adhesive tape surrounding an "island" of foam. Highly absorbent foams allow less frequent dressing changes. Foams that absorb exudate and keep it off the wound can decrease maceration of surrounding tissue. Often used on heavily exudating wounds, deep-cavity wounds, and weeping ulcers. See *dressing*.

foam stability test; **index**—a determination of maturity of the fetal lungs, as demonstrated by the ability of pulmonary surfactant in the amniotic fluid to form a stable foam in ethanol after being vigorously shaken. Also called *shake test*.

foamy esophagus—radiographic feature of *Candida albicans* esophagitis, seen on double contrast esophagograph, particularly in patients with scleroderma. It is caused when numerous tiny bubbles intermingle with barium suspension along the top of the barium column, producing a layer of foam.

foamy macrophages—a descriptive term used in pathology. Usage: "Panbronchiolitis is characterized histologically by mononuclear cell inflammation of respiratory bronchioles and the presence of foamy macrophages in the bronchiolar lumina and adjacent alveoli."

FOB (fiberoptic bronchoscopy).

Fobi pouch—transected vertical gastric bypass with Silastic ring band and gastrostomy performed for severe obesity. Developed by Dr. Mathias A. L. ("Mal") Fobi, Bellflower, California.

FOBT (fecal occult blood test).

focal and diffuse lung texture analysis (Radiol).

focal cortical resection—surgical procedure of the brain for patients with

focal *(cont.)*
epilepsy. It involves removing epileptic brain tissue. Once thought to be a procedure of last resort, studies reportedly show that focal cortical resection may offer the best outcome for a seizure-free patient.

focal expansion technology—a means by which direct pressure is "focalized," e.g., applying pressure only to the site of blockage or disease, thereby treating the site of the disease while lessening risk of damage to the surrounding healthy arterial wall. This is the technology used in the FACT line of catheters.

focality—a coined term derived from *focal*. Usage: "No gross focality was noted on neurological exam."

focal nodular hyperplasia (FNH).

FocalSeal—a liquid sealant used to seal air leaks in patients undergoing lung volume reduction surgery.

Focalseal-L—a hydrogel synthetic absorbable sealant applied in two steps, a primer step and the sealant proper.

FocalSeal-S—a surgical sealant used in neurosurgical procedures.

focal segmental glomerulosclerosis (FSGS).

focal vestibulitis vulvae—see *vulvar vestibulitis syndrome.*

focal vulvitis—see *vulvar vestibulitis syndrome.*

focused heat technology—new method of nonsurgical minimally invasive tumor ablation using heat alone.

Fodéré sign—swelling of the lower eyelids in patients with kidney disease.

Foerster capsulotomy knife—used in plastic and reconstructive procedures on the breast to remove spherical contractures from the breast pocket during re-do breast implant procedures.

Foerster sponge forceps.

fog artifact (Radiol)—caused by radiation scatter.

Fogarty adherent clot catheter—used in removing clots or other material adherent to synthetic bypass grafts. Also, *Fogarty balloon biliary catheter.*

FOLFOX4 colorectal cancer trial (oxaliplatin).

folinic acid rescue—see *leucovorin rescue.*

Folstein Mini-Mental Status Examination (MMSE)—a method of grading the cognitive state of patients. This is one of the tests administered to patients with symptoms suggestive of Alzheimer disease.

Fonar Stand-Up MRI—designed for full-body imaging in the weight-bearing position.

Fonar-360 MRI scanner—open sky MRI which is, from the patient's point of view, a full-size room with two circular structures projecting from the ceiling and floor. There are no structures between the patient and the walls of the scanner room in any direction.

Fontan modification of Norwood procedure—for hypoplastic left-sided heart syndrome. See *Norwood; Gill/Jonas; Sade.*

Fontan procedure—anastomosis of the right atrial appendage to the pulmonary artery, to separate the left and right heart circulations in patients with levotransposition of the great vessels, single ventricle, atrial septal defect, coarctation of the aorta, and small left atrium.

FoodSCAN—a food allergy test that uses the IgG ELISA technique from a single drop of the patient's blood.

FOOSH (fall on outstretched hand)—an acronym which should be expanded in transcription.

footballs—see *Zandy bars*.

football sign (Radiol)—a large pneumoperitoneum outlining the entire abdominal cavity.

foot drop—passive plantar flexion of the foot due to paralysis of dorsiflexor muscles.

foot pound—a unit of measurement related to work, i.e., stress placed upon the extremities.

FOP (fibrodysplasia ossificans progressiva).

foramen of Luschka—opening at the side of the fourth ventricle of the brain communicating with the subarachnoid space.

foramen ovale (*not* O'Valley, although it sounds like that)—an opening in the sphenoid bone through which pass a branch of the trigeminal nerve and some blood vessels (foramen ovale basis cranii), and also an opening in the septum secundum of the heart of the fetus between the atria (foramen ovale cordis).

foraminal compression test (FCT)—another name for *Spurling maneuver, test,* or *sign*.

Force balloon dilatation catheter.

forced beat—a beat or complex dependent in some way on the preceding conductant beat.

forced expiratory volume (FEV).

forced midexpiratory flow ($FEF_{25\text{-}75}$)—a measure of the rate at which the patient can expel air from the lungs. Flow is measured in liters per second during the median half of forced expiration—that is, from the time that 25% of total volume has been expelled to the time that 75% has been expelled. This study is more sensitive to mild airway obstruction than other tests of pulmonary function. Usage: "Spirometry obtained at this time reveals a normal examination, with the exception of the $FEF_{25\text{-}75\%}$ which is reduced to 50% of predicted. These findings are sometimes considered indicative of some degree of small airway disease."

Forrest classification of gastroduodenal ulcer.

forced oscillation technique (FOT)—a noninvasive test used to measure the limitation of air flow in the respiratory system.

forced vital capacity (FVC).

forceps—an instrument with a pair of blades and handles, used in surgery to grasp tissue, and also surgical sponges, etc. Why do we give this well-known term? Forceps, though it sounds plural, can be either singular or plural and should always retain the *s* on *forceps*. An example of *incorrect* use: "This was resected with a double action bone forcep." But grasping with a single blade would be like clapping with one hand or eating with one chopstick. So, "forceps" it is. When the article *a* is used in front of a phrase with *forceps*, it takes a singular verb; without an article, it takes a plural verb. Usage: "A Takahashi forceps was then used to remove this tissue." "Takahashi forceps were then used to remove this tissue." "This was removed with a combination of sharp dissection with a Rosen needle and removed with a cupped forceps."

Examples:

ACMI Martin endoscopy

Acufex straight and curved basket

alligator grasper/forceps

forceps *(cont.)*
ASSI bipolar coagulating
Barraquer
bayonet bipolar
Bechert lens-holding
Bonaccolto utility and splinter
bone-cutting
Brown-Adson tissue
Caesar grasping
Calibri
Castroviejo-Colibri
DeJuan
Dodick Nucleus Cracker
Drews
end-biting
Englert
Ernest-McDonald soft IOL folding
Foerster sponge
Fujinon biopsy
Graspit nitinol stone retrieval
Grieshaber manipulator
Halsted hemostatic mosquito
Hardy microbipolar
Hartmann
Hildebrandt uterine hemostatic
HotMaxx reusable hot biopsy
Iselin
Jacobson hemostatic
Jaffee capsulorrhexis
Jawz endomyocardial biopsy
Kraff nucleus splitter
Kraff-Utrata tear capsulotomy
Lalonde delicate hook
Lalonde extra fine skin hook
Laurer
Livernois lens-holding
Livernois-McDonald
Llorente dissecting
Max Fine tying
Maxum reusable
Mazzariello-Caprini
McKerman-Adson
McKerman-Potts
McPherson
microbipolar

forceps *(cont.)*
MicroFrance bipolar neuro-otology coagulating
MIC Thermal Option
Moolgaoker
Neville-Barnes
Ogura tissue and cartilage
Olympus FBK 13
Peyman intraocular
Pierse corneal
Pierse tip
pike-jawed
Pilling Weck Y-stent
Puntenney
Quadripolar cutting
Quire mechanical finger
Radial Jaw single-use biopsy
ring
Rowe disimpaction
Russian
Seitzinger tripolar cutting
serrated ear-vessel
Shark disposable biopsy
Sinskey
spoon
SureBite biopsy
Therma Jaw (or Thermajaw) hot urologic
Tischler cervical biopsy punch
Toffel angled thru-cutting
Tricep hooked-prong grasping
Twisk
upbiting
Utrata capsulorrhexis
Vickers ring tip
vulsellum
Walsham
Yeoman uterine biopsy

Fordyce granules—an ectopic collection of sebaceous glands or choristomas in the oral cavity that requires no treatment and causes no untoward effects.

foregut—bronchi, stomach, and proximal portion of duodenum. See *midgut* and *hindgut*.

foreign material artifact (MRI and Radiol)—In MRI, small ferromagnetic objects, accidentally within the magnet bore, produce a scrambled image. These may include hearing aids, hairpins, buttons, paper clips, clothing with metal objects, such as zippers or buttons, cigarette lighters, political buttons, or make-up or hair coloring made with ferromagnetic substances, or metal objects within the body as a result of surgery or trauma. In plain film radiography, buttons, zippers, bra underwires, necklaces, earrings, metal mesh in a toupee or wig, rings, watches, pens, tooth fillings, or results of surgery such as shunts and probes produce images difficult or impossible to interpret.

Forel—scc *space of Forel.*

ForeRunner—automatic external defibrillator device.

Forma water-jacketed incubator—for use in in vitro fertilization. This incubator fosters an embryo's growth by recreating the body's optimal temperature, humidity, and pH level.

forme fruste—an atypical, prematurely arrested, or incompletely expressed form of a disease. From a French phrase meaning incomplete, truncated, or botched form. Also, a mild expression of a genetic trait, of no clinical significance.

formication—a sensation of insects crawling over the skin; most commonly seen in cocaine or amphetamine intoxication. Cf. *fornication.*

formication sign—a tingling sensation in the distal end of a limb when percussion is made over the site of a divided nerve. It indicates a partial lesion or the beginning regeneration of the nerve. Called also Tinel sign, DTP sign, and distal tingling on percussion. *Not* fornication.

formin cells (GEMM-CFC).

fornication—sexual intercourse between unmarried people. Cf. *formication.*

fortification spectrum—a jagged formation of bright lines, sometimes seen as an aura of migraine headache and in other conditions. See *scintillating scotoma.*

Fortigel (testosterone gel)—a transdermal gel for men that delivers physiologic levels of testosterone. It is applied to the inner thigh. In clinical trials, this drug was named Tostrex; the name was changed because it was too similar to other products on the market.

49er brace—knee brace; probably first used by that football team.

forward shift—used to describe conditions of the cornea after keratoplasty and implantation of intraocular lenses and in conditions of the ciliary body. For example, when the ciliary body contracts, a flexible implanted intraocular lens shifts forward. See also *corneal forward shift.*

Foscan (temoporfin) **mediated photodynamic therapy**—a nonsurgical minimally invasive technique that uses light (usually from a laser) to activate light-sensitive drugs (photosensitizers) in treatment of cancer and other diseases.

fossa (pl., fossae)—a depression, hollow, or channel. Usage: "The pain radiates into both tonsillar fossae."

FOT (forced oscillation technique).

Fouchet reagent ("foo-shay").

Foundation shoulder prosthesis—for shoulder arthroplasty.

founder effect—a high frequency of a genetic mutation among a population whose members are all descended from a single ancestor in which the mutation first occurred.

fourchette (Fr., fork)—a fork-shaped object or area; usually refers to the frenulum labiorum pudendi. Usage: "At surgery a small amount of scar was seen at the posterior fourchette."

four-dimensional (4-D) ultrasound—see *real-time 4-D ultrasound.*

four E's—a term referring to the triggers for pain of angina pectoris: **e**ating (particularly a heavy meal), **e**motion (anxiety or anger precipitated by some sudden event), **e**xertion (walking uphill, shoveling snow), or **e**xposure to cold.

four-flap Z-plasty—for thumb web deepening, in surgery for repair of syndactyly.

Fourier analysis of electrocardiogram—in exercise-induced myocardial ischemia.

Fourier transform infrared spectroscopy—a technique used in forensic pathology to examine plastic, paint coating, automobile lenses, paper, etc., to determine manufacturer or origin. See *Fourier transform Raman spectroscopy.*

Fourier transform Raman spectroscopy—a technique used in forensic pathology to supply complementary or confirmatory information about a substance under investigation. Cf. *Fourier transform infrared spectroscopy.*

Fournier gangrene—a polymicrobial necrotizing fasciitis of the perineal, perirectal, or genital area. Diagnosed by CT scan. Also, *Fournier syndrome.*

four-slice coronal CT scan of sinuses—see *coronal CT scan of sinuses.*

"14 C"—see ^{14}*C-urea* in the C's.

14-3-3 assay—see *beta isoform, 14-3-3.*

four-view chest x-ray—PA and lateral, and both oblique views.

FOV (field of view)—MRI term.

fovea centralis retinae—a tiny pit in the center of the macula, composed of slim, elongated cones; it is the area of clearest vision.

foveal avascular zone (FAZ).

Fowler-Stephens orchiopexy (orchidopexy)—a staged laparoscopic procedure for locating undescended testicles and moving them to their normal position. Testicles not moved are at risk for developing cancer.

Fox shield—placed over the eye after ophthalmic surgery.

FPA (fibrinopeptide A)—a substance released as part of the clotting process, an elevated level indicating an abnormal clotting process such as disseminated intravascular coagulation (DIC).

FPG (fasting plasma glucose).

FPIES (food protein-induced enterocolitis syndrome), infantile.

FPL (flexor pollicis longus).

FPSA vs. TPSA—ratio of FPSA (free [floating] prostate-specific antigen) to TPSA (total prostate-specific antigen) used to diagnose cancer. If the ratio of FPSA to TPSA is less than 0.19, the patient is more likely to have prostate cancer.

fractionated stereotaxic radiation therapy—combines the advantages of conventional fractionation (where the total radiation a patient receives is divided into smaller dosages delivered at different times) with radiosurgery. See *stereotactic radiosurgery* (SRS).

Fractura Flex—elastic plaster of Paris bandage. In applying the bandage to form a cast, the bandage material is first moistened in water and then applied in bandage-fashion to the extremity, rubbing each layer of the bandage into the layer beneath it. The cast is said to set within four minutes.

fracture
- Bennett
- blow-in
- blow-out
- boxer's
- burst
- Cedell
- Chance
- circumferential
- closed
- collicular (of the medial malleolus)
- corner
- diastatic
- Ellis
- finger
- fulcrum
- Galeazzi radial
- hangman's
- Kapandji radial
- LeFort I, II, III
- Malgaigne
- march
- pillion
- ping-pong
- ring
- sacral insufficiency (SIF)
- Salter I through VI
- seat belt
- SER-IV
- Zingg
- zygomatic-malar complex (ZMC)

fragile X syndrome (refers to X chromosome)—a form of retardation that males may inherit from the maternal side of the family.

fragmentation phase of Legg-Calvé-Perthes (LCP) disease—a period ranging from two months to three years (mean eight months) during which the developing femoral head fragments and collapses. Preservation of the periphery of the bone tends to maintain the shape and functional integrity of the femoral head even when the central portion is severely fragmented. Collapse of the lateral rim is associated with flattening of the head and an unfavorable prognosis.

fragment-in-notch sign (Ortho)—used in association with meniscal displacement of knee joint.

fraise, diamond—an instrument used in dermabrasion.

frameshift mutation (Genetics)—a gene mutation involving deletion or insertion of a number of base pairs other than three or a multiple of three; as a result all succeeding base pairs in the gene are out of phase and protein synthesis is accordingly deranged.

Framingham criteria for heart failure.

Franceschetti-type freeblade (Oph).

Francisella tularensis—organism that causes tularemia.

frank—fully developed, obvious, unequivocal, as in "frank pus," "frank breech."

Frank-Starling law of the heart—the heart pumps out of the right atrium all the blood returned to it without letting any back up in the veins. Named for Otto Frank (German) and Ernest Henry Starling (British), physiologists who, in the early 20th century, formulated the concept upon which the law of muscle contraction is based. Also called *Frank-Starling principle.*

Frank vaginal construction—creation of a new vagina in patients with congenital vaginal aplasia, or in males having a sex change operation. Other techniques include McIndoe and Davydov. See also *colocolponeopoiesis*.

Franseen needle—used in stereotactic fine needle aspiration biopsy.

frappage—clapping with a cupped hand on the patient's chest and back to loosen pulmonary secretions so they can be coughed up or suctioned out. See *percussion, chest PT.*

fraternal twins—dizygotic twins, resulting from the fertilization of two oocytes.

Fraxel SR laser—laser used to help remove age spots as well as lessen wrinkles. This laser treatment may replace deep chemical peels and laser skin resurfacing, which often leave the skin raw and take more than a week to heal.

FRC (functional residual [or reserve] capacity).

freckled—spotted, speckled. Usage: "There was a major intrasellar component that was a typical soft, freckled gray adenoma."

FRED (fog reduction/elimination device)—used on endoscopic instruments.

Fredrickson classification of lipid disorders.

free air (Radiol)—air or gas in a body cavity where it does not belong, usually after escape from the gastrointestinal tract. Cf. *air-fluid level*.

free beta test—a screening test that detects a specific protein marker for Down syndrome at 14-17 weeks of gestation.

Freedom arthritis support—protects and supports the arthritic hand to maintain joint alignment and mobility without bulkiness.

Freedom prosthetic foot—artificial foot for lower limb amputees.

Freedom knife—a diamond knife blade used during intraocular surgery.

FreeDop—hands-free Doppler monitor for obstetrical use.

free-floating testis—can occur as a result of bell-clapper deformity (see *bell-clapper deformity*). The free-floating testis is more likely to twist on its cord and strangulate its blood supply through intravaginal torsion.

free-GEPA graft—a procedure in which the gastroepiploic artery is separated entirely from the greater curvature of the stomach at both ends. One end is anastomosed proximally to either the aorta, a saphenous vein graft, or another arterial inflow source. The remaining end is anastomosed distally to the coronary artery. See also *gastroepiploic artery graft*.

Freehand system (Neuro, Rehab)—a surgically implanted neuroprosthetic device that allows people with quadriplegia to regain use of a paralyzed hand. The implanted components work in tandem with an external controller using radio waves and electrical stimuli.

free induction decay (FID)—MRI term.

free induction signal—MRI term.

Freeman cookie cutter areola marker—used in reduction mammoplasty.

Freeman femoral component with a Rotalok cup.

Freeman Punctum Plug—a small, bullet-shaped plug made of silicone that is inserted in the opening of the tear duct at the inner aspect of the lower eyelid. It prevents tears from being drained from the eye and is used to treat dry eyes.

free perforator flaps
DIEP (deep inferior epigastric [artery] flap)
SIEP (superior gluteal artery perforator) flap
lumbar artery perforator
anterolateral thigh flap
medial thigh flap

free PSA (prostate-specific antigen)—Some PSA clings to protein in the blood; some floats freely. The free form of PSA is key to identifying who really needs a prostate biopsy.

free radicals—some oxygen molecules turn into free radicals which can cause damage and even cancer. Diets to lessen or eliminate free radicals exist.

Freer elevator (Oph, ENT).

Freestanding Tissue Retraction Bridge system—free-standing balloon dissection system to maintain the dissected operative working space without tissue retractors. In dictation, you may hear just the word *Bridge* used in reference to this system.

FreeStyle—glucose monitoring device that allows people with diabetes to obtain a blood sample from places other than fingertips, such as the upper arm, thigh, calf, or hand.

Freestyle aortic root bioprosthesis—a stentless aortic porcine valve that comes in a full-root configuration designed to improve blood flow.

free thyroxine index (FTI).

free tie—a suture that is not connected to any other suture; by itself (free).

free-tissue transfer (FTT)—used in major skull-base resections, with wide surgical excision of dura and skull-base structures that normally separate the intracranial and extracranial cavities.

free toe transfer—construction of a finger, often the thumb, by transplanting a toe to the hand.

free/total PSA (prostate-specific antigen) **index**—a test that can better distinguish between men who have benign prostatic hypertrophy and those who have prostatic carcinoma, when PSA levels are less than 10 ng/mL or lower.

Freeway PTCA catheter.

Freezor cryoablation catheter—used to treat AVNRT (atrioventricular node reentry tachycardia).

Freezor Xtra surgical cardiac cryoablation device.

Freiberg disease—avascular necrosis of metatarsal head, treated with DuVries arthroplasty.

French-eye needle—the eye of the needle has a split, or spring, at the end with a little slot for the suture material to slip into, rather than the customary way, through the eye.

French scale—used for denoting size of catheters, sounds, and other tubular instruments, each unit being roughly equivalent to 0.33 mm in diameter.

frequency domain imaging (FDI)—in ultrasound.

fresh frozen plasma (FFP).

Freund complete adjuvant (FCA)—a water-in-oil emulsion of antigen which, when injected, induces antibody formation. Cf. *Freund incomplete adjuvant*.

Freund incomplete adjuvant—water-in-oil emulsion of antigen, without mycobacteria. Cf. *Freund complete adjuvant*.

FRF (filter replacement fluid).

fria—pelvic muscle-training aid for women with urinary incontinence.

friable—crumbly; fragmenting or bleeding easily on touch or manipulation. It is usually said of diseased tissue.

Frialoc transgingival threaded dental implant.

Frick test—used to diagnose tibiofibular syndesmosis sprain of the ankle.

friction knot—see *surgeon's knot*.

Friedländer bacillus—see *Klebsiella pneumoniae*.

Friedländer marker—used during corneal surgery. Types: arcuate; optical zone; transverse incision.

Friedman curves (Ob-Gyn)—when each determination of dilatation and station is made during labor, it is plotted on a graph. The patterns of changes in these parameters are referred to as Friedman curves or "labor curves."

Friedman Splint—polypropylene hip abduction brace for treating hip dysplasia in toddlers up to 2½ years of age.

Frigitronics probe—used in freeze-thaw cryotherapy.

frogleg view—a radiographic study of one or both hip joints for which the patient lies on his back with thighs maximally abducted and externally rotated and knees flexed so as to bring the soles of the feet together.

Frohse, arcade of—in the elbow. Sports medicine physicians have found that some windsurfers develop compression of the median interosseous nerve over the head of the radius in the arcade of Frohse.

Froment sign—a simple test of ulnar nerve function. The patient puts the tips of his thumb and index finger together, and if the resulting circle is askew, this is a positive Froment sign and points to ulnar nerve damage and loss of thumb adductor function.

fronds, sea—description of neovascularization seen on eye examination.

frondy—see *fronds*.

frontal irregular rhythmic delta activity (FIRDA)—in electroencephalogram.

frontal release sign (Neuro).

frontal sinus obliteration—a surgical treatment for frontal sinusitis using materials such as muscle, bone, fascia, osteoneogenesis (auto-obliteration), hydroxyapatite cement, and bioactive glass.

Frontier biventricular cardiac pacing system.

Frontier stent delivery system—designed to treat atherosclerotic lesions in native coronary arteries at the site of a bifurcation.

Frontier 3 x 2—multi-chamber stimulation device that uses ventricular resynchronization therapy rather than a standard drug-based regimen to treat congestive heart failure. See *ventricular resynchronization therapy*.

frontotemporal dementia (FTD)—the second most frequent cause of young-onset dementia. It is characterized by profound character changes and alterations in social behavior.

Frontrunner XP CTO (chronic total occlusion) **catheter**—combines with the Outback reentry catheter to facilitate treatment of chronic total occlusions in peripheral arteries.

frost—see *synovial frost*.

Frostline—linear cryoablation system for treatment of atrial flutter.

froth—see *meibomian froth*.

frown incision (Oph)—a downward curved incision above the superior

frown *(cont.)*
limbus of the eye, patented by Dr. Pallin. Much controversy and litigation exist over the right to patent an incision method.

frozen section (Path)—a technique by which tissue removed in an operation is quickly frozen and pathology identified (while the patient is still on the operating table) so that the surgeons will know what they are dealing with; this will then determine their options in proceeding with the operation. Cf. *paraffin section, permanent section.*

Frykman classification—of hand fractures.

FSAD (female sexual arousal disorder).

F-scan—with a combination of computer technology and a sensor pad in the patient's shoe, an orthotist uses the F-scan to identify high-pressure areas in the foot of a diabetic patient where a nonhealing wound is likely to start. Using this information, the orthotist can design a shoe insert that will shift the pressure to areas less likely to have tissue breakdown.

FSD (female sexual dysfunction).

FSD (Fletcher-Suit-Delclos).

FSE (fast spin echo)—MRI term.

FSE-T2 with fat suppression (MRI)—used to detect ligamentous abnormalities.

FSGS (focal segmental glomerulosclerosis).

FSH (facioscapulohumeral) **muscular dystrophy**.

FSH (follicle-stimulating hormone).

FTA-ABS—fluorescent treponemal antibody absorption test for syphilis.

FTD (frontotemporal dementia).

FTI (free thyroxine index). Usage: "The FTI was normal at 2.6, and all other thyroid function tests were within normal limits."

F to N (sounds like *F2N*)—finger-to-nose test.

FTP (flexible transgastric peritoneoscopy).

FTT (failure to thrive).

FTT (free-tissue transfer).

Fuchs phenomenon—a paradoxical lid retraction associated with eye movements during third nerve regeneration. While the eye may be adducted and lid elevated, no movement up or down occurs when the vertical recti contract together. It occurs classically in exophthalmic goiter, but also due to trauma or tumor at the base of the skull, anterior poliomyelitis, or vascular lesions of the brain stem, with regenerating fibers growing to wrong muscles. Also, *Fuchs sign.*

fudge factor—arbitrary adjustment of quantitative test result to support a desired interpretation.

fugue state ("fyoog")—a period of days, weeks, or years, in which a person loses memory and takes flight from a painful or untenable situation and may start a new life, new job, new marriage, etc., without memory of the past.

Fuji AC2 storage phosphor computed radiology system—eliminates many artifacts noted with earlier CR systems.

Fuji FCR9000 computed radiology (CR) **system**.

Fujinon biopsy forceps—used in endoscopic biopsies.

Fujinon Sonoprobe—system for endoscopic procedures.

Fujita snake retractor (Neuro).

Fukuda test—an enhanced Romberg test in which the patient is asked to stand upright with the eyes closed, then to march on the spot; if the patient tends to rotate toward the side

Fukuda *(cont.)*
of the lesion, the test is positive. Also called *Unterberger test.*

Fukushima C-clamp (Neuro).

Fukushima cranial retraction system.

Fukushima-Giannotta instruments—includes curettes, dissectors, needle holders, and scissors for use in keyhole eye surgery.

FUL (functional urethral length).

fulcrum fracture—seat belt fracture. See *Chance fracture.*

full-bladder technique (Radiol)—ultrasound examination of the pelvic region performed while the subject's bladder is distended with urine. This is done to improve the recognition of the bladder outline, which cannot be distinguished adequately when the bladder is empty.

full colon—dictated punctuation indicating the need for a colon mark, as opposed to a semicolon.

full-column barium enema (Radiol)—barium enema examination in which the contrast medium is injected into the colon under full pressure by elevation of the barium reservoir to the maximum safe height.

Fuller shield—a rectal dressing.

full Monti—a technique in which two Monti tubes may be anastomosed end-to-end ("full Monti") to provide additional length in patients with a long distance between the reservoir and the abdominal wall (older patients and those with a generous distribution of subcutaneous fat). See *Yang-Monti.*

full stop—dictated punctuation indicating the need for a period.

full-thickness skin graft (FTSG).

Functional Capacity Evaluation (FCE) (Rehab)—a comprehensive objective test of a person's ability to perform work-related tasks. Used for guidelines for physical restrictions and return-to-work suitability.

functional endoscopic sinus surgery (FESS)—can help people suffering from chronic fatigue caused by sinusitis. It requires minimal cutting and is directed through a very localized area in the nose.

Functional Independence Measure (FIM)—commonly referred to in the dictation of rehabilitation and physical medicine patients.

1 = Complete dependence
2 = Maximal assistance
3 = Moderate assistance
4 = Minimal assistance
5 = Supervision
6 = Independent with equipment use
7 = Complete independence

functional intact fibrinogen (FiF) **test**—a fibrinogen determination test in blood coagulation conditions, such as disseminated intravascular coagulation, cardiovascular disease, and primary fibrinolysis.

functional MRI (fMRI)—an advanced imaging system currently used only for research purposes; high-speed functional MRI imaging has been able to document the presence of fibromyalgia.

functional urethral length (FUL).

fundal height—the distance from the symphysis pubis to the top (dome or fundus) of the uterus. After the twentieth week of pregnancy, the fundal height in centimeters equals the number of weeks of pregnancy. If the fundal height increases more than this, it may indicate a multiple pregnancy or a fetus that is large for dates. Usage: "The fundal height is approximately 31 cm."

fundoplication (see also *operations*)
Belsey Mark IV
Collis-Nissen
Hill gastropexy
laparoscopic Nissen and Toupet
ligamentum teres cardiopexy
Nathanson liver retractor
Nissen
Toupet hemifundoplication

fundus oculi—the posterior inner part of the eye as seen with the ophthalmoscope.

funduscopic—*not* fundoscopic.

fungating—growing rapidly and irregularly, like a fungus, usually said of a neoplasm.

fungemia—systemic fungal infection.

fungus—see *pathogen*.

funicular suture—used in interfascicular or grouped fascicular repair.

funnel chest or pectus excavatum repair—a technique that reconstructs the chest wall in one operation by using plastic mesh bands instead of a metal plate with a body brace. The condition is caused by excessive growth of the cartilage that joins the ribs to the breastbone. The excess cartilage forces the ribs to curve in a manner that pushes the breastbone, or sternum, inward. To correct the problem surgically, the excess cartilage is removed. Then, using the plastic mesh bands, the straightened ribs and breastbone are brought together in a way that pushes the sternum out.

Funston syndrome—congenital cervical rib.

Furnas otoplasty technique—for correction of lop ears. The depth of the concha is altered by placing mattress sutures from the full thickness of the posterior conchal cartilage to the mastoid fascia. These sutures compress the posterior wall of the concha against the mastoid prominence, reducing conchal projection.

furrier's lung disease—extrinsic allergic alveolitis caused by exposure to animal fur and hair dust.

fusion—coordination of images seen by both eyes into one image.

fusion inhibitors—a new class of drugs that works specifically on a virus to prevent it from fusing with the cell and prevent viral replication. Fusion inhibitors are said to have great promise as anti-HIV drugs. Also called *HIS fusion inhibitors*.

fusion protein—a biotechnologic product that targets malignant cells and some normal lymphocytes that contain interleukin-2 (IL-2) receptors, for treating patients with advanced or recurrent cutaneous T-cell lymphoma.

futile cycles—high levels of cytokines causing fat to be stored as triglycerides, instead of being available for energy. Thought to cause some of the weakness and wasting in HIV disease. Futile cycles also exist for glucose and protein metabolism.

Futura resectoscope sheath—used in transurethral resection and ablation procedures within the urethra, prostate, and bladder.

Fuzeon (enfuvirtide)—anti-HIV drug called a *fusion inhibitor.* It is designed to block HIV before it enters the human immune cell.

FVC (forced vital capacity).

FVL (flexible video laparoscope).

FX miniRAIL RX PTCA catheter—indicated for balloon dilatation of the stenotic portion of a coronary artery, including in-stent restenosis, to improve myocardial perfusion. The miniRail catheter is a flexible tube

FX *(cont.)*
containing an inflatable balloon and external stainless steel wires. The inflatable balloon is attached to a segment of the tube near its end. This end is inserted into a small opening in an artery in the arm or the leg and gently advanced over a guide wire to the area of the blockage in the coronary artery. The balloon is inflated, pushing the wires into plaque. This causes the plaque to crack and break up, thus reopening the coronary artery.

FyBron alginate wound dressing.

G, g

GABEB (generalized atrophic benign epidermolysis bullosa).

gabexate mesylate—synthetic protease inhibitor drug that may help prevent ischemic/reperfusion injuries after liver resection.

GABHS (group A beta-hemolytic streptococcus)—the pathogen causing pharyngitis, rheumatic fever, toxic strep syndrome, and cellulitis.

gadolinium-enhanced subtracted MR angiography, 3-D—can detect graft complications such as occlusions, stenoses, and aneurysms.

gadolinium-enhanced T1-weighted images—MRI term.

Gaenslen test—for evaluation of sacroiliac joint disease. The patient lies supine with the lumbar spine flat against the table to eliminate the curvature. The patient then flexes the hip and knee on affected side, holding the knee with both hands, while the examiner hyperextends the opposite thigh over the side of the table. Pain on thigh hyperextension suggests sacroiliitis.

GAF (Global Assessment of Functioning)—one of the axis categories in psychiatric diagnoses; it is usually followed by a numeric value (e.g., Axis V).

Gaffney joint—orthosis for ambulation in children with cerebral palsy and myelomeningocele. Made of stainless steel vacuformed into polypropylene in seven sizes for use in a hinged ankle joint.

gag reflex—contraction of the pharyngeal musculature in response to stimulation of the pharyngeal mucosa.

GAHM (genioglossal advancement with hyoid myotomy).

gait and station—a term used in the physical examination. *Gait* refers to the way a patient walks, and the pattern of it. *Station* is a test for coordination problems. When the patient stands with feet close together and the body sways, this is one sign of incoordination.

gait cycle—the series of movements of the leg and foot between one touch of the heel on the ground and the next time the same heel touches.

gait lock splint (GLS) **brace**—maintains the leg in extension when the patient is weightbearing, without worry about the knee giving way.

GAIT (great toe arthroplasty implant technique) **spacer**—augments the Keller arthroplasty for class 3 Regnauld-type degeneration of the first metatarsophalangeal joint.

galactography—a pre-excision x-ray study of women with spontaneous nipple discharge, using contrast medium to outline breast ducts.

galactose-1-phosphate uridyl transferase test—a screening test for galactosemia.

Galand disc lens—a rigid one-piece intraocular lens made from PMMA (polymethyl methacrylate).

galantamine hydrobromide—see *Reminyl*.

GA LAW (pronounced "Georgia law") —acronym to describe a particular set of symptoms. A surgical resident might say, "The patient is positive for Georgia law," with *GA LAW* standing for **g**lucose, **a**ge, **L**DH, AST, **W**BC.

Galeazzi fracture of radius.

Galeazzi sign—indicates dislocation of hip. Lying supine, with the knees bent, if one knee is lower than the other, there is dislocation of the hip, or a shortened femur.

Galen—see *vein of Galen*.

Galida (tesaglitazar)—drug for the treatment of type 2 diabetes.

Galileo intravascular radiotherapy system—automated treatment designed to reduce or minimize restenosis in coronary arteries.

Gallavardin phenomenon (Cardio).

galling—chafing of apposed skin surfaces, as in the groin; intertrigo.

gallium-arsenide (GaA) **laser**—often used in acupuncture.

gallium scan (Radiol)—the intravenously introduced ^{67}Ga localizes in areas of granulocyte concentration, such as in osteomyelitis, thus revealing hidden infections.

gallop—see *summation gallop*.

GALOP syndrome (Neuro)—characterized by ataxia, positive Romberg test, and polyneuropathy.

G gait disorder
A autoantibody
L late-age
O onset
P polyneuropathy

GALT (gut-associated lymphoid tissue).

galvanic body sway test (GBST)—detects retrolabyrinthine disorder of the vestibular system.

galvanic stimulation—see *high-voltage stimulation and iontophoresis*.

galvanic vestibular stimulation (GVR) —maneuver used to study the vestibular system.

Galveston metacarpal brace—to treat fractured second through fifth metacarpals.

Galveston Orientation and Amnesia Test (GOAT)—a neuropsychological test given to patients with cognitive deficiencies following brain injury.

Gambee method, Gambee technique —a single-layer suture technique used in GI surgical procedures. Usage: "An end-to-end jejunojejunostomy was created by hand, using the Gambee method." "The distal end of the pouch was anastomosed end-to-end by hand to the distal gastric remnant using the Gambee method."

Gambee ("gam-bay") **suture**.

Gambro Lundia Minor—brand of artificial kidney (hemodialyzer), parallel plate type.

gamekeeper's thumb—instability of first metacarpophalangeal joint due to ligament tear.

game leg—impaired by injury or disease.

gamete—a sex cell (sperm or oocyte) having the haploid chromosome number (23 single chromosomes)

gamete intrafallopian transfer (GIFT).

gamete provider—one of the biological parents of an embryo; may not necessarily have legal custody of the embryo or the authority to make decisions regarding its disposition.

gamma counter probe—used intraoperatively to assess radionuclide uptake in tumors.

gamma glutamyl transferase (GGT).

gamma-herpesvirus—a virus of the family *Gammaherpesvirinae*, which includes Epstein-Barr virus and HHV-8.

Gamma Knife—not a knife, but a radiosurgical instrument used in radiation therapy. The gamma rays are fired with such accuracy that only the diseased cells are destroyed, leaving the adjacent healthy tissues intact. Thus, more radiation can be administered to the tumor if that is indicated. Cf. *roentgen knife*.

Gamma locking nail system—includes both the trochanteric locking nail and the long locking nail.

Gamma nailing—orthopedic procedure performed with the Gamma locking nail.

gamma-ribbon radiation therapy—used for reduction of restenosis in patients with reoccluded or narrowed coronary artery stents. A closed-end lumen catheter with a tiny ribbon containing 6, 10, or 14 seeds of ^{192}Ir is inserted into the stenosed vessel.

Gammex RMI DAP meter—real-time dose area product (DAP) meter that continuously measures accumulated radiation dose throughout fluoroscopic examination.

Gamna-Gandy body of the spleen—organized focus of hemorrhage, caused by portal hypertension. Contains fibrous tissue, hemosiderin, and calcium. Also called *siderotic nodules* or *bodies*.

ganglioglioma—a rare variety of tumor composed of ganglion cells and glial cells; prevalent in first three decades of life.

ganglion impar—a solitary retroperitoneal structure, located at the level of the sacrococcygeal junction, that marks the termination of the paired paravertebral sympathetic chains. Presacral blockade of the ganglion impar is an alternative means of managing intractable perineal pain, especially those with significant sympathetic component.

ganglioside GM1—a natural component of cells in the central nervous system. Has been found to allow damaged nerves to regrow. Along with the now-standard treatment of methylprednisolone following spinal cord injury, the use of ganglioside GM1 produces an increase in neurologic function one year status post injury.

gantry angulation—in CT-guided percutaneous biopsies.

Ganz periacetabular osteotomy—a procedure for the treatment of dislocated hip.

Ganzfeld sphere (Oph).

gaposis—slang term or nonce word for having one or more undesirable gaps. Examples: gap between front teeth, gap in clothing in an obese

gaposis *(cont.)* patient, gap in the closure of a hernia, gap in a patient's health insurance coverage.

Garcin syndrome—unilateral paralysis of all or most of the cranial nerves due to a tumor at the base of the skull or in the nasopharynx. Called also *half base syndrome*.

Garden classification of femoral neck fractures—uses the degree of dislocation as the criterion, which seems to be more accurate in terms of prognosis than Pauwels classification. Cf. *Pauwels classification*.

Gardner chair—used as an operating table, with the patient in the sitting position, in neurological surgery.

Gardnerella vaginalis—newer name for the bacterium formerly called *Haemophilus vaginalis*. Normal vaginal flora, but thought perhaps to be the cause of vaginitis infections.

Garin-Bujadoux-Bannwarth syndrome—see *Lyme lymphocytic meningoradiculitis*.

Garrett dilator—used in kidney transplant surgery.

GAS (group A streptococcus).

GasBGon filter seat cushion—incorporates a carbon filter and acoustical foam technologies to muffle the sound and absorb the odors of flatulence.

gas-bloat syndrome—complication of Nissen fundoplication for gastroesophageal reflux.

gas chromatography—an analytic technique with many applications in medicine, particularly in screening serum and urine for poisons and drugs of abuse.

gas density line (Radiol)—a linear band of maximal radiolucency, representing or appearing to represent a narrow zone of air or gas on x-ray.

gas-forming liver abscess.

gas-forming organism in bowel wall.

gasless anterior neck skin lifting method—video-assisted endoscopic surgery of the neck, used for lymph node dissection for papillary carcinoma of the thyroid.

Gastaut syndrome—HEE syndrome (hemiconvulsion, hemiplegia, and epilepsy).

gastric antral vascular ectasia (GAVE). See *watermelon stomach*.

gastric electrical stimulation—therapy for patients with gastroparesis. The stimulating device delivers high-frequency, low-amplitude stimulation via electrodes implanted in the gastric muscle.

gastric neobladder procedure—uses a wedge of stomach in bladder replacement surgery.

gastric retention (GR)—end-designation on drugs designed to improve the absorption and bioavailability of oral drugs through controlled release high in the gastrointestinal tract. Metformin GR and ciprofloxacin GR are examples of drugs in the GR formulation.

gastrinoma—hormonally active tumor of pancreas or stomach.

gastrinoma triangle—90% of gastrinomas are found within this area. The three points that define this region are (1) the confluence of the cystic and common bile ducts, (2) the junction of the second and third portions of the duodenum, and (3) the junction of the neck and body of the pancreas.

Gastroccult—lab test for gastric occult blood as well as pH.

gastrocnemius reflex. Cf. *Achilles reflex and ankle jerk*.

gastroduodenal intussusception due to Peutz-Jeghers syndrome in infancy—treated with a combination of endoscopy and laparotomy/laparoscopy.

gastroenteroanastomosis—see *retrocolic submesocolic approach for creating gastroenteroanastomosis.*

gastroenterostomy—see *operation.*

gastroepiploic artery (GEPA) **graft**—a graft in which the gastroepiploic artery is freed from the greater curvature of the stomach and the distal end anastomosed into the coronary artery. The proximal end remains attached to native circulation. See also *free-GEPA graft.*

gastroesophageal reflux (Radiol)—on upper GI series, abnormal backflow of material from the stomach into the lower esophagus.

gastroesophageal reflux disease (GERD).

Gastroesophageal Reflux Disease–Health-Related Quality of Life (GERD-HRQL) symptom severity scale.

gastrointestinal cross—intentional ingestion of a metallic foreign body. Inmates reportedly have swallowed such objects to create an emergency surgical condition.

gastroplasty—see *operation.*

gastrostomy—see *operation.*

gastrulation—a process during embryonic development whereby the inner cell mass of the blastocyst differentiates into the three germ layers (ectoderm, mesoderm, and endoderm).

GAT (Goldmann applanation tonometry).

gatch—from height of setting of Gatch bed, as "45° gatch."

Gatch bed.

gated blood (pool) **cardiac wall motion study**—a radionuclide study.

gated view (in multiple gated acquisition scan, or MUGA)—an image obtained by a technique synchronized with motions of the heart to eliminate blurring.

Gatekeeper reflux repair system—a noninvasive treatment of GERD.

gating—timing of images (MRI term). See *electrocardiographic gating, MUGA, spirometric gating.*

gauge (noun)—standard measure, as of wire or needle diameter; (verb)—to find the exact measurement of. Cf. *gouge.*
Dacomed snap gauge
Holladay-Godwin cornea
mercury-in-Silastic strain gauge
Preston pinch gauge

gauss ("gowse")—see *tesla* (MRI).

gaussian ("gow'-zee-en") **mode profile laser beam**—MRI term.

Gauss sign—the marked degree of mobility of the uterus, seen in the early weeks of pregnancy.

Gautier ureteroscope.

GAVE (gastric antral vascular ectasia). See *watermelon stomach.*

"GAY-gen-hal-ten"—phonetic for *gegenhalten.*

Gaynor-Hart position—positioning the patient for an axial radiographic projection of the carpal tunnel. See *carpal tunnel syndrome.*

Gazayerli endoscopic retractor—lifting device used in conjunction with CO_2 insufflation in laparoscopic procedures. A retractor with three prongs in the closed position is inserted into the abdomen and the prongs then splayed out in a fan or triangular shape. The fan retractor is then elevated by a powered mechanical arm, thus creating an enlarged laparoscopic cavity, avoiding the tenting of the cavity that occurs with

Gazayerli *(cont.)*
other lifting schemes. Two "fans" attached to a cross-bar may be inserted into the abdomen and lifted by a single arm for obese patients.

gaze—see *disconjugate gaze*.

G banding—technique of chromosome staining.

G bands (Genetics)—light and dark transverse bands disclosed in chromosomes after treatment with Giemsa stain.

GBC-590—a carbohydrate lectin inhibitor, which is a new class of anticancer drugs that specifically interfere with cellular interactions. This drug is currently being tested in patients with pancreatic carcinoma and may also be indicated for cancers of the colon, liver, and prostate.

GBM (glioblastoma multiforme).

GBST (galvanic body sway test).

GCA (giant cell arteritis).

G-CFC (granulocyte colony-forming cells).

G-CSF (granulocyte colony-stimulating factor, filgrastim)—a naturally occurring growth factor produced by epithelial cells and monocytes that acts on the bone marrow to increase the production of neutrophils. Used in chemotherapy and in treating bone marrow depression in AIDS patients. See *filgrastim*. Cf. *GM-CSF*.

GCT (germ cell tumor) of the central nervous system.

GDC (Guglielmi Detachable Coil).

GDC SynerG Detachment System—for endovascular treatment of brain aneurysms.

GDM A-1 (gestational diabetes mellitus, insulin controlled, type 1).

GDNF (glial cell-derived neurotrophic factor).

GDS (Global Deterioration Scale).

GDx, GDx Access—confocal scanning laser polarimeter for measuring and analyzing the retina.

GEA (gastroepiploic artery) **graft**—used instead of saphenous veins in coronary artery bypass surgery.

Geenan cytology brush.

Geenan Endotorque guidewire—used for cannulation of tortuous or strictured biliary ducts.

gegenhalten ("GAY-gen-hal-ten")—seen in cerebral cortical disorders, when the patient involuntarily resists passive movement. Usage: "Gegenhalten increase in tone is present and noticeable during the examination."

gelatin compression boot—used in the treatment of venous ulcer and stasis dermatitis. Works on the principle of even pressure on the veins, protecting them from further trauma. See *Unna boot*.

gelatin-resorcin-formalin glue—a tissue glue used instead of staples or sutures to repair dissected tissues.

gelatin sponge slurry—used like Gelfoam in arterial embolization.

gelbe cell—a cell in the mucosa of the gastrointestinal tract. Cf. *helle cell*.

Gelfoam—a purified gelatin product the body tissues will absorb. Used for hemostasis in surgery, and also used, in some forms, for treatment of gastric ulcer. See *Gelfoam cookie*.

Gelfoam cookie—used in neurosurgery. Usage: "A Gelfoam cookie was placed over the craniotomy." See *Gelfoam*.

Gellhorn pessary—a reduction device used to correct bladder prolapse.

gelling phenomenon—a term used to describe joint stiffness after inactivity.

Gelocast—a cast material.

Gelocast Unna boot compression dressing or wrap.

gel pads—used on the operating table to prevent or relieve pressure on shoulders, chest, or knees during surgery.

Gelport—a laparoscopic hand access device with a special port affixed to the patient so that surgeons can insert a hand into the operative field through a small incision.

Gem DR—implantable defibrillator that provides dual chamber pacing according to circulatory needs of the patient as well as detection and discrimination of ventricular and atrial tachyarrhythmia.

Gemini paired helical wire basket—used for ureteral stone retrieval in laparoscopic procedures.

gemistocytes—swollen astrocytes, either reactive or part of tumor.

GEMM-CFC (granulocyte, erythrocyte, monocyte, megakaryocyte colony-forming cells).

GEM-Premier analyzer—a 150-sample testing cartridge that can be used over a seven-day period, analyzing seven critical values from a single blood sample.

GEMSS (glaucoma, lens ectopia, microspherophakia, stiffness of the joints, and shortness) **syndrome.**

GEM II DR/VR implantable cardioverter-defibrillator (ICD).

GEM III AT dual-chamber implantable cardioverter-defibrillator (ICD).

GEN, GEIN (gradual elongation [intramedullary] nailing).

gene—a functional unit of heredity, consisting of a specific sequence of DNA and occupying a specific position (locus) on a specific chromosome. Each gene codes for the synthesis of a specific protein.

gene and **oncogene**—see also *tumor marker* and *tumor suppressor gene.*
- AH 1
- APC (adenomatous polyposis coli) tumor suppressor
- Bcl-2 oncogene
- BRCA1 (breast cancer one)
- BRCA2 (breast cancer two)
- c-erb B-2 oncogene
- DCC (**d**eleted in **c**olon **c**arcinoma) tumor suppressor
- env
- gag
- hERG (human ether-a-go-go related)
- HER-2-neu oncogene
- HLA-DR3
- MCC (mutated in colorectal carcinoma)
- MLH_1
- MSH_2
- mutant
- myosin heavy chain 9 gene (MYH9)
- nef
- NF1 (neurofibromatosis) tumor suppressor
- NF2 (neurofibromatosis) tumor suppressor
- p22 phox
- p53 adenoviral
- pol
- PTEN
- RB1 (retinoblastoma) tumor suppressor
- recessive
- recombinant DNA (artificial gene)
- RET proto-oncogene
- rev
- silent
- structural
- suicide
- tat
- TP53 (p53) tumor suppressor
- tumor suppressor
- VHL (von Hippel-Lindau) tumor suppressor

gene *(cont.)*
vif
von Hippel-Lindau (VHL)
vpr
vpu
WT1 (Wilms tumor) tumor suppressor

GeneAmp PCR (polymerase chain reaction) **test**—detects early HIV infection and also childhood leukemia (chronic myeloid and acute lymphocytic). It is said to be one thousand times more sensitive than previous leukemia tests and weeks faster. See *polymerase chain reaction.*

gene amplification—formation of an excessive number of copies of a gene; occurs most often in malignant cells.

GeneChip system—see *Affymetrix GeneChip system.*

gene flow—the gradual diffusion of genes from one population to another as a result of geographic migration and interbreeding of different racial stocks.

gene map—a graphic representation of the human karyotype showing the positions (loci) of genes on specific chromosomes.

gene pool—the sum of all the genes present at a given locus in the population.

General Electric CT/T 8800 scanner—analyzes stereotaxic data to obtain X, Y, and Z coordinates for each target lesion.

GE 0.5 Tesla Double-Doughnut Magnet—an MRI machine.

generalized atrophic benign epidermolysis bullosa (GABEB)—a form of nonlethal junctional epidermolysis bullosa, characterized by generalized blistering after birth, atrophic healing, and patchy bodywide atrophic alopecia with onset in childhood.

generalized nephrographic (GNG) **phase imaging**.

Generation 6—integrated radiotherapy system that provides high-resolution intensity modulated radiation therapy (IMRT) treatment for patients with breast, head, neck, pancreatic, and other cancers where precise beam targeting and dose delivery are needed.

GeneRx—nonsurgical gene therapy product developed for the treatment of patients with stable exertional angina due to coronary artery disease.

genes in colorectal carcinoma—identified as DCC (deleted in colorectal CA), APC (adenopolyposis coli), and MCC (mutated in colorectal CA). These do not follow the usual naming methods of genes.

GenESA System—combines a drug and computer-controlled drug administration system for use in the diagnosis of coronary artery disease in conjunction with electrocardiography, echocardiography, and radionuclide imaging for patients who cannot exercise adequately.

gene-silencing therapy (GST)—a genetic "message" that halts proliferation of tumor cells. While there are believed to be naturally occurring GSTs in the human body, drug companies have developed genetically engineered GSTs to fight cancer.

Genesis arthroplasty hardware.

Genesis 2000—a carbon dioxide laser used in "laser tooth whitening."

GenesisXP—implantable pulse generator for spinal cord stimulation.

gene therapy—the therapeutic or medical application of somatic genetic transfer.

genetic—pertaining to transmission of traits or defects by genes.

genetically modified or transgenic pigs—bred for the expression of a human complement-regulatory protein to limit rejection in xenotransplantation.

genetic code—the system according to which various base triplets in a strand of nucleic acid specify or "code for" a specific amino acid to be added to a polypeptide chain in the synthesis of protein.

genetic counseling—providing information, advice, and emotional support to persons or their relatives, including prospective parents, who are at risk of a genetic disorder.

genetic death—extinction of a genetic mutation, which is not passed on to the next generation.

genetic drift—a random fluctuation in the distribution of a given gene in a limited population.

genetic engineering—intentionally altering the genetic composition of an organism.

genetic marker—any observable or measurable feature that can be used to detect the operation of a given gene in an individual.

genetic screening—testing of apparently normal persons to assess the risk of their having a specific genetic disorder or of producing a child with such a disorder.

genetics terms for quick reference

acentric
acrocentric
allele
amplification
aneuploid
anticipation
antisense
association

genetics terms for quick reference *(cont.)*

autosomal dominant
autosomal recessive
autosome
banding
burden
carrier
centimorgan (cM)
chromosomal aberration
chromosomal satellite
concordant
contig
crossover (crossing over)
dicentric
discordant
divergence
dominant
duplication
empiric risk
expressivity
forme fruste
frameshift mutation
G bands
heterogeneity
heteroploid
heterozygote
heterozygous
homologous
homozygote
homozygous
inversion
isolate
karyotype
kindred
lethal equivalent
linkage
locus
map unit
mendelian inheritance
missense mutation
monosomy
monozygotic twins
mosaic
nondisjunction

genetics terms for quick reference *(cont.)*
nonpenetrance
nonsense mutation
pedigree
phenocopy
phenotype
pleiotropy
polygenic
polyploid
proband
propositus
recombination
recurrence risk
repressor
ring chromosome
segregation
selection
simplex
trisomy
wild type

geniculum—sharp, knee-like bend in a structure or organ.

genioglossal advancement with hyoid myotomy (GAHM)—surgical procedure for obstructive sleep apnea.

genome—the full complement of genetic information possessed by the chromosomes of an individual organism or species.

genotype—the genetic composition of an individual. Cf. *phenotype*.

Gen-Probe—hybridization kit.

Gensini cardiac device.

GenStent biologic—gene-based therapeutic designed to help reduce restenosis in patients following angioplasty or stent placement procedures.

Gentell alginate wound dressing.

Gentell foam wound dressing.

Gentiva Health Services—provider of home health care services.

GentleLASE Plus—a laser system for removal of hair and purpura-free treatment of vascular lesions in large leg veins.

GentlePeel skin exfoliation system—removes old or damaged skin cells.

Gentle Touch—postoperative colostomy appliance.

gents—slang for *gentamicins*. Usage: "Blood cultures grew *E. coli* which is susceptible to cefotetan, ceftazidime, gents, levofloxacin, and tobramycin."

genuine stress incontinence (GSI).

genupectoral position (knee-chest position)—a position for examination or therapeutic procedures in which the subject kneels on the examining table and bends forward so that the weight of the upper body rests on the chest.

Genutrain P3—active knee support for patellar realignment.

Geo-Mattress—a line of therapeutic mattresses, many of which are designed to hold patients who weigh up to 600 pounds.

geographic tongue—a condition of the tongue in which irregular zones of redness appear and create an appearance somewhat like a map.

geophagia artifact (Radiol)—shows up radiologically as increased opacity in bowel and bands in fatty tissue. It is evidence of patients who eat dirt, paint, etc. Also *pica*.

Georgiade visor—halo fixation apparatus.

GEO Structure spinal implant—a titanium geometric device that is implanted into the lumbar or thoracic spine to restore the integrity of the anterior, middle, and posterior spinal columns for a prolonged period, even in the absence of fusion.

GER (gastroesophageal reflux).

GERD (gastroesophageal reflux disease).

Gerdy tubercle in the knee.

Geriatric Depression Scale (GDS)—to assess depression in the elderly.

Geriatric *(cont.)*
It is available in short-form or long-form questionnaire, and may be administered in oral, written, or on-line format.

Geristore—anhydrous nonacidic glass ionomer-based composite dental restorative.

germ cell—a gamete (sperm or oocyte) or a primordial cell that can mature into a gamete.

germination tube—see *germ tube*.

germ layer—any of the three primitive layers—endoderm, mesoderm, and ectoderm—into which the inner cell mass of an early embryo (blastocyst) divides as a preliminary to further development.

germ line—the line of primordial cells, identifiable in the late embryonic stage of development, that will eventually differentiate into gametes (sperm or oocytes, depending on the sex of the embryo).

germ tube test (brief form for *germination tube*)—a quick lab test to distinguish *Candida albicans* from other yeasts. Usage: "The patient had a yeast growing also, thought not to be *Candida albicans* by two-hour germ tube."

Gerson therapy—a dietary approach that has been used by some to treat cancer and other diseases. It focuses on the role of minerals, enzymes, hormones, and other dietary factors in restoring health and well-being. The daily regimen calls for drinking 13 glasses of juice prepared from fresh organic fruits and vegetables, and eating vegetarian meals prepared from organically grown fruits, vegetables, and whole grains. Various supplements and enemas are given. Gerson therapy was named after Dr. Max B. Gerson, who initially developed this approach to treat his migraine headaches.

Gerstmann syndrome—agraphia.

GE Senographe 2000D—fully digital mammography system.

get-up-and-go test—a measure of mobility that involves timed standing from an armless chair, walking fast for 10 yards, returning, and sitting down.

Gey balanced salt solution—a fixative solution used in multiple applications.

GFAP (glial fibrillary acidic protein)—a test for identifying some types of brain tumors.

GFR (glomerular filtration rate).

GFS Mark II inflatable penile prosthesis.

GFX coronary stent.

GGT (gamma glutamyl transferase).

GGTP (gamma glutamyl transpeptidase)—a liver function test.

Ghajar guide—for intraventricular catheter placement. Used in trauma, in reduction of intracranial pressure; for placement of shunts in hydrocephalus; for placement of pharmacologic agents directly into cerebral ventricles.

Gherini-Kauffman Endo-Otoprobe—laser probe used in ear surgery.

GHLs (glenohumeral ligaments).

Ghon complex—a peripheral calcified granuloma and lymph node in the lung, diagnostic of old tuberculous infection.

ghost vessels—in the cornea.

GHz (gigahertz).

Giampapa suturing technique—plastic surgical technique developed by Dr. Vincent C. Giampapa. It treats sagging neck and jaw muscles by tightening the underlying platysma muscle.

Giannestras step-down procedure—to lengthen post-traumatic shortness of the metatarsals.

Gianotti-Crosti syndrome—papular acrodermatitis of childhood.

giant anorectal condyloma acuminatum—giant anal wart caused by human papillomaviruses, and often oncogenic human papillomaviruses, with over 30% case rate of malignant transformation.

giant cell arteritis (GCA)—a systemic disease of unknown etiology; characterized by vasculitis in branches of the carotid artery, with narrowed vascular lumen and thickened intima. The artery may be occluded by thrombosis. This may be an immune-mediated abnormality. See *von Willebrand factor*.

Gianturco expandable (self-expanding) **metallic biliary stent**; **prosthesis**—a metal stent used to treat biliary and esophageal strictures; its wires are crisscrossed in a Z pattern. Also called *Z stent*.

Gianturco-Roehm—bird's nest vena cava filter.

Gianturco-Roubin flexible coil stent—an intracoronary stent used after a failed or suboptimal PTCA. Also used in hepatic revascularization.

Gianturco-Rösch Z-stent—an esophageal stent with an impermeable polyethylene film, inside and outside, to deter tumor ingrowth and seal fistulae.

Gianturco wool-tufted wire coil—used in embolization treatment of arteriovenous fistulae or pseudoaneurysms.

Giardia lamblia—a protozoan parasite virulent in AIDS patients. Can be transmitted in drinking water and through sexual contact.

GIA stapler—transects and staples. (GIA, gastrointestinal anastomosis.)

gibbous deformity—humped, humpbacked, protruding. Cf. *gibbus*.

Gibbs phenomenon (MRI term)—"ripples" parallel to sharp edges separating areas of different densities. See also *edge ringing artifact* and *truncation band artifact*.

gibbus (noun)—a hump. Cf. *gibbous*.

Gibson inner ear shunt—used to reduce inner ear pressure in patients suffering from Ménière disease.

giddy headache—an old lay name for a headache preceded by vertigo.

Giebel blade plate—used in supratubular (or tubercular) wedge osteotomy.

GIFT (gamete intrafallopian transfer).

gift-wrap suture technique—the anatomic structure is wrapped on four sides with suture, and tied off at the top, resembling a gift-wrapped package.

gigahertz ("gig'-uh-herts") (GHz)—unit of frequency that equals 1 billion hertz (cycles per second); 10^9 Hz.

Gigli saw ("gee-lee," "jig-gly," or "gig-lee").

GIK (glucose, insulin, and potassium)—drug given to patients within 24 hours of experiencing heart attack symptoms. When administered, it is said the death rate from heart attack falls by half.

Gilbert-Rutkow-Robbins classification of groin hernias (types 1-7).

Gilles de la Tourette syndrome—see *Tourette syndrome*.

Gillette joint—orthosis for ambulation in children with cerebral palsy and myelomeningocele. Made of rubber vacuformed into polypropylene to provide a plantar-flexion stop and free dorsiflexion.

Gilliam suspension of the uterus.

Gillies elevation—procedure for fractured zygoma.

Gillies horizontal dermal suture.

Gill/Jonas modification of Norwood procedure—for hypoplastic left-sided heart syndrome. See *Fontan; Sade*.

Gill laminectomy—a procedure for spondylolisthesis, which consists of removing the involved loose lamina and decompressing the exiting nerve roots by removing hypertrophic fibrocartilage in the pars inarticularis defect. Because of the risk of slip progression, a concurrent fusion procedure in adults to prevent late symptomatic instability, especially in the setting of degenerative disk disease, has been recommended.

Gilvernet ("Jheel-vehr-nay") **retractor**.

Gimmick elevator—used in otologic surgery. "When opening posterior fossa dura, put a Gimmick in and cut with Belucci scissors over the top, always pulling outward to look for vessels."

gimpy—pejorative term for a lower extremity in which pain, spasm, or deformity causes a limp.

Gingrass and Messer pins—used in sagittal split ramus osteotomy.

Giraffe Spot PT Lite—a phototherapy system for the treatment of infant jaundice. The compact light box allows for easy portability, while the flexible light pipe positions and focuses the light exactly where it's needed. The Giraffe Spot PT Lite provides high-intensity natural white light with a long-lasting metal halide bulb, and is cooler than traditional spotlights to reduce the risk of thermal stress on the infant.

Girard Fragmatome—a fragmentation probe used in cataract extraction.

Girdlestone-Taylor procedure (Ortho).

Gitelman syndrome—variant of hypokalemic-hypomagnesemic tubular disorder with hypocalciuria.

GITS (gastrointestinal therapeutic system)—a drug-delivery system that protects the GI tract.

gitter cell—not to be confused with *glitter cell*.

Gittes urethral suspension procedure (Dr. Ruben F. Gittes).

Given diagnostic imaging system—utilizes the swallowable M2A imaging capsule for endoscopic procedures.

GKA (glucokinase activator).

glabellar tap (Neuro)—a test for brain damage. With the extended index finger, the examiner taps the patient's forehead in the midline at the level of the supraorbital ridges. The patient blinks. This maneuver is then repeated. Normally the patient, knowing what is happening, does not again blink. However, a patient with certain central nervous system pathology blinks every time the glabella is tapped. A positive glabellar tap after infancy is a sign of brain damage.

"glackoff"—phonetic for *Glagov*.

GLAD (glenolabral articular disruption [of shoulder]).

Glagov phenomenon—the outward compensatory remodeling (increased external elastic lamina) in diseased coronaries, allowing the vessel to accommodate the plaque and maintain physiological shear stress. Sometimes sounds like "Glackoff."

glandular atypia—atypical glandular cells of undetermined significance.

Glasgow classification of choledocholithiasis.

Glasgow Coma Scale (GCS)—assesses the prognosis of patients with head injuries by describing the patient's level of consciousness. It is divided into three parts:
Eyes open:
spontaneously
to speech
to pain
do not open
Best verbal response:
oriented
confused
inappropriate words
incomprehensible sounds
no verbal response
Best motor response:
obeys commands
localizes pain
flexion to pain
extension to pain
no motor response
Each of the parameters is scored on a scale of 1 through 5. The total of the values added together indicates the patient's level of consciousness. Normal would be 14 or 15; 7 or less would be considered coma. A score of 3 would be considered brain death (but is not conclusive). See *EMV grading*.

Glasgow Outcome Scale
Good recovery
Moderate disability
Severe disability
Permanent vegetative state
Death

Glasscock dressing (ENT).

glass eye artifact (Radiol)—appears on x-ray because of inadequate history given to radiologist.

Glassman clamp—used in thoracoscopy for compression and repositioning of the lung to facilitate stapling technique.

Glassman stone extractor—for removal of impacted common duct stones.

Glaucoma Wick—for long-term treatment of glaucoma.

glaukomflecken—yeast-shaped opacities that form following acute glaucoma attack.

Gleason score—for carcinoma of the prostate: a grading for prognosis, on a scale of 1 through 5, from well differentiated to poorly differentiated. The test is done twice, in different areas, and the results added together. A score of 10, for example, would give a grave prognosis.

Glenn anastomosis procedure—in hypoplastic left heart syndrome.

glial cell-derived neurotrophic factor (GDNF).

glial fibrillary acidic protein (GFAP) —a test for identifying some types of brain tumors.

GliaSite—radiation therapy system implanted in the brain during the surgical procedure conducted to remove a tumor. The device is later filled with a liquid radiation source that places a high dose of radiation directly into the tissue most likely to contain residual cancer cells.

glide—a surgical instrument for intracapsular cataract extraction when the lens is subluxated.

GlideCath—a brand name for a number of instruments used in cardiovascular surgery; namely, guidewire, torque device, syringe, entry needle, dilator and sheath.

Glidewire—trade name of a coated, kink-resistant guidewire used in endourology procedures. Also, Microvasive Glidewire. See also *long taper/stiff shaft Glidewire.*

glioblastoma multiforme—malignant tumor usually occurring in the cerebrum of adults.

Glisson capsule—connective tissue covering of the liver.

glissonean sheath—a connective tissue sheath surrounding the glissonean triad (portal vein, hepatic artery, common bile duct) at the hepatic hilum, an extension of the glissonean (Glisson) capsule enclosing the liver.

glistenings—tiny clear-to-white sparkling areas within an implanted intraocular lens that may or may not affect vision.

glitter cell—not to be confused with *gitter cell.*

Global Assessment of Functioning (GAF).

Global Deterioration Scale (GDS)—for assessment of primary degenerative dementia.
Level 1: no cognitive decline.
Level 2: very mild cognitive decline.
Level 3: mild cognitive decline.
Level 4: moderate cognitive decline.
Level 5: moderately severe cognitive decline.
Level 6: severe cognitive decline.
Level 7: very severe cognitive decline.
Stages 4-7 are considered the dementia stages.

Global total shoulder arthroplasty.

globus hystericus—the sensation of having a lump in the throat, sometimes accompanied by choking, due to emotional upset. See also *globus pharyngis.*

globus pallidus—a structure in the brain, sometimes referred to simply as pallidus. It can be seen on an MRI.

globus pallidus internal (GPi) **segment**—area of the brain that contributes to fine control of voluntary movement. An electrical lead implanted in this area can block abnormal nerve signals that cause tremors and other symptoms of Parkinson disease. See also *subthalamic nucleus (STN)*.

globus pharyngis—sensation of having a lump in the throat, often associated with esophageal motility disorder or stress (called *globus hystericus*).

Glo Germ—a liquid and a powder used with ultraviolet light for demonstrations to medical personnel of proper handwashing techniques.

glomerular filtration rate (GFR).

glomerulonephritis, acute poststreptococcal (APSGN).

glomus tumor—rare benign vascular tumor composed of a mass of arteriovenous anastomoses with a rich nerve supply and surrounded by special muscle cells known as glomus cells. Seventy-five percent of such tumors occur in the hand. Intraosseous (within bone) are rare.

glomus vagale—paraganglioma of the vagus nerve. Also called *glomus intravagale* or *nonchromaffin paraganglioma.*

glottic chink—see *posterior glottic chink.*

glove-juice technique—a method for obtaining culture samples from hands. The subject's hand is placed in a plastic bag containing a sampling solution that neutralizes any residual antiseptic on the skin and disperses colonies of microorganisms into single cells. The hand is massaged through the bag for one minute, and the bag is then transported to the laboratory for culture.

GLS (gait lock splint) **brace**.

Glucatell test kit—laboratory blood test to help diagnose severe fungal infections. It tests for beta-glucan in the blood, which may indicate a fungal infection.

Gluck rib shears—an autopsy instrument used to cut through the costosternal joints.

Glucometer DEX blood glucose monitor—a self-monitoring blood glucose system that allows diabetics the ability to test 10 times in a row through a self-calibrating 10-test cartridge.

Glucometer II—a home glucose monitoring system.

Glucoprime—a skin ulcer repair compound.

Gluco-Protein—a self-test for glycated protein for use by patients with diabetes.

glucose, insulin, and potassium (GIK).

glucose-6-phosphate dehydrogenase (G-6-PD) deficiency—a hereditary sex-linked enzyme defect that results in the breakdown of red blood cells when the person is exposed to the stress of infection or certain drugs.

GlucoWatch—bloodless glucose monitor, worn like a wristwatch, and measuring glucose automatically through intact skin every 30 minutes, 24 hours a day.

GlucoWatch G2 Biographer—diabetes monitoring system.

glue—see *adhesive*.

glue ear—a term for middle ear effusion in which the secretions are glue-like.

glue-footed gait—an ataxic gait in which the patient seems unable to lift either foot from the floor.

glutaraldehyde cross-linked collagen injections—used to treat urinary incontinence in women. The material is biocompatible, biodegradable, sterile, nonpyrogenic, purified bovine dermal collagen which is cross-linked with the glutaraldehyde and dispersed in saline. The substance completely degrades in 9 to 19 months, resulting in the need for repeat injections to sustain efficacy.

glutaraldehyde-tanned umbilical vein graft—used for lower limb revascularization.

glutaraldehyde-tanned porcine heart valve—xenograft or heterograft.

gluteal bonnet—gluteus maximus and minimus.

glycol methacrylate—an embedding medium for pathology specimens.

Glycosal diabetes test—rapid doctors' office test to assist in the identification and management of diabetes.

glycosylated hemoglobin—an assay of diabetic control; glucose stays attached to the red cell for the life of the cell and can be measured.

Glynase Pres Tab (glyburide)—an oral antidiabetic drug, also marketed as DiaBeta and Micronase.

GM-CSF (granulocyte/macrophage colony-stimulating factor)—also regramostim, sargramostim, molgramostim).

GMS stain (Gomori, or Grocott, methenamine silver)—a stain used to establish the diagnosis of *Pneumocystis carinii* pneumonia.

GNG (generalized nephrographic) **phase imaging**—used on CT scan to detect acute renal infection.

GnRH (gonadotropin-releasing hormone). See *LHRH* (luteinizing hormone-releasing hormone).

GOAT (Galveston Orientation and Amnesia Test).

Goeckerman regimen—treatment for psoriasis including application of tar and tar-based medications, shampoos with tar, and two types of light treatment (shortwave ultraviolet light in increasing doses daily, and quartz light in increasing doses).

Goetz cardiac device.

goiter—see *diffuse toxic goiter; lithiumogenic goiter*.

Golaski graft—a knitted Dacron graft used during carotid endarterectomy and carotid-subclavian artery bypass.

Golay coil—MRI term.

GOLD clinical trial—Global Strategy for the Diagnosis, Management, and Prevention of Chronic Obstructive Pulmonary Disease.

Goldenberg footplate shoe—designed to slip over the end of an incudostapedial prosthesis.

Goldenberg Snarecoil bone marrow biopsy needle.

Goldenhar syndrome—oculoauriculovertebral dysplasia. A congenital anomaly involving the eye, ear, vertebrae, and mandible, temporal and zygomatic bones, and the muscles used in facial expression and mastication.

Goldman cardiac risk index score—a clinical scoring system used to predict cardiac morbidity.

Goldman-McNeill blepharostat—see *McNeill-Goldman corneal transplant ring*.

Goldmann applanation tonometer—used to measure intraocular pressure.

Goldmann campimeter—used to evaluate the visual fields; may also be used to assess pupil diameter.

Goldmann lens—a three-mirror contact lens used in photocoagulation procedures for detached retina, or in lattice degeneration.

Goldmann visual fields—refers to Goldmann perimetry or perimeter.

Goldman procedure—a nasal tip reconstructive technique.

Gold Probe bipolar hemostasis catheter.

Goldstein Microspike approximator clamp (Urol)—a clamp with tiny spikes on its surface to aid in gripping the vas deferens to assist in anastomosis during vasovasostomy.

gold weight—a weight used in surgery for Bell palsy.

Golgi complex—a collection of vesicles in the cell cytoplasm where products of cell metabolism are placed into vacuoles for excretion.

Goligher retractor—modification of the Berkeley-Bonney self-retaining 3-blade abdominal retractor for use in abdominal surgery.

GoLytely (polyethylene glycol-electrolyte solution)—gastrointestinal lavage drug prep for improved visualization in bowel examination.

gomer (acronym for "get out of my ER")—a disparaging slang term for a difficult patient, particularly an elderly male with many chronic, complicated problems and much psychological overlay.

Gomori (or Grocott) **methenamine silver** (GMS)—a stain used to establish the diagnosis of *Pneumocystis carinii* pneumonia.

gonad—an organ (testis or ovary) that produces sex cells (sperm or oocytes).

gonadal ridge—embryonic structure from which the gonads develop.

gonadotropin-releasing hormone (GnRH). See *goserelin acetate*.

gonial angle—of the mandible.

goniometry—a standardized testing procedure to determine the mobility of a joint, irrespective of the strength of the surrounding muscles, their nerve supply, or the subject's coordination and ability to follow directions. Goniometry measures the passive range of motion.

gonioscope—an optical instrument for direct visualization of the anterior chamber through the use of a goniolens; e.g., Sussman gonioscope.

Gonzales blood group—a blood group character (antigen Goa) for which the antibody was reported in a mother (Mrs. Gonzales) of a newborn infant with erythroblastosis fetalis. This is an antibody apparently found only in individuals who are of African-American parentage, and it is distinct from all previously classified blood group systems.

Goodale-Lubin cardiac device.

Goodell sign—softening of the cervix because of an increased blood supply, an early clue to pregnancy.

Goodenough test—a draw-a-man test to estimate intelligence. The name of the test does not refer to the performance; it is named for Florence Goodenough.

GoodKnight 418A, 418G, 418P—home care CPAP system for treatment of patients suffering from obstructive sleep apnea.

Good Nights Sleep—sleep aid throat spray.

Goodwin sound—a sound (an instrument) used in the endoscopic treatment of obliterated membranous urethral strictures.

Gordon-Sweet staining—used to determine the growth pattern of tumors (follicular or follicular and diffuse).

Gore cast liner—waterproof cast liner that breathes.

Gore 1.5T Torso Array—MRI surface coil for imaging of chest, abdominal, and pelvic regions.

gore pattern—created by cutting the surface of a sphere along longitudinal lines to change the radius of curvature. See *Hendel correction of scaphocephaly.*

Gore Smoother Crucial Tool—used as a trial graft and replacement tool in cruciate replacement operations.

Gore-Tex—nonabsorbable surgical suture and a graft material; also used for many other purposes. Examples:
bifurcated vascular graft
cardiovascular patch
catheter
knee prosthesis
limb
shunt
soft tissue patch
stretch vascular graft
surgical membrane
tapered vascular graft
vascular graft

Gore-Tex FEP-Ringed vascular graft.

Gore-Tex nasal implant—used to augment the nasal dorsum or base in the rhinoplasty procedure.

Gore-Tex Propaten—vascular graft with a proprietary heparin coating.

Gore-Tex SAM (subcutaneous augmentation material) **facial implants** (Plas Surg)—made of expanded polytetrafluoroethylene (PTFE) that is reinforced with fluorinated ethylene propylene to make a rigid, but soft, material that is easy to carve or shape. It is easier to shape than nonreinforced PTFE, and its structure permits cellular ingrowth and incorporation of connective tissue.

Gore-Tex strips—used in plastic surgery as implants to augment soft tissue in facial contouring.

gorilloid—resembling a gorilla. You might hear this in radiology dictation in reference to the navicular bone.

GOS (Glasgow Outcome Scale).

Gosling pulsatility index.

Gosset—see *spiral band of Gosset*.

gossypiboma (cotton)—a term applied to a laparotomy pad left in at previous surgery and recovered by laparoscopy.

Gottschalk Nasostat—a rubber cannula used to stop epistaxis (nosebleed).

Gott shunt—used in liver transplantation.

gouge—(noun) a hollow chisel used for cutting or removing bone or cartilage; (verb) to scoop out, as with a gouge. Cf. *gauge*.

Gould electromagnetic flowmeter—records arterial blood flow rates.

Gould polygraph—device for measuring gastric motility.

Goulian mammoplasty.

Gowers maneuver—patients with weakness may find it necessary to "climb" up their legs with their hands, to rise from a sitting position.

Gowers sign—classical sign of Duchenne muscular dystrophy; also called *tripoding*.

GPC (giant papillary conjunctivitis).

GPi (globus pallidus internal) **segment**.

GPMAL (obstetrical history): gravida, para, multiple births, abortions, live births.

GR (gastric retention).

graciloplasty—see *dynamic graciloplasty*.

grade—see *classification*.

gradient coil—MRI term.

gradient magnetic field—MRI term.

gradient-recalled echo (GRE)—MRI term.

gradual elongation (intramedullary) nailing (GEN, GEIN)—leg-lengthening procedure that does not require external fixation.

graft, **graft material** (see also *flap* and *graft, skin*)
- Advanta SST
- Advanta SST PTFE vascular
- Advanta Super-Soft
- Advanta Super-Soft vascular
- Advanta V12 stent
- Advanta VS
- Advanta VS vascular
- Advanta VXT vascular
- AlloAnchor RC allograft
- AlloDerm processed tissue
- allograft
- AlloMatrix injectable putty bone graft substitute
- amniotic membrane transplantation
- AneuRx stent
- AneuRx tube graft
- aortofemoral bypass (AFBG)
- Apligraf (Graftskin)
- Aria coronary artery bypass
- arthroscopic autologous chondrocyte transplantation
- autologous fat
- BAGF (brachioaxillary bridge graft fistula)
- Bard Composix mesh
- Bard Sperma-Tex preshaped mesh
- Bard Visilex mesh
- batten
- Biobrane/HF
- Biograft bovine heterograft
- BioPolyMeric
- bone graft substitute—CHAG
- BonePlast
- Bonfiglio
- bovine heterograft
- BPTB (bone-patellar tendon-bone)

graft *(cont.)*
brachiosubclavian bridge
BSGF (brachiosubclavian bridge graft fistula)
CABG (coronary artery bypass)
Calcitite
Capset (calcium sulfate) bone graft barrier
carbon fiber synthetic ligament
Carbo-Seal
Cardiopass
cavum conchal cartilage
CHAG (coralline hydroxyapatite Goniopora)
Collagraft bone graft matrix
Cotton cartilage
Cragg endoluminal
cultured epithelial autograft
cymba conchal cartilage
Cymetra tissue replacement material
Dacron synthetic ligament material
Dardik Biograft
delayed xenograft rejection (DXR)
denatured homograft
Dermagraft human-based dermal replacement
Dermagraft-TC (transitional covering)
Diastat vascular access
discordant cellular xenograft
discordant organ xenograft
Distaflo bypass
doubled semitendinosus and gracilis autograft (DST&G)
DTAFA (descending thoracic aorta-to-femoral artery) bypass
DualMesh biomaterial
DuraGen
Durapatite
E-CABG (endoscopic coronary artery bypass graft)
Edwards woven Teflon aortic bifurcation
EndoFit aortic endovascular
endovascular stent

graft *(cont.)*
epidural blood patch
Exxcel ePTFE soft vascular graft
flap
Fluoropassiv thin-wall carotid patch
free-GEPA
full-thickness skin
GEA (gastroepiploic artery)
glutaraldehyde-tanned umbilical vein
glutaraldehyde-tanned porcine heart valve
Golaski
Gore-Tex
Gore-Tex FEP-Ringed vascular
Gore-Tex Propaten
Gore-Tex stretch vascular
Gore-Tex tapered vascular
Grafton DBM (demineralized bone matrix) bone
Graftpatch
Graftskin (Apligraf)
Hapset bone graft plaster
Healos synthetic bone-grafting material
Hedrocel bone substitute material
Hemashield
Hemashield Gold branch graft
Hemashield Gold Microvel knitted double velour graft
Hemashield Vantage vascular graft
Hemobahn endovascular prosthesis
heterografts, bovine and porcine
HTO Wedge
human meniscal allograft
hydroxyapatite
IEA (inferior epigastric artery)
IMA (inferior mammary artery)
infrarenal aortobifemoral bypass
Infuse bone graft LT-Cage
inlay
InterGard Knitted collagen coated
Interpore
Ionescu-Shiley pericardial xenograft
isograft
ITA (internal thoracic artery)

graft *(cont.)*
Jostent
Kimura cartilage
LIMA (left internal mammary artery)
Lyodura dura mater graft
Marlex synthetic
Martius
MD-111 bone allograft
Meadox Microvel arterial
Microknit vascular
mitral valve homograft
MycroMesh biomaterial
myocutaneous
Ne-Osteo bone morphogenic protein (BMP)
Nicoll
onlay
paddle
Paritene mesh
PepGen P-15 (peptide-enhanced bone graft)
Perma-Flow coronary bypass
PermaMesh
Perma-Seal dialysis access
PFTE (polyfluorotetraethylene)
pigskin
porcine xenograft
portacaval H
postage-stamp type skin
ProOsteon 500 bone implant
Proplast
PTFE (polytetrafluoroethylene)
pulmonary autograft (PA)
Pyrost
Rapidgraft arterial vessel substitute
rib cartilage
Sauvage
sentinel skin paddle
seromuscular intestinal patch
skin
Slider GDS (graft deployment system)
Solvang
Sperma-Tex preshaped mesh

graft *(cont.)*
spiral vein grafts
spreader
stem cell autograft
subcutaneous polytef patch (Gore-Tex)
Sure-Closure skin-stretching system
Surgipro prolene mesh
Surgisis Gold hernia repair
Surgisis Gold mesh graft
SurgiSis sling/mesh
sutured in place, shield-shaped tip
Synergraft
Thiersch
Thoralon biomaterial
TransCyte skin substitute
transplanted stamp
Trelex mesh
Ultramax coated knitted velour vascular
Unigraft bone graft material
Unilab Surgibone
Vascu-Guard bovine pericardial surgical patch
vascularized fibula
VascuLink
Vascutek
Vectra vascular access (VAG)
Venaflow vascular
Weavenit vascular
Wesolowski vascular
Wolfe
XenoDerm
xenograft
Zenith AAA (abdominal aortic aneurysm) endovascular
Zenotech

GraftAssist vein and graft holder—reduces the chance of narrowing at the anastomosis site.

GraftCyte—a gauze wound dressing containing copper peptide. It is used particularly in hair restoration procedures.

Grafton DBM (demineralized bone matrix) **bone graft**. Also, Grafton DBM gel, putty, and flex strips.

Graftpatch—used in general surgical procedures to reinforce soft tissue.

graft seeding technique—see *cell seeding*.

graft, skin

split thickness—.010 to .035 inch thick

full thickness—greater than .035 inch thick

free graft—does not have its own blood supply; gets blood from capillary ingrowth from underlying tissue

pedicle—gets its blood supply from subcutaneous vessels that came with the pedicle portion of the graft

Graftskin—a manufactured human skin product used to treat chronic wounds that do not respond well to traditional treatment.

graft versus host disease (GVHD)—caused by reaction to an allograft, from marrow transplant, etc. Following is the GVHD grading system (written as clinical grade 1, etc.):

1 Mild skin rash (generally maculopapular). No gastrointestinal or liver function abnormalities.

2 Moderately severe skin rash. Mild gastrointestinal symptoms. Slight increase in bilirubin and perhaps also in liver enzymes.

3 Moderately severe skin rash, gastrointestinal symptoms, and liver function abnormalities.

4 Severe peeling and flaking of the skin, severe gastrointestinal symptoms, and liver function abnormalities.

graft versus host reaction—see *graft versus host disease*.

Graham plication—an omental patch sutured over a perforated ulcer site.

Graham Steell heart murmur (no hyphen).

gram-negative organisms—*Haemophilus, Neisseria, Pseudomonas*. See *Gram stain; gram-positive*.

gram-positive organisms—*Clostridium, Corynebacterium, Staphylococcus, Streptococcus*. See *Gram stain; gram-negative organisms*.

Gram stain (named for Hans Christian Joachim Gram)—a stain using the bacterial property of stain retention or loss to help in classification and subsequent treatment. The smears are fixed to a slide by heat and stained with a solution of crystal violet, which stains all bacteria. An iodine solution then fixes the dye to the gram-positive organisms. The specimen is decolorized by washing with a mixture of acetone and alcohol, and then counterstained with a dye of another color (usually safranin). Gram-positive organisms retain the original purple stain; gram-negative organisms, however, turn pink (if safranin was used). Note: Capitalize *Gram stain*, but lowercase *gram-negative* and *gram-positive*. See *gram-negative; gram-positive*.

GraNee needle (Riza-Ribe grasper needle)—single-use device used in laparoscopic surgical procedures for grasping free ends of a suture ligature for intracorporeal or extracorporeal tying.

granulocyte colony-stimulating factor—see *G-CSF*.

granulocyte/macrophage colony-stimulating factor (GM-CSF)—a natu-

granulocyte *(cont.)* rally occurring growth factor which stimulates myeloid progenitor cells in the bone marrow to divide and differentiate into granulocytes and macrophages. Also stimulates mature granulocytes and macrophages to higher levels of migration towards pathogens, phagocytosis, and cytotoxic activity, thus enhancing the effectiveness of the immune system. Used in chemotherapy and in conjunction with AZT in treatment of AIDS. See *sargramostim.* Cf. *G-CSF.*

granulocyte transfusions—may have a greater effect on survival rates compared to use of broad-spectrum antibiotics in neutropenic patients with cancer.

granuloma—see *pyogenic granuloma* (granuloma pyogenicum).

granuloma gravidarum—gingival pyogenic granuloma of pregnancy.

granulomatous mastitis—a very rare lesion somewhat similar to duct ectasia, except that it is always peripheral and confined to the breast lobule. See *duct ectasia.*

graphesthesia—relates to the perception and identification of letters or numbers written on the skin with a blunt object.

graphospasm—writer's cramp.

Graspit nitinol stone retrieval forceps.

grasp reflex—the reflex of an infant who will automatically grasp a finger placed against the palmar surface of its hand.

GRASS (gradient recalled acquisition in a steady state)—technique for cardiac MRI test.

gravida—the number of pregnancies a woman has had: *gravida 4,* having been pregnant 4 times; *gravida 5, para 3, ab 2,* five pregnancies, three live births, two abortions or miscarriages. See also *GPMAL*; *para.*

Gravindex—relatively sensitive pregnancy test used in physician offices.

gray (Gy)—the International System unit of absorbed dose, equal to the energy imparted by ionizing radiation to a mass of matter corresponding to 1 joule per kilogram. Used in radiotherapy. See *joule.*

Gray bone drill—developed by Frank B. Gray, M.D.

gray line—in the eye.

Grayson ligament in hand—it keeps the skin sleeve from twisting around the bones of the digit. You may hear this referred to in operative procedures for Dupuytren contracture. See also *Cleland ligament*; they are *not* synonymous.

GRE (gradient-recalled echo). Usage: "three-dimensional GRE MR imaging of TFC (triangular fibrocartilage) tears and triangular fibrocartilage complex (TFCC)."

great vessels—on chest x-ray, the major vascular trunks entering and leaving the heart: the superior and inferior venae cavae, the pulmonary arteries and veins, and the aorta.

Green and O'Brien wrist function score—combines both subjective and objective data in assigning a score for wrist function.

Greene needle—a biopsy needle used for aspiration and also for removal of solid tissue specimens.

Greenfield IVC filter—a permanent inferior vena cava filter, placed via the right jugular vein into the inferior vena cava to filter out emboli that might otherwise reach the lung.

green lizard—GI cocktail.

Greenwald cutting loop—used with Storz resectoscope.

Greenwald flexible endoscopic electrodes.

Greenwald retractor—used in bladder surgery.

Green-Waterman osteotomy—a procedure for the treatment of dislocated hip.

Greenwich grading system—a system developed to quantify the effect of electrodiagnostic testing on diagnosis, investigation, and treatment in ophthalmology patients.

Greig cephalopolysyndactyly syndrome—a relatively rare condition in which fingers, toes, or other body parts are completely or partially webbed, with craniosynostosis sometimes present. It is caused by a chromosomal translocation thought to involve chromosome 7.

grenz ray—long wave irradiation; used in treatment of localized neurodermatitis and in lichen simplex chronicus; a low-energy x-ray.

Greulich and Pyle, bone age—for measurement of bone age and for staging skeletal maturation. Also referred to as *G & P*.

GRFoma—a rare pancreatic endocrine tumor.

Grice-Green procedure—to correct hindfoot valgus deformity.

Grieshaber manipulator—multi-function instrument used in vitreous surgery. It has a light source, a suction forceps, and a coagulator.

Griesinger sign—swelling and pain in the neck on rotation, easily mistaken for meningitis, but in this case due to thrombophlebitis of the mastoid emissary vein.

Grignolo-Tagliasco-Zingirian projection campimeter—used to evaluate visual fields.

Grinfeld cannula—a triple-lumen cannula that accommodates cardioplegia, arterial return, and aortic clamping during coronary artery bypass surgery.

Gripper needle.

grip tester—see *Jamar*.

Grocott (or Gomori) **methenamine silver** (GMS) **stain**. See *Gomori*.

Grollman catheter.

Groningen voice prosthesis.

Groshong catheter—used in central venous lines for administration of intravenous chemotherapeutic agents.

gross description (Path)—description of tissue as it appears to the unaided eye prior to fixation and paraffin embedding.

Grosse and Kempf locking nail system—femoral and tibial nails. There are two types: static locking (complete locking) and dynamic locking (partial locking). Stabilizes and controls fragment rotation and maintains desired bone length.

ground-glass cells—pathology as seen in chronic hepatitis B.

group A beta-hemolytic streptococcus (GABHS)—the pathogen that causes pharyngitis, rheumatic fever, toxic strep syndrome, and cellulitis. See *streptococcal A infection*.

Grover disease—temporary skin disorder that consists of small, firm, raised red lesions on the skin. Small blisters containing a watery liquid are present, which tend to group and have a swollen red border around them. Its cause is unknown but is thought to be related to trauma to sun-damaged skin, and it occurs mainly in men over the age of 40.

Gruentzig—see *Grüntzig*.

grunting—involuntary noise made by newborns with respiratory distress to try to keep lungs adequately inflated.

Grüntzig (Gruentzig) **balloon catheter**—used in percutaneous transluminal dilatation and angioplasty. (An umlaut is required over the "u" in *Grüntzig*; if an umlaut is not available on the keyboard, the spelling is *Gruentzig*.)

GSI (genuine stress incontinence).

G6PD (glucose-6-phosphate dehydrogenase)—X-linked enzyme. Used as a cell marker to study possible origin of different neoplastic disorders.

GST (gene-silencing therapy).

G-suit—an external counterpressure device used to control hemorrhage; provides tamponade of pelvic fracture-induced hemorrhage.

GTD (gestational trophoblastic disease).

GTS great toe system—two-piece implant designed to provide anatomic movement for the first metatarsophalangeal joint.

GTV (gross tumor volume).

GII (Generation II) **unloader knee brace**—provides symptomatic relief of pain caused by unicompartmental degenerative joint disease or osteoarthritis.

guaiac test of occult blood in the stool (blood in too small an amount to be detected by naked-eye observation). Usage: "Stool is guaiac negative." See also *fecal occult blood test*; *Hemoccult Sensa*; *Hemoccult II*; and *occult blood*.

guanine—a purine (symbol G), one of the four bases found in DNA and RNA; in the formation of a double-stranded nucleic acid, it always pairs with the purine adenine (A).

GUARD—saphenous vein graft intervention using AngioGuard for reduction of distal embolization.

Guardsman femoral screw—interference screw and delivery system used in endoscopic femoral fixation and orthopedic procedures where graft protection is required. Also used in knee arthroscopy.

GuardWire angioplasty system—seals one end of a bypass graft with a balloon to prevent debris from floating downstream into the coronary artery. A second balloon inflated at the site of blockage presses material that caused the blockage against the vessel wall within the bypass to restore blood flow to the heart. A low-pressure vacuum aspiration catheter then draws out remaining debris from inside the vessel. Also, *PercuSurge GuardWire system*.

Gudden atrophy—retrograde degeneration of the thalamus after cortical lesions. Named for German neurologist, Bernhard Aloys von Gudden. Also, *Gudden commissure, Gudden tract, nucleus of Gudden*.

Gudden tract—mammillotegmental tract in the brain.

Guepar II hinged knee prosthesis.

guerney—see *gurney*.

guggul, guggulsterone, Gugulipid—an herbal antischistosomal drug that appears to be effective for the treatment of elevated cholesterol. It contains a chemical that blocks the action of the cell receptor protein FXR, causing the body to eliminate more cholesterol. Guggul refers to a tree from which gum resin is extracted that contains the active agent guggulsterone. Gugulipid is a standardized preparation for OTC use.

Guglielmi Detachable Coil (GDC)—used to treat intracranial aneurysms that are considered inoperable or at high-risk for surgery. The GDC is delivered to the aneurysm site by a microcatheter. The coil fills the

Guglielmi *(cont.)*
aneurysm, isolating it from the circulation.

Guibor Silastic tube—used in surgery of the lacrimal system.

Guidant Multi-Link Tetra coronary stent system.

Guidant TRIAD three-electrode energy defibrillation system (Cardio) —said to reduce the amount of energy needed for defibrillation.

Guidant Ventak Prizm defibrillator.

Guidant Vigor-DR pulse generator.

guidewire (see also *Glidewire*)
ACS Hi-Torque Balance Middleweight
Amplatz Super Stiff
Athlete coronary
Extra Sport coronary
FasTrac
floppy
Geenan Endotorque
HPC
Intercept-Vascular
Lumina
Lunderquist
Magnum
Microvasive Glidewire
Mirage
Mustang steerable
QuickSilver hydrophilic-coated
Radiofocus Glidewire
ROTACS
Sensor PTFE-nitinol guidewire with hydrophilic tip
Silk
steerable guidewire system
Terumo
WaveWire

Guilford brace.

Guillain-Barré syndrome—acute idiopathic polyneuritis, an acute, rapidly progressive nerve inflammation, with weakness of the muscles of the legs, then weakness in the arms and face, and may also affect the muscles of respiration. It appears to be self-limiting in 90 to 95% of patients, with complete recovery, but it can result in flaccid quadriplegia or respiratory failure. Also called *infectious polyneuritis, Landry-Guillain-Barré-Strohl syndrome, Landry-Guillain syndrome,* and *Landry paralysis.*

Gullstrand slit lamp—see *biomicroscope*.

gull-wing incision—a midcolumellar transverse incision that looks like the drawings of birds we all did in grade school. Used in nasal tip reconstructive surgery.

gumma—a rubbery nodule of inflammation and necrosis, characteristic of tertiary syphilis.

gum sculpting—grafting procedure in which sections of gum in one area of the mouth are inserted into a receded area. This produces teeth that appear even in length.

Gunderson conjunctival flap.

Gungor test—for evaluation of anterior displacement of the talus from the ankle mortise. Similar to the *anterior drawer test*.

Gunn crossing sign (Cardio).

GunSlinger shoulder orthosis—for correct positioning and immobilization of the shoulder and arm following surgery.

Gurd criteria—for diagnosing fat embolization syndrome.

gurney (guerney)—high wheeled cot for moving patients.

Gusberg hysterectomy clamp—with Kapp-Beck serrations.

Gustilo-Kyle cementless total hip arthroplasty.

Gustilo ("gus-TILL-oh") **fracture classification**—a fracture classification, named for Ramon B. Gustilo,

Gustilo *(cont.)*
who wrote a manual called *The Fracture Classification Manual.*

gut-associated lymphoid tissue (GALT).

gut-hormone profile—a pattern of hormone release that may help to distinguish celiac disease from other abdominal problems.

Guttmann subtalar arthrodesis.

Guyon canal—anatomical landmark in operative procedures designed to reduce ulnar nerve compression which occurs as the ulnar nerve passes behind the medial epicondyle, between the heads of the flexor carpi ulnaris, or along Guyon canal from the pisiform bone to the hook of the hamate.

guy sutures (*not* Guy)—a steadying or guiding suture, to prevent movement. Also, *guy wire.* Cf. *guidewire.*

GVHD (graft-versus-host disease) (or reaction). See *graft-versus-host disease.*

GVR (galvanic vestibular stimulation).

GVR (growth velocity ratio).

gymnast's wrist—ulnar pain, ulnar variance of several millimeters, prominence of the ulnar head with either full or limited range of motion. These findings are due to repetitive compression of the bones of the forearm during handstands and other gymnastic maneuvers. The bones of the wrist may show abnormalities in the growth plates.

Gynecare TVT—a tension-free urethral sling for the treatment of incontinence in women. A sling composed of tape or mesh is placed beneath the urethra to provide support and help control involuntary leakage.

Gynecare Versascope hysteroscopy system—fiberoptic technology for diagnostic and operative hysteroscopy procedures.

Gynemesh PS—a polypropylene mesh indicated specifically for pelvic floor repair in cases of cystocele, rectocele, and vaginal vault suspension.

Gypsona—a rapid-setting cast material.

gyromagnetic ratio—MRI term.

Gyroscan ACS NT MRI scanner.

gyrus—a folding in the surface (cortex) of the cerebrum.

Gyrus endourology system—uses PlasmaKinetic radiofrequency energy delivery for minimally invasive endoscopic treatment of urethral obstructions in men secondary to an enlarged prostate.

H, h

HA (hydroxyapatite)—coating for load-bearing implants.

HAART (highly active antiretroviral therapy)—used for the treatment of HIV/AIDS to aggressively suppress viral replication and progress of HIV disease. HAART has been shown to reduce the amount of virus so that it becomes undetectable in a patient's blood.

HAB (Histoacryl Blue).

habenula ("hah-ben´u-lah")—a small protuberance at the dorsal and posterior edge of the third ventricle, adjacent to the pineal body. It is part of the epithalamus.

HAC (hydroxyapatite cement).

HACEK—an acronym for a group of gram-negative bacilli, including *Haemophilus aphrophilus* (and other *Haemophilus* species), *Actinobacillus actinomycetemcomitans, Cardiobacterium hominis, Eikenella corrodens,* and *Kingella kingae*, which are usually associated with infectious endocarditis, but can also occur with other infections.

H-Ae interval (retrograde conduction) —in electrophysiologic studies of supraventricular tachycardia.

Haemonetics Cell Saver—collects a patient's blood for transfusion at the end of an operative procedure.

Haemonetics V-50—used to reduce volume and deplete red cells in harvested bone marrow.

Haemophilus ducreyi—the cause of soft chancres or chancroids on the genitalia of humans. Also called *Ducrey bacillus*.

Haemophilus vaginalis—see *Gardnerella vaginalis*.

Hafnia alvei—new name of *Enterobacter hafnia*, associated with enteritis.

Hageman factor—factor XII of blood coagulation factors.

Haglund deformity—causes traumatic inflammation of Achilles tendon and bursa.

HAI (hepatic arterial infusion).

Haid Universal bone plate system—titanium, MRI-compatible plate and screw system for treating fracture traumas, postlaminectomy instability, and degenerative spinal disease.

hair apposition technique (HAT)—using hair from both sides of a scalp wound. In the procedure the surgeon twists it and then apply tissue glue to hold the hair and scalp together.

hair-on-end sign—abnormal finding on skull x-ray. The "hair" represents accentuated trabeculae extending between the inner and outer skull tables in the expanded diploic marrow spaces. It appears to be "on end" because the trabeculae are oriented perpendicular to the inner and outer tables of the skull. The term is now classically associated with the radiographic changes seen in hemolytic anemia.

hairy-cell leukemia (HCL)—first described in 1958. On electron micrographs, the cells have projections radiating from their walls.

Hakim-Cordis pump—used in neurological surgery procedures.

Halban culdoplasty.

Halbrecht syndrome—ABO erythroblastosis.

half and half nails—a dull-white proximal half of the fingernails meets a reddish-brown distal half. A sign of possible renal disease that may precede symptoms of renal disease.

half base syndrome—see *Garcin syndrome*.

half-dose enhanced MRI with MT (magnetization transfer). Cf. *standard-dose enhanced conventional MR imaging*.

half-Fourier acquisition single-shot turbo spin-echo (HASTE)—technique for MRU (magnetic resonance urography).

half-hitch—the simplest knot that can be tied in the two ends of a single looped strand; the first half of a square knot. Used in surgery.

half-moon mark artifact—see *kink artifact*.

Halifax interlaminar clamp system—provides stabilization of the posterior cervical spine with placement from C1 through C7 at multiple levels.

Hall dermatome—an oscillating blade type.

Haller layer—the vascular layer of the choroid of the eye.

Hallpike caloric stimulation test (ENT)—see *caloric testing of vestibular function*.

Hallpike-Dix maneuver—a maneuver in which the direction of the vertical component of nystagmus is observed in patients with benign paroxysmal positional vertigo affecting the posterior canal.

Hallpike test—see *Dix-Hallpike test*.

hallucinosis—pathological entity characterized by hallucination. Types: alcoholic and drug-induced.

hallux abductovalgus—the deformity which causes the great toe to be abducted and everted (abductovalgus) and usually is corrected surgically with a bunionectomy.

hallux extensus—a deformity in which the great toe is held in the extended position.

Hall valve—a prosthetic heart valve by Medtronic.

Hall valvulotome—used to disrupt the valves in a vein and make the valve leaflets incompetent. This allows the vein to be used in distal saphenous vein bypass procedures.

halo test—a bedside test for cerebrospinal fluid rhinorrhea. In this test, a drop of bloody fluid from the nose is placed on a cloth surface. If present, the CSF will diffuse in a radial pattern along with the blood; however, the CSF will migrate farther

halo *(cont.)*
than the blood, forming a "halo" effect.

halo traction—see *cervical support*.

HALS (hand-assisted laparoscopic surgery).

Halstead-Wepman Aphasia Screening Test.

Halsted hemostatic mosquito forceps (straight/curved).

Halsted inguinal herniorrhaphy (*not* Halstead).

HAMA (human antimurine antibody) **response**.

Hamman-Rich syndrome—diffuse interstitial pulmonary fibrosis.

Hamman sign—a sign of pneumopericardium, an acute medical emergency. The physician hears a loud clicking or crunching sound in time with the heart beat.

Hammer mini-tubular external fixation system.

hammer toe—clawlike flexion contracture of the second and distal phalanges.

hammer toe repair—see *DuVries hammer toe repair*.

hammock-like fashion—flap fixation in breast reconstruction surgery.

Hampton hump—a pleurally based, triangular lung infiltrate.

Hamus wrist arthroplasty.

Hancke-Vilmann biopsy handle instrument—see *Vilmann-Hancke*.

Hancock M.O. bioprosthesis—a tissue valve for the small aortic root; used instead of a porcine valve.

Hancock M.O. II bioprosthesis porcine valve.

Hancock II tissue valve—porcine prosthetic heart valve indicated for both aortic valve and mitral valve replacement. Special features include a stent and a scalloped sewing ring to facilitate placement and implantation.

hand—see *Myobock hand* and *Utah artificial arm*.

Handages—specially designed dressings for the burned hand that are shaped like a glove and feature a Velcro opening on the back for easy application and removal. The bandage gloves consist of three layers, including a breathable transparent film barrier that protects the wound from contamination, an absorbent middle layer, and a nonadherent wound contact layer. Handages can be removed without soaking. Because they do not adhere to the wound, changing them is not as painful as traditional bandages are.

hand-assisted laparoscopic sigmoidectomy—a technique that reportedly has a minimum learning curve yet retains the benefits of a laparoscopic procedure.

hand-assisted laparoscopic surgery (HALS)—combines advantages of open surgery with minimal invasiveness and rapid recovery of laparoscopy; ideally suited to remove malignant kidney tumors and to repair renal, ureteral, and bladder abnormalities. Provides for minimally invasive kidney donation, reducing recovery time for donors (17 vs. 60 days) and a kidney that has suffered a minimal period of interrupted blood flow.

hand-assisted Miami pouch, laparoscopic.

H&E stain (hematoxylin and eosin).

H&H—abbreviation for hemoglobin and hematocrit. Should be expanded in medical reports.

hand movements (HM).

Hands Free knee retractor system.

hand-sewn ileoanal anastomosis—as compared with stapled anastomosis

hand-sewn *(cont.)* with or without mucosectomy in restorative proctocolectomy.

hand surgery graft—see *flap*.

hang-back technique—ophthalmic surgical method for performing bimedial rectus recession for correction of strabismus and exotropia. May also be called *anchored hang-back* or *adjustable hang-back technique*.

Hanger ComfortFlex—socket system that combines with a computerized knee prosthesis, allowing an amputee to have maximum control and command over the lower limb.

hanging panniculus—see *apron*.

hangman's fracture—sometimes the result of injury to the neck in motorcycle or automobile accidents, in which there is rupture of the anterior and posterior longitudinal ligaments, leading to anterior luxation of C2 over C3, with crushing of the intervertebral disk.

Hanks balanced salt solution (HBSS) —used in bone marrow transplantation.

Hansel stain—used in microscopic examination of eosinophils.

Hantavirus pulmonary syndrome (HPS)—identified in 1993 in an outbreak in the American Southwest. The virus was named for the Hantaan River of Korea in 1978. HPS is caused by the Sin Nombre virus (SNV) and transmitted by rodents.

Ha-1A—a human monoclonal antibody found to be effective against gram-negative sepsis (a virulent and deadly multisystem disease caused by the endotoxins released in the bloodstream by gram-negative bacteria). Ha-1A binds to the endotoxins, inactivating them. See *Centoxin*.

HAP (hepatic arterial-dominant phase) **images** (CT scan).

haploid ('simple')—the number of chromosomes in a gamete; 23 unpaired chromosomes in human beings.

HappySkin acne light—uses blue and red light waves. The blue light leads to photoexcitation of porphyrins to produce oxygen that destroys the bacteria. The red light appears to have an anti-inflammatory effect on inflamed skin pores.

Hapset—HA (hydroxyapatite) bone graft plaster also used for periodontal defects and tooth extraction sites. The plaster itself absorbs, leaving only an HA scaffold for bony ingrowth.

haptens—the little loops on implant cataract lens through which the sutures are passed to keep the lens in place. Used interchangeably with *haptics*.

haptics—see *haptens*.

HAR (hyperacute rejection).

hardware disease—traumatic pericarditis.

Hardy-Sella punch—a small punch used to create an osteotomy in the lacrimal fossa.

Harmonic Scalpel—see *UltraCision ultrasonic knife*.

Harmonic Scalpel probe—ball-tipped ultrasonic cutting and coagulating surgical device

Harmony breast pump—maximizes milk flow with two-pattern pumping.

Harpoon suture anchor.

Harrell Y stent—Y-shaped stent with posts for short-term management of airway obstructions.

Harrington retractor (Ortho)—called "sweetheart," probably because the tip of the blade is somewhat heart-shaped. Used in acetabular fracture repair.

Harrington rod—used to correct scoliosis.

Harris-Galante porous-coated femoral component.

Harris hip score (scale)—a numerical rating scale for hip function. Four areas are surveyed: pain, function, deformity, and motions. Scores for each area are totaled, and in this scale, the lower the number, the more severe the disability.

Harrison groove—a horizontal groove along the lower thorax; seen in children with rickets, or in people who have had rickets.

Harrison-Nicolle polypropylene pegs—used in hand surgery.

Hartmann hemostatic mosquito forceps (straight/curved).

Hartmann solution (Ringer lactate) — a physiologic salt solution.

Hartzler ACX-II or RX-014 balloon catheter.

Hartzler Micro II balloon—used in coronary angioplasty.

Harvard Criteria for Brain Death—including unreceptivity and unresponsiveness, total unawareness to externally applied stimuli and inner need, and complete unresponsiveness, in addition to:

No movements or breathing—no spontaneous muscular movements or spontaneous respirations or response to stimuli such as pain, touch, sound, or light for at least one hour. After a patient has been on a mechanical respirator, the total absence of spontaneous breathing may be established by turning off the respirator for three minutes and observing for any effort by the patient to breathe spontaneously.

No reflexes—fixed and dilated pupils that do not respond to a direct source of light, and absence of ocular movement, blinking, swallowing, yawning, vocalization, and corneal and pharyngeal reflexes.

Harvard pump—an infusion device which continually injects medication at a preset rate.

Harvard 2 dual syringe pump—a multiple syringe infusion pump that can deliver two drug agents simultaneously and alert clinicians to blockages in infusion lines.

harvest—to remove tissue or organs from a donor for transplantation; to take skin, bone, or cartilage from the patient for an autologous graft. See also *evisceration*, *recovery, stem-cell marrow harvesting*, *total abdominal evisceration*.

Harvey hospital prognostic nutritional index.

Hasson blunt-end cannula—used in laparoscopic procedures.

Hasson graspers—used in endoscopic procedures.

Hasson open laparoscopy cannula.

Hasson SAC (stable access cannula)—for use in laparoscopic procedures.

Hasson trocar—used in laparoscopic procedures.

HASTE (half-Fourier acquisition single-shot turbo spin-echo)—a fast, breath-hold, magnetic resonance imaging sequence.

Hastings frame—frame attached to the operating table to keep the patient in a flexed knee-chest position for surgery on the spine. Cf. *Andrews spinal frame/table*.

HAT (hair apposition technique).

HAT (hepatic artery thrombosis).

HAT (humanized anti-TAC).

Hauser procedure—medial transplantation of the patellar tendon insertion, with reefing of the vastus medialis.

HAV (hepatitis A virus).

Haverhill fever (also, *ratbite fever*)—named for Haverhill, Massachusetts, where the first epidemic of this disease occurred. It is usually transmitted by the bite of an infected rat, but occasionally by the bite of infected dog, cat, or squirrel. The responsible organism is *Streptobacillus moniliformis*. The symptoms include high fever; enlarged regional lymph nodes; red, painful, and swollen joints; and there may also be a rash and back pain. Responds to treatment with antibiotics.

haversian canal—a microscopic feature of bone.

Hawkeye suture needle—used arthroscopically for soft tissue repair and anchoring.

Hawkins-Bell retractor.

Hawkins breast localization needle, with FlexStrand cable—used for marking nonpalpable lesions. These needles are designated I, II, and III. Number III can be used to inject dye, or for aspiration. They come in 5, 7.5, 10, and 12.5 cm lengths.

"hay-nee"—see *Heaney clamp*; *Heaney suture*. *Not* Haney.

Hays retractor—used in hand surgery.

HbAg, HB Ag ("H-bag")—hepatitis B antigen.

HBcAb—hepatitis B core antibody (not to be confused with HBcAg, which is hepatitis B core antigen).

HBeAb—hepatitis B *e* antibody.

HBeAg—the soluble *e* antigen in hepatitis B antigen.

HBIG (hepatitis B immune globulin).

HBsAb—hepatitis B surface antibody.

HBsAg—hepatitis B surface antigen.

H_2 blockers—a class of drugs that block H_2 receptors in the stomach to stop release of histamine that stimulates gastric acid secretion; e.g., Tagamet (cimetidine) and Zantac (ranitidine).

HBS (headless bone screw) **system**—used for the fixation of most small bone fractures and small joint fusions. The screws are both inert and nonprotrusive and thus do not have to be removed, making them an ideal implant for use within or adjacent to a joint.

HBSS (Hanks balanced salt solution).

HBV (hepatitis B virus).

HBV test—see *Hybrid Capture II HBV test*.

HCC (hepatocellular carcinoma).

hCFHrp (human complement factor H-related protein).

hCG, HCG (human chorionic gonadotropin).

HCPCS (Healthcare Common Procedure Coding System).

HCT, HCTZ (hydrochlorothiazide)—a diuretic.

HC II test (Hybrid Capture II test).

HCV Super Quant RT-PCR assay.

HCV 3.0 Strip Recombinant Immunoblot Assay.

HD (hemodialysis).

HDI 1000—software-based, all-digital ultrasound system that can perform routine ultrasound as well as color imaging and tissue-specific imaging. It is equipped to provide Internet/Intranet access to digital images stored in the system's memory. Also, HDI 5000.

HD II (or 2) **total hip prosthesis**.

HDL (high-density lipoprotein)—the so-called good cholesterol that protects from arteriosclerosis and heart attacks. HDL levels are high in those who exercise, run, walk, etc., and HDL is thought to reduce the risks of heart disease. Cf. *LDL*.

HDL-C (high-density lipoprotein cholesterol).

HDPEB (high-dose PEB protocol)—chemotherapy protocol.

HDR (high-dose-rate) **brachytherapy**.

HDRA (histoculture drug response assay)—a cancer test.

Head Injury Rehabilitation Centers (HIRE) Center.

Healey classification, Healey segments—classification system used in hepatic resection.

Healey revision acetabular component.

healing by secondary intention—referring to an incision or wound that heals by itself rather than being closed surgically. For example, drain wounds are often left open and heal by secondary intention (by themselves) rather than being sutured closed (closed primarily).

Healos—synthetic bone-grafting material for use in spinal fusions.

Healthcare Common Procedure Coding System (HCPCS).

Health Insurance Portability and Accountability Act of 1996 (HIPAA).

health-related quality of life (HRQoL, HRQL).

HealthShield antimicrobial mediastinal wound drainage catheter.

hearing aid (see also *implant)*
- Argosy Cameo CIC (completely-in-the-canal)
- CIC (completely-in-the-canal) completely-in-the-ear
- InSound XT
- Prisma digital
- ReSound Digital 2000
- RetroX hearing system
- Songbird disposable
- Soundtec
- Triano digital

hearing aid *(cont.)*
- Unitron Esteem CIC (completely-in-the-canal)
- Vibrant Soundbridge

heart and hand syndrome—Holt-Oram atriodigital dysplasia.

HeartBar—edible granola bar-type "medical food" for the dietary management of cardiovascular disease. See *medical food*.

HeartBar Orange Drink—a "medical food" drink that purports to offer the same benefits as the HeartBar. See *medical food*.

HeartCard—a cardiac event recorder the size of a credit card. When the patient experiences cardiac symptoms, the HeartCard is placed directly on the chest and it records and stores EKG information that can be transmitted over the telephone to the hospital or doctor's office.

Heart Failure Knowledge Test—assesses the patient's knowledge of the causes, symptoms, medications, food selection, actions to take if there are side effects, and self-management relative to weight monitoring and physical activity, and worsening symptoms.

heart-hand syndrome—an autosomal-dominant heart disease usually associated with hypoplastic thumb and short forearm. Also Holt-Oram syndrome.

Health Failure Self-Care Behavior Scale, revised—measures a patient's activities relating to self-care.

Heaney (*not* Haney) **clamp**—pronounced "hay-nee."

Heaney (*not* Haney) **suture**—pronounced "hay-nee."

Heart Laser for TMR (transmyocardial revascularization)—used to drill 1

Heart *(cont.)*
mm channels in the myocardium of the left chamber of the heart in order to get in fresh blood.

HeartMate—air-driven implantable left ventricular assist system (LVAS) utilized in patients awaiting heart transplant whose damaged or diseased heart is unable to function adequately on its own. It is implanted alongside the natural heart and takes over the pumping function of the left ventricle.

HeartMate SNAP-VE LVAS (sutures not applied-vented electric left ventricular assist system)—formerly approved for short-term treatment, and newly approved for long-term treatment for severe heart failure in patients who are not candidates for heart transplants. The HeartMate system includes an implanted pump and a controller and power supply worn outside the body.

HeartMate vented electric LVAS (left ventricular assist system)—portable LVAS, consisting of a blood pump implanted in the abdominal area, connected by a cable through the skin to a small external computer worn at the waist. The computer can be powered by a base unit that is plugged into the wall or by batteries worn at the waist or under the arms.

Heartport Port-Access system—used with less invasive heart valve replacement and repair.

HeartSaver VAD—an artificial heart that is remotely powered and monitored.

Heartsbreath test—used along with a traditional endomyocardial biopsy to measure possible organ rejection in heart transplant patients.

Heartscan heart attack prediction test—ultrafast CT scanner used to identify narrowed coronary vessels. It is said to be greater than 95% effective in ruling out obstructive coronary artery disease.

HEARTS (healthy early alarm recognition and telemonitoring system) **project**—links continuous monitoring of health behavior through noninvasive wearable sensors with decision support. HEARTS offers support to healthy, ill, and high-risk people.

HeartStart home defibrillator.

Heartstream ForeRunner automatic external defibrillator.

Heartstring proximal seal system—a temporary seal for use in vascular and cardiovascular surgery. *Not* Heartstrings.

HeartView CT—a noninvasive method of cardiac imaging that includes visualization of soft plaque. Used in conjunction with a general purpose multislice CT, it allows users to perform highly specialized cardiac imaging.

HearTwave EP—measures Microvolt T-wave alternans in patients undergoing electrophysiology testing.

heater probe thermocoagulation—an alternative treatment to injection therapy for bleeding peptic ulcers.

heat-moisture exchanger (HME)—a device, attached to a tracheostomy tube, that collects a patient's expired heat and moisture and returns it during the following inspiration. Also called *artificial nose*.

HeatProbe—trade name of a water irrigation/lavage device.

heat shock protein 72 (HSP-72)—induction of this material may prevent neutrophil-mediated human endothelial cell necrosis.

heave and lift—often used interchangeably; a diffuse lifting impulse along the left sternal heart border with each heartbeat.

heavy-chain deposition—rare malignant neoplasms, indistinguishable from light-chain deposition by clinical features but detectable by using heavy-chain antibodies in biopsy studies, sometimes occurring in patients with renal symptoms associated with myeloma. Cf. *light chain deposition.*

heavy ion irradiation—helium is usually used for this therapy.

heavy-metal screening—lab test for poisoning from heavy metallic elements such as arsenic, iron, lead, and mercury. *Heavy* refers to the atomic weight, not to the physical weight of the metal.

HED (hypohidrotic ectodermal dysplasia).

hedgehog molecule—used to generate brain tissue for treatment of Alzheimer and Parkinson diseases.

Hedrocel biomaterial—a trabecular metal material used in orthopedic implants.

HEE—see *Gastaut syndrome*.

Heel Float gel insert—suspends sensitive heels over an air cavity to prevent pressure sore formation or aid in the healing of existing sores.

heel pad sign (Radiol)—a grossly enlarged and thickened calcaneal heel pad seen on lateral radiograph of foot. A heel pad thickness greater than 23 mm may indicate acromegaly.

heelstick hematocrit—blood obtained from the heel of infants for hematocrit test.

heel-to-shin test—a test of cerebellar function. The patient is asked, while in the supine position, to place the heel of one foot on the knee of the other leg, and then to "run" the heel down the shin. This test is done bilaterally and provides an assessment of the patient's cerebellar function, as indicated by the smoothness and coordination with which it is performed.

Heffington lumbar seat spinal surgery frame—a table on which the patient is placed, kneeling on a little shelf extending out from the end, with the chest flat on the table. This position helps to decrease epidural venous bleeding.

Heimlich maneuver—a technique for removing foreign matter from the trachea of a choking victim.

Heineke-Mikulicz pyloroplasty.

Heinz body—seen in unstable hemoglobin disease (a congenital hemolytic anemia).

Heister valve—redundant cystic duct mucosal folds, which cause a valve-like obstruction of the cystic duct.

HeLa cells—cells from the first continuously cultured strain of human malignant tissue derived from the cervical carcinoma of Henrietta Lacks in Baltimore in 1951.

helical CT—see *spiral CT.* Cf. *electron-beam CT technology.*

helical wrap—see aortomyoplasty.

Helicobacter hepaticus *(H. hepaticus)* —a species of bacterium related to *H. pylori.*

Helicobacter pylori *(H. pylori)* (formerly classified as *Campylobacter pylori*)—believed to be the cause for up to 90% of duodenal ulcers and 80% of stomach ulcers, and now recently found to be associated with non-Hodgkin lymphoma of the stomach. No cause for the association can as yet be proved.

***Helicobacter pylori* breath test**—used to confirm the presence of *Helicobacter pylori* prior to treating a peptic ulcer with antibiotics. A dose of urea labeled with the radionuclide carbon-14 is given orally. The breath test indirectly measures urease activity. Urease, an enzyme produced by the bacteria, acts on urea to produce ammonia which can be measured in the breath. See *Helicobacter pylori*, *^{14}C-urea breath excretion test*.

Helios diagnostic imaging systems.

Helioseal—titanium dioxide particles suspended in polymer containing a photoinitiator that cures under illumination with a blue light. Used as a diffuser with lasers.

heliotrope infraorbital discoloration—purplish discoloration under the eye (*not* ecchymosis).

Helisal rapid blood test—a minimally invasive whole-blood test to detect the presence of antibodies to *Helicobacter pylori* (*H. pylori*) bacteria.

Helistat—absorbable collagen hemostatic sponge.

Helitene—absorbable collagen hemostatic agent, in fibrillar form.

helium-neon laser—see *HeNe laser*.

heliX knot pusher—for extracorporeal knot tying during laparoscopic surgery.

Hellberg-Kupka scissors—cardiovascular microscissors with ergonomic handle.

helle cell—a cell in the mucosa of the gastrointestinal tract. Cf. *gelbe cell*.

Heller-Belsey operation—for achalasia of esophagus.

Heller-Dor procedure—laparoscopic surgical procedure for treatment of esophageal achalasia (swallowing difficulty) by reducing the resistance of the esophageal sphincter.

Heller esophagomyotomy—minimally invasive surgery.

Heller-Nissen operation—for achalasia of the esophagus.

HELLP syndrome—a manifestation of preeclampsia. *HELLP* is an acronym for hemolysis, elevated liver enzymes, and low platelets.

helmet-molding therapy—cranial orthotic therapy following endoscopic strip craniectomy to manipulate cranial growth so that normocephaly will be attained. It is used for 3 to 4 months postoperatively.

Helmholtz coil—MRI term.

heloma durum—a callosity on the hand or the foot.

heloma molle—a soft corn.

helper cell—also called helper/inducer cell and T-4 cell; these are the lymphocytes that the AIDS virus specifically attacks and converts into a tool for making additional virus, and this is done much more quickly than with other viruses.

helper-suppressor cell ratio—used to describe the disappearance of functioning T-4 helper cells. This ratio changes in AIDS and the change is diagnostic. It may be dictated as the ratio of T-helper to T-suppressor cells or of T-4 to T-8 cells, or you may hear that "the ratio of OKT4 to OKT8 is less than 1.0," OKT4 and OKT8 being monoclonal antibodies to T-4 and T-8.

Hemaflex PTCA sheath with obturator—collagen hemostat specifically designed to stop blood flow from vessels in cardiovascular surgery, as it is easy to wrap around vessels. Placed percutaneously in the femoral artery in PTCA. Cf. *Hemaquet*.

"hem/ahnk/room"—phonetic for the heading *hematology/oncology/rheumatology*.

hemangiolymphangioma—mixed cavernous hemangioma and cystic lymphangioma.

hemangioma
choroidal
circumscribed choroidal (CCH)
diffuse choroidal (DCH)

hemangiopericytic meningioma—a vascular neoplasm that is sometimes malignant. Also known as *hemangiopericytoma meningioma*.

hemangiopericytoma—a rare vascular neoplasm, usually benign.

Hemaquet PTCA sheath with obturator—see *Hemaflex*.

Hemaseel HMN—biological tissue glue for control of bleeding during surgical and orthopedic procedures.

Hemashield—a woven vascular graft enhanced with collagen which promotes intimal development and may reduce thrombogenicity. Used to replace diseased segments of the aorta or iliac arteries.

Hemashield Gold branch graft.

Hemashield Gold Microvel knitted double velour graft.

Hemashield Vantage vascular graft.

HemaStrip-HIV 1/2—whole blood test for HIV 1 and 2.

Hemasure r/LS red blood cell filtration system—designed to reduce leukocytes in donated blood. Leukocytes can transmit a number of bacteria and viruses and cause reactions in patients receiving blood transfusions.

hematoma—see *DTICH* (delayed traumatic intracerebral hematoma).

hematometrocolpos—progressive accumulation of menstrual blood in the uterus due to obstruction of the genital tract.

hematopoiesis—the body's mechanism for replacing cells.

hematopoietic progenitor clonogenic assay—assesses bone marrow viability.

hematopoietic stem cell (HSC)—a stem cell from which all red and white blood cells develop; found in adult bone marrow, umbilical cord blood, peripheral blood, and fetal liver. Adult hematopoietic stem cells can replace bone marrow that has been destroyed by disease or radiation therapy and can continue to produce mature blood cells.

hematoporphyrin derivative (HpD)—a drug when given intravenously is a photosensitizing agent that is absorbed only by malignant cells, which can then be destroyed by laser surgery.

hemicallotasis—surgical procedure for arthritic knees.

hemiepiphysiodesis—a surgical procedure in which the hemivertebrae are fused for the correction of scoliosis.

hemi-Fontan procedure—involves an atriopulmonary patch that directs superior vena caval blood flow into both pulmonary arteries and the inferior vena caval flow into the ventricle. Atrial conduction may be affected by the atrial suture lines with resulting arrhythmia. The procedure is performed to repair certain congenital heart defects.

"heminose"—phonetic for *HME nose*. See *HME* (heat-moisture exchanger).

Hemi Sling—designed to reduce shoulder subluxation.

hemi-T augmentation—a bladder augmentation technique for continent urinary diversion in pediatric patients. It is used when the appendix is unavailable and is a modification of the double-T pouch urinary diversion.

hemizygous—referring to the genes on the X chromosome in a male.

Hemobahn endovascular prosthesis—nitinol stent-graft.

hemodialyzed—a coined term for underwent hemodialysis.

Hemoccult Sensa—enhanced system for detecting hidden blood in stool. It is said to be easier to read than the standard Hemoccult test.

Hemoccult II—a test for fecal occult blood.

Hemochron high-dose thrombin time (HiTT)—a whole-blood assay for monitoring high-dose heparin anticoagulation. Used in monitoring coagulation time following coronary artery bypass procedures.

Hemoclip—a ligating clip; it comes in titanium and also in tantalum.

HemoCue photometer—for a quick office test for hemoglobin determination done on a drop of blood.

Hemo-Dial—dialysate additives.

hemodialyzer—apparatus used in the hemodialysis of kidney patients to remove toxic elements. There are three types of hemodialyzers: the coil, the hollow fiber, and the parallel plate.

HemoDoppler device—checks for diastolic augmentation of the anastomosis in beating heart surgery.

hemofiltration—a technique by which waste products of hemodialysis are removed from the blood along with plasma water by rapid ultrafiltration, and then the blood is reconstituted with a solution, either before or after hemodialysis. The technique appears to reduce side effects of dialysis and seems to assure better tolerance of fluid removal, particularly in patients with high vascular instability. See *continuous arteriovenous hemofiltration* (CAVH); *continuous renal replacement therapy* (CCRT).

HemoGlide dialysis catheter.

Hemolink—a hemoglobin replacement product, or red blood cell substitute, for use in blood transfusions.

Hem-o-lok—polymer ligating clip.

hemolytic uremic syndrome (HUS)—a complication of the pathogen *E. coli* 0157:H7, occurring mostly in children and resulting in acute renal failure. Successful treatment depends on strict attention to fluid and electrolyte balance.

Hemopad—absorbable collagen hemostat, which comes as nonwoven pads that can be cut, folded, or wrapped around a bleeding site. It can be peeled away easily, but any remaining bits are soon absorbed.

hemophilia A—factor VIII deficiency (classical hemophilia).

hemophilia B—factor IX deficiency. See *Christmas disease*.

Hemophilus—see *Haemophilus*. With a lowercase "h," may refer generically to any bacterium of the genus *Haemophilus*. Also used for the Hemophilus B conjugate vaccine. If you are typing genus and species in a report, you should use the Latin spelling.

Hemopump—temporary external pump which completely supports circulation, used in the treatment of cardiogenic shock. This device is an improvement over the intra-aortic balloon pump which provides only 25% circulatory assistance.

Hemospan and Hemospan PS—an oxygen carrier or blood substitute.

Hemo-Split long-term hemodialysis catheter—features a fixed split-tip design that reduces the risk of excess tunnel bleeding and infection.

Hemo-Split *(cont.)*
It also reduces the risk of lumen damage from the tip being split too far apart.

hemostatic eraser (Oph)—used for pinpoint hemostasis in anterior and posterior segment surgery.

hemostatic material—see *collagen*.

Hemotene—absorbable collagen hemostat to control bleeding during surgery when sutures are not practical.

Hemotherapies liver dialysis unit—liver-assist technology used for treatment of patients with liver disease or liver impairment due to hepatitis, cirrhosis, overdose, drug toxicity, aggressive drug therapies, or other causes.

Hendel correction of scaphocephaly—uses a gore pattern to alter the shape of individual sections of the skull by changing the radius of curvature.

HeNe (**he**lium-**ne**on) **laser** (Oph)—has a visible low power red beam and is often used in conjunction with the carbon dioxide (CO_2) laser. The advantage of the HeNe is that the beam is visible and the surgeon can see its location.

Henning meniscal retractors—used in knee surgery.

Henning system—technique for arthroscopic meniscal repair. Also, *Henning instruments*.

Henoch-Schönlein—also *Schönlein-Henoch purpura*.

Hensen cells—in the organ of Corti.

Hepamed-coated Wiktor stent—see *Wiktor stent*.

heparin anti-XA assay—laboratory test to monitor therapeutic heparin levels.

heparinized CeeOn intraocular lens.

heparin lock (Hep-Lock)—an intermittent infusion reservoir; permits periodic infusion of drugs without continuous fluid infusion. A heparin solution injected into the reservoir between infusions will keep the I.V. patent without the necessity of a continuous fluid drip. Although the heparin lock was first used for administration of heparin, it is also used for transfusion therapy and in the administration of a number of drugs, including chemotherapeutic agents and antibiotics. See also *Hep-Lock*, a trade name.

hepatic arterial-dominant phase (HAP) **images** (CT scan).

hepatic arterial infusion (HAI) **chemotherapy**—high-dose chemotherapy performed under hepatic venous isolation by direct hemoperfusion (HVI-DHP). The hepatic vein is isolated by double balloon technique with an occlusion catheter and balloon catheter. This procedure allows higher doses than standard systemic chemotherapy in nonresectable hepatic carcinoma. Standard hepatic arterial infusion that does not occlude the hepatic vein from the systemic circulation is dose-limited due to systemic side effects of chemotherapy.

hepatic artery thrombosis (HAT).

hepatic resection—treatment for metastatic neuroendocrine cancers.

hepatic segmentectomy—a therapeutic approach for small hepatocellular carcinomas and in patients with chronic liver disease and impaired liver function.

hepatic venous isolation by direct hemoperfusion (HVI-DHP)—see *hepatic arterial infusion chemotherapy*.

hepatic venous web disease (in Budd-Chiari syndrome).

hepatic web dilation—to establish hepatic vein outflow (in hepatic venous web disease).

hepatitides ("heh-puh-tih´-tih-dees")—plural form of *hepatitis*.

hepatitis—inflammation of the liver caused by viral and bacterial infection and parasitic infestation. See related entries: *hepatitis A, B, C, D, E,* F, *NANB hepatitis*, *peliosis hepatitis*.

hepatitis A (infectious hepatitis)—an acute, self-limited infection, generally causing mild symptoms. The virus is transmitted chiefly by the fecal-oral route.

hepatitis B (serum hepatitis)—a more severe infection which, in some cases, becomes chronic and is transmitted chiefly via the bloodstream and also by sexual contact. After recovery some patients become carriers.

hepatitis B antigen (HbAg).

hepatitis C—the major cause of post-transfusion hepatitis, typically causing a mild clinical illness but becoming chronic in at least half of all cases. Formerly called *non-A, non-B hepatitis*.

hepatitis D—occurs only in persons previously infected with hepatitis B, although it is due to a distinct virus. Also called *delta hepatitis*.

hepatitis E—occurs chiefly in the tropics. Resembles hepatitis A in that it is transmitted by the fecal-oral route and does not become chronic or lead to a carrier state, but has a much higher mortality.

hepatitis F—the newer name for non-A, non-B, non-C hepatitis.

hepatization—transformation into a liver-like mass, as the solidified state of the lung in lobar pneumonia.

hepatobiliary scintigraphy—used in children to assess liver disease.

hepatocellular carcinoma (HCC)

hepatofugal flow—flowing away from the liver. Usage: "Angiography for esophageal varices was done and revealed hepatofugal flow."

hepatojugular reflux—swelling of the jugular vein caused by applying pressure over the liver. This swelling indicates right heart insufficiency.

hepatopancreatoduodenectomy.

hepatopetal flow—flowing toward the liver. Usage: "Angiography for esophageal varices was done and revealed hepatopetal flow."

hepatoprotection—a coined word denoting factors that protect the liver against toxicity.

Hepcon system—device useful in OPCAB patients as heparin metabolism is increased with the patient at normothermia. Reversal is accomplished by the calculations provided from the Hepcon machine, and protamine is administered accordingly.

Hep-Lock—a trademarked device for the administration of heparin and other intravenous fluids. See *heparin lock*.

Heprofile ELISA (enzyme-linked immunosorbent assay)—lab test for hepatitis B.

heptacarboxyl—a radical occurring in porphyrin, found in quantitative urine studies for hepatitis.

herald patch—a single lesion that is seen before the eruption of pityriasis rosea.

Herbert bone screw.

Herbert classification—a method of describing fractures of the scaphoid bone, one of the carpal bones of the wrist. Screw fixation of a scaphoid fracture is generally preferred over

Herbert *(cont.)*
conservative therapy and may involve the use of a Herbert screw.

Herbert-Whipple bone screw—used for reduction and compression of small bone and intra-articular fractures.

HercepTest—HER2 protein expression system for the guidance of breast cancer therapy.

Herculon suture—synthetic material.

hereditary sensory and autonomic neuropathy type IV (HSAN-IV)—an autosomal recessive hereditary disorder characterized by recurrent episodic fever, inability to sweat, absence of reaction to noxious stimuli, self-mutilating behavior, and mental retardation. Also referred to as *congenital insensitivity to pain with anhidrosis* (CIPA).

hereditary nonpolyposis colorectal cancer (HNPCC)—see *Lynch syndrome*.

Herellea vaginicola—included in the genus of gram-negative coccobacilli *Acinetobacter*.

hERG (human ether-a-go-go related gene)—a potassium channel.

hERG blocker—a class of drugs that blocks hERG; a potassium channel blocker. Cf. *calcium channel blocker.*

Hering, nerve of—carotid sinus nerve.

heritability—a statistical measure of the degree to which a trait is genetically tranmissible.

Heritage Panel—a patented genetic screening test, currently available only to high-risk Ashkenazi Jews affected with breast or ovarian cancer or who are related to a known mutation carrier. It can detect hereditary breast and ovarian cancers in the BRCA1 and BRCA2 genes.

Herpasil—an over-the-counter topical drug for patients with oral or genital herpes. The active ingredient is *Prunella vulgaris*.

Herp-Check—antibody test for herpes simplex virus which provides results in four hours, rather than up to seven days, as before.

herpes encephalitis.

herpes simplex virus (HSV)—can disseminate in AIDS.

herpesvirus (one word).

herpes whitlow—herpesvirus infection, occurring in hospital workers and dentists, that can be transmitted through contact with the patient's oral mucous membrane or saliva. It involves the folds of tissue around the fingernail and consists of pyogenic and vesicular paronychia. Related terms: *paronychia, felon*.

herpes zoster virus (HZV)—can disseminate in AIDS.

Herplex Liquifilm (idoxuridine).

hersage ("air-SAHZH")—the surgical separation of scarred peripheral nerve fibers by splitting the sheath and separating the nerve into a ribbon of fine free fibers.

HER-2-neu—an oncogene that is a potential prognostic marker for breast cancer.

hertz (Hz)—a unit of frequency, equal to one cycle per second; measurement used in audiograms.

heterogeneity (Genetics)—the production of a given phenotype by two distinct genotypes or genetic mechanisms.

heterografts, bovine and porcine—used as valves in cardiac surgery; they are specially prepared so they are not rejected as foreign bodies.

heterokaryon—a cell containing two nuclei of different genetic composition.

heterologous (Genetics)—pertaining to a mixed or nonuniform group or population.

heteromorphism—variation in size or shape between the two chromosomes forming a pair.

heteroploid (Genetics)—a number of chromosomes other than the normal 23 pairs.

heterozygote (Genetics)—an individual who has two different alleles at corresponding gene loci, or with respect to a given trait.

heterozygous (Genetics)—having different alleles for a given trait.

Hewlett-Packard ear oximeter—used to record oxygen saturation continuously. See *ear oximeter*. (Note: *Hewlett-Packard* has a hyphen.)

Hewlett-Packard phased-array imaging system—MRI term.

hexagonal keratotomy surgery—includes an intracorneal implant (Kerato-Gel) made from lidofilcon A.

hexagonal phospholipid assay—a test for hypercoagulable state.

Hexcelite—intermediate phase casting and thermoplastic light mesh immersed briefly in 80°C water and then wrapped around the extremity to be casted; hardens quickly.

Hexcel total condylar knee system—femoral and tibial components, and patellar dome.

Hex-Fix—a fracture fixation system.

Heyer-Schulte tissue expander.

HFCWO (high-frequency chest wall oscillation)—see *ABI Vest airway clearance system* and *ThAIRapy Vest*.

HF infrared laser.

H5N1 virus—strain of influenza A originating in birds (usually poultry) and believed to be responsible for flu deaths in Hong Kong in 1997. Investigations are being conducted to determine how the virus is transmitted from avians to humans.

H. flu—slang for *Haemophilus influenzae*.

HFU, HIFU (high-intensity focused ultrasound).

HGD (high-grade dysplasia).

HGE (human granulocytic ehrlichiosis).

hGH (human growth hormone)—see *Protropin*.

HGSIL (high-grade squamous intraepithelial lesion)—corresponds to Pap smear changes that were formerly called moderate and severe dysplasia or CIN 2 and CIN 3.

HHH or **triple-H** (hypertensive hypervolemic hemodilution) **therapy** after subarachnoid hemorrhage.

HHV-8 (human herpesvirus-8).

HI (hypopnea index).

HIAA—see *5-HIAA* (hydroxyindoleacetic acid) laboratory test.

Hib or **HIB** (pronounced "hib") (*Haemophilus influenzae* type B) **disease**—a leading cause of bacterial meningitis.

Hibbs retractor.

HIB (*Haemophilus influenzae* type b) **polysaccharide vaccine**—used to treat HIB disease in children. See *HIB disease*.

Hickman catheter—indwelling right atrial catheter used in treatment of patients receiving bone marrow transplants and those whose medical care requires frequent access to their circulation, e.g., drawing blood, administering blood, for total parenteral nutrition. Also used for withdrawing blood for plasmapheresis and for central venous pressure monitoring. Its use eliminates the need for frequent venipuncture.

HIDA ("high-dah") (**h**epato**i**mino**d**iacetic **a**cid) **scan**—a technetium scan.

HIDA *(cont.)*
Also given as TcHIDA, or technetium-HIDA, for biliary tract imaging. See *PIPIDA*.

HIDA-CCK scintigraphy—an imaging study of the gallbladder using simultaneous injections of hepatobiliary iminodiacetic acid (HIDA) and cholecystokinin (CCK).

Hieshima coaxial catheter—used in some interventional procedures in radiology.

HIFI (High-Frequency Ventilation in Premature Infants) study.

HIFU (high-intensity focused ultrasound).

Higgins technique for ureterointestinal anastomosis.

high-density linear array—term used in B-scan, Doppler, and color Doppler imaging. See *B-scan*.

high-density lipoprotein (HDL).

high-density lipoprotein–cholesterol (HDL-C).

high-dose-rate (HDR) **brachytherapy**—a treatment for prostate cancer in which very tiny plastic catheters are placed into the prostate gland. A series of radiation treatments are given through these catheters. The catheters are then easily pulled out, and no radioactive material is left in the prostate gland. This temporary brachytherapy is in contrast to the usual permanent seed placement.

high-energy lasers, hot lasers—used to make surgical incisions or destroy tumors.

higher integrative functions (HIF).

Highet and Sander criteria of Mackinnon and Dellon, modified—for measuring sensory recovery following nerve repair.

Highet and Sander criteria of Zachary and Holmes, modified—for measuring motor recovery following nerve reconstruction.

high field strength scanner—MRI device using a static magnetic field of maximal intensity.

high-frequency jet ventilation (Pulm)—the delivery of very small tidal volumes at extremely rapid rates (150 to 900 breaths per minute), allowing significant reduction in mean airway pressure and possible reduced risk of barotrauma. Volumes delivered are smaller than the physiologic dead space. May be related to bronchopleural fistulas and major volume-losing pneumothoraces when used in children with parenchymal lung disease. A similar technique is called *high-frequency oscillatory ventilation*.

high-frequency oscillatory ventilation—see *high-frequency jet ventilation*.

High-Frequency Ventilation in Premature Infants (HIFI) **study**.

high-grade squamous intraepithelial lesion (HSIL).

high-intensity focused ultrasound (HFU, HIFU)—used to treat benign prostatic hypertrophy. Administered via transrectal probe.

highly active antiretroviral therapy (HAART).

high McCall suspension—a vaginal vault repair procedure.

high myope—one who has a high degree of myopia (nearsightedness).

high normal—a quantitative test result that is near the upper limit of normal, though within the normal range.

high nuclear-to-cytoplasmic ratio—description of a finding in a biopsy diagnosed as oat cell carcinoma.

high-osmolar media (Radiol)—controversial use of high-osmolar (or ionic)

high *(cont.)*
versus low-osmolar (or nonionic) contrast media. The media lower in osmolality are much more expensive but are thought to be less dangerous to some patients, particularly cardiac, asthmatic, or allergic patients.

high-resolution computed tomography (HRCT).

high-resolution multileaf collimator—computerized mechanical device that uses individually controlled leaves or fingers to sculpt a radiation beam to the shape of a tumor when delivering intensity modulated radiotherapy treatments in radiation oncology. See also *intensity modulated radiation therapy*.

high-resolution storage phosphor managing—reportedly may replace conventional chest radiography in detection of subtle interstitial lung diseases.

High-Risk Hybrid Capture II HPV test—DNA-based technology designed to detect the 13 key types of human papillomavirus that cause cervical cancer.

high shear blood flow—used to describe blood flow through arteries that may cause plaque to break off from the walls of the arteries.

high-speed rotational atherectomy (RA)—percutaneous procedure for treatment of coronary stenoses by plaque abrasion. It is an alternative to PTCA for complex lesions, especially those with extensive calcification.

high-velocity, low-amplitude (HLVA) maneuvers—a traditional chiropractic manipulation. Also HLVA technique.

high-voltage pulsed galvanic stimulator—controls pain and increases circulation following injury or surgery.

high-voltage stimulation (HVS)—delivers electrical energy to deep tissues without damage to superficial tissues. It is believed to relieve pain and accelerate wound healing. Similar to TENS. May be incorrectly referred to as *galvanic stimulation*.

Hildebrandt uterine hemostatic forceps—has a split in the jaws of the forceps that permits suturing with the forceps in place and then removing the forceps without disturbing the sutures.

Hilgenreiner line—between the inferior edges of the triradiate cartilage and the line tangential to the medial ossified edge of the proximal metaphysis of the femur.

Hilger facial nerve stimulator—used for clinical evaluation of the facial nerve, clinical testing of muscle tissue viability, and for nerve identification and testing during surgery.

Hill cluster harvest technique—micrograft technique.

Hill repair—for esophageal reflux.

Hill-Sachs lesion; **deformity** (Ortho).

Hill-Sachs sign (Radiol)—represents deformity of the superior-posterior border of the humeral.

HIM (health information management) —formerly known as *medical record management*.

hindgut—distal colon and rectum. See *foregut* and *midgut*.

Hinds repair of subcondylar fracture —modified surgical approach for repair of subcondylar fractures, using an incision parallel to the posterior border of the mandible, just below the earlobe. It is believed to have good cosmetic results without facial nerve paresis.

HIPAA (*not* HIPPA)—the Health Insurance Portability and Account-

HIPAA *(cont.)* ability Act of 1996, which sets forth specific standards for the protection of individually identifiable health information. Although the primary intent of HIPAA is to protect medical information that is electronically transmitted, the law as enacted applies to individually identifiable health information in all forms—electronic, written, oral, and any other. The HIPAA Privacy Rule requires each provider of healthcare to adopt specific policies and procedures, including physical safeguards, to protect the confidentiality of all medical information in its keeping and to provide information to patients about their privacy rights and how their medical information can be used and transmitted.

hip arthrodesis—with the cobra head plate and pelvic osteotomy.

HIPciser abduction splint—for use as a hip abduction splint and an isometric exercise device.

hip dysplasia measurements in cerebral palsy
AA (acetabular anteversion)
AAI (axial acetabular index)
AD/FHD (ratio of acetabular depth to femoral head diameter)
AI (acetabular index)
CEA (center-edge angle) of Wiberg
FA (femoral anteversion)
MI (migration index)
NSA (neck-shaft angle) of femur
SMAI (superior-medial acetabular index)

Hi-Per cardiac device.

hip hiking—gait modification where the pelvis is lifted on the side of the swinging leg by contraction of the spinal muscles and the lateral abdominal wall.

HipNav process—a computer-assisted hip navigation system used in hip replacement surgery to improve accuracy when implanting a replacement for the acetabulum.

HipSaver—protective underwear for elderly at risk for hip fractures. It incorporates a soft thin pad over each hip bone to absorb and dissipate the impact of a fall.

hip spica cast—used after surgery for correction of congenital hip dysplasia.

hippocampus (Greek *hippokampos*, sea horse)—area of cortex in bottom of inferior (temporal) horn of the lateral ventricle; it has the appearance of a seahorse, thus the name.

Hippocrates manipulation—for anterior dislocation of the shoulder joint. The physician exerts traction on the patient's arm and at the same time places his heel (with the shoe removed first!) in the patient's axilla to give countertraction, thus forcing the head of the humerus from beneath the acromion.

hippocratic wreath—seen in men with male pattern baldness, the rim of hair surrounding the bald area. Cf. *male pattern baldness*.

Hirano bodies—structural changes revealed by pathological examination of brains of Alzheimer disease victims. Also, *Hirano inclusion body.*

HIRE Center—an acronym for Head Injury Rehabilitation Centers.

Hirschberg measurement of esotropia.

Hirschsprung disease—congenital megacolon (giant colon).

hirudin—see *recombinant desulfato-hirudin*.

HIS fusion inhibitors—a new class of drugs that works specifically on a

HIS *(cont.)*
virus to prevent it from fusing with the cell and prevent viral replication. Fusion inhibitors are said to have great promise as anti-HIV drugs. Also called *fusion inhibitors.*

HiSonic—an ultrasonic bone conduction hearing device placed behind the ear on the mastoid bone. Allows profoundly deaf patients to perceive sounds.

Hi Speed Pulse Lavage—for debridement of bone surfaces during knee and hip replacements.

His-Purkinje conduction ("hiss pur-kin´gee") (Cardio)—as in bundle of His and Purkinje fibers.

Hiss, angle of—anatomic site encountered in laparoscopic gastric bypass procedure. Usage: "The root of the left diaphragmatic crus was exposed by caudad traction on the stomach fundus by the assistant to the patient's left, and the phrenogastric ligament was incised at the level of the angle of Hiss." Do not confuse with *His bundle of the heart*.

Histoacryl Blue (HAB)—tissue adhesive used in closure of incisions and lacerations.

Histoacryl glue (cyanoacrylate)—a tissue adhesive used to seal some perforating-type corneal wounds as may be seen in stromal herpetic keratitis. Also used to close incisions in blepharoplasty procedures.

histocompatibility—the ability of a host to accept, rather than reject, a graft from a donor containing no antigens that the host lacks.

histoculture drug response assay (HDRA)—to detect certain cancers.

Histofreezer cryosurgical wart treatment—cryotherapy device for the treatment of benign skin lesions: verruca vulgaris, verruca plantaris, human papillomavirus, acrochordon, molluscum contagiosum, seborrheic keratosis, verruca plana, actinic keratoses, and lentigo.

Histoplasma—the fungus which causes histoplasmosis. Disseminated histoplasmosis was recently added to the growing list of once very rare (in disseminated form) infections which are now often seen in AIDS.

Histoplasma capsulatum—pathogen associated with sinusitis in AIDS patients.

***Histoplasma capsulatum* polysaccharide antigen** (HPA)—detection of HPA, a rapid method for detecting histoplasmosis.

HI (hemagglutination inhibition) **titer**—a rubella screening test.

Hitzelberger sign (Derm).

HIV (human immunodeficiency virus) —the official name for the AIDS virus, changed because of the unwieldiness of the earlier terms and the debate over who discovered the virus first. HIV is a retrovirus, of the cytopathic lentivirus group.

HIV AC-le—potential AIDS vaccine by Bristol-Myers.

HIVAGEN—lab test for HIV.

HIV antibody—antibodies to the virus thought to lead to AIDS. Most AIDS tests are tests for the HIV antibody. Some very sophisticated ones test for part of the virus itself, such as the p24 antigen test, which is widely used in some areas.

HIV-associated thrombocytopenia—treated with high-dose intravenous immune globulin therapy.

HIV classification for children—the Centers for Disease Control and Prevention classification for HIV-infected or exposed children is as follows:

HIV *(cont.)*

P0: Asymptomatic infants to 15 months of age in whom definitive HIV infection has not been diagnosed.

P1: Asymptomatic infants and children regardless of age in whom HIV infection has been established by HIV p24 antigen or HIV culture with or without laboratory evidence of immunodeficiency.

P2: Symptomatic HIV-infected child. Includes subgroups A-F based on disease manifestations.

HIV disease—infection with the HIV virus, as shown by p24 antigen or HIV antibody test. HIV disease itself is not AIDS. Whether all cases go on to full-blown AIDS is not known at this time.

HIV encephalitis—see *AIDS dementia complex*.

HIV-1E—a virus subtype prevalent in Thailand, that grows much more efficiently in the cells that line the vagina than subtypes prevalent in the U.S. and elsewhere. May explain the rapid spread of AIDS among heterosexuals in Southeast Asia.

HIV phenotype test—still a research tool and not yet available through private physicians. Can detect which variants of the virus a patient has and whether the nonsyncytium inducing (NSI) variant has mutated to the more dangerous SI variant. See *NSI, SI*.

HKAFO (hip-knee-ankle-foot orthosis) —ambulation aid for children with cerebral palsy and myelomeningocele. Orthosis is in three forms: parapodium, reciprocating gait, and swivel walker.

HLA (human lymphocyte antigen)—a designation used in tissue typing for organ transplants.

HLA-A—see *locus of HLA*.

HLA-DR (histocompatibility antigen-DR)—a marker protein for the development of coronary artery disease in heart transplant patients. See also *ICAM-1*.

HLA-DR3 gene—associated with development of anti-HLA class II antibodies.

HLA-DR4—a genetic marker that has a correlation to the severity of the rheumatoid arthritis process in a patient.

HLHS (hypoplastic left heart syndrome).

HLVA (high-velocity, low-amplitude) maneuvers.

HM (hand movements) (Oph).

HMB-45 melanosome (a melanoma antibody)—a test for melanoma and other tumors.

HME (heat-moisture exchanger).

HME nose ("hemi" nose)—a somewhat redundant slang term for a heat-moisture exchanger.

HMFG1 (human milk fat globule 1)—an antigen found in prostate cancer.

hMSCs (human mesenchymal stem cells).

HNP (herniated nucleus pulposus).

HNPCC (hereditary nonpolyposis colorectal cancer)—see *Lynch syndrome*.

hockey-stick appearance of catheter tip (Cardio).

HOCM-like ("HOCUM-like")—hypertrophic obstructive cardiomyopathy (HOCM). Usage: "HOCM-like left ventricular outflow obstruction."

Hoehn and Yahr scale—for Parkinson disease staging.

Hoehne sign (Ob-Gyn)—failure to respond to oxytocic drugs, a sign of uterine rupture.

Hoek-Bowen cement removal system by Micro-Aire.

Hoffa tendon shortening—a procedure in which gathering stitches are run up a portion of the tendon, and then the suture is tightened to the appropriate length.

Hoffman and Mohr procedure—technique for repair of unicoronal cranial synostosis.

Hoffman-Clayton procedure—podiatric procedure to treat rheumatoid arthritis.

Hoffmann external fixation device—developed by Swiss surgeon Raoul Hoffmann.

Hoffmann mini-lengthening fixation device.

Hoffmann reflex—twitching of the thumb when the middle finger is snapped, one of the signs of upper neuron damage. Named for Johann Hoffmann, German neurologist.

Hofmeister gastroenterostomy.

Hohmann retractor (Ortho)—used in acetabular fracture repair. Also, *Mini-Hohmann*.

Hohn central venous catheter, single- and double-lumen.

Holdrinet method—calculates the fraction of bone marrow nucleated cells that come from peripheral blood.

Holinger anterior commissure laryngoscope.

Holladay formula (Oph)—a formula for calculating the depth of the anterior chamber of the eye.

Holladay-Godwin cornea gauge—a set of two double-sided instruments designed to measure the horizontal corneal diameter. It allows the technician to measure corneal diameter while performing the A-scan and keratometry.

Hollande solution—used as a fixative for some types of pathology specimens.

Hollenhorst plaques—yellow-orange cholesterol plaques which, when seen on examination of the optic fundi, indicate the presence of atherosclerosis. Usage: "His optic fundi were closely inspected and were benign for Hollenhorst plaques, for papilledema and hemorrhage."

Hollingshead Four Factor Index—a measure of socioeconomic status.

hollow bandage contact lens—a protective contact lens with a 6-mm central opening that allows the intraocular pressure to be monitored without removing and replacing the lens.

holmium laser—a pulsed noncontact laser similar to a carbon dioxide laser in that its wavelength is absorbed by water-containing tissues. It can operate in a fluid (liquid) medium and it can coagulate bleeding vessels. It can also resect and vaporize tough cartilaginous tissues.

holmium:YAG (yttrium-argon-garnet) **laser**—a laser used in endoscopic laser cholecystectomy and in angioplasty. Also known as *Ho:YAG*.

Hologic QDR 1000W—dual energy x-ray absorptiometry scanner.

Holt-Oram atriodigital dysplasia—heart and hand syndrome.

HOM (high-osmolar media) (Radiol). See *ionic contrast media*. Cf. *LOM, nonionic contrast media*.

HomMed monitor—a home monitoring system for patients with congestive heart failure. It works by measuring the patient's weight, blood pressure, pulse, and oxygen saturation, and transmits the data via telephone lines from the patient's home directly to specially trained personnel.

Homans sign—forced dorsiflexion of the foot causes discomfort behind the knee in thrombosis in the leg.

home ambulatory inotropic therapy—allows patients awaiting heart transplants to leave the hospital and enjoy a more normal lifestyle at home. The patients self-administer a regimen of medications through a tunneled subclavian Silastic catheter, using a syringe pump and syringe driver. Medication regimen is directed at maintaining hemodynamics and includes ACE inhibitors, digoxin, vasodilators, and amiodarone.

HomeChoice Pro with PD Link—home-based dialysis treatment with advanced computer technology to communicate therapy data to clinicians via data card or modem. The system allows clinicians to monitor patient data on a daily basis so that they can adjust prescriptions and identify potential problems between clinic visits.

home O_2 (oxygen)—in dictation it sounds like "homo-2." Usage: "The patient was discharged on home O_2."

Homer-Wright rosette (Neuro)—sometimes seen on histologic examination of medulloblastomas. Also, *Homer-Wright pseudorosette.*

HomeTrak Plus—compact cardiac event recorder about the size of a pager, designed for cardiac patients with transient symptoms that cannot be captured via standard Holter monitor or 12-lead EKG.

HomMed Monitoring System—a patient-friendly, cost-effective method of monitoring congestive heart failure patients from their homes.

homocysteine—a sulfur-containing homolog of the amino acid cysteine, normally found in small amounts in plasma. Elevation, which occurs in dietary deficiency of folic acid, inherited deficiencies of certain enzymes, and some chronic diseases (renal failure, hypothyroidism), is a risk factor for premature cardiovascular disease and, in pregnant women, for fetal neural tube defects such as spina bifida. Most dictators pronounce this term in exactly the same way as homocystine, a related but chemically distinct substance. The following rule of thumb will virtually always guide the transcriptionist to the correct spelling: Blood is tested for homocysteine. Urine is tested for homocystine. Cf. *homocystine.*

homocysteine testing—standard testing for homocysteine done on blood (plasma). Physicians may refer to "plasma homocysteine." Not to be confused with *urine homocystine.* See *homocystine, homocystinuria.*

homocystine testing—standard testing for homocystine done on urine. Physicians may refer to "urine homocystine." Not to be confused with *plasma homocysteine.* See *homocysteine, homocystinuria.*

homocystinuria—rare genetic disorder of metabolism in which a specific enzyme deficiency leads to a buildup of homocysteine in the plasma and to the appearance of its oxidation product, homocystine, in the urine. See also *homocysteine* and *homocystine.*

homogeneous gene assay system—uses a fluorescent technique with bound probes to isolate and amplify the nucleotides (segment of DNA or RNA) of interest in a specimen. See *polymerase chain reaction.*

homograft—see *denatured homograft.*

homologous—similar or uniform; in genetics, a perfectly matched pair of chromosomes, one from each parent.

homologous recombination—a laboratory technique of inactivating ("knocking out") a given gene in an experimental animal or in a stem cell colony by substituting for it a synthetic, nonfunctioning DNA sequence of similar configuration.

"homo-2"—phonetic for *home* O_2 or *home oxygen.*

homozygote (Genetics)—an individual who has a pair of identical alleles at a given locus.

homozygous (Genetics)—possessing identical alleles at a given locus.

Honan balloon—used in phacoemulsification of cataracts. Usage: "After ascertaining adequate akinesia and anesthesia, and after the Honan balloon was set at 30 mmHg for 15 minutes, the left face was prepared and draped in the usual sterile ophthalmic fashion."

Honan manometer—used in lowering intraocular pressure.

H1 receptors—histamine receptors in the respiratory tract which are blocked by antihistamines.

honeycomb mucosa—seen in the jejunum of patients with celiac disease.

honk, precordial—an abnormal heart sound.

Hoodia (*Hoodia gordonii*)—a natural appetite suppressant made from an African cactus plant.

hood O_2—humidified oxygen administered in a clear hard plastic container encasing the baby's head with an opening for the neck. Due to small air leaks around the neck it can attain only about 40% oxygen concentration.

Hood stoma stent—a device that utilizes a valve to allow a patient with a tracheostomy to speak without first having to put a finger over the stoma.

hookah—a traditional Arabic device for smoking hashish, marijuana, and later tobacco, or indeed any other smokeable substance, operating on the principle of a water pipe. Also spelled *huka.* Also known as *sheesha, kalian,* or *hubble-bubble.*

hook-fist positioning—postoperative exercise for tendon repair.

Hoover sign—for unilateral leg paralysis in suspected hysteria. The physician allows the patient to think he is testing the unaffected leg, but places a hand underneath the heel of the "paralyzed" leg. When the good leg is raised, an individual with normal muscle strength will be unable to refrain from pressing down on the bed with the heel of the other leg. Lack of such pressure indicates organic paresis.

Hopkins 70° rigid telescope—used in laryngoscopy.

hordeolum—acute inflammation of a sebaceous gland of the eyelid. See *sty (stye).*

Horizon—see *CD Horizon Sextant spinal system.*

Horizon AutoAdjust CPAP system—a respiratory care product designed to provide patients suffering from obstructive sleep apnea (OSA) with relief through nightly therapy.

Horizon prostatic stent—for relief of bladder outlet obstruction.

horizontal adduction test—see *cross-chest adduction test.*

Hormodendrum—an inhalant antigen.

hormone
- Biotropin (human growth hormone)
- follicle-stimulating (FSH)
- Genentech biosynthetic human
- gonadotropin-releasing (GnRH)
- growth (Protropin)
- human growth (Biotropin)
- Humatrope human growth
- hypothalamic luteinizing hormone-releasing
- Innofem (estradiol tablets)
- Leuprolide
- long-acting thyroid-stimulating (LATS)
- luteinizing hormone-releasing (LHRH)
- parathyroid (parathormone)
- placental growth (PGH)
- Protropin human growth
- secretin

Horn Endo-Otoprobe—a laser probe used in ear surgery.

Hoskins nylon suture laser lens (Oph)—used to cut subconjunctival nylon sutures in postoperative situations such as trabeculectomies, sutures in cataract wounds causing astigmatism, and flap sutures that are too tight to permit filtration. This is a noninvasive procedure.

Hospital Anxiety and Depression (HAD) **scale**—used to evaluate patient anxiety and depression.

hospitalist—a physician whose chief professional activity is general inpatient care; usually a primary care physician who assumes responsibility for the observation and treatment of hospitalized patients and returns them to the care of their private physicians when they are discharged from the hospital. A hospitalist may be an employee of a hospital or HMO, a contractor, or a private practitioner; about 75% of hospitalists are general internists.

hospital johnny—a hospital gown.

hostile—an English word used in a medical context to mean unfriendly or not amenable to. Usage: "The peritoneal cavity was hostile (due to adhesions)" or "Operating conditions were hostile." See also *hostile neck*.

hostile neck—a neck which makes catheterization for the purposes of angiography or some other procedure difficult. Causes include such things as a high internal carotid artery, previous radiation, total laryngectomy, or creation of a tracheotomy.

HOT (hypertension optimal treatment).

Hot and Cold Sensory System—designed to enhance upper extremity prostheses. It contains a fingertip temperature probe in the prosthetic hand. The temperature readings are sent to circuitry inside the prosthesis and then to a pair of corresponding electrodes that touch the patient's residual limb. The electrodes become warm or cool depending on the voltages received, and the patient registers the sensation of hot or cold in the prosthesis.

Hot/Ice Cold Therapy Cooler—portable cold therapy device for outpatient or home treatment. It delivers continuous cold therapy needed after orthopedic procedures such as foot, ankle, or knee surgery.

Hot/Ice System III—for controlled cold therapy following orthopedic procedures.

HotMaxx reusable hot biopsy forceps—used to obtain gastrointestinal mucosal samples for microscopic examination and removal of sessile polyps.

hot potato voice—hollow voice caused by edema or paralysis of the soft palate; most commonly observed in severe pharyngitis or peritonsillar abscess.

Hot Sampler—used to obtain gastrointestinal mucosal tissue samples for microscopic examination and removal of sessile polyps.

Hotsy Cautery—a disposable surgical cautery.

Houget maneuver—used in inguinal hernia repair.

Hough ("huff") **hoe**—elevator with an angled tip and handle.

Hounsfield unit—density measurement indicative of calcium (on CT scan).

hourglass biceps—hypertrophy of the tendon of the long head of the biceps brachii that makes it impossible for the tendon to slide into the bicipital groove during elevation of the arm; frequently associated with a rotator cuff tear.

hourglass constriction of hip capsule—radiographic finding in developmental dysplasia of the hip.

House and Pulec otic-periotic shunt—for treatment of progressive endolymphatic hydrops (Ménière disease).

House-Brackman facial nerve grading system—a scale that ranges from grades I (normal) through XI (total loss of function). A scale point of 1 is assigned for each 0.25 cm of motion up to 1 cm for both eye brow and commissure movement. The points are then added together. Thus, a total of 8 points can be obtained, if each structure moves 1 cm. Grade I is the equivalent of a score of 8 out of 8; grade VI a score of 0 out of 8 possible points.

House-Brackmann grading scale—for facial nerve function in paralysis due to Wegener granulomatosis. Usage: "This patient's facial nerve function at this time would be considered to be House-Brackmann grade 3."

Housecall—transtelephonic monitoring system that uses a telephone to download diagnostic data and programmed parameters from an implanted cardioverter-defibrillator.

housemaid's knee—older term for *prepatellar bursitis*, seen in patients who repeatedly traumatize the bursa by kneeling.

Houston Halo—to treat cervical spine disorders.

Howell biopsy aspiration needle.

Howmedica Osteonics bone cement.

Howmedica Universal compression screw (Ortho)—available in cancellous and cortical thread types.

Howship lacuna—a pit or cavity resulting from resorption of calcium from bone. Named for John Howship (1781-1841), English surgeon.

Ho:YAG (holmium:yttrium-argon-garnet) **laser**.

Ho:YAG LTK (noncontact holmium: YAG laser thermal keratoplasty)—technique for correction of low hyperopia.

Hoyer lift transfer.

HPA (*Histoplasma capsulatum* polysaccharide antigen).

HPA (hypothalamic-pituitary-adrenal) **axis suppression**—a syndrome that occurs following systemic absorption of significant amounts of topically applied corticosteroids. This may occur from prolonged use or extensive use (over a large body area) of topical corticosteroids. Symptoms include Cushing syndrome and elevated blood glucose levels.

HPCD (hemostatic puncture closure device)—used after interventional or diagnostic vascular procedures to seal the arteriotomy.

HPC guidewire—a flexible hydrophilic guidewire used to cannulate the biliary duct. Produces less trauma than other methods, in the presence of tight strictures.

Hp Chek—screening system for serological detection of *H. pylori* antibodies.

HpD (hematoporphyrin derivative).

Hpfast—an agar gel test for *Helicobacter pylori*.

HPRC (hereditary papillary renal cancer) **syndrome**—hereditary familial cancer syndrome.

HPS (hematoxylin, phloxine, and safranin)—histochemical stains.

HP (Hewlett-Packard) **SONOS 5500** ultrasound imaging system.

HPV (human papillomavirus).

HRARE (hybrid rapid acquisition with relaxation enhancement)—MR imaging to evaluate small bowel involvement in Crohn disease. Cf. *HASTE*.

HRCT (high-resolution computed tomography).

H reflex study—electromyography, given in milliseconds (msec). Through an electrically induced spinal reflex, a determination can be made as to the presence of unilateral S1 radiculopathy.

HRL (Hardy-Rand-Littler) **screening plates**—test charts composed of dots of different colors. Geometric figures can be seen among the dots. The charts are used to test color vision.

HRQL, HRQoL (health-related quality of life).

HRS (hepatorenal syndrome).

HRT (hormone replacement therapy) **patch**—drug for treatment of vasomotor symptoms related to menopause.

Hruby lens ("ruby")—slit-lamp biomicroscopy.

HS, h.s. (hora somni)—half-strength; bedtime.

HSAN-IV (hereditary sensory and autonomic neuropathy type IV)

HSC (hematopoietic stem cell).

HSC (Hospital for Sick Children) **Scale**—a scale used to measure pain experienced by patients undergoing Ilizarov limb-lengthening procedures. Measures pain for an extended period. Cf. *APPT*.

HSCT (hematopoietic stem cell transplantation).

HSIL (high-grade squamous intraepithelial lesion).

H-SLAP (human stromelysin aggregated proteoglycan)—an ELISA diagnostic test to evaluate stromelysin inhibitors that degrade cartilage, leading to osteoarthritis and rheumatoid arthritis.

HSM—slang for *hepatosplenomegaly*.

HspBcor—a vaccine for chronic HBV infection; it is a CoVal fusion protein engineered from HBV core (HBc) antigen and Hsp65 from *Mycobacterium bovis* BCG.

HSP-72 (heat shock protein 72).

HSSG (hysterosalpingosonography).

HS-tk gene therapy—for treatment of malignant brain tumors in children.

HSV (herpesvirus; herpes simplex virus).

hTERT (human telomerase reverse transcriptase).

HTLV-I retrovirus (human T-cell leukemia/lymphoma virus).

HTLV-III (human T-cell lymphotropic virus).

HTO Wedge—human donor tissue allograft used to correct malalignment of the knee. The wedge can be customized to precise shape and size in the operating room.

HT receptor blockers—see *5-HT receptor blockers*.

HTR-MFI implants—onlay facial augmentation implants for aesthetic facial surgery for augmentation of malar, paranasal, premaxillary, ramus, and chin regions.

H-TRON insulin pump.

Hubbard hydrotherapy tank—treatment for psoriasis.

Huber needle—a specially designed needle for use with ports. The sharply angled bevel leaves a line-like tear (in the rubber-covered entry site) which self-seals easily. Comes in straight or 90° angle design, the latter being used for continuous infusion because it will lie flat when taped to the skin.

Hudson-Stahli line—a linear subepithelial deposit of iron pigment on the surface of the cornea.

"huff" hoe—see *Hough hoe*.

Hughston knee evaluation (or score) —divides the patient's clinical performance into three categories: subjective, functional, and objective, yielding a combined score.

Hughston view—x-ray view of the flexed knee to demonstrate subluxation of the patella or fracture of the femoral condyle.

Hulka tenaculum.

Humalog Mix 75/25 Pen—75% insulin lispro protamine suspension, 25% insulin lispro injection (rDNA origin); first premixed insulin containing a rapid-acting insulin. Helps patients control blood glucose levels more easily throughout the day, at mealtime, between meals, and at nighttime.

human antichimeric antibody (HACA) —can develop after receiving infliximab. HACAs are associated with an increased rate of infusion reactions.

human chorionic gonadotropin (hCG or HCG).

human cloning—see *cloning, human*.

human diploid cell strain rabies vaccine (HDRV).

human fibroblast growth factor-I (FGF-I)—genetically engineered human protein that can induce growth of new blood vessels when injected into diseased heart tissue. A dense capillary network appears around the site of injection and brings about an increase in blood supply through the newly formed functional vessels.

human embryonic stem cell—a pluripotent stem cell derived from the inner cell mass of the blastocyst stage of a human embryo.

human ether-a-go-go related gene (HERG)—a potassium channel.

Human Genome Project—cooperative international project to map the entirety of human DNA, including all 23 chromosomes and an estimated 100,000 genes.

human granulocytic ehrlichiosis (HGE) —a tick-borne disease, with some fatalities reported.

human growth hormone (hGH).

human herpesvirus 6 (HHV-6)—one of the most widespread members of the family of human herpesviruses, infecting up to 90% of most populations during infancy. Primary infection is either asymptomatic or manifests itself as a febrile illness that may include exanthem subitum. While severe or fatal complications are rare in immunocompetent pa-

human *(cont.)* tients, the virus poses an additional health risk for immunodeficient patients, particularly those who have undergone organ or bone marrow transplants or who are HIV seropositive.

human immunodeficiency virus (HIV).

human insulin—see *Humulin.* Cf. *semisynthetic human insulin.*

humanized anti-TAC (T-cell activated antigen) **monoclonal antibody**—an anti-inflammatory agent used in treatment of Behçet disease, uveitis, and other eye conditions.

human lymphocyte antigen (HLA).

human mammary tumor virus (HMTV)—primitive retrovirus identified in human breast cancer tissues.

human meniscal allograft—used in knee surgery to repair large, complex tears of the meniscus, reestablishing normal load-bearing at the knee and delaying degenerative changes that follow total meniscectomy. The allografts are securely fixed by implantable bone anchors.

human mesenchymal stem cells (hMSCs).

human papillomavirus (HPV)—cause of genital warts, a sexually transmitted disease and a risk factor for cancer of the cervix.

human parvovirus B19 (HPV B19)—the virus that causes erythema infectiosum (fifth disease), a common mild febrile exanthem of children. Less often it causes chronic anemia, neutropenia, myocarditis, vasculitis, or encephalitis, particularly in immunodeficient persons or pregnant women.

human stromelysin aggregated proteoglycan (H-SLAP).

human T-cell lymphotropic virus (HTLV-III)—name given to the virus isolated by Robert Gallo, the American researcher who thought he was the first to isolate the AIDS virus. The researchers at the Pasteur Institute in Paris were actually the first by a considerable margin. HIV (human immunodeficiency virus, now the official name for the AIDS virus), is one of the lentiviruses. See *HIV.*

Humatrix Microclysmic gel—wound filling material.

HumatroPen—reusable growth hormone delivery device for administration of Humatrope as treatment for growth hormone deficiency and short stature associated with Turner syndrome.

humeral—pertaining to the humerus bone. Cf. *humoral, humorous.*

humerus—the long arm bone between the shoulder joint and the elbow joint. Cf. *humeral, humoral, humorous.*

HumidAire heated humidifier.

Humira (adalimumab)—a self-injectable therapy for rheumatoid arthritis.

HUMI uterine manipulator/injector.

Hummer—a powered microdebrider designed originally for temporomandibular joint surgery. It is also now used as a sinus surgery instrument. It consists of a power unit, a foot-switch pedal, a handpiece, and a disposable blade.

Hummingbird wand—used for ablation and excision of soft tissue in well-defined channels or submucosally in ENT procedures.

humoral—pertaining to the immunity provided by antibodies in the blood. Cf. *humeral, humorous.*

humorous—funny or witty in character. Cf. *humerus*.

hump—see *diaphragmatic hump*.

Humphrey frequency-doubling perimeter—used for visual field testing.

Humphrey Systems ablation planner topography—a method to identify appropriate treatment sites in the eye by analyzing where off-centered corneal irregularities exist.

Humulin—a human insulin (of recombinant DNA origin).

Humulin 70/30, Humulin R, and **Humalog Pens**—prefilled disposable insulin drug delivery devices that hold 300 units of insulin and fit in pocket or purse. A dose knob can be dialed backward or forward in single-unit increments.

Hunner interstitial cystitis (*not* Hunter)—a severe, chronic inflammation of mucosa and muscularis of the urinary bladder, associated with ulcers of the bladder. Also, *Hunner ulcer*.

Hunner ulcer (Urol)—see *Hunner interstitial cystitis*.

Hunt and Hess neurological classification—to predict the prognosis in patients with subarachnoid hemorrhage and intracranial aneurysms, grades 1-4.

Hunter canal (canalis adductorius)—contains the femoral vessels and saphenous nerve.

Hunter-Sessions balloon—used in inferior vena cava to intercept a venous embolus.

Hunter tendon rod insertion—a treatment for deep venous insufficiency (DVI) of the lower extremities which causes symptoms of chronic edema and pain because the valves in the veins of the lower leg are incompetent. An incision is made at the back of the leg in the popliteal fossa. The Hunter tendon rod (made of Dacron) is sewn to the gracilis tendon at the side of the leg, woven through the popliteal artery and vein deep inside the leg, sutured to the biceps tendon on the other side of the leg, and drawn up snugly as a sling. This device then acts as a substitute valve by periodically occluding the popliteal vein as it passes tightly across it. When the patient stands or sits, the popliteal vein remains unoccluded. However, when the knee is actively flexed and the gracilis and biceps muscles retract, the popliteal vein is occluded to prevent venous reflux and venous stasis in the leg. Results are said to be superior to those obtained with other techniques.

Hunt-Lawrence pouch—a modification of the Roux-en-Y esophagojejunostomy reconstruction after total gastrectomy for carcinoma. This pouch is constructed to replace the gastric reservoir (removed in the Roux-en-Y procedure), to relieve symptoms of feelings of fullness, nausea, vomiting, dumping, and abdominal discomfort.

Hürthle cell neoplasm.

Hurwitz dialysis catheter.

HUS (hemolytic uremic syndrome).

Hutchinson teeth—older term for one of the manifestations of congenital syphilis, now rare; the teeth are broad at the base and the biting surface is narrow and notched. Also, *hutchinsonian molars*.

HVI-DHP (hepatic venous isolation by direct hemoperfusion).

HVO (hallux valgus orthosis) **splint in a bag**—a forefoot splint used to treat hallux valgus either pre- or postoperatively. The splint is placed in a

HVO *(cont.)*
bag, and boiling water is added to make it moldable for custom fitting.

HVS (high-voltage stimulation).

HVS (hyperventilation syndrome).

hyaloid corpuscle—see *Mittendorf dot*.

hyaloid membrane peel.

Hyams grading system (or criteria)—for esthesioneuroblastoma.

Hybrid Capture cytomegalovirus DNA test—provides clinicians with a cost-effective and timely aid for diagnosing CMV infection in solid organ transplant, bone marrow transplant, and HIV-positive/AIDS patients.

Hybrid Capture II—DNA-based test to detect the human papillomavirus.

Hybrid Capture II HBV test—a laboratory test for hepatitis B virus.

Hybrid Capture II HPV test—a laboratory test that can detect all 13 forms of the human papillomavirus associated with cervical cancer; said to be more reliable than the Pap test.

Hybrid Capture II *Neisseria gonorrhoeae* test.

hybrid cell—a cell resulting from the junction of two cells of different origins, whose nuclei have fused into one.

hybridization—pairing of an RNA strand and a DNA strand, or of two different DNA strands.

hybridoma—a cell line formed in the laboratory by the fusion of normal immune cells (e.g., lymphocytes) and tumor cells (e.g., myeloma). Such cells retain the ability of their immune ancestors to produce monoclonal antibody and the capacity of their neoplastic ancestors to replicate indefinitely in culture.

Hybritech Tandem PSA ratio (free PSA/total PSA) (PSA, prostate-specific antigen)—a test to distinguish between prostate cancer and other conditions that are non-cancerous but involve an enlarged prostate.

Hycor rheumatoid factor (RF) IgA ELISA autoimmune test—for early diagnosis of rheumatoid arthritis.

hyCure G hydrogel dressing.

Hydrasorb foam wound dressing.

Hydrasorb Plus—a hydrophilic polyurethane wound dressing.

hydrazine sulfate—an alternative cancer therapy to promote weight gain and appetite in patients with incurable colorectal carcinoma.

HydroBlade keratome—Microjet device used to produce hinged corneal flaps and to alter the shape of the cornea for vision correction.

HydroBrader irrigating/aspirating dermabrader—a rotating diamond bur with aspiration ports that uses coarse or fine grit for polishing the skin and simultaneously evacuates debris from operative site.

HydroBrush keratome—used in the debridement of epithelium from the cornea.

Hydrocol—see *hydrocolloid dressing material*.

Hydrocollator—a silica gel pack used in applying localized heat. The silica gel is encased in a canvas bag. The pack is immersed in water and heated to 140 to 160°F. The pack is then wrapped in several layers of terry cloth before applying to the area to be heated. The pack maintains its heat for approximately 20 to 30 minutes, which gives it an advantage over the hot water bottle.

hydrocolloid dressing—combines absorbent colloid materials with adhe-

hydrocolloid *(cont.)* sive elastomers for application to wounds with light to moderate exudate. Most hydrocolloid dressings react with wound exudate to form gel-like coverings that protect the wound bed and maintain a moist wound environment. Hydrocolloid is available in occlusive and wafer-type dressings, as well as in powder and paste forms. See also *dressing*.

hydrofiber dressings.

HydroFlex—arthroscopy irrigating system.

hydrogel dressing—wound gel that helps create or maintain a moist wound environment. Some hydrogels provide absorption, desloughing, and debriding of necrotic and fibrotic tissue. See *dressing*.

hydrogel sheet—cross-linked polymer gels in sheet form for wound dressing. These materials help create or maintain a moist wound environment and may also provide absorption, desloughing, and debridement of necrotic and fibrotic tissue. See *dressing*.

hydrography, MR—see *MR hydrography.*

Hydrolyser microcatheter—used in thrombectomy systems to negotiate tortuous arterial curves.

Hydromer—coated bipolar coagulation probe.

Hydromer Aquatrix II—hydrogel technology for biosurgery applications. It is based on chitosan, a structural analog to hyaluronic acid derived from chitin, a natural biopolymer, and polyvinylpyrrolidone (PVP), a synthetic polymer.

Hydron Burn Bandage.

hydrophilic—water-loving. Used in medicine to refer to stains. Cf. *lipophilic*, fat-loving.

hydrophilic semipermeable absorbent polyurethane foam dressing (Surg) —provides a moist wound environment with a petrolatum gauze dressing for donor sites. It is said to produce less initial patient donor site discomfort and to produce more complete donor site healing by postoperative day 14.

HydroPlus—a coating material for stents that helps prevent restenosis.

Hydro-Splint II—used to immobilize fractures of upper or lower extremities. It is not only a splint, but also a cold (or warm) compress, and provides soft tissue compression for chronic or acute swelling.

HydroSurg laparoscopic irrigator.

HydroThermAblator—system to treat excessive uterine bleeding.

Hydroview intraocular lens—implant for correction of vision following cataract extraction procedures.

hydroxyapatite (or *hydroxylapatite*) (HA)—dense ceramic material manufactured from coral found in the ocean. It is porous, like human bone. Used as an adjunct to bone grafting in cranial defects, to restore normal contour. In ophthalmology, it can be formed into a sphere and used as an ocular implant after enucleation of the eye. Also, *Biomatrix ocular implant, Durapatite, Interpore.*

hydroxyapatite cement (HAC)—used in repairing large traumatic defects of the craniofacial skeleton and in surgery on the paranasal sinuses and bones.

hydroxyindoleacetic acid (5-HIAA).

hydroxylapatite—see *hydroxyapatite*.

HyFil hydrogel dressing.

Hyfrecator—a desiccator-fulgurator-coagulator.

hygroma—a fluid-filled cystic mass, often seen in the necks of children.

Hylaform (hylan polymer)—viscoelastic gel for correction of facial wrinkles and depressed scars.

Hylaform gel—a skin filler made from a highly purified form of hyaluronic acid that mimics the effects of natural hyaluronic acid. When injected just below the surface of the skin, Hylaform adds volume to the skin, smoothing unwanted lines and wrinkles.

Hylaform Plus—a hyaluronic acid wrinkle treatment that lasts from three months to one year.

Hylagel-Nuro—viscoelastic gel for the reduction of postoperative scarring and adhesions secondary to lumbar surgery. It is administered via injection of the spinal area immediately following surgery.

Hylashield and **Hylashield Nite** (hylan A)—provides an elastoviscous shield and protects the surface of the eye from noxious environmental conditions.

HylaSine—viscoelastic gel device injected into anatomical compartments of the sinus during and following sinus surgery in order to coat surgically altered tissue, control intraoperative and postoperative bleeding, reduce postsurgical scarring and adhesions, minimize patient discomfort, and shorten postoperative rehabilitation time.

hymenal ring (*not* hymeneal, as it is often mispronounced).

hyoscyamine sulfate—anticholinergic drug for irritable bowel syndrome and other GI conditions. See *NuLev*.

hyoid bone suspension—surgical procedure for obstructive sleep apnea.

Hypafix—nonwoven tape with a low-allergy adhesive used to hold dressings in place.

hyper-, prefix meaning *excessive, above, beyond*. Cf. *hypo-*.

hyperacute—having a very abrupt onset or very brief course.

hyperacute rejection (HAR)—graft rejection immediately after transplantation.

hyperal'd—slang for *given hyperalimentation*.

hyperbaric chambers—increasingly seen in hospital inventories because of oxygen's capacity to aid healing. Trainers for major sports teams also have the chambers on hand for athletes, and celebrities are touting them as age-defying devices.

hyperbaric oxygen therapy—high-pressure therapy used in treatment of cyanide poisoning, exceptionally high blood loss anemia, decompression sickness, and as adjunctive therapy in osteomyelitis, radiation injury, acute cerebral edema, and injury to the head and spinal cord. Also used as adjunctive therapy in the treatment of rhinocerebral mucormycosis. The fungi, when they infect immunosuppressed patients, can be highly invasive, causing a rapidly progressive infection.

Hypercare (aluminum chloride [hexahydrate] 20% in anhydrous ethyl alcohol)—a medication for the treatment of hyperhidrosis of the palms and soles.

hyperesthesia of the vulva—see *vulvar vestibulitis syndrome.*

Hypergel hydrogel dressing.

Hyperion LTK (laser thermal keratoplasty)—holmium laser-based system for the performance of laser thermal keratoplasty.

hyperlexia—an autism-like syndrome that has been identified in some language-disordered children, char-

hyperlexia *(cont.)* acterized by difficulty understanding verbal language and difficulty socializing and interacting appropriately. What is unusual is that these children exhibit a precocious ability to read words far above what would be expected at their chronological age and show an intense fascination with letters or numbers.

hyperlipoproteinemia (HLP).

hyperopia—farsightedness.

hyperoxia—used for treating carbon monoxide poisoning, chronic nonhealing ulcers, acute traumatic and chronically ischemic wounds, and refractory osteomyelitis.

hyperprosody—excessive variation in voice features such as pitch, loudness, tempo, intonation, as occurs in manic patients. In patients with Broca aphasia, hyperprosody manifests as their using the very few words at their disposal to convey to the utmost their attitudes and emotions. Cf. *dysprosody*.

hyperreflectile granular sparkling appearance of the myocardium—the appearance on echocardiogram of the heart in a patient with stiff-heart syndrome.

hyperreninemia—a condition of elevated levels of renin in the blood, which may lead to aldosteronism and hypertension.

hypersensitivity syndrome—see *drug reaction with eosinophilia and systemic symptoms* (DRESS).

hypertelorism—abnormally increased distance between two organs, as in Crouzon disease.

hypertension optimal treatment (HOT) —a five-year study begun in 1992 to determine precisely how far high blood pressure should be lowered to minimize cardiovascular morbidity and mortality. It also examines the effects of adding low doses of aspirin to the antihypertensive regimen. The HOT study involves patients from 26 countries on four continents and includes both male and female hypertensives.

hypertension standard—changed from 140/80 to 135/85, resulting in many more patients requiring medication.

hyperthermia, whole body—used in the therapy regimen of patients with certain types of tumors, some bone metastases, and Ewing sarcoma. These cancer cells are particularly sensitive to heat; therefore, heat increases the effectiveness of chemotherapy and radiotherapy. When the patient's body is heated to 108°F after irradiation, the cancer cells cannot readily repair themselves. When the patient is given hyperthermia before chemotherapy is introduced, the cancer cells are more susceptible to the effects of chemotherapy agents.

hypertrophic cardiomyopathy (HCMP).

hypertrophic obstructive cardiomyopathy (HOCM).

hypertrophic obstructive cardiomyopathy (HOCM).

hypertrophied nasal turbinate—enlargement of the inferior turbinate due to repeated infection. The enlargement may be allergic or due to an increase in circulation. There may be huge pools of blood in the turbinate, or there may be a physical swelling due to this enlargement that blocks breathing. See *empty nose syndrome.*

hypertrophy, asymmetric septal (ASH).

hypertylosis of the palms—callosities.

hypesthesia—diminished sensitivity to stimulation, feeling, sensation or perception. Also, *hypoesthesia.*

hypnagogic startle—a sleep start or sudden body jerk, observed normally just at sleep onset and resulting in at least momentary awakening.

hypnosis, focused open neurosensory induction of—a self-hypnotic method using vision, hearing, and kinesthetic sensations.

hypnotic—a drug used to induce sleep.

hypo-, prefix meaning *deficient, decrease, under, beneath, below*. Cf. *hyper-*.

hypoaeration (Radiol)—on chest x-ray, abnormal reduction in the amount of air in lung tissue.

hypoattenuating—coined word applied to CT scan findings of low attenuation.

hypoechoic ("hi-po-e-ko´-ic")—a term used in ultrasonography, when only few echoes are given off as the ultrasound waves bounce off structures or tissues at which they are directed. Usage: "The patient had a hypoechoic area in the right lobe of the prostate."

hypohidrotic ectodermal dysplasia (HED)—a rare hereditary congenital disease that affects several ectodermal structures.

hypokinesis—abnormal reduction of mobility or motility; reduced contractile movement in one or both cardiac ventricles.

hypophysis—pituitary gland (hypophysis cerebri); pharyngeal hypophysis (a mass in the wall of the pharynx similar in appearance to the hypophysis). Cf. *apophysis, epiphysis, hypothesis*.

hypoplastic left heart syndrome (HLHS).

hypopyon—a complication associated with postoperative corneal graft infection.

hypotensive shock bowel—see *abnormal bowel wall enhancement*.

hypothalamic-pituitary-adrenal axis (HPA).

hypothalamus—the portion of the brain that controls the autonomic mechanism.

hypothenar hammer syndrome—a disorder of the hand characterized by thrombosis, spasm, or aneurysm of the ulnar artery as a result of minor repetitive trauma. Often the narrowing occurs adjacent to the hook of the hamate. It occurs when workers repeatedly use the palm of the hand (especially the hypothenar eminence) as a hammer to grind, push, and twist objects. These activities can damage certain blood vessels of the hand, especially the ulnar artery.

hypothermia blanket—used for cooling patients to 28 to 30°C for open heart and brain surgery; reduces normal oxygen requirements.

hypothesis—a theory that appears to explain certain phenomena and is used as the basis of experimentation and reasoning to prove the theory. Cf. *apophysis, epiphysis, hypophysis*.

hysterectomy (see *operations*)

hysteroscopic sterilization—a method of plugging the fallopian tubes to prevent conception. This technique involves inserting a nickel-titanium and stainless steel springlike device into the fallopian tubes using a hysteroscope. The metal device encapsulates and holds in place white polyester fibers able to cause scarring and thus block the fallopian

hysteroscopic *(cont.)*
tubes within 12 weeks, preventing the possibility of future pregnancy. This method is less expensive than laparoscopic tubal ligation and requires minimal sedation and no surgical incision because the surgeon enters via the vagina.

hysterosonography—the infusion of saline into the uterus through a catheter while a transvaginal ultrasound is performed. This procedure is used to identify lesions undetected by endometrial biopsy.

hysterosalpingosonography (HSSG)—a diagnostic ultrasound technique used to assess uterine cavity defects and patency of the fallopian tubes.

Hy-Tape—waterproof, medicated tape safe for direct use on skin and especially used by ostomy patients.

HY-TEC—automated diagnostic system designed to perform tests for both allergy and autoimmune disease.

HZA (hemizona) **assay**—for the evaluation of sperm binding to the zona pellucida, with high predictive value for in vitro fertilization.

HZV (herpes zoster virus).

I, i

IAET (International Association of Enterostomal Therapists) **stages**—a staging system for grading chronic wounds by their depth, stages I through IV.

IABC (intra-aortic balloon counterpulsation).

IABP (intra-aortic balloon pump).

Ialo photocoagulation—of the whole retina.

Iamin Gel wound dressing—a hydrogel dressing used in the management of various types of wounds, including skin abrasions, first and second degree burns, diabetic and venous stasis ulcers, pressure sores, and surgical incisions.

I&D (incision and drainage). Cf. *IND*.

I&O, I/O (intake and output)—intake of liquid (intravenous, per mouth, per tube) and output (urine, tube, drain) plus insensible output, in a 24-hour period. Measured in cubic centimeters or milliliters. Usage: "The patient's I&O was monitored." See *INO; insensible output*.

iatrogenic illness—caused (inadvertently) by a physician. Cf. *nosocomial*.

IBD (inflammatory bowel disease).

iBOT wheelchair—raises vertically to eye level, balances on two wheels, climbs stairs, and traverses rough terrains.

ibotenic acid—one of the poisons from the deadly mushroom *Amanita muscaria*.

ICA (intracranial aneurysm).

ICAM-1 (intercellular adhesions molecule-1)—a marker protein for the development of coronary artery disease in heart transplant patients.

ICBI (intact cortical bone index).

ICCE (intracapsular cataract extraction).

ICD (implantable cardioverter-defibrillator). See *AICD*.

ICD-9, ICD-10 (International Classification of Diseases) (coding).

ICE (intracardiac echocardiography).

ice-ball—a term used to describe the area of freezing in cryoablation of a tumor as seen on ultrasonography.

ice cream headache—a sensation of sudden head pain upon biting into very cold ice cream.

ICE disorders—immunoglobulin-complexed enzyme disorders.

IceSeeds—see *SeedNet System.*

ICE syndrome—iridocorneal-endothelial syndrome.

ICEUS (intracaval endovascular ultrasonography).

IC-Green (indocyanine green) **fluorescein angiography**.

ICIT (infrared coagulation of the inferior turbinate).

ICL (idiopathic CD4+ lymphocytopenia).

ICL (implantable contact lens)—refractive lens that is implanted over the natural lens of the eye for correction of myopia and hyperopia.

ICLH apparatus (Ortho)—by Imperial College, London Hospital.

ICM (inner cell mass).

i.com Comfort Shield—preservative-free viscoelastic ophthalmic solution for the treatment of dry eyes.

ICP catheter (intracranial pressure)—used with Tele-Sensor monitor after brain surgery. See *Cosman ICP Tele-Sensor*.

ICR (intrastromal corneal ring) or **KeraVision ICR**—an implant composed of two thin, transparent half-rings made of polymer material that are inserted into the periphery of the cornea, reshaping the clear tissue of the eye, to correct myopia. The procedure, which requires no cutting or removal of tissue, is designed to be a permanent implant, though it may be removed and replaced as vision changes.

ICS—intracellular-like, calcium bearing crystalloid solution. See *cardioplegic solution*.

ICSI (intracytoplasmic sperm injection).

ICSRA (intercompartmental supraretinacular artery).

ictal fear—an aura of anxiety or fear preceding temporal lobe seizures in some patients. May be more or less intense, with some patients reporting only uneasiness or nervousness and others intense fear and horror.

IDEA (Inventory for Déjà Vu Experiences Assessment)—prolonged or frequent episodes of déjà vu have clinical significance in patients with complex partial seizures and psychotic relapses.

ideal body weight (IBW).

Ideal (trademark) **cardiac device**.

ideation (noun)—the process of forming ideas or images. Usage: "He has no suicidal or homicidal ideation."

idée fixe ("ee-day'-feeks")—an obsessively fixed idea.

IDET (intradiscal electrothermal) **procedure**.

IDIF (indirect immunofluorescent assay). The usual abbreviation for this assay is IFA.

idiojunctional rhythm, junctional or nodal rhythm—a phenomenon in which the AV node becomes the pacemaker for the heart. When effective electrical impulses are no longer generated by the sinoatrial (SA) node, the atrioventricular (AV) node (located near the junction of atria and ventricles) becomes the pacemaker for the heart.

idiopathic CD4+ lymphocytopenia (ICL)—name given by the Centers for Disease Control and Prevention for controversial cases where patients seem to have AIDS-like symptoms in the absence of HIV.

idiopathic (cryptogenic) **epilepsy**—a condition of recurring seizures for which no cause can be assigned.

idiopathic hypertrophic subaortic stenosis (IHSS).

idiopathic thrombocytopenic purpura (ITP).

idiosyncratic asthma—asthma characterized by the following factors: (1) the person has no history of allergic diseases, (2) symptoms usually begin after age 30, (3) it is difficult to distinguish from chronic bronchitis, and (4) attacks often begin with minor respiratory symptoms.

IDIS angiography system (intraoperative digital subtraction).

IDI-Strep B—detects group B streptococcus in pregnant women in less than an hour. Can be used in all phases of pregnancy, including the time of delivery.

IDSS (internal decompression for spinal stenosis).

IEAP (Individual Employee Assistance Program).

IDXrad—a radiology information system that includes multi-organizational scheduling, patient tracking, and diagnostic reporting.

IEA (inferior epigastric artery) **graft**—may be used instead of saphenous veins in coronary artery bypass.

IECRT (intraoperative endoscopic Congo red test).

I-E ratio ("I to E ratio," inspiratory-expiratory ratio)—the ratio between the duration of inspiration and that of expiration. Usage: "Lungs: Normal I-E ratio, and no rales, rhonchi, or wheezes."

I-FABP (intestinal fatty acid-binding protein), **human serum.**

IFA test—indirect fluorescent antibody test for *Legionella pneumophila*. See also *DFA*.

IFL (internal facelift).

I-Flow nerve block infusion kit—for the continuous infusion of local anesthesia as a regional nerve block for pain management before and after orthopedic and general surgical procedures.

IFN-alpha (interferon alfa).

IFT (interferential current therapy).

IGF-BP3 complex (SomatoKine).

IGF-1 (insulin-like growth factor 1)—women under 50 with high blood levels of this factor appear to have a greater risk for breast cancer. However, for postmenopausal women, there is no association between IGF-1 and breast cancer risk.

IgG, platelet-associated (PAIgG).

IgG 2A monoclonal antibody (ImmuRAIT-LL2)—labeled with iodine 131; a drug used to treat B-cell lymphoma and leukemias.

Iglesias fiberoptic resectoscope.

IGM (inheritable genetic modification).

IgM-RF antibody (rheumatoid factor).

IGRT (image-guided radiation therapy).

IGS (implantable gastric stimulator)—see *Transcend*.

I-HAST (In-Home Alzheimer Screening Test).

IHSS (idiopathic hypertrophic subaortic stenosis). Now called *ASH* (asymmetric septal hypertrophy).

^{125}I iothalamate GFR (glomerular filtration rate)—a test of glomerular filtration rate using renal clearance of I-125 iothalamate.

^{131}I, ^{132}I—radioactive iodine with atomic weights of 131 and 132. Also written I-131, I-132.

II ("eye eye")—abbreviation for *image intensifier.*

IKDC (International Knee Documentation Committee) **Subjective Knee Form.**

ILA stapler—has three interchangeable heads and a long handle, giving access to deep operative sites.

ILC (interstitial laser coagulation).

IL4-PE (interleukin-4-*Pseudomonas* exotoxin fusion protein)—blood-cell-derived growth factor drug used for treatment of malignant brain tumors.

ileal conduit (*not* ileoconduit or ileo conduit)—a segment of ileum formed into a new bladder in patients who have undergone total cystectomy. The ends of the ureters are then anastomosed to the new ileal "bladder." See also *reservoir*.

ileal neobladder—see *W-stapled urinary reservoir*.

ileal pouch design—various designs (J pouch, S pouch, W pouch) related to the length of intestine used and thus the volume the pouch will hold. The J pouch, the simplest design, is the most common one performed.

ileoanal pouch anastomosis (IPAA).

ileocystoplasty—see *operation*.

ileosigmoid knot—condition where loops of ileum wrap around the base of a redundant sigmoid loop. The closed proximal loops of the ileum become congested and gangrenous within a few hours. Surgical intervention is required. Also known as *compound volvulus*.

ileostomy—see *operation*.

ileovesicostomy—see *Monti procedure*.

Ile-Sorb absorbent gel—introduced into ileostomy pouch to transform liquid into semi-solid gel in order to keep pouch contents away from stoma, reduce sloshing and pouch noise, and provide easier emptying.

ileum—the part of the small intestine located between the jejunum and the large intestine. Cf. *ilium*.

ileus—small-bowel obstruction due to failure of peristalsis.

Ilfeld-type abduction brace—a brace used in the treatment of chronic dislocated hip (CDH) in infants.

iliac crest pad—to pad pressure points while patient is on the operating table.

iliopopliteal bypass—the bypass of a stenotic femoral artery, with the graft passing from the common iliac or one of its branches to the popliteal artery.

iliopsoas test—for an inflammatory process. On abdominal examination, if pain is elicited when the patient flexes his thigh against pressure of the examiner's hand, there is an inflammatory process in contact with the iliopsoas muscle.

iliotibial band—a fibrous reinforcement of the fascia lata on the lateral surface of the thigh extending from the tensor muscle downward to the lateral condyle of the tibia. Usage: "The iliotibial band and tensor fasciae latae were identified next."

ilium—the superior portion of the hip bone. Cf. *ileum*.

Ilizarov limb lengthening procedure ("eh-liz´-a-rov").

Ilizarov system—instruments used to facilitate limb lengthening, fracture fixation, and nonunion of long bones.

illicit—unlawful, improper, not permitted. Usage: "The patient denies use of illicit drugs." Cf. *elicit*.

Illi intracranial pressure monitoring and fixation device—for ICP monitoring in children and adolescents in pediatric neurotraumatology, hydrocephalus, and craniofacial surgery. Designed by Dr. O. E. Illi, it has two movable components compressing the skull from inside and outside and is fully compatible with a range

Illi *(cont.)*
of fiberoptic or pneumatic transducer systems.

illness, food-borne (FBI).

Illness Severity Instrument—for use in determining extent of HIV-infected patient's illness.

Illumen-8 guiding catheter.

Illumina PROSeries—laparoscopy system.

illusion—an unreal or misleading image or perception. Usage: "He was suffering from the illusion that there were insects crawling over him." Cf. *allusion, elusion*.

iloprost—see *Ventavis*.

ILUS catheter (intraluminal ultrasound) (GI).

IMA (internal mammary artery) **graft**. Also, inferior mesenteric artery.

IMA (inferior mesenteric artery) **retractor**—used in cardiac bypass.

IMAB (internal mammary artery bypass).

image acquisition time—MRI term.

Imagecast—an imaging management system that integrates Picture Archiving and Communication Systems (PACS), Radiology Information System (RIS), and other technologies.

ImageChecker—computer-aided detection system for mammography.

image-guided radiation therapy (IGRT).

image-guided surgery—using a robotic microscope (SurgiScope) and a surgical digitizer (The Viewing Wand).

image intensifier (II).

imaging—see also *operation*
- breast imaging technique
- bubble study (contrast echocardiography)
- chase bolus

imaging *(cont.)*
- digital tomosynthesis
- electronic portal imaging
- fecalogram
- HIDA-CCK scintigraphy
- magnetic resonance spectroscopic (MRSI)
- multi-slab and cine techniques for single breath-hold cardiac-synchronized angiography
- SEE IT substernal epicardial echocardiography
- stress Myoview nuclear
- TDOG (tissue Doppler gated) dynamic three-dimensional ultrasound imaging
- 3-D CEMRA (three-dimensional, contrast-enhanced MR angiography)

imaging agent—see *medication*; *radioisotope; technetium*.

imaging system (see also *scan, scanner, ultrasound*)
- Advantx LC+ cardiovascular
- Biad SPECT
- CathScanner ultrasound
- Convergent color Doppler imaging technology
- Delta 32 TACT (tuned aperture computed tomography)
- DICOM (digital imaging and communications in medicine)
- Digirad 2020 TC imager
- digital Add-On Bucky image acquisition
- digital fundus imager
- Digitron digital subtraction imaging
- DirectView CR 900
- DTU-one UltraSure
- dynamic optical breast imaging (DOBI)
- EchoEye 3-D ultrasound
- electronic portal imaging device (EPID)

imaging *(cont.)*
Ensemble contrast imaging (ECI)
EnSite 3000
FluoroPlus Cardiac digital imaging
functional MRI (fMRI)
Given diagnostic imaging
HeartView CT scan
Helios diagnostic
HP SONOS 5500 ultrasound
Imagecast
Isocam SPECT
Luma cervical
Magnes 2500 WH (whole head) imager
Micro-Imager
MIMCOM (multimode imaging confocal optical microscope)
multislice computed tomographic angiography (MSCTA)
MyoSight
Nicolet Elite Doppler ultrasound
Photopic Imaging ultrasound
pulse inversion harmonic
real-time 4-D ultrasound
Reveal XVI PET/CT
Rotograph Plus
SAMBA
Selenia
Senographe 2000D digital mammography imaging
SenoScan full-field digital mammography system
Sens-A-Ray 2000 dental
Sequoia ultrasound system
SieScape imaging technology
Signa SP/i 0.5T MR imaging unit
SonoCT real-time compound imaging
Site-Rite and Site-Rite II ultrasound systems
SoftScan laser mammography system
SonoCT
SONOLINE Sierra ultrasound imaging

imaging *(cont.)*
SPECT/MRI
tissue harmonic imaging
transcranial color-coded sonography
transperineal ultrasonography
turbo spin-echo T2-weighted sequence
UBIS 5000 ultrasound bone sonometer
ultrasonic pachymetry
UltraSure DTU-one
Velocity
videomicroscopy
virtual colonoscopy
virtual cystoscopy
Virtuoso
Voluson ultrasound system
VScore with AutoGate
Xplorer

Imagyn microlaparoscope (Oph)—a very small laparoscope used in eye surgery.

Imatron Ultrafast CT scanner—uses electron beam technology. It is used for general purpose CT scanning, as well as for noninvasive diagnosis of coronary artery disease.

IMax or **IMAX**—brief form for internal maxillary artery. Usage: "Angiography was performed, and IMax was embolized." The brief form should be expanded when transcribed.

iMedConsent Ophthalmology—software program that assists ophthalmologists in educating and informing their patients about a number of serious eye disorders and conditions.

IMED infusion device—for intravenous fluids.

IMEX scleral implants—solid silicone, sponge silicone, and Miragel

IMEX *(cont.)*
buckling components. See *Miragel*; *implant*.

imidazotetrazines—a new class of drugs that works by damaging DNA in cancer cells, causing them to self-destruct. Noncancerous cells are not harmed and, unlike most cancer treatments, it can filter through the brain's protective barrier.

IMIG (International Mesothelioma Interest Group) **classification**—newer staging method for malignant mesothelioma.

immersion foot—the third stage of trauma due to exposure to cold; first stage—frostbite; second stage—trench foot.

imminent—about to occur in the near future; immediately threatening. Cf. *eminence*.

Immix bioabsorbable implant—bioabsorbable tissue scaffolds for regeneration and repair of bone and cartilage defects.

immobilize—prevent from moving. Cf. *mobilize*.

immortal—referring to a cell line that is capable of indefinite propagation; see telomerase.

immotile cilia syndrome—a condition more formally known as primary ciliary dyskinesia (PCD), a rare genetic birth defect that involves the blocking of respiratory passages. Patients with PCD have abnormal or absent cilia, the tiny hair-like structures that move mucus out of the respiratory passages. Also known as *Kartagener syndrome*.

Immulite assays and confirmatory kits for hepatitis
Immulite HBsAg
Immulite 2000 HBsAg
Immulite Anti-HBc IgM

Immulite *(cont.)*
Immulite 2000 Anti-HBc IgM
Immulite Anti-HBc
Immulite 2000 Anti-HBc
Immulite Anti-HBs
Immulite 2000 Anti-HBs

Immulite PSA assays—for the detection of prostate cancer.

immune globulin—see *antibody molecules*.

immune system modulator (Imreg-1).

immunobead assay—measurement of platelet-associated and plasma autoantibody. Also, a test to check for sperm antibodies.

ImmunoCard STAT! Rotavirus—a one-step test that can detect rotavirus, using a stool specimen.

ImmunoCyt—noninvasive diagnostic test that uses a urine sample for the detection of superficial bladder cancer and transitional cell carcinoma.

immunofixation in agar (Agar-IF)—of blood serum.

immunoisolating microreactors—implantable cell systems, or microreactors, containing living cells that produce a therapeutic molecule, e.g., insulin. The cells are encapsulated and injected into the body where they release the needed substance. Under study are microreactor treatments for hemophilia, Huntington chorea, Parkinson disease, Alzheimer disease, cancer, and AIDS.

immunoliposomes—a combination of liposomes (small synthetic particles used to carry potent anticancer drugs) and antibodies that can recognize and bind to cancer cells. Immunoliposomes can selectively target and kill cancer cells while avoiding normal cells.

immunomodulation—manipulation of donor tissue antigens prior to transplantation to deter host rejection; may allow long-term cellular transplant survival without immunosuppression.

Immuno 1 complex PSA (cPSA) **test**—aids in detection of prostate cancer.

immunoperoxidase stain—used in immunologic testing. Usage: "Immunoperoxidase stains were performed in formalin-fixed, paraffin-embedded sections, using the peroxidase-antiperoxidase technique."

immunoproliferative small intestinal disease (IPSID)—also known as *small intestinal malignant lymphoma* or *Mediterranean lymphoma*, most prevalent in developing countries.

immunoreactive parathyroid hormone (iPTH) (lowercase *i*).

immunoscintigraphy—a study using technetium 99m-labeled antigranulocyte antibodies, when echocardiographic findings are equivocal. May also be used to monitor antibiotic therapy and to detect melanoma.

immunosuppressant cocktail—a combination drug in which several immunosuppressant drugs are given together.

immunosuppressive therapy (IST).

Imount instruments (Ortho)—used in total knee replacement.

Impact assays—disposable rapid-test kits that detect amphetamines, methamphetamine, and other drugs in a saliva sample.

Impact total hip system.

impactor—see *vertebral body impactor*.

impar—odd, single, unpaired.

IMP-Capello arm support—provides stability and access to the patient's arm to monitor I.V., blood pressure. (IMP stands for Innovative Medical Products.)

impedance plethysmography (IPG)—a noninvasive test to determine the presence and degree of deep vein obstruction in venous thrombosis. It evaluates patency of the veins by measuring venous volume changes.

impingement—contact or pressure, generally abnormal, between two structures.

impingement sign—produces pain in rotator cuff tendinopathy and tear.

implant—consisting of metal orthopedic implants used mainly for total joint replacement, Silastic silicone rubber implants used in plastic surgery, and silicone orthopedic implants used for hand and foot; also, breast, dental, ear, and eye implants.
- AbioCor implantable replacement heart
- Acticon Neosphincter
- Alcon SA60AT intraocular lens
- Alpha 1 penile
- anterior chamber acrylic
- Arenberg-Denver inner-ear valve
- Arrow LionHeart heart assist
- attic defect plate of ear
- autologous osteochondral transplantation
- autologous ovarian transplantation
- Avanta joint skeletal
- Baerveldt glaucoma
- Biocell RTV saline-filled breast
- Biocoral
- BioCuff bioresorbable screw and spiked washer
- Biodel
- Bio-eye
- Biomatrix ocular
- Bionx SmartNail bioresorbable
- Bio-Oss
- bioresorbable
- BrachySeed Pd-103

implant *(cont.)*
Branemark endosteal
Cerestore
Clarion multi-strategy cochlear
cochlear
Codere orbital floor
collagen meniscus (CMI)
Compliant pre-stress bone
Contigen Bard cochlear
Contigen collagen continent
Contigen glutaraldehyde cross-linked collagen
Contour Profile anatomically shaped silicone breast
CosmoDerm (1 and 2) human-based collagen
CosmoPlast human-based collagen
Dicor
DISA S-Flex coronary stent
double plate Molteno
Dura-Guard patch
Durapatite
Durasul polyethylene material
Empress
Envision TD
Envoy middle ear
expanded polytetrafluoroethylene (ePTFE) facial
Fortress
Frialoc transgingival threaded
GEO Structure spinal
Gore-Tex facial contouring strips
Gore-Tex nasal
Gore-Tex SAM facial
Graftpatch
GTS great toe system
Healos autograft bone replacement material
Hedrocel biomaterial
Heyer-Schulte
Hi-Ceram
HTR-MFI
Hydroview intraocular lens
hydroxyapatite (HA)
ICL (implantable contact lens)

implant *(cont.)*
ICR (intrastromal corneal ring)
IMEX scleral
Immix bioabsorbable
IMZ endosteal
InSound XT
Intacs
Integral Omniloc
Interpore
intracorneal (Kerato-Gel)
islet cell
K-Centrum anterior spinal fixation system
Kerato-Gel (intracorneal)
KeraVision ICR
Kinetik great toe
Krupin-Denver eye valve
K2 hemi toe implant system
LARSI (lumbar anterior-root stimulator)
Macroplastique continent
McCutchen
McGhan facial
methylmethacrylate, beads of
Micronail intramedullary distal radius
middle ear (MEI)
Mini-Med continuous glucose sensor
Miragel
Natural-Knee system
Nexus
NovaGold breast
NovaSaline inflatable saline breast
Nucleus 24 Contour cochlear
Nucleus 24 multichannel auditory brainstem
Oasis burn matrix
Oasis wound matrix
OP–1 (osteogenic protein 1)
Optec
Optimed glaucoma pressure regulator
Osteonics-HA coated
Oxonium (oxidized zirconium)

implant *(cont.)*
palatal
Pelvicol collagen
peripheral bulging ring
PhacoFlex II SI-30NB
PharmaSeed (palladium Pd 103 seeds)
PhotacFil
ProOsteon Implant 500
ProstaSeed ^{125}I radiation treatment
prosthetic disk nucleus (PDN)
Radiesse
radioactive seed
Restore dental
retropharyngeal
SAM (subcutaneous augmentation material)
Sculptra wrinkle filler
segmentally demineralized bone technology
silicone
SmartNail (Bionx SmartNail)
SoftForm facial
STAAR Toric implantable contact lens
STOP (selective tubal occlusion procedure) permanent contraception device
Suspend sling
SutureGroove Gold eye weights
Syed template interstitial
System-S soft skeletal
Tear-Trough
TheraSeed
ThinProfile eyelid implants
3Dknee
titanium rib
Trilucent breast
UltraFix RC
Unilab Surgibone
vertical expandable titanium rib (VEPTR)
Vitrasert intraocular
Wedge, The

implantable cardioverter-defibrillator—see *AICD*.

implantable contact lens (ICL)—refractive lens that is implanted over the natural lens of the eye for correction of myopia and hyperopia.

implantable gastric stimulator (IGS)—a relatively new approach of electrical gastric stimulation to treat obesity. It consists of a stimulation lead implanted in the gastric wall connected to an electric programming unit implanted under the skin of the abdomen. See *Transcend implantable gastric stimulator*.

implantation (Embryology)—the attachment of a blastocyst to the uterine lining.

implantation response—reperfusion injury of the postischemic lungs, as seen in lung or heart and lung transplant patients. It resolves within 3 to 5 days. If a pathologic pulmonary process following lung transplantation takes longer to resolve, another process is probably responsible.

Implast bone cement.

Import vascular access port with BioGlide—features new hydrophilic properties on the catheter component of the access port.

impossible meningioma—physicians' term for a meningioma just anterior to the optic foramen; it is very difficult to detect by visualizing tests. The physician needs a high index of suspicion.

Impress Softpatch—incontinence care product from UroMed.

impulse, apical—MRI term.

I-MRI (interventional MRI).

IMRT—see *intensity-modulated radiation therapy* or *radiotherapy.* See also *intensity-modulated arc therapy*.

IMT (inspiratory muscle trainer).

IMT (intima media thickness).

IMV (intermittent mandatory ventilation).

IMZ endosteal implants (ENT).

inactivation technique, psoralen.

Inappropriate Sleep Composite Score—indicative of obstructive sleep apnea.

inborn error of metabolism—a genetic disorder in which a specific genetic defect leads to a specific biochemical abnormality.

inbreeding—the mating of closely related individuals.

INCA (infant nasal cannulae assembly)—an oxygen delivery system consisting of nasal prongs and flexible oxygen tubing connected by fasteners to a knit cap on the infant's head.

incentive spirometer—a device into which you blow, to measure the volume of air taken into the lungs. It registers on a vertical cylindrical plastic meter that works much like one of those games you see at county fairs, where you hit a metal plate with a heavy hammer and the plate goes up and rings a bell and you get a prize. When a nurse was asked what the prize is with the spirometer, she replied: "The prize is that you don't get pneumonia."

Incert—a bioabsorbable, implantable sponge designed to prevent post-surgical tissue adhesions. Placed over the surgical site and surrounding tissues and organs, it provides a physical barrier to prevent internal tissue surfaces from sticking together.

In Charge diabetes control system—handheld monitor for personal use. It performs both a rapid glucose test and a test for glycated protein.

incidence—in medicine, the number of new cases of a disease that occur in a given population in a certain period of time. Cf. *incidents*.

incidentaloma—a coined word for a finding on sonography of a nodule that is unrelated to a palpable mass.

incidents—events, happenings, occurrences. Cf. *incidence*.

incipient—just beginning to appear; initial or early stage.

Incise Pouch—plastic bag affixed with adhesive tape over a laparotomy site to collect lavage fluid in a delayed abdominal closure.

incision—a cut or a wound made by a sharp instrument. Cf. *excision*.
Types of incisions include:
bayonet-type
Bevan
Bruser skin
Cherney
chevron
clamshell
cross-tunneling
cruciate
curvilinear
frown
gull-wing
intercartilaginous
Kocher collar (thyroidectomy)
LaRoque herniorrhaphy
lazy H
lazy Z
minilaparotomy
muscle-splitting
Owens-type
relaxing
Rethi
Rockey-Davis
scoring
smiling
watchband
Wilde
Y
York-Mason

incisura dextra of Gans—deep groove on the inferior surface of the liver near the bed of the gallbladder.

inclusion body—see *body*.

Incomplete Sentence Blank Test (ISB) —mental status examination.

incontinence ring—a bladder support prosthesis.

increment—amount by which a dose or value is increased. Usage: "Steroids were increased in weekly increments of 5 mg to a maximum dose of 25 mg."

IND (investigational new drug)—a drug which may be used in clinical testing by licensed researchers with the permission of the FDA, but not yet approved by the FDA for marketing. Cf. *I&D*.

independent beam steering, electronic —a feature of advanced ultrasound units that allows the sonographer or clinician to separately manipulate B-scan, color flow, and pulsed-wave Doppler in real time. This makes it possible to keep a constant perpendicular angle of the beam with an artery in vascular examinations and maximize the arterial interface to obtain the best images.

Indermil—topical tissue adhesive used in wound closure.

index (see also *test)*
- amniotic fluid (AFI)
- apnea/hypopnea (AHI)
- BASMI (Bath Ankylosing Spondylitis Metrology Index)
- Broders
- ChAM (charcoal alveolar macrophage)
- Dermatology Index of Disease Severity (DIDS)
- Euler-Byrne
- Ferrans and Powers Quality of Life Index, Cardiac Version

index *(cont.)*
- fetal-pelvic
- Fick cardiac
- foam stability
- free/total PSA
- FTI (free thyroxine)
- Gosling pulsatility
- Gravindex
- Growth Potential Realization
- Harvey hospital prognostic nutritional
- HI (hypopnea index)
- Hollingshead Four Factor Index
- indirect immunofluorescent assay (IDIF)
- Insall-Salvati
- intact cortical bone (ICBI)
- lipid-laden macrophage (LLMI)
- Mengert pelvimetry
- Mohtadi Quality of Life Index
- Penetrating Abdominal Trauma Index (PATI)
- penile-brachial pressure (PBPI)
- Pittsburgh Sleep Quality Index
- prognostic nutritional (PNI)
- PSA (prostate-specific antigen)
- PSA free/total
- Psoriasis Area Severity Index (PASI)
- Quetelet BMI
- respiratory disturbance (RDI)
- short increment sensitivity (SISI)
- Stanford Dependency Index
- umbilical coiling

Indiana pouch—an ileocolic continent urinary diversion used in patients who require cystectomy for carcinoma or trauma, or patients who have a neurogenic bladder, bladder dysfunction, or congenital anomaly. Other procedures for continent urinary diversion: Camey ileocystoplasty, Kock pouch, Mainz pouch urinary reservoir, and Mitrofanoff. See also *operation*; *pouch*; *reservoir*.

Indiana Tome system—for endoscopic carpal tunnel release surgery.

Indiclor—an indium (In 111, ^{111}In) radioimaging agent used with OncoScint CR/OV to identify location and extent of colorectal and ovarian cancers.

indifferent electrode—an ECG or EEG electrode whose input is used to balance the input of the recording electrode. Cf., recording electrode.

Indigo LaserOptic treatment system—for the treatment of symptoms of benign prostatic hyperplasia. The Indigo system combines fiberoptics with diode laser fiber technology. Using direct visualization, a surgeon employs a diode laser to quickly destroy a precise area of the prostate by interstitial laser coagulation.

indiplon—a nonbenzodiazepine GABA modulator for the treatment of insomnia.

indirect fluorescent antibody test (IFA).

indirect laser ophthalmoscope—used for treatment of ROP (retinopathy of prematurity).

indium-111-labeled human nonspecific immunoglobulin G (^{111}In IgG)—a radiopharmaceutical for imaging focal inflammation in febrile granulocytopenic patients.

indium 111 scintigraphy scan (^{111}In).

indocyanine green dye—for detection of intracardial shunt.

induced hypothermia—a folk remedy in which drug overdose victims are immersed in ice water in the hopes of preserving consciousness and brain function until medical help arrives.

inducer cell—a name for the T-4 helper lymphocyte, the specific target of the AIDS virus; also called *helper/ inducer cell*; it plays an important role in activating other parts of the immune system.

indurated plantar keratoma (IPK).

Inerpan—a special dressing for burn patients that requires less frequent changing. This decreases pain for the patient and allows the donor site to heal more completely.

In-Exsufflator—cough machine that assists patients in removal of bronchial secretions.

in extremis—at the point of death.

InfaCare infant formula—incorrect spelling for EnfaCare.

Infamyst aerosol spray device—a device for pulmonary delivery of drugs to infants.

infant distraction test—a pediatric hearing test that is carried out at 7 to 8 months of age.

Infant Flow nasal CPAP system.

infantile food protein-induced enterocolitis syndrome (FPIES, "effpies")—a severe, cell-mediated gastrointestinal food hypersensitivity typically provoked by cow's milk or soy. Solid foods are rarely considered a cause. Some of the expressions seen in conjunction with this disease are "solid-food-FPIES," "cow's-milk-FPIES," "soy-FPIES."

infarcts, shower of.

In-Fast—a bone screw system used in transvaginal cystourethropexy and sling procedures.

infection—see *disease*.

inferior mesenteric artery (IMA).

inferior sagittal mandibular osteotomy—surgical procedure for obstructive sleep apnea.

inferior turbinate blade—used in ENT surgery for volumetric reduction to the inferior turbinate while avoiding

inferior *(cont.)*
unpredictable collateral thermal damage to surrounding tissue.

infibulation (also referred to as "pharaonic circumcision")—the most extreme form of female genital mutilation consisting of removal of clitoris, adjacent labia (majora and minora), and joining of scraped sides of the vulva across the vagina, where they are secured with thorns or sewn with catgut or thread. A small opening is left to allow passage of urine and menstrual blood. Area is cut open to allow intercourse on the wedding night and closed again afterward to ensure marital fidelity. See also *clitoridectomy* and *Sunna circumcision.*

infiltrate, 5-lobe—a pulmonary infiltrate involving all lung lobes (3 right, 2 left).

infiltrating endometriosis (*not* infiltrated).

Infiniti catheter (Cardio).

Infinity hip system—modular hip replacement implant.

InFix interbody fusion system—standalone lumbar fusion device that is inserted through an anterior approach. Height, width, and lordotic angle can be independently adjusted during implantation to match patient anatomy.

inflamed (one *m*, unlike *inflammation*, *inflammatory*).

inflammation—classic signs of inflammation are rubor (redness), calor (heat), dolor (pain), tumor (swelling), and loss of function.

influenza vaccine—may be administered as a nasal spray offering protection against flu. It has the ability to immediately block the growth of influenza viruses that cause disease, in addition to, and apart from, its ability to induce antibody formation. It is an attenuated live influenza virus but one which can block the growth of other influenza viruses. Other vaccines against the flu require two weeks to adequately stimulate the body's antibody defenses to produce immunity; this flu vaccine provides almost instantaneous protection—a real plus when a flu epidemic strikes. Of note, influenza is still the sixth leading cause of death in this country.

Inform—a HER-2/neu gene-based test for breast cancer recurrence. Using the original breast cancer tissue sample, the Inform test identifies the presence or absence of increased copies of the HER-2/neu gene. This indicates whether breast cancer is likely to recur.

infra-, prefix meaning under, beneath, below. Cf. *inter-, intra-, inner-*.

infracted—to be broken off. Cf. *infractured.*

infractured—fractured inward, as opposed to outward. Not to be confused with "infracted," which means to be broken off.

infranate—material that settles to the bottom of a liquid. Cf. *supernate.*

infrared coagulation of the inferior turbinate (ICIT)—provides relief of nasal obstruction.

infrarenal aortobifemoral bypass graft—procedure for aortoiliofemoral reconstruction in atherosclerotic occlusive disease.

Infusaid—an implantable drug infusion pump.

InfusaSleeve II catheter—designed for coronary drug delivery, using "over-the-balloon" technology to track over a standard angioplasty balloon catheter.

Infuse-A-Cath—a central venous catheter for the infusion of medications and other solutions or blood products.

Infuse-a-Port—implantable vascular access system. Used for administration of chemotherapeutic agent via cephalic vein (or possibly other veins).

Infuse bone graft LT-Cage.

Infuse bone graft device—a metal cage that contains a genetically engineered protein called rhBMP-2 that stimulates new bone growth at the site of a degenerated disk.

infusion—the slow therapeutic introduction of fluid other than blood into a vein. Cf. *effusion*.

Ingram regimen for psoriasis—similar to Goeckerman regimen. See *Goeckerman regimen*.

inhalant antigens (major outdoor allergens), including the fungi:
Alternaria
Cladosporium
Hormodendrum

inhaler—see *device; medication*.

inheritable genetic modification (IGM) (germline genetic modification, germline engineering)—a technique of altering the genetic composition of gametes (oocytes and sperm) in which viral vectors are used to insert new genes. Since these changes are inheritable, they are passed on to offspring and become part of the human gene pool.

inherited—genetically transmitted.

injection technique—an alternative method to use on a thigh tourniquet for creation of a bloodless field in operations for anterior cruciate ligament reconstruction. The injection technique uses lidocaine and epinephrine with bupivacaine. As these operations are lengthy, the tourniquet must be applied for long periods of time, which can cause muscular, vascular, and systemic problems postoperatively, and which puts pressure on the surgeon to rush, once the tourniquet is inflated.

injector—see *HUMI uterine*.

InjecTx—customized cystoscope which shrinks prostate tissue by injecting purified alcohol, killing prostate cells without painful swelling. The prostate then shrinks as the body eliminates the cells.

Injex—single-use disposable needle-free injector.

Injury Severity Scale (ISS)—a system used to describe multiple trauma injuries.

ink-potassium hydroxide test—a test using India (writing) ink. The principle involved is similar to that of the Schiller test for cancer of the cervix—a negative stain. The ink is not absorbed by *Acanthamoeba* cysts, and they appear as light structures on a dark background of the ink. Usage: "Ink-potassium hydroxide preparation of corneal scrapings showed *Acanthamoeba* cysts in the corneal stroma." Cf. *onlay graft*. See *Schiller test*.

inlay graft—a bone graft, not to be confused with onlay graft. Both are used in craniofacial surgery. Skin can also be used as an inlay graft.

inner cell mass (ICM)—a small group of cells within the cavity of a blastocyst (a very early embryo), which will give rise to the embryonic disk, then the three germ layers, and finally to all the cells and tissues of the fetus except the placenta and fetal membranes. Embryonic stem cell lines are derived from cells isolated from the inner cell mass.

inner rims of the fluorescein ring—used in discussing applanation tonometry.

InnerVasc—sheath for percutaneous vascular access in cardiology, radiology, neuroradiology, and critical care.

InnerVision transillumination system—lights organs from within to help identify anatomic landmarks during laparoscopic and open procedures.

Innofem (estradiol tablets)—hormone replacement drug therapy.

Innova home therapy system—for urinary incontinence.

InnovaTome microkeratome device—used by refractive surgeons in ophthalmology to perform LASIK (laser in situ keratomileusis).

Innovator Holter system (Cardio).

INO (intranuclear ophthalmoplegia). Cf. *I&O*.

inotropic therapy—medication regimen designed to preserve hemodynamics in patients with cardiomyopathy who are awaiting cardiac transplantation. See *home ambulatory inotropic therapy*.

Inoue balloon techniques.

InPath—a device for cervical cancer screening.

INRO surgical nails—used for nail bed injuries. These prosthetic nails protect the nail bed and prevent adhesion of the eponychial fold to the nail bed. Note: You may want to capitalize all the letters (as the manufacturer does), or simply the first letter.

Insall/Burstein II system—total knee replacement.

Insall-Salvati index—ratio of the length of the patellar tendon to the length of the patella.

Insemi-Cath—an intrauterine insemination catheter.

insensible fluid output—fluid loss that cannot be measured, such as by respiration and through the skin, without visible perspiration, as differentiated from measurable fluid output such as urine.

"in-sep"—phonetic for NCEP (National Cholesterol Education Program).

insertion—a chromosomal aberration in which part of one chromosome is inserted into another, nonhomologous chromosome.

insidious—gradual or subtle development.

in situ—in the natural or normal place; confined to the site of origin without invasion of neighboring tissues, e.g., carcinoma in situ.

in situ hybridization—laboratory technique in which a single-stranded DNA probe of known sequence, radioactively or fluorescently labeled, is made to seek out and fuse with a corresponding nucleic acid sequence in a specimen.

InSound XT—designed for all hearing-impaired patients except those with a profound loss, and worn invisibly and continuously without removal deep inside the ear canal for up to four months.

Inspiration ventilator.

Inspirator—an implantable device for treating chronic pulmonary obstructive disorders.

inspiratory muscle trainer (IMT)—a small device used to exercise and strengthen respiratory muscle endurance.

Inspiron—small inspiratory training device to strengthen the muscles used in breathing.

inspissated—a thickened or dried out secretion within a duct or cavity.

Instat—collagen absorbable hemostatic agent. Cf. *INSTAT MCH*.

INSTAT MCH (microfibrillar hemostat)—used as an aid in hemostasis when bleeding cannot be controlled by usual methods, or when the bleeding site cannot be reached. It looks something like building insulating material. It can be removed in this form if necessary; in contact with blood, it becomes a gelatinous mass which can be removed in that state. It is absorbable and, if indicated, may be left in situ, although the long-term effect is not known. Not recommended in urology, neurosurgery, or orthopedic surgery.

InstaTrak—a device that provides intraoperative localization during endoscopic sinus surgery.

InStent—developer of self-expanding and balloon-expandable stents used in a variety of medical therapies.

InStent CarotidCoil stent—resists compression after placement in the neck arteries to maintain blood flow to the brain.

in-stent restenosis—reduced by application of coronary radiation therapy with a gamma source (beta emitter 90-Yttrium).

instill—administration of a liquid, drop by drop. Do not confuse with *install*, although some dictators use these words interchangeably.

instrument—see type of instrument, e.g., clamp, forceps.

Insuflon—indwelling device for delivering insulin. It consists of a small needle inserted subcutaneously and allowed to remain in place for up to one week. The needle is connected to a small catheter which is easily accessible on the surface of the skin. The patient injects the insulin dose into the catheter. Insuflon eliminates multiple injections for patients whose diabetes requires one or more shots each day.

insulin detemir—a long-acting insulin analog that evens out the hills and valleys in glucose control by other forms of insulin.

insulin-like growth factor I—developed as an outgrowth of research by Genentech on Protropin (human growth hormone). It has an insulin-like chemical structure but is actually being studied for its ability to preserve and restore muscle mass in patients with AIDS. The etiology of body wasting from AIDS is not understood, and it is thought that this drug, also known as somatomedin C, could be useful because of its protein-sparing attributes.

insulinotardic—when insulin comes out too slowly and in insufficient quantity.

insulinotropin—a naturally occurring peptide hormone which stimulates insulin release in response to increase in blood sugar levels.

insulin resistance syndrome—a condition that may lead to type 2 diabetes and also may predispose patients to coronary heart disease. Exercise can play an important role in preventing and treating the syndrome.

!nSure—a fecal occult blood test. (Note the use of an exclamation mark in the trade name.)

InSurg—laparoscopic stone baskets, used for common bile duct stone retrieval during intraoperative cholangiograms: Segura CBD basket, Pursuer CBD basket; these come in 2, 4 and 3.0 French sizes, Helical, and the Mini-Helical basket which comes in 1.9 French.

InSync—a multisite cardiac stimulator implanted transvenously in patients suffering from heart failure. It is able to synchronize right and left sides of the heart.

Intacs—flexible micro-inserts that provide a nonlaser option for surgical correction of mild myopia. Intacs does not require cutting or removing tissue from the eye's central optic zone. It can be removed and exchanged for a new prescription if a person's vision changes because of age.

intact cortical bone index (ICBI)—used with simple functional assessment in predicting fracture s in patients with long bone metastases.

intake and output (I&O). See *I&O*.

Integra artificial skin—used in conjunction with the Dermal Regeneration Template. Together they are used for treatment of patients with life-threatening, full-thickness, or deep partial-thickness burns in situations where conventional autografts are not available or contraindicated due to the patient's condition.

Integral Omniloc implants—used for oral and maxillofacial surgery.

integrated parallel acquisition technique (IPAT).

Integrated Wound Manager—Internet-based wound management technique including tools for digital photo documentation, wound measurement, advice, supply integration, and outcome-based data.

Integris 3-D RA (rotational angiography)—provides reconstructed 3-D images of the patient's vascular morphology for use in planning neurointerventional surgical procedures.

Integrity AFx AutoCapture pacing system.

Integrity AFx pacemaker.

Intelect laser system—orthopedic/physical therapy device that provides topical heating for temporary increase in local blood circulation, temporary relief of minor muscle and joint aches, pain and stiffness, and muscle spasm.

Intelligent Dressing—contains Acemannan hydrogel to keep a wound at optimum moisture level, donating moisture to dry wounds and absorbing moisture from wounds that contain too much exudate.

intense pulsed light source (IPLS)—a pulsed photothermal device used to treat small leg varicosities.

intensifying screen artifacts (Radiol)—can include dust, hair on screen, rough handling of film when placing screen, static electricity, rivets in film carriers damaging screen, or warped cassette preventing film surface from being in direct contrast with screen.

intensity-modulated radiation therapy or **radiotherapy** (IMRT)—advanced mode of high-precision radiotherapy utilizing computer-controlled x-ray accelerators to deliver precise radiation doses to a malignant tumor or specific areas within the tumor. The radiation dose is designed to conform to the three-dimensional (3-D) shape of the tumor by modulating—or controlling—the intensity of the radiation beam to focus a higher radiation dose to the tumor while minimizing radiation exposure of surrounding normal tissues. Typically, combinations of several intensity-modulated fields coming from different beam directions produce a custom tailored radiation dose that maximizes tumor

intensity *(cont.)*
dose while also protecting adjacent normal tissues. IMRT is used to treat cancers of the prostate, head and neck, breast, thyroid and lung, as well as in gynecologic, liver and brain tumors and lymphomas and sarcomas. IMRT is also beneficial for treating pediatric malignancies. See also *high-resolution multileaf collimator*.

Intensive Narcotic Detoxification—patented anesthesia-assisted one-day detox procedure for heroin addiction and dependencies on methadone, pain medications, and other opiates.

intentional transoperative hemodilution—a blood transfusion method. When a patient is prepared for surgery, up to 3 units of blood are taken from the patient and stored in regular blood donor bags. Blood expanders are then administered to the patient to restore the blood volume. Thus, during surgery, the patient loses only diluted blood. Then, near the end of the operative procedure, the previously removed blood is infused. This reduces the need for blood transfusion, with all its attendant risks.

inter-, a prefix meaning *between*. Cf. *intra-*.

interatrial septum—referring to the septum between the atria of the heart. *Not* intra-atrial septum.

Interax—a total knee system.

intercalary defect of the pollical ray—see *pouce flottant*.

intercartilaginous incision—used in rhinoplasties.

Interceed Adhesion Barrier—a pliable, biodegradable cellulose fabric that is used to prevent adhesions between tissues and organs following surgery, and specifically to prevent or reduce the possibility of pelvic adhesions. The knitted absorbable fabric becomes a gelatinous coating (over the organs just under the incision) which is absorbed in less than a month. Also known as *Interceed (TC7) Absorbable Adhesion Barrier.*

Intercept—oral fluid drug test.

Intercept Esophageal Internal MR Coil.

Intercept Platelet System—designed to inactivate viruses, bacteria, and other pathogens in platelets intended for transfusion.

Intercept Vascular guidewire—a tiny magnetic resonance coil that can be threaded into a patient's artery or vein to detect early signs of blood vessel disease.

Intercept Vascular 0.030-inch Internal MR Coil—a loopless or balloon-expandable transesophageal probe to obtain high-resolution vascular images.

intercompartmental supraretinacular artery (ICSRA)—actually a branch of the radial artery. You may see the branches designated as the 1,2 ICSRA and the 2,3 ICSRA.

interdigital clavus—a corn (clavus) between the fingers or toes, usually in the fourth interspace.

interferential current therapy—a method of pain relief which involves the application of alternating-current sine waves of differing frequencies via four electrodes applied in such a way as to generate a beat pulse in the area of interest. Interferential current may also be referred to as beat pulse or alternating modulation frequency. Studies have shown this therapy effective in relieving pain due to lateral epicondylitis, knee osteo-

interferential *(cont.)* arthritis, sprains, and jaw dysfunction.

interferential stimulator—controls pain and increases circulation following injury or surgery.

interferometer—see *Takata laser interferometer*.

interferometry—a method that measures the path of reflected light.

interferon—glycoproteins produced by some cells in response to viral infections, which also seem to have anti-tumor properties. See *IL-2*.

interferon, low-dose—see *low-dose interferon*.

Inter Fix—a titanium threaded spinal fusion cage for treatment of degenerative disk disease. The hollow, threaded cage is packed with small pieces of bone taken from another part of the body; the cage is then capped and implanted between adjacent vertebral structures.

Inter Fix RP (reduced profile) **threaded spinal fusion cage**—designed to be used in conjunction with the Inter Fix device. Both are cylindrical in shape, but the RP has a "C" cut out of one side that enables interlocking of the two devices, saving space while providing necessary vertebral support.

InterGard—knitted collagen coated grafts and patches.

Intergel adhesion prevention solution—used following laparotomy and laparoscopy.

interloop abscess—seen in the mesentery of distal ileum with extensive inflammation on CT scan in patients with Crohn disease.

intermittent exotropia—a common form of childhood strabismus that has a late onset. It may be treated with IM injections of botulinum toxin type A into the extraocular muscles, which is considered a safe, effective, and noninvasive drug alternative to surgical treatment of strabismus in adults.

intermittent mandatory ventilation (IMV)—used in weaning a patient from long-term ventilator use. While the patient remains on the ventilator, the number of mandatory breaths is gradually reduced. In between the mandatory breaths, the system allows the patient to breathe independently. With this method, the muscles used in breathing are gradually strengthened until the patient can breathe independently.

internal mammary artery bypass (IMAB).

International Association of Enterostomal Therapists (IAET) **stages**.

International Knee Documentation Committee (IKDC) **Subjective Knee Form**—a knee-specific, rather than a disease-specific, measure of symptoms, function, and sports activity.

international normalized ratio (INR)—a system for reporting the results of blood coagulation (clotting) tests.

International Mesothelioma Interest Group (IMIG) **classification**.

International Prostate Symptom Score (IPSS)—used extensively around the world to quantify the level of lower urinary tract symptoms in a standardized manner. The seven symptoms assessed include (1) the sensation of not having emptied the bladder completely after urination; (2) the urge to urinate again within two hours; (3) the urge to stop and start again several times during urination; (4) difficulty in postponing urination; (5) weak uri-

International *(cont.)*
nary stream; (6) the need to push or strain to begin urination; (7) the need to get up at night to urinate. The frequency of each symptom is quantified by the patient on a scale from 1 to 5, the maximum total score being 35. Patients with a total score of less than 7 are classified as having mild symptoms, whereas those with total scores of 8 to 19 and more than 20 have moderate and severe symptoms. Inconvenience caused by urinary symptoms is registered by a corresponding, almost identical questionnaire, which yields a separate score (called the "bother" score).

International System of Measuring Units (SI, the initials for Système International d'Unités in French, is used internationally). In the U.S., the American Medical Association and the College of American Pathologists are sponsoring its use. We are already using gray (Gy) as the unit of measuring absorbed radiation dose, equal to 100 rads; becquerel (Bq) as the unit of radioactivity; joule (J) as the unit of energy; hertz (Hz) as the unit of frequency equal to 1 cycle per second.

International 10-20 System—for placing electrodes on the scalp when performing electroencephalograms. The electrodes are placed in predetermined positions that are 10 to 20 percent of the distance between certain pairs of skull reference points.

Inter-Op acetabular prosthesis—hip prosthesis from Sulzer that was found to be defective and has been removed from the market. Over 17,500 people were implanted with the Inter-Op before its discontinuation.

interphase—the interval between two successive cell divisions.

interpleural analgesia—a technique for providing pain management in patients with multiple rib fractures, or who have undergone thoracotomy. Interpleural analgesia provides prolonged analgesia and is administered via a percutaneously placed epidural catheter in the interpleural space (between the parietal pleura and the visceral pleura).

Interpore—a form of hydroxyapatite. See *hydroxyapatite*.

interrupted near-far, far-near sutures.

interscapulovertebral arterial bruit—an arterial bruit that may be heard between the spine and one or both scapulae in coarctation of the aorta, Takayasu disease, aortic dissection, or interventricular septal defect.

InterStim—a neurostimulation device designed for patients with urinary control problems. It sends mild electrical impulses to sacral nerves in the lower back that control bladder function, alleviating symptoms of urinary urge incontinence, urgency-frequency, and urinary retention. Based upon the electrical stimulation technology used for pacemakers.

interstitial cystitis (IC)—a chronic, progressive, and debilitating urinary bladder disease afflicting primarily women. Characterized by severe bladder and pelvic pain, and urinary frequency. See *Elmiron*.

interstitial markings—the radiographic appearance of lung tissue, as opposed to the appearance of air contained in the lung.

interstitial laser coagulation (ILC).

interventricular septum—referring to the septum between the ventricles of the heart. *Not* intraventricular septum.

Inter-Vial drug delivery system—consists of a syringe that stores powdered medication in a standard vial and sterile diluent in a separate mechanically connected cartridge, enabling the user to mix wet and dry in one motion just prior to injection.

intestinal fatty acid-binding protein (I-FABP), **human serum**—a biochemical marker of erythrocyte origin. Establishes a useful diagnostic marker for acute ischemic disease of the small bowel.

in-the-bag implantation—implantation of an intraocular lens in the capsular bag.

in the magnet—said by radiologists, when they are working in the MRI unit. They say they're "in the magnet."

intima media thickness (IMT).

intra-, a prefix meaning *within*. Cf. *inter-*.

intra-aortic balloon counterpulsation (IABC).

intra-aortic balloon pump (IABP) —effective for short-term support of cardiac patients. (Dictionaries retain a hyphen between the two *a*'s in *intra-abdominal*, *intra-aortic*, and *intra-atrial*, although some publications omit a hyphen.) Cf. *intra-atrial baffle*.

intra-aortic endovascular sonography —used in detecting aortic invasion by esophageal carcinoma.

intra-atrial baffle—used in repair of atrial septal defect.

Intrabeam intraoperative radiotherapy (IORT) **system**—uses a miniature x-ray source to deliver x-rays inside a tumor cavity.

intracardiac amobarbital sodium procedure—used to evaluate intractable epilepsy.

Intracath catheter.

intracaval endovascular ultrasonography (ICEUS)—a sonogram in which an intravascular ultrasonographic catheter is passed through the right femoral vein into the suprahepatic inferior vena cava under fluoroscopic guidance. From there it is gradually withdrawn, while recording cross-sectional ultrasonographic images. It is used for detecting intravascular tumor thrombi and is more diagnostic than conventional CT or cavography.

intracavernous injection test—a diagnostic procedure for impotence. The erectile response is observed following intracavernous administration of vasoactive agents with or without supplementary manual, vibratory, or audiovisual sexual stimulation. A positive test is a full and maintained erection.

Intracell—a device that treats myofascial trigger points due to repetitive strain injuries, cumulative trauma, overuse syndromes, or carpal tunnel syndrome. It is a nonmotorized device that can be operated by the patient. Moved over the affected area, it rolls, stretches, twists, and compresses the muscles, diffusing barrier trigger points and rehabilitating noncompliant muscles.

intracisternal tPA (tissue plasminogen activator)

IntraCoil self-expanding nitinol stent —used to maintain a patent lumen in the femoral and popliteal arteries of the leg in the treatment of peripheral vascular disease.

intracoronary artery radiation—procedure to reduce restenosis after angioplasty.

intracoronary Doppler flow wire—measures rate of blood flow through coronary arteries and assists clinicians in evaluating the severity of blockage and effectiveness of therapeutic treatment.

intracoronary ultrasonography—uses a mechanically rotated transducer contained within a monorail catheter to determine vessel diameter for selection of angioplasty balloon size. The catheter tip is delivered over a coronary guidewire, and automated pullback of the ultrasound device is performed. Images are recorded on videotape and then digitized into a computer.

intracorporeal shock wave lithotripsy (ISWL)—procedure to treat choledocholithiasis, in which energy is delivered either through probes to achieve electrohydraulic lithotripsy or through laser fibers.

intracranial pressure (ICP) **catheter**; **monitor**.

intracranial temperature monitoring —see *brain temperature monitoring*.

intracytoplasmic sperm injection (ICSI) (Ob-Gyn)—a technique used in couples with severe male factor infertility due to low or poor quality sperm. Cumulus-corona cells are enzymatically removed from the oocytes, and a single sperm is microscopically injected into each oocyte, all of which are then transferred into the uterine cavity 72 hours after ICSI.

intradermal neurilemomas—cutaneous lesions that may occur as firm papules on the chin and lower extremity. Multiple localized (agminated) intradermal neurilemomas often clinically mimic a granulomatous dermatitis and are thus difficult to diagnose.

intradermal tattoo—used in areola reconstruction.

intradiscal electrothermal (IDET) **anuloplasty**—minimally invasive procedure for the treatment of severe low back pain secondary to degenerative disk disease.

IntraDop—intraoperative Doppler probe used for blood vessel identification during laparoscopic surgery.

IntraDose-CDDP injectable gel—used to treat head and neck cancers and accessible tumors.

intraductal papillary-mucinous neoplasm (IPMN).

intraepidermal blistering diseases (pemphigus)—skin diseases characterized by detachment of epidermal keratinocytes, commonly referred to as acantholysis. Forms include:
bullous pemphigoid (BP)
cicatricial pemphigoid (CP)
epidermolysis bullosa acquisita (EBA)
herpes gestationis (HG)
linear IgA bullous dermatosis (LABD)
paraneoplastic pemphigus (PNP)
pemphigus foliaceus (PF)
pemphigus vulgaris (PV)

intrahepatic cholangioenterostomy (of 2-5 intrahepatic ducts)—a procedure using a Roux-en-Y loop and internal stents across the anastomosis. It involves pancreatogastrostomy, gastrojejunostomy in an end-to-end manner, and cholangiojejunostomy.

IntraLASIK procedure—uses the Pulsion FS (femtosecond) laser to create a corneal flap as part of LASIK vision correction surgery, providing

IntraLASIK *(cont.)*
a bladeless alternative to the microkeratome currently being utilized.

intralesional therapy—used for treatment of benign hemangiomas in children and adults. With the patient under general anesthesia, a laser fiber is threaded into the lesion, allowing laser energy to pulsate into the tumor.

intralocular—within the locules of a structure. Cf. *intraocular*.

intraluminal brachytherapy (with or without endoluminal laser treatment) —used in treatment of non-small cell lung carcinoma (or cancer).

intramedullary skeletal kinetic distractor (ISKD)—intramedullary nail for lengthening the femur and tibia. This leg-lengthening technique is said to cause less pain, infection, and joint contracture than external devices.

intramural duodenal hematoma after blunt abdominal trauma—treated by conservative therapy, with bowel rest and parenteral nutrition; it resolves spontaneously.

Intran—disposable intrauterine pressure measurement catheter.

intranuclear ophthalmoplegia (INO).

intraocular—within the eye. Cf. *intralocular*.

intraocular lens—see *lens*.

intraocular pressure (IOP)—the pressure of aqueous humor within the eye, as measured with a tonometer. IOP above 20 or 21 indicates the presence of glaucoma.

Intra-Op autotransfusion—a system for collecting and reinfusing autologous blood during surgery.

intraoperative autologous transfusion (IOAT).

intraoperative cholangiography (IOC).

intraoperative digital subtraction angiography (IDIS system).

intraoperative endoscopic Congo red test (IECRT)—used to assess completeness of vagotomy.

intraoperative high-dose-rate (IOHDR) **brachytherapy**—placement of radioactive material inside, or close to, a tumor during a surgical procedure.

intraoperative hippocampal cooling—a procedure during epileptic surgery in which iced liquid is irrigated into the temporal horn of the lateral ventricle until the hippocampus is "cooled." May be useful in determining the risk of postoperative memory disorder among patients who had epileptic surgery.

intraoperative hourglass test (Ortho). In a positive test, the hypertrophic intra-articular portion of the biceps tendon will buckle as the arm is elevated, and the hypertrophied tendon cannot slide in the bicipital groove. Treatment requires removal of the hypertrophic segment and tenodesis.

intraoperative lymphatic mapping—injection of radiocolloid and blue dye to identify sentinel nodes in the axilla of a patient with breast cancer.

intraoperative navigation (iON) **system**—a virtual fluoroscopy device that permits surgeons to view multiple images in real time.

intraoperative radiation therapy (IORT)—removal or debulking of tumor mass, followed by direct irradiation of site with electron beam radiation.

intraoperative radiofrequency microbipolar coagulation—used in atrial ablation.

intraoperative radiolymphoscintigraphy—combined with blue dye map-

intraoperative *(cont.)*
ping during lymphadenectomy for melanoma.

intraoperative transmyocardial revascularization (ITMR).

intraoperative ultrasonography (IOUS)—biliary exploration during a laparoscopic cholecystectomy.

intraosseous glomus tumor—see *glomus tumor*.

intraosseous pneumatocyst, cervical spine (Radiol)—a finding on x-ray that mimics susceptibility artifacts from metallic hardware within the vertebral body.

intraperitoneal hyperthermic chemotherapy (IPHC).

intraperitoneal hyperthermic perfusion (IPHP).

intraperitoneal onlay mesh (IPOM)—laparoscopic hernia repair technique for small- to moderate-sized indirect hernias.

intraportal endovascular ultrasonography (IPEUS)—a high-frequency, high-resolution, intravascular ultrasound catheter is inserted into the portal vein. The catheter is then withdrawn slowly for sequential observation of the cross-sectional images, providing precise information about the portal vein walls and any existing tumors.

intraretinal microangiopathy (IRMA).

intraretinal microvascular abnormalities (IRMA).

IntraSite gel—a sterile hydrogel for treatment of dry wounds and wounds with slough by creating and maintaining an optimal moist environment.

IntraStent DoubleStrut biliary endoprosthesis—balloon-expandable stainless steel stent used to open and support obstructed lumina or vessels. Investigation is currently being done to determine the safety and effectiveness of this stent in the iliac artery, the main artery supplying blood to the lower extremity.

IntraStent DoubleStrut LD stent—a stent for use in vessels with wide lumens.

intrastromal photorefractive keratectomy (IPRK).

intrathoracic rib—a rare anomaly that may be diagnosed from chest radiographs and recognized as a benign lesion.

intrauterine growth retardation (IUGR).

intrauterine pregnancy (IUP).

intravaginal ring (IVR)—delivery system for hormone replacement drug therapy.

intravascular MRI—experimental catheter-based MRI technique used to identify components of coronary artery plaques and assess their potential for rupture which may result in heart attack or stroke.

intravascular oxygenator (IVOX)—artificial lung designed for temporary use in patients whose respiratory failure is caused by infection or trauma. It consists of a number of very thin 24-inch hollow tubes which are inserted together through the femoral vein into the vena cava. The tubes are then connected to a catheter which supplies oxygen. The oxygen diffuses through the tubes into the bloodstream. The IVOX helps reduce demands on the patient's lungs temporarily until they can again function fully.

intravascular red light therapy (IRLT)—uses a diode laser source to reduce neointimal hyperplasia and avoid restenosis following balloon-induced injury and coronary stenting.

intravascular signal intensity in MR angiography.

intravascular ultrasound (IVUS).

intravenous drug abuse (IVDA).

intravenous drug abuser (IVDA)—Usage: "This 24-year-old IVDA was admitted for right-sided MSSA endocarditis." See also *MSSA*.

intravenous fluorescein angiography (IVFA).

intravenous pyelogram (IVP) or **intravenous urogram** (IVU)—evaluation of the urinary system by introduction of contrast material into a vein, and by x-ray films observing the concentration of the contrast material in the renal pelves, renal calices, ureters, and urinary bladder. The procedure demonstrates the presence of tumors, stones, or structural abnormalities.

intraventricular block—referring to a block within the ventricles of the heart. *Not* interventricular.

Intrel 3 spinal cord stimulation system—to control chronic pain.

Intrepid PTCA catheter (percutaneous transluminal coronary angioplasty).

intrinsic sphincter deficiency—urethral cause of urinary incontinence.

introducer—see *catheter*.

Introl bladder neck support prosthesis—used in urinary stress incontinence. When placed in the vagina, the flexible, ring-shaped prosthesis elevates the urethrovesical junction to its normal position. It can be used as a temporary alternative to surgery, or a permanent one if surgery is not a choice. This is also a good indication if surgery would bring a permanent solution.

intron—a gene segment that does not transmit genetic information. Introns are copied during the formation of messenger RNA, but are then enzymatically removed and the remaining sequences spliced together to form mature messenger RNA.

intubation—see *CAGEIN*.

InVance male sling procedure—a urologic procedure in which six titanium bone screws are implanted into the pubic bone, three on each side of the urethra, and sling material is attached to the screws. The sling is pulled tight to form passive compression and support for the urethra. This procedure is said to offer immediate relief of incontinence, is minimally invasive, and can be performed in about one hour on an outpatient basis.

invasive procedure—defined by the Centers for Disease Control and Prevention as surgical entry into tissues, cavities, or organs, or repair of major traumatic injuries associated with any of the following: (1) an operating or delivery room, emergency department or outpatient setting, including both physicians' and dentists' offices; (2) cardiac catheterization and angiographic procedures; (3) a vaginal or cesarean delivery or other invasive obstetric procedure during which bleeding may occur; or (4) the manipulation, cutting, or removal of any oral or perioral tissues, including tooth structure, during which bleeding occurs or the potential for bleeding exists.

inventory—see *test*.

inversion (Genetics)—a chromosomal aberration in which a fragment broken off from a chromosome rotates end-for-end before reattaching.

inversion-ligation appendectomy—the appendix is inverted or intussuscepted using a blunt probe with a tie

inversion *(cont.)*
(ligature) placed around the base of the inverted appendix; principally used on children.

inversion-recovery technique—MRI term.

inverted L capsulotomy—a portion of an Austin bunionectomy procedure.

inverted Napoleon hat sign—indicative of spondylolisthesis of the L5 vertebral body on x-ray of the lumbar spine. The deformity appears as an upside-down (or inverted) Napoleon hat.

inversion time (TI)—MRI term.

inverted schneiderian papilloma—see *schneiderian papilloma, inverted.*

inverted U-pouch ileal reservoir—a technique for conversion of straight ileoanal pull-through used in surgical treatment of ulcerative colitis.

Invisalign—proprietary method of straightening teeth without braces or brackets.

in vitro (L., in glass)—in the laboratory in glass dishes. Cell growth can be observed in vitro in scientific investigation in the laboratory. Cf. *in vivo*. See *GIFT; LAK; ZIFT.*

in vitro fertilization (IVF)—an assisted reproductive technique for infertile couples in which fusion of a sperm and an oocyte is carried out in a laboratory rather than within the female reproductive tract. After the resulting zygote has developed to the blastocyst stage, it is implanted in the uterus of the mother for further development. See *GIFT; ZIFT.*

in vivo (L., vivus, living)—within the living body. Cf. *in vitro.*

in vivo optical spectroscopy (INVOS) —uses low-intensity visible and near-infrared light to quantify various characteristics of human blood and tissue.

involuntary smoking—the newest term for second-hand smoke or exposure to environmental tobacco smoke.

INVOS (in vivo optical spectroscopy).

INVOS cerebral oximeter—noninvasive monitoring system that continuously measures changes in the blood oxygen level in the adult brain.

INVOS 2100—an early warning test for breast cancer, using optical spectroscopy to detect growths before mammography.

INVOS 3100 (and **3100A**) **cerebral oximeter**—monitors regional blood oxygen saturation (rSO_2) in microvascular structures of the brain by noninvasive means.

INX stainless steel stent—used for treatment of occluded and tortuous vessels deep in the brain secondary to atherosclerotic disease. The neurovascular stent is used to improve blood flow in areas of the brain where surgery is not possible and when medical therapy has failed.

IOAT (intraoperative autologous transfusion).

Ioban antimicrobial incise drape (*not* loban)—an iodine drape used in surgery.

IOCM (isosmolar contrast medium).

Iodamoeba buetschlii—intestinal protozoan parasite.

iodinated contrast medium—contains iodine rather than a metallic salt and is used in angiography, intravenous pyelography, oral cholecystography, and other studies.

iodine I 131 MIBG, iodine I 123 MIBG (I 131 MIBG, I 123 MIBG; ^{131}I MIBG, ^{123}I MIBG)—radioactive imaging agents used in CT scan and scintigram to demonstrate the primary tumor of neuroblastoma and metastasis. ^{131}I MIBG (metaiodobenzylguanidine) theoretically has

iodine *(cont.)*
the possibility of delivering to the primary and metastatic sites of neuroblastoma a fatal dose of radiation, doses easily tolerated by the whole body. Synthetic MIBG is a guanethidine derivative similar to norepinephrine.

Iodoflex absorptive dressing.

iodoform gauze.

iodophor—an iodine compound used in preoperative skin preparation and postoperative skin closure for protection against infection by controlling skin bacteria. Cf. *iodoform gauze*.

iodophor-impregnated adhesive drape.

Iodosorb absorptive dressing.

IOHDR (intraoperative high-dose-rate).

IOL (intraocular lens).

iON (intraoperative navigation system).

I/1 size test object—roman numeral I relates to luminescence, I to V; arabic numeral 1 relates to size in millimeters, 1 to 5.

Ionescu-Shiley pericardial xenograft; valve.

Ionescu tri-leaflet valve (Cardio).

ionic contrast media (Radiol)—also known as *high-osmolar media,* HOM; the singular is *medium*, which is often misdictated. Relatively inexpensive contrast agents can cause lethal allergic reactions in some patients and are illegal in several countries. Cf. *LOM, nonionic contrast media.*

iontophoresis—a way to administer narcotics for pain relief, using galvanic current to drive charged particles into or through a biologic membrane. Weak solutions of both water- and lipid-soluble drugs may be iontophoresed, including anesthetics, antibiotics, corticosteroids, and salicylates. Not to be confused with *electrophoresis*.

IOP (intraocular pressure).

IOP (intensive outpatient program) **criteria**—a system for evaluating drug abuse and mental health patients.

IORT (intraoperative radiation therapy).

Iowa trumpet—guiding instrument used in the administration of a pudendal block.

IPAA (ileal pouch-anal anastomosis).

IPAA (ileoanal pouch anastomosis).

IPAP (inspiratory positive airway pressure).

IPAT (integrated parallel acquisition technique) (Radiol).

IPEUS (intraportal endovascular ultrasonography).

IPG (impedance plethysmography).

IPHC (intraperitoneal hyperthermic chemotherapy).

IPHP (intraperitoneal hyperthermic perfusion).

IPK (indurated plantar keratoma).

I-Plant (iodine I 125) **brachytherapy seeds**—radioactive ^{125}I seed (small encapsulated radiation sources approximately half the size of a grain of rice) used for primary brachytherapy drug treatment of early-stage prostate cancer.

IPLS (intense pulsed light source).

IPM Wound Gel—a sodium hyaluronate wound gel (a dressing and ointment) to treat foot and leg ulcers, pressure ulcers, and abrasions. *Wound Gel* (initial capitals) is a trademarked part of the brand name. Formerly called *LAM ulcer matrix*.

IPMN (intraductal papillary-mucinous neoplasm).

IPOM (intraperitoneal onlay mesh).

IPP (inflatable penile prosthesis).

IPRK (intrastromal photorefractive keratectomy).

IPSID (immunoproliferative small intestinal disease)—see *Mediterranean lymphoma.*

ipsilateral—on the same side.

IPSS (International Prostate Symptom Score)—also known as AUA-SI (American Urological Association Symptom Index). See *International Prostate Symptom Score*.

iPTH (immunoreactive parathyroid hormone) (yes, lowercase *i*).

IRAF (first recurrence of atrial fibrillation [after cardioversion]).

Iressa (gefitinib)—a drug to treat lung cancer. It is legal in Japan, is currently undergoing FDA review in the U.S., and has managed to find its way to the U.S. and into dictation.

IR-guided pigtail catheter placement—the placement of a catheter guided by interventional radiology technique.

iridectomy—excision of a portion of the iris, either surgically or through laser photocoagulation.

iridencleisis (*not* iridenclysis)—an operative procedure to reduce intraocular pressure. It creates a permanent drain which filters the aqueous from the anterior chamber to the subconjunctival tissue.

irides, plural of *iris*.

iridis—see *rubeosis iridis*.

iridocorneal-endothelial syndrome (ICE).

IRIS (Intensified Radiographic Imaging System)—used in STS lithotripsy system.

iris bombé ("bom-bay")—curving or swelling outward of the iris.

IRIS coronary stent—a tubular stent made of stainless steel.

iritis—an acute or chronic inflammation of the iris.

IRK-151 infrared coagulator—used in atrial ablation.

IRMA (intraretinal microangiopathy).

IRMA (intraretinal microvascular abnormalities).

irofulven—investigational anti-cancer drug compound.

iron storage disease—see *bronze disease.*

irradiation—see *heavy ion irradiation*.

irregularly irregular cardiac rhythm—abnormal cardiac rhythm without any discernible pattern, beats occurring at random intervals.

Irrijet DS—system for debridement and irrigation of wounds.

irritant-induced vocal cord dysfunction (IVCD).

IRS (impaired regeneration syndrome).

Iscar—a derivative of mistletoe, a popular cancer remedy in Europe. It is a complementary cancer therapy in the U.S.

ISCs (irreversible sickled [red] cells).

ischemic penile gangrene—a disease in diabetics with end-stage atherosclerosis and renal disease.

ISD (intrinsic sphincter deficiency).

iseganan hydrochloride—oral broad-spectrum, fast-acting antibiotic drug that substantially reduces the likelihood of microbial resistance. It is the first in a new class of antibiotic peptide drugs known as protegrins. Iseganan is also in clinical development for prevention of ventilator-associated pneumonia.

Iselin forceps (Plas Surg).

ISG (immune serum globulin).

Ishihara plates—test for color vision.

ISI laparoscopic instruments.

ISIS (International Spinal Injection Society) **guidelines**—guidelines for spinal injection.

ISKD (intramedullary skeletal kinetic distractor).

island of Reil—structure in the brain.

island wound dressing—a patch-type dressing with the medication in the center part of the bandage surrounded by nonmedicated material or adhesive.

islet cell (*not* eyelet)—the cells that compose the islets of Langerhans in the pancreas.

islet cell antibodies (ICA)—a screening test for persons at high risk for developing type 1 insulin-dependent diabetes mellitus. High levels of ICA indicate that the person's immune system is attacking the insulin-secreting islets of Langerhans in the pancreas.

islet cell implant—technique of injecting islet cells from a cadaver into the portal vein of patients with diabetes. The islet cells migrate to the pancreas, where they begin to produce insulin.

Isletest and **Isletest-ICA**—kit that detects islet cell autoantibodies. It is used to identify individuals at high risk of developing type 1 diabetes several years before actual onset of the disease.

isobutyl 2-cyanoacrylate (IBC)—a tissue adhesive used to occlude an unresectable aortic aneurysm after axillofemoral grafting. Also, bucrylate.

Isocam SPECT imaging system.

isochromosome—an abnormal chromosome, one of whose arms is duplicated by a second arm bearing the same loci in reverse sequence.

isodose line (Radiol)—a term used in Gamma Knife radiosurgery.

isoechoic ("i-so-eh-ko´-ic")—refers to the even distribution of echoes in ultrasonography as the ultrasound waves bounce off structures or tissue. Usage: "The seminal vesicles were small and isoechoic."

isoenzymes—see *CPK isoenzymes*.

isoflurane—drug used with oxygen for anesthesia. Usage: "When IV lines were in place, the anesthesiologist continued anesthesia induction with oxygen, air, and isoflurane."

isograft—a tissue graft from a donor having the same genotype as the recipient.

Isola spinal instrumentation system. The connectors and hooks have a patented V-groove which allows force to be applied to all four sides of the rod, creating additional gripping force, making this system more stable than other systems in which force can be applied from only two directions.

isolate (Genetics)—a population (e.g., religious, ethnic, or regional) in which matings take place exclusively with other members of the same population.

isolated heat perfusion of an extremity—therapy for malignant melanoma of the extremities. The vessels of the extremity are cannulated and the cannulae attached to the cardiopulmonary bypass machine. The temperature of the limb is elevated and perfusion carried out with melphalan included in the perfusate. The limb temperature may be elevated to about 40°C. The extremity vessels are washed out and perfused with fresh blood.

Isolex system—extracts and purifies stem cells for reinfusion into cancer patients to rebuild their immune systems after high-dose chemotherapy.

IsoMed—implantable drug pump used to deliver chemotherapy directly to the liver. Also delivers morphine sulfate to the spinal fluid as treatment for chronic pain.

isosmolar contrast medium (IOCM).

Isospora—the protozoan parasite causing isosporiasis, which can cause an unusually virulent diarrhea in AIDS patients.

isotactic—reduces peak pressures by increasing the surface contact area to distribute force (a term related to gait).

isotopic cisternography—a test used to determine the presence of normal pressure hydrocephalus.

isovaleric acidemia—an inborn error of metabolism in which there is marked elevation in the isovaleric acid levels in the serum because of an inability to metabolize protein-rich foods. Manifested by severe metabolic acidosis and coma, slight intention tremor, slight psychomotor retardation, retinal vessel tortuosity, nonspecific mottling of the retina, and a locker room odor of the body, urine, and breath of patients with this entity. Also called *locker room syndrome.*

ISRA (intercompartmental supraretinacular artery).

ISS (Injury Severity Scale).

Isshiki thyroplasty type I (ITTI)—a procedure to treat unilateral vocal cord paralysis. It uses a Silastic implant placed in a window of the thyroid ala between the inner and outer perichondrium causing lateral compression of the vocal cord.

IST (immunosuppressive therapy).

Istalol (timolol)—once-daily topical drug for treatment of glaucoma.

i-STAT—a handheld analyzer used at patient's bedside or in emergency departments or StatCare.

i-STAT system—a handheld analyzer that performs a panel of critical blood tests at patient's bedside or in emergency departments.

isthmusectomy—also *isthmectomy*.

ISWL (intracorporeal shock wave lithotripsy).

it's, its—the first a contraction, the second a pronoun. How to use *it's* and *its* correctly seems to present problems for many people; I see them misused all too often. Put as simply as I can, *it's* is a contraction of *it is*; use of the apostrophe indicates that a letter has been omitted. Its meaning changes when the apostrophe is omitted; *it's* then the possessive form, *its*. It might be helpful, when you use the word *it's*, to read the sentence aloud and substitute *it is*; you will then hear whether the sentence says what you mean to say.

ITA (internal thoracic artery) **graft** (also called *internal mammary artery*)—the use of an artery from the chest rather than the leg in heart bypass surgery. One end of an artery near the collarbone is stitched into the downstream end of the cardiac artery clogged by disease. As a result, blood pumped out of the heart through the aorta is detoured into the cardiac muscle. See *IEA and GEA*.

ITC balloon catheter—inserted through the carotid artery. This radiopaque catheter has a silicon balloon that is inflated to temporarily occlude a cerebral artery during operations for aneurysms, arteriovenous malforma-

ITC *(cont.)*
tions, or tumors. (ITC stands for Interventional Therapeutics Corporation.)

ITE (in-the-ear) **hearing aid**—*ITE*, not the translation, is typed in medical reports.

iteration—the process by which multiple computerized images converge to make an increasingly accurate image.

ITP (idiopathic thrombocytopenic purpura).

Itrel 3 spinal cord stimulation system—a pulse generator implanted surgically in the abdominal area to control angina pain. The implanted system delivers mild electrical stimulation to the spinal cord to override pain signals to the brain.

IttI (Isshiki thyroplasty, type I).

IUdR (idoxuridine, iododeoxyuridine) —halogenated thymidine analogue, a radiosensitizer.

IUGR (intrauterine growth retardation).

IUP (intrauterine pregnancy).

IVAC electronic thermometer.

IVAC volumetric infusion pump—a positive pressure infusion device for delivery of intravenous solutions or drugs. IVAC is the manufacturer.

IVB (intraventricular block).

IVC (inferior vena cava).

IVCD (irritant-induced vocal cord dysfunction).

IVDA (intravenous drug abuser).

I.V. or **IV drip**—intravenous administration of drugs in which the drug is mixed with the fluid in the I.V. bag or bottle and administered over several hours as the I.V. runs in slowly. Cf. *I.V. push*.

Ivemark syndrome—splenic agenesis syndrome.

IVF (in vitro fertilization).

IVFA (intravenous fluorescein angiography) (Oph).

IVH (intraventricular hemorrhage).

ivory phalanx sign—increased radiographic density throughout the osseous structures of the involved digit in a person with psoriatic arthritis.

ivory vertebra sign—a uniformly white vertebra with no abnormality of its contour or adjacent disks. The vertebra stands out against the adjacent normal, or darker, vertebral bodies. While the list of possible etiologies of ivory vertebrae is extensive, the most common causes of ivory vertebrae are metastatic malignancy and Paget disease.

IVOX (intravascular oxygenator).

IVP (intravenous pyelogram).

I.V. (or **IV**) **piggyback**—see *piggyback*.

I.V. (or **IV**) **port**—see *port*.

I.V. (or **IV**) **push**—a method of administering drugs in which the entire dose of a drug is given intravenously by manually injecting it directly into a port in the I.V. line. The therapeutic effect is felt immediately. This method is often used in emergency situations. Cf. *I.V. drip*. See also *bolus*.

IVR (idioventricular rhythm).

IVR (intravaginal ring).

IVUS (intravascular ultrasound) **catheter**—for viewing the interior of an artery or vein to determine the degree of stenosis or plaque formation.

Ivy bleeding time—the number of minutes it takes for a small incision in the skin (by puncture of the forearm), made with a lancet, to stop bleeding. Cf. *Duke bleeding time*.

Ivy Block—poison ivy, poison oak, and poison sumac topical drug used as a skin protectant and available without a prescription.

iWALKfree—a hands-free crutch that enables people who must be non-weightbearing due to pathology of the lower leg to maintain mobility and self-sufficiency.

Ixodes dammini—a species of tick, the carrier of Lyme disease.

Ixodes pacificus—western black-legged tick, implicated as a carrier in tularemia on the West Coast. Cf. *erythema migrans; Ixodes dammini; Lyme disease*.

J, j

JACE-STIM electrotherapy unit—provides high-voltage, pulsed-current stimulation.

JACE W550—continuous passive motion wrist device.

jackknife position—The patient lies on his stomach with shoulders elevated and thighs at right angles to the abdomen. Used for rectal and coccygeal procedures. Also, *Kraske position.*

Jackman orthogonal catheter (Cardio).

Jackson epilepsy (possessive eponym), but *jacksonian* epilepsy, march, or seizure. Note: An adjective formed from an eponym is not capitalized.

jacksonian march—progression of a jacksonian seizure from one muscle group to adjacent areas or to a generalized motor seizure.

jacksonian seizure—focal seizure (also rolandic). Usually starts as a spasm in the face, a hand, or a foot, and then spreads to other muscles.

Jackson rod insertion technique—used in spinal instrumentation procedures.

Jackson sign—the wheezing produced by foreign bodies lodged in the bronchus or trachea, similar to that of asthma, audible without a stethoscope.

Jackson spinal surgery and imaging table—has the capability of rotating the patient 180° without the necessity of moving for repositioning.

Jackson-Weiss syndrome—craniostosis, broad big toes, tarsal-metatarsal conditions, and sometimes syndactyly. Caused by a mutation in the fibroblast growth factor receptor 2 (FGFR2).

jackstone calculus—a calcium oxalate dihydrate stone shaped like the 6-pointed metal jacks that children play with. Found primarily in the bladder and rarely in the upper urinary tract.

Jacobson hemostatic forceps.

Jacobson organ—an obscure structure in the nose of all mammals except porpoises, with its own nerve supply. It is thought to be important in chemoreception to pheromones.

Jacquemier sign—the bluish-violet color seen in the vagina and cervix at 8 to 12 weeks of pregnancy. Also known as *Chadwick sign.*

Jadassohn-Dössekker disease—atypical tuberous myxedema.

Jaeger eye chart—Findings on examination are given as *J* and a number, indicating the line on the chart with the smallest letters the patient can see.

Jaeger lid plate.

Jaffe-Campanacci syndrome—café au lait spots.

Jaffee capsulorrhexis forceps—forceps with blunt tips to hold the capsular bag and to tear a continuous curvilinear capsulorrhexis.

Jahnke anastomosis clamp.

Jako facial nerve monitor—for middle ear and mastoid surgery, enabling the surgeon to judge the depth of the nerve beneath the exposed tissue bed.

jamais vu (Fr., never seen)—the incorrect feeling that one has never seen or experienced a certain thing before, in contrast to déjà vu, already seen, the incorrect feeling that one has seen or experienced something before.

Jamar dynamometer—a device used to measure hand strength by calibrating the hand grip. Three readings are made for each hand, measured in pounds. Usually higher readings are seen on tests of the dominant hand, unless there has been an injury on that side. Also, *Jamar grip test*.

James fibers—in AV nodal area of the heart.

Jameson calipers—used to measure the lid crease in blepharoplasty.

Janeway lesions—erythematous macules that may be seen on the palms and soles in infective endocarditis.

Janus syndrome—see *Brett syndrome*.

jargon—unintelligible language, gibberish.

Jarit P.E.E.R. retractor—used in laparoscopic surgery.

Jarit Rotator—reusable instrument line for endoscopic surgical procedures.

Jatene arterial switch procedure and **valve** (*not* Jantene)—for correction of transposed great arteries in the neonate.

jaw bra—a compressive dressing placed on the jaw after surgery to provide stability and minimize swelling. See *Jobst jaw bra*.

Jawz—endomyocardial biopsy forceps.

Jay seating system—for positioning patients.

Jedmed/DGH A-scan (Oph).

jejunization of the ileum—alteration of the mucosal pattern so that it resembles that of the jejunum. See *comb sign*.

Jelco intravenous catheter.

jelling—in arthritis, becoming stiff and "fixed" in any position in which movement does not occur for a prolonged period (e.g., overnight).

jersey finger—an injury sustained to the finger of a football player when a gripped jersey is forced out of the tackler's hand.

Jerusalem syndrome—psychological phenomenon in which religious visitors to holy sites assume the identities of various biblical figures. Many stricken with this mental illness have no previous history of psychological problems; symptoms usually disappear within days of leaving the holy site that originally triggered the illness.

Jessner-Kanof lymphocytic infiltration of the skin—treated with thalidomide.

Jeter lag screws or position screws—in sagittal split ramus osteotomy.

jet lesion—usually an autopsy finding. A valvular or septal cardiac defect allows a strong jet of blood, over time, to produce an area of endocardial fibrosis or even an endocardial pocket.

Jet-X internal fixator.

Jewel AF implantable defibrillator—all-in-one arrhythmia management device.

Jewett brace—used for spondylitis, spinal fusion, compression fractures.

Jewett classification of bladder carcinoma:
- O noninfiltrating (in situ)
- A infiltrating submucosa
- B invading muscle
- C involvement of surrounding tissue
- D distant involvement

J-FX bipolar head—prosthesis for use in cemented or uncemented hip surgery.

jiroveci—new species name for *Pneumocystis carinii*.

jittery—describes involuntary jerky muscle movements of extremities of babies with hypoglycemia or drug addiction.

JJ Aligner—a new grid device that will help orthodontists accurately place and guide mini-orthoscrews without damaging the teeth.

J lift (jowl lift)—a technique in cosmetic surgery to achieve minimal facelifting, using a J-shaped incision in front of the ear, with sparing of the hairline and maximum scar camouflage, and using tissue glue to close the incision. A jowl implant lifts the jowl, avoiding the stretched look of other face-lift surgeries.

JL4 catheter—Judkins left 4 cm curve catheter.

JL5 catheter—Judkins left 5 cm curve catheter.

JNC 7—report of the Joint National Committee on the Prevention, Detection, Evaluation, and Treatment of High Blood Pressure.

J needle—named for its shape, it is a modification of the nonswaged fishhook needle used for hernia repair.

Jobst jaw bra—see *jaw bra*.

Jobst stockings (Vasc Surg).

Jocath Maestro coronary balloon catheter.

Joe's hoe—a retractor, also known as the *Weinberg retractor*.

Joffroy sign—absence of brow wrinkling in Graves disease when the patient suddenly looks up.

Jography angiographic catheter.

Joguide coronary guiding catheter.

Joint-Jack finger splint—provides steady, nonelastic force to correct flexion deformities of the fingers.

joint mice—loose fragments of cartilage or other material within the synovial capsule of a joint.

joint position sense (JPS).

joker—operating room slang for an instrument; in different services it could refer to different instruments.

Jonas modification of the Norwood procedure—for hypoplastic left-sided heart syndrome. See *Fontan; Gill/Jonas; Sade*.

Jones criteria, revised—used as a guide in the diagnosis of rheumatic fever. If there has been an earlier strep infection, the presence of one major and two minor manifestations, or of two major manifestations of the disease, makes the diagnosis of rheumatic fever likely. Minor manifestations include history of rheumatic fever or evidence of preexisting rheumatic heart disease, fever, arthralgias, abnormal erythrocyte sedimentation rate or C-reactive protein, or EKG

Jones *(cont.)*
changes. Major manifestations include subcutaneous nodules, carditis, chorea, polyarthritis, erythema marginatum.

Jonnson maneuver—a modified Valsalva maneuver; produces maximal distention of the hypopharynx by holding the patient's nose and mouth closed while he makes forcible expiratory efforts. Note: Jo**nn**son.

Jo-1 antigen—a marker for polymyositis and dermatomyositis.

Joplin bunionectomy.

Josephs-Diamond-Blackfan syndrome —see *Blackfan-Diamond syndrome*.

Jostent—polytetrafluoroethylene-covered coronary stent-graft.

Joubert ("zhoo-bear") **syndrome**—see *AH 1 gene*.

joule ("jewel") (abbreviation, J)—unit of electric power. Usage: "The heart was defibrillated with a single shock of 40 joules." Named for J. P. Joule, an English physicist.

Joystick—used in laparoscopic surgery to retract the gallbladder.

J point—on an EKG tracing, the junction between the end of the QRS complex and the beginning of the ST segment.

J sign (Ortho)—indicates humeral avulsion of the glenohumeral ligament.

Juberg-Marsidi syndrome—rare X-linked inherited disorder that affects males only and is apparent at birth or during the first few weeks of life. Affected children exhibit severe mental retardation, developmental delays, muscle weakness, diminished muscle tone, often delayed bone growth as well as growth retardation, hearing loss, microgenitalism, and/or abnormalities of the craniofacial area.

Judd repair—postoperative ventral hernia repair.

Judet ("joo-day") **grading classification**—a grading system (grades 1, 2, 3, 4a, 4b) for fractures of the epiphysis of the neck of the radius. The grade assigned correlates to the degree that the fracture fragment tilts as compared to its normal horizontal position.

Judet ("joo-day") **hip prosthesis**—a prosthesis which does not require the use of cement; the femoral and acetabular components are made to fit tightly.

Judkins 4 diagnostic catheter—used as a dilator in an artery.

Judkins selective coronary arteriography (*not* Judkin's). Also, *Dotter-Judkins technique*.

jugulodigastric nodes—deep cervical nodes in the area of the jugular trunk and the digastric muscle.

Juquitiba virus—a variation of hantavirus pulmonary syndrome found in Brazil.

juxtaposition—see *apposition*.

Juzo knee-high compression hosiery.

J-Vac closed wound drainage system —consists of a Blake silicone drain and a J-Vac suction reservoir.

JVP (jugular venous pressure).

J-wire—used in a procedure to support extracorporeal membrane oxygenation (ECMO) in infants with severe pulmonary insufficiency and pulmonary hypertension. Usage: "The chest tube catheter was then withdrawn, and we then used a J-wire which we passed down the jugular vein into the inferior vena cava. With this, we were able to slip the venous cannula over the J-wire into the right atrium, and the J-wire was then removed."

K, k

Kadish staging of esthesioneuroblastoma (Neuro).

KAFO (knee-ankle-foot orthosis).

Kairos—rate-adaptive single and dual chamber pacemakers.

Kalginate alginate wound dressing.

Kallassy ankle brace (*not* Kalassy).

kallikrein inhibitor unit (KIU).

kallikrein-kinin (KK) **system**—refers to possible mediator function in vasogenic brain edema.

Kaltostat—hydrofiber wound packing material which is highly absorbent.

Kambin and Gellman instrumentation—used in percutaneous lumbar diskectomy.

KAM Super Sucker—for arthroscopic surgery. Will accept particles of bone without clogging.

Kanavel brain-exploring cannula.

Kandahar sore—a sandfly-borne infection caused by the parasite *Leishmania tropica*. Afghanistan experienced an outbreak among citizens and aid workers, and it conceivably could be brought back to USA by volunteers. There are multiple synonyms, including Alibert disease II, Borovskii disease, and cutaneous leishmaniasis.

Kaneda (ka-NAY´da) **device** (Kioshi Kaneda, M.D.)—anterior spine stabilizing system used in the treatment of burst fracture of the spine. See *Cotrel-Dubousset instrumentation*.

kangaroo care—used to treat premature infants (the name referring to kangaroos nurturing their helpless young in a pouch). With kangaroo care, a medically stable infant can be kept with the mother, lying on the mother's chest, skin to skin, rather than spending hours in an Isolette. This seems to result in fewer breathing problems and faster weight gain.

Kangaroo Kids NutraPops—vitamin and mineral supplement in a popsicle for children.

Kantor-Berci video laryngoscope—replaces the surgical microscope in laryngeal surgery, which has limited view in microsurgical operations on the larynx due to the laryngoscope spatula and its limited depth of focus. The Kantor-Berci instrument uses an endoscope connected to a

Kantor *(cont.)*
video camera with a focus range from a few millimeters to infinity. The camera is connected to a video with better viewing and the ability for permanent documentation of findings.

Kao Lectrolyte—electrolyte replenisher used to treat dehydration in children.

Kapandji fracture of radius—a rare inferior dislocation of the distal radioulnar joint caused by spontaneous post-fracture epiphysiodesis of the radius.

Kapandji-Sauve technique—allows restoration of forearm deviation caused by a radioulnar joint dislocation in which the radius stopped growing and the ulna slowed but did not stop. The procedure provides maintenance of wrist stability and restores normal range of hand movement. Eponyms for the same procedure include *Baldwin Bowers, distal radioulnar joint repair, Milch, Moore-Darrach.*

Kaplan-Meier survival curves—used in the prognosis of cancer.

Kaplan PenduLaser 115—surgical CO_2 laser system for skin resurfacing.

kaposiform hemangioendothelioma—a rare, aggressive vascular proliferation in children that is clinically and histologically distinct from hemangioma of infancy. It has no known association with the Kaposi sarcoma related to HIV infection.

Kaposi sarcoma (KS)—no longer considered to be one of the criteria included in the diagnosis of AIDS, but simply another of the opportunistic diseases a person with AIDS is likely to get.

Kappa 400 Series—the first of a new generation of pacemakers, featuring a unique integrated dual sensor combination (activity and minute ventilation) to provide patients with heart rate support regardless of activity level or exercise tolerance. The activity sensor is best for tracking low-level transient activities, while the minute-ventilation sensor increases heart rate at higher, sustained exertion levels.

Karapandzic flap—innervated musculocutaneous arterial lip and cheek flap used in lip reconstruction. It is named for Modrag Karapandzic.

karate chop phaco technique—for emulsification and removal of cataracts.

Karickhoff laser lens—used for panretinal photocoagulation.

Karl Storz Calcutript—for use with the Karl Storz ureteropyeloscope in upper urinary tract procedures.

Karl Storz flexible ureteropyeloscope—used to visualize the upper urinary tract and perform retrograde intrarenal surgery.

Karnofsky performance rating scale—for patients with malignant neoplasms.

100 normal, no complaint or evidence of disease
90 normal activity, with minor symptoms
80 normal activity, with effort, and some symptoms
70 cares for self, unable to do normal activity
60 requires occasional assistance
50 requires considerable assistance and care
40 disabled, requires special care and assistance
30 severely disabled; requires supportive measures
20 very sick
10 moribund

Karydakis flap or **operation**—excision of pilonidal cyst and sinus with asymmetric flap advancement repair, developed by Dr. G. E. Karydakis.

karyotype (Genetics)—the full chromosomal complement of an individual, as demonstrated by photographing a microscopic preparation of a cell in mitosis, stained to show banding, and arranging the photographic images in pairs in a standard array.

Kasabach-Merritt syndrome—occurs in infants and is marked by giant hemangiomas of the skin and spleen associated with thrombocytopenic purpura and afibrinogenemia.

Kasai peritoneal venous shunt—for biliary atresia in infants, to deal with accumulated ascitic fluid.

Kaster mitral valve prosthesis. Also, *Hall-Kaster*.

Katena cannula—for hydrodissection and hydrodelineation of the lens nucleus.

Katena spoon and spatula.

KaVo reusable dental handpieces.

Kawasaki disease—mucocutaneous lymph node syndrome; usually occurs in infants and small children.

Kaycel towels—absorbent sterile towels used in the operating room as a drape. They have adhesive areas for sealing at the wound site and also for holding the drape in place.

Kaye tamponade balloon catheter—a method of controlling severe nephrostomy tract bleeding. Allows for continued drainage, which may be important if there is a perforation in the upper collecting system.

Kayser-Fleischer ring (Oph)—seen in the corneas of patients with Wilson hepatolenticular degeneration, a completely or partially pigmented ring which is green, and which encircles the cornea near the limbus.

Kazangia and Converse classification—for facial fractures involving the jaw.

Kazanjian midline forehead flap—used in nasal reconstruction procedures.

Kaznelson syndrome—see *Blackfan-Diamond syndrome*.

kb (kilobase)—a unit of 1000 bases in a strand of DNA or RNA.

K-Blade—disposable ophthalmic microsurgical blades, including keratome, slot, scleral, lamellar, miniature, and super-sharp blades.

K-Caps—protective caps to cover the sharp ends of Kirschner wires and similar types of fixation devices used in orthopedic and podiatric procedures.

KCD (kinestatic charge detector).

K-Centrum anterior spinal fixation system—implant for treatment of thoracolumbar instability secondary to burst fractures and tumors.

KCl—abbreviation for potassium chloride drug used for diuretic therapy. The trade drug Kay Ciel is one of many KCl drugs. When "KCl" is dictated, the abbreviation should be transcribed as dictated or translated as potassium chloride. A trade name should not be substituted for "KCl."

K channel openers—see *potassium channel openers*.

$K_{(ATP)}$ channel openers—adenosine triphosphate (ATP)-sensitive potassium channel openers. See *potassium channel openers*.

K complex—a sharp, negative, high-voltage EEG wave that is followed by a slower, positive component.

KDF-2.3 intrauterine catheter—trade name for catheter used for artificial insemination.

K diet, K+2 diet—low-fat, high-protein, low-carbohydrate ketogenic diets designed to provide dangerously obese children and adolescents with a rapid, healthy means of losing weight.

Kearns-Sayre syndrome—progressive ophthalmoplegia, with pigmentary retinopathy, ptosis, and heart block. Also, *Kearns-Sayre-Shy syndrome*—ophthalmoplegia plus oculocraniosomatic neuromuscular disease, mitochondrial cytopathy.

Kech and Kelly osteotomy—surgery for Haglund foot deformity.

keel and wing—phrase used in joint replacement procedures.

keel excision—an excision for diagnostic or therapeutic purposes in which the excised tissue is shaped like the keel of a boat. May be dictated in video-assisted thoracoscopy of lung.

keel punch—a bone punch.

Kegel exercises—to strengthen the pelvic/vaginal muscles, for control of stress incontinence.

k82 ImmunoCap—a blood test that can determine allergy to latex. The k82 ImmunoCap is combined with the patient's serum to measure the level of immunoglobulin E (IgE) antibodies to latex-specific proteins.

Keith bundle—a bundle of fibers located in the right atrial wall of the heart, between the openings of the venae cavae. Also called *sinoatrial bundle.*

Keith-Wagener (K-W) classification of hypertensive retinopathy, roman numerals I through IV. (Not to be confused with *Kimmelstiel-Wilson disease*, also abbreviated *K-W.*)

Keith-Wagener-Barker stages of hypertensive retinopathy.

Kelikian modified Z osteotomy.

Kell—blood antibody type; factor in agglutination. Also *Duffy, Kidd, Lewis, Lutheran*.

Kellan hydrodissection cannula—used for intraocular hydrodelineation and hydrodissection in cataract surgery.

Keller arthroplasty.

Keller bunionectomy.

Kelman phacoemulsification—used in cataract extraction.

kelvin (K). The kelvin is a unit of absolute temperature in the International System (SI) on a scale in which the zero point corresponds to absolute zero. When using the Kelvin scale, you do not use a degree sign—just the numerals followed by *K*. To convert temperatures from the Kelvin scale to the Celsius system, add 273.16. Named for Lord Kelvin, a British physicist. (Note that the unit *kelvin* is lowercase, and *Kelvin scale* is capitalized.)

Kempf internal screw fixation—used in sagittal split ramus osteotomy.

Kendall AV Impulse—a sequential compression device for the foot.

Ken nail—used in hip fracture repair.

Kennedy pack or **splint**—used in sinus surgery.

Kent bundle—atrioventricular bundle in the heart. See *AV bundle*.

Keofeed feeding tube—used in nasogastric feeding.

Keppra (levetiracetam)—a drug for treatment of epileptic patients who experience partial-onset seizures.

Keramos ceramic total hip system—an alumina ceramic artificial hip replacement system, surgically implanted to completely replace a diseased hip joint.

keratectomy—see *operation*.

keratin—a highly insoluble protein (scleroprotein) in epidermis, hair,

keratin *(cont.)*
nails, and part of the teeth. Cf. *carotene, creatine, creatinine*.

keratinocyte growth factor (KGF)—an epithelial cell-specific mitogen.

keratin whorls (*not* whirls)—layers of squamous cells spiraled onto each other, producing a spherical body rich in the protein keratin.

keratitic precipitates; **keratic precipitates**; **keratoprecipitates** (KPs) (Oph).

keratitis, microbial—may be caused by extended-wear soft contact lenses, including disposable lenses.

keratoconus—a conical protrusion of the center of the cornea, without inflammation. Occurs most often in pubescent females.

keratome—see *Jaeger keratome*.

keratometer—see *Terry keratometer*.

keratomileusis, laser in situ (LASIK).

keratoplasty (see also *operation*)
automated lamellar therapeutic (ALTK)
conductive (CK)
CorneaSparing LTK (laser thermal)
deep lamellar endothelial (DLEK)
deep lamellar (DLK)
endokeratoplasty (EKP)
endothelial lamellar
endothelial lamellar (ELK)
Ho:YAG LTK (noncontact holmium:YAG laser thermal)
Hyperion LTK (laser thermal)
LTK (laser thermal)
PLK (posterior lamellar)
radial thermokeratoplasty
S-PK (synthetic penetrating)
Sunrise LTK (laser thermokeratoplasty)
ViewPoint CK (conductive keratoplasty)

keratosis—production of keratin, producing a horny growth such as a wart or callosity. See *solar keratosis*.

KeraVision Intacs intracorneal ring—a tiny device consisting of two very small plastic arcs that are placed in the peripheral cornea, slightly stretching and flattening the cornea so that light rays are focused on the back of the eye, thereby correcting myopia, or nearsightedness. The implant is removable should a patient be dissatisfied or wish to take advantage of a future development in visual correction technology.

KeraVision ring—a tiny, insertable (and removable), clear polymer ring designed to replace glasses, contact lenses, and vision correction surgery techniques that permanently alter the eye's central optical zone.

Kerckring folds—scalloped duodenal folds diagnostic for celiac disease.

kerfs—grooves or channels placed in bone grafts (e.g., in cranial synostosis surgical repair) to allow for bending or contouring of the graft.

Kerley A (B or **C) lines** (*not* curly)—on chest x-ray: *A*, centrally located horizontal linear densities; *B*, horizontal linear densities in the bases of the lungs; *C*, fine linear shadows interlaced throughout the lung, giving a spiderweb appearance.

Kernohan grading—malignant astrocytoma of the spinal cord, given in roman numerals.

Kernohan notch—indentation and necrosis of the brain caused by pressure on the brain by the free edge of the tentorium cerebelli; this is sometimes associated with tentorial herniation.

Kestenbaum repair of nystagmic torticollis.

ketolides—see *Ketek (telithromycin)*.

KetoSite—quantitative test for B-hydroxybutyrate (ketones) to monitor the status of ketoacidosis.

ketotifen (Zaditen)—oral (non-inhalation) antiasthmatic drug used to prevent bronchial asthma attacks.

keyhole resection (ENT)—a surgical technique to decrease the width and length of the tongue in patients with congenital macroglossia, resulting in improved cosmesis and improved function of the oropharyngeal airway, with no change in speech and feeding.

keyhole surgery—a surgical technique to treat patients with blocked coronary arteries. It is a minimally invasive heart bypass technique and uses only four Band-Aid-sized incisions.

Key-Med dilator.

Keystone last—used in management of hyperkeratotic lesions of the foot. See *last*.

KGF (keratinocyte growth factor).

kHz (kilohertz).

kick counts—a picture of the activity of the fetus. If there are enough kicks by the fetus, this is an indication of a healthy baby.

Kicker Pavlik harness—polypropylene hip abduction brace for treating hip dysplasia in toddlers up to 2$^1/_2$ years of age.

Kidd—blood antibody type; factor in agglutination. Also, *Duffy, Kell, Lewis, Lutheran*.

Kid-Kart—for children ages 1-10 with moderate to severe disabilities, and designed to be pushed by an attendant rather than self-propelled by the child.

Kidney Internal Splint/Stent (KISS) **catheter**. See *KISS*.

Kiel classification of non-Hodgkin lymphoma.

Kienböck lunatomalacia disease—refers to the lunate bone in the wrist. It is thought to be caused by vascular interruption or by fracture of the lunate bone.

Kifa catheter.

Killian dehiscence—a splitting open. Usage: "The Zenker diverticulum is a herniation of pharyngeal mucosa through the weakened area of Killian dehiscence just proximal to the cricopharyngeal muscle."

Killian-Jamieson area—a fat-filled lateral dehiscence that transmits the inferior laryngeal nerve and artery forward between the cricopharyngeus muscle above and the upper esophageal fibers below.

Killian-Lynch laryngoscope.

Killip classification—a classification of heart failure ranging from grade I (no failure) to grade IV (frank heart failure).

Killip wire—inserted to give the heart a shock during cardiac arrest.

kilobase (kb).

kilohertz (kHz).

kilopascal (kPa)—a blood gas pressure measurement, equaling 1000 pascals; an SI unit of measurement.

Kimmelstiel-Wilson disease—not to be confused with Keith-Wagener, for both are often given as "K-W."

Kim-Ray Greenfield caval filter—a metallic filter inserted into the inferior vena cava for prevention of pulmonary embolism; transvenous insertion is the approach used. See also *Mobin-Uddin umbrella filter*, which is *not* synonymous.

Kimura cartilage graft—split-thickness costal cartilage graft for management of tracheal stenosis. Cartilage is an ideal material for this type of graft because it is semirigid and obtains its nutrients by diffusion and thus is not dependent on direct vascular supply.

kindred (Genetics)—an extended family.

Kinematic rotating hinge—knee prosthesis.

kinestatic charge detector (KCD)—a motion-compensated scanning device for computerized imaging of the breast. The primary difference between KCD and all other x-ray imaging methods is that KCD reduces the noise associated with the MR technology, and ultimately reduces the radiation dose required for a given signal-to-noise ratio.

Kinetec hip CPM (continuous passive motion) **machine**.

Kinetik great toe implant—a total joint replacement for the first metatarsophalangeal joint.

kinetin—used for treatment of aging- and photodamaged skin.

Kinetix instruments—including Surgenomic and AccuSharp endoscopic instruments used in carpal tunnel release.

KinetiX (capital *X*) **ventilation monitor**—handheld, compact monitor, used when single expired breath or maximum voluntary ventilation tests are needed.

kinetochore—a structure adjacent to the centromere of a chromosome to which the spindle fibers are attached.

King-Armstrong unit—measurement of alkaline phosphatase. Also *Bodansky unit, Bessey-Lowry unit*.

King cardiac device.

kink artifact (Radiol)—may be caused by rough handling of film. Static discharge, bending, or abrasion of film during processing can cause streaks or crescents which can resemble a fracture. This can be dangerous in the case of a skull film, causing an unnecessary admission to rule out fracture with other studies. Also, *crescent artifact, crinkle artifact, half-moon mark artifact, wrinkle artifact,* and *pseudofracture.*

Kinsey atherectomy catheter.

Kinyoun stain—for acid-fast bacilli.

Kiricuta reconstructive breast operation.

Kirklin fence—area of mediastinal pleura used to retract the lung in thoracic surgery.

Kirschenbaum foot positioner—foot rest that positions leg in flexion, used in total knee surgery.

Kirsch laser welding technique—using a protein solder consisting of human albumins, hyaluronic acid, and indocyanine green dye.

Kirschner Medical Dimension—hip replacement system.

Kirschner Modular IIC shoulder prosthesis—for shoulder arthroplasty.

Kish urethral illuminated catheter set.

Ki-67—an immunophenotypic marker on the cells of patients with multiple myeloma; it is being evaluated for its correlation with relapses and overall survival.

KISS (kidney internal splint/stent)—a catheter believed to provide more reliable urinary drainage after pyeloplasty in children. The KISS catheter prevents occlusion because the segment of the tube draining the ureter/pelvis is constructed as a trough. The catheter is passed in a retrograde manner through the renal cortex using the trocar tip, and the trough is positioned in the pelvic ureter. After pyeloplasty, the catheter drains externally for 24 hours, and after a week is clamped and removed.

kissing spines—see *Baastrup syndrome.*

kissing-type artifact (Radiol)—results when there are too many films in the processor tank, and some get unequal amounts of developer.

Kistler force plate—used to measure ground reaction force as the subject walks across it.

Kitano knot—used in laparoscopic procedures.

KIU (kallikrein inhibitor unit).

Kiwi vacuum extraction cup—a vacuum extractor device for fetal delivery, consisting of a rigid plastic Malmström-type cup attached by a wire to a unique combined handle/pump, especially useful for cases involving cranial deflexion/malpositioning.

KJ (knee jerk).

Klagsbrun technique—to harvest chondrocytes which are used to provide a template for new cartilage formation in vivo.

Klatskin needle—for liver biopsy.

Klatskin tumor—a tumor classification system.

Klebsiella oxytoca—newer name for *K. pneumoniae.*

Klebsiella pneumoniae*, *Friedländer bacillus—a component of the normal flora of the oropharynx and GI tract in patients with functioning immune systems, but in AIDS it can cause a fatal sepsis.

kleeblattschädel (German)—cloverleaf skull.

Kleihauer-Betke test (K-B test)—used in assessing hemolysis.

Kleihauer test—of fetal-maternal hemoglobin.

Kleinert flexor-tendon protocol.

Klein pump—used in liposuction.

Kleinsasser anterior commissure laryngoscope.

Klinefelter XXY syndrome.

Kling—adhesive dressing.

Kling fluff rolls and sponges—all-purpose wound dressing.

Klintmalm clamp—used in liver transplantation surgery.

Klippel-Feil syndrome—congenital fusion of the cervical vertebrae.

KLS centre-drive screws—for application of rigid fixation devices.

Knack—exercise technique consisting of rapid pelvic floor muscle contractions performed immediately prior to and during any action that might cause leakage of urine by increasing intra-abdominal pressure.

knee—see *housemaid's knee.*

Kneed-It kneeguard—for relief of minor knee pain associated with arthritis and tendinitis.

knee jerk (KJ).

Knee Signature system (KSS)—used to measure anterior tibial displacement and the angle of knee flexion. Manufactured by Acufex.

Kniest dysplasia or **syndrome**—genetic disorder characterized by dwarfism; flat facies; ears, nose, and throat disorders; and musculoskeletal deformities.

knife (see also *blade*)
A-K diamond
A-OK ShortCut
bladebreaker
Edgeahead phaco slit
Foerster capsulotomy
Freedom
Gamma radiosurgical
Harmonic Scalpel
Lebsche
Lorenz PC/TC scissors ultra-sharp
Neoflex bendable
NeoKnife electrosurgical instrument
Paufique
Rein rib-cutting

knife *(cont.)*
roentgen radiosurgical
ShortCut
sickle
Tiemann Meals tenolysis
UltraCision ultrasonic
Visitec circular
Visitec crescent
Visitec EdgeAhead phaco slit
Visitec stiletto

Knee Society Score—a measure of knee function. Usage: "Knee Society Score was greater than 80 after supracondylar varus osteotomy stabilized with a blade plate."

K9 Scooter—an alternative to crutches. It is steered with the knee, freeing up hands and arms.

knockout—referring to a cell line or experimental animal from whose genome a gene has been deliberately deleted by homologous recombination.

Knodt rod—not easy to find in references unless you know it begins with a silent *K*; also may be erroneously heard as a *knot rod*.

knot
Aberdeen
convertible slip
double-twist
Endoknot
lark's head
Roeder loop slipknot
square
surgeon's (also *friction knot)*
syncytial knot formation
Tennessee slider
Topel

Knuttsen bending roentgenograms.

Ko-Airan maneuver—a technique for controlling bleeding due to early division of the posterior cystic artery in laparoscopic cholecystectomy.

Koala intrauterine pressure catheter.

Kocher collar incision—used in thyroidectomy.

Kocher interval—the interneural interval between the anconeus and the extensor carpi ulnaris (ECU) in a posterolateral approach for operative release of posttraumatic contracture of the elbow (Kocher approach). Usage: "The standard lateral approach to the elbow was made. An incision was made approximately 10 cm laterally over the lateral epicondyle. The incision was taken down through the Kocher interval, and the lateral and collateral ligament, superior half, was protected. Dissection was taken down along the lateral column in the humerus."

Kocher-Langenbeck—ilioinguinal approach in repair of acetabular fracture; it is the most frequently used posterior approach for this procedure.

Koch node—see *sinoatrial node*.

Koch nucleus hydrolysis needle—used in cataract surgery.

Koch phaco manipulator/splitter—used in phacoemulsification to push and fracture the nucleus in cataract surgery.

Koch technique—a technique for intraocular lens insertion using a 4-5 mm incision and closure with the suture knots buried.

Kock nipple valve (Urol).

Kock ("coke") **pouch modified procedure**—to enable women who are postcystectomy to urinate through the rectum. The Kock pouch is connected to the kidneys via the ureters and then surgically attached to the sigmoid colon just above the rectum. Urine collects in the pouch and subsequently is eliminated through the rectum. Backflow is prevented by

Kock *(cont.)*
two valves. In a similar procedure for men, a Kock pouch is connected to the urethra, permitting normal elimination. Called *continent ileostomy*, *reservoir ileostomy.*

Koebner phenomenon (koebnerization) —psoriasis at the site of an injury. Also, pseudo-Koebner phenomenon.

Koenig MPJ implant and arthroplasty—two-component system for replacement of the first MPJ (metatarsophalangeal joint).

KOH colpotomizer system—a device used in laparoscopic hysterectomy that provides improved visualization of anatomical landmarks.

Köhler lines—used to grade hip protrusion. If, on a radiograph, the femoral head is medial to the ilioischial line, protrusio is present.

KOH mount (potassium hydroxide)—a test used in diagnosing cutaneous fungal disease. Scrapings are taken from the skin in the affected area. A few drops of 15 to 20% potassium hydroxide (KOH) are added to the scrapings on a slide. The slide is heated over a flame several times and can then be examined for fungal organisms.

koilocytotic—characteristic of a wart cell.

Kold Kap—plastic bag with a frozen gel, applied to scalp of patient undergoing chemotherapy to decrease hair loss. Also, *ChemoCap*.

Kollagen—purified bovine collagen derivative that promotes wound granulation.

Kommerell diverticulum, normal variant—see *diverticulum*

König disease—osteochondritis dissecans (*not* dessicans) of the knee. Also, *Koenig*.

Konno procedure—patch enlargement of ascending aorta.

Konsyl ("council")—a bulk laxative.

Kontron catheter—used to position intra-aortic balloon pump.

Köper Knit—thin-wall carotid patch.

Koplik spots—an indication of measles; tiny gray-white spots with a rim of erythema, appearing on the buccal mucosa before the skin rash of measles appears.

Korotkoff sounds—the sounds heard through the sphygmomanometer which, properly calibrated, indicate blood pressure. Usage: "The first and fifth phase Korotkoff sounds were taken as systolic and diastolic pressures, respectively."

Kousseff syndrome—condition caused by deletion of chromosome 22q11-13, the main features of which are conotruncal heart defects, neural tube defects, and dysmorphic facial features.

Kostuik internal spine fixation system.

kPa (kilopascal)—a blood gas pressure measure, equaling 1000 pascals; an SI unit of measure.

KPs (keratoprecipitates, keratic precipitates, or keratitic precipitates)—large white keratic precipitates that resemble drops of solidified mutton fat; they are seen on corneal endothelium.

Krackow point—orthopedic landmark in the knee.

Krackow suture—a suture technique used in ligament-tendon fixation, particularly ACL reconstruction. Developed by Dr. K. A. Krackow.

Kraff nucleus splitter—fine forceps with serrated tips used to grasp and fracture the nucleus during cataract surgery.

Kraff-Utrata tear capsulotomy forceps—used to make the circular tear in the anterior capsule when performing capsulorrhexis.

Kraske approach—a posterior sagittal (transsacral or transcoccygeal) approach for surgery on the rectum.

Kraske position in surgery—the jackknife position used for rectal and coccygeal procedures.

K-ras mutations—oncogene mutations implicated in human malignancies.

kraurosis vulvae—progressive atrophy of the vulva in postmenopausal women.

"kre-day"—phonetic for *Credé (maneuver)*.

Kreiselman unit—apparatus used in resuscitation of newborn infants; provides oxygen, heat, suction, etc.

Kreuscher bunionectomy.

Krimsky measurement—of exotropia.

Kropp bladder neck reconstruction—to create bladder outlet competence.

"kro-shay-tahj"—phonetic for *crochetage*.

Krukenberg spindle—an opacity on the posterior surface of the cornea which is vertical, spindle-shaped, and brownish-red in color.

Krukenberg tumor—carcinoma of the ovary, usually metastatic from cancer of the intestinal tract, stomach, or breast.

Krupin-Denver eye valve—surgically implanted for control of glaucoma (made by Storz).

Krupin valve with disc—for treatment of uncontrolled glaucoma. Usage: "In 1991 she underwent a Krupin valve with disc implant to the inferonasal quadrant."

Kruskal-Wallis test—for acoustic neuroma.

krypton (red) **laser photocoagulation**—used in treating choroidal neovascular membrane, and pigment epithelial detachment.

krypton, inhalation of—in positron scanning technique for measuring cerebral blood flow.

KS—see *Kaposi sarcoma*.

KS 5 ACL brace—a functional brace designed to inhibit tibial translation.

KSHV (Kaposi sarcoma-associated herpesvirus).

K-Sponge—sterile hydrocellulose sponge used during ophthalmic or microvascular surgical procedures.

KTP (potassium-titanyl-phosphate) **laser**—used in laparoscopic laser cholecystectomy.

K2 hemi toe implant system—a one-piece surface replacement system/big toe.

K-Tube—trade name for a silicone jejunostomy tube designed to facilitate easy surgical placement for use in enteral nutritional support in patients who are in bed or are ambulatory.

KUB (kidneys, ureters, and urinary bladder) (Radiol).

Kugelberg-Welander disease—juvenile hereditary motor neuron disease.

Kuhn frontal sinus curette.

Kuhn-Bolger angled curette (ENT)—used in frontal sinus surgery.

Kurz tube—ventilation tube and trocar for myringotomy surgery.

Kuske breast template—a device that allows precision guidance during interstitial accelerated partial breast irradiation.

L, l

LABA (laser-assisted balloon angioplasty).

Labbé ("lab-bay"), **vein of**.

label—to render a substance radioactive by incorporating a radionuclide in it; also, to cause a tissue or organ to take up radioactive material. Cf. *sensitize; tag*.

la belle indifférence—seen in certain patients with strokes or conversion disorders who show an inappropriate lack of concern about their disabilities.

labial (adj.)—(1) referring to the labia majora and labia minora, the fleshy structures in the genital area just anterior to the vagina (Gyn); (2) the surface of the incisor and canine teeth directly opposite the lips (Dental). Cf. *labile.*

labile—an adjective describing a condition or emotion easily or spontaneously changed; unstable. Examples: labile hypertension, labile affect.

labor—see *arrest of labor*; *stages of labor*.

labor curves—see *Friedman curves*.

labrum-ligament complex (LLC)—a structure involved in shoulder dislocations and instability of the shoulder joint.

Lachman test—used to determine the presence of a tear in the anterior cruciate ligament.

"lack"—phonetic for *lac*, slang for *laceration*. Usage: "Lac was treated with TAC ('tack')." See *TAC*.

lacrimal scintigraphy (Oph).

lactamase—see *beta-lactamase*.

lactated Ringer solution—a physiologic salt solution used for irrigation in surgery. *Lactated* does not refer to milk, but to lactic acid solution.

Lactobacillus casei—a "helpful" bacteria present in yogurt and milk products that are partially fermented.

lactobezoar—concretion of milk products in the stomach or intestines of infants. Some children manifest abdominal distention, palpable mass in the left upper quadrant of the abdomen, or nonbilious emesis. Surgical intervention is sometimes necessary.

lactoferrin—a protein found in a number of human secretions (bile, saliva, milk, tears). It is an iron-binding protein and has been found to retard fungal and bacterial growth, possibly by depriving these organisms of iron.

Lactomer material—used for absorbable subcuticular skin staples.

Lactosorb—an advanced resorbable plating system used in correcting craniomaxillofacial deformities in infants and children.

lacunar limbectomy—microsurgical reconstruction of the corneal limbus as a treatment for glaucoma.

lacy trabecular pattern—a finding on x-ray indicative of bone resorption.

LAD (left anterior descending) **artery**.

LADAR (laser detection and ranging).

LADARVision Custom Cornea—a customized laser treatment of lower and higher order aberrations (visual imperfections in the eye's optical system). Unless these aberrations are addressed during laser vision correction, the quality of the vision may not be ideal, even with postoperative vision of 20/20.

LADARVision system—for treatment of myopia, with or without astigmatism, using LASIK.

LADARWave Custom Cornea Wavefront System—see *LADARVision Custom Cornea*.

Ladd bands—tight peritoneal folds that pass over and across the second part of the duodenum, often seen associated with malrotation.

Ladd procedure—for correction of malrotation of the bowel (freeing up the duodenum and Ladd bands, and bringing up the small bowel over to the right side of the abdomen and leaving the colon on the left side of the abdomen, thus broadening the base of the mesentery).

LADD (lacrimoauriculodentodigital) **syndrome**—genetic disorder characterized primarily by malformations of the upper limbs and inherited through an autosomal dominant trait. Other symptoms may include malformations in the lacrima, abnormalities of the teeth, small cupped ears, absent or underdeveloped salivary glands, hearing loss, abnormalities of the genitourinary system, and/or unusual skin ridge patterns.

Laerdal resuscitator—a right-angled nonrebreathing valve.

LAF (lymphocyte activating factor)—see *interleukin-1*.

Lafora body disease—the malignant form of Unverricht-Lundborg syndrome, a progressive myoclonus epilepsy associated with progressive dementia. See *Unverricht-Lundborg syndrome*.

LAG (lymphangiogram).

lagophthalmos—incomplete closure of the palpebral fissure when an attempt is made to shut the eyelids. May be caused by involvement of the facial nerve. It results in exposure and injury to the bulbar conjunctiva and cornea.

lag screw.

Laguna Negra virus—a variation of hantavirus pulmonary syndrome found in Paraguay.

Laimer triangle—Laimer-Haeckerman V-shaped area of the esophagus. It is a potential site of herniation of esophageal or pharyngeal mucosa.

Laimer-Haeckerman V-shaped area of esophagus.

Laing concentric hip cup.

LAIS laser—excimer laser for coronary angioplasty.

Laitinen CT guidance system and stereotactic head frame (Neuro).

LAK (lymphokine-activated killer) **cells**—cells capable of killing tumor cells in vitro. LAK cells are produced by incubation of peripheral blood lymphocytes with interleukin-2 for three days. Although LAK cells are capable of killing a great many autologous and allogenic tumor cells, they do not affect normal cells. LAK cells are used in treatment of gliomas and some other types of cancers, sometimes in combination with interleukin-2.

Lakeside cotton dressing.

Lalonde delicate hook forceps—combines the advantages of needleholder jaws and overlapping skin hooks for two-handed closures. Used for skin closure in plastic surgery procedures.

Lalonde extra fine skin hook forceps—used in delicate surgery like hypospadias repair. It is considered to be less traumatic because it gently grasps with overlapping hooks instead of crushing teeth. Scarring is minimal, and postoperative healing is improved.

LAL (*Limulus* amoebocyte lysate) **test**—gauges the presence of endotoxins such as *E. coli* by exposing the blood of horseshoe crabs (a limulus species) to the endotoxin, which causes the blood to clot. The amoebocytes in the crab blood are similar to human white blood cells. The cells are then spun in a centrifuge and intentionally ruptured to create a "lysate," the essence of the LAL test. The lysate is subsequently freeze-dried and looks like grains of salt. Pharmaceutical and medical device manufacturers use the LAL test to ensure that injectable products and invasive devices are endotoxin-free. Also known as *Bang horseshoe-crab blood test*.

LAM (lymphangioleiomyomatosis).

LAMA (laser-assisted microvascular anastomosis or laser-assisted microanastomosis).

Lambda Plus PDL 1 and **Lambda Plus PDL 2 laser systems**—used to activate Photofrin in a two-step treatment system called photodynamic therapy for palliation of certain esophageal cancers.

LAMB syndrome—acronym for lentigines, atrial myxomas, mucocutaneous myxomas, and blue nevi. Now included in the Carney complex. See *Carney complex*.

lamellar body number density—an effective and inexpensive test for rapid identification of a fetus at high risk for respiratory distress syndrome. This test assesses fetal lung maturity by using an electronic cell counter.

laminar air flow—a technology used in clean air surgical suites for orthopedic surgery, especially with knee and hip replacements, and in burn treatment units, in conjunction with environmental suits, hood devices, and double gloves.

laminaria (L., lamina, blade)—a sterile applicator made of kelp, used to dilate the cervix. See *Dilapan*; *Laminaria*.

Laminaria—a genus of seaweed (kelp). The dried *Laminaria digitata* is often used in induced abortion, since, as it absorbs fluids, it expands, thus dilating the cervix. See *Dilapan*; *laminaria*.

Laminar needle (Oph)—a surgical needle used in cataract surgery.

lancinating pain—stabbing, piercing.

L&L panel—a panel of tests for liver enzymes and lipids.

Landolt pituitary speculum.

Landolt ring—a device for testing vision. It is like a letter *C* with a very small opening. The opening is moved up, down, and to each side and is used to test vision in the same way as the E chart.

L&W—jargon for *living and well*, usually referring to parents and siblings in the family history. Expand when encountered in dictation.

Landry-Guillain-Barré-Strohl syndrome—acute idiopathic polyneuritis. See *Guillain-Barré syndrome*.

Landry vein light Venoscope—a fiberoptic illumination device. It has two arms, separated by a few inches, which, when pressed to the skin of the patient, transilluminate the skin and reveal the location of veins. It facilitates the visualization of veins which are deep seated or difficult to find so that an intravenous line can be quickly inserted.

Landsmeer ligament—a deep fascial band in the hand. Reference is made to this structure in operative procedures for correction of Dupuytren contracture.

Lane bone-holding clamp (Ortho).

Langer lines—linear clefts in the skin indicative of direction of its fibers. Do not confuse with Langerhans cells or islet.

Lange skin-fold calipers—used to measure fat in certain areas of the body in diet and weight assessment.

Lange tendon lengthening and repair.

LANS-RH—see *liposuction-assisted nerve-sparing radical abdominal hysterectomy*.

Lanz—low-pressure cuff endotracheal tube.

lap—brief form for laparotomy. See *lap tape*.

lap appy—slang for laparoscopic appendectomy.

LAP (laser ablation of the prostate).

Laparofan—used in conjunction with Laparolift as an alternative to pneumoperitoneum produced by CO_2 gas insufflation.

Laparolift system—an Airlift balloon retractor for use in gasless laparoscopy. It is a doughnut-shaped cushion inserted and inflated to allow free access to abdominal organs without requiring gas insufflation. It is an instrument for stone fragmentation in laparoscopic cholecystectomy.

LaparoSAC single-use obturator and cannula—used in laparoscopic surgery.

laparoscopically assisted—see *laparoscopic-assisted* or *laparoscopy*.

laparoscopic appendectomy—minimally invasive alternative, which cannot be performed if rupture or abscess is suspected. See *lap appy*.

laparoscopic-assisted abdominoperineal pull-through procedure—for treatment of high anorectal malformations.

laparoscopic-assisted bowel resection—laparoscopy used to perform a major part of the dissection of the bowel, allowing for a smaller incision. The mobilization and dissection of the bowel is carried up to the transection of the mesenteric pedicle, and resection is then completed and anastomosis performed through a small incision.

laparoscopic-assisted colorectal resection—performed for colorectal carcinoma, both curative and palliative.

laparoscopic-assisted ileocystoplasty and ileovesicostomy—see *Monti procedure.*

laparoscopic-assisted vaginal hysterectomy (LAVH).

laparoscopic biopsy of liver—an alternative to open wedge biopsy of the liver.

laparoscopic bladder neck suture suspension procedure—anchors a suture in Cooper ligament and transvaginally in the anterior vaginal wall to provide upper and lower suspension points.

laparoscopic Burch procedure.

laparoscopic cholecystectomy—laparoscopic gallbladder removal requiring only four small incisions, resulting in rapid recovery time. Acute inflammation may require conversion to the open procedure.

laparoscopic contact ultrasonography (LCU)—a viable alternative to intraoperative cholangiography. Used in the detection of ductal stones but less reliable in the disclosure of anomalous biliary anatomy.

laparoscopic donor nephrectomy (LDN).

laparoscopic Doppler probe—useful in identifying arteries during laparoscopic surgery.

laparoscopic fundoplication—see *Nathanson liver retractor.*

laparoscopic hand-assisted Miami pouch—see *Miami pouch.*

laparoscopic Heller myotomy—used for treatment of dysphagia and gastroesophageal reflux, as an alternative to open surgery.

laparoscopic intracorporeal ultrasound (LICU)—used in place of cholangiography to examine biliary duct system.

laparoscopic laser-assisted autoaugmentation (Urol)—performed in children for neurogenic bladder dysfunction.

laparoscopic laser cholecystectomy (LLC)—laparoscopic gallbladder removal utilizing laser instead of electrocautery technique.

laparoscopic lysis—a procedure for lysis of adhesions and placement of a peritoneal dialysis catheter.

laparoscopic Nissen and Toupet fundoplication—surgical treatment of complicated GERD (gastroesophageal reflux disease).

laparoscopic pelvic lymph node dissection and extraperitoneal pelvioscopy—operative staging procedures.

laparoscopic pneumodissection—dissection technique used in laparoscopic surgery that uses short bursts of high-pressure carbon dioxide as a dissection medium.

laparoscopic radical prostatectomy—performed on men with localized prostate cancer, low-volume tumors, and favorable pelvic anatomy. Surgeons performing this procedure are better able to visualize the prostatic apex and urethra, facilitating reconnection of the bladder neck to the urethra and offering the possibility of better postoperative continence.

laparoscopic sigmoid colectomy—surgical treatment for diverticulitis.

laparoscopic surgeon's thumb—area of paresthesia in the distribution of the lateral digital nerve due to holding laparoscopic instruments for long periods. Generally resolves within hours, but sometimes takes days.

laparoscopic total extraperitoneal hernioplasty.

laparoscopic transcystic duct exploration—used to treat common bile

laparoscopic *(cont.)*
duct stones and allows for open choledochotomy.

laparoscopic transcystic papillotomy—for endoscopic bile duct stone removal in laparoscopic cholecystectomy.

laparoscopic ultrasonography (LUS).

laparoscopic ultrasound (LUS).

laparoscopic urinary diversion procedure—for intestinal urinary conduit.

laparoscopic uterine nerve ablation (LUNA).

laparoscopy under local anesthesia (LULA).

LaparoSonic coagulating shears for autograft harvesting.

laparotomy—see *second-look*.

Lap-Band adjustable gastric banding (LAGB) **system**—see *Lap-Band system*.

Lap-Band system—rigid silicone band or prosthesis used in adjustable gastric banding for the laparoscopic treatment of severe obesity. The Lap-Band procedure consists of several small incisions of 5-10 mm and application of the adjustable band around the upper part of the stomach. It is then inflated or deflated according to the patient's needs. By creating a smaller gastric pouch, the Lap-Band system limits the amount of food that the stomach will hold at any time. The inflatable ring controls the flow of food from this smaller pouch to the rest of the digestive tract. The surgery is reversible by removing the band.

lap chole—slang for laparoscopic cholecystectomy.

Laplacian mapping—see *body surface Laplacian mapping*.

lap Nissen (laparoscopic Nissen fundoplication)—may be done with esophageal lengthening variation for treatment of gastroesophageal reflux with short esophagus. (A short esophagus is the end result of severe, long-standing GE reflux.)

Lapro-Clip—ligating clip system.

Lapro-Flex—self-forming laparoscopic retractor.

Lap Sac—used to enclose larger organs or masses of resected tissue, which are then morselized for removal through a small laparoscopic incision. See *Pleatman sac*.

lap tape (pad or sponge)—a large laparotomy sponge used in major abdominal (laparotomy) surgery. A small one is called "appy" tape (for appendectomy). Usage: "The wound was packed with a moist lap tape."

LAP (leukocyte alkaline phosphatase) **test**—a test for chronic myelogenous leukemia. Result is given as a score, with normal being greater than 20.

LapTie—endoscopic knot-tying instrument.

Lapwall—trade name of a laparotomy sponge and wound protector.

LAR/CAA (low anterior resection in combination with coloanal anastomosis)—for primary rectal cancer.

large clothing artifact (Radiol)—caused by wrinkles in gowns that are too large, imitating calcified arteries on film. Also, rolled-up pants may have radiopaque objects such as stones in the folds, confusing the radiologists.

large-core needle biopsy (LCNB)—such as that done with a Mammotome.

large loop excision of the transformation zone (LLETZ)—an alternative to colposcopically directed punch biopsy for diagnosing cervical intraepithelial neoplasia (CIN). It is also

large *(cont.)*
used as an alternative to the carbon dioxide laser in the treatment of CIN.

large skull-implant surgery—used to repair the skulls of persons who have undergone brain surgery or have suffered serious head trauma, including gunshot wounds. Previously, only defects 3 cm or smaller could be covered by traditional surgery.

Larmor equation; **frequency**—terms used in MRI.

LaRoque herniorrhaphy incision.

Larrey hernia—a herniation through the subcostosternal space. More commonly known as a Morgagni hernia. Named for Dominic John Larrey, Napoleon's surgeon general, who described the surgical approach to the pericardial cavity through the anterior diaphragmatic defect.

LARS (laparoscopic antireflux surgery).

LARSI (lumbar anterior-root stimulator implants).

laryngeal framework surgery (LFS) (also called *thyroplasty* or *phonosurgery*)—a procedure to change or improve the voice.

laryngeal web (ENT)—a congenital anomaly, malformation; it can be either a thin membrane or a thick one, most often at the level of the vocal cords. This membrane compromises the airway and may require surgery.

laryngomalacia—treated by unilateral supraglottoplasty or epiglottoplasty.

laryngoplastic phonosurgery (ENT)—laryngeal framework surgery to treat voice disorders. Includes medialization laryngoplasty and the arytenoid adduction procedure for unilateral paralysis.

laryngospasm—persistent, long-lasting vocal cord dysfunction during inspiration.

laryngotracheal reconstruction—technique to save the larynx in patients suffering from vocal cord cancer. Five centimeters of the trachea is stretched out and put in place of the part of the larynx which was removed. In order to maintain a sufficient blood supply, a bit of tissue is taken from the forearm and wrapped around the trachea to connect it with the blood vessels in the neck. Following such an operation, patients can breathe as before through the mouth and nose, and they still have their sense of smell.

LAS (lymphadenopathy syndrome).

LASE (laser-assisted spinal endoscopy).

Lasègue sign ("la-segz")—straight leg raising test. A positive Lasègue sign is indicative of nerve root irritation or possible low back pathology.

laser (light amplification by stimulated emission of radiation)—used in many procedures for everything from brain surgery to cleaning out clogged arteries to disintegrating stones in the biliary duct and kidney. See individual entries:
AccuLase excimer
acupuncture
alexandrite (solid-state)
AlexLAZR
Allegretto Wave excimer
Apex Plus excimer
ArF excimer
argon
argon/krypton
ArthroProbe
Aura desktop ENT
Aurora diode-based dental

laser *(cont.)*
Aurora diode soft-tissue
biocavity
BriteSmile
Candela 405 nm pulsed dye
carbon dioxide (CO_2)
Centauri Er:YAG dental
CHRYS CO_2
ClearView CO_2
Coherent CO_2 surgical
Coherent UltraPulse 5000C
CoolGlide
copper-vapor pulsed
CorneaSparing LTK system
coumarin pulsed dye
CTE:YAG (CrTmEr:YAG)
Derma K
DermaLase
Derma 20
DIAGNOdent
diode
Dodick Laser Photolysis System
dye
Eclipse TMR
ELCA
endolaser venous therapy (ELVT)
endoscopic
Epic ophthalmic 3-in-1
EpiLaser
EpiStar Diode Laser System
EpiTouch
erbium:YAG (Er:YAG)
ErCr:YAG
excimer
FCPA2
FeatherTouch CO_2
femtosecond laser keratome
Fiberlase
FiberScan
flashlamp-pulsed Nd:YAG
flashlamp-pumped pulsed dye
Flexlase 600
flying spot excimer
Fraxel SR
gallium-arsenide (GaA)

laser *(cont.)*
Genesis 2000
GentleLASE Plus
Gherini-Kauffman Endo-Otoprobe
Heart Laser (for transmyocardial revascularization)
HF infrared
high-energy
holmium
holmium:YAG (yttrium-argon-garnet)
Horn Endo-Otoprobe
hot
Hyperion LTK
Indigo LaserOptic
Intelect
Kaplan PenduLaser 115
Kirsch
krypton (red)
KTP (potassium-titanyl-phosphate)
LADARVision excimer
LAIS excimer
Lambda Plus PDL 1 and PDL 2
laparoscopic
laser Doppler flowmetry (LDF)
Laserscope
Laser Lancet
laser scanning cytometry (LSC)
LaserSonics EndoBlade
LaserSonics Nd-YAG Laserblade
LaserSonics Surgiblade
Laserthermia
LaserTripter MDL 3000
Lasertrolysis
LaserTweezers
Lasette laser finger perforator
LightSheer (and LightSheer SC) diode
Lightstic 180 and Lightstic 360
LPI (Laser Photonics, Inc.)
LTK (laser thermal keratoplasty)
LX 20
Lyra
Mainster retina
Maloney Endo-Otoprobe

laser *(cont.)*
Microlase transpupillary diode
Microprobe
mid-infrared
Multi-Operatory Dentalaser (MOD)
Nerve Fibre Analyzer Gdx
Niagara PV
Nidek EC-5000 excimer
Nlite nonablative
NovaLine Litho-S DUV excimer
NovaPulse CO_2
Nuvolase 660
OcuLight SL diode
OLM (ophthalmic laser micro-endoscope)
OmniPulse-MAX holmium
Opmilas 144 Plus
Opmilas CO_2
Optical Biopsy System
OptiVision
OtoLAM
Palomar SLP1000 (super long-pulse) diode
Pegasus Nd:YAG surgical
PhotoGenica V-Star
PhotoPoint
Polaris 1.32 Nd:YAG
Prima
Prostalase
pulsed-dye (PDL)
PulseMaster
Pulsion FS (femtosecond)
Pulsolith
Q-LAS 10 YAG
Q-switched neodymium:YAG
Q-switched ruby
Revitalase erbium cosmetic
scanning laser polarimetry
ScleroLaser
ScleroPlus
ScleroPLUS HP
Selecta 7000
Sharplan SilkTouch flashscan surgical
SilkLaser aesthetic carbon dioxide

laser *(cont.)*
Silk Touch laser skin resurfacing
Skinlight erbium YAG
SLS (Spectranetics laser sheath)
Smoothbeam
SoftLight
Softscan
SolarGen 2100s
SPTL-1b vascular lesion
STATLase-SDL diode
Surgilase Nd:YAG
Surgilase 150
THC (thulium, holmium, chromium):YAG
Topaz CO_2
TruPulse CO_2
2040 erbium SilkLaser
UltraFine erbium
UltraPulse CO_2
Urolase fiber
Vbeam pulsed dye
Vectra Genisy
VersaLight
VersaPulse holmium
Versatome
Visulas Nd:YAG
VISX excimer
VISX Star S2 excimer
VISX Star 3 excimer
Vitesse Cos
Xanar 20 Ambulase CO_2
XeCl (xenon-chloride)
XTRAC
YAG (yttrium-aluminum-garnet)
YagLAZR *or* YagLazr
Zeiss Visulas 690s
Zyoptix
Zyoptix Infinity

laser ablation of the prostate (LAP).

laser acupuncture—used to promote analgesia locally or systemically.

laser-assisted balloon angioplasty (LABA)—a thermal laser delivery system that creates a small channel in the artery (particularly the femoral

laser *(cont.)*
artery), followed by balloon angioplasty to dilate the residual stenosis, thereby allowing sufficient blood flow for symptom relief.

laser-assisted internal fabrication (L.I.F.T.) **technique**—creates a "bra" that holds breast tissue up and in place internally, helping to extend the results of mastopexy, breast reduction, and breast augmentation procedures.

laser-assisted microanastomosis or **laser-assisted microvascular anastomosis** (LAMA)—use of a laser instead of sutures to seal small vessels at anastomotic site.

laser-assisted spinal endoscopy (LASE) —a less invasive technique for automated percutaneous lumbar diskectomy. Laser fibers are inserted through 18 or 20 gauge needles for vaporization of lumbar disk material. Using the holmium:YAG (Ho:YAG) laser, a flexible cannula is inserted, through which a malleable and directable laser fiber is inserted under visual control via optical fibers also within the cannula. Constant irrigation through the same cannula keeps the disk space cool, decreasing the risk of thermal injury.

laser-assisted tissue welding technique —bladder augmentation or enterocystoplasty method.

laser-assisted uvulopalatoplasty (LAUP)—for treatment of snoring, but not sleep apnea. See *LAUP*.

laser biomicroscopy (Oph)—provides visualization and photographic record of vitreoretinal structures at the macula.

Laser bra procedure—see *L.I.F.T.*

laser correlational spectroscopy (LCS) —method for diagnosing malignant diseases by blood plasma analysis.

laser Doppler flowmetry (LDF)—noninvasive measure of cochlear blood flow through the intact otic capsule bone.

laser detection and ranging (LADAR).

Laserflo blood perfusion monitor (BPM)—for evaluating or monitoring in situ microvascular circulation invasively or noninvasively.

laser image custom arthroplasty (LICA).

laser in situ keratomileusis (LASIK).

Laser Lancet—laser device for capillary blood draws for screening purposes. It eliminates the need for needle sticks, thereby making the procedure safer for patients and healthcare workers.

laser midline glossectomy—partial glossectomy of the tongue base.

laser myringotomy—for treatment of serous otitis media. A small hole is created in the tympanic membrane (myringotomy) without the insertion of ventilation tubes. The opening allows for drainage and endoscopic evaluation of the middle ear space, which remains open for several weeks, followed by spontaneous and complete healing of the tympanic membrane. The procedure may be done in a physician's office under local anesthesia on patients age six years or older.

laser nucleotomy—a surgical technique for correction of a herniated disk. Under local anesthesia, the VersaPulse holmium laser is inserted into the nucleus pulposus of the disk, and a portion of the disk vaporized.

laser photoablation.

laser plume—the toxic by-product of laser and electrosurgical procedures, composed of chemicals, bacteria, and viruses.

laser scanning cytometry (LSC)—a microscope-based device that combines the advantages of flow cytometry and image analysis.

laser sclerostomy (Oph)—use of the laser to produce an outflow channel in treatment of glaucoma.

Laserscope—manufacturers of a line of medical lasers and advanced fiberoptic devices.

LaserSonics EndoBlade—for laparoscopic use.

LaserSonics Nd:YAG Laserblade scalpels.

LaserSonics Surgiblade—for colposcopic procedures.

laser speckle—used to assess degree of night myopia. When light from a laser is reflected from a granular surface, a speckled pattern is seen; and when a patient with night myopia looks at this pattern and moves his head, the speckles seem to move, and move opposite to the direction of head movement if the eye is myopic at that distance. Correcting the refractive error with lenses will neutralize the pattern's movement.

laser stapedotomy (ENT)—the procedure of making a small opening by a laser into the footplate of the stapes (instead of removing the entire stapes) to correct deafness caused by otosclerosis.

laser thermal keratoplasty (LTK)—a laser treatment performed through the lens of a specially modified slit-lamp biomicroscope. With use of an infrared laser, the corneal collagen is changed from a double-helix conformation to a partly coiled state, resulting in contraction of the fibers and change in the curvature of the cornea.

laserthermia—see *transurethral balloon laserthermia prostatectomy.*

laser trabeculodissection (LTD)—glaucoma surgery ablation technique using a scanning excimer laser.

lasertripsy—an endoscopic procedure using a laser, such as the Candela pulsed-dye laser or a holmium-YAG laser, to fragment calculi in the ureters.

LaserTripter MDL 3000—provides precise destruction of calculi with least thermal effect.

Lasertrolysis—proprietary name for hair removal using the EpiLaser to heat and disable the hair follicle without causing harm to the surrounding skin.

LaserTweezers—for optical trapping. It uses the pressure of a laser to isolate particles or cells and move them.

laser uterosacral nerve ablation (LUNA).

laser welding—sutureless tissue welding using a diode laser and protein solder. Used with anastomoses of the blood vessel, bowel, ureter, and nerve.

Lasette laser finger perforator—used for sampling capillary blood for glucose and other blood chemistry readings. It is reportedly less painful to patients than needle sticks, but also eliminates accidental fingersticks and the possibility of cross-contamination from the patient.

Lash hysterectomy technique.

LASIK (laser in situ keratomileusis) (Oph)—a corneal procedure for vision correction. A flap of anterior corneal stroma is dissected, the deeper layers are partially ablated with the laser, and the hinged superficial flap is then replaced.

Lassa fever—a highly virulent disease found in some central and western African countries, named for Lassa, Nigeria, where it was first recognized.

last—a metal or plastic form shaped like the human foot and over which a shoe is shaped or repaired. See *bunion last* and *Keystone last*.

Latarjet, Andre—a French anatomist. See *nerve of Latarjet*. Also, *Latarjet vein* (vena prepylorica).

Latarjet nerve—see *nerve of Latarjet*.

late-life depression (LLD).

late luteal phase dysphoric disorder (LLPDD)—the most debilitating form of premenstrual syndrome.

lateral acetabular shelf operation (Ortho).

lateral crural steal (LCS)—a technique for nasal tip reconstruction that involves advancing (in essence, "stealing") the lateral crura onto the medial crura to project the nasal tip anteriorly.

lateral hypopharyngeal pouch (LHP).

lateral mamillary nucleus of Rose (Neuro).

lateral transverse thigh flap (LTTF).

latissimus dorsi demand dynamic wrapping—an aortomyoplasty technique in which the latissimus dorsi muscle wrap is stimulated to provide active systolic assistance. See *aortomyoplasty*.

latissimus dorsi muscle (LDM).

latissimus dorsi myocutaneous flap—a method of breast reconstruction utilizing the latissimus dorsi muscle, and skin transferred from the back. It can be combined with a breast implant to produce a larger breast mound.

LATS (long-acting thyroid-stimulating) **hormone**.

lattice degeneration (retinal)—a sharply demarcated circumferential lesion that is located at, or somewhat anterior to, the equator, characterized by an interconnecting network of fine white lines, and may be associated with numerous round, punched-out areas of retinal thinning or actual retinal holes. May lead to retinal detachment.

Lattimer, manner of—an adjunct to orchiopexy that places the testis in a subcutaneous scrotal pocket external to the dartos layer and uses a gentle testis traction regimen to diminish the chances of testis retraction after orchiopexy, described by J.K. Lattimer.

Latzko vesicovaginal fistula repair.

Lauge-Hansen classification of ligamentous ankle fractures.

LAUP (laser-assisted uvulopalatoplasty) —alternative surgical procedure to UPPP (uvulopalatopharyngoplasty) for treating snoring. It is not recommended for obstructive sleep apnea due to unpredictable response.

Laurence-Moon-Biedl syndrome—hereditary syndrome characterized by obesity, retinitis pigmentosa, mental retardation, polydactyly and hypogonadism. Other abnormalities may include ataxia, dwarfism, heart defects, and ocular complications.

Laurer forceps.

Laurin x-ray view.

LAVH (laparoscopically assisted vaginal hysterectomy).

Lawrence Add-A-Cath—sharp-tipped, bevelled trocar and peel-off sheath for suprapubic insertion into the bladder.

Lazaro da Silva technique—the creation of a continent perineal colostomy following abdominoperineal

Lazaro *(cont.)*
resection of the rectum for low rectal cancer.

Lazarus-Nelson technique—generally used for peritoneal lavage that may be adapted for creating a pneumoperitoneum for laparoscopy. Generally felt to be safer, especially in obese patients, than other blind methods for introducing pneumoperitoneum.

lazeroids—in cerebral hypoxia-ischemia.

LazerSmile—a tooth-whitening system for home use. It uses a light source embedded within a battery-operated toothbrush and clear, nonabrasive tooth-whitening gel.

lazy H incision.

lazy leukocyte syndrome (LLS).

lazy Z incision.

LBP (low back pain).

L-Camipure (L-carnitine tartrate)—a natural supplement.

L-Cath—peripherally inserted neonatal catheter.

LCD (liquor carbonis detergens).

LCF (left circumflex) **coronary artery**.

LCIS (lobular carcinoma in situ).

LCNB (large-core needle biopsy).

LCS (laser correlational spectroscopy).

LCSD (left cardiac sympathetic denervation).

LDF (laser Doppler flowmetry).

LDL (low-density lipoprotein).

LDL Direct—a test for LDL (low-density lipoprotein) using a process called *immunoseparation*. It does not require a triglyceride measurement and can be performed on nonfasting patients. In the past, tests were based on a mathematical equation using the results of total cholesterol, HDL, and triglycerides.

LDM (latissimus dorsi muscle).

LDN (laparoscopic donor nephrectomy).

LDR (low-dose-radiation) **brachytherapy**.

LDR (labor, delivery, and recovery) **room**, where the expectant mother goes through labor, delivery, and recovery in the same room.

LDX System—see *Cholestech LDX System.*

leading bar—a device by which a surgeon can guide the tape or the thread to the outside of the abdomen, facilitating extracorporeal lifting of the round ligament and gallbladder for exposing Calot triangle during laparoscopic surgery.

Leadbetter-Politano ureterovesicoplasty—submucosal tunnel technique.

lead line—a blue line which is observed on the gums in lead poisoning cases.

leaf of the broad ligament—the area where the ligament fans out and widens, resembling a leaf. The broad ligament supports and stabilizes the uterus and associated reproductive organs. There are both an anterior leaf and a posterior leaf.

Lea Shield—a barrier contraceptive device with a cup-shaped design, intended to cover the cervix without actually being held by the cervix. It has a valve to place it in the vagina and a loop to remove it between uses. The thick lip of the device is designed to fill the area surrounding the cervix.

leather-bottle stomach—a kind of gastric carcinoma (also called *linitis plastica*). The tumor is hard (scirrhous) and the stomach wall becomes thick and rigid.

Le Bag reservoir—an ileocolic urinary reservoir for urinary diversion in total cystectomy patients.

Leber ("lay-ber") **disease**—hereditary optic atrophy occurring in young men between the ages of 20 and 30. The optic nerve degeneration is rapidly progressive, but finally stabilizes, and some vision remains.

Leber miliary aneurysms (Oph).

Lebsche knife—a heavy knife with a curved end (to hook under the xiphoid process) and a T-shaped handle; used for splitting the sternum for quick entry into the thoracic cavity.

lecithin/sphingomyelin ratio—see *L/S ratio*.

Leder stain (chloracetate esterase) (LAB)—used in identifying granulocytic sarcoma by differentiating that entity from lymphoma, embryonal rhabdomyosarcoma, Ewing sarcoma, and undifferentiated carcinoma.

LeDuc anastomosis—a method of ureteral reimplantation used in urinary diversion procedures.

LeDuc-Camey ileocystoplasty—antireflux implantation of the ureters, for patients with bladder cancer.

leech—see *mechanical leech*.

Leeds-Keio ligament prosthesis—an open-weave tube of polyester mesh that can be fixed to bone at each end with bone plugs. New ligament tissue forms along the scaffold of the mesh, providing a sound new ligament within two years.

LEEP (loop electrosurgical excision procedure).

LeFort I apertognathia repair.

LeFort II fracture—pyramidal fracture of the maxilla.

LeFort III fracture—craniofacial disjunction and transverse facial fracture.

LeFort urethral sound.

LeFort uterine prolapse repair.

left anterior descending (LAD) **artery**.

left brain, left face, left heart, etc.—when dictated, edit to left side or part of the brain, face, heart, etc.

left cardiac sympathetic denervation (LCSD)—a 40-minute surgical procedure that cuts part of the nerves to the heart and reduces the heart's control from the sympathetic nervous system. It is used in treatment of long QT syndrome. See *acquired long QT syndrome* and *long QT syndrome*.

left circumflex (LCF) **coronary artery**.

left face—left side of the face.

left shift—see *shift to the left*.

left ventricular end diastolic pressure (LVEDP).

left ventricular outflow tract obstruction (LVOTO).

Legacy Phaco-Emulsifier—aspirator used in cataract extractions.

Legasus Sport CPM (continuous passive-motion) **device**—used for sports medicine rehabilitation.

Legionella pneumophila—gram-negative organism causing legionnaires' disease and Pontiac fever. Can be devastating in AIDS patients. Other species include:

L. bozemanii
L. dumoffii
L. feeleii
L. gormanii
L. jordanis
L. longbeachae (serogroups 1 and 2)
L. micdadei

Legionella Urinary Antigen (LUA) **ELISA test**—adjunct to culture for presumptive diagnosis of past or current legionnaires' disease.

legionnaires' disease—pulmonary form of legionellosis, resulting from infection with *Legionella pneumophila*. Called legionnaires' disease because

legionnaires *(cont.)*
of an outbreak at a 1976 convention of the American Legion in Philadelphia, when the causative agent was first identified. Patients with this disease have very high fevers, abdominal pain, headaches, and pneumonia. They may also have kidney, liver, and nervous system involvement. According to the CDC, legionellosis is spread with breathing water mists in air conditioner cooler towers, whirlpool spa and showers, but not from household or car air conditioner units.

Lehman cardiac device.

Leibinger miniplate system—see *E-Z Flap*. Also, *Leibinger plate.*

Leibinger Profyle system—a titanium hand and small bone fragment fixation system. This is a plating system for rigid internal fixation of hand fractures.

Leiden factor—see *factor V Leiden.*

LEIs (lower extremity injuries).

Leishmania donovani—an opportunistic parasite found in the GI tract of patients with AIDS. It causes leishmaniasis.

Lejeune syndrome—see *cri du chat.*

Lejour-type breast reduction, modified—breast reduction technique that utilizes a vertical scar. Reportedly, the result is a better breast shape with significantly reduced scars.

Leksell stereotaxic frame—used to place electrodes.

Lemaire reconstruction—extra-articular reconstruction technique using fascia lata.

LeMaitre Glow 'N Tell tape—radiopaque tape with centimeter markings placed on the leg to pinpoint the site of saphenous branches.

lemon sign—concave deformity of the fetal frontal bones seen in association with spina bifida.

LENI (lower extremity noninvasive)—an acronym (usually plural) used to refer to patients checked for emboli in legs. Usage: "LENIs were positive."

Lenke classification of adolescent idiopathic scoliosis—named for Dr. Lawrence Lenke.

Lennox-Gastaut syndrome—mixed seizure disorder.

Lenox Hill brace (*not* Lennox)—knee orthosis.

lens, lenses
AcrySof acrylic foldable intraocular
AcrySof ReSTOR intraocular
Adaptar contact
Alcon MA 60 BM
AMO Array IOL
Artisan intraocular
Bagolini
Baron
BioComFold foldable intraocular
Boston Scleral Lens
CeeOn heparinized intraocular
Cilco Slant
Coburn equiconvex
Collamer foldable intraocular
Dulaney intraocular implant
etafilcon A
Galand disc
Goldmann
heparinized CeeOn intraocular
hollow bandage contact
Hoskins nylon suture laser
Hruby ("ruby")
Hydroview intraocular
ICL (implantable contact lens)
IOL (intraocular)
Karickhoff laser
Leiske
Lieb-Guerry cataract implant

lens *(cont.)*
Mainster retina laser
MemoryLens intraocular
Monoflex
Morgan
Oculaid capsular tension ring
Paragon CRT (paflufocon B)
Paragon CRT 100 (paflufocon D)
Paragon Quadra RG (paflufocon B) contact
Paragon Quadra RG 100 (paflufocon D) contact
PC-IOL
Pearce Tripod implant cataract
PhacoFlex
PMMA (polymethylmethacrylate) contact
Prokop intraocular
Quadra RG (paflufocon B)
Quadra RG 100 (paflufocon D)
RGP (rigid gas permeable) contact
Sauflon PW (lidofilcon B)
SeeQuence II disposable
Sensar intraocular, The
Silsoft extended wear contact
Single-Stitch inserter for PhacoFlex
Slant
SN60AT AcrySof soft foldable
Staar foldable IOL
Staar implantable contact (ICL)
Stableyes capsular tension ring
STAAR Toric implantable contact
TICL contact
T lens
Toric intraocular
Unfolder intraocular, The
Volk Pan Retinal
Volk Quadraspheric fundus
Volk SuperPupil XL
Worst gonioprism contact

lenses, intraocular (IOL). Styles:
anterior chamber IOL (secured in front of iris)
iridocapsular/iris fixation lens or iris plane lens (sewn to iris)

lenses *(cont.)*
posterior chamber IOL (secured in back of iris)

lens lasso—for repositioning of dislocated posterior chamber intraocular lens.

lens-sparing external beam radiation therapy (LSRT)—treatment for patients with diffuse choroidal hemangiomas. Cf. *episcleral plaque brachytherapy.*

lenticular nuclear sclerosis.

lentivirus—a retrovirus.

Leonard Arm (first assistant)—a pneumatic action support device for laparoscopy and endoscopy.

LEOPARD syndrome—acronym for multiple **l**entigines, **e**lectrocardiographic conduction abnormalities, **o**cular hypertelorism, **p**ulmonic stenosis, **a**bnormal genitalia, **r**etardation of growth, and sensorineural **d**efects.

Lepper-Trier formula—a formula for calculating the depth of the anterior chamber of the eye.

leptomeninges—inner two membranes covering the brain and spinal cord.

Leriche syndrome—intermittent claudication of the buttocks and inability to maintain an erection, due to insufficiency of the external iliac arteries.

Lermans-Means scratch—a systolic grating sound heard in the second left intercostal space during expiration in hypertension. It is due to friction between the pleural and pericardial surfaces. Also may refer to a rub heard at the left sternal edge in thyrotoxicosis, possibly due to increased blood flow.

"ler-meet"—phonetic for *Lhermitte* (sign).

LES (lesser esophageal sphincter).

Lesch-Nyhan syndrome—hereditary hyperuricemia.

LES incompetence—lower esophageal sphincter incompetence, which can cause severe esophagitis.

lesion (see also *disease*)
Antopol-Goldman
bull's eye
condylomatous atypia
cyclops
dendritic
DREZ
dysplasia-associated
Essex-Lopresti
frondy
herald patch
hereditary nonpolyposis colorectal cancer (HNPCC)
high-grade squamous intraepithelial (HGSIL)
Hill-Sachs
intradermal neurilemomas
intraductal papillary-mucinous neoplasm (IPMN)
Janeway
jet
low-grade squamous intraepithelial (LGSIL)
Lynch and Crues type 2
macro-orchidism
melanocytic lesions in conjunctiva
micro-crust formation
multifocal choroidal melanoma
osteochondral lesions of the talar dome
PCNSL (primary central nervous system lymphoma)
phlyctenule
pinguecula
satellite
shagreen
SLAP
squamous intraepithelial (SIL)
synchronous airway lesions (SALs)
target (of Lyme disease)

lesioning—a radiofrequency procedure using electrical impulses to interrupt nerve conduction on a semipermanent basis.

Leslie Parachute stone retrieval device.

LESP (lower esophageal sphincter pressure).

Lester Martin modification of the Duhamel procedure—a treatment for Hirschsprung disease.

LET (lidocaine, epinephrine, tetracaine)—acronym for a topical anesthesia mixture.

lethal equivalent (Genetics)—a gene carried in the heterozygous state which, if homozygous, would be lethal.

Letterer-Siwe disease—a fulminant disease with multisystem manifestations, including skin, bone, pulmonary, central nervous system and endocrine features, and hepatosplenomegaly.

lettering artifact (Radiol)—lettering or designs picked up on film from some Band-Aids or underwear marketed for children.

leucine aminopeptidase test.

leucine zipper—investigational chain of amino acids which "zips" up to half of the AIDS virus, preventing replication.

leucovorin rescue—used to decrease the toxicity of folic acid antagonist chemotherapy drugs such as methotrexate and fluorouracil. It rescues normal cells, but not malignant cells, from the toxic effects of the chemotherapy. Also known as *citrovorum factor rescue* and *folinic acid rescue*.

leukanakmesis—arrest of maturation of white cell series.

leukemia
acute lymphoblastic (ALL)
acute lymphocytic (ALL)
acute monoblastic (AMOL)
acute myeloblastic (AML)
acute myelomonoblastic (AMMOL)
acute promyelocytic (APML)
Burkitt-type acute lymphoblastic
chronic lymphocytic (CLL)
chronic myelocytic (CML)
hairy-cell
monoblastic
null cell lymphoblastic

leukemia classification
FAB, M1 (myeloblastic, with no differentiation)
FAB, M2 (myeloblastic, with differentiation)
FAB, M3 (promyelocytic)
FAB, M5 (monocytic)
FAB, M6 (erythroleukemia)

leukemia inhibitory factor (LIF)—a naturally occurring protein (so named because it suppresses development of mouse leukemia cells) that has been used to inhibit differentiation in a stem cell line.

leukocyte alkaline phosphatase test (LAP).

leukocyte esterase—test to detect the presence or absence of white blood cells in the urine. A negative test means that an infection is unlikely and that, without additional evidence of urinary tract infection, microscopic exam and/or urine culture need not be done to rule out significant bacteriuria.

leukocyte-poor red blood cells—red blood cells from which at least 70% of the leukocytes have been removed by a saline-washing process or by centrifuge. Used for patients who have had severe, febrile nonhemolytic reactions to blood transfusion. Also, *leuko-poor red cells*.

leukocyte reduction filter—used during blood products transfusion. It prevents nearly all leukocytes from entering the patient's bloodstream, thus reducing the potential for sensitization in transplant patients.

leukomalacia—degenerative softening of the white matter of the brain.

LeukoNet Filter—removes leukocytes from blood components.

leuko-poor—slang for *leukocyte-poor* (packed red blood cells). Example: "He was immediately transferred to the ICU and received 20 cc/kg of packed RBCs—leuko-poor—as an emergency transfusion due to severe high output cardiac failure from the hemolytic anemia." See *leukocyte-poor red blood cells*.

leuko-reduced platelet product for transfusion—see *Amicus separator*.

Leukotrap RC (red cell) **storage system**—used to reduce transfusion reactions and HLA sensitization by removing the white cells prior to red cell storage.

leukovirus—an RNA virus causing leukemia and tumors.

levatorplasty—surgical approach to physiological reconstruction of the velopharyngeal sphincter.

LeVeen peritoneal shunt—used in peritoneal venous shunt for portal venous drainage in Budd-Chiari syndrome.

lever arm—a term used in orthopedic surgery and positioning.

Levitra (vardenafil HCl)—a medication for the treatment of erectile dysfunction and associated depression.

levonorgestrel and ethinyl estradiol—see *Aviane-28*.

Lewis blood antibody type—a factor in agglutination. Also *Duffy, Kell, Kidd, Lutheran*.

Lewis Pair-Pak needle—a needle with a double-armed suture used in intraocular surgery.

Lewis-Tanner procedure—a subtotal esophagectomy and reconstruction.

Lewis upper limb cardiovascular disease—a congenital disorder.

Lewis-X antigen—urinary marker for transitional cell carcinoma.

"lew-ko-ma-LAY-sha"—phonetic for *leukomalacia.*

Lewy body dementia—a syndrome including dementia, parkinsonism, cognitive fluctuations, and visual hallucinations. It responds to treatment with acetylcholinesterase inhibitors but not to neuroleptics.

Lewy inclusion body—in Parkinson disease.

Lewy suspension laryngoscope.

Lexer gouge (Ortho).

Leydig cells—endocrine cells of the testis, producing testosterone. When Leydig cells are found with Reinke crystals on testicular biopsy of prepubertal boys, they are indicative of precocious puberty.

Lezak Malingering Test (Psych).

LFS (laryngeal framework surgery).

LFS (Li-Fraumeni syndrome).

LFTs (liver function tests).

LGD (low-grade dysplasia).

LGSIL (low-grade squamous intraepithelial lesion)—the term for squamous cellular changes seen on Pap smear that were formerly called mild dysplasia or CIN 1, including cellular atypia characteristic of human papillomavirus infection.

LHE (light- and heat-based electrical) **apparatus**—a device for treating pigmented and vascular lesions and facial skin aging effects, and for acne clearance and hair removal, for medical and aesthetic purposes.

Lhermitte-Duclos disease—dysplastic gangliocytoma of the cerebellum, an uncommon condition seen usually in young and middle-aged adults. It is a benign mass lesion of the cerebellum, probably hamartomatous.

LHMT (low-range heparin management test)—measures lower doses of heparin and is used primarily in diagnostic and interventional cardiology procedures.

LHPs (lateral hypopharyngeal pouches) —protrusions of the lateral hypopharyngeal wall that appear in the intradeglutitive phase of swallowing and disappear in the same or postdeglutitive phase, as seen on radiological studies.

LHRH (luteinizing hormone-releasing hormone)—polypeptide hormone also known as *GnRH* (gonadotropin-releasing hormone). This hormone is used in research on contraception, including contraceptives to be taken by males. It has been used in treatment of precocious puberty, delayed puberty, cryptorchidism, endometriosis, acute intermittent porphyria, and hormone-dependent tumors.

Liberty CMC thumb brace—a hand therapy product.

Liberty One splint—a one-size, ambidextrous wrist splint.

LICA (laser image custom arthroplasty).

lichen planus—a skin disorder.

Lich-Gregoire repair—used in kidney transplant surgery.

Lich technique—for ureteral implantation in transplantation surgery or neobladder construction following total cystectomy.

Lichtenstein hernia repair—tension-free technique consisting of a circumferentially sutured onlay patch. Cf., *mesh plug hernioplasty.*

Lichtenstein open tension-free mesh hernioplasty.

Lichtman radiographic classification of Kienböck disease

Stage 1: Normal except for the possibility of either a linear or compression fracture.

Stage 2: Definite density changes apparent in the lunate.

Stage 3a: Collapse of entire lunate without fixed scaphoid rotation.

Stage 3b: Collapse of entire lunate with fixed scaphoid rotation (significance of stage 3b is that the load is significantly shifted over to the lunate, which will further hasten the collapse).

Stage 4: Stage 3 with generalized degenerative changes in the carpus.

Licox monitoring device—for continuous quantitative regional monitoring of dissolved oxygen and temperature in body fluids and tissues.

LICU (laparoscopic intracorporeal ultrasound).

lid lag—abnormally sluggish movement of the upper eyelid over the eye in exophthalmos. Commonly seen in thyroid disease.

lid margin vascular dilation (brush marks) (Oph).

lidocaine, epinephrine, and tetracaine (LET) **anesthesia**.

Lido Lift—simulates actual work functions, for testing and rehabilitation.

lie (noun)—the relative position of the long axis of a fetus with respect to that of the mother: longitudinal or transverse.

Lieb-Guerry cataract implant lens.

LIF (leukemia inhibitory factor).

LifeCare PCA Plus II infusion system—a patient-controlled analgesia pump.

life-flighted—transported by air ambulance.

LifeGuide system—handheld blood glucose monitor for use by diabetics.

LIFE-Lung fluorescence endoscopy system—allows identification of areas of abnormal fluorescence that may not be visible on white-light examination.

Life-Pack 5 cardiac monitor.

LifePoint Impact—a rapid, noninvasive on-site drug and alcohol test.

LifeShirt—a comfortable shirt with embedded sensors that provide ongoing analysis of vital signs during a patient's waking and sleeping hours.

LifeSite hemodialysis access system—provides dialysis access through the use of a valve implanted below the skin. Reportedly minimizes the pain associated with insertion and removal of a standard dialysis fistula needle. The valve closes immediately after use, providing immediate hemostasis.

Lifestream coronary dilatation catheter.

Lifestream personal cholesterol monitor—a home cholesterol testing device that is connected to a computer. It uses Microsoft Windows-based Smart Card operating system.

LifeVest—a wearable cardiac defibrillator.

Li-Fraumeni syndrome (LFS)—predisposes carriers of the syndrome to cancers including rhabdomyosarcoma, osteosarcoma, brain tumors, leukemia, adrenocortical carcinomas, and breast carcinoma.

LiftMate—patient transfer device.

lift-off test—an orthopedic test to assess partial versus full-thickness tear of subscapularis muscle.

LiftStation—simulates actual work functions, for testing and rehabilitation.

L.I.F.T. (laser-assisted internal fabrication) **technique**.

Ligaclip—used in minimally invasive procedures for surgical dissection.

ligamentization—a process by which a graft transforms into a structure that is similar histologically to the normal anterior cruciate ligament (ACL), particularly after ACL reconstruction with bone-patellar tendon-bone) (BPTB) graft or quadrupled hamstring tendon autograft.

ligamentum teres cardiopexy—also called *esophageal sling procedure*. Entails complete mobilization of the ligamentum teres (round ligament), which is passed behind the esophagus and anchored to the lesser curvature of the stomach. This secures the lower esophageal sphincter in the abdomen. Intraoperative manometry is used to adjust the sphincter pressure. This procedure is done in an attempt to avoid the complications associated with total fundoplication.

ligand (L., to bind)—organic molecules (chemical "superglue") used to bond therapeutic agents to monoclonal antibodies.

ligase chain reaction—uses a thermostabile enzyme ligase to detect a known DNA or RNA sequence in a specimen. See *polymerase chain reaction*.

LigaSure—a hemostasis tool. Not to be confused with ligature; the terms sound similar and can be used similarly in a sentence.

ligature—see *suture ligature*.

light-chain deposition—a disease process closely related to light-chain amyloidosis that can occur in patients with immunoproliferative disorders. Cf. *heavy-chain deposition*.

light reflection rheography—imaging procedure that detects deep vein thrombosis using near-infrared light. The light is beamed from diodes to a depth of 1-2 mm into the skin. In the absence of disease, dorsiflexion of the foot will empty the venous plexus of the calf, reduce the amount of light absorbed, and result in an increased signal. In chronic venous insufficiency, light absorption is reduced to 10-15 seconds. In deep vein thrombosis, light absorption is reduced to less than 10 seconds, showing significantly reduced venous emptying.

light reflex—constriction of the pupil in response to light striking the retina.

LightSheer and **LightSheer SC**—high-performance diode laser hair removal system.

Lightstic 180, Lightstic 360—fiberoptic lasers that diffuse the laser light laterally rather than out the end of the fiber. This reportedly allows physicians to heat and destroy diseased cells in a less invasive and therefore less costly procedure.

Light Talker—a computerized communication device (designed by Dr. Janice Light) which enables patients who are unable to speak (due to neurological or traumatic injuries) to convey messages. With a movement even as slight as raising an eyebrow, the patient can indicate a selection which is spoken by a speech synthesizer or printed out on paper.

"lig-sill"—phonetic for *LGSIL* (low-grade squamous intraepithelial lesion).

LILI (low-intensity laser irradiation).

Liliequist membrane—located near the pituitary gland and stalk.

Lilliput—neonatal oxygenator for use in ECMO.

LILT (low-intensity laser therapy).

LIMA (left internal mammary artery) **graft**—used in coronary artery surgery. Usage: "He underwent quadruple coronary artery bypass grafting, including LIMA."

LIMA-Lift—used to provide a window into the chest cavity, allowing the surgeon to efficiently harvest the left internal mammary artery (LIMA) for use as a bypass conduit around the blocked area in MIDCAB, minimizing incisions.

LIMA-Loop—enables the surgeon to reach into the chest to help isolate the left internal mammary artery (LIMA) for harvest during MIDCAB.

limbal groove.

limbectomy—surgical excision of any limbus (anatomic rim or margin), used in both orthopedics and ophthalmology. Acetabular limbectomy is used to treat congenital hip dislocation, and lacunar limbectomy to treat glaucoma.

Limberg flap closure—used (in addition to rhomboid excision) in treatment of sacrococcygeal pilonidal sinus.

limb length discrepancy developmental causes
- avascular necrosis of hip
- hip dislocation
- idiopathic
- Klippel-Trenaunay-Weber syndrome
- linear scleroderma
- local tumor
- melorheostosis
- neuromuscular
- osteomyelitis
- slipped capital femoral epiphysis
- talectomy
- trauma

limb-sparing technique—see *rotationplasty.*

limbus corneae—the edge of the cornea where it joins the sclera.

Limitrol-DM—a fat-free chewable wafer form of the herb fenugreek (*Trigonella foenum-graecum*) that assists diabetic patients in achieving tight blood glucose control.

***Limulus* amoebocyte lysate** (LAL) **test**—see *LAL test*.

LINAC or **linac radiosurgery** (Neuro) —a coined word or acronym referring to *linear accelerator*. It is written in all capitals in some medical journals and in lowercase letters in others. Its form as a word will probably follow the pattern of *laser* and *radar*, terms which came into the language as initialisms and quickly became accepted as acronyms.

Lindholm operating laryngoscope.

Lindorf lag screws or **position screws** —used in sagittal split ramus osteotomy.

Lindseth modified technique—treatment of spinal deformity in patients with myelomeningocele with kyphectomy with wire fixation and posterior and anterior spinal fusion. In modification of Lindseth technique, the wires are crisscrossed posteriorly, said to result in better stability at the osteotomy site.

Lindstrom arcuate incision marker (Oph).

line, lines
- arterial
- Beau
- bite
- Cantlie
- cell
- Commander PTCA wire
- Cyma
- Fine Lines
- Fleischner
- gas density

line *(cont.)*
germ
gray
Hilgenreiner
Hudson-Stahli
isodose
Kerley A (B or C)
Köhler
Langer
lead
Lorentzian
Mees
Muehrcke
Sampaolesi
scorbutic white
subcutaneous fat
Toldt
TPN (total parenteral nutrition)
trough
Vogt
white line of Toldt
Whiteside
Zahn

lineage—the descendants of a common ancestor.

linear accelerator (LINAC or linac) **radiosurgery**—*not* radiotherapy. A single exposure of multiple radiation beams is used to eradicate tumor tissue. Cf. *Gamma Knife*.

linear cutter stapler.

line imaging—MRI term.

line of Zahn—a phenomenon due to the layering of fibrin and blood cells in a clot.

line scanning—MRI term.

lines of election—the lines of skin tension that surgeons use when they plan incisions in facial or cosmetic surgery.

line width—MRI term.

linezolid—see *Zyvox*.

lingoscope—an endoscope (modified laryngoscope) used to facilitate visualization of the base of the tongue and excision of the lingual tonsils.

lingualplasty—partial glossectomy of the tongue base.

linguine sign—multiple wavy lines in the breast seen on MRI scan as the classic sign of silicone implant rupture.

linitis plastica—see *leather-bottle stomach*.

linkage (Genetics)—the nearness of two gene loci on the same chromosome, a measure of the likelihood of their being transmitted together.

linkage disequilibrium—the tendency of two linked alleles to occur together on the same chromosome more frequently than would be expected.

Link cementless reconstruction hip prosthesis.

Link Endo-Model rotational knee—total knee replacement prostheses.

Link Lubinus SP II—anatomically adapted total hip replacement system.

Link Stack Split splint—finger splint with a split down the middle, for ease of application and removal.

Linton procedure—treatment of varicose veins using open subfascial division technique.

Linvatec cannulated interference screw—used in knee arthroscopy.

Linvatec microdebrider—power instrument used for sinonasal tract surgery.

LINX-EZ cardiac device.

LionHeart left ventricular assist device (LVAD)—totally implantable device.

lion jaw tenaculum (Ortho).

LIP (lymphocytic interstitial pneumonitis).

lipid-associated sialic acid—a nonspecific tumor-associated marker seen on serum assays for the presence of gynecological malignancies.

lipid-laden macrophage index (LLMI) —a laboratory test performed on bronchoalveolar lavage (BAL) fluid in the diagnosis of aspiration pneumonia.

lipid storage disease—see *Fabry disease.*

lip lift—a plastic surgery procedure in which skin is removed at the base of the nostril, hiding the incision directly in the nasal sill. This procedure may or may not be performed as an adjunct to corner mouth lift. See *corner mouth lift*.

lipoid nephrosis—see *nil disease*.

lipophilic—fat-loving, in reference to stains. Cf. *hydrophilic*, water-loving.

liposhaver—a handheld device with a sharp orifice and sharp edges that oscillates and takes rapid "bites" of tissue, which are then suctioned away. Originally designed for use in sinus surgery, the liposhaver is now being used to remove fat from the neck and chin without the trauma associated with liposuction. See *XPS Sculpture System.*

liposomes, encapsulated—particles of water surrounded by a membrane of phospholipids. They hold (or encapsulate) certain drugs such as amphotericin B (to treat severe systemic fungal infections), doxorubicin (to treat various types of cancer), and TLC G-65 (an antibiotic to treat MAI infection), reducing drug toxicity and unwanted side effects.

Liposorber LA-15 System—a machine that removes LDL cholesterol by filtering all the blood in a patient's body. The blood slowly passes from a tube placed in one arm, through a machine which separates plasma from other cells, through the Liposorber which filters the bad cholesterol out of the plasma, and then is returned to the body via a tube in the patient's other arm. Used in patients with severe hypercholesterolemia uncontrolled by medicine or diet. The procedure is not a cure and must be repeated indefinitely.

liposuction-assisted nerve-sparing radical abdominal hysterectomy (LANS-RH)—a procedure in which potentially tumor-bearing pelvic tissue is resected. It may improve the detection of occult tumor cell deposits.

liquid crystal thermography (LCT).

Liquiderm liquid healing bandage—for treatment of minor cuts and abrasions. It creates a moist wound-healing environment and provides a barrier to infection.

Liquid Ice—reusable cooling and compression wrap that needs no refrigeration and provides cooling for up to 2 hours.

LIS (lung injury score).

Lisch spots—nodules on the iris seen on slit lamp exam.

Liss CES device—see *cranial electrical stimulation.*

LISS (less invasive stabilization system) **plating**.

listening areas for auscultation of heart murmurs—A (aortic), P (pulmonic), T (tricuspid), and M (mitral) valves.

***Listeria* meningitis**—often seen in neonates but also in the immunocompromised and the elderly.

Listerine PocketPaks—oral care strip that dissolves instantly on the tongue to reportedly kill germs and freshen breath.

Lister tubercle—located in the wrist, near the posterior interosseous nerve.

listing gait—leaning toward one side when walking.

LiteNest portable seating system—for wheelchairs, chairs, or 3-wheel scooters.

lithiumogenic goiter—caused by lithium therapy, which is used to treat bipolar affective disorders, major depression, and schizoaffective disorders.

LithoCatch immobilization device.

Lithostar—a lithotriptor. With the Lithostar, the patient is treated on a table and requires no anesthesia. In earlier lithotripsy treatment, the patient was immersed in water, and the shock waves that disintegrated the stones were conducted through the water.

lithotripsy—ultrasonic lithotripsy, electrohydraulic lithotripsy, and laser lithotripsy. The medium used in laser lithotripsy is coumarin dye (*not* Coumadin).

lithotripsy, extracorporeal shock wave—procedure for treating upper urinary tract stones. See *lithotriptor*.

lithotriptor (or *lithotripter*)—an extracorporeal stone-disintegrating machine. It generates shock waves that are focused on the kidney stones to break them up. The patient is immersed in water while the shock waves are generated. The disintegrated stones are then passed in the urine over a several-day period.

Calcutript lithotripter
DoLi S extracorporeal shock wave
Dornier gallstone lithotriptor
Lithostar lithotriptor
Modulith SL 20 lithotriptor
Piezolith-EPL (extracorporeal piezoelectric lithotriptor)
Sonolith Praktis
Swiss lithoclast

lithotrite—an instrument used to grasp and crush large stones occurring in the bladder.

litmus test—for acidity and alkalinity. Cf. *Titmus test*.

LITT (laser-induced thermotherapy).

Littleford-Spector introducer—allows the rapid and atraumatic insertion of one or more permanent pacemaker electrodes into the heart using a peel-away sheath in the subclavian vein. Also known as *subclavian peel-away sheath, permanent lead introducer*.

Little League elbow (also *pitcher's elbow*)—a condition that affects professional baseball players. It is now seen in children ages 7 to 15 years whose coaches and parents encourage more training time. Little League players are at greater risk than professionals because they overtrain when they throw, relax their elbows less quickly, and do not have the arm strength of older players.

littoral cell angioma—benign vascular tumor unique to the spleen. Patients present clinically with splenomegaly, thrombocytopenia, or anemia. In many cases the tumor is discovered incidentally during abdominal surgery performed for another reason.

Littre, glands of—glands in the distal urethra of the male where gonococcal infection usually begins.

live flesh—a term used by patients to describe their condition of having multiple fasciculations.

liver-directed ex vivo gene therapy—treatment for homozygous familial hypercholesterolemia.

liver flap—asterixis; a coarse flapping tremor of the hands, so called because it is often seen in hepatic failure.

liver function tests (LFTs).

Livernois lens-holding forceps—having thin jaws for use in insertion of thin soft intraocular lenses.

Livernois-McDonald forceps—for use in ophthalmic surgical procedures.

liver palms—intense redness of the hypothenar and thenar eminences, suggestive of cirrhosis of the liver on physical examination.

liver panel plus 9 (LAB)—a reagent disc product that is designed to measure hepatic function.

liver span (the size of the liver)—the distance between the upper and lower limits of hepatic dullness, as determined by percussion. Normal range is 6 to 12 cm, depending upon the age, sex, and size of the patient.

Livewire Duo-Decapolar—electrophysiology catheter.

Livewire TC ablation catheter—electrophysiologic catheter for diagnosis and treatment of supraventricular tachycardia.

LLC (labrum-ligament complex).

LLD (late-life depression).

LLETZ (large loop excision of the transformation zone).

LLMI (lipid-laden macrophage index).

Llorente dissecting forceps—used with EndoMed laparoscopic systems.

Lloyd-Davies scissors.

LLPDD (late luteal phase dysphoric disorder).

LLS (lazy leukocyte syndrome).

LMA-Unique—a disposable laryngeal mask airway used in elective surgery and for emergency cases.

LMR (localized magnetic resonance)—MRI term.

LNOP Neo (Low Noise Optical Probe Neonatal Y) **adhesive sensor**.

load arm—a term used in orthopedic surgery and positioning.

loading dose—an initial dose of a medication, larger than the subsequent maintenance doses, given in order to achieve effective blood and tissue levels promptly.

loath (adj.)—reluctant, unwilling. Usage: "The patient is loath to undertake surgery at this time, so we will follow her closely for a while longer." Cf. *loathe*.

loathe (verb)—dislike intensely; hate; detest. Cf. *loath*.

lobules (plural of lobule).

localizing or **focal neurological signs**—indicate the location of a lesion to the neurologist. See *soft neurological signs*.

Locke clamp—used in podiatric surgery to grasp the phalanx, metatarsal, or sesamoid.

locked-in syndrome—a rare neurological disorder characterized by complete paralysis of voluntary muscles in all parts of the body except for those that control eye movement. Possible causes are traumatic brain injury, circulatory system diseases, myelin sheath destruction, or medication overdose. Patients are conscious and can think and reason, but cannot speak or move. Some communication may be possible with eye-blinking.

locker room syndrome—see *isovaleric acidemia*.

loculated effusion—on chest x-ray, a collection of fluid in the pleural space; its distribution is limited by adjacent normal or abnormal structures.

locus (plural, loci) (Genetics)—the normal position of a gene on a particular chromosome. A chromosome consists of a short arm and a long arm, which are joined at the cen-

locus *(cont.)*
tromere. Genes are arrayed in linear sequence along each arm of each chromosome. Differential staining of chromosomes allows genes to be grouped in regions, bands, subbands, and sub-subbands. A locus designation (e.g., 3q21.12) consists of the following elements: (1) chromosome number (or, for a sex chromosome, X or Y); (2) chromosome arm (p for short arm, q for long arm); (3) region and band numbers, written together as a 2-digit numeral; (4) a period; (5) subband and sub-subband numbers, written together as a 2-digit numeral.

locus of HLA (human leukocyte antigen)—used in tissue typing for transplants. Each HLA locus (A, B, C, D, or DR) contains multiple alleles. Some 19 alleles have thus far been identified at locus A, 20 at locus B, 8 at locus C, 10 at locus D, and 10 at locus DR. These are written HLA-C8, HLA-DR2, etc. (no subscript or superscript).

Löffler syndrome (also Loeffler)—chronic eosinophilic pneumonia.

logorrhea—extreme loquacity; a copious flow of talk, often incoherent.

loin pain hematuria syndrome (LPHS)—occurs mostly in women. Symptoms of LPHS include loin pain and hematuria, usually bilateral, and often accompanied by dysuria and low-grade fever. LPHS is difficult to diagnose because renal function is normal, urine cultures are negative, and IVPs and renal biopsies are negative. The true cause is unknown and the diagnosis is made by excluding other pathologies. The pain can become so severe that nerve blockade, nephrectomy, and even renal transplantation have been tried as treatments. Narcotics for pain relief remain the only effective therapy.

LOL—jargon for *little old lady*. (Instant messagers use "LOL" for *laughing out loud*.)

LOM (low-osmolar media) (Radiol). Cf. *HOM, ionic contrast media*. See *nonionic contrast media*.

lone AF (atrial fibrillation)—the appearance of atrial fibrillation in young individuals (under 60 years of age) without clinical or echocardiographic evidence of cardiopulmonary disease. Cf. *nonvalvular AF*.

Lone Star retractor—used to facilitate surgical access during a mucosal proctectomy and said to eliminate the need for anal dilatation and the use of a Gelpi retractor. Produced by Lone Star Medical Products of Houston, Texas, this self-retaining retractor encircles the anus and uses eight elastic holders, or stays, around the anal circumference (which gives the instrument a star-shaped appearance) to hold back all edges of the anal canal.

long-acting thyroid-stimulating hormone (LATS).

long-echo-train fast spin-echo sequence—MRI term.

long-edge medullary nail (Ortho).

Long45 endocutter—has a shaft 4 inches longer than other endocutters that allows easier access during laparoscopic weight loss surgery, such as gastric bypass, where longer instruments are needed to reach inside to the stomach area of morbidly obese patients (those 100 pounds or more overweight or with a body mass index of more than 40).

long Gamm locking nail—used in repair of complex femoral fractures.

longitudinal magnetization; **relaxation**—MRI terms.

longitudinal melanonychia—a mole-like lesion of the nail matrix that mimics the appearance of malignant melanoma. Excision is usually performed to rule out malignancy. It is rare and more common in non-Caucasians.

Longo hemorrhoidectomy—uses a supra-anodermal resection stapling technique to treat prolapsing hemorrhoids.

long PFN (proximal femoral nail)—a modified reconstruction nail which can be inserted percutaneously in patients with femoral metastases.

long QT syndrome (LQTS)—an inherited or acquired disorder of the heart's electrical system. The syndrome gets its name from a characteristic markedly elongated QT interval on an electrocardiogram. People with LQTS are prone to develop an extremely rapid heart rhythm, often brought on by exercise, emotion, or loud noise. This improper rhythm interferes with blood flow to the brain and can result in fainting or cardiac arrest. See *acquired long QT syndrome* and *left cardiac sympathetic denervation*.

long taper/stiff shaft Glidewire—used in coronary artery imaging.

long-term nonprogressors—individuals with HIV who have had at least 10 years of seropositivity, without symptoms or T-cell depletion, in the absence of therapy.

long-term self-renewal—the persistence of a stem cell line for months or years due to repeated divisions forming the same undifferentiated cell types.

long tract—the main spinal nerve fibers and their pathways connecting the spinal cord and the brain. See *long tract signs*.

long tract signs—seen in patients with upper neuron damage. Include the upgoing great toe on the Babinski, twitching of the thumb on the Hoffmann, and twitching of the chin on the palmomental test.

long TR/TE (also, *T2 weighted*)—MRI term. TR (repetition time); TE (echo time).

"loo-ee"—phonetic for *Luys, body of*.

loop—oval, closed or nearly closed turn in a tube, suture, rope, or figure. Example: loop of bowel, sentinel loop. Cf. *loupe*.

loop electrosurgical excision procedure (LEEP)—used to treat precancerous lesions of the cervix, in addition to laser and cryosurgery techniques. A wire loop through which radio waves are conducted is used to excise cervical tissue. LEEP allows cervical specimens to be excised and examined by the pathologist.

loopogram—ileostogram.

loopostomy—a contraction of "loop ileostomy." It should be transcribed as dictated. This is an excellent illustration of how new medical words are coined and eventually weave their way into common use.

Looser zones—in insufficiency fractures.

lop ears repair—see *Furnas otoplasty technique*.

LoPro—right angle ArthroWand.

LORAD StereoGuide stereotactic breast biopsy system.

Lord total hip prosthesis—uses no cement; instead, its rough surface

Lord *(cont.)*
stimulates growth of new bone in the medullary canal, and the growth of new cancellous bone incorporates the prosthesis into the structure of the limb. Also known as *madreporic hip*.

Lorentzian line—MRI term.

Lorenz PC/TC scissors ultrasharp knife (Surg).

Lortat-Jacob hepatic resection—used to gain initial vascular control prior to liver resection by ligating the hepatic artery, the portal vein, and the hepatic veins, followed by liver parenchymal transection.

Lotronex (alosetron, "ah-LOW-se-tron")—a serotonin antagonist used to treat irritable bowel syndrome (IBS) in women who have diarrhea as their main symptom.

lottery fantasy syndrome—a form of psychological depression that can occur in lottery purchasers when they think they will win and don't.

Louis-Bar syndrome—ataxia telangiectasia.

loupe ("loop")—convex lens in a short tube, used for magnifying or for concentrating light on an object. Used by ophthalmologists, microsurgeons, and jewelers. Cf. *loop*.

Lovaas program—behavior modification technique for the treatment of autism, based on the work of Ivar Lovaas.

Lovibond angle—the angle at which the fingernail meets the finger, normally less than 180°, but exceeding this in clubbing of the fingers.

Low-Beers projection (Radiol).

low-density lipoprotein (LDL)—the so-called bad cholesterol linked with arteriosclerosis and myocardial infarctions. This is a plasma protein which carries cholesterol through the blood. At high levels it increases risk of arteriosclerosis and heart attack. Cf. *high-density lipoprotein*.

low-dose interferon—a less costly and less toxic alternative to high-dose interferon. Interferon plays a critical role in immune system modulation. Low-dose interferon is used or under study in the treatment of AIDS, hepatitis, Sjögren syndrome, lupus, and more.

low-dose screen-film technique—a radiographic technique designed to provide adequate imaging with less radiation than conventionally.

low-energy lasers (LELs)—used in sports medicine to promote healing and reduce pain associated with tendinitis, bursitis, tennis elbow, and other musculoskeletal injuries. May be used to stimulate cellular repair and treat wounds and soft tissue disorders, arthritis, and peripheral neuropathies. The infrared gallium arsenide and the visible helium-neon (HeNe) lasers are the most common LELs. Also called *cold, low-power*, or *soft lasers, low-intensity laser therapy*.

lower extremity injuries (LEIs)—surgically treated with pedicled flap and microsurgical free-tissue transfer technique.

lower extremity noninvasive (LENI).

lower soft-tissue attenuation of the accordion sign (Radiol)—represents marked thickening of the haustral folds due to intramural edema.

Lowe syndrome—inborn error of metabolism resulting in mental retardation, cataracts and glaucoma, muscular dystrophy, and renal tubular defect for amino acids.

low-grade squamous intraepithelial lesion (LGSIL).

low-grade temp—edit to "low-grade temperature" or, for accuracy, "low-grade fever." Dictators often erroneously say "temperature" when they mean "fever."

low-intensity laser therapy (LILT)—see *low-energy lasers*.

low-intensity pulsed ultrasound—found to promote fracture healing. This is the diagnostic range ultrasound, not the usual higher-frequency therapeutic ultrasound.

Lown-Ganong-Levine syndrome—a combination of short P-R interval and short QRS complex demonstrated by electrocardiography, and including paroxysmal tachycardia.

low normal—a quantitative test result that is near the lower limit of normal, though within the normal range.

low-osmolar media—see *high-osmolar media*.

low-range heparin management test (LHMT).

low-resistance rolling seal spirometer.

low signal intensity—MRI term.

low-surface reactive bioglass—a bioceramic joint replacement material.

low-tension glaucoma (Oph)—occurs with a sudden increase in pressure in the eye, with resulting damage to the optic nerve.

low urethral pressure (LUP).

low-velocity, variable-amplitude (LVVA) **maneuvers**—a chiropractic joint mobilization technique.

low-voltage microampe stimulation (LV-MS, microcurrent)—similar to TENS, considered experimental for the relief of pain.

Lp(a)—an apolipoprotein (cholesterol-carrying protein) that has been found to be a separate and distinct risk factor (besides total serum cholesterol and triglycerides, smoking, hypertension) for premature atherosclerotic peripheral vascular disease. Lp(a) levels, measured by electroimmunoassay, greater than 30 mg/dL, are considered a risk factor.

LPI (Laser Photonics, Inc.) **laser system**—an excimer laser system for treatment of psoriasis.

LPPS (low-pressure plasma spray) **hydroxyapatite**—for cementless fixation.

LR (length ratio)

LRT (living related transplant).

LRUT (locally made rapid urease test) —a test for detecting *Helicobacter pylori*, the pathogen that can cause duodenal ulcers.

LSC (laser scanning cytometry).

L-shaped trocar.

LSIL (low-grade squamous intraepithelial lesion).

LSKMT, no—slang for no liver, spleen, kidney masses or tenderness.

L/S ratio—a test on amniotic fluid (by amniocentesis) to determine the maturity of the fetal lungs. Lecithin and sphingomyelin are the two phospholipids which comprise surfactant. Low levels of surfactant contribute to hyaline membrane disease in premature infants. Cf. *lamellar body density count*.

LSRT (lens-sparing external beam radiation therapy).

LSU (Louisiana State University) **reciprocation-gait orthosis**—bracing device for use by paralytic patients or patients who would otherwise be confined to wheelchairs. It gives structural support to the trunk and lower extremities and consists of a system of cables and joint-locking devices.

LTAC (long-term acute care) **facility**.

LTACH (long-term acute care hospital).

LT-Cage lumbar tapered fusion device—used with InFuse bone graft in spinal fusion surgery.

LTD (laser trabeculodissection).

LTK (laser thermal keratoplasty).

LUA (Legionella Urinary Antigen).

Lubri-Flex stent—a hydrophilic-coated urologic stent with inner lumen hydrogel coating to ensure ease of placement over a guidewire.

lucent defect—abnormal zone of decreased resistance to x-rays.

Lucentis (ranibizumab), formerly AMD-Fab—an anti-VEGF antibody fragment drug for the treatment of the wet form of age-related macular degeneration.

LUCs (large undifferentiated cells)—may be dictated in the differential leukocyte count.

Ludington test—to determine a rupture of the long head of the biceps tendon. The patient is seated and clasps both hands on top of the head, supporting the weight of the upper limbs. The patient then alternately contracts and relaxes the biceps muscles. The test is positive if the examiner cannot palpate the long head of the biceps tendon of the affected arm during the contractions.

Ludloff fleck—intercondylar notch line.

Ludwig angina—infection of the deep tissues of the neck and floor of the mouth. The resultant swelling can push the tongue up and back, interfering with breathing. Edema of the glottis can occur and the process can be fatal before fluctuation or redness of the neck occurs. Antibiotics have made this a rare condition.

Luhr fixation system.

Lukes-Collins classification—of non-Hodgkin lymphoma.

Luki aspirating tube (ENT).

"luko-malasha"—phonetic for *leukomalacia*.

LULA (laparoscopy under local anesthesia).

Luma cervical imaging system—helps to determine areas of possible cancerous lesions. Without touching the patient, a 12-second optical scan of a woman's entire cervix is carried out. Areas of the cervix with high-grade precancerous lesions are identified and displayed on a color video image of the patient's cervix. The clinician uses the image of high-grade disease areas in combination with colposcopy to select locations to biopsy.

lumbar anterior-root stimulator implant (LARSI)—a surgically placed device that stimulates the roots of the lower spinal nerves supplying the muscles of the leg. It is hoped the LARSI implant will enable some paraplegic patients to stand with support and walk short distances.

Lumina guidewire—coated guidewire with radiopaque gold markings.

Lumiscan 150 scanner.

Lumiwand—light used in eye examination.

LUNA (laparoscopic uterine nerve ablation)—procedure for treatment of pelvic pain by disruption of the uterine nerves.

LUNA (laser uterosacral nerve ablation).

lunate prosthesis—for the lunate bone of the wrist, fashioned of acrylic cement.

Lund Browder burn diagram, modified—diagram of the anterior and

Lund *(cont.)*
posterior aspects of the human body, divided into segments; used in estimating the percentage of burned body tissue area. One of these diagrams is made at each surgery, to show the areas covered with skin, skin grafts, donor sites, biosynthetic grafts, or xenografts. These will provide a continuous picture of the progress of the coverage of the burn wounds. Note: No hyphen in *Lund Browder.*

Lunderquist guidewires (*not* Linderquist)—used with a Chiba needle for percutaneous stone manipulation, and in catheter cholangiography. Also, *Chiba needle, fine needle, Skinny needle*.

Lunderquist-Ring torque guide—used in catheter cholangiography, and in maintaining long-term percutaneous antegrade biliary drainage.

lung diffusion test—measures how well oxygen passes from the air sacs in the lungs into the blood. The patient inhales a single breath from a volume of gas containing a known small amount of carbon monoxide, holds the breath for 10 seconds, then rapidly exhales. The exhaled gas is then analyzed to determine the amount of carbon monoxide that was absorbed during the breath.

lung volume reduction surgery (LVRS)—involves an innovative surgical stapling technique for removing emphysematous lung tissue, using bovine pericardium strips to reinforce surgical staple lines and thus prevent persistent air leaks along the staple lines.

lunula (pl., lunulae)—crescent-shaped light-colored area at the base of the fingernail. Usage: "Examination of the thumb reveals swelling and tenderness over the lunula and paronychial margin medially, with some pus seen under the nail."

LUP (low urethral pressure) (Urol).

lupus pernio—seen in sarcoidosis as violaceous, shiny patches on the skin of the face, fingers, and toes.

Luque rods and sublaminar wires—used in spinal fusion for scoliosis.

LUS (laparoscopic ultrasound; ultrasonography).

Lusk instruments—for pediatric endoscopic sinus surgery.

lutein—yellow pigment from the corpus luteum. Lutein change in the ovary is revealed by the amount of lutein remaining of an egg cell which secretes hormones to support a pregnancy.

lutein and zeaxanthin—a formulation of two carotenoids, which are found in some vegetables. There is some evidence that intake of carotenoids can reduce the risk of age-related macular degeneration and cataracts.

luteinizing hormone-releasing hormone. See *LHRH, GnRH.*

Lutrin—photosensitizer drug for photodynamic therapy of patients with recurrent breast cancer to the chest wall.

Luxtec fiberoptic system—a fiberoptic light source for diagnostic and surgical visualization; used with arthroscopes and endoscopes.

luxury perfusion (Neuro)—abnormally increased flow of blood to an area of the brain, leading to swelling. Causes include trauma, nearby cerebral infarction, and epileptogenic focus.

Luys ("lou-ee")—see *body of Luys.*

LVAS (left ventricular assist system) **implantable pump**. See *HeartMate; Novacor.*

LVgram—slang for *left ventriculogram.*

LVOTO (left ventricular outflow tract obstruction).

LVRS (lung volume reduction surgery).

LVVA (low-velocity, variable-amplitude) **maneuvers**.

LX 20 laser—used in skin rejuvenation procedures.

Lyme disease ("lime")—named for Old Lyme, Connecticut, where the disease, transmitted by the bite of the deer tick, was first recognized. The infectious agent is the spirochete, *Borrelia burgdorferi*. The first manifestations of Lyme disease are a skin rash at the site of the bite, chills, fever, flu-like symptoms, drowsiness, fatigue, joint swelling, headache, which responds to antibiotics. There may be a second stage of the disease, with cardiac irregularities, meningitis symptoms, and, rarely, paralysis. Third-stage symptoms are arthritis, and occasionally skin and neurologic manifestations.

Lyme lymphocytic meningoradiculitis—causes respiratory failure in patients with Lyme disease. Also called *Garin-Bujadoux-Bannwarth syndrome.*

lym-1 monoclonal antibody—labeled with iodine 131. Used to treat B-cell lymphoma.

lymphadenopathy syndrome (LAS)—considered by some to be a prodrome to development of AIDS.

lymphangioleiomyomatosis (LAM)—lung disease that affects only women; abnormal muscle cells invade the lung and airways, as well as blood and lymph vessels, causing them to become obstructed.

lymphapheresis—removal of peripheral blood lymphocytes; used on an experimental basis as pretreatment in rejection of liver transplants.

lymphatic mapping—a staging tool for breast cancer and melanoma.

Lymphedema Alert bracelet—worn by breast cancer survivors to protect them from receiving treatment to their affected arm or arms that could trigger onset of lymphedema. Treatments triggering the problem include blood pressure measurements, injections, blood draws, and chemotherapy.

lymphedema praecox—the classic form of primary lymphedema, seen mostly in young women in their early twenties.

lymph node location system of the neck—developed by the Memorial Sloan-Kettering Group:

Level I—submental group and submandibular group
Level II—upper jugular group
Level III—middle jugular group
Level IV—lower jugular group
Level V—posterior triangle group
Level VI—anterior compartment group

lymphocyte activating factor (LAF)—see *interleukin-1.*

lymphocytic choriomeningitis virus (LCMV)—arenavirus seen in intrauterine LCMV infection, causing fetal or neonatal death, as well as hydrocephalus and chorioretinitis in infants. LCMV may be a frequent cause of central nervous system disease in newborns.

lymphocytic colitis—see *microscopic colitis.*

lymphocytic interstitial pneumonitis (LIP)—once a rare pulmonary disease and now seen more frequently in AIDS patients.

lymphogranuloma venereum (LGV)—caused by a strain of *Chlamydia.* Also called *fifth venereal disease.*

lymphokines—a group of substances produced by various stimulated cells of the immune system, which include interferons and interleukin-2. See *interleukin-2*.

lymphoplasmacytic lymphoma—cellular classification of one type of lymphoma.

lymphoscintigraphy—peritumor injection of filtered technetium sulfur colloid, followed by gamma camera scanning. It is used to document nodal basins at risk for metastatic breast cancer. Images are obtained of the breast, sternum, and axilla.

Lynch and Crues Type 2 lesion—seen in the knee on MRI scan when the subchondral plate is interrupted.

Lynch syndrome I and **Lynch syndrome II**—also known as hereditary nonpolyposis colorectal cancer (HNPCC). The Lynch syndromes are rare hereditary disorders that cause cancer to develop in the colorectal area, but it can occur in other sites.

Lyodura dura mater graft—harvested from cadavers and processed.

LYOfoam dressing—its gas-permeable design reduces wound maceration. Also, *LYOfoam C* and *LYOfoam tracheostomy dressings*.

lyophilized—freeze-dried, as in frozen corneal tissue used for lamellar keratoplasty.

LyP (lymphomatoid papulosis).

Lyra laser system—for treatment of leg veins. The extended pulse duration technology may be used for hair removal.

Lyrica (pregabalin capsules)—for the management of neuropathic pain associated with diabetic peripheral neuropathy and postherpetic neuralgia.

Lysholm knee score—a subjective evaluation system with eight categories: instability, pain, locking, swelling, support, limp, stairs, and squatting. Used in association with tests like Lachman, drawer, pivot-shift.

lyssa inclusion body (lowercase *l)*—found in rabies. Also, *Negri body*.

lytic lesion (or osteolytic)—a disease or abnormality resulting from or consisting of focal breakdown of bone, with reduction in density.

M, m

m (meta-stable)—in technetium, as in ^{99m}Tc or Tc 99m.

MAb, MoAb, MCAb (monoclonal antibody).

MaBeX, Mabex—a mixture of Maalox, Benadryl, and Xylocaine.

MAC (Miami Acute Care) **collar**—for cervical support.

MAC (minimal alveolar concentration) of an anesthetic agent.

MAC (monitored anesthesia care).

MAC anesthesia—bupivacaine (Marcaine), adrenaline, and cocaine.

MacConkey agar—culture medium.

MACE (major adverse cardiac events).

MACE (Malone antegrade continence enema.

Macewen ("mak-u´enz") **sign**—written with lowercase first *e*. See *cracked pot sign*.

machinery murmur—a rumbling cardiac murmur, continuous through systole and diastole with only slight variation in pitch and intensity. It is heard in patent ductus arteriosus.

MAC (*Mycobacterium avium* complex) **infection**—frequently seen in AIDS patients. Also called *Battey-avium complex*.

Mackay-Marg tonometer—measures intraocular pressure.

Mackinnon-Dellon Disc-Criminator—an instrument used to assess two-point discrimination.

macro-, a prefix meaning large or abnormally big in size. Cf. *micro-*.

macrodacryocystography—see *digital subtraction macrodacryocystography.*

macrolides—a class of antibiotics similar in effectiveness to penicillin and erythromycin but with fewer side effects. Particularly effective against *Mycoplasma pneumoniae* and resistant strains of *Haemophilus influenzae.*

macrometastasis—a grossly evident metastasis.

macro-orchidism (Urol).

macrophage colony-forming cells (M-CFC).

Macroplastique implant—placed between the midurethra and the bladder neck to resolve or diminish stress urinary incontinence by augmenting the function of the bladder neck sphincteric mechanism.

macroscopic magnetization vector.

Macrotec (technetium ^{99m}Tc albumin).

Macugen (pegaptanib sodium injection)—drug for the treatment for neovascular ("wet") age-related macular degeneration, the leading cause of severe vision loss in patients over the age of 50. It is the first in a new class of ophthalmic drugs known as vascular endothelial growth factor (VEGF) inhibitors.

macula—a spot or area which can be distinguished by color or other characteristic from surrounding tissue; often refers to the macula retinae.

macular degeneration—see *dry age-related macular degeneration* and *wet age-related macular degeneration.*

macular fan; macular star—a fan- or star-shaped folding or pleating of the retina due to edema.

macular rash (Derm).

MAD (mandibular advancement device).

Madayag biopsy needle—used for fine-needle percutaneous aspiration/biopsy, percutaneous pancreatic aspiration biopsy, renal cystic puncture, and soft tissue biopsy.

mad cow disease—see *bovine spongiform encephalopathy*.

Maddacrawler—an adjustable tubular crawler frame with attached pad. It supports the abdomen of a child while the legs and arms are free to touch the floor and initiate movement. Assists crawling motions for children in therapy.

Madden technique—for repair of incisional hernia.

Maddox rod test (Oph)—assesses the degree of muscle dysfunction.

MADD panel—a victim impact panel first initiated by the Mothers Against Drunk Driving. Usage: "The patient is court-ordered to attend a MADD panel."

Madigan prostatectomy—a procedure in which adenomatous tissue is removed from outside the urethra which is preserved intact, so that the urinary tract is not entered.

madreporic coral (Madrepora group, genus *Porites*)—a substitute for autologous bone in cranial reproduction, in bur holes, and even larger implants. A coral graft can be at least partially ossified, and with its use, incisions for harvesting rib or iliac crest grafts are unnecessary (thus obviating the pain and the risk of infection), and the operative procedure takes less time to perform. The coral is prepared for use by ultrasonic treatment and is then cut into cone-shaped plugs for bur holes, and in various-sized blocks which can be cut and shaped intraoperatively. See *Biocoral.*

madreporic hip prosthesis—see *Lord total hip prosthesis* and *madreporic coral*. Also called *madreporic trochanterodiaphysary support system.*

Madura foot—a rare fungal infection of the feet, seen in farm workers who work without shoes.

Maffucci syndrome—characterized by enchondromatosis, hemangiomatosis, and malignant tumors.

MAFH (multicentric angiofollicular hyperplasia).

mag cit—brief form for magnesium citrate.

Magerl technique—for screw placement in lower cervical spine.

magic angle artifact (MRI)—noted to occur when curving structures such as tendons assume an angle of 55° to the bore of the magnet. Other views can confirm that the "lesion" seen is artifactual.

magic angle effect—intermediate signal intensity on T1-weighted images on MRI scan of the ankle.

Magic Bullet (bisacodyl 10 mg)—a suppository for the treatment of constipation with spinal cord injury.

Magic Wallstent—self-expanding coronary stent.

MagnaPod—pain relief magnets. The system features thin magnets that are said to increase blood circulation; they are marketed with elastic braces for application on arms, wrists, legs, and back.

MAGneedle controllers.

Magnes 2500 WH (whole head) **imager**.

Magnetic Controlled Suturing (MCS) (trademark).

magnetic field gradients (MFG).

magnetic resonance angiography (MRA)—gated inflow technique.

magnetic resonance cholangiography (MRC)—uses three-dimensional fast spin-echo technology. Used increasingly in neonates and infants to detect biliary atresia, congenital choledochal dilatation, and biliary complications in hepatic transplantation.

magnetic resonance cholangiography with HASTE (half-Fourier acquisition single-shot turbo spin-echo).

magnetic resonance cystometry—using MRI to calculate bladder volume. The use of ultrasonography to measure bladder volume is dependent on the accuracy of the sonographer. The catheterization method can cause injury and infection. Also, *magnetic resonance hydrometry*.

magnetic resonance elastography (MRE)—combines MR and the application of acoustic waves (i.e., propagation of shear waves) to painlessly image the breasts. It could replace painful mammography. Just as palpation measures the stiffness of certain tissues (breast, prostate), MRE can quantitatively assess the stiffness of breast, prostate, muscle, and brain tissues.

magnetic resonance hydrometry—see *magnetic resonance cystometry*.

magnetic resonance imaging (MRI)—noninvasive radiologic procedure for imaging tissues of high fat and water content that cannot be seen with other radiologic techniques. An MRI image gives information about the chemical makeup of tissues, thus making it possible to distinguish normal, cancerous, atherosclerotic, and traumatized tissue masses in the image. It can measure vessel flow and does not involve ionizing radiation. Formerly called *nuclear magnetic resonance imaging* (NMR). For a quick-reference list of terms, see *MRI terms*.

magnetic resonance mammography (MRM)—useful in detecting silicone rupture, the need for biopsy for cancer, and in cancer staging.

magnetic resonance neurography (MRN).

magnetic resonance spectroscopy (MRS)—a noninvasive technique to study the body chemistry, using magnetism and radio waves, without radiation or needles. The patient is placed within a large circular magnet (as in magnetic resonance imaging), and radio waves are beamed toward the patient. The body's atoms are excited by these waves, and the radiofrequency of each chemical is interpreted by computer, which thus maps out the chemical components

magic *(cont.)*
of each area. Chemical changes caused by heart attack or stroke can be detected quickly. The MRS may prove useful in studying changes in muscle of patients with multiple sclerosis and could lead to new forms of therapy.

magnetic resonance tomography (MRT)—investigation of the inner organs of the body, including the blood vessels, using a high-power magnetic field. High-performance computers attached to this device can rebuild three-dimensional images of any part of the investigated structure, allowing visualization of obstructions or dilatations of the arteries.

magnetic resonance urography (MRU).

magnetic source imaging (MSI)—uses ultrasensitive antenna to detect the magnetic field in the human body and provides noninvasive information about neurological and cardiac functions. Also called *3-D MSI*.

magnetic stimulation—a treatment for nonunion of fractures in which electric, or magnetic, currents stimulate more rapid regrowth of bone in cases of failure of healing in fractures of long bones. A noninvasive means of treatment that may avoid the necessity of surgery and possible bone grafting. See *EBI bone healing system, OrthoGen/OsteoGen*.

Magnetic Surgery System—uses external magnetic fields to direct a magnet-tipped flexible catheter to a target within the brain along a specific route planned by the surgeon. The surgeon can thus map out a pathway that maneuvers around vital brain areas instead of going through them, in order to perform such procedures as tissue biopsy.

magnetic susceptibility artifact—an air-tissue interface, such as at the sella turcica or temporal bones, can produce a bright band or focal distortion.

magnetoencephalogram (MEG)—used in the diagnosis of epilepsy. MEG technique can record the location, depth, orientation, and polarity of magnetic spike field strength in epileptic patients.

Magnetom MRI system—open design that eases the anxiety often caused patients by a closed system. It permits kinematic joint studies and allows for visualization of blood flow and cardiac motion.

Magnum guidewire—used in coronary angioplasty.

MAGPI (meatal advancement, glanuloplasty, penoscrotal junction meatotomy) **operation**—an acronym for a procedure to correct hypospadias. Pronounced “magpie,” like the bird.

Ma-Griffith end-to-end anastomosis—repairs a lacerated Achilles tendon.

Magrina-Bookwalter vaginal retractor—provides exposure of the vagina for surgical procedures; it can expand for use in multiple surgical fields. See *Bookwalter retractor*.

Mahaim bundle in the heart—a term used in electrophysiologic studies of supraventricular tachycardia.

Maico Gamma programmable hearing aids.

Maico-MA 20 audiometer—used to perform bedside audiography.

MAID (monoclonal acute inflammatory demyelination).

MAI (*Mycobacterium avium-intracellulare*) **infection**—a TB variant once considered not to be a pathogen in

MAI *(cont.)* humans, but now appearing as disseminated tuberculosis in AIDS patients. Usage: "The patient was referred for ongoing management of HIV-related issues, including MAI bacteremia." Cf. *MAC infection*.

main d'accoucheur ("obstetrician's hand")—the position in tetany that the hand assumes after a positive Trousseau sign (carpopedal spasm). See *Trousseau sign*.

main magnetic field inhomogeneity artifact (Radiol)—a hardware artifact in which poor shimming of the MRI magnet can produce distortions of image appearance. A square-appearing object can thus appear barrel-shaped, cushion-shaped, or trapezoidal.

Mainstay urologic soft tissue anchor.

Mainster retina laser lens—for panretinal photocoagulation and focal laser therapy.

maintain—to control or limit the effects of an illness or abnormal state with diet, medicine, or other means.

Mainz pouch urinary reservoir—a urinary pouch made from a com- bination of cecum and ileum. Pronounced "mintz" with a long *i*.

MAIPA (monoclonal-antibody-specific immobilization of platelet antigens) **assay**.

major adverse cardiac events (MACE).

Makler insemination device—for intrauterine insemination.

malacoplakia of kidney—rare granulomatous disorder of unknown etiology simulating malignancy.

maladie-de-Roger (Fr., "ro-zhay," Roger disease)—congenital defect of the interventricular septum of the heart.

malaria—infectious febrile disease characterized by periodic paroxysms of fever, chills, and sweating. It is caused by four species of protozoa of the genus *Plasmodium* (*P. vivax, P. falciparum, P. malariae*, and *P. ovale*), parasitic in the red blood cells, and transmitted to the bloodstream of humans by the bite of Anopheles mosquitoes. Cf. *miliaria*.

***Malassezia furfur* pustulosis**—nonfollicular pustulosis of the newborn, caused by a pathogenic yeast. Cf. *neonatal acne*; *sebaceous miliaria*.

Malbran approach—in transscleral fixation of intraocular lens.

Malcolm-Lynn C-RXF cervical retractor frame—a system of cervical retractors made of a carbon composite that is radiolucent rather than radiopaque as are standard metal retractors. These retractors are used during neurosurgical procedures that require intraoperative x-ray visualization of fixation devices.

male menopause—see *Andractim*.

male pattern baldness—characteristic thinning of hair along the temples, front, and back of the head in men. Also called *male pattern alopecia*. See also *hippocratic wreath*.

Malgaigne fracture—bilateral vertical pelvic fracture.

malignant mixed mullerian tumor (MMMT)—a highly malignant tumor of the uterus.

malignant mixed tumor—see *carcinoma ex pleomorphic adenoma*.

Malis CMC-II bipolar coagulator—used with Malis irrigation forceps, and irrigation module, for irrigation, coagulation, and cutting.

Mallampati classification—a classification used in airway assessment. It relates to tongue size compared to pharyngeal airway. It is used by

Mallampati *(cont.)*
anesthesiologists to predict difficulty of intubation. Also called *Mallampati score* or *test*.

malleable retractor (Surg).

Malleoloc anatomic ankle orthosis—used to prevent excessive inversion and eversion.

malleolus—the rounded lateral projections of the bone at the ankle. See *malleus*.

mallet toe—flexion contracture of the distal joints of the second, third, fourth, and fifth toes.

malleus—the outermost of the three small bones in the ear. Cf. *malleolus*.

malleus nipper—a surgical instrument used in ear surgery.

Mallinckrodt Laser-Flex tube—stainless steel, laser-resistant endotracheal tube.

Mallinckrodt sensor systems—for in vitro diagnostic blood gas and electrolyte evaluation.

Mallory-Azan stain—a special stain for collagen fiber.

Mallory-Head modular calcar system.

Mallory PTAH (phosphotungstic acid-hematoxylin)—see *PTAH*.

Mallory-Weiss tear—a tear in the mucosa at the cardioesophageal junction, generally caused by retching or vomiting, resulting in upper GI bleed.

Malmstrom cup (Ob-Gyn)—attached to a vacuum source to facilitate vacuum-assisted vaginal deliveries.

Malone antegrade continent enema (MACE)—a surgical procedure in which the appendix is used to form a cutaneous cecostomy for fluid irrigation. Usage: "All patients had an antireflux Mitrofanoff channel constructed using distal part of the appendix with its divided mesothelium. The proximal half of the appendix was preserved as a modified MACE." Also, *Malone antegrade colonic enema*.

Malone conduit—the tubularized ileum used for urinary diversion.

Malone principle—a method of continent urinary diversion, as in "antegrade continent enema was constructed using the Malone principle."

Malone stoma—an enterostomy. A reversed appendicocecostomy is performed.

Maloney Endo-Otoprobe—laser probe used in ear surgery.

malpighian corpuscles—urine-forming units in renal cortex of kidneys; aggregations of lymphoid tissue in white pulp of spleen.

MALT (mucosa-associated lymphoid tissue) **lymphoma** or **MALT tumor**. See *MALToma*.

MALToma—mucosa-associated lymphoid tissue lymphoma, a low-grade B-cell lymphoma.

mammaplasty—see *mammoplasty*.

mammastatin—a protein that controls abnormal cell growth in breast tissue. Found in healthy breast tissue but absent or reduced in breast cancer patients, mammastatin is being developed for use in the treatment of advanced-stage breast cancer.

Mammex TR—computer-aided mammography diagnosis system.

mammography (see also *system*)
contoured tilting compression
CT laser (CTLM)
GE Senographe 2000D digital
diffraction-enhanced imaging (DEI)
Egan
ImageChecker
magnetic resonance (MRM)

mammography *(cont.)*
Mammex TR computer-aided scintimammography (SMM)
Selenia full-field digital
SenoScan full-field digital
SoftScan laser
step-oblique

Mammomat Novation—a full-field digital mammography system used with an x-ray system. The device passes x-rays through the breast tissue to the digital receptor which converts the x-ray energy to numbers, processes the numbers, and produces an image that can be viewed at a work station or sent to a film printer. It is used to screen and diagnose breast cancer just as regular film mammography.

mammoplasty—plastic augmentation or reduction reconstruction of the breast. Also spelled *mammaplasty*.

MammoSite RTS (radiation therapy system) **catheter**—single-use catheter and radiation solution source used to deliver local radiation therapy to the tissue surrounding a resected malignant breast tumor. After the tumor is resected, the catheter is inserted into the tumor cavity before surgical closure. Once the patient has recovered from surgery, the radiation liquid (Iotrex) is delivered through the catheter to provide local radiation therapy directly to the tumor cavity. When the treatment is completed, the radiation source and catheter are removed. See also *balloon brachytherapy*.

Mammotest system—a breast biopsy system by Fischer Imaging that allows accurate localization of small breast lesions for placement of a core biopsy needle for histologic sampling.

Mammotome—a handheld version of a minimally invasive breast biopsy device. It employs computer technology to replace open surgical procedures.

Mancini plates—referred to in quantitation of immunoglobulins. Usage: "Mancini plates showed IgA 72 g/L, IgG 2.5 g/L."

mandibular advancement osteotomy (MAO)—surgical procedure for obstructive sleep apnea.

Mandibular Excursiometer—for measuring mandibular excursion on the X and Y axis in the coronal plane during active opening during temporomandibular joint treatment.

mandibular repositioning oral appliance—for treatment of sleep apnea.

mandrin, wire—a probe, stylet, or guide for a catheter. Examples:
coudé curve
Guyon-Benique curve
malleable tip
Van Buren curve

maneuver—see *operation*.

Man facelift expander and technique—a small balloon-like device, which is inserted under the skin for several minutes during facelift surgery to stretch the skin circumferentially. The excess skin is excised and the skin flaps sutured into place. The procedure reduces tension on the skin flaps during closure and minimizes hair loss around the temple and ears. Named for Dr. Daniel Man.

manic-depressive—see *bipolar affective illness*.

manifest refraction spherical equivalent (MRSE)—a practical measure of the refractive capacity of an eye, calculated from both spherical and cylindrical refractive errors, if any.

manipulated autologous structure (MAS) cells.

manofluorography (MFG)—simultaneous fluoroscopy and manometric evaluation of pharyngeal swallowing and dysphagia. The swallowing events (as seen by fluoroscopy) and the pressure generated during swallowing (manometry) are displayed simultaneously on a screen. See *deglutition mechanism, peristaltic wave.*

Mantoux test—an intradermal tuberculin test. Read at 48 to 72 hours after injection, induration of more than 10 mm in diameter at the injection site is considered positive.

MAP (mean arterial pressure).

MapCath catheter—a specialized catheter for locating the position of another catheter or other medical device disposed within a patient's body.

maple bark stripper's disease—extrinsic allergic alveolitis caused by exposure to moldy maple bark.

maple leaf flap—used in gynecological reconstruction of vulvar deformities.

maple-syrup urine disease (MSUD)—caused by a defect in metabolism of the ketoacid analogs of leucine, isoleucine, and valine. The maple-syrup odor in the urine is caused by the presence of these compounds.

maplike color interference fringes—color bands in a maplike pattern caused by interference or diffraction of white light; used to describe a finding on applanation tonometry.

MAPs (microtubule-associated proteins).

map unit (Genetics)—a measure of the distance between two gene loci on a single chromosome, based on the percentage frequency of recombination between them; one map unit is equivalent to one centimorgan (or 1% likelihood of recombination).

Maquet ("muh-kay'") **technique**—advancement of the tibial tuberosity by elevation of the tibial crest.

marantic—pertaining to cachexia or wasting.

Marathon guiding catheter—used during coronary angioplasty.

Marburg fever—Ebola-like hemorrhagic fever currently active in Africa. See also *Ebola virus*.

marche à petits pas—short-stepped, wide-based, shuffling gait, seen in patients with parkinsonism.

march fracture (not an eponym)—a fracture of the shaft of the second or third metatarsal bone without a history of injury.

Marchiafava-Bignami disease—uncommon demyelination of the corpus callosum.

Marcus Gunn syndrome ("jaw winking")—unilateral ptosis of the eyelid, with association of movements of the affected upper eyelid with those of the jaw. Named for Robert Marcus Gunn, an English ophthalmologist. Note: There is no hyphen in the name.

Mardis firm stent with HydroPlus coating.

Marie ataxia—a hereditary disease of the nervous system.

marital—pertaining to marriage, as in "marital relationship" or "marital introitus." Cf. *martial*. These are often confused. It is, of course, entirely possible that both adjectives could apply to the same relationship.

marker—see also *gene marker; tumor marker; markers, refractive surgery.*
acanthosis nigricans (AN)
AFP (alpha-fetoprotein)

marker *(cont.)*
ALZ-50 (Alzheimer disease)
anti-CCP antibody
antiendomysial antibody
Arrowsmith corneal
Berkeley optic zone
beta isoform, 14-3-3
bone mineral density
Bores radial
CA1-18 tumor
CA 15-3 tumor
CA 19-9 tumor
carotid intima-media thickness (c-IMT)
CA 72-4 tumor
cathepsin D
CEA (carcinoembryonic antigen)
chromosome tumor 14q
C-reactive protein (for arteriosclerotic disease)
DNA polymerase-alpha
DSM
Freeman cookie cutter areola
Friedländer arcuate
Friedländer transverse incision
G6PD cell
HLA-DR4 genetic
Ki-67
Lewis-X antigen urinary
Lindstrom arcuate incision
lipid-associated sialic acid
McDonald optic zone
nicked free beta subunit of human chorionic gonadotropin
NMP22 urinary
Nordan-Ruiz trapezoidal
oncomarker
perinuclear antineutrophil cytoplasmic antibody (pANCA)
P-glycoprotein gene
PLAP serum
Polo-like kinase (PLK)
PSA (prostate-specific antigen)
RET proto-oncogene
sigmaS serum tumor

marker *(cont.)*
Storz radial incision
Thornton 360° arcuate
tripe palm
tumor

markers, refractive surgery (Oph):
Arrowsmith corneal
Berkeley optic zone
Lindstrom arcuate incision
Lindstrom small incision
McDonald optic zone
Nordan-Ruiz trapezoidal

Mark IV Moss—decompression-feeding catheter.

Markov chain Monte Carlo technique—a method of probability calculation rather than an imaging technique. You may hear this in the future as PACS workstations become more commonplace.

Marlex—synthetic graft material used in hernioplasties and in other abdominal surgery where the tissues need reinforcement.

Marlex methylmethacrylate sandwich.

Marlow Primus instrument collection—handles, shafts, and tips used for minimally invasive surgery.

Marquest Respirgard II nebulizer—for aerosolized pentamidine.

MARS (Modular Acetabular Revision System) (trademark).

MARSA (methicillin-aminoglycoside-resistant *Staphylococcus aureus*)—a strain of *S. aureus* which is resistant to methicillin and the aminoglycoside class of antibiotics (gentamicin, kanamycin, tobramycin). See *MRSA*.

Marshall and Tanner pubertal staging—see *Tanner Developmental Scale*.

Marshall syndrome—a rare pediatric skin disease that is characterized by acquired, localized neutrophilic der-

Marshall *(cont.)*
matitis, followed by loss of elastic tissue in the dermis and cutis laxa. The cause of this syndrome is unknown.

marshmallows—marshmallow-shaped pieces of dressing material. They are used as padding, to anchor a dressing, or to keep a dressing from sticking to a wound.

Mark VII cooling vest—worn by some patients with multiple sclerosis to decrease body temperature and temporarily alleviate symptoms of fatigue and poor coordination. The vest was originally designed for NASA astronauts and is attached via a cord to a battery-operated cooling unit.

Mark II Chandler retractor—used to retract soft tissue away from bone during hip and knee surgery.

Mark II Kodros radiolucent awl—used with image intensifier to locate holes in interlocking nails.

Mark II Sorrells—hip arthroplasty retraction system to expose the acetabulum.

Marsupial—an adjustable terry-cloth belt with an attachable pouch, used by postmastectomy patients to free their hands from the dangling drains. The pouch-like product can also be used to help patients recovering from cardiac and orthopedic surgeries.

martial—pertaining to war or battle. Cf. *marital*.

Martius flap and fascial sling—used to cover a urethral repair and create a continent urethra.

Martius graft—used in urethral reconstruction.

Martius labial fat pad flap.

Martorell hypertensive ulcer.

Marx bridging plate system—low-profile system that minimizes soft tissue dehiscence on mandibular fixation.

Marx classification of microtia.

Marx protocol—for treatment of osteoradionecrosis.

Maryland dissector.

MAS (manipulated autologous structure)—living human cells manipulated outside the body and returned to the patient for structural repair or reconstruction. See *Carticel*.

MAS (meconium aspiration syndrome).

Mascot indirect ophthalmoscope.

MASE (microsurgical extraction of sperm from epididymis).

Masimo SET (signal extraction technology)—pulse oximetry designed for accuracy during conditions of low perfusion, bright ambient light, and electrosurgical interference.

Masket technique—a technique for intraocular lens insertion using a 4-7 mm incision with closure involving multiple small, interlaced stitches with the suture knots buried.

mask facies—the expressionless appearance of the face seen in patients with Parkinson disease.

masking technology—involves the treatment of the donor cells prior to transplantation to prevent T-cell activation. Alteration of initial T-cell recognition confers T-cell anergy and long-term acceptance of the graft.

Mason abdominotranssphincteric resection.

Mason shunt—used in bariatric surgery.

Mason vertical-banded gastroplasty.

Masaoka staging system, modified—for thymic carcinoma.

mass effect—the radiographic appearance created by an abnormal mass in or adjacent to the area of study.

massive genital prolapse—mainly affects elderly women.

mass lesion—anything that occupies space within the body and is not normal tissue.

Masson tumor—papillary endothelial hyperplasia (PEH); also, Masson vegetant intravascular hemangioendothelioma, Masson pseudoangiosarcoma, intravascular endothelial proliferation, and intravascular angiomatosis. Now you know why *PEH* seems to be the preferred term.

mast cell—a type of inflammatory cell which releases histamine and is important in allergic reactions.

Master Flow Pumpette—a disposable I.V. pump that maintains I.V. flow rate under changing conditions, i.e., bed height, patient position, and fluctuations in venous pressure.

masterly inactivity—same as *benign neglect.*

Master two-step test—a timed stress test in which the patient climbs and descends two 9-inch steps a given number of times; indicates the degree of decreased coronary artery blood flow and the consequent degree of ischemic heart disease.

MAST (military antishock treatment) **suit**—a pneumatic antishock garment that reverses the effect of shock on the body's blood distribution by applying external counterpressure to the legs and abdomen. Also called *medical antishock trousers.* One company has trademarked the acronym *MAST.* See *DMAST.*

maternal blood clot patch therapy—a procedure in which maternal blood is given under ultrasonic guidance to produce a clot patch when amniocentesis is complicated by amniorrhea (escape of amniotic fluid).

maternal serum alpha fetoprotein (MSAFP)—screening performed to identify presence of twins, erroneously dated pregnancies, or fetal demise, and to identify fetal anomalies such as spina bifida and abdominal wall defects.

Matles test—aids in the determination of an Achilles tendon rupture.

matricectomy ("may-tris-sec'tum-ee") —excision of nail matrix (nail plate) for chronic nail disease or deformity.

Matritech NMP22—a test kit for bladder cancer.

matrix metalloprotease inhibitor (MMPI)—used orally in cancer treatment. Matrix metalloproteases (MMPs) are natural body chemicals that break down material between cells to make room for new cellular growth. When produced or present at the wrong time, they can break down extracellular matrix that holds cells together, allowing growth of unhealthy tissue, such as cancer and rheumatoid arthritis, by contributing to three processes that lead to progression of cancer: invasion, metastasis, and angiogenesis. An oral MMPI can block these processes, while limiting damage resulting from broad suppression of MMPs. See *Galardin.*

Matroc femoral heads—used for long-term implantation. Utilizes Zyranox Zirconia or Vitox alumina ceramic materials.

Matsner median episiotomy and repair.

Mattox maneuver—extensive mobilization of the left colon, left kidney, spleen and tail of the pancreas, and stomach, and reflecting these structures to the midline, in exposure of the suprarenal aorta. Used in treating

Mattox *(cont.)*
patients with vascular injuries (hematoma or active hemorrhage) from penetrating abdominal wounds.

mature cataract—a cataract in which the lens is completely opaque or ripe for surgery.

maturity-onset diabetes of the young (MODY).

Maverick over-the-wire balloon catheter.

Maverick Monorail balloon catheter.

Maverick2 Monorail catheter—a coronary balloon dilatation catheter.

Mauriceau-Smellie-Veit maneuver—method of delivery of the aftercoming head, with the infant resting on the physician's forearm. Also, *Smellie-Veit, Smellie method, Mauriceau method*.

MaxCast—fiberglass casting tape consisting of a knitted fiberglass fabric impregnated with a water-activated polyurethane resin. Cf. *Fractura Flex, Gypsona*.

Max Fine tying forceps (Oph)—Max Fine, M.D., ophthalmic surgeon.

Max Force catheter—balloon catheter used to dilate biliary stenosis.

Maxilift Combi patient-lifting system.

maxillomandibular osteotomy—surgical procedure for obstructive sleep apnea.

Maxima Forté blood oxygenator.

Maxima II TENS unit—see *TENS*.

Maxim modular knee system.

maximum predicted heart rate (MPHR).

maximum urethral closure pressure (MUCP).

Maxon polyglyconate monofilament suture.

Maxorb alginate wound dressing.

Maxum reusable forceps—used to obtain endoscopic mucosal tissue biopsies and/or for foreign body retrieval.

Maxx Impulse—an energy supplement.

May anatomical bone plates—used to repair proximal humeral fractures.

Mayday distal first metatarsal osteotomy for hallux valgus—a surgical modification of the spike osteotomy of the neck of the first metatarsal. It has the advantages of simplicity, no shortening of the first metatarsal, and no risk of dorsal displacement of the distal fragment.

Mayer-Rokitansky-Kuster-Hauser syndrome—congenital aplasia of the vagina and uterus in women with normal female phenotype and with anatomically and functionally normal ovaries.

Mayfield-Kees headholder (Neuro).

Mayfield three-pin skull clamp—used intraoperatively with a halo ring in cervical spine stabilization in cervical fractures.

Mayo Clinic system for primary biliary cirrhosis—a set of evaluation criteria to determine prognosis for patient survival.

Mayo culdoplasty—fixation of the vaginal vault to the sacrospinous ligament or to the uterosacral ligament.

Mayo-Gibbon heart-lung machine—artificial cardiopulmonary support in extracorporeal membrane oxygenation.

maze cut-and-sew protocol—see *maze procedure*.

maze procedure (Cardio)—a surgical procedure performed on the left and right atrium for treatment of atrial fibrillation. Its name is based on the concept of a puzzle. The incisions made create barriers and several blind alleys, allowing for only one

maze *(cont.)*
major route for an electrical impulse to travel from the top to the bottom of the heart. The original laborious "cut-and-sew" technique is being replaced by a variety of newer techniques that can be performed on a beating heart, using radiofrequency energy, microwave energy, or cryotherapy to create the "maze" paths. Microwave energy allows the surgeon to produce long narrow lesions without gaps, is very reproducible in terms of ablation depth and length, uses a flexible ablating probe, and is capable of creating transmural lesions, with no surface sticking or charring. Also called *Cox maze III procedure* and *maze cut-and-sew protocol.*

Mazzariello-Caprini forceps.

MB bands of CPK—the number relates to the amount of myocardial damage in myocardial infarction, or suspected myocardial infarction.

MBO (malignant bowel obstruction).

MBP (myelin basic protein) **assay**—a test on cerebrospinal fluid of patients with various kinds of tumors, including malignant tumors, using radioimmunoassay.

MBTS (modified Blalock-Taussig shunt).

mc, mCi (millicurie).

MC (multifocal choroiditis).

MCA (middle cerebral artery).

MCAG (multiple colloid adenomatous goiter).

MCC (*Mycobacterium* cell wall complex).

MCC (mutated in colon cancer) **gene**—seems to be involved with the regulation of growth in normal and cancer cells and may suggest a way in which a new class of chemotherapy drugs might be developed. Damage to four different genes has been linked to the development of colon cancer: the MCC gene on chromosome 5, the p53 gene, the DCC gene, and the RAS oncogene. See also *MSH_2 gene.*

McCain TMJ arthroscopic system—includes cannulas, trocars, probes, scissors, forceps, files, scalpels, curets, switching stick, and monopolar and bipolar cautery probes.

McCall modified posterior culdoplasty—see *culdoplasty*.

McCarey-Kaufman (M-K) **medium**—used to store excised cornea with scleral rim attached. This preserves the corneal endothelium for grafting purposes.

McCort sign—one of the radiologic criteria of the presence of ascites.

McCoy facial tri-square (Plas Surg).

McCraw gracilis myocutaneous flap—for vaginal reconstruction.

McCune-Albright syndrome—triad of fibrous dysplasia of long bones and cranium, irregular café au lait spots, spurious episodes of precocious sexual development accompanied by ovarian follicular activity.

McCutchen implant—press-fit titanium femoral implant with longitudinal grooves that enhance rotational stability.

McCutchen SLT hip prosthesis.

McDonald bone plates—used in sagittal split ramus osteotomy.

McDonald optic zone marker (Oph).

McDonald procedure—cervical cerclage.

McDougal prostatectomy clamp—used for dissection of the dorsal vein complex during radical retropubic prostatectomy procedures.

M-CFC (macrophage colony-forming cells).

MCFSR (mean circumferential fiber-shortening rate) (Cardio).

McGaw volumetric pump—used for continuous nasogastric feedings.

McGee platinum/stainless steel piston—used in ear reconstruction.

McGhan ("muh-GAN") **breast implant study**.

McGhan facial implants (Plas Surg).

McGhan tissue expander (Plas Surg).

McGill pain questionnaire—method used in pain management programs to rate pain.

McGlamry elevator (*not* McClamary).

McGovern nipple—a type of airway through which a baby with bony choanal atresia can breathe. A large nipple is modified by having its end cut off and then ties are attached to the nipple and placed around the occiput.

McIvor mouth gag—used in tonsillectomies.

McKenzie extension exercises—an exercise regimen designed to relieve back pain. Also *Robin McKenzie exercises*.

McKernan-Adson forceps.

McKernan-Potts forceps.

McKinley EpM pump—designed for epidural infusion of analgesic pain medications.

McKrae strain—herpes simplex virus.

McLeod blood phenotype—reported in patients with chronic granulomatous disease.

McMurray maneuver, sign, test—to assess the knee for torn cartilage. To demonstrate, flex the knee and turn the foot out and feel knee cartilage; flex the knee and turn the foot in and feel knee cartilage. A clicking indicates a torn knee cartilage.

McNaught keel—laryngeal prosthesis.

McNeill-Goldman corneal transplant ring—a combined scleral ring and blepharostat. Some references give the eponym as Goldman-McNeill, but the designer is James I. McNeill and Ken N. Goldman publicized it for him, thus the compound name. Note that Ken Goldman's name has only one *n*, although there is another ophthalmologist named Goldmann, whose name is attached to a number of instruments.

McNemar test—a test for the presence of ascites.

M-component—see *M-protein*.

McPherson forceps.

McRoberts maneuver—used in vaginal delivery to deliver the infant's shoulders.

MCS (Magnetic Controlled Suturing).

MCS (mesocaval shunt).

M-CSF (macrophage colony-stimulating factor).

MCT (Motor Control Test).

MCTD (mixed connective tissue disease).

MCT (medium-chain triglyceride) **oil**—a source of extra calories, given in formula to premature infants.

MCV (molluscum contagiosum virus).

MDAC (multiple dose activated charcoal)—for drug overdose.

MDCT (multidetector computed tomography)

MDI (metered-dose inhaler), as in Proventil MDI inhaler. The term *MDI inhaler* is redundant but is frequently dictated.

MDILO—portable electronic device that monitors the medication intake of patients using metered dose inhalers. It records the date, time, and quality of dispensing (patient shaking, dispensing, and inhaling of medication).

MD-111—bone dowel and interference screw allograft, machined from cortical bone.

MDR (multidrug resistance)—to chemotherapy agents.

MDR-TB (multidrug-resistant tuberculosis).

MDS (myelodysplastic syndrome).

MDS system—scanning microscopy platform used by pathologists in detection and classification of specific rare cancer cells in bone marrow specimens.

MDX-240—used to treat HIV-infected patients.

MEA (multiple endocrine adenopathies, or abnormalities).

Meadox Microvel arterial graft material—double velour knitted Dacron.

meat wrapper's asthma—from inhalation of the isocyanate fumes caused by heat used in cutting and sealing plastic wrapping for meat.

meaty—having the appearance or texture of raw meat.

mechanical leech—experimental device that performs essentially as a medicinal leech to relieve venous congestion following replantation procedures but without the increased possibility of infection via the medicinal leech's gut contents.

meconium aspiration syndrome (MAS).

meconium stain—fecal material produced by the fetus, which stains the placenta and membranes when decreased oxygen is present.

Mectra Tissue Sample Retainer—for the collection of resected tissue during endoscopy or laparoscopy. See *Pleatman sac* and *Lap Sac*.

Medela breast pump—collects breast milk in presterilized plastic bags for refrigeration or freezing.

Medelec DMG 50 Teflon-coated monopolar electrodes—used in body plethysmography.

medevac'd, medevaced—transported by air ambulance.

Medfusion 2001 syringe infusion pump.

Medgraphics body plethysmograph.

medial olivocochlear bundle (MOCB).

medial tibial stress syndrome (MTSS)—injuries such as shin splints that occur following continuing physical stress to the bones and muscles in the lower leg, inner aspect.

median percent shortening—a measure of the degree to which the length of a stent is reduced as its diameter is increased.

median sternotomy (*not* medium, medial, or mediosternotomy)—a midline incision into the sternum. See *mediastinotomy* and *mediastinum*.

mediastinotomy—incision into the mediastinum, an anterior mediastinotomy or cervical mediastinotomy, or a dorsal or posterior mediastinotomy. Cf. *median sternotomy*.

mediastinum—a group of tissues and organs separating the sternum in front and the vertebral column behind, containing the heart and large vessels, trachea, esophagus, thymus, lymph nodes, and other structures and tissues. It is divided into anterior, middle, posterior, and superior regions.

medical food—defined by the FDA as "a food that provides nutritional support specifically modified for the unique nutrient needs that result from the specific disease or condition, as determined by medical evaluation."

medical holography—an innovative, newly designed imaging technology

medical *(cont.)*
that permits three-dimensional visualization of complex anatomic structures, the translucent images of which are amenable to viewer interaction. Because the images can be viewed from a variety of angles, this technology allows a surgeon to study surgical anatomy and topographical relationships in order to format planning and rehearsal of complex surgical procedures. The technology also provides an educational tool for surgical residents.

Medical Outcomes Study–Social Support Network—used to assess social network and social support. It is a 19-item survey that assesses emotional, informational, tangible, affectionate, and positive social interaction, focusing on the perceived availability, if needed, of various components of functional support.

medicated urethral system for erection (MUSE) **urethral suppository** (alprostadil)—noninvasive transurethral system for treatment of male impotence, composed of a prefilled plastic applicator for delivery of alprostadil in suppository form.

medications—a quick-reference list of pharmaceuticals defined in main entries throughout the book, including AIDS drugs, chemicals, chemotherapy drugs and protocols, investigational drugs, natural substances, prescription and over-the-counter drugs, and radioisotopes. See also *dietary supplements; drug categories; imaging agents.*
ABCD (amphotericin B colloid dispersion)
Abilify (aripiprazole)
Abraxane (albumin nanoparticle paclitaxel)

medications *(cont.)*
acamprosate calcium
ACE (angiotensin-converting enzyme) inhibitor
ActHIB (*H. influenzae* type B vaccine)
activated charcoal
Advexin
Affinitac
Aftermath nutritional supplement
Alcar (L-acetylcarnitine)
Alinia (nitazoxanide) oral suspension
Alista
Allovectin-7 (DNA/lipid complex)
alosetron
Aloxi (palonosetron)
Altastaph (*Staphylococcus aureus* immune globulin [human])
Altocor (lovastatin)
Alvesco (ciclesonide)
Alzhemed
AMD-Fab
Amin-Aid nutritional supplement
amphotericin B colloid dispersion (ABCD)
Andractim (dihydrotestosterone gel)
AngioMark contrast agent
Antabuse (disulfiram)
Antagon (ganirelix acetate)
A_1-PI (alpha$_1$-proteinase inhibitor)
Apo-Zidovudine (Canadian name for Retrovir)
Aqua Glycolic
Artecoll
Arthro 7
Arouse-All combination of herbs
Aslera (prasterone)
Astringedent
atazanavir
ATO (arsenic trioxide)
Atrovent (ipratropium bromide)
Avastin (bevacizumab)
Aviane-28 (levonorgestrel and ethinyl estradiol)

medications *(cont.)*
Avlimil (salvia rubus)
AZT (azidothymidine changed to zidovudine)
balanced salt solution (BSS)
banana bag detox cocktail
BDNF (brain-derived neurotrophic factor)
BeneJoint
Beneprotein instant protein powder
BiDil
biliopancreatic diversion
Biofreeze with Ilex
BMX mouthwash
bone wax
BPM (bioabsorbable polymeric material)
BrachySeed
Brompton solution (cocaine, morphine sulfate, Compazine, ethyl alcohol, syrup)
BSS Plus
BTX-A (botulinum toxin, type A)
bucrylate
Burow solution
Calahist Clear
Cal Mag Fizz
Campral (acamprosate calcium)
capravirine
CardioTec (^{99m}Tc teboroxime)
Carlesta
Cartilade (shark cartilage)
CCB (calcium channel blocker)
CDA (chenodeoxycholic acid)
CD4-IgG
cefazolin and dextrose
Cellegesic (nitroglycerin ointment)
CellSpray
Ceretec (technetium Tc-99m exametazime) contrast agent
Choletec (technetium ^{99m}Tc mebrofenin) contrast agent
ciclesonide
cilantro
cinacalcet HCl (Sensipar)

medications *(cont.)*
Cipro XR
cisplatin
Climara Pro
cloretazine
Clolar (clofarabine)
coal tar shampoo
colloidal bismuth subcitrate
Commit lozenge
conjugated estrogen (CE)
corticotropin-releasing factor (CRF) receptor antagonist class of drugs
Cosamine DS
crude coal tar
crystalloids
Cs131 (Cesium-131) Seed isotope
Dacogen (decitabine)
DAP/TMP (dapsone plus trimethoprim)
dapsone plus trimethoprim (DAP/TMP)
darusentan
DCS (D-cycloserine)
decitabine (Dacogen)
Deflux injectable gel
Dermagran ointment
desulfatohirudin (hirudin)
Detour bar
Diabetes Plus
Digitek
dipyramidole (Canadian)
dipyridamole (U.S.)
doripenem
DOT (deodorized opium tincture)
doxorubicin (Adriamycin)
Dryvax smallpox vaccine
Duac (clindamycin and benzoyl peroxide)
Duodopa (levodopa/carbidopa)
DuraPrep surgical solution
EleCare infant formula
Elestat (epinastine HCl)
Embol-78

medications *(cont.)*
EMLA (eutectic mixture of local anesthetics [lidocaine and prilocaine]
enalapril maleate
endostatin
Endur-acin (sustained release nicotinic acid)
EnfaCare infant formula
Enjuvia
Entereg (alvimopan)
Entero Vu (barium sulfate for suspension)
epi-ADR
epi-Adriamycin
Epivir/Retrovir (lamivudine/zidovudine)
Epzicom (abacavir sulfate 600 mg and lamivudine 300 mg)
esprolol plus Viagra (sildenafil citrate)
EstroLogic
Eular (extended release oxymorphone)
Evacet (liposome-encapsulated doxorubicin)
Exubera (inhaled insulin)
farnesoid X receptor (FXR) agonist
Ferriprox (deferiprone)
Festalan (pancrelipase)
Fiblast (trafermin)
Fibrel (injectable porcine derivative collagen)
flax seed oil
Flex-A-Min (glucosamine chondroitin MSN) tablets
Flexeril (cyclobenzaprine)
fluasterone
fluorosilicone oil
Fortigel (testosterone gel)
Fuzeon (enfuvirtide)
gabexate mesylate
Galida (tesaglitazar)
GeneRx
Glo Germ

medications *(cont.)*
Glucoprime
Good Nights Sleep
Hartmann solution
HCT, HCTZ (hydrochlorothiazide)
HeartBar nutritional supplement
HeartBar Orange Drink
Hemospan
Hemospan PS
Herpasil
Hib polysaccharide vaccine
hirudin (recombinant desulfato-hirudin)
Hoodia (*Hoodia gordonii*) appetite suppressant
HspBcor vaccine
Humira (adalimumab)
Humulin (recombinant insulin)
Hylaform gel
Hylaform Plus
Hypercare (aluminum chloride [hexahydrate] 20% in anhydrous ethyl alcohol)
IC-Green (indocyanine green)
IFN-A (interferon alfa)
IIb/IIa ("to be to a") platelet inhibitor
implantable gastric stimulation (IGS)
Indiclor imaging agent
indium In 111-labeled human non-specific immunoglobulin G imaging agent
Infasurf surfactant
Innofem (estradiol tablets)
insulin detemir
iodine 123 MIBG
iodine 131 MIBG
I-Plant (iodine I 125) brachytherapy seeds
IPM Wound Gel ointment
Iressa (gefitinib)
irofulven
iseganan hydrochloride
isoflurane

medications *(cont.)*
Istalol (timolol formulation)
IUdR (idoxuridine, iododeoxyuridine)
Ivy Block
kinetin
Konsyl bulk laxative
lactated Ringer solution
L-Camipure (L-carnitine tartrate)
LET (lidocaine, epinephrine, tetracaine)
Levitra (vardenafil HCl)
lidocaine, epinephrine, and tetracaine (LET)
Listerine PocketPaks
Lucentis (ranibizumab)
lutein and zeaxanthin
MaBeX, Mabex
MAC (Marcaine, adrenaline, and cocaine) bupivacaine
Macrotec (technetium ^{99m}Tc albumin) imaging agent
Macugen (pegaptanib sodium injection)
Magic Bullet (bisacodyl 10 mg) suppositories
Maxx Impulse nutritional supplement
Melacine (melanoma cell lysate vaccine)
Mestinon (pyridostigmine)
metaiodobenzylguanidine (MIBG)
MethyPatch (methylphenidate)
MicroGuard antifungal powder
Mifeprex (mifepristone, RU-486)
MigraHealth nutritional supplement
Mirapex
MN rgp120 AIDS vaccine
monarsen
MPL (monophosphoryl lipid A) vaccine adjuvant
Mycobacterium phlei cellular extract
NasalGuard allergen screen topical gel

medications *(cont.)*
NeuroCharge hardcore concentration/reaction time formula
NeutroSpec imaging agent
Niaspan
Nichols-Condon bowel prep
Nitrol (nitroglycerin) ointment
nitrospray 0.4
Novitra (zinc)
Numby Stuff (lidocaine and epinephrine)
Omni-Pac
Onyx
Optibond Solo bonding agent
Optisol GS corneal storage medium
Oxilan-300, Oxilan-350 (ioxilan) contrast medium
oxycodone and acetaminophen capsules
oxymetholone
palladium 103 (103Pd)
Paxceed (micellar paclitaxel for injection)
Paxil (paroxetine)
Pegasys plus Copegus (peginterferon alfa-2a plus ribavirin) protocol
pegylated liposomal doxorubicin
percutaneous myocardial channeling (PMC)
Perfan I.V. (enoximone)
perfluoropropane (C_3F_8) gas
Periogard oral rinse
Perlane (animal hyaluronic acid)
Permacol injection (injectable porcine dermal collagen matrix)
Phenoptin (sapropterin hydrochloride)
phenoxodiol
Photrex (rostaporfin)
PlasmaGel (patient-derived plasma emulsion with vitamin C complex)
PolyGlycopleX (PGX)

medications *(cont.)*
potassium hydroxide (KOH)
Prestara (prasterone)
Prevacare moisturizing cream
Preven
Prialt (ziconotide intrathecal infusion)
Primovist (gadolinium EOB-DTPA) imaging agent
Prochieve 4%, Prochieve 8% (progesterone gel)
prostaglandin E-1 (PEG-1)
Provenge vaccine
Pseudomonas exotoxin
Pulmicort Turbuhaler (budesonide)
PVAC therapeutic vaccine
pyranocarboxylic acid
Radiance (calcium hydroxylapatite, [CaHA] microspheres suspended in polysaccharide gel)
Radiogardase (insoluble Prussian blue)
radiolabeled peptide alpha-M2 imaging agent
Raskin DHE-45 protocol
RepHresh vaginal gel
RESOURCE Beneprotein instant protein powder
Restylane Fine Lines injectable gel
Restylane injectable gel
retrocolic submesocolic gastro-enteroanastomosis (RIRS)
Revatio (sildenafil citrate)
Reviderm
Ringer lactate solution
Ringer solution
Rituxan (rituximab)
rofecoxib
rosiglitazone
RU-486 (now Mifeprex)
ruboxistaurin Sanvar IR (vapreotide)
Ryna-12 S (phenylephrine tannate/pyrilamine tannate)
Rythmol (propafenone)

medications *(cont.)*
SA-IGIV (*Staphylococcus aureus* immune globulin intravenous [human])
Schlesinger solution (morphine and scopolamine)
Seasonale (ethinyl estradiol and levonorgestrel)
Segard (afelimomab)
selenium-75 (^{75}Se) imaging agent
Sensipar (cinacalcet HCl)
sestamibi Tc-99m imaging agent
17-beta-Estradiol
SF-ELS (sulfate-free electrolyte lavage solution)
S-fluoxetine (racemic fluoxetine)
Similac Alimentum Advance protein hydrolysate formula with iron
sivelestat
Snorenz
Soothe-N-Seal
Stalevo
Staphylococcus aureus immune globulin intravenous [human] (SA-IGIV)
sterile talc powder
subureteric Teflon injection (STING)
sulfur hexafluoride (SF_6)
Surgifoam
sweet oil
Symmetra ^{125}I brachytherapy seed
TAC (triamcinolone cream)
talc slurry
Tannihist-12
Tc 99m or ^{99m}Tc (technetium)
TCA (trichloroacetic acid)
TcHIDA imaging agent
TCN-P (triciribine phosphate)
TCR (T-cell receptor) peptide vaccine
tecadenoson
TechneScan MAG3 imaging agent
technetium pertechnetate (Tc 99m)

medications *(cont.)*
tegaserod
Testim (testosterone)
TEVs (tissue-engineered blood vessels)
thallium 201 imaging agent
Thelin (sitaxsentan sodium)
TheraCLEC-Total
TheraSeed
13-cis retinoic acid (13-cRA)
TNKase (tenecteplase)
Tonalin (conjugated linoleic acid)
t-PA (tissue plasminogen activator)
TRA (all-trans-retinoic acid)
transdermal testosterone gel
Trelstar Depot (triptorelin pamoate)
triamcinolone cream (TAC)
trichloroacetic acid (TCA)
Trinovin
Triseptin
Trufill n-BCA
Truvada (tenofovir disoproxil fumarate 300 mg and emtricitabine 200 mg)
IIb/IIa ("to be to a") platelet inhibitor
Ultracal HN Plus nutritional supplement
Unna paste
ursodeoxycholic acid (ursodiol)
VBMCP (vincristine, BCNU, melphalan, cyclophosphamide, prednisone)
Velcade (bortezomid)
Veletri (tezosentan)
Ventavis (iloprost)
Vicks VapoRub
Vicotuss (guaifenesin with hydrocodone)
vidarabine (adenine arabinoside, Ara-A, Vira-A)
Vytorin (ezetimibe/simvastatin)
Warheads candy for salivary gland stimulation

medications *(cont.)*
water-soluble contrast medium (WSCM)
WDE (wound dressing emulsion)
Xenaderm (trypsin, balsam, castor oil)
Xcytrin (motexafin gadolinium)
Zaditen (ketotifen)
Zaditor (ketotifen fumarate)
Zanfel
ZDV (zidovudine)
Zelapar (selegiline HCl)
Zelnorm (tegaserod maleate)
Zemaira (A1-PI, alpha$_1$-proteinase inhibitor)
Zetia (ezetimibe)
zidovudine (AZT, azidothymidine)
Zimycan
Zirpursky regimen

Med-ic ECP (electronic compliance monitor).

medicinal botanicals—term used for therapeutic natural products ignored by medical providers for many years but perceived by many to be more cost-effective and gentle, with fewer side effects, than traditional prescription medications. Some botanicals and their purported uses include bilberry (strengthens vessels, improves night vision), *Echinacea* (enhances immune system, prevents colds), kava kava and valerian (relaxants), garlic (improves HDL/LDL ratios, lowers blood pressure), ginseng (increases endurance), *Gingko biloba* (increases blood flow to brain and extremities), feverfew (treats migraine headache), ginger (acts as an antinauseant), hawthorne (improves heart, blood, and oxygen flow), St. John wort (reduces anxiety and depression). Most are now sold as dietary supplements.

medicine
complementary and alternative (CAM)
cytogenetics
darwinian
evolutionary
regenerative

Medicon instruments—for vascular and cardiac surgery.

Medifil—collagen hemostatic wound dressing.

Mediflex-Bookler—holding and positioning devices.

Mediflex-Gazayerli retractor—endoscopic retractor-dissector that can be introduced through a rigid straight port and then reshaped.

Medigraphics 2000 analyzer—used in testing exhaled gases in cardiopulmonary exercise study.

Medi-Jector Vision needle free insulin injection system.

mediolysis—a coined term, meaning destruction of a segment of artery.

Medipore Dress-it—a precut surgical dressing of a porous material with a cloth backing.

Medi-Ject—needle-free insulin injection system.

Medi-Jector Choice—needle-free insulin injector.

MediPort—a totally implanted vascular access device for continuous or intermittent outpatient delivery of fluids and medications. May be used with externalized catheters.

Medisense Pen 2—self blood glucose monitor. See *SBGM*.

Medisorb drug delivery system—allows controlled, sustained release of injectable drugs.

Mediterranean lymphoma—small intestine malignant lymphoma. The disease is characterized by a diffuse, intense plasma cell infiltrate in the lamina propria of the small intestine that may give rise to a malignant lymphoma. See *IPSID*.

MedJet microkeratome—a cutting device for vision correction and corneal transplant procedures.

Medline—medical bibliographical computer database, through which a search of the current literature on almost any medical subject can be conducted.

MedNext bone dissecting system—a high-speed system used in neurosurgery, otolaryngologic surgery, and plastic-craniofacial surgery.

Medoff sliding fracture plate.

Medrad automated power injector—injects a set amount of iodinated contrast medium at the therapist's discretion.

Medrad MRInnervu endorectal colon probe.

meds—brief form for *medications*.

MEDS (microsurgical extraction of ductal sperm)—in infertility.

MedSpeak/Radiology—with Windows NT, a real-time continuous speech recognition system developed by IBM.

Medstone STS shock wave generator—used to produce shock waves for dissolving kidney stones and gallstones. Also, *Medstone STS lithotripsy system*.

MED (microendoscopic diskectomy) **system**.

Medtronic Activa tremor control therapy—uses an implanted device to suppress essential tremor and tremor associated with Parkinson disease. The implanted system delivers mild electrical stimulation to block brain signals that cause tremor.

Medtronic distal perfusion kit—provides aorto-coronary blood flow via an olive-tipped arteriotomy cannula.

Medtronic Gem automatic implantable defibrillator—protects survivors of cardiac arrest and others whose hearts beat dangerously fast.

Medtronic Hancock II—tissue valve, available in both aortic and mitral models.

Medtronic Hemopump—a cardiac assist device used in minimally invasive heart surgery. This system allows the surgeon to perform some procedures without stopping the heart completely. In addition, blood does not actually leave the body as it does in more conventional perfusion techniques.

Medtronic Inspire—a system of implantable devices that deliver electrical stimulation to the hypoglossal nerve for control of obstructive sleep apnea.

Medtronic InSync implantable cardioverter-defibrillator.

Medtronic Jewel AF—implantable arrhythmia management device.

Medtronic Micro Jewel II—very small implantable defibrillator, about the size of a small pager.

Medtronic Octopus—a tissue stabilizing system used in coronary artery bypass graft surgery. It stabilizes the beating heart in order to facilitate suture placement.

Medtronic Pisces Quad Plus lead.

Medtronic Pulsor Intrasound—pain reliever using sound vibrations.

Medtronic Sprint lead for cardioverter-defibrillators.

Medtronic SynchroMed pump—implantable subcutaneous infusion pump used to deliver chemotherapy drugs.

Medtronic temporary pacemaker.

Medtronic tremor control therapy device—an implanted device, similar to a cardiac pacemaker, that delivers electrical stimulation to block or override brain signals that cause tremor.

medullaris—conus medullaris.

medulloscopy—used for visualization and irrigation of sepsis or nonunion of the tibia and femur when access to the intramedullary canal is necessary.

MedX physical therapy device.

Mees lines—transverse lines on the fingernails, strongly suggestive of arsenic poisoning. Cf. *Beau line*.

MEG (magnetoencephalogram).

MegaDyne all-in-one hand control—used in laparoscopic surgery for aspiration, irrigation, and cauterization.

MegaDyne E-Z clean laparoscopic electrodes—Teflon-coated electrodes that do not have to be removed from the operating port for cleaning after coagulation.

megahertz (mHz)—thousand cycles per second, used as measurement in audiograms. See *hertz*.

megakaryocyte growth and development factor (MGDF)—reduces the duration and severity of thrombocytopenia in cancer patients following chemotherapy.

Megalink biliary stent—for the treatment of malignant obstructions of the biliary duct.

mega-OATS (osteochondral autologous transfer system)—repair of large osteochondral defect of the femoral condyle by transplantation of a single osteochondral piece taken from the autologous posterior femoral condyle, providing better approximation of the femoral cartilage curvature and joint congruence.

MEI (metastatic efficiency index).

meibomian cyst—see *chalazion*.

meibomian froth (Path).

meibomian gland—one of the sebaceous glands of the eyelid.

Meige ("mezh'uhz") **disease**—dystonia of facial and oromandibular muscles with blepharospasm, grimacing mouth movements, and protrusion of the tongue. Primarily affects middle-aged and elderly adults, women more often than men. Also called *Meige syndrome*, *Brueghel syndrome*, illustrated in Brueghel's painting *De Gaper*. First described by Dr. Henry Meige in 1910. Do not confuse with *Meigs syndrome*.

Meigs ("megz") **syndrome**—ascites and hydrothorax, seen with pelvic tumors, including ovarian fibromas. Named for Dr. Joe Vincent Meigs, an American surgeon. Do not confuse with *Meige syndrome.*

meiosis—the special type of cell division in the formation of gametes whereby the diploid chromosome number (26 pairs) is reduced to the haploid number (26 single chromosomes); occurs in two stages, meiosis I and II; reduction division takes place during stage I.

meiotic drive—the tendency of one allele in a heterozygote rather than the other allele to be passed on to offspring.

melanin—the dark brown to black pigment normally present, predominantly in the hair, skin, the choroid coat of the eye, and substantia nigra of the brain. Also in some tumors, e.g., melanoma. Cf. *melena*.

melanocytes—see *cultured autologous melanocytes.*

melanocytic lesions in conjunctiva.

melanonychia—see *longitudinal melanonychia*.

melanotic—referring to the presence of melanin. Often confused with *melenic*. *Melenic* stools, not *melanotic* stools. Cf. *melenic*.

melanotic stool—incorrect dictation for melenic stool, which pertains to melena (tarry black color of stools). Not to be confused with melanotic which pertains to melanin.

MELAS (mitochondrial myopathy, encephalopathy, lactic acidosis, and stroke-like episodes).

MELD (Model for End-Stage Liver Disease) **score**—a model end-stage liver disease score. Cf. *PELD score.*

melena—passage of dark, tarry stools, indicating bleeding in the lower gastrointestinal tract. Cf. *melanin*.

melenic—referring to or marked by melena, as in *melenic stools*. Cf. *melanotic*.

melenic stool—pertains to melena, tarry black color of stools. Not to be confused with melanotic which pertains to melanin. Dictators erroneously dictate "melanotic stools" instead of the correct "melenic stools."

Melastatin—test kit for detecting early malignant melanoma. It works by detecting the presence or absence of Melastatin, a gene found in normal skin and in nonmetastatic melanoma.

melolabial flap—a flap from the medial cheek, used as a transposition flap, to repair a defect on the side of the nose. It is used for deep nasal defects, providing thick sebaceous skin and subcutaneous fat for rebuilding tissue lost in surgery and, folded on itself, can recreate an alar rim. Erroneously referred to as *nasolabial flap*.

meloplasty—face-lift; plastic surgery of the cheek.

melorheostosis—an uncommon bone disorder characterized by cortical thickening of the bone with irregular dense hyperostosis along the cortex. It most often affects the lower limbs but can affect the hands. The cause is still unknown, although it was first described in 1922.

memapsin 2—protein-cutting enzyme, or protease, believed to be directly responsible for Alzheimer disease. Also known as *beta-secretase*.

membrane delamination wedge (Oph) —an instrument that allows the surgeon to separate proliferative membranes from the retina effectively and safely. Used to decrease the risk of iatrogenic retinal tears that may complicate procedures to treat proliferative vitreoretinal diseases.

membrane stripping—used to induce labor at term, thus avoiding oxytocic drugs or amniotomy. It is done by digital separation of the membranes from the lower uterine segment.

membranous croup—the bacterial cause of serious airway obstruction in children. Also called *membranous laryngotracheobronchitis* or *bacterial tracheitis*.

Memorial Sloan-Kettering Cancer Center, New York. Also, MSK Cancer Center.

Memorial Sloan-Kettering protocol—a chemotherapy protocol.

MemoryLens—a foldable intraocular lens (IOL).

MemoryTrace AT—ambulatory cardiac monitor which automatically records an EKG when it senses an arrhythmia in the patient's heart. The EKG is stored electronically and can be transmitted over the telephone to a cardiologist.

Memotherm—a nitinol self-expanding stent used for peripheral artery procedures.

MEN (multiple endocrine neoplasia).

mendelian inheritance (Genetics)–the ideal pattern of single-gene inheritance, as first described by Gregor Mendel in 1865. According to Mendel's laws, derived from experiments with peas, parental alleles separate during gametogenesis and non-allelic genes are distributed to offspring independently of one another.

Mendelian Inheritance in Man—an exhaustive and monumental atlas of inherited traits, normal and abnormal, compiled by Victor McKusick and continually updated by him and his associates; accessible in print format and on the World Wide Web.

Mengert index—in pelvimetry.

meningococcal supraglottitis—a recent clustering of cases caused by *Neisseria meningitidis* suggests this may be an emerging infectious syndrome.

meninx—the singular form of the membrane covering the brain and spinal cord; meninges (plural) consist of the dura, pia, and arachnoid.

meniscal (*not* menisceal) (adj.)—usually refers to one of the crescent-shaped structures of the knee joint.

Menke steely hair syndrome.

MEN 1 (multiple endocrine neoplasia, type 1) **syndrome**.

mental status examination—see *test*.

mentis—see *non compos mentis*.

Mentor Alpha 1 inflatable penile prosthesis.

Mentor BVAT—computer screen chart used in testing visual acuity.

Mentor saline-filled testicular prosthesis—a cosmetic replacement for a

Mentor *(cont.)*
missing testicle. It is silicone rubber, oval shaped, and contains saline.

MEP (motor evoked potential)—used to monitor descending pathways in neurosurgery.

MEP (multimodality evoked potential) —a combination of visual, somatosensory, and brain stem auditory evoked potential.

Mepitel contact-layer wound dressing.

Mepore absorptive dressing.

mEq (milliequivalent).

meralgia paresthetica—a neuropathy, usually due to compression of the lateral femoral cutaneous nerve, producing pain, paresthesias, and sensory disturbances. See *Roth-Bernhardt disease*, which is synonymous.

M/E ratio (myeloid/erythroid).

Mercator atrial high-density array catheter—used in the right atrium for diagnosing and mapping complex arrhythmias that may be difficult to identify using conventional mapping systems alone.

Mercedes tip cannula—used for liposuction.

Merci Retriever—a wire with a corkscrew-like twist in the middle, the first medical device cleared by the FDA to remove blood clots from the brain in patients experiencing ischemic stroke. The device was evaluated in the MERCI (mechanical embolus removal in cerebral ischemia) trial. The Merci Retriever is also used to remove foreign bodies in the peripheral, coronary, and neurologic vasculature.

mercury artifact (Radiol)—mercury seen in unexpected places in the body, after the breaking of a Cantor tube that was weighted with mercury to stay in the stomach.

mercury-in-Silastic strain gauge (Vasc Surg)—used for determination of the blood flow.

meridian therapy—acupuncture, identifying 14 main meridians running vertically up and down the surface of the body. Acupuncture points are specific locations where the meridians come to the surface of the skin and are easily accessible by "needling," moxibustion, and acupressure: Yuan-Source points, Xi-Cleft points, Back-Shu and Front-Mu points, Luo-Connecting points, Eight Influential points.

Merindino procedure—distal esophagectomy, 50% gastrectomy, jejunal interposition, with esophagojejunostomy, pyloroplasty and vagotomy, and jejunojejunostomy.

Merkel cell carcinoma (MCC)—rare and aggressive neuroendocrine tumor of dermal origin.

Merlin bendable blade (ENT).

Merocel sponge—a compressed, lint-free, nonfiber sponge that expands when in contact with nasal secretions, used in postoperative nasal packing. It may be used in other settings.

MeroGel nasal dressing and sinus stent—a postoperative mucosal dressing following functional endoscopic sinus surgery.

MERRF (myoclonus epilepsy associated with ragged-red fibers).

Merry Walker ambulation device—a device modeled on a baby walker and designed for adults with ambulation problems.

Mersilene (*not* Mersiline)—a braided nonabsorbable suture that becomes encapsulated in the body tissues. Used in cardiovascular, general, and

Mersilene *(cont.)*
plastic surgery as retention sutures. Colors: green and white.

Mersilk—a braided silk suture.

MESA (microepididymal sperm aspiration or microsurgical epididymal sperm aspiration)—used in infertility treatments.

Mesalt dressing—crystalline sodium chloride-impregnated dressing used to cleanse infected wounds.

Mesalt impregnated absorbent dressing.

mesenchymal stem cell (MSC)—a multipotent cell found in embryonic connective tissue and, much more rarely, in adult bone marrow and connective tissue; capable of differentiating into bone, cartilage, and fat cells.

mesenteric fat stranding—finding on CT scan indicative of inflammation.

mesh (see also *graft*)
Bard Composix mesh graft material
Bard Sperma-Tex preshaped
Bard Visilex
Composix E/X
Devex
Dexon
DualMesh
Emerge
Gynemesh PS
intraperitoneal onlay (IPOM)
Monarc
MycroMesh biomaterial
Parietex composite
PelviSoft
PerFix Marlex mesh plug
PermaMesh
Sepramesh
Sperma-Tex preshaped mesh
Supramesh
Surgipro Prolene
Surgisis Gold mesh graft
SurgiSis sling/mesh

mesh *(cont.)*
Tanner mesher
tantalum
TiMesh
Trelex
Ventralex
Visilex

mesh plug hernioplasty—a hernia repair procedure using a cone-shaped plug of Marlex mesh to close the hernia defect. See *PerFix*.

mesoderm—the middle one of the three germ layers of the early embryo, derived from the inner cell mass of the blastocyst. As fetal development progresses it gives rise to muscle, connective tissues including bone and fat, and blood cells.

messenger RNA (mRNA)—a strand of RNA transcribed from the DNA of a gene, which provides a template for protein synthesis.

Messerklinger sinus endoscopy set.

Mestinon (pyridostigmine) —a myasthenia gravis therapy that appears to be effective for the treatment of orthostatic hypotension.

met, mets—unit of measurement for treadmill scoring; 1 met = 3.5 ml O_2/kg/min. Cf. *mets, "Metz."*

metabolic equivalent—the amount of oxygen required while sitting very quietly at rest (approximately 3.5 milliliters of oxygen per kilogram of body weight).

metabolic syndrome—a constellation of physiologic disorders, including obesity, hypertension, insulin resistance, high triglycerides, and low HDL cholesterol, that are found together in as many as one-fourth of adults in the U.S. Each of the disorders that compose the metabolic syndrome is an independent risk factor

metabolic *(cont.)* for cardiovascular disease. The syndrome may be partly genetic but is made worse by overweight and physical inactivity. Also called *metabolic syndrome X* and *insulin resistance syndrome.*

metabolically obese but normal weight (MONW)—a term applied to young women who are potentially at increased risk for development of metabolic syndrome despite their young age and normal body mass index. MONW women have a higher percentage of body fat, higher plasma cholesterol levels, lower insulin sensitivity, lower fat-free mass, lower physical activity energy expenditure, and lower peak oxygen uptake than non-MONW women.

metacarpal—refers to the bones of the metacarpus, that part of the hand between the wrist and the fingers. Cf. *metatarsal*. The above words are often confused, even by the dictators, so be aware of the anatomic area referred to.

metachronous seeding—metastases occurring from a secondary tumor rather than directly from the primary tumor.

metacyte—a popular brief form for metamyelocyte among hematologists and oncologists. It should be transcribed as metamyelocyte.

Meta DDDR pacemaker.

metaiodobenzylguanidine (MIBG).

metallic stent placement—used to relieve acute colonic obstruction secondary to colorectal carcinoma.

metaphase—the stage of mitosis or meiosis at which the chromosomes align themselves on the equatorial plane of the cell; the stage at which chromosomes are most readily examined and photographed for karyotyping.

metaphyseal lesion of the distal femur —a common site to indicate abuse in an infant.

metaphysis—the wide part at the end of the shaft of a long bone, adjacent to the cartilaginous disk of the epiphysis. In childhood, this is composed of spongy bone and contains the growth zone. In the adult, it is continuous with the epiphysis. Cf. *metastasis*.

metastasis—spread of cancer from one organ or part of the body to another not necessarily contiguous with it; it may spread through the lymphatic system or venous system, etc. See *metaphysis*. Cf. *met, mets*.

metastatic efficiency index (MEI). Usage: "The MEI value for the eye is by far the highest, indicating a very favorable environment for the growth of cancer cells."

Metasul—metal-on-metal hip prosthesis.

metatarsal—refers to the bones of the metatarsus, that part of the foot between the ankle articulation and the toes. See *metacarpal*.

methemoglobin (metHb)—does not carry oxygen through the blood. A small amount of methemoglobin is normally present in the blood, but if hemoglobin is converted to excess methemoglobin through injury or exposure to toxic agents, cyanosis can result.

methicillin-resistant *Staphylococcus aureus* (MRSA, "mer'sa")—a strain of *S. aureus* that is resistant to methicillin, gentamicin, and ciprofloxacin. Now treated with vancomycin. This resistant gram-positive bacterium often inhabits the nares of healthy individuals. See *MARSA*.

methicillin-sensitive *Staphylococcus aureus* (MSSA).

method (see also *operation)*
- Albert-Lembert
- bench
- C-CAP (custom contoured ablation pattern)
- Cherry-Crandall
- Credé
- CSQI
- flow cytometry
- flush
- Holdrinet
- interferometry
- Ionescu
- Ko-Airan bleeding control
- Lown and Woolf
- Mauriceau-Smellie-Veit
- Mosley
- moving-bed infusion-tracking MRA
- moving platform posturography
- myofascial release
- NDT (neurodevelopmental techniques)
- Numby Stuff needle-free method
- Oliver-Rosalki
- Parker-Kerr closed method
- Pfeiffer-Comberg method
- photothermal sclerosis
- piggybacking
- Pilates method of exercise
- polydioxanone plating
- Pulvertaft weave
- Raman spectroscopy
- Roche Microwell Plate Hybridization
- Sigma CPK serum testing
- Smellie
- Sub-Q-Set
- Syed-Neblett brachytherapy
- Turner-Warwick
- Wheeless
- Wroblewski testing serum LDH

methylmalonic acidemia—a nutritional deficiency thought to be responsible for certain skin diseases.

methylmethacrylate—a cement used in orthopedics and neurosurgery.

methylmethacrylate beads—a method of providing an antibiotic to prevent postfracture osteomyelitis. Impregnated with an antibiotic, the beads of methylmethacrylate are strung on a surgical wire, implanted in the area of an open fracture (following surgical debridement and irrigation with an antibiotic solution). The beads dissolve, releasing the antibiotic in situ at therapeutic levels over several weeks.

methylphenidate—see *Metadate CD.*

methyl tertiary butyl ether (MTBE).

MethyPatch (methylphenidate)—transdermal drug patch that delivers methylphenidate, for the treatment of attention-deficit hyperactivity disorder. The patch is changed daily.

Metricath catheter/transducer—device used to measure the size or compliance of a vessel.

Metrix atrial defibrillation system—an implantable device designed specifically for patients suffering from recurrent symptomatic episodes of atrial fibrillation.

metrology score summarizing cervical rotation (in sitting position)—term used in assessing ankylosing spondylitis.

METRx system—for minimally invasive spinal surgery.

mets (plural of met)—unit of measurement in treadmills. See *met.*

mets—slang for metastases. Cf. *meds, met, "Metz."*

Metz—slang for Metzenbaum scissors. Cf. *mets.*

Meuli arthroplasty.

Meurmann classification of congenital aural atresia.

MFG (magnetic field gradients).

MFG (manofluorography).

MFH (malignant fibrous histiocytoma).

MGBG—a polyamine synthesis inhibitor for treatment of brain tumors.

MGDF (megakaryocyte growth and development factor).

MG II total hip system.

MHA-TP (microhemagglutination test for *Treponema pallidum*, the organism that causes syphilis).

MHz (megahertz) (1 million hertz)—a term often used in radiology and audiology. A hertz equals 1 cycle per second.

MI (migration index).

Miami Acute Care (MAC) **collar**—for cervical support.

Miami J collar—cervical immobilization for ICU patients restricted to the supine position.

Miami pouch—a reconstructive technique for continent urinary diversion after pelvic exenteration.

MIAS (minimal incision aortic surgery).

MIBG (metaiodobenzylguanidine).

MIC—see *minimal inhibitory concentration*.

MIC disposable cytology brush.

MIC gastroenteric tube—a dual lumen catheter which allows access to the stomach and the jejunum, for use in patients who need both gastric decompression and jejunal feeding. (MIC, Medical Innovations Corp.)

Michaelis-Gutmann bodies—lamellar inclusion bodies found in the cytoplasm of Von Hansemann cells, consistent with diagnosis of malacoplakia of kidney.

Michelangelo factor—a reference to the skill of the ultrasound examiner (sonologists are artists). Detection is inversely proportional to patient's obesity and directly proportional to the ability of the examiner (sonographer, sonologist, radiologist, urologist).

Michel deformity—complete failure of development of the inner ear.

MIC-Key G and **MIC-Key J** (pronounced "Mickey")—gastrostomy tubes.

Micral chemstrip—urine test for microalbuminuria.

Micral urine dipstick test—detects low levels of albumin.

micro-, prefix meaning small or abnormally small. Cf. *macro-*.

Micro-Aire pulse lavage system—for debriding bone surfaces in hip and knee implantation procedures.

microbial keratitis—see *keratitis*.

microbipolar forceps—electronic forceps in straight and curved versions; used in microsurgery.

Microblator—small joint ArthroWand.

microbubble contrast agent for color Doppler ultrasound on breast masses—a minimally invasive technique that enables accurate differentiation of benign masses from carcinomas through the use of anatomic and dynamic features.

microcalcification—very small deposit of calcium in breast tissue, as seen in a mammogram. Clustered microcalcifications are highly suggestive of malignancy.

microchimerism—findings related to the presence of donor cells in a graft recipient that can mimic infection.

Micrococcus sedentarius—a coagulase-negative organism. Can be confused with *Staphylococcus epidermidis*, but *S. epidermidis* ferments glucose and micrococci do not.

microcrust formation—skin lesions after epidermal injury.

microdebrider—a powered rotary dissection device with suction assistance, now approved for removal of pediatric airway lesions including stenoses, granulation tissue, and cysts.

Micro Diamond-Point microsurgery instruments.

microdots—panstromal occurrence of fine, highly reflective structures appearing in the eyes of chronic contact lens wearers.

Microdot technique for precision suture placement.

microendoscopic diskectomy (MED) **system**—used in herniated disk surgery. This microsurgical instrumentation is used to perform back surgery through a one-half-inch incision.

Microflo test strip—used with Precision QID glucose monitoring system.

Microfoam surgical tape (*not* Microform).

MicroFrance Angot-Vanecloo retractor.

MicroFrance Backbiter (ENT).

MicroFrance bipolar neuro-otology coagulating forceps.

MicroFrance minimally invasive surgical instruments—including the MicroFrance BackBiter and pediatric BackBiter.

MicroFrance Selesnick lateral skull base instrument set.

micrognathia-glossoptosis syndrome. See *Pierre Robin syndrome*.

MicroGuard antifungal powder.

Micro-Imager—high-resolution digital camera.

Microjet-based cutting and debriding devices—used as alternatives to scalpel and laser surgery approaches for common ophthalmic procedures.

microkatals (μkat) **per liter**—a katal is a unit of measure proposed to express enzymatic activity. The abbreviation for *katal* is *kat*.

MicroKlenz wound cleanser.

Microknit vascular graft prosthesis—a fine-knit, thin-walled Dacron prosthesis that comes as a straight tube or patch graft. It is said to handle much like normal arterial tissue. It has also been marketed under the names of *Weavenit* and *Wesolowski* prostheses.

MicroLap and MicroLap Gold—a microlaparoscopy system used in diagnosis and treatment of pelvic pain, infertility, and tubal ligation.

Microlase transpupillary diode laser (Oph).

Microlight 830 laser—a hand-held, battery-operated, nonsurgical laser device that uses photo-biostimulation to treat carpal tunnel syndrome.

microlumbar diskectomy (MLD)—a rigid microsurgical operative technique which uses microscopic-aided dissection throughout rather than just at the point of disk dissection.

MicroLYSUS—ultrasound-enhanced drug delivery system used to treat patients suffering from ischemic stroke by delivering thrombolytic drugs directly into the area of a brain clot.

MicroMed DeBakey ventricular assist device—for use in patients with heart failure who are refractory to other treatment modalities.

micrometastasis—a microscopic metastasis.

MicroMewi multiple sidehole infusion catheter—a microcatheter used to deliver drugs into the peripheral vasculature for therapeutic emboli-

MicroMewi *(cont.)* zation. Named for Mark Mewissen, M.D., interventional radiologist.

Micro Minix pacemaker—a smaller version of the Minix pacemaker. The term *Micro* is part of the trade name.

Micronail intramedullary distal radius implant—minimally invasive system that provides immediate fracture stabililization utilizing fixed-angle locking screws.

Micron bobbin ventilation tubes—made of titanium; used in surgery.

Micron Res-Q—implantable cardioverter-defibrillator.

Microny K SR—a unipolar single-chamber rate-responsive pacemaker.

Microny II SR+—single-chamber, rate-responsive pulse generator.

Microny II SR Plus (or **Microny II SR+**)—a single-chamber rate-responsive pacemaker.

Microplaner blade—part of the XPS 2000 Microresector system instrument set, used in plastic surgery.

Microplaner soft tissue shaver—used to shave facial soft tissue. It is said to be less traumatic than conventional tissue aspiration techniques.

Microprobe laser (Oph)—ophthalmic laser microendoscope that provides both laser function and illumination in one instrument. It is used to visualize and treat retinal or choroidal vascular disease, retinal tears or detachments and also treats the ciliary processes in intractable neovascular glaucoma.

Micro-Probe tip—used for microdissection.

Micropuncture Peel-Away introducer—used to introduce balloon, electrode, and other catheters. Knobs allow the sheath to be peeled away and removed.

microscope, microscopy
- atomic force (AFM)
- biomicroscope (slit lamp)
- confocal
- dark-field
- DIC (differential interference contrast)
- scanning acoustic (SAM)
- Wild operating

microscopic colitis—chronic diarrheal syndrome that is caused by inflammation in the large intestine. It is called microscopic colitis because the inflammation can be detected only with a microscope. During colonoscopy or sigmoidoscopy, the colon looks normal. The presence or absence of a specific feature within the colonic inflammatory process as seen under the microscope (thickened collagen under the surface of the biopsy) has led to use of two other names for this syndrome: *collagenous colitis* and *lymphocytic colitis*.

microSelectron-HDR (high-dose-rate)—an afterloader used in radiation therapy.

MicroSmooth probe—a vitreoretinal probe for attachment to an ocutome.

microsomal triglyceride transfer protein (MTP).

MicroSpan microhysteroscopy system—a 1.6 mm hysteroscope and MicroSpan sheath that allow atraumatic access to the uterus without cervical dilatation.

microsurgery—see *transanal endoscopic microsurgery*.

microsurgical denervation of the spermatic cord—an effective testicular-sparing surgical alternative for treatment of chronic orchialgia.

microsurgical DREZ-otomy—a procedure to treat spasticity and pain in

microsurgical *(cont.)*
lower limbs. (DREZ, dorsal root entry zone.)

microsurgical epididymovasostomy (MSEV)—for congenital and acquired vasoepididymal obstruction.

microsurgical extraction of sperm from epididymis (MASE)—an infertility procedure.

microsurgical tubal reanastomosis (MTR)—used to reverse surgical sterilization in women.

Microtaze—microwave tissue coagulator.

MicroTeq portable belt—device worn for home treatment as augmentation for TENS.

microtome—see *Stadie-Riggs microtome.*

microtubule-associated proteins (MAPs).

MicroVas vascular treatment system—a device used for the treatment of ischemia that generates ionic impulses which pass through the body, or an extremity, using strategically placed carbon emitter pads. The pads are positioned 180° from each other in groups of up to eight pairs. The ionic impulses pass completely through the limb or body, creating circulation in the treated area through neuromuscular stimulation of the venous muscle pump, and by upregulating metabolic processes. MicroVas stimulates autolytic debridement and alleviates pain.

microvascular anastomotic coupler system—sutureless polyethylene/stainless steel coupler (mechanically pinned rings) that produces a more uniform and reproducible vessel anastomosis than can be achieved with conventional sutures.

microvascular angiopathy (MVA).

microvascular free tissue transfer—a procedure used in near-total or total glossectomy following reconstruction with a latissimus dorsi flap modified to create a muscle sling attached to pterygoid and masseter stumps. The flap is then reinnervated by anastomosis of the hypoglossal nerve stump to the nerve of the latissimus dorsi.

microvascular therapy (MVT)— physical therapy for ischemia, working directly and mechanically to elevate blood flow through neuromuscular stimulation of the venous muscle pump.

Microvasive Glidewire—see *Glidewire.*

Microvasive stiff piano wire guidewire.

Microvit cutter—used in vitreoretinal surgery in cutting the vitreous, in posterior segment surgery.

microwave cardiac ablation system—a minimally invasive system used to treat cardiac arrhythmias.

microwave endometrial ablation (MEA) system—a surgical device that uses microwave energy to treat excessive menstrual bleeding by destroying tissue lining the uterus. A long slender tube that delivers microwave energy is inserted into the uterus to destroy tissue. Treatment typically lasts three minutes and is usually painless.

microwave nonsurgical treatment—for benign prostatic hypertrophy. Performed under local anesthesia. Ultrasound defines the size and shape of the prostate gland, and the physician uses a computer to guide the procedure. A catheter is inserted through the urethra to the prostate. Microwave energy from an antenna inside the catheter heats and destroys enlarged cells in the gland. The

microwave *(cont.)* equipment has a cooling and flushing provision. Heated cells dissolve and are absorbed by the body, with resultant shrinkage of the prostate and return of normal urinary function.

microwave thermoradiotherapy (Oph) —used to treat uveal melanoma.

Micro-Z—wearable, high-volt-pulsed, galvanic neuromuscular stimulator.

MIC Thermal Option—disposable biopsy forceps.

MIC-TJ—transgastric jejunal tube.

MID (multi-infarct dementia).

Midas Rex pneumatic instruments—used in working on bone and articular cartilage; in cement removal and in polyethylene and metal cutting.

MIDCAB (minimally invasive direct coronary artery bypass) **procedure**.

middle cerebral artery (MCA).

middle ear implantable (MEI) **system**—for restoration of hearing.

middlescence—an inexact period of time in which people are between the ages of 26 to 45 years (the parenting years). Do not confuse with *middle-age*.

middlescent—the adjective form of middlescence; see *middlescence*.

midface sling procedure—plastic surgery procedure in which a sling of prosthetic (Gore-Tex) or autogenous (tendon or fascia) material is placed through the cheek mass. The sling is secured medially to the infraorbital rim. As variable tension is applied laterally toward the superficial temporal fascia, the sling functions as a fulcrum to return the cheek mass to a more youthful anatomical position. Elevating the cheek mass in this fashion fills the infraorbital hollow and results in amelioration of deep nasolabial folds and jowling.

midgut—distal duodenum, jejunum, ileum, and right colon. See *foregut* and *hindgut*.

mid-infrared laser—alternative to excimer, which uses ultraviolet light.

midline shift—displacement of a structure that is normally seen at or near the midline of the body, such as the pineal gland or the trachea.

midparental height—a term used in discussion of patients with possible growth hormone deficiency. One of the factors which must be taken into consideration is the height of the patient's parents, as short stature might simply be a familial characteristic. Therefore, the heights of both parents are added together and divided by 2 (the midparental height), and if this is low, it indicates that the patient's short stature is normal for that family and not necessarily a growth hormone failure. Conversely, if the midparental height is relatively high, consideration might be given to institution of supplemental growth hormone therapy.

Miescher cheilitis granulomatosa—noncaseating granulomas of the lips, a manifestation of Melkersson-Rosenthal syndrome.

Mighty Bite Zimmon lateral biopsy cup—used to obtain gastrointestinal mucosal tissue biopsies for microscopic examination.

MigraHealth—a dietary supplement containing riboflavin, magnesium, and feverfew for the treatment of migraines.

migraine equivalent—symptom-complex of migraine (aura, autonomic instability, transient neurological deficits, aphasia, or other features) without the headache component.

Migre Lief—a patented formula of feverfew, magnesium, and riboflavin. It is used to support cardiovascular tone and reduce platelet aggregation.

MigraSpray—an herbal remedy for migraine available in a saline solution containing the herb feverfew (*Tanacetum parthenium*). It is sprayed under the tongue or inside the cheek, allowing instant absorption of the herb and direct passage into the blood stream, bypassing the GI tract and eliminating the need to swallow bulky pills.

migration index (MI)—hip dysplasia measurement in children with cerebral palsy.

Mijnhard electrical cycloergometer—a device for measuring the heart rate under stress; a type of exercise tolerance test.

mil—unit of measurement equals 0.001 inch. Often used to express diameter of wire sutures.

milestones—see *developmental milestones*.

miliaria—heat rash. Cf. *malaria*.

militate—to affect, to carry weight, used with the word "against." Usage: "His long smoking history would militate against a very good prognosis." Cf. *mitigate*.

milk leg disease—the edematous, uniformly swollen, white extremity seen in femoroiliac thrombophlebitis.

milk scan—a series of scans that track the journey of a liquid after it is swallowed.

Millard R-A cleft lip repair—the use of a rotation flap to return a malpositioned philtral unit to its normal position and use an advancement flap to advance the lateral lip to fill the remaining defect.

Millard rotation flap advancement technique—rotation advancement flap repair of unilateral cleft lip.

Millar MPC-500 catheter—a high-fidelity microtipped catheter used in transesophageal echocardiography.

Millenia balloon catheter—for use during percutaneous transluminal coronary angioplasty.

Millen technique retropubic prostatectomy—a transverse row of sutures, with the "smile" removed from upper margin of bladder neck.

Miller-Abbott tube—a double-lumen long gastrointestinal tube.

Miller Galante I condylar total knee system.

mill-house murmur—a loud, continuous churning sound heard over the precordium (sometimes even without the use of a stethoscope). May be diagnostic of a venous air embolism.

millicurie (mCi, mc) (1/1000th of a curie)—the unit of measurement of radioactivity.

milliequivalent (mEq)—the unit of measurement used in writing electrolyte values and dosage of potassium chloride.

Milligan-Morgan technique—for treatment of hemorrhoids.

millijoule (mJ) ("mil-e-jul") (1/1000th of a joule)—measurement used in YAG laser and argon laser applications.

Millikan modified mesh-plug hernioplasty—a technique for primary unilateral inguinal herniorrhaphy. It is associated with minimal postoperative pain and permits an early return to normal activities and manual labor, with a minimal documented early recurrence rate.

milliliter (mL).

millimoles per liter (mmol/L).

milliner's needle—a straight needle with an eye, used primarily for suturing skin or readily accessible tissue.

milliosmole (mOsm).

Millon reagent—a nitric acid/mercuric nitrate solution that reacts with tyrosine and other phenols, turning red or orange in the presence of proteins. Since tyrosine is present in most proteins, Millon reagent is a good indicator of the presence of protein in urine.

Milroy disease—manifested by congenital lymphedema; the patient has an inborn error of development of the lymphatic channels.

Miltex surgical instruments.

Mima polymorpha—see *Acinetobacter lwoffi*.

MIMCOM (multimode imaging confocal optical microscope)—a class of optical microscopes providing novel imaging modalities, including biological imaging.

Mimix bone replacement cranioplasty.

MindSet toe splint—a plastic toe splint for broken or injured toes that can be worn inside a regular shoe. Allows the patient to remain active and in less pain.

Minerva neurosurgical robot.

Minerva-type cast—used for odontoid fracture.

Mini-Acutrak—a small-bone fixation system.

miniarousals (*not* many arousals)—a term used in sleep studies.

MINI Crown stent—specifically engineered for smaller vessels.

mini-FES (functional endoscopic sinus) **surgery** (ENT)—made possible by the use of microdebriders. Reportedly causes few complications in patients, especially children, undergoing sinus surgery.

mini Hoffmann external fixation system.

Mini-Hohmann podiatric retractor.

minilap—minilaparotomy.

minilaparotomy pelvic lymph node dissection—found to be significantly cheaper, but just as successful, as laparoscopic pelvic lymph node dissection in surgically staging prostate cancer.

minilaparotomy incision—used in vesicolithotomy, ureterolithotomy, suprapubic tube insertion, and bladder neck suspension.

minilaparotomy staging pelvic lymphadenectomy.

minimal change disease—a disorder of the kidneys that affects the structures (glomeruli) which include small capillaries surrounded by membranes through which the blood is filtered to form urine. Also known as minimal change nephrotic syndrome; nil disease; lipoid nephrosis; idiopathic nephrotic syndrome of childhood.

minimal incision aortic surgery (MIAS)—for treatment of high-risk patients with infrarenal aneurysms.

minimal inhibitory concentration (MIC)—an indication of antifungal susceptibility, determined by a change from pink (indicating growth) to blue or purple (growth inhibition) in the broth mixture used to grow the fungus.

minimally invasive surgery—an all-inclusive term used for procedures including laparoscopy, thoracoscopy, or percutaneous diskectomy. Generally employs a number of tiny incisions through which trocars are placed. Retractors, dissecting instruments, scopes, graspers, and suturing de-

minimally *(cont.)* vices are all inserted through strategically placed incisions, and any resected organs or tissue is removed via the same incisions. Minimally invasive surgery, properly performed, results in quicker recovery, fewer complications and side effects, shorter hospital stays, and more rapid return to normal activities.

minimally invasive video-assisted thyroidectomy (MIVAT).

Mini-Med continuous glucose sensor—implanted device that continuously records patient's glucose levels, then downloads data to an external computer for analysis.

Mini-Mental State Examination (MMSE)—a formal mental status test used to evaluate Alzheimer disease. A score of 10-26 correlates with Alzheimer of mild to moderate severity.

minimum alveolar concentration (MAC)—the potency of a given anesthetic, measured as minimum alveolar concentration (MAC). Technically, MAC is the alveolar partial pressure of a gas at which 50% of humans will not move to a painful stimulus (e.g. skin incision). Injected liquid anesthetics have a "MAC equivalent" which is the blood concentration of the liquid anesthetic that provides the same effect. Using MAC as a guideline, the amount of anesthetic given to a patient depends on that particular patient's needs.

Miniquant assay—test to detect D-dimer (a degradation product of fibrin), which is used as a marker or prognostic factor in various thrombotic diseases.

MiniSite laparoscope with 2 mm access site.

Minnesota antilymphoblast globulin—given to post-transplantation patients experiencing allograft rejection.

Minnesota Multiphasic Personality Inventory (MMPI)—mental status examination.

Minnesota Test for Differential Diagnosis of Aphasia (MTDDA)—a test to assess neurological deficit following such incidents as a subarachnoid hemorrhage. The test consists of seven subtests, including reading comprehension, reading rate, oral reading, describing a picture, writing letters dictated by the examiner, writing sentences dictated by the examiner, and arithmetic problems.

minor vestibular adenitis—see *vulvar vestibulitis syndrome.*

miotic—(1) an agent that causes the pupil to contract; (2) pertaining to, or causing, contraction of the pupil.

MIP (maximum intensity projection)—a term used in MRI and CT scans.

MIP (maximal inspiratory pressure).

Mirage Guidewire—used to access arteriovenous malformations in the brain for interventional treatment.

Miragel—hydrophilic sponge material used in the IMEX scleral implant.

Mirage nasal ventilation mask system—used for treatment of obstructive sleep apnea.

Miraluma—nuclear medicine test used in breast imaging.

Mirapex—a medication used but not approved for restless leg syndrome.

Mirena IUD—an intrauterine device that releases small amounts of a synthetic progesterone hormone to decrease the excessive bleeding and cramping that some women have with an IUD.

Mirizzi syndrome—common hepatic duct obstruction caused by extrinsic compression from an impacted stone in the cystic duct.

mirror image breast biopsy—a biopsy of the same spot in the opposite breast as the location of an earlier lesion (the same, but opposite, as in a mirror).

mirror-imaging—can affect a physician's sense of orientation within the cavity being operated. It occurs in laparoscopy due to the placement of viewing port and instrumentation port such that the instrument comes toward the viewer, rather than both pointing in the same direction.

mirroring—a phenomenon in which one extremity cannot move without the other moving in an identical manner.

Miser tube—a device for delivering contrast media in angiographic procedures.

Miskimon cerebellum retractor.

misregistration artifact—major cause of image degradation in digital subtraction angiography.

missed ostium sequence (MOS)—caused by the inadequate surgical removal of the most anterior portion of the uncinate process during endoscopic sinus surgery. It is postulated to be the cause of FES (functional endoscopic sinus) surgical failure.

missense mutation (Genetics)—a genetic mutation that replaces a codon specific for one amino acid with a codon specific for a different amino acid.

Mississippi Scale for Combat-Related Posttraumatic Stress Disorder—a psychiatric test for measuring posttraumatic stress disorder.

Mississippi 3-class system—a scoring system for HELLP syndrome that is based on the mother's platelet count. HELLP syndrome (hemolysis, elevated liver enzymes, low platelets) is a severe form of preeclampsia/eclampsia that can lead to pleural effusion, ascites, and even liver necrosis and is thought to have a genetic origin.

mist stick—emergency department term for a device that delivers humidified oxygen.

misty mesentery—an imaging term indicating an increased density of the mesenteric fat due to increased cellularity, fluid accumulation, tumor deposition, or fibrosis.

Mitchell distal osteotomy—to correct hallux valgus.

Mitchell technique—for epispadias repair.

Mitek anchor system—used in medial canthoplasty for reattaching the medial canthal tendon to the medial orbital wall. The operation can be performed through a small incision as well and may not be as invasive as other conventional procedures. It also has the advantage of being an easy technique with very accurate placement of the anchor and, consequently, reduced operating time.

Mitek BioKnotless anchor.

Mitek side effect electrode.

mitigate—to make milder, less severe. Usage: "We might attempt to mitigate his symptoms with phototherapy." Cf. *militate*.

mitochondria—organelles that synthesize ATP (adenosine triphosphate) and are the principal site of cellular energy metabolism through the oxidation of foodstuffs (carbohydrates, fats, and proteins).

mitochondrial DNA—genetic material in mitochondria that codes for synthesis of mitochondrial proteins and enzymes independently of nuclear DNA. Virtually all of the mitochondrial DNA in a cell is derived from the cytoplasm of the oocyte (maternal gamete).

mitosis—division and reapportionment of chromosomes in the nucleus in preparation for cell division; each chromosome makes a copy of itself, so that each daughter nucleus contains the full (diploid) complement of 23 pairs of chromosomes.

mitotic chromosomes.

Mitraflex wound dressing—sterile multilayer wound dressing which is very thin and can be used over the entire face or around the shoulder, for example.

mitral regurgitation artifact (cineangiography)—induced if the catheter is too close to the mitral valve in left ventricular angiography.

mitral valve homograft—mitral valves taken from cadavers, reducing chance of rejection that occurs with animal or mechanical valves. Valves are taken from young organ donors and can be preserved for up to 10 years, thus making use of hearts that are not suitable for whole-heart transplants. Transplant of human valves does not require lifelong use of blood thinners, and it is expected that these valves will last longer than animal valves.

mitral valve prolapse (MVP).

Mitrofanoff appendicovesicostomy—a technique for continent urinary diversion.

Mitrofanoff catheterizable stoma—a bladder reconstruction technique for urinary incontinence.

Mitrofanoff channel—a channel created for continent urinary diversion. Also conduit.

Mitrofanoff neourethra procedure—creates a neourethra for a continent abdominal stoma. A neourethra is developed by implanting a tubular segment into the bladder, which, when brought out through the skin, creates a continent, catheterizable neourethra.

Mitsuo scale—used in ophthalmology. Usage: "Anterior chamber pigment was measured on a modified Mitsuo scale."

mittelschmerz—pain midway between the menstrual periods.

Mittendorf dot—also known as *hyaloid corpuscle*. Represents the attachment of a hyaloid vessel to the posterior capsule.

Mityvac cup (Ob-Gyn)—a rigid traction handle attached to a semirigid cup, with the vacuum port located at the end of a traction handle. Shaped like a Dixie cup.

MIVAT (minimally invasive video-assisted thyroidectomy).

MIVR (minimally invasive valve repair or replacement).

mixed angina—a widely used term with controversial definitions. The simplest definition seems to be "the coexistence of effort angina and rest angina, without any judgment as to the etiology." Also called *variable threshold angina*.

mixed connective tissue disease (MCTD).

mixed leukocyte culture (MLC).

Miya hook ligament carrier—used in sacrospinous ligament suspension.

Miyazaki-Bonney test—for stress incontinence. It duplicates the effects of the Burch bladder neck suspen-

Miyazaki *(cont.)*
sion procedure to determine if surgery will help the patient. See also *Bonney test*.

mJ (millijoule).

MKM AutoPilot stereotactic system—allows the operator to visualize navigation during surgery.

M-K (McCarey-Kaufman) **medium**.

mL (milliliter)—unit of liquid measure equivalent to a cubic centimeter (cc). Usage: "Estimated blood loss was 200 mL." (*Not* cc, even if dictated.)

MLC (mixed leukocyte culture)—a trial in a test tube to determine in advance if donor and recipient tissues are compatible.

MLD (microlumbar diskectomy).

MLD (minimum lethal dose)—refers to ingestion of poisons or toxins.

MLG (midline glossectomy)—see *laser midline glossectomy*.

MLH_1 gene—the second defective gene linked to colon cancer discovered by the team that discovered MSH_2. See *MSH_2*.

M listening—see *A, P, T, M*.

MLNS (mucocutaneous lymph node syndrome).

MLS (mini lag-screw)—see *Alphatec*.

MMCM (macromolecular contrast medium)—MRI term.

MMEF (maximum midexpiratory flow rate).

MMMT (malignant mixed mullerian tumor).

M-mode echocardiogram.

mmol/L (millimoles per liter)—an SI (International System) unit of measurement of serum values.

MMSE (Mini-Mental State Examination).

MMS-10 tympanic displacement analyzer—a device to measure the perilymphatic pressure in patients with Ménière disease.

MND (motor neuron disease).

MN rgp120—an AIDS vaccine that has shown encouraging results by inducing HIV-1 MN antibody production. A protein associated with HIV, *rgp120* stands for recombinant gp120 protein.

MNTI (melanotic neuroectodermal tumor of infancy)—rare neoplasm occurring most often in the first year of life.

MOAB, MoAb, MAb (monoclonal antibody).

mobes—slang which should be expanded to mobilizations. Mobilizations may be administered in various gradations or degrees of pressure. Very gentle "mobes" are used for very sensitive or acute patients to initiate more normal movement. These are called "Grade One" mobes. "Grade Two's" are administered for pain relief. They are slightly stronger than Grade Ones. "Grade Three" mobes both relieve pain and gently improve the range of motion of stiff joints. "Grade Four's" are for stretching tight tissues and restoring range in more chronic situations.

Mobetron intraoperative radiation therapy (IORT) **treatment system**—a mobile, self-shielded electron linear accelerator that directly delivers IORT to patients as they are undergoing cancer surgery.

mobilize—move. Cf. *immobilize*.

Mobin-Uddin umbrella filter—for transvenous vena cava interruption in prevention of pulmonary emboli. See also *Kim-Ray Greenfield filter*, which is *not* synonymous.

MOBS (Montefiore Organic Brain Scale).

MOCB (medial olivocochlear bundle).

moccasin-type tinea pedis—characterized by scaling, hyperkeratosis, minimal inflammation, particularly refractory to topical therapy and usually requiring an oral antifungal agent.

MOCNI ("mock-ney") (method of collection not indicated) (Path).

Model for End-Stage Liver Disease (MELD) and Pediatric End-Stage Liver Disease (PELD)—numerical scales that are currently used for liver allocation. The MELD and PELD scores are based on a patient's risk of dying while waiting for a liver transplant, and are calculated from objective and verifiable medical data. The MELD score is used for adult liver patients and is based on bilirubin, INR, and creatinine. Liver transplant candidates under the age of 18 are assigned a PELD score. The PELD score is based on bilirubin, INR, albumin, growth failure, and age when listed for transplant, factors which better predict mortality in children. These scores do not determine the likelihood of getting a transplant, which is based upon organ availability and the distribution of MELD/PELD scores for patients in a local area or region.

Modic classification of disk abnormality—numbered 1, 2, 3, 4, 4A, 4B, and 4C; based on MRI findings.

modified endoventricular circularplasty—see *endoventricular circular patchplasty*. Also known as the *Dor procedure.*

modified Hughes procedure—reconstruction of large defects of the lower eyelid.

modified Isshiki type 4 thyroplasty—used in treatment of unilateral cricothyroid muscle paralysis.

modified Linton procedure—treatment of varicose veins using endoscopic subfascial division technique.

modified Pereyra bladder neck suspension.

modified Rodnan total skin-thickness score technique—used to determine skin thickness in scleroderma.

modified Stahl classification of Kienböck disease

Stage 1: Normal structure of the lunate, with evidence of compression fracture usually appearing as a radiodense or radiolucent line.

Stage 2: Rarefaction along the line of previous compression fractures developing within the first 3 months.

Stage 3: Changes of stages 1 and 2 together with sclerosis of the proximal pole occurring at about 3 months.

Stage 4: Fragmentation or flattening of the lunate.

Stage 5: Changes of arthrosis of radiocarpal and intercarpal joints.

MODS (multiple organ dysfunction syndrome)—thought to be a more accurate term than *MOF (multiple organ failure)*.

Modulap—reusable electrosurgical cutting and coagulation probe for use in general laparoscopic surgical procedures.

Modulith SL 20—a third-generation lithotriptor equipped with fluoroscopic and ultrasound localization systems.

Modulock posterior spinal fixation.

MODY (maturity-onset diabetes of the young)—a distinct form of non-insulin-dependent diabetes mellitus.

Moe—instrumentation and wiring of the spinous processes for scoliosis.

Moebius sign—in exophthalmos, one or both eyes fail to converge on attempting to look at an object close to midline.

Moersch-Woltmann syndrome—progressive neurological disorder characterized by constant painful contractions and spasms of voluntary muscles, particularly the muscles of the back and upper legs, in response to stimuli such as loud noises. Also known as *stiff-man syndrome* and *stiff-person syndrome.*

MOF (multiple organ failure)—see *multisystem organ failure*.

mohel (Hebrew)—the person who performs the Jewish circumcision ceremony known as a bris. Also, moyel in Yiddish.

Mohs fresh tissue chemosurgery—used primarily in basal cell carcinoma. After fixation in vivo with zinc chloride paste, the tumor is then excised under microscopic control. Named for surgeon Dr. Frederick E. Mohs.

Mohtadi Quality of Life Index—outcome measure for anterior cruciate ligament deficiency.

moiré artifact (Radiol)—a pattern, sometimes seen in expensive silks, caused by the superimposition of two grids with linear patterns running in almost the same direction; the slight variation causes the moiré phenomenon.

Moire topographic assessment—scoliosis screening test that is more expensive and time-consuming than the Adams test.

moisture vapor permeability (MVP).

molar pregnancy—refers to a hydatidiform mole, an abnormal pregnancy which results from an ovum which has been converted to a mole. (This has nothing to do with molar teeth.)

molars—see *mulberry molars*.

molding—the shaping of the fetal head by the birth canal. Also, *moulding*.

molecular coincidence detection (MCD) **imaging**—imaging technology that is able to detect lung cancer and show the location and extent of the disease.

molecular recognition unit (MRU)—pharmacologic technology based on monoclonal antibodies but physically much smaller. MRUs link with drugs or diagnostic radiology agents and allow them to reach more fully into body tissues. See *ThromboScan MRU*.

mole syndrome—see *atypical mole syndrome*.

Molina band—a dual-mesh gastroplasty banding technique.

molluscum contagiosum virus (MCV) —a poxvirus that results in persistent skin infection, often manifesting itself in AIDS patients.

Molnar disk—plastic disk to anchor a nephrostomy tube in place.

Molteno filtering bleb (Oph).

Molteno implant drainage device (Oph).

Molteno seton—a tube which allows aqueous humor to flow from the anterior chamber to the subconjunctival space to decrease intraocular pressure.

Molt periosteal elevator.

molybdenum—see *SMo*, stainless steel with molybdenum.

MOM (milk of magnesia).

Monaghan 300 ventilator—a pressure-cycled ventilator that forces air into the lungs until an airway pressure (which has previously been determined) is obtained.

Monarc mesh.

Monarc subfascial sling—repair of female urinary incontinence using Monarc mesh.

Monarc transobturator tape sling—for stress incontinence.

monarsen—a medication for the treatment of myasthenia gravis.

Monday crust—the phenomenon of patients being less open to analysis after a weekend.

Mondini dysplasia.

Mondor disease—superficial thrombophlebitis of the skin of the breast, usually occurring spontaneously in the upper outer quadrant. The condition often mimics the appearance of cancer.

mongoloid fissure—groove in the lateral canthus of the eyelid.

monitor
- Accu-Chek InstantPlus
- Accu-Chek II Freedom
- AccuGuide injection
- actocardiotocograph
- Acuson V5M
- Androflo
- Androsonix biological sound
- A1cNow
- Appraise
- AtLast blood glucose
- Appraise diabetes
- Biotrack coagulation
- BioZ system
- blood perfusion (BPM)
- Brackmann facial nerve
- brain or intraventricular temperature monitoring
- Bravo pH monitoring
- CA (cardiac-apnea)
- CardioBeeper CB-12L
- Cardiocap 5
- CareLink
- CDI 2000 blood gas
- Cenflex central

monitor *(cont.)*
- Chronicle implantable hemodynamic
- Companion 2 self blood glucose
- Corometrics maternal/fetal
- Crit-Line
- Cueva cranial nerve electrode
- C-VEST system
- Diascan glucose
- Dinamap blood pressure
- Dopplette
- DynaPulse 5000A blood pressure
- EFM (electronic fetal monitoring)
- endotracheal cardiac output monitoring (ECOM)
- Excel GE glucose monitoring strip
- FastTake electrochemical blood glucose
- Glucometer DEX blood glucose
- HomMed
- Housecall transtelephonic
- Illi intracranial pressure
- Jako facial nerve
- KinetiX ventilation
- Laserflo blood perfusion (BPM)
- Licox monitoring device
- LifeGuide blood glucose
- Life-Pack 5 cardiac
- Lifestream personal cholesterol
- MDILO medication intake
- Med-ic ECP (electronic compliance monitor)
- Medisense Pen 2 blood glucose
- MyoTrac and MyoTrac 2 EMG
- Nicolet Nerve Integrity Monitor-2 (NIM-2)
- NIM-Spine system neural integrity
- OnLineABG
- OxiFirst fetal oxygen
- Paradigm Link blood glucose
- Persona monitoring kit
- Polar Vantage XL heart rate
- PressureSense
- Prestige IQ blood glucose
- Propaq Encore vital signs
- PSC fertility

monitor *(cont.)*
Pulse Pro heart rate
Pushita bloodless glucose
Silverstein facial nerve
Sof-Tact glucose
Stryker compartment pressure
Stryker Intracompartmental Pressure
TD Glucose monitoring system
Tracer Blood Glucose Micromonitor
UPlink
Vasotrax
VentCheck ventilator
Vigilance CCO/SvO_2/CEDV
virtual labor (VLM)
Vitatron Selection Afm
WinABP ambulatory blood pressure

monkeypox—an orthopox virus with an appearance and behavior very similar to smallpox. One of its most interesting features is that it appears to have both human-to-human and animal-to-human transmission. Outbreaks of this disease, which was thought to have been eradicated many years ago, have occurred in the Republic of Congo (formerly Zaire) in what has been described as epidemic proportions.

monochromatization—filtering technique that permits the passage of only certain x-rays that fall within a narrow band of energy levels.

monoclonal antibody (MAb; MoAb; MOAB)—an antibody produced by a hybridoma (a clone of cells derived from the fusion of an immune cell and a tumor cell). Monoclonal antibodies to T-cells are called *OKT antibodies* and are used to study the T-cell populations (or T-cell subsets) in patients. See also *antibody*; *medication*.

monoclonal antibody-based enzyme immunoassay.

monoclonal antibody-specific immobilization of platelet antigens (MAIPA) **assay**.

Monocryl suture (polyglecaprone 25) —a pliable, synthetic, absorbable, monofilament suture.

monodrug therapy—treatment of a condition such as hypertension or malignancy with a single drug rather than a combination of drugs.

Monoflex lens—intraocular lens made of PMMA.

Monojector—see *fingerstick devices for blood glucose testing*.

Monolyth oxygenator—extracorporeal membrane oxygenation system used during cardiac bypass procedures.

Monoscopy locking trocar with Woodford spike—a locking trocar which features an intra-abdominal locking mechanism. Used in laparoscopic procedures.

monosomy (Genetics)—an abnormal condition in which one chromosome of a pair is missing.

monosomy 7 syndrome.

Monospot test—a rapidly performed serum agglutination test for infectious mononucleosis. Note: *Monospot* is one word, *not* two.

Monostrut cardiac valve prosthesis.

monozygotic twins (Genetics)—identical twins, derived by splitting of a single fertilized ovum (zygote).

Monro, foramen of—brain anatomy.

Monsel solution—a hemostatic drug solution. Usage: "There was a small amount of oozing from the cervical biopsy site, and Monsel solution was used to stop this bleeding."

monster rongeur.

monstrocellular—composed of giant cells. This is a term you will likely hear in pathology dictation.

Montefiore Organic Brain Scale (MOBS).

Monteggia fracture-dislocation—fracture of the ulna, with a radial head dislocation.

Montevideo units—measurement of the length and strength of uterine contractions.

Montgomery Safe-T-Tube—used in patients with acute tracheal injuries, to support the trachea post reconstruction, and also to support an intrathoracic tracheal stenosis.

Monticelli-Spinelli system—a circular external fixation system for fractures of the leg and for leg lengthenings.

Monti-Malone, left—a combination of the Monti and Malone procedures for continent urinary diversion in combination with antegrade colonic enema for fecal incontinence. The "Malone continent cecostomy for antegrade colonic enema (ACE) and the Monti intestinal conduit, as an alternative conduit to replace the appendix, are two major improvements in incontinence surgery."

Monti procedure—a technique for bladder augmentation with autologous bowel (a segment of ileum instead of the appendix) for continent urinary diversion. The mobility of the appendix is restricted by the length of its mesentery, whereas the Monti tube can be placed wherever suitable along the digestive tract. Also *continent ileovesicostomy*, and *laparoscopy-assisted ileocystoplasty and ileovesicostomy*.

MONW (metabolically obese but normal weight)

Moolgaoker forceps—for spontaneous vaginal delivery assist.

Moon Boot brace—used as an external support to brace fracture of the distal tibia and fibula.

moon face (or *facies*)—a pronounced rounding of the cheeks in Cushing syndrome or prolonged adrenocortical therapy.

Moran repair—an inguinal hernia repair technique.

Moraxella lwoffi—see *Acinetobacter lwoffi*.

morcellation—see *morselize*.

More-Flow catheter—a double-lumen hemodialysis catheter.

Moretz Tab—ventilation tube used for tympanoplasty procedure.

Morgagni ("mor-gah-nyee") **appendix**.

Morgagni crypt.

Morganella morganii—newer name for what was called *Proteus morganii*.

Morgan lens—for use in ocular irrigation, especially for the treatment of eye trauma and ocular chemical injury. It consists of a small lens-shaped plastic piece attached to thin tubing, which is then hooked up to an irrigant. The lens part is placed directly onto the eye after topical anesthetic eyedrops are instilled, the eyelids are closed over the lens, and the irrigant is delivered via the tubing.

Morganstern continuous-flow operating cystoscope.

moribund—dying.

Moro reflex—seen normally in infants up to 3 or 4 months of age. An infant is placed supine, and a sudden noxious stimulus is made (usually a loud noise by slapping the table alongside). The child will respond by extending and then flexing the arms (in a protective or embracing attitude) and flexing the hips and knees. Also called *embrace* or *startle reflex*.

Morris—incorrect spelling of *Morse (taper stem)*.

Morscher titanium cervical plate—for treatment of complex cervical spine disorders.

morselize (verb)—to take small pieces (morsels) of bone or cartilage in nasal surgery or orthopedic surgery. Usage: "The distal fibula was morselized and the bone chips packed tightly into the arthrodesis site laterally after the fibrous tissue had been curetted out." (English dictionaries have *morsel, and* medical dictionaries have *morcellation* as main entries. The need for the verb form frequently used in surgical dictation is not recognized in nonmedical dictionaries.)

Morse taper stem (*not* Morris)—used in orthopedic surgery. Usage: "The hip was then redislocated and the trial head was taken off and the final cobalt chromium head was placed on the Morse taper. It was pounded into position using ten taps."

morsicatio buccarum—the nervous habit of biting or chewing the buccal mucosa.

mortise—a slot, or wedge-shaped cut into bone (or timber) into which will fit a tenon. This is also a carpenter's or furniture-maker's word. Cf. *Webster's* definition of *tenon* (*not* tendon). The ankle mortise is the normal articulation between the talus and the distal tibia and fibula.

morula—a stage of embryonic development preceding the blastocyst stage; the morula is a spherical mass of undifferentiated cells.

MOS (missed ostium sequence).

mosaic (Genetics)—an individual or tissue containing at least two cell lines that differ in genotype or karyotype, but are derived from a single zygote.

mosaic perfusion (Radiol)—used in radiologic description of lung in bronchiolitis and other conditions.

mosaicplasty—technique to repair talar injuries resulting from osteochondritis dissecans, which generally strikes active children, young adults, and athletes. Mosaicplasty has also been used to repair knee joints.

Mosaic porcine bioprosthesis—stented tissue heart valve.

Mosaic valve—a bioprosthetic heart valve designed to reduce valve calcification and maintain the natural shape and function of the valve, reducing mechanical stress on the tissue.

Moschowitz procedure—obliteration of the cul-de-sac.

Mosley method—for anterior shoulder repair.

Moses sign—the presence of pain with compression of the calf against the tibia. Some patients with deep vein thrombosis will have more pain with this maneuver than with transverse compression of the gastrocnemius. Also, *Bancroft sign*.

mOsm (milliosmole).

mosquito clamp.

Moss G-tube PEG kit—for PEG and laparoscopic procedures. Rigid introducer for simplified duodenal placement of J-wire and G-tube. For simple gastric feeding without decompression.

Moss Miami load-sharing spinal implant system—provides anterior column support in balancing natural forces of spine.

Moss nasal tube, Mark IV—esophageal/duodenal decompression device for enteral hyperalimentation.

Moss Suction Buster tube—see *Suction Buster catheter*.

Moss T-anchor needle introducer gun—used to implant nylon T-anchors in the Moss percutaneous endoscopic gastrostomy regimen.

-most—commonly used in medical dictation to form an adjective, as in *medialmost margin*; also, topmost, hindmost, innermost, outermost.

MOST Options—a line of modular instruments for hip and knee reconstruction.

moth-eaten appearance—radiologic appearance reflecting increased density and rarefaction in the long bones of children with congenital syphilis.

mother and baby endoscope—same as *mother-daughter scope*; physicians may refer to each scope separately as *motherscope* and *babyscope*.

Mother2Be—line of natural skin and body care treatments designed to soothe, heal, and protect the skin of pregnant women.

Motor Control Test (MCT)—used in conjunction with computerized dynamic posturography.

motorcyclist's knee—see *O'Donoghue unhappy triad* (OUT).

motor evoked potential (MEP).

motor meal barium GI series—shows transit time, stomach to colon (normal transit time, 60 minutes).

motor-sensory 5/5—a hyphen between *motor* and *sensory* is essential, for correct meaning.

Motrin Migraine Pain (ibuprofen)—an over-the-counter ibuprofen drug product developed for migraines.

MOTT (*Mycobacterium* other than tuberculosis).

Mouchet syndrome—paralysis of the cubital nerve following fracture of the external humeral condyle.

moulding—see *molding*, which seems to be the preferred spelling.

mouse units (MU)—used in an endocrinology test to measure levels of circulating pituitary hormones.

mouth gag
- Dingman
- Dingman-Denhardt
- Dott
- Dott-Dingman self-retaining cleft palate
- McIvor

moving-bed infusion-tracking MRA—method for imaging the entire peripheral vascular tree with only one bolus of Magnevist over a scanning time of four minutes.

moving platform posturography—method of quantifying a patient's sense of equilibrium, and often used to determine whether a disorder is getting better or worse.

moxa—shredded artemisia that is burned on or near the body to produce local heating, as well as to generate an additional influence from the moxa material itself, perhaps imparting borneol and other active constituents to the body. See *moxibustion* and *sparrow-picking technique*.

moxi—slang for amoxicillin.

moxibustion—treatment of disease by applying heat to acupuncture points. Used for ailments such as bronchial asthma, bronchitis, certain types of paralysis, and arthritic disorders.

moyamoya ("puff of smoke")—angiographic diagnosis of bilateral stenosis or occlusion of the internal carotid arteries above the clinoids.

moyel (Yiddish)—the person who performs the Jewish circumcision ceremony known as a bris. Also mohel in Hebrew.

MPC scissors—automated intravitreal scissors.

MPD (main pancreatic duct) **stent**.

MPGR (multiplanar gradient-recalled) **echo.**

MPHR (maximum predicted heart rate) —a term used in exercise tolerance tests. See *Bruce protocol, ETT*.

MPIF-1 (myeloid progenitor inhibitory factor-1).

MPL (monophosphoryl lipid A) **vaccine adjuvant**—vaccine adjuvant for use in preventing various infectious diseases and allergies.

MPM hydrogel dressing.

mPower PET scanner—by Positron.

MPR (multiplanar reformation).

MP-RAGE (magnetization prepared three-dimensional gradient-echo) **sequences**—MRI term.

M-protein, M-component—used in reference to chemotherapy response in patients with multiple myeloma (and perhaps other diseases).

MRA (magnetic resonance angiography)—gated inflow technique. See *3DCE MRA technique*.

MRC (magnetic resonance cholangiography).

MRCP (magnetic resonance cholangiopancreatography).

MRCP using HASTE with a phased array coil—noninvasive technique for revealing the pancreaticobiliary tract in young children. See *HASTE*.

MRE (magnetic resonance elastography).

MR enteroclysis (MRE).

MR hydrography—technique that displays static or slow-moving fluids as bright structures against the dark background of the rest of the body. The images show fluid-containing structures, such as ducts, cysts, sacs, and spaces, as white on black; thus, calculi can be readily identified as filling defects.

MRI (magnetic resonance imaging) **terms** for quick reference
- acquisition time
- adiabatic fast passage
- A-FAIR
- AMT-25-enhanced MR images
- analog-to-digital converter
- angular frequency
- angular momentum
- antenna
- array processor
- artifact
- axial proton-density-weighted image
- axial T2-weighted image
- Bloch equation
- Boltzmann distribution
- bone marrow edema pattern
- breath-hold fast spin-echo images
- bright signal
- Carr-Purcell-Meiboom-Gill sequence
- Carr-Purcell sequence
- chemical shift
- chemical shift imaging (CSI)
- cine study
- coherence
- coil
- continuous wave
- contrast enhancement
- conventional spin-echo images
- coronal SPIR image
- coronal T1-weighted MR image (spin echo)
- crossed coil
- cryomagnet
- cryostat
- demodulator
- detector
- diamagnetic
- diffusion
- diffusion tensor magnetic resonance imaging
- digital-to-analog converter
- echo, echoes
- echo planar imaging

MRI terms *(cont.)*
echo time (TE)
eddy currents; eddies
edge detection (ED)
endorectal coil
endovaginal coil
excitation
Exorcist respiratory compensation technique
Faraday shield
fast-Fourier transform
fast spin-echo acquisition, 2-D or 3-D
fat- and water-suppressed T2-weighted images
ferromagnetic
field gradient
field lock
field of view (FOV)
filling factor
filtered-back projection
FLAIR (fluid-attentuated inversion recovery)
flip angle
flow artifact
flow-compensated 2D T1-weighted spin-echo
flow-compensated 2D T2-weighted spin-echo
flow-compensated respiratory-triggered 3D turbo spin-echo
flow-related enhancement
flow-related phase shifts
fMRI (functional MRI)
FNH (focal nodular hyperplasia)
Fonar Stand-Up
Fourier transform
free induction decay (FID)
free induction signal
frequency
FSE-T2 (fast spin echo) with fat suppression
functional
gadolinium-enhanced T1-weighted images

MRI terms *(cont.)*
gauss
Golay coil
gradient coil
gradient-echo pulse sequence
gradient magnetic field
gyromagnetic ratio
half-dose enhanced MRI with MT (magnetization transfer)
half-Fourier acquisition single-shot turbo spin-echo (HASTE)
HASTE (half-Fourier acquisition single-shot turbo spin-echo)
Helmholtz coil
hertz (Hz)
homogeneity
HRARE (hybrid rapid acquisition with relaxation enhancement)
image acquisition time
inductance
inhomogeneity
interface
interpulse time
intravascular signal intensity in MR angiography
inversion
inversion recovery
inversion time (TI)
IPAT (integrated parallel acquisition technique)
kilohertz (kHz)
Larmor equation
Larmor frequency
lattice
line imaging
line scanning
line width
LMR (localized magnetic resonance)
long echo train fast spin-echo sequence
longitudinal magnetization
longitudinal relaxation
Lorentzian line
macroscopic magnetization moment

MRI terms *(cont.)*
macroscopic magnetization vector
magnetic dipole
magnetic field
magnetic gradient
magnetic induction
magnetic moment
magnetic resonance signal
magnetic susceptibility
magnetization
magnetization transfer (MT) saturation
MIP (maximum intensity projection)
MMCM-enhanced MR imaging
MP-RAGE (magnetization prepared 3-D gradient-echo) sequences
MRCP using HASTE with a phased array coil
multiple line-scan imaging (MLSI)
multiple plane imaging
multiple sensitive point
multishot spin-echo echo-planar imaging
nidus patency
no phase wrap function
nuclear magnetic resonance
nuclear signal
nuclear spin
nuclear spin quantum number
nucleon
number of excitations
nutation
opposed loop-pair quadrature magnetic resonance coil
orientation
  axial
  coronal
  sagittal
  transverse
oversampling
paramagnetic
partial saturation
PASTA (polarity-altered spectral selective acquisition) imaging
PC (phase-contrast) technique

MRI terms *(cont.)*
pelvic floor MRI
percentage signal intensity loss (PSIL)
permanent magnet
permeability
phantom
phase
phase contrast
phase imaging
phase sensitive detector
phase shift
pixel (picture element)
planar spin imaging
point imaging
point scanning
precession
precessional frequency
proton density
PSIL (percentage signal intensity loss)
pulsed gradients
pulse length
pulse, radiofrequency
pulse sequences
pulse width
quality factor
quenching
radian
rapid acquisition with relaxation enhancement (RARE)
rapid imaging
RARE (rapid acquisition with relaxation enhancement) technique
readout delay
receiver
receiver coil
reconstruction
reduced signal intensity
relaxation rate
relaxation time
repeated FID (free induction decay)
rephasing gradient
resistive magnet
resolution, spatial

MRI terms *(cont.)*
resonance
resonant frequency
respiratory triggered fast SE technique
respiratory triggering
RF (radiofrequency) coil
RF (radiofrequency) pulse
ROC (receiver operating characteristic)
ROPE (respiratory ordered phase encoding)
rotating frame of reference
saddle coil
sagittal T1-weighted image
saturation recovery
saturation transfer
selective excitation
selective irradiation
sensitive plane
sensitive point
sensitive volume
sequence time
sequential plane imaging
sequential point imaging
shaded surface display (SSD)
shim coil
shimming
signal-to-noise ratio (SNR or S/N ratio)
simultaneous volume imaging
single shot fast spin echo (SSFSE)
single slice fast dynamic in vivo
skin depth
solenoid coil
spectrometer
spectrum
spin
spin density
spin echo
spin-echo imaging
spin-lattice relaxation time
spin-spin relaxation time
spin-warp imaging
SPIR (selective partial inversion-recovery)

MRI terms *(cont.)*
SPIR fat-suppression images
SPIR-FLAIR images or sequences
split renal function (SRE)
SSD (shaded surface display)
standard-dose enhanced conventional T1-weighted images
steady state free precession (SSFP)
STEAM (stimulated echo acquisition mode) sequence
STIR (short inversion time inversion-recovery) sequence
superconducting magnet
surface coil
tagged red blood cell nuclear scan
TE (echo time)
tesla (T)
three-dimensional Fourier
3-D TOF (time-of-flight) MR angiographic sequences
THRIVE (T1 high resolution isotropic volume examination) technique
TI (inversion time)
time-of-flight (TOF) echoplanar imaging
time-of-flight (TOF) method
TOF (time of flight)
T1 (spin-lattice or longitudinal relaxation time)
TR (repetition time)
transform imaging
transverse magnetization
TRIADS (time-resolved imaging by automatic data segmentation)
T1-weighted fat-suppressed gadolinium-enhanced SE images
T1-weighted gadolinium-enhanced SE images
T2 (spin-spin or transverse relaxation time)
T2-weighted fast SE images
T2-weighted turbo SE images
true FISP (true fast imaging with steady-state precession)

MRI terms *(cont.)*
- tuning
- tunnel
- 2-D or 3-D fast spin-echo acquisition
- 3-D CEMRA (three-dimensional, contrast-enhanced MR angiography)
- 3D heavily T1-weighted dynamic gradient-echo sequence
- 3-D Turbo FLAIR (fluid-attenuated inversion-recovery)
- transaxial fat-saturated 3-D images
- triple-dose gadolinium-enhanced MR imaging without MT (magnetization transfer)
- turbo spin-echo sequences
- turbo STIR images
- two-dimensional Fourier
- UBOs (unidentified bright objects)
- vector
- velocity encoding
- venetian blind artifacts
- volume acquisition
- volume analysis
- volume imaging
- volume rendering
- volumetric
- voxel (volume element)
- zeugmatography, Fourier transformation

MRM (magnetic resonance mammography).

MRN (magnetic resonance neurography).

mRNA (messenger RNA).

MRP (magnetic resonance pancreatography).

MR peritoneography—a study in which the imaging agent is instilled into the peritoneal cavity, magnetic resonance scanning is performed with the peritoneal cavity filled, and after complete drainage of the contrast material, a scan is again performed. Images are reviewed for evidence of peritoneal leaks, hernias, loculated fluid collections, and adhesions. MR peritoneography is particularly useful in continuous ambulatory peritoneal dialysis.

MRS (magnetic resonance spectroscopy).

MRSA (methicillin-resistant *Staphylococcus aureus*).

MRSE (manifest refraction spherical equivalent).

MRSI (magnetic resonance spectroscopic imaging)—detects a chemical marker to diagnose breast cancer. The diagnostic technique produces pictures of choline within breast tumors. MRSI of the breast is not yet cost-effective as a routine screening tool for breast cancer but may prove to be a noninvasive alternative to biopsy in cases with positive mammography or clinical breast exam results.

MRT (magnetic resonance tomography).

MRU (magnetic resonance urography).

MRU (molecular recognition unit).

MSAFP (maternal serum alpha-fetoprotein).

MSBP or **MSP** (Munchausen syndrome by proxy).

MS Classique catheter—balloon dilatation catheter for angioplasty.

MSCTA (multislice computed tomographic angiography)

MSEV (microsurgical epididymovasostomy).

MSH_2 gene—the gene responsible for the most common forms of inherited colon cancer. Identification of this gene may lead to a broadly used genetic cancer screening. The MSH_2 gene normally "corrects" mistakes that occur when cells are damaged

MSH_2 gene *(cont.)*
or divide. However, a flawed gene may allow mistakes to accumulate, thus triggering the growth of cancerous neoplasms.

MSI (magnetic source imaging).

"m-site"—phonetic for *Emcyt*.

MSLT (multiple sleep latency test).

MSP, **MSBP** (Munchausen syndrome by proxy).

M spike—monoclonal proteins seen as a sharp spike on serum protein electrophoresis.

MSSA (methicillin-sensitive *Staphylococcus aureus*).

MSTRs (multiple signal transduction regulators)—a new class of anticancer drugs.

MSTS (Musculoskeletal Tumor Society) **staging system**—for soft-tissue sarcomas.

MSUD (maple syrup urine disease)—difficult only because the MT cannot believe the dictator is really saying "maple syrup urine."

MTBE (methyl tertiary butyl ether)—a drug instilled under local anesthesia to dissolve large cholesterol stones in the gallbladder. Via transhepatic catheter, the bile is aspirated from the gallbladder, and 5 to 10 ml of MTBE is instilled in the gallbladder. As the stone dissolves, the MTBE containing dissolved cholesterol is removed, and more MTBE instilled. This process is continued until fluoroscopy reveals complete dissolving of the stones.

MTD (maximum tolerated dose).

MTM (modified Thayer-Martin medium, a culture medium)—used in culturing *Neisseria gonorrhoeae*.

MTP (microsomal triglyceride transfer protein)—a protein linked to low levels of LDL and thus indicative of low risk for heart attack or stroke.

MTP-PE—see *muramyl-tripeptide*.

MTR (microsurgical tubal reanastomosis).

MT (magnetization transfer) **saturation**—MRI term.

MTSS (medial tibial stress syndrome).

M2A capsule—a capsule used in the Given diagnostic imaging system.

M2A Swallowable Imaging Capsule—contains a camera-in-a-capsule and is swallowed as a regular pill, transmitting images of the GI tract to an external device worn on a belt. The capsule travels via normal peristalsis over a period of six to eight hours and then leaves the body naturally.

Much ("mooks") **granules**—found in the sputa of patients with tuberculosis. They are visible on Gram stain but not on stain for acid-fast bacilli or by other methods.

mucocutaneous lymph node syndrome (MLNS)—affects prepubertal children almost exclusively, mostly males, with a peak incidence during the first 18 months. See *Kawasaki disease*.

mucolipidosis III (pseudo-Hurler deformity)—a rare congenital abnormality which includes clawhand, ground-glass corneas, aortic valvular disease, and other orthopedic and biochemical abnormalities. Onset is around age three.

mucopus—a mixture of mucus and pus.

mucormycosis—rare and often fatal mycotic infection caused by one of the sporophytic fungi of the order Mucorales. It is known to affect patients who are immunocompromised. The most common form is rhinocerebral, although primary infections of the skin, lungs, and GI

mucormycosis *(cont.)*
tract have also been reported. Involvement of the GU tract is primarily limited to the kidneys. Mucormycosis (*not* mucomycosis) may also be referred to as *phycomycosis* or *zygomycosis*.

mucosa (pl., mucosae)—the mucous membrane. See *mucous, honeycomb mucosa*.

mucosal ileal diaphragms—diaphragm-like mucosal strictures of GI tract, associated with use of nonsteroidal anti-inflammatory drug use.

mucous (adj.)—pertaining to mucus, or secreting mucus, as *mucous membrane*; the epithelium-covered membrane that lines certain organs, such as the eyes, nose, mouth, throat, and vagina. Cf. *mucus*.

MUCP (maximum urethral closure pressure) (Urol).

mucus (noun)—viscid secretion produced by mucous membranes. See *mucous*.

Muehrcke lines—seen on the fingernails and toenails in patients with hypoalbuminemia. The lines run across the nail and are parallel to each other.

Mueller (Müller) **muscle**—in the upper and lower eyelids; involved in correction of eyelid retraction in Graves ophthalmopathy.

MUGA (multiple gated acquisition) **scan**—a blood pool radionuclide study of cardiac shape and dynamics in which a radionuclide is introduced into the circulation. Radioactive emissions from the heart are electronically monitored, stored, and analyzed, resulting in a composite scan consisting of a series of successive images all taken at the same point in the cardiac cycle.

mulberry molars—five-pointed molars are a sign of congenital syphilis. Also, *Hutchinson teeth and hutchinsonian molars*.

Mulder sign—a click felt between the metatarsal heads when diagnosing Morton neuroma in the web space of the toes.

Mullen prognostic nutritional index.

Mullins cardiac device.

Multibite biopsy forceps—biopsy forceps that allow the surgeon to obtain multiple samples with only one pass through the scope.

MultiBoot—an orthosis that provides pressure-free positioning of the ulcerated heel.

Multicath catheter—trade name for a multifunction catheter.

multicentric angiofollicular hyperplasia (MAFH)—a disease characterized by diffuse lymphadenopathy, splenomegaly, anemia, polyclonal hypergammaglobulinemia, and constitutional symptoms. It is the multicentric form of Castleman disease, a localized form of mediastinal lymphoid hyperplasia. See *Castleman disease.*

Multiclip—a disposable surgical ligating clip device.

multidetector computed tomography (MDCT)—performs rapid 3-D scanning with thin slices or rapid whole body images for accurate diagnosis in trauma or ovarian cancer. It takes four different images at the same time and potentially reduces the need for repeat scans, overlapping radiation exposure, additional doses of contrast media, and missed diagnoses.

Multidex wound-filling material.

multidrug-resistant tuberculosis (MDR-TB).

multi-echo images—a series of spin echo images obtained with various pulse sequences in MRI scans.

multifactorial—caused or determined by several independent factors, genetic or nongenetic, each of which contributes only a minor effect by itself.

Multifire Endohernia clip applier—used in laparoscopic herniorrhaphy.

Multifire GIA, Multifire Endo GIA (30 or 60)—stapling device used in laparoscopic surgery.

multiflanged Portnoy catheter—for hydrocephalus shunts.

Multi-Flex stent—a hydrophilic-coated urologic stent with inner lumen hydrogel coating to ensure ease of placement over a guidewire.

multifocal chorioretinitis—small, multifocal retinal lesions with intraocular inflammatory cells. Usually classified as one of the white dot syndromes.

multifocal choroidal melanoma—may be related to underlying ocular melanocytosis.

multigenic carcinogenesis—involvement of multiple genes in the origin of carcinomas and other malignant neoplasms.

multi-infarct dementia (MID).

Multileaf Collimator (MLC)—a device used in radiation oncology that allows the radiation beam to automatically follow the shape of a tumor, irradiating only cancerous tissue and not adjacent healthy tissue.

multilineage dysplasia—the presence of two or more cytopenias; often seen with acute myeloid leukemia.

Multi-Link Duet—noncoated coronary stent.

Multi-Link Penta—coronary stent system.

Multi-Link Tetra—coronary stent system.

Multi-Link Vision RX and OTW (over-the-wire) **coronary stent system**—a stent and delivery system designed to treat coronary artery disease in small vessels in patients with abrupt or threatened abrupt closure. The small latticed metal tubes are made from L-605 cobalt chromium (CoCr) alloy. The delivery system, used to deliver the stent through a blood vessel, is a catheter, a thin flexible wire-like tube with a small balloon attached. The stent is intended to stay in place permanently and help hold the blood vessel open, improving the flow of blood and relieving the symptoms of coronary heart disease.

Multilok hand operating table.

multiple magnet ingestion by children—requires immediate surgical removal. Left inside the children, the magnets can attract each other through opposing intestinal walls, which can lead to obstruction, necrosis, and perforation of the intestines. If the possibility of magnets in the abdomen exists, magnetic resonance imaging is to be strictly avoided.

multimer assay.

multimode imaging confocal optical microscope (MIMCOM).

multinucleated giant cell—an abnormally large cell, having several nuclei, such as may be detectable in certain viral infections.

Multi-Operatory Dentalaser (MOD)—used for composite curing and teeth whitening.

Multipad absorptive dressing.

multiplanar gradient-recalled (MPGR) **echo**—MRI term.

multiplanar mode; **technique**—MRI terms.

multiplanar reformation (MPR).

multiple endocrine adenopathies, or **abnormalities** (MEA).

multiple endocrine neoplasia (MEN), **type 2b**—a syndrome, often familial, characterized by medullary carcinoma of the thyroid, pheochromocytoma, mucosal neuromas, Marfan body structure, and ophthalmologic manifestations.

multiple evanescent white dot syndrome—seen usually in young adults, mostly women. It is characterized by unilateral visual loss, occasionally preceded by viral-like symptoms. It appears to be self-limiting, with recovery in approximately seven weeks. The syndrome takes its name from the widespread white dots seen at the posterior pole, deep in the retina or at the level of the retinal pigment epithelium.

multiple gated acquisition scan—see *MUGA*.

multiple organ dysfunction syndrome (MODS).

multiple organ failure (MOF).

multiple signal transduction regulators (MSTRs)—a new class of anticancer drugs.

multiple sleep latency test (MSLT)—used to diagnose the sleep apnea syndrome, narcolepsy, and other sleep disorders.

multiple sort flow cytometry—a flow cytometer used in detection and identification of cancer cells.

Multi Podus (boot) **system**—bracing device for the treatment of foot and ankle abnormalities including contractures, foot drop, pressure sores, spasticity, inversion and eversion, rotation, tendinitis, sprains, and stress fractures. It is also used postoperatively after ligament and tendon repairs.

multipotent—referring to stem cells that can develop into at least two types of mature, more differentiated cell, but not into a wide range of cell types.

multipotent adult progenitor cells (MAPC)—cells derived from adult bone marrow that can be differentiated into various connective tissue cells.

Multipurpose-SM catheter.

multi-slab and cine techniques for single breath-hold cardiac-synchronized angiography—techniques designed to improve the yield of cardiac-synchronized gadolinium-enhanced magnetic resonance angiography of the coronary arteries. Conventional cardiac-synchronized MRA acquires data only during the rest period of the coronary arteries, or about one-fourth of each cardiac cycle. Multi-slab acquisition provides ECG-synchronized imaging of the entire heart, while cine acquisition yields a series of images with a narrower focus but representing various phases of the cardiac cycle. Both techniques permit acquisition of more data without an increase in the duration of breath-holding or a deterioration in image quality.

multislice computed tomographic angiography (MSCTA)—an imaging technique that reportedly provides excellent results in assessing vascular involvement by neoplasms arising from the liver, biliary tract, pancreas, kidneys, and all other abdominal organs.

multisystem organ failure (MSOF)—the most common cause of death in

multisystem *(cont.)* patients in the ICU. Multisystem organ failure, by definition, involves the simultaneous failure of two or more of these body systems: lungs, liver, kidneys, GI tract, circulatory system, or central nervous system.

MultiVac—suction ArthroWand.

MultiVysion PB assay—a genetic test that can be used to identify chromosomal abnormalities in genetic material released by the ovum prior to, and immediately following, fertilization.

Mumford-Gurd procedure—arthroplasty used in separation of the acromioclavicular joint.

mummification—necrosis of tissue (as in gangrene) or of a dead body accompanied by extreme drying and shriveling, with only slight evidence of putrefaction.

Munchausen syndrome—named for the fictional Baron Munchausen, who told greatly exaggerated tales. In this syndrome the patient gives exaggerated and dramatic symptoms of a disease he does not have. Because the book about the fictional baron was written in English and his name spelled with a single *h* and no umlaut, *Munchausen* is the spelling used today in a medical context.

Munchausen syndrome by proxy (MSP, MSBP)—a bizarre variation of Munchausen syndrome involving a mother (or other caregiver) and a child. The mother (often a healthcare professional) seems concerned and caring, while actually causing physical symptoms in the child or sometimes reporting the unconfirmed occurrence of such symptoms. The child may suffer through numerous medical and surgical interventions. This is a serious and potentially lethal form of child abuse which apparently has its psychological roots in the mother's need for a relationship with a physician due to her own profound sense of early abandonment as a child. This syndrome presents a confusing number of symptoms but may result in the child's death, if undiagnosed. See *Munchausen syndrome*.

murmur grades—may use either roman or arabic numerals:
- grade I or 1, barely audible, must strain to hear
- grade II or 2, quiet, but clearly audible
- grade III or 3, moderately loud
- grade IV or 4, loud
- grade V or 5, very loud; may be heard with the stethoscope partly off the chest
- grade VI or 6, so loud that it can be heard with the stethoscope just off the chest wall

Murphy skid (Ortho).

muscimol—one of the poisons from the deadly mushroom *Amanita muscaria*.

muscle balance [was] **ortho** (Oph)—short for muscle balance was orthophoric, not orthopedic.

muscle-splitting incision.

MUSE (medicated urethral system for erection) **urethral suppository**.

Musgrave pedobarograph—a floor-mounted system for measuring pressure underneath the foot.

mushroom worker's disease (or **lung**) —pulmonary symptoms caused by exposure to *Thermoactinomyces* organisms in the compost in which mushrooms grow.

mushrooms—refers to the projections on the closure sheet that attaches through the loop sheet of a Velcro

mushrooms *(cont.)* closure. The Velcro fasteners are used for temporary abdominal closure.

Mustang steerable guidewire—used to introduce and place catheters during angioplasty procedures.

mustard—see *L-phenylalanine mustard.*

Mustardé otoplasty technique—flap otoplasty for repair of lop ears. Permanent mattress sutures are placed posteriorly through the full thickness of the scaphoid and conchal cartilage on either side of the antihelix. The sutures are tied only tight enough to create the fold, not to have the cartilage surfaces meet. Cf. *Mustard procedure.*

Mustard procedure—for transposition of the great vessels. Cf. *Mustardé procedure.*

MUSTPAC—a portable medical ultrasound 3-D communications system that can be carried as a backpack. It enables a technician in a remote location to scan patients and transmit 3-D images many miles away.

mutagen—a substance that increases the likelihood of genetic mutation by altering DNA.

mutagenicity—the tendency of a substance to promote genetic mutations by altering DNA.

mutant—a gene, or the individual in which it is expressed, that has undergone mutation.

mutation—a permanent, inheritable change in the sequence of chromosomal DNA.

mutation rate—the rate at which mutations occur at a given gene locus, expressed as mutations per gamete per locus per generation.

mute toe signs—equivocal Babinski reflexes.

mutton fat KPs (keratitic precipitates)—clusters of inflammatory cells and white cells that adhere to the corneal endothelium. Found in patients with uveitis.

MVA (microvascular angiopathy).

MVP (mean platelet volume).

MVP (mitral valve prolapse).

MVP (moisture vapor permeability).

MVST (multi-vessel small thoracotomy).

MVV (maximal voluntary ventilation).

myalgic encephalomyelitis (ME)—the British term for what in the U.S. is called *chronic fatigue syndrome.* Also called *postviral fatigue syndrome* and *yuppie flu.*

mycelium—a mat of fungal growth consisting of hyphae.

MycoAKT latex bead agglutination test—used for the identification of *Mycobacterium* species, needed because of the increasing frequency of nontuberculous mycobacterial diseases associated with AIDS.

Mycobacterium abscessus—a rapidly growing, opportunistic organism, known to cause disease by inoculation after trauma. It is the suspected cause of refractory post-tympanostomy tube otorrhea.

***Mycobacterium avium* complex**—see *MAC infection.*

***Mycobacterium avium-intracellulare* infection**—see *MAI infection.*

***Mycobacterium* cell wall complex** (MCC)—anticancer technology prepared from the nonpathogenic *Mycobacterium phlei (M. phlei).* It interacts synergistically with chemotherapeutic agents, thus significantly enhancing their ability to inhibit growth of malignant melanoma cells.

Mycobacterium gordonae—has been cultured from tap water, soil, sputum, and gastric lavage specimens.

***Mycobacterium phlei* cellular extract**—used to treat carcinoma in situ of the bladder.

***Mycobacterium* strains**—difficult to locate:

M. alvei
M. bohemicum
M. branderi
M. confluentis
M. conspicuum
M. genavense
M. goodii
M. hassiacum
M. heckeshornense
M. heidelbergense
M. immunogenum
M. interjectum
M. intermedium
M. kubicae
M. lentiflavum
M. mageritense
M. mucogenicum
M. novocastrense
M. palustre
M. phlei
M. triplex
M. tusciae
M. wolinskyi

mycosis fungoides—lymphoma (white blood cell malignancy) which occurs in the skin.

mycosis fungoides palmaris et plantaris—an infection that manifests primarily on the palms and soles and clinically may mimic various inflammatory palmoplantar dermatoses.

mycotic aneurysm—an aneurysm due to local infection with a fungus. Although this is the literal meaning of the term, in practice it usually refers to local infection caused by bacteria carried in the circulation from another site.

MycroMesh biomaterial—inert, expanded polytetrafluoroethylene material used in repair of hernias.

myelodysplastic syndrome (MDS)—hematopoietic stem cell disorders characterized by bone marrow dysplasia and various combinations of anemia, leukopenia, and thrombocytopenia.

myeloid/erythroid (M/E) **ratio**.

myeloid progenitor inhibitory factor-1 (MPIF-1)—a human protein in development that may allow cancer patients to be treated with more potent chemotherapy.

myelomere—spinal cord segment.

Myers-Briggs Personality Inventory.

MYHIIA (myosin heavy chain Iia) **syndrome**—a name proposed to encompass the disorders caused by nonmuscle myosin heavy chain 9 gene (MYH9) mutation, that is, May-Hegglin anomaly and Fechtner, Sebastian, Epstein, and Alport syndromes.

Myhre syndrome—rare inherited disorder characterized by mental retardation, short stature, unusual facial features, and skeletal abnormalities. Other findings may include hearing impairment, muscular hypertrophy, and/or joint stiffness. The syndrome is thought to be inherited as an autosomal dominant genetic trait.

Myobock artificial hand—the Utah artificial arm, a myoelectric prosthesis for amputations above the elbow. Available with either a hook or an artificial Myobock hand.

myocardial adrenergic signaling—the normal physiological stimulation of heart function. It is generated when chemical transmitters known as catecholamines bind with certain receptors on the surfaces of heart cells, triggering a series of events which results in increased heart rate and force of contraction of the heart. In congestive heart failure, the heart is

myocardial *(cont.)*
often unable to respond adequately to catecholamines.

myocardial remodeling—a feature in the progression of myocardial failure involving changes in the structure and function of the myocardium.

myochosis—muscular hypertrophy.

myoclonus epilepsy associated with ragged-red fibers (MERRF).

myocutaneous graft.

myodesis—procedure to affix or anchor muscle to bone; often performed during an amputation of the leg.

myofascial release—a physical therapy method of light-touch techniques designed to release tight fascial restrictions throughout the body. It is often used in conjunction with other therapies such as NDT (neurodevelopmental techniques) and SI (sensory integration).

MyoSight—a dedicated nuclear cardiology imaging system.

myosin heavy chain 9 gene (MYH9) —believed to be cause of several autosomal dominant platelet disorders.

myositis ossificans (MO)—benign muscle tumor, mostly of young men. This is difficult for radiologists, orthopedic surgeons, and pathologists to differentiate from much more serious conditions. Plain films are the most reliable method of making the diagnosis, as MRI scans, radionuclide scans, and smears from biopsies can offer misleading information. This condition has a string sign. See *string sign*.

Myosplint device—an implantable medical device designed to improve cardiac performance and efficiency in heart failure patients by changing the size and shape of the heart. See *ventricular geometry change*.

Myotherm XP cardioplegia delivery system.

MyoTrac and **MyoTrac 2 EMG monitoring**—a biofeedback medical device used to help prevent repetitive strain injury. EMG electrodes are placed on the back and shoulders to measure muscle tension and relaxation. The device can be worn all day to maintain healthy working and resting positions.

Myself female incontinence device—over-the-counter pelvic floor muscle trainer for at-home use. It consists of a pneumatic bulb for insertion into the vagina, a series of pelvic floor strength training exercises, and a visual display for monitoring progress and offering biofeedback.

myxoma—a tumor of mucoid (mucous) material.

N, n

Nabi-HB (hepatitis B immune globulin [human])—for treatment of acute exposure to blood containing HB_sAg (hepatitis B surface antigen), perinatal exposure of infants born to HB_sAg-positive mothers, sexual exposure to HB_sAg-positive persons, and household exposure to persons with acute hepatitis B virus (HBV) infection. Administration by intramuscular injection.

NAC (nipple-areola complex)—integral part of breast reconstruction.

NAD (no appreciable disease).

Nadbath akinesia—facial nerve block given behind the ear in preparation for cataract surgery.

nadir—the lowest point; in hematology-oncology, the lowest point reached by the white cell count after chemotherapy has been administered. When the WBC count falls below 1000, the chemotherapeutic agent may be discontinued until the white cell count rises. Pronounced like (Ralph) Nader.

NAE (no ankle edema)—an abbreviation used in reporting findings on the examination of the extremities.

NAET (Nambudripad allergy elimination technique).

NAFLD (nonalcoholic fatty liver disease)—in obese children.

Nagahara phaco chopper and phaco chop technique—nucleus emulsification device and technique developed by Dr. Kunihiro B. Nagahara for removal of cataracts.

NAI (Nuremberg Activities Inventory.

nail—see *device*.

nail bed (*not* nailbed)—the skin surface just under the nail.

nail fold (nailfold) **capillaroscopy**—test to rule out connective tissue disorders such as scleroderma and Raynaud phenomenon. It is performed by placing a small drop of oil on the nail fold and looking at it under the microscope. A positive finding shows enlarged, dilated capillaries.

Nakao snare I and **II**—a snare that combines the actions of polyp transection and retrieval into one. It snares and transects a polyp while the polyp is in the capture pouch.

Nambudripad Allergy Elimination Technique (NAET)—acupuncture

Nambudripad *(cont.)* technique that eliminates allergies by use of muscle testing. The patient holds a vial of allergen; the practitioner then applies pressure to see if the muscles weaken. If they do, the patient is allergic, and acupuncture is then done to eliminate the allergic reaction.

NAME syndrome—acronym for nevi, atrial myxoma, myxoid neurofibroma, and ephelides.

NANB hepatitis (*not* NA&B)—non-A, non-B hepatitis (now called hepatitis C), an acute viral hepatitis that does not have antibodies or antigens of either hepatitis A or B.

nanogram (millimicrogram)—used in plasma testosterone measurement, growth hormone assay results; given in nanograms per cubic centimeter (ng/cc).

NanoWalker—three-legged device with a probe that can measure and image a surface with nanometer precision over a large area.

N-ANP (N-terminal fragment atrial natriuretic peptide).

naproxen (Anaprox, Naprosyn, Naprelan)—nonsteroidal anti-inflammatory drug.

NAR (nipple-areola reconstruction).

Nardi test (morphine-Prostigmin)—for ampullary stenosis of pancreaticobiliary sphincters.

narrowband UV-B (NBUVB)—therapeutic light exposure of narrowband ultraviolet B light in the treatment of psoriasis. Narrowband has been found to facilitate faster clearing and more complete disease resolution than broadband UV-B.

narrowed pulse pressure—the difference between the systolic and diastolic pressures.

nasal flaring—involuntary outward movement of nasal alae in newborns with respiratory distress and in patients with some types of heart disease. Also called *alar flaring*.

NasalGuard allergen screen topical gel.

nasal septal crossover flap technique—choanal atresia micro-endoscopic surgical repair.

nasal T-cell/natural killer cell lymphoma—a locally destructive disease typically presenting with obliteration of the nasal passages and maxillary sinuses. Involvement of the adjacent alveolar bone, hard palate, orbits, and nasopharynx is found in more than 50% of cases and is associated with extensive soft-tissue masses. Presence of bone erosion on x-ray is suggestive but not diagnostic of the disease.

NASH (nonalcoholic steatohepatitis)—the most severe form of nonalcoholic fatty liver disease in obese children.

Nashold TC electrode—for making dorsal root entry zone (DREZ) lesions in the spinal cord.

nasogastric (NG) **feeding tube**.

nasojejunal (NJ) **feeding tube**.

nasometry—in speech analysis, a few words or sentences are spoken into a microphone and analyzed by a computer for resonance (percentage of nasalance). Too much nasality (whiney sound) may indicate insufficient or inefficient soft palate. Not enough nasality (congested sound) may indicate an upper airway obstruction.

NAT (nucleic acid testing)—can detect HIV and hepatitis C in donated blood.

natatory ligament—a term used in surgery of the hand, particularly in the context of Dupuytren contracture.

"natho-dye-nia"—gnathodynia (silent *g*).

National Cholesterol Education Program (NCEP) **guidelines**.

National Institute for Allergy and Infectious Diseases (NIAID).

National Institutes of Health Stroke Scale (NIHSS).

Nathanson liver retractor—used in laparoscopic fundoplication.

National Notifiable Disease Surveillance System (NNDSS)—an arm of the Centers for Disease Control and Prevention. States submit annual reports on incidence of certain diseases in order to assess effectiveness of vaccination programs and need for additional preventive measures.

National Organizations Responding to AIDS (NORA).

native tissue harmonic imaging (NTHI)—used in echocardiography on difficult-to-image patients. It allows for deep penetration while maintaining high resolution images of the body's native tissue.

natriuresis—excretion of abnormal amounts of sodium in the urine.

natriuretic peptides—elevated in patients with congestive heart failure and asymptomatic left ventricular dysfunction.

Natural-Hip prosthesis.

Natural-Knee system—implants used to surgically manage the arthritic knee.

natural supplements—see *dietary or natural supplements*.

Naughton cardiac exercise treadmill test—used for patients who cannot stand for prolonged periods as required in traditional treadmill tests.

Navarre—devices for interventional radiology.

navel sign (Oph)—slang term for a certain area within the eye that looks like a belly button.

NAVF—slang abbreviation for *normal antegrade vertebral flow*.

Navigator flexible endoscope.

Naviport deflectable tip guiding catheter—has open lumen or tube designed for delivery of diagnostic or therapeutic microcatheters into the chambers and/or the coronary vasculature of the heart.

NaviStar DS (dual sensor) **diagnostic/ablation deflectable tip catheter**—a steerable thin flexible catheter (tube) containing multiple electrodes. The catheter can transmit RF (radiofrequency) current through an electrode at the catheter tip for the purpose of ablation (destruction) of a small segment of heart tissue responsible for abnormal impulse conduction.

Navitrack—computer-assisted surgery system used in total hip and knee replacements, anterior cruciate ligament procedures, and spinal surgeries.

Navratil retractor (Ob-Gyn). Also, *Breisky-Navratil retractor*.

NBD (nasobiliary drainage).

NBIH cardiac device.

NBTE (nonbacterial thrombotic endocarditis).

NB200 vascular access device—a device for determining type and location of blood vessels via transmission and reception of ultrasound energy.

n-butyl cyanoacrylate (n-BCA)—a permanent liquid embolic material and tissue adhesive for use in cerebral arteriovenous malformations.

NCEP (National Cholesterol Education Program) **guidelines**.

NCM (neurocutaneous melanosis).

NCP (NeuroCybernetic Prosthesis) **system**—vagal nerve stimulation device for treatment of epilepsy that has proven refractory to antiseizure medication and surgical therapy.

NC-Stat—nerve conduction monitoring system used to evaluate entrapment and systemic neuropathies involving the median and ulnar nerves.

NCV (nerve conduction velocity).

NDT (neurodevelopmental techniques) —a physical therapy method to facilitate active, functional movement of patients suffering from lack of muscle tone, sensory loss, and diminished range of motion.

Nd:YAG (neodymium:yttrium-aluminum-garnet) **laser**. See *neodymium.*

Nd:YAG CTLC (contact transscleral laser cytophotocoagulation)—used in treatment of glaucoma.

Nd:YLF (neodymium:yttrium-lithium fluoride) **laser**.

near-infrared spectroscopy (NIRS).

near-miss—adjective describing near-fatal occurrence, e.g., *near-miss SIDS, near-miss drowning*.

nebs—slang for nebulizations (high flow nebulizations).

NEC ("neck") (necrotizing enterocolitis)—develops in premature infants unable to tolerate formula.

necrotizing enterocolitis (NEC).

necrotizing fasciitis—a fulminating group A streptococcal infection beginning with severe or extensive cellulitis that spreads to involve the superficial and deep fascia, producing thrombosis of the subcutaneous vessels and gangrene of the underlying tissues. A cutaneous lesion usually serves as a portal of entry for the infection, but sometimes no such lesion is found. Also called *flesh-eating bacteria*. See *streptococcus A infection.*

NED (no evidence of disease).

needle
- Accucore II biopsy
- Arachnophlebectomy
- Atraloc surgical
- Baldwin perineum
- B-D spinal
- B-bevel
- Bierman
- Biopty cut
- Boynton needle holder
- Brockenbrough
- butterfly
- Cardiopoint
- Charles flute
- Chiba
- Cibis ski
- CIF-4
- coaxial sheath cut-biopsy
- Cobb-Ragde
- Colapinto curved
- Colorado microdissection
- Control-Release pop-off
- Cook endoscopic curved
- Core aspiration/injection
- Core CO_2 insufflation
- C-type acupuncture
- cut-biopsy
- Dieckmann intraosseous (IO)
- docking
- Dos Santos
- D-TACH removable
- Echo-Coat ultrasound biopsy
- Endopath Ultra Veress
- Ethalloy TruTaper cardiovascular
- Franseen stereotactic
- French-eye
- GraNee (Riza-Ribe grasper)
- Goldenberg Snarecoil bone marrow biopsy
- Greene biopsy

needle *(cont.)*
Gripper
Hawkeye suture
Hawkins breast localization
Howell biopsy aspiration
Huber
J
Keith
Klatskin
Koch nucleus hydrolysis
Laminar surgical
Lewis Pair-Pak
Madayag biopsy
milliner's
Nottingham colposuspension
PC-7
PD Access
Pencan spinal
PercuCut cut-biopsy
Pereyra
Plum-Blossom
Protect Point
Punctur-Guard
Quincke spinal
Riza-Ribe
Rosen
Rosenthal
Rotunda perineum
Sabreloc spatula
SafeTap tapered spinal
Safety AV fistula
SafetyGlide
Sahli
SC-1
Seldinger gastrostomy
self-aspirating cut-biopsy
Sensi-Touch anesthesia
side-cutting spatulated
Skinny
SmallPort
SmartNeedle
Solitaire
spatulated half-circle
Stamey
steel-winged butterfly

needle *(cont.)*
Steis
stereotactic biopsy
Stifcore aspiration
Teflon-coated hollow-bore
Terry-Mayo
THI
Thomas
Tru-Cut
T12
Tuohy
Turner biopsy
Unimar J
Veress
Visi-Black surgical
Voorhees
Waterfield
Weiss fixed wing epidural
Westcott biopsy
Westerman-Jensen
Whitacre spinal
Wright

Neer classification of shoulder fractures—I, II, III.

Neer hemiarthroplasty.

negative hepatosplenomegaly—erroneous dictation. Transcribe: "Negative for hepatosplenomegaly" or "No hepatosplenomgaly."

negative stroke margin—a term used on fine-needle biopsy in which breast is compressed before the needle is inserted. However, breast compression to 3.5 cm or less may pass the needle through the back wall of the breast. This danger is termed "negative stroke margin."

negative symptoms of schizophrenia—apathy, depression, emotional unresponsiveness, social withdrawal. Cf. *positive symptoms of schizophrenia.*

Negri body (inclusion body found in rabies).

Neiguan point—acupressure point P6, which is located approximately three

Neiguan *(cont.)* fingerwidths up from the wrist crease, between the flexor tendons on the medial aspect of the forearm.

Neisseria—now split between the genus *Branhamella* and the genus *Neisseria.*

Neisseria meningitidis—the cause of meningococcal meningitis.

Nélaton dislocation of the ankle.

Nélaton rubber tube drain.

Nellcor Symphony—blood pressure monitoring system.

NEMD (nonspecific esophageal motility disorder) (Radiol, GI).

neoadjuvant hormonal therapy (NHT) —drug therapy in conjunction with radiation therapy, which is reported to offer significantly improved clinical outcomes.

neochoana—artificially created choana.

Neocontrol—magnet technology embedded in the seat of a chair. The patient who is treated for urinary incontinence sits in the chair with clothes on for 20 minutes, twice a week for 8 weeks. As the magnetic field pulsates at a controlled rate, muscles contract in the pelvic floor, improving muscle strength and bladder control.

neodymium:yttrium-aluminum-garnet laser (Nd:YAG laser)—used in glaucoma procedure combining a nonpenetrating trabeculectomy with a Nd:YAG trabeculectomy. It forms through-and-through filtration under a scleral flap without actually entering the anterior chamber. See *laser.*

Neo-EpCAM cancer detection kit—used for the detection of cancers of epithelial origin such as lung, breast, colon, prostate, head and neck, stomach, ovary, pancreas, esophagus, and larynx.

Neoflex bendable knife—electrocautery with a flexible pencil-like device that provides the surgeon access to difficult-to-reach areas.

NeoKnife electrosurgical instrument —for cutting, fulguration, and desiccation.

neonatal acne—nonfollicular pustulosis of the newborn; recent findings indicate it is caused by *Malassezia furfur* yeasts. Cf. *Malassezia furfur pustulosis.*

NeoNaze—nasal function restoration device for laryngectomy patients.

neon particle protocol—focal radiation therapy.

Neoprobe 1000 detector—handheld gamma-detection probe, used for lymphatic mapping in patients with breast cancer.

Neoprobe 1500 portable radioisotope detector—handheld device that detects gamma rays and can be used externally and intraoperatively to track an injected radiopharmaceutical within the body.

neoscrotum—constructed, using skin flaps or a split-thickness graft fashioned into a neopouch, after blunt trauma has damaged the scrotum.

Neo-Sert umbilical vessel catheter insertion set—used in neonates.

Ne-Osteo bone morphogenic protein (BMP)—a combination of bone factors within a collagen matrix, used as an alternative to autograft and the necessity for bone harvesting. Ne-Osteo is used with the BAK interbody-fusion system. Additionally, Ne-Osteo BMP may be used in dental applications, e.g., the treatment of bone loss due to periodontal disease.

Neotrend system—provides multiparameter blood gas monitoring in premature infants without drawing blood.

neoumbilicus—the creation of a new umbilicus after surgery for bladder exstrophy, which destroys the native umbilicus. The procedure is also called neoumbilicoplasty. Usage: "A V-shaped flap was raised and buried subcutaneously. The flap eventually became a tube around the cystotomy tube and the cicatrix formed the umbilical dimple. . . . The technique evolved into a tubularized U-shaped flap. A rubber tube was placed indwelling as a stent to maintain inward projection of the neoumbilicus."

neovascularization of disk (NVD)—refers to new vessel formation in the optic disk.

neovascularization elsewhere (NVE)—refers to new vessel formation elsewhere other than the optic disk.

nephrectomy—see *laparoscopic donor nephrectomy* (LDN).

nephritogenic—causing or relating to causing nephritis.

nephrostomy-type catheter.

nephrotic syndrome—defined as serum albumin greater than 3.0 gm/dl and proteinuria of 3.5 gm or more in 24 hours.

nephroureterectomy—a procedure consisting of en bloc removal of a cuff of bladder around the ipsilateral ureteral orifice. Traditional management of transitional cell carcinoma of the renal pelvis. Now replaced by local surgical resection alone or in combination with other local therapies.

NERD (nonerosive reflux disease).

nerve block infusion kit—provides continuous infusion of local anesthetic near a nerve for regional pain management during orthopedic and general surgery.

nerve conduction velocity (NCV)—a diagnostic test which may be performed along with an EMG. It tests the integrity of peripheral nerves by measuring the time it takes for an impulse generated by an electric stimulator, placed over a nerve, to travel over a segment of it.

Nerve Fibre Analyzer GDx, The—a laser used for scanning laser polarimetry.

nerve growth factor (NGF)—a substance produced in the brain. Levels of nerve growth factor may be decreased in patients with Alzheimer disease. Without NGF, neurons die; future therapy for Alzheimer disease may involve supplementation with NGF.

nerve of Latarjet ("LAT´ar-zhay")—continuation of the vagus nerve along the stomach. In a proximal gastric vagotomy procedure, tiny branches of this nerve to the stomach are divided, which decreases the acid output of the stomach and protects against ulcer disease.

nerve of Wrisberg—there are two nerves with the same name: the medial cutaneous nerve of the arm and the intermediate nerve. Named for an 18th century German anatomist.

NervePace—noninvasive nerve conduction testing machine that measures sensorimotor latencies to assess compression neuropathies, as in carpal tunnel syndrome.

nesidiodysplasia—large hyperchromatic islet cell nuclei.

network—see *artificial neural networks (ANNs)*.

neural stem cell—a stem cell occurring sparsely in the adult brain that can differentiate into neurons and neuroglial cells.

neural tube defects (NTD)—birth defects such as spina bifida. Some research indicates that obese women are twice as likely to have children with neural tube defects.

neurapraxia (*not* neuropraxia)—a conduction block (either partial or total) of a segment of nerve fiber, causing a temporary paralysis. Usage: "The patient has a right ulnar nerve neurapraxia."

neurilemmoma (schwannoma)—proliferation of cells forming a nerve sheath; a common peripheral nerve tumor.

neuroacanthocytosis—a frontosubcortical type of dementia.

neuro-Behçet disease.

Neurobehavioral Cognitive Status Examination—neurological test.

NeuroCharge hardcore concentration/reaction time formula—an acetylcholine and Gingko biloba supplement used by body builders and exercise enthusiasts.

neurocutaneous melanosis (NCM)—a rare congenital neurocutaneous syndrome in which benign and malignant melanocytic tumors of the leptomeninges develop, along with large or numerous congenital melanocytic nevi.

NeuroCybernetic Prosthesis System (NCP)—new indication for use of this vagus nerve stimulation device. Previously approved for the treatment of epilepsy, it is now also used to treat depression. A stopwatch-sized generator is implanted in the left chest, and a nerve stimulation electrode is attached to the vagus nerve in the neck in a 1-2 hour outpatient procedure. The NCP delivers preprogrammed intermittent electrical pulses to the vagus nerve 24 hours a day. This has been shown to significantly reduce the number and severity of depressive episodes in half of those tested.

neuroendovascular interventional procedures (Radiol).

neurofibrillary tangles—snarled neurofilaments of cortical neurons, seen on biopsy, diagnostic of Alzheimer disease.

Neuroform microdelivery stent system—designed to prevent the rupture of brain aneurysms.

neurogastroenterology—medical field that deals with the enteric nervous system, which refers to a "second brain" in the human body, located in the gut. The central nervous system brain and the gut's brain function independently but also react to each other. Many gastrointestinal problems, such as colitis and irritable bowel syndrome, can be attributed to the gut's brain. Also, many links exist between the two brains, as seen in certain food allergies as well as autoimmune diseases like Crohn disease and ulcerative colitis.

neurogram—see *pudendal neurogram.*

neuroimmune dysfunction—increased density of nerve fibers reactive to immune system neuropeptides associated with production of pain linked to inflammation. Investigators think that this triggers the pain associated with appendicitis, without the usual inflammation, leading to a normal-appearing appendix at the time of operation.

NeuroLink II—an EEG data acquisition system that converts analog brain wave data into digital signals.

neurological signs—see *localizing* or *focal neurological signs*, *soft neurological signs.*

NeuroMate—robotic technology for use in stereotactic brain surgery. NeuroMate consists of a robotic arm assembly and a PC-based positioning system.

Neuromed Octrode—implantable device for chronic pain management.

Neuromeet nerve approximator—single-use clamp used in reattachment of damaged nerve endings. Once aligned, entire nerves may be sutured concentrically by rotating the approximator.

neuronal apoptosis inhibitory protein (NAIP)—naturally occurring protein that has been found to prevent brain cell death and holds promise in human clinical trials.

neuron specific enolase (NSE)—a tumor marker.

Neuroperfusion pump—used to treat stroke victims. Oxygenated blood is pumped from an artery in the groin to the brain through a catheter or hollow tube to a vein in the neck to the damaged region of the brain.

Neuroprobe—a pain management system said to be able to modulate pain at every known level of the nervous system. It uses five modes of stimulation and is laser compatible.

neuroretinopathy, acute macular.

NeuroSector—trade name for an ultrasound system. See *real-time ultrasonography.*

Neuroshield cerebral protection device—a percutaneous transluminal intra-arterial filtration system.

NeutroSpec imaging agent—a radiolabeled monoclonal antibody that binds to a type of infection-fighting white blood cell, for use in patients five years and older who have inconclusive symptoms of appendicitis.

neurotmesis—complete transection of a nerve, which results in cell death.

Neuro-Trace—an instrument that provides pulsating low current stimulation for location of nerves during operative procedures.

Neurotrend—system designed for continuous monitoring of blood gases for determination of cerebral ischemia and/or hypoxia in patients suffering from closed-head trauma and during surgical intervention.

neutrophil attachment level.

neutrophil elastase-releasing capacity.

NEV (noninvasive extrathoracic ventilator)—similar to the old "iron lung."

Neville-Barnes forceps—for spontaneous vaginal delivery assist.

Neville tracheal and **tracheobronchial prostheses**—for tracheal reconstruction in patients with benign tumor, primary or secondary carcinoma, or stenosis caused by intubation or other trauma.

newton—SI unit representing the amount of force needed to impart an acceleration of 1 m/sec/sec to a mass of 1 kg.

Nevyas drape retractor—a disposable stick-on arched frame, which is placed over the patient's forehead, and the sterile surgical drape is placed over it, thus permitting the patient to breathe more easily.

New England Baptist acetabular cup—used for total hip arthroplasty.

new knit—misspelling for *Nu-Knit*. See *Surgical Nu-Knit*.

New Mind Set toe splint—for ambulation during healing process.

Newport MC hip orthosis—a brace consisting of pelvic and femoral braces linked by a metal rod. It is used to keep the leg in abduction

Newport *(cont.)*
following total hip arthroplasty, while permitting ambulation. *MC* stands for *maximum control*.

new variant Creutzfeldt-Jakob disease (nvCJD)—name given to the type of bovine spongiform encephalopathy that is transmitted to humans. It is a subject of debate whether nvCJD is truly any different from standard CJD.

Newvicon vacuum chamber pickup tube—for video camera used in arthroscopy. Also, *Circon video camera, Saticon vacuum chamber pickup tube, Vidicon*.

NexGen complete knee replacement—femoral components for total knee arthroplasty.

NexStent carotid stent—a nitinol-based continuous-mesh carotid stent.

Nextep—a line of walkers and braces used to treat foot, ankle, and lower limb injuries. Functional knee brace with a bipivotal hinge.

Nexus implant—a cemented chrome cobalt femoral implant.

Nexus 2 linear ablation catheter—used in treatment of atrial arrhythmias.

Nezelof syndrome—see *DiGeorge syndrome*.

Nezhat-Dorsey Trumpet Valve hydrodissector—includes SmokEvac electrosurgical probe for hydrodissection of tissue, aspiration of fluids, lavage, blunt dissection, smoke evacuation, and the delivery of laser and electrical energy. For precise fingertip control of suction and irrigation in laser surgery.

NF-ATc—proteins that have been found to play a key regulatory role in the immune response and in cardiac hypertrophy; also referred to as "NFAT-3."

NG (nasogastric) **feeding tube**.

N-geneous HDL cholesterol test—measures how much high-density lipoprotein cholesterol is present in a patient's serum.

NGF (nerve growth factor).

N High Sensitivity CRP (C-reactive protein) **assay**—offers physicians the ability to assess risk of cardiovascular and peripheral vascular disease many years before its occurrence by detecting low levels of C-reactive protein in the blood, allowing the opportunity for implementing preventive health measures.

NHL (non-Hodgkin lymphoma) **tumors**.

NHSR—slang abbreviation for *no hemodynamically significant stenosis recorded* (by Doppler).

NHT (neoadjuvant hormonal therapy).

Niagara PV laser for benign prostatic hypertrophy.

NIAID (National Institute for Allergy and Infectious Diseases).

Nibbler—a device for dissection, morcellation, suction, and irrigation.

Nibblit—laparoscopic device that provides for aquadissection, sharp and blunt dissection for lysis of adhesions, biopsy, and specimen retrieval in one instrument.

NicCheck-I—a test that measures the level of nicotine and its metabolites in the urine, classifying nicotine usage as high or low.

NicCheck-II—a more sensitive version of NicCheck-I, this test is able to detect passive exposure to smoke.

Nichols-Condon bowel prep.

Nichols procedure—a vaginal suspension procedure for urinary stress incontinence.

nicked free beta subunit of human chorionic gonadotropin—a poten-

nicked *(cont.)*
tial marker for Down syndrome screening.

"nick-yoo"—phonetic for *NICU* (Neonatal Intensive Care Unit).

Nicolet Elite Doppler ultrasound—an imaging system to aid in the detection of peripheral vascular disease and to listen to blood flow in the fetal heart.

Nicolet Nerve Integrity Monitor-2 (NIM-2)—used in surgery to locate and identify the facial and other cranial nerves quickly. It also helps to map the course of each nerve and to ascertain whether it is functioning.

Nidek EC-5000 excimer laser system—used in LASIK procedures.

Nidek MK-2000 keratome system—ophthalmic keratome system for the creation of a lamellar flap on the cornea during keratoplasty and other refractive procedures.

nidus ("nest")—the point of origin or focus of a morbid process. Usage: "The nidus of infection was identified."

Niebauer prosthesis—Silastic metacarpophalangeal joint.

Niemann-Pick disease—a rare form of familial lipidosis, resulting in mental retardation, growth retardation, and progressive blindness.

NightBird nasal CPAP (continuous positive airway pressure)—for treatment of obstructive sleep apnea. (No space in NightBird.)

night nurse's paralysis—a variant of the narcolepsy/cataplexy syndrome, also called *cataplexy of awakening*. A temporary paralysis which quickly disappears.

NightOwl pocket polygraph—a small recording device used to diagnose sleep disorders.

NIHSS (National Institutes of Health Stroke Scale).

nil disease—synonym for lipoid nephrosis, so-called because so little evidence of disease is seen on light microscopy of a renal biopsy in a case of lipoid nephrosis.

NIM-Spine system neural integrity monitor—a surgeon-guided device for locating and identifying peripheral motor nerves during spinal surgery.

NIM-2 (Nicolet Nerve Integrity Monitor-2).

ninety-ninety (90/90) **intraosseous wiring**—used to obtain rigid fixation for digital replantation or for transverse fractures. Two intraosseous wires are placed perpendicular to each other (hence, 90° angle or 90/90).

Nipah virus—human pathogen identified in recent outbreaks of disease and death in Malaysia.

nipple-areola reconstruction (NAR)—uses a modified S dermal-fat flap technique. Also, arrow flap and rib cartilage graft for long-lasting nipple projection.

nipple slippage—a complication in continent urinary diversion procedures.

NIRflex coronary stent.

Niroyal Elite Monorail—coronary stent system.

NIR Primo Monorail stent system—coronary stent system used in PTCA procedures for the treatment of coronary artery disease.

NIRS (**n**ear-**i**nfrared **s**pectroscopy)—a device which uses light to assess and quantify various characteristics of human blood and tissue.

Nirschl scratch test—orthopedic test for identifying degeneration of the rotator cuff. Several methods have

Nirschl *(cont.)*
been proposed for identifying degenerative pathologic changes of the rotator cuff, such as direct palpation over the critical zone, probing the superficial surface of the rotator cuff, performing a blush test with a dilute solution of methylene blue, and performing the Nirschl scratch test.

NIR with SOX—over-the-wire coronary stent system for treatment of coronary artery disease. The SOX system stent sleeves protect the proximal and distal ends of the stent for a smooth interface between the stent system and arterial wall.

Nissen fundoplication—procedure to control gastroesophageal reflux.

Nissen laparoscopic fundoplication—surgical procedure for the treatment of reflux esophagitis and gastroesophageal reflux disease.

Nissl granules—cytoplasmic bodies in nerve cell bodies. (Franz Nissl, German neuropathologist.)

Nissl stain (Path).

nitazoxanide—see *Alinia.*

nitinol mesh-covered frame—used for laparoscopic herniorrhaphy.

nitinol mesh stent.

nitric oxide (NO)—a gas sometimes used for newborns in respiratory distress and for patients status post heart procedure.

nitroglycerin ointment—see *Cellegesic.*

nitrogen-13 ammonia—a radioactive tracer used to perform a PET scan to evaluate heart function at rest and during stress. Nitrogen-13 ammonia has a longer half-life than rubidium-82. Therefore, the stress portion of the test may be done with an exercise bike or treadmill.

nitroglycerin—a vasodilator administered as sublingual tablets or spray, by injection, or topically (as an ointment) to treat angina pectoris. See *"nitro paste."* See also *Cellegesic.*

Nitrol ointment—a brand of the drug nitroglycerin in ointment form. See *"nitro paste."*

"nitro paste" (Cardio)—careless jargon widely used by physicians for nitroglycerin ointment. The dosage of this coronary vasodilator is measured in inches of ointment (or fractions thereof) as it comes from the tube. The patient is supplied with disposable ruled applicators, with which the ointment is measured out and smeared over the skin in much the same way as one spreads mucilage or wallpaper paste—hence, probably, the popular misnomer "paste." When "nitro paste" is dictated, "nitro" should be expanded to "nitroglycerin," and "paste" should be translated "ointment"—unless departmental rules forbid using the right words when the dictator uses the wrong ones. Note that the name of one brand of nitroglycerin, Nitrol, is easily mistaken for "nitro" in dictation.

nitrospray 0.4—slang for Nitrolingual Spray (First Horizon) 0.4 mg/spray.

nitrous oxide—see N_2O.

Nizoral (ketoconazole)—an oral treatment for stubborn fungal dermatitis, often used for 2-4 months or more.

NJ (nasojejunal) **feeding**.

NK (natural killer) **cell**—evaluated in specific and nonspecific immunotherapy and in cytotoxicity assays.

NLite—nonablative laser used to remove wrinkles around the eyes. It reportedly stimulates the production of collagen under the skin; as new

NLite *(cont.)* collagen forms under the treated area, it begins to fill in and reduce wrinkles around the eyes.

NLP (no light perception).

NMES (neuromuscular electrical stimulation) **protocol**—see *ReAct device.*

N-methyl-D-aspartate (NMDA) **receptor antagonists**—drugs that are said to protect the brain from toxic neurotransmitters released after stroke or head injury.

N-MID osteocalcin ELISA test—to test for blood levels of osteocalcin. Osteocalcin is synthesized by the bone-forming cells (osteoblasts) and is therefore a marker of bone formation.

NMP (nuclear matrix protein).

NMP22 test—urinary marker for the early detection of transitional cell carcinoma of the bladder.

NMR (nuclear magnetic resonance) **scan**—early term for what is now called MRI (magnetic resonance imaging) scan. The name is said to have been changed because of patients' resistance to the word *nuclear*.

NNDSS (National Notifiable Disease Surveillance System).

N_2O (nitrous oxide)—an alternative to carbon dioxide (CO_2) for creating a pneumoperitoneum for laparoscopic surgery.

no ankle edema (NAE).

Nocardia—the fungus causing nocardiasis, more devastating than usual in the AIDS patient.

nocturnal polysomnography.

nodal rhythm—any rhythm generated by the atrioventricular node acting as pacemaker.

node
- Aschoff-Tawara
- Bouchard
- Flack
- jugulodigastric
- Koch
- Osler
- Rouviere
- SA or S-A (sinoatrial)
- sentinel
- shotty
- signal
- singer's (of a vocal cord)
- Sister Mary Joseph
- Troisier
- Virchow

node of Rouviere—situated in retropharyngeal space.

nodo-Hisian (or nodohisian) **bypass tract**—an abnormal accessory pathway in the cardiac conduction system between the atrioventricular node and the bundle of His, predisposing to paroxysmal supraventricular tachycardia.

nodules—see *siderotic nodules of the spleen.*

Nogo protein—a protein known for its ability to regulate nerve regeneration. It may control the progression of Alzheimer disease.

Noiles posterior stabilized knee prosthesis.

Noiles rotating hinge total knee prosthesis.

no LSKMT—slang for no liver, spleen, or kidney masses or tenderness.

no man's land in the hand—the area between the distal palmar crease and the proximal interphalangeal joints (the web space between the thumb and index finger). Until modern microsurgical techniques were developed, tendon repair in the palm was usually unsuccessful, as the swelling of the newly sutured tendon in this tight part of the hand led to is-

no man's *(cont.)* chemia. Hand microsurgeons are now able to do primary tendon repair in no man's land in the hand.

nomogram—a graphic representation of three interdependent quantities or values on three scales. Used, for example, to calculate body surface area (BSA) when height and weight are known. The West nomogram is widely used to calculate BSA in children.

Nomos—pin-free attachment stereotactic system.

non-A, non-B hepatitis—now called hepatitis C.

nonalcoholic fatty liver disease (NAFLD)—in obese children. It demonstrates clearly different patterns and locations of liver scarring and inflammation in children as compared to that typically seen in adults.

nonalcoholic steatohepatitis (NASH)—a chronic disorder characterized by steatosis, mixed-cell-type inflammation, focal hepatocyte degeneration, and perivenular or pericellular fibrosis. The disease is slowly progressive, occasionally resulting in cirrhosis, portal hypertension, liver failure, or hepatocellular carcinoma.

non-Alzheimer dementias—account for 50% of all dementias: dementias with a vascular cause, neurodegenerative dementias, and others.

nonbacterial thrombotic endocarditis (NBTE).

nonballoon therapies—used for treatment of ischemic heart disease in suitable coronary anatomy. They include *stents* (Palmaz-Schatz and Gianturco-Roubin), *atherectomy* (directional, rotational, and extraction), and *excimer laser angioplasty*.

noncholecystokinin—a substance that is thought to be important in regulating gallbladder contraction and emptying.

noncomitant—see *comitant*, *concomitant*.

noncompliant—said of patients who do not follow their physician's directions and advice regarding diet or medicinal treatment.

non compos mentis—a psychiatric and legal term for a patient not of sound mind and in need of guardianship.

nondisjunction (Genetics)—the failure of a chromosome pair to separate during meiosis, so that both chromosomes are passed to one daughter cell and none to the other.

nonerosive reflux disease (NERD)—the presence of typical symptoms of gastroesophageal reflux disease (GERD) due to intraesophageal acid but in the absence of visible esophageal mucosal injury on endoscopy.

noninvasive extrathoracic ventilation (NEV).

nonionic contrast media (Radiol)—more expensive but safer than low-osmolar media (ionic media). Nonionic contrast media are almost universally used in the U.S., and radiologists invariably indicate thus in their dictation for medicolegal reasons. The words *nonionic contrast medium* begin more sentences, by a large margin, in reports involving contrast than the name of the pharmaceutical itself or the dose. See *ionic contrast media*, *low-osmolar contrast media*.

nonischemic dilated cardiomyopathy (NIDCM)—a chief cause of congestive heart failure.

nonmuscle myosin heavy chain IIa (MYHIIA) **mutations**—believed to

nonmuscle *(cont.)* be cause of several autosomal dominant platelet disorders.

non-nasal CD56+T/NK (natural killer) **cell lymphoma**—uncommon tumors that show predominantly extranodal presentation, high-stage disease, a highly aggressive course, and strong association with Epstein-Barr virus.

nonpenetrance (Genetics)—failure of a gene to be expressed in an individual possessing it.

non-Q-wave myocardial infarction (NQWMI).

nonrapid eye movement (NREM).

nonrheumatic valvular aortic stenosis.

nonseminomatous germ cell tumor (NSGCT).

nonsense mutation (Genetics)—a genetic mutation in which a codon coding an amino acid is replaced by a chain-termination codon, so that a protein in process of formation is prematurely ended.

non-small cell lung carcinoma (or **cancer**) (NSCLC)—all types of lung cancer other than small cell lung carcinoma (SCLC). This group of cancers includes adenocarcinoma, squamous cell carcinoma, and large cell carcinoma. See *Navelbine*.

NonSpil drug delivery system—a spill-resistant liquid that can be used with a wide variety of both over-the counter and prescription drugs.

non-STEMI (non-ST-segment elevation myocardial infarction).

nonsustained ventricular tachycardia (NSVT)—risk factor for sudden cardiac death in some patients.

nonsyncytium-inducing (NSI) **variant of the AIDS virus**—not as virulent as the SI (syncytium-inducing) strain. This quickly changing virus can mutate into a more aggressive strain. See *SI* and *HIV phenotype test.*

nonspecific esophageal motility disorder (NEMD).

nonspecific urethritis (NSU).

nonvalvular AF (atrial fibrillation)—atrial fibrillation in which the rhythm disturbance occurs in the absence of rheumatic mitral valve disease or a prosthetic heart valve. Cf. *lone AF*.

nonweightbearing—see *weightbearing*.

no phase wrap function to eliminate aliasing artifacts—see *anti-aliasing techniques* (MRI terms).

NoProfile balloon catheter (Cardio).

Norco ulnar deviation support—hand therapy product.

Nordan-Ruiz trapezoidal marker—used in refractive eye surgery.

NordiPen—a pen system used to deliver Norditropin.

Norditropin (somatropin [rDNA origin] for injection)—a liquid formulation of the human growth hormone drug delivered in a pen system, NordiPen, designed to make daily injections more convenient.

no-reflow phenomenon—failure of a significant proportion of capillaries within the tissue to re-perfuse upon restoration of blood flow in the arteries supplying the tissue, such as might occur in reconstructive surgery. Oxygen free radicals such as human manganese superoxide dismutase that scavenge or inhibit formation of reactive O_2 metabolites are being investigated as possible treatment.

norgestimate/ethinyl estradiol—see *Ortho TriCyclen Lo*.

Norian SRS (skeletal repair system)—an injectable bone substitute paste or cement used in fracture treatment procedures.

Norland bone densitometry.

normal axis deviation—incorrect dictation for *no axis deviation* or *normal axis*. In an electrocardiogram, axis deviation is a shift from the normal axis; thus, "normal axis deviation" makes no sense. Edit to *no axis deviation* or *normal axis.*

normal perfusion pressure breakthrough syndrome—massive multifocal bleeding after the technically successful removal of a cerebral arteriovenous malformation.

normal pressure hydrocephalus (NPH).

normal sinus rhythm—normal heartbeat.

normal spontaneous vaginal delivery (NSVD).

Normigel hydrogel dressing.

normoactive—a term coined from "normal active," applied to bowel sounds as well as to deep tendon reflexes and children who are not hyperactive.

Norrie syndrome—inherited neurodevelopmental disorder characterized by blindness in both eyes at birth. Some children with this disorder may experience varying degrees of mental retardation. Other symptoms may include mild to profound hearing loss, growth delays, and/or diabetes. Cataracts may develop during early infancy, and the eyeball may shrink. The gene responsible for Norrie syndrome is inherited as an X-linked recessive genetic trait.

Norwood operation—performed for hypoplastic left-sided heart syndrome. See *Fontan; Gill/Jonas; Sade.*

nosocomial disease—disease originating in a hospital.

No Sting barrier film—provides sting-free, alcohol-free protection for wound care.

notch or notching—see *crochetage.*

notochord *(not* notocord) (chorda dorsalis)—seen in the embryo; in adults the nuclei pulposi are the vestigial notochord.

no-touch technique—used to perform vascular anastomoses that avoid vascular traction during implantation.

Nottingham colposuspension needle—for bladder neck elevation. Malleable tipped, colposuspension needle that is adjustable to any angle for use in Stamey bladder neck suspension procedures.

Nottingham introducer—used to place a tube as a palliative procedure in patients with esophageal cancer. See *Atkinson tube stent.*

NovaCath multi-lumen infusion catheter.

Novacor left ventricular assist system (LVAS)—an implantable pump that keeps blood circulating in patients with end-stage heart disease. It is designed as both a "bridge" to heart transplant and a long-term alternative to transplant.

Novafil suture (*not* Novofil). See *Sutureloop*.

NovaGold breast implant—water-based (PVP-hydrogel-based) breast implant that contains radiolucent biocompatible polymer filling.

NovaLine Litho-S DUV excimer laser—provides high spectral purity.

NovaPulse CO_2 laser—for cosmetic skin resurfacing facial cosmetic surgery to remove blemishes, scars, and birthmarks.

NovaSaline inflatable saline breast implant—for breast augmentation and breast reconstruction surgery. Also, *NovaSaline pre-filled breast implant*.

NovaSure endometrial ablation—a permanent endometrial ablation

NovaSure *(cont.)* method to treat menorrhagia. Performed in a physician's office, the procedure takes approximately 90 seconds, with a 2-hour recovery period for the patient. In a single treatment, the lining of the uterus is permanently removed and the cells responsible for regeneration are eliminated.

Novel erythropoiesis stimulating protein (NESP)—a recombinant protein that stimulates red blood cell production. It is used to treat anemia in patients with chronic renal failure.

no-view cataract (also, no-view lens) —a condition in which the cataract lens cannot be viewed because of corneal scarring or other eye condition.

Novitra—an over-the-counter zinc preparation for the treatment of cold sores.

NovolinPen device—holds cartridges of insulin. A patient can select and inject correct dose without need for syringes or insulin vials.

Novoste Beta-Cath system (brachytherapy).

Novus Verdi diode-pumped green photocoagulator—for treatment of retinal diseases and glaucoma.

NOX (number of excitations)—MRI term. The initialism *NOX* is often dictated.

N.P. or **NP**—nurse practitioner.

NPH (normal pressure hydrocephalus).

NPPV (noninvasive positive pressure ventilation).

NREM sleep—non-rapid eye movement in which the heart rate is slowed and regular, the blood pressure is low, the brain waves are slow and of high voltage, and sleep is dreamless, interspersed with occasional periods of REM sleep. See *REM sleep*.

NRSI (nonrapid sequence induction)—orotracheal intubation.

NRT (nicotine replacement therapy).

NSAIDs (nonsteroidal anti-inflammatory drugs)—a category of drugs commonly used for treatment of rheumatoid arthritis and osteoarthritis are acetylsalicylic acid (aspirin) and ibuprofen (Motrin). Pronounced "en´sayds" or "en´seds." Not to be confused with the trade name *Ansaid,* an NSAID.

NSA (neck-shaft angle) **of femur**—hip dysplasia measurement in children with cerebral palsy.

NSCLC (non-small cell lung carcinoma, or cancer).

NSE (neuron specific enolase).

NSI (nonsyncytium-inducing) **variant of HIV.**

NSO (non-nutritive sucking opportunities)—used to stimulate premature babies suffering from lack of stimulation. They were given pacifiers four times a day and did better than other high-risk infants.

NSR (normal sinus rhythm).

NSRA—abbreviation for *nonspecific repolarization abnormalities*.

NSSTWA—abbreviation for *nonspecific ST and T-wave abnormalities*.

NSTE ACS (non-ST-segment elevation acute coronary syndrome).

NSTE acute coronary syndrome—myocardial infarction without any associated ST-segment elevation.

NSTEMI (non-ST-segment elevation myocardial infarction).

NSU (nonspecific urethritis).

NSVT (nonsustained ventricular tachycardia).

NSVD (normal spontaneous vaginal delivery).

NTD (neural tube defects).

N-Terface—contact-layer wound dressing.

N-terminal fragment atrial natriuretic peptide (N-ANP).

NTG (normal-tension glaucoma).

NTHI (native tissue harmonic imaging).

NTM (nontuberculous mycobacterium).

NT-pro-BNP (N-terminal fragment brain natriuretic peptide).

NT-proBNP immunoassay—a diagnostic test used to assess left ventricular function. NT-proBNP is a peptide secreted almost exclusively by the heart and indicative, when elevated, of congestive heart failure. See also *Elecsys proBNP Immunoassay.*

NTx assay—see *Osteomark test.*

nuchal cord—umbilical cord wrapped around the neck of the fetus can result in hypoxia or even death.

nuchal translucency—ultrasound appearance of fluid accumulation in neck of a fetus that may indicate Down syndrome.

nuclear contour index (NCI) **on blood lymphocytes**—used as the criterion for differential diagnosis of erythrodermic actinic reticuloid vs. Sézary syndrome.

nuclear grade—an assessment of malignant potential based on the size, shape, and staining characteristics of the nuclei of tumor cells. The higher the nuclear grade, the more likely the tumor recurrence.

nuclear magnetic resonance imaging (NMR)—see *magnetic resonance imaging*.

nuclear matrix protein (NMP)—used to enable detection and monitoring of prostate, cervical, colorectal, breast, and bladder cancers using urine, serum, and cell-based NMP.

nuclear molding—description of a finding in a biopsy diagnosed as oat cell carcinoma.

nuclear signal; spin; spin quantum number—MRI terms.

nuclear-tagged red blood cell bleeding study (Radiol).

nuclectomy—excision of nucleus pulposus.

nucleic acid-based crosslinking assay—a laboratory test for HBV.

nucleic acid sequence-based amplification—a rapid research-targeted method for isolating DNA or RNA sequence in a specimen that has excellent specificity. Cf. *polymerase chain reaction.*

nucleic acid testing (NAT).

nucleolar pattern of ANA (antinuclear antibodies)—associated with scleroderma.

nucleolus (pl., nucleoli)—a part of the nucleus which is spherical and more hyperchromatic than the nucleus.

nucleoplasty—a minimally invasive treatment for contained herniated disks.

nucleotide—a molecule consisting of a purine or pyrimidine base, a 5-carbon sugar (ribose or deoxyribose), and a phosphate group; DNA and RNA are polymers (very long chains) of nucleotides.

Nucleotome—an instrument used to cut away herniated disk during an endoscopic microdiskectomy. This instrument includes a light source, the visual imaging of a steerable, flexible endoscope, and the cutting ability of a Nucleotome.

Nucleotome Flex II—a flexible cutting probe for removing herniated nucleus pulposus material during spinal surgery. Its flexible probe can rotate from 0 to 90° within the disk

Nucleotome *(cont.)* space. Used in percutaneous diskectomy.

Nuclepore prep (Path).

Nucletron—radiotherapy products for the treatment of cancer.

nucleus (pl., nuclei)—a dense, usually solitary body suspended in the cytoplasm of a cell, which contains the genetic material of the cell in the form of chromosomes. See *stippled salt-and-pepper nuclei*; *Westphal-Edinger nucleus.*

nucleus lateralis of Le Gros Clark—dorsal portion of the lateral mammillary nucleus of Rose.

nucleus of Darkschewitsch—located in the rostral part of the midbrain. See *Darkschewitsch.*

nucleus of Gudden—dorsal tegmental nucleus.

nucleus of Luys—see *body of Luys.*

nucleus of Perlia—central nucleus of the oculomotor nerve.

nucleus of Rose—also *lateral mammillary nucleus of Rose.* See *nucleus lateralis of Le Gros Clark.*

nucleus pulposus *(not* pulposis)—the semifluid inner portion of the intervertebral disk.

Nucleus 24 Contour—cochlear implant system.

Nucleus 24 multichannel auditory brainstem implant (multichannel ABI)—for use in patients suffering from neurofibromatosis type 2 (NF2), which is characterized by development of tumors on cranial and spinal nerves. When these tumors are removed, it is often necessary to remove parts of the auditory nerve, leaving the patient with total deafness. This device bypasses the auditory nerve and cochlea to transmit sound signals directly to the brain.

Nu-Derm—hydrocolloid dressing material.

NUG (necrotizing ulcerative gingivitis).

Nu Gauze dressing (marketed by Johnson & Johnson). *Not* Nu-gauze.

Nu-Gel—clear hydrogel wound dressing for wounds with light to medium exudate, burns, and skin reactions to oncological procedures.

nuisance fistulas—enteroenteric fistulas that are clinically silent and are detected on intestinal contrast radiographs done for reasons other than obstruction or inflammatory masses. The fistulas do not require surgical therapy by their mere presence.

Nu-Knit—see *Surgical Nu-Knit.*

null cell lymphoblastic leukemia.

null-type non-Hodgkin lymphoma.

number of excitations (NOX)—MRI term. *NOX* is often dictated.

Numby Stuff—needle-free method for delivering local anesthesia in children. It uses lidocaine HCl 2% with epinephrine 1:100,000, and drug delivery electrodes that penetrate the skin 10 mm deep within 7 to 10 minutes.

Numeric Rating Scale (NRS, NRS-101)—measures patient's perceived level of pain on a scale of 1 to 100, one being "no pain at all" and 100 being "worst pain imaginable."

Nuport PEG tube—a percutaneous endoscopic gastrostomy tube.

Nuremberg Activities Inventory (NAI).

Nurolon suture—a braided nylon suture with extremely low tissue reaction (made by Ethicon).

Nuss repair—a minimally invasive procedure for the repair of pectus excavatum, a depression of the sternum and anterior chest. Through small

Nuss *(cont.)*
incisions lateral to the sternum and with the aid of a thoracoscope placed in a third small incision, a bar, individually curved for each patient, is passed underneath the sternum and affixed to the ribs on either side, sometimes with the addition of a plate to aid in fixation. The bar remains in place for a minimum of two years and is removed when the deformity has been corrected.

nutcracker esophagus (Radiol).

Nu-Tip disposable scissor tip—with reusable handle and shaft.

nutmeg appearance of liver (Radiol).

nutratherapy—vitamin and/or mineral supplementation.

Nutricath—silicone elastomer catheter.

NuTech Plexipulse—a sequential compression device for the foot.

Nu-Trim—dietary fat substitute said to be good for the heart. It contains a high concentration of beta-glucans, the soluble fibers found in oats and barley and known to lower LDL cholesterol and total cholesterol; they may also play a role in lowering blood sugar levels.

NutriMan TNT (*Tribulus terrestris* extract)—a natural sexual stimulant said to have the libido-enhancing properties of Viagra without the dangerous side effects. It works by helping to regulate secretion of hormones, increases muscle tone and sexual endurance, and is a natural testosterone precursor.

nutritional supplement (see *medications*)

Nuvolase 660—medical laser system used in the treatment of benign cutaneous vascular and pigmented lesions.

Nuzyme—a dietary supplement.

nvCJD (new variant Creutzfeldt-Jakob disease).

NVD (neovascularization of disk).

NVE (neovascularization elsewhere).

NVE (native valve endocarditis).

NWB (nonweightbearing).

NWRR—slang abbreviation for *no wheezes, rales, rhonchi*.

NWS (nonwithdrawal [alcohol-related] seizures).

Nycore cardiac device.

nyctalopia—night blindness.

NYHA (New York Heart Association) classification of congestive heart failure:
class I, asymptomatic
class II, slightly symptomatic
class III, congestive heart failure symptoms
class IV, severe congestive heart failure

Nyhus-Nelson tube—gastric decompression and jejunal feeding tube which permits gastric decompression and enteral feeding simultaneously.

Nyhus procedure—posterior preperitoneal mesh hernioplasty.

Nylen-Bárány maneuver (Neuro).

Nylok self-locking nail (Ortho).

Nymox urinary test—used (in addition to brain and spinal fluid studies) to diagnose Alzheimer disease.

Nyquist limit (Cardio).

nystagmus—a rhythmic horizontal or vertical oscillation of (usually both) eyeballs, generally more pronounced when looking in certain directions. See *periodic alternating nystagmus* and *optokinetic nystagmus*.

O, o

OA (osteoarthritis).

O&P test (ova and parasites)—examination of stool, urine, or other material for parasites or their ova (eggs). Usage: "Stools for O&P x 2 [times two] were obtained and were negative."

Oasis burn matrix—a product that provides a supportive environment for healing of first-degree and second-degree burns and graft donor sites. Based on SIS technology, it is a naturally derived extracellular matrix created from the submucosal layer of porcine small intestine.

Oasis thrombectomy system—catheter-based system which removes blood clots that develop in access grafts of dialysis patients. Uses a low-pressure water jet to break up the clot and remove fragments from the occluded graft.

Oasis wound matrix—a natural matrix which supports the management of all partial- and full-thickness wounds.

Oasis wound dressing—for management of full-thickness skin injuries.

Obecalp (*placebo* spelled backwards)—a non-drug given as a medication.

Ober-Barr brachioradialis transfer—for weakness of the triceps muscle.

obliterative bronchiolitis—not the same as bronchiolitis obliterans. The pathologic hallmark of this disease is the presence of submucosal and peribronchiolar fibrosis. It is less common than bronchiolitis obliterans with organizing pneumonia (BOOP).

OBS (organic brain syndrome).

obsessive-compulsive disorder (OCD)—a psychiatric disorder characterized by persisting or recurring thoughts or impulses (obsessions) and repetitive, ritualized, stereotyped acts (compulsions), such as hand washing, touching all the posts of a fence, or carrying out a series of actions in a certain order. Sometimes these symptoms overlap with the tics (with the absence of intention), twitching of the face, blinking, throat-clearing, hyperactivity, tearing hair, gnashing teeth, etc., of Tourette disease.

Obsessive Compulsive Drinking Scale (OCDS)—a 14-item quick and reliable self-rating instrument that provides a total and two subscale scores that measure some cognitive aspects of alcohol "craving." It is used as an alcoholism severity-and-treatment outcome instrument.

obstructive sleep apnea syndrome (OSAS)—a disorder characterized by repeated episodes of reductions or cessation in breathing during sleep, which is associated with clinical complications such as daytime sleepiness, hypertension, heart disease, increased risk for stroke, and an increased risk for early death.

obstructive sleep apnea oral appliances
- A.M.E. tongue retaining device
- Ameflow
- dental anti-snoring device
- Dr. B's mouthpiece
- EMA (elastic mandibular advancement)
- EMA-T (elastic mandibular advancement-titration)
- elastomeric sleep appliance
- equalizer airway device
- H&M anti-snoring device
- Klearway
- NAPA (nocturnal airway patency appliance)
- OSAP (obstructive sleep apnea prosthesis)
- Perl-Rad sleep disorder aid
- PM positioner, also adjustable PM positioner
- Silencer
- Silent Nite, Silent Nite soft oral appliance
- Silent Nightshirt sleep kit
- Sleep-In bone screw system
- SNOAR (sleep nocturnal obstruction airway repositioner) open airway appliance

obstructive *(cont.)*
- Snore Aid Plus
- Snore Peace
- Snore Tec
- Snoremaster snore remedy
- Snorex
- Snore-Cure
- Snore-Ezzer
- Snore-No-More
- Snore-X mouth guard
- snoring control device
- soft palate lifter, adjustable
- TheraSnore, also adjustable TheraSnore
- TOA (Thornton oral appliance)
- tongue stabilizer device

obturator—a rod or wire placed inside a catheter, trocar, endoscope, or other tubular instrument to close the opening in its tip during insertion. Usage, in an arthroscopic temporomandibular joint procedure: "A sheath with a sharp obturator was inserted into the superior joint space. After the space was entered, the sharp obturator was replaced with a dull one to further direct the sheath into the joint."

obturator hernia—hernia through the obturator foramen, a cause of small bowel obstruction.

obturator sign—may be positive in appendicitis or when there is fluid or blood in the pelvis. The flexed thigh is rotated both internally and externally, and hypogastric pain is elicited when there is an inflammatory process in contact with the obturator externus muscle.

obtuse marginal (OM) **coronary artery**.

obtuse marginal branch (OMB)—one of the coronary arteries.

Obwegeser-Dalpont internal screw fixation—used in sagittal split ramus osteotomy.

Obwegeser sagittal mandibular osteotomy technique—Salyer and Bardach modifications.

O-Cal f.a.—prescription oral multivitamin with calcium and folic acid.

OCB (optical coherence biometry).

occipitofrontal circumference (Peds)—a term used in measurement of the head.

occult—in medicine, something that is present in such a tiny quantity that it is effectively hidden. Usage: "We still must rule out the possibility of occult neoplasm." See also *fecal occult blood test* and *occult blood*.

occult blood—blood present in stool, urine, or other material in too small an amount to be detected by naked-eye observation, but detectable by chemical testing or microscopic examination. See *fecal occult blood test*.

occupational contact dermatitis.

occur, occurred (past tense); **occurring**. Frequently misspelled.

OCD (obsessive compulsive disorder).

OCD (osteochondral defect).

OCG (oral cholecystogram).

OCG—see *osteochondral graft*.

OCR (optical coherence reflectometry)—a device used to diagnose vascular occlusions.

OCT (optical coherence tomography).

OCT (optimal cutting temperature).

OCT (oxytocin challenge test).

Octopus retractor—used in cardiac surgery.

octopus test—measures peripheral vision. The patient is seated before a large screen, holding a counter. Each time the patient sees a light reflected at any angle on the screen, he presses the hand counter, which is monitored in another room by a technician.

Octopus 2+ tissue stabilization system.

Oculaid capsular tension ring—intraocular lens.

ocular adnexal lymphoma—a malignant lymphoproliferative tumor that occurs in the eye.

ocular melanocytosis—may be the underlying cause of multifocal choroidal melanoma.

ocular rosacea—involvement of the eye secondary to acne rosacea, which affects facial skin and the eye. It may result in mild blepharoconjunctivitis or in blindness.

OcuLight SL (Oph)—diode laser.

oculogyric crisis—occurs when the eyeballs become fixed in one position for a considerable period of time, minutes to hours. It is seen in encephalitis or postencephalitic parkinsonism. Usage: "She is having an acute extrapyramidal reaction. She is drooling, unable to speak coherently; no evidence of oculogyric crisis."

oculoplethysmography/carotid phonoangiography (OPG/CPA)—examination used in evaluating suspected intracranial cerebrovascular disease. A noninvasive test, serial angiography of the internal carotid artery, using the OPG-Gee instrument, to determine thc degree of occlusion of the internal carotid. The ophthalmic systolic pressure is correlated with the brachial systolic pressure (as determined by arm cuff and auscultation) which is measured immediately after the OPG study.

Ocutech vision enhancing system—autofocusing glasses that allow distance vision for patients whose eye conditions cannot be corrected with regular glasses.

ocutome—a device to remove vitreous; e.g., O'Malley ocutome.

O.D. (*oculus dexter*, right eye).

o.d. (*omni die*)—every day (also *q.d.*).

OD (overdose).

OD'd—slang for overdosed.

O_2 (oxygen) **debt** —when available oxygen is less than oxygen requirements, in reference to resuscitation of newborns and in exercise physiology.

O'Donoghue unhappy triad (OUT) —a triple injury of damage, with joint cartilage and both outside and inside knee ligaments being torn. Also called *motorcyclist's knee.*

odontoid view of cervical spine—x-ray view of the odontoid process of the second cervical vertebra, also called the *dens*.

OD (ocular or optical density) **values**—antibody titer determination on amniotic fluid for erythroblastosis fetalis.

Odyssey phacoemulsification system (Oph).

off-center ablation—can occur after a second laser surgery to correct vision. It can cause glare, double vision, and a halo effect.

off-pump coronary artery bypass (OPCAB)—see *beating heart surgery.*

off-pump coronary revascularization with endoscopic saphenous vein harvesting (OPCRES).

Ogden anchor—used to anchor soft tissue to bone.

Ogilvie syndrome—pseudo-obstruction or adynamic ileus of colon.

Ogura tissue and cartilage forceps.

Ohashiatsu—a form of shiatsu massage developed by the Ohashi Institute of New York City, consisting of techniques to alleviate symptoms common to pregnancy (fatigue, aching, general discomfort) and the delivery process through the use of pressure to specific body areas.

OHSS (ovarian hyperstimulation syndrome).

oil drop change—a localized brown color, a sign of psoriasis in the nail bed.

oil droplet reflex—seen on retinoscopy.

oil red O stain (Oph)—a dye used in histologic demonstration of neutral fats. Usage: "Oil red O stain for intracytoplasmic fat was present."

Ojemann cortical stimulator—a device used in intraoperative functional cortical mapping.

Oklahoma ankle joint—orthosis for ambulation in children with cerebral palsy and myelomeningocele. Made of polypropylene vacuformed in plastic.

OKN (optokinetic nystagmus) (Neuro).

OKT3—see *Orthoclone OKT3.*

OKT4—monoclonal antibody to human T-4 cells. Also, *antihuman T-4 cell, antihuman inducer/helper T-cell.*

OKT8—the monoclonal antibody to human T-8 cells. Also called *antihuman T-8 cell*, and *antihuman suppressor/cytotoxic T-cell.*

Olean (olestra)—a fat-based substitute for conventional fats, used in certain snack foods. It adds no fat or calories to food, but it may cause abdominal cramping and diarrhea in some people and inhibits the absorption of certain vitamins and nutrients.

Olerud and Molander fracture classification.

olestra—see *Olean.*

oligoclonal bands.

oligodendroglioma—derived from cells forming and maintaining the myelin sheaths in the central nervous system.

OligoDetect—test kit for West Nile virus.

oligopotent progenitor cells—progenitor cells that can differentiate into a limited number of mature cell types.

oligoteratoasthenozoospermia syndrome—spermatozoa reduced in number with poor motility and an increased number of abnormal shapes.

oligozymes—catalytically interactive oligomers used to treat diseases and to aid in pharmaceutical or genomic research.

Oliver-Rosalki method of testing serum CPK—see also *Sigma*.

olive wire; ring—used in Ilizarov limb lengthening procedure.

Ollier disease—enchondromatosis.

OLM (ophthalmic laser microendoscope)—see *Microprobe*.

Olsen cholangiogram clamp.

OLT (orthotopic liver transplantation).

Olympia VACPAC—a support device used in back surgery that is able to be molded under the patient during inspiration and hardened by suction while an inflated urologic irrigation bladder is under the abdomen. After hardening, the irrigation bladder is deflated and a vacant space is left under the abdomen that decreases extradural venous pressure. Lumbar respiratory movements are also minimized by the technique. Cf. *Andrews spinal frame/table, Hastings frame*.

Olympus CF-1T100L—forward-viewing video colonoscope.

Olympus CF-200Z colonoscope—provides high-power magnified observation of the surface of colorectal neoplasms.

Olympus CYF-3 OES cystofiberscope—used in urinary endoscopy.

Olympus ENF-P2 scope—flexible laryngoscope.

Olympus EU-M30S endoscopic ultrasonography receiver.

Olympus EVIS 140—endoscope reprocessing system.

Olympus EVIS Q-200V—video endoscope.

Olympus FBK 13 forceps—endoscopic biopsy forceps.

Olympus GF-UM3 and **CF-UM20 ultrasonic endoscope**—designed to allow a limited visual exam of upper GI tract and endoscopic ultrasonography of organs adjacent to esophagus, stomach, and duodenum.

Olympus GIF-EUM2 echoendoscope—side-viewing gastroscope or duodenoscope with ultrasound probe.

Olympus GIF-1T10 and **GIF20 echoendoscope**—forward-viewing gastroscope with ultrasound probe.

Olympus JF1T10 fiberoptic duodenoscope.

Olympus JF-UM20 echoendoscope—endoscopic ultrasonography instrument for ERCP and pancreatic-biliary ultrasonography.

Olympus One-Step Button—short gastrostomy tube (the thickness of the stomach wall) with an internal button to hold it in place and an external opening with an attached plastic plug. Inserted endoscopically and used for tube feedings.

Olympus OSF scope—flexible sigmoidoscope.

Olympus SIF10 enteroscope.

Olympus TJF-100 endoscope—with reusable biopsy channel caps.

Olympus UM-1W endoscopic probe—transendoscopic ultrasound probe to be used with regular endoscopes, rather than with specially made ultrasonograph endoscopes.

Olympus URF-P2 translaparoscopic choledochofiberscope—used in the management of biliary tract disease including removal of cystic and common bile duct stones.

Olympus VU-M2 and **XIF-UM3 echoendoscope**—a side-viewing gastroscope with ultrasound probe.

Olympus XQ230 gastroscope.

OMB (obtuse marginal branch).

Omed bulldog vascular clamp—for atraumatic occlusion of vessels.

omega-shaped epiglottis—shaped like the Greek letter *omega* (Ω).

Omega splinting material—used in hand therapy.

Omiderm—transparent adhesive film dressing.

Ommaya reservoir.

OmniCath atherectomy catheter.

omni die (o.d.)—every day.

OmniFilter—mounted on a guidewire, it prevents blood clots from reaching various organs of the body.

Omnifit HA hip stem—prosthesis of hydroxyapatite.

Omnifit Plus—enhanced offset cemented hip system.

Omni-Flexor—a handheld physical therapy device that allows for all six ranges of wrist movement. Because it is small, the patient can use it at home after proper instruction.

Omni Flush shape—Accu-Vu catheter design that allows opacification of the aorta from distal vessels without obscuring the image by superior mesenteric artery filling.

Omni-Link .018 and **.035**—a biliary stent system.

Omniloc dental system—used in tooth restorations.

Omni-Pac—a unit dose packaging for Omnicef.

OmniPulse-MAX holmium laser—a pulsed laser system for use in lithotripsy procedures.

Omni retractor.

Omniscience—single leaflet cardiac valve prosthesis.

OmniStent—a stent used in angioplasty and atherectomy procedures. Used to reduce restenosis in blood vessels.

Omni-Tract—adjustable wishbone retractor.

omphalodiverticular band.

"on block" or **"ahn block"**—see *en bloc.*

oncogene—a gene that can induce malignant change in cells; it may arise by mutation of a normal gene or be introduced by a virus. See *gene*.

oncomarker—a coined term synonymous with tumor marker, for substances within the body that are indicators of the presence of cancer.

On-Command catheters (male and female)—used to treat urinary incontinence and retention.

oncovirus—an RNA virus capable of inducing malignant change in a cell infected by it.

Ondine curse—periodic breathing. Chronic alveolar hypoventilation together with unresponsiveness of the carotid body to hypoxemia.

1+ to 2+ pitting edema—the proper way to transcribe "one to two plus" pitting edema, when dictated (no hyphen; plus sign used with each numeral). Do not use *1 to 2+* or *1-2+*, which is properly used in relation to motor strength: "Motor strength in the upper extremities 3 to 3+ bilaterally," and "Motor strength in the upper extremities 3- to 3 bilaterally." In the latter examples of the alternative number scale, the plus sign functions as an incre-

1+ *(cont.)*
ment and the minus sign functions as a decrement.

one-shot anastomotic instrument— allows the surgeon to complete a vascular anastomosis, as in coronary artery bypass grafting, in two minutes with one squeeze of the handle (compared to 20 to 25 minutes for hand sewing). It is based on the VCS vascular clip technology, which allows the surgeon to join two vessels by individually placing a series of titanium clips to complete the anastomosis. The one-shot automates this process by simultaneously placing 12 clips.

One Touch blood glucose meter—for self-testing by diabetics.

1,2 intercompartmental supraretinacular artery—the 1,2 stands for the 1st and 2nd branches of the intercompartmental supraretinacular artery (ISRA).

onlay graft—a bone graft, not to be confused with inlay graft. Both are used in craniofacial surgery. Cf. *inlay graft*.

OnLineABG monitoring system—attached to the patient to deliver arterial blood gas values within 60 seconds.

"ONP"—see *O&P* (ova and parasites).

ON-Q—an anesthesia delivery system.

Ontario Prehospital Advanced Life Support Study (OPALS).

On-X prosthetic heart valve—a mechanical heart valve with two movable half-disks (bileaflets), contained within a housing surrounded by a man-made fabric-covered ring. It is used to replace diseased, damaged, or malfunctioning natural or prosthetic aortic valves.

onychopachydermoperiostitis—see *psoriatic onychopachydermoperiostitis*.

Onyx—a nonadhesive liquid embolic agent (ethylene vinyl alcohol copolymer [EVOH]) used for treatment of spinal dural AV fistula (DAVF) where penetration into the proximal radicular vein is required, and for cerebral aneurysms.

Onyx finger pulse oximeter.

oocyte—a female gamete (sex cell); this term is now preferred to *ovum*.

OOKP (osteo-odontokeratoprosthesis).

"oona boot"—phonetic for *Unna boot*.

ooplasmic transfer (cytoplasmic transfer)—an experimental technique of injecting cytoplasm from an oocyte of a woman known to be fertile into an oocyte of an infertile woman. The oocyte thus modified is then fertilized in vitro and implanted into the uterus of the infertile woman.

ooplasm—the cytoplasm of an oocyte; its mitochondria possess genetic material (mitochondrial DNA) that functions independently of nuclear (chromosomal) DNA and is the principal source of mitochondrial DNA in a zygote.

opacification—increase in the density of a tissue or region, with increased resistance to x-rays.

opacities—see *snowball opacities* (Oph).

Opal Photoactivator—used with Visudyne (verteporfin for injection) therapy for treatment of the wet form of age-related macular degeneration.

OPALS (Ontario Prehospital Advanced Life Support Study).

OPART—open MRI with access to all four sides.

OPCAB (off-pump coronary artery bypass)—surgery performed while the heart is still beating. Uses a stabilizer

OPCAB *(cont.)*
arm attached to the device that holds the chest open during surgery. The arm touches the heart and temporarily stops movement in one spot, allowing the surgeon to attach grafts to the arteries without stopping the entire heart.

OPCRES (off-pump coronary revascularization with endoscopic saphenous vein harvesting).

OpenAnchor—for securing mesh in laparoscopic hernia repair.

open-book injury—pelvic trauma consisting of both fracture or dislocation involving the pubic arch and unstable fracture or dislocation of a sacroiliac joint.

opening snap—an important finding on physical examination because an audible opening snap in mitral or tricuspid stenosis implies a flexible valve.

open mesh-plug hernioplasty—used for preperitoneal hernioplasty and femoral hernia repair. Mesh is inserted through the trocar; the plug has a fluted outside layer combined with an inside arrangement of mesh "petals" that expand or contract to fit the hernia defect.

open-mouth odontoid view—a view of the odontoid process of the second cervical vertebra for which the x-ray beam is aimed through the patient's open mouth.

open reduction and internal fixation (ORIF)—an orthopedic procedure to correct a severely fractured bone.

OpenSail—balloon catheter used to clear blockages from coronary arteries.

open sky MRI—see *Fonar-360 MRI scanner*.

open-sky vitrectomy—operative procedure to remove vitreous from the eye by first removing a button of cornea. The vitreous is then removed through the pupil, after the lens has been extracted.

OPERA (outpatient endometrial resection/ablation)—minimally invasive alternative procedure to hysterectomy for patients suffering from abnormal uterine bleeding (AUB).

OPERA STAR SL—a hysteroscope used in OPERA (outpatient endometrial resection/ablation) procedures. STAR is an acronym for **s**pecialized **t**issue **a**spirating **r**esectoscope.

Operating Arm system—mechanical arm used as a pointer in image-guided and intraoperative navigation for neurosurgery (i.e., during surgical procedure).

operation or procedure—a quick-reference list of diagnostic procedures and studies (invasive and noninvasive) and surgical procedures, approaches, maneuvers, techniques, and treatments of all kinds. See individual entries in alpha order throughout the book for descriptions.
Abbe repair
Abbe-McIndoe vaginal construction
abdominal-sacral colpoperineopexy
ab-externo laser sclerotomy
ab-interno laser sclerotomy
ACAT (automated computerized axial tomography)
acetabular limbectomy
acetabuloplasty
acupressure without needles
Acuson computed sonography
adenosine echocardiography
advanced cardiac mapping
affinity chromatography
agarose gel electrophoresis (AGE)
air contrast barium enema

operation *(cont.)*
Albizzia procedure
alcohol ablation
Alfieri mitral valve
Allgower-Donati technique
Alliston GE reflux repair
ALT (argon laser trabeculoplasty)
Altemeier perineal recto-
sigmoidectomy
ALT-RCC (autolymphocyte-based
treatment for renal cell
carcinoma)
amnioinfusion
anconeus arthroplasty
Ancure endovascular repair
antecolic anastomosis
antecolic gastrojejunostomy
anterior pelvic exenteration
Antia
Antia-Buch chondrocutaneous
advancement flap
Antia-Buch helical rim
advancement flap
anthropometry
anti-aliasing technique on x-ray
antifibrin antibody imaging
antiperistaltic technique
aortobifemoral reconstruction
aortomyoplasty
apheresis
APLD (automated percutaneous
lumbar diskectomy)
appendicocecostomy
appendicovesicotomy
appendogram
applanation tonometry
arachnophlebectomy
argon laser trabeculoplasty (ALT)
Aries-Pitanguy correction of
mammary ptosis
arrested heart surgery
arrow flap reconstruction of nipple
arterial switch
A-scan ultrasound
aspheric custom ablation

operation *(cont.)*
aspiration biopsy cytology (ABC)
astigmatic keratotomy
Atavi atraumatic spine fusion
Auchincloss modified radical
mastectomy
Aufranc-Turner arthroplasty
auricular acupuncture
autoaugmentation
autologous augmentation of breasts
following mastectomy
autologous osteochondral transplantation
autologous ovarian transplantation
autologous transfusion
automated lamellar therapeutic
keratoplasty (ALTK)
automated percutaneous lumbar
diskectomy (APLD)
auxiliary transplant
Avesta laparoscopic procedure
axillofemoral bypass
Bacon-Babcock rectovaginal fistula
BAK interbody fusion surgical
procedure
Baldy-Webster correction of uterine
retrodisplacement
balloon catheterization
Ball treatment of pruritus ani
band-snare technique
Bankart shoulder dislocation repair
banner transposition flap for ear
reconstruction
Barcat modified technique
Bardenheuer modified bifurcation
procedure
barrel-stave osteotomy
Bassini inguinal hernia repair
Batchelor modified procedure to
correct hindfoot valgus deformity
Batista left ventriculectomy
Batista ventricular reduction
surgery
BEAM (brain electrical activity
mapping)

operation *(cont.)*
beating heart surgery
Belsey Mark IV fundoplication
Benirschke approach
Bennett quadriceps plastic procedure
Bernese periacetabular osteotomy (PAO)
biliopancreatic diversion with duodenal switch
Billroth gastroenterostomy
biosurgery
Bishop-Koop ileostomy
bladder neck closure (BNC)
Blalock-Hanlon cardiac surgery
Blalock-Taussig cardiac surgery
blind esophageal brushing (BEG)
Blumgart hepaticojejunostomy
Blythe uvulopalatoplasty
body floss access
Boerema hernia repair
Bohlman triple-wire technique
bolus-chase technique
bone density measurement
Booth wire osteotomy
Bosker transmandibular reconstructive surgery
bow-tie repair
brachioplasty
Brackin ureterointestinal anastomosis
Brandt-Daroff exercises
Braun enteroenterostomy
breast reduction technique
breath-hold MR cholangiography
Bricker ureteroileostomy
Bristow repair of shoulder dislocation
bronchial artery embolization
bronchial sleeve
bronchopleuromediastinal fistulectomy
Brooke ileostomy
Broström ankle repair
brow-lift
Brown two-portal endoscopic carpal tunnel release

operation *(cont.)*
Bruhat laser surgery neosalpingostomy
bubble ventriculography
bundle-nailing treatment of bone shaft fractures
bunionectomy
bunionplasty (bunionectomy)
Bunnell tendon transfer
Burch
Burch colposuspension for stress incontinence
Burch iliopectineal ligament
Burch laparoscopic procedure
Burhenne stone basket
butterfly flap technique
button cecostomy
buttonpexy fixation of stomal prolapse
callus distraction technique
Camey ileocystoplasty
Camitz palmaris longus abductorplasty
canalith repositioning maneuver (CRP)
capillary electrophoresis (CE)
capnography
can-opener capsulotomy
capsulorrhexis
cardiac hybrid revascularization
cardiokymography
Cardiolite scan
cardiomyoplasty
CardioTec scan
cardiotocography
carotid angioplasty with stenting
carotid endarterectomy (CEA)
Casale vesicostomy
Casola cecostomy
catheter balloon valvuloplasty
catheter-directed thrombolysis and endovascular stent placement
Cavitron ultrasonic surgical aspiration of tumor

operation *(cont.)*

CECT (contrast enhancement of computed tomographic) head and body imaging
celiacography
cementless surface replacement arthroplasty (CSRA)
cervicectomy
cervicography or cervigram
Chait percutaneous cecostomy
channel osteotomy
cheilectomy
chemoprevention
chevron osteotomy
Chiari medial displacement pelvic hysterectomy
cholescintigraphy
Chonstruct chondral repair
chorionic villi biopsy
Chow technique
Chrisman and Snook correction of ankle instability
chromopertubation
chymonucleolysis
cine CT (computed tomography)
circularplasty
circumduction-adduction shoulder maneuver
cisternography
Clagett-Barrett esophagogastrostomy
Clark perineorrhaphy
classic abdominal Semm hysterectomy (CASH)
claviculectomy
clitoridectomy
closed intramedullary pinning (CIMP)
closing base wedge osteotomy (CBWO)
club sandwich tympanoplasty
coagulum pyelolithotomy
Coblation
Coblation Channeling
Coblation tonsillectomy
Cody tack

operation *(cont.)*

Coffey ureterointestinal anastomosis
Cohen reimplantation
cold cup biopsy
cold-dissection technique
Collin-Beard resection of levator muscle
Collis-Nissen fundoplication
Collis-Nissen gastroplasty
colocolponeopoiesis
color Doppler sonography
colostomy shift en masse
colpocystourethropexy (CCUP)
computed dental radiography (CDR)
computed tomographic angiography (CTA)
computed tomography angiographic portography (CTAP)
computed tomography laser mammography (CTLM)
computer-assisted minimally invasive surgery
computerized dynamic posturography (CDP)
computerized phonoenterography
conductive keratoplasty (CK)
conjunctivodacryocystorhinostomy (CDCR)
contact transscleral laser cytophotocoagulation (CTLC)
continent catheterizable appendicovesicostomy using the Mitrofanoff principle
continent ileovesicostomy
continent supravesical bowel urinary diversion
continent vesicostomy
continuous arteriovenous hemofiltration (CAVH)
continuous circular capsulorrhexis technique
continuous curvilinear capsulorrhexis (CCC)
continuous wave Doppler examination

operation *(cont.)*
contoured tilting compression mammography
contrast echocardiography
contrast material enhanced scan
corner mouth lift
coronary artery bypass graft (CABG)
coronary artery scan (CAS)
coronary atherectomy
coronary remodeling
corpus cavernosum penile electromyography
corset platysmaplasty
corticomedullary junction (CMJ) phase imaging on CT scan
Cosgrove-Edwards anuloplasty
Costello laser ablation of prostate
Cotton cartilage graft to cricopharyngeal area
cough CPR
counterflow centrifugal elutriation
counterstaining technique
coupled suturing
Cox maze III
Crawford-Adams arthroplasty
Crawford graft inclusion reattachment
cribogram
Crikelair otoplasty
Cröhnlein
crossed-swords technique
crowncork tympanoplasty
crural steal procedure
crush technique in balloon angioplasty
cryoablation for prostate cancer
cryosurgery
cryosurgical ablation of hepatic tumor
CT (computed tomography)
CTHA (CT during hepatic arteriography)
CTLM (computed tomography laser mammography)

operation *(cont.)*
CT/SPECT fusion
CT with slip-ring technology
culdolaparoscopy
cupping (acupuncture)
Cushieri maneuver
custom contoured ablation pattern (C-CAP) method
Cutler-Beard eyelid
Cyclops reconstruction to cover defect
cystocolpoproctography
cytoreductive surgery
dacryocystorhinostomy (DCR)
Damus-Kaye-Stansel congenital heart defect repair
Darrach ulnar tenodesis
Davies Z-plasty repair
Davydov vagina construction
deep lamellar endothelial keratoplasty (DLEK)
deep lamellar keratoplasty (DLK)
Dennis-Varco pancreaticoduodenostomy
Dennyson-Fulford extra-articular subtalar arthrodesis
DentaScan
DePalma staple
dermabrasion
dermoscopy using epiluminescent microscopy
detubularization principle
De Vega tricuspid anuloplasty
DEXA radiographic technique
DEXA (dual energy x-ray absorptiometry) scan
diaphanography
Dibbell unilateral cleft lip nasal reconstruction
diffraction-enhanced imaging (DEI)
diffusion-weighted ultrafast MRI imaging
digital image fusion (DIF)
digital radiography
digital subtraction angiography (DSA)

operation *(cont.)*
digital subtraction macrodacryocystography
distraction laminoplasty
distraction osteogenesis surgery
DioPexy probe
dipyridamole echocardiography
directional coronary angioplasty (DCA)
directional coronary atherectomy (DCA)
direct myocardial revascularization (DMR)
direct vision internal urethrotomy (DVIU)
distal tibial osteotomy
distortion product otoacoustic emission (DPOAE)
dobutamine stress echocardiography (DSE)
Döderlein (or Doederlein) laparoscopic hysterectomy
Dohlman endoscopic repair of Zenker diverticulum
donor island harvesting
donor-specific transfusion
Doppler echocardiography
Doppler-guided hemorrhoidal artery ligation (DGHAL)
Doppler tissue imaging (DTI)
Dotter-Judkins PTA
double contrast arthrography
double contrast barium enema
double freeze-thaw sequence
double-orifice repair
double-T pouch urinary diversion
double-twist knot (DTK) technique
douglasectomy
DREZ-otomy
DS (duplex sonography)
dual photon densitometry
Duecollement hemicolectomy
Duhamel pull-through anastomosis, laparoscopic
duodenal seromyectomy

operation *(cont.)*
duodenal switch
duplex ultrasound
Duval pancreaticojejunostomy
DuVries hammer toe repair
DVIU (direct vision internal urethrotomy)
Dwyer correction of scoliosis
Dwyer osteotomy
dynamic computerized tomography
dynamic graciloplasty
dynamic nasopharyngoscopy
dynamic spiral CT lung densitometry
echocardiography
Eckhout vertical gastroplasty
ECMO (extracorporeal membrane oxygenation)
EDAS (encephaloduroarteriosynangiosis)
Egan mammography
egg shelling procedure
ELAS (endoluminal laser ablation of the greater saphenous vein)
ELCA (excimer laser coronary angioplasty)
elective lymph node dissection (ELND)
electrocardiographic gating with electron-beam CT technology
electrocochleography
electrocorticography
electroejaculation
electrohydraulic lithotripsy (EHL)
electron beam angiography of coronary arteries
electron beam computed tomography
electron beam tomography (EBT)
electro-oculogram
electroretinogram
electrothermally assisted capsulorrhaphy (ETAC)
electrothermal procedure
Elmslie triple arthrodesis

operation *(cont.)*
embryoscopy
Emmet-Studdiford perineorrhaphy
en bloc transplantation of small pediatric kidneys into adult recipients
en bloc vein resection
encephaloduroarteriosynangiosis (EDAS)
Endocare renal cryoablation
endokeratoplasty (EKP)
endometrial ablation
endometrial resection and ablation (ERA)
endopyelotomy
endoscopic aspiration mucosectomy
endoscopic band ligation (EBL)
endoscopic biliary endoprosthesis
endoscopic brow lift
endoscopic division of incompetent perforating veins
endoscopic laser cholecystectomy
endoscopic laser dacryocysto-rhinostomy
endoscopic ligation
endoscopic mucosal resection (EMR)
endoscopic mucosectomy
endoscopic papillectomy (EP)
endoscopic plantar fasciotomy (EPF)
endoscopic posterolateral fusion (PLF)
endoscopic retrograde cholangi-ography (ERC)
endoscopic retrograde cholangio-pancreatography (ERCP)
endoscopic sewing machine technique
endoscopic sphincterotomy (ES)
endoscopic strip craniectomy
endoscopic transpapillary catheteri-zation of the gallbladder (ETCG)
endoscopic ultrasonography
endoscopic ultrasound-assisted band ligation

operation *(cont.)*
endoscopic ultrasound-guided fine needle aspiration (EUS-FNA)
endoscopic variceal ligation (EVL)
endosonography
endothelial lamellar keratoplasty (ELK)
endovascular coil embolization
endoventricular circular patchplasty
end-stage coxarthrosis
enhanced external counterpulsation (EECP)
enlargement of Beck drill hole
EnSite cardiac mapping procedure
enteroenterostomy
Entero-Test
Enteryx
enucleation
epididymovasostomy
epidural neuroplasty
EpiFilm club sandwich technique for tympanoplasty
ErecAid treatment of erectile impotence
esophageal sling
esophageal stretching
esophagodiverticulostomy, endoscopic, staple-assisted
ethoxysclerol procedure
ETS (endoscopic thoracic sympathectomy)
EVac CAT procedure
EVAL embolization
Evans tenodesis
EVAR (endovascular aortic repair)
Eve transfer
evisceration
exenterative surgery for pelvic cancer
excimer laser coronary angioplasty (ELCA)
EXIT (ex utero intrapartum treatment)
Exogen SAFHS (sonic accelerated fracture healing system)

operation *(cont.)*
exposure osteotomy
Exorcist respiratory compensation
extended right hepatectomy
external cephalic version (ECV)
extracorporeal photoimmune therapy
extracorporeal shock wave lithotripsy
extracranial-intracranial (EC-IC) bypass
extradural clinoidectomy
extraperitoneal excision of lower one-third of ureter with bladder cuff without an initial vesicotomy
facet denervation
facial resurfacing
facilitated angioplasty
Faden retropexy
Falcinelli OOKP (osteo-odonto-keratoprosthesis)
falloposcopy
fascia lata suburethral sling
fast spin-echo acquisition technique
FDG (18-fluorodeoxyglucose) positron emission tomography
feather-lift
female genital mutilation (FMG)
fetal magnetocardiography
fetal neuron allotransplantation
fetal pig cell transplantation
fetal tissue transplant
fetal ventral mesencephalic tissue transplantation
fiberoptic bronchoscopy
fibroid embolization
fibula free flap
Fick sacculotomy
Finesse Dacron patch angioplasty
flap surgery
flap tracheostomy
flap valve principle
flexible transgastric peritoneoscopy (FTP)
flicker electroretinogram (ERG)

operation *(cont.)*
fluorescein angiography
fluoroscopic cystocolpoproctography
flush aortogram
FOAM (fluorescence overlay antigen mapping)
Fobi pouch procedure
focal cortical resection
focused heat technology
Fonar Stand-Up MRI
Fontan anastomosis
Fontan-Kreutzer repair
four-flap Z-plasty
Fourier transform infrared spectroscopy
Fourier transform Raman spectroscopy
Fowler-Stephens orchiopexy (orchidopexy)
Frank nonsurgical perineal autodilation for vaginal construction
free toe transfer
frontal sinus obliteration
full-bladder ultrasound
full-column barium enema
full Monti
functional endoscopic sinus surgery (FESS)
functional MRI technique
Furnas otoplasty technique
Furniss ureterointestinal anastomosis
gadolinium-enhanced subtracted MR angiography, 3-D
galactography
gallium scan
galvanic vestibular stimulation (GVR)
Gambee technique
gamete intrafallopian transfer (GIFT)
Gamma nailing
Ganz periacetabular osteotomy
gas chromatography
gastric neobladder

operation *(cont.)*
gastroenteroanastomosis
gastroplasty banding of Molina
gating
generalized nephrographic (GNG) phase imaging
GenESA System pharmacological stress test
genioglossal advancement with hyoid myotomy (GAHM)
Giampapa suturing technique
Giannestras step-down modified
Gillies elevation
Gill laminectomy
Girdlestone-Taylor
Gittes urethral suspension
Glenn anastomosis
Goldman
Goulian mammoplasty
gradual elongation (intramedullary) nailing (GEN, GEIN)
granulocyte transfusion
great toe arthroplasty implant (GAIT)
Green-Waterman osteotomy
Grice-Green correction of hindfoot valgus deformity
gum sculpting
Gustilo-Kyle arthroplasty
hair apposition technique (HAT)
Halban culdoplasty
HALS (hand-assisted laparoscopic surgery)
Halsted inguinal herniorrhaphy
hammer toe repair
hammock-like fashion of flap fixation
hand-assisted laparoscopic sigmoidectomy
hand-assisted laparoscopic surgery (HALS)
hand-sewn ileoanal anastomosis
hang-back technique
harvesting
Hauser transplantation of patellar tendon insertion

operation *(cont.)*
heater probe thermocoagulation
heavy ion irradiation
Heineke-Mikulicz pyloroplasty
Heller-Belsey correction of achalasia of esophagus
Heller-Dor laparoscopic procedure
Heller-Nissen correction of achalasia of esophagus
hematopoietic stem cell (HSC) transplant
hemicallotasis
hemicolectomy
hemi-Fontan
hemofiltration
hemi-T bladder augmentation
Henning arthroscopic meniscal repair
hepatic resection
hepatic segmentectomy
hepatobiliary scintigraphy
hepatopancreatoduodenectomy
hexagonal keratotomy
HIDA scan
Higgins ureterointestinal anastomosis
high McCall suspension
high-resolution storage phosphor managing
high-speed rotational atherectomy (RA)
high-voltage pulsed galvanic stimulation
Hill cluster harvest micrograft
Hill esophageal antireflux repair
Hill gastropexy fundoplication
Hinds repair of subcondylar fracture
Hoffa tendon shortening
Hoffman and Mohr repair of unicoronal cranial synostosis
Hoffman-Clayton podiatric treatment of rheumatoid arthritis
Hofmeister gastroenterostomy
Hofmeister-Shoemaker gastro–jejunostomy

operation *(cont.)*
Ho:YAG LTK (noncontact holmium:YAG laser thermal keratoplasty)
HRARE (hybrid rapid acquisition with relaxation enhancement)
Hunter open cord tendon implant
Hunter tendon rod insertion
Hunt-Lawrence pouch
hyoid bone suspension
hyperoxia
hypertension optimal treatment (HOT)
hyperthermia, whole body
hysterectomy
hysterosalpingosonography (HSSG)
hysteroscopic sterilization
hysterosonography
IC-Green (indocyanine green) fluorescein angiography
ICSI (intracytoplasmic sperm injection)
IDET (intradiscal electrothermal) procedure
ileal pouch-anal anastomosis (IPAA)
ileoanal pouch anastomosis (IPAA)
ileovesicostomy
Ilizarov limb lengthening
iliopopliteal bypass
image-guided surgery
immunoscintigraphy
impedance plethysmography (IPG)
incentive spirometry
indium 111 scintigraphy scan
indocyanine green (IC-Green) fluorescein angiography
inferior sagittal mandibular osteotomy
infibulation
injection technique
Integris 3-D RA (rotational angiography)
Intensive Narcotic Detoxification
intentional transoperative hemodilution

operation *(cont.)*
interferometry
intermittent exotropia
interpleural analgesia
in-the-bag IOL lens implantation
intra-aortic endovascular sonography
intracardiac amobarbital sodium procedure
intracaval endovascular ultrasonography
intracoronary artery radiation
intracoronary ultrasonography
intracytoplasmic sperm injection (ICSI)
intradiscal electrothermal (IDET) anuloplasty
intrahepatic cholangioenterostomy
IntraLASIK procedure
intraluminal brachytherapy
intramedullary skeletal kinetic distractor (ISKD)
intraoperative cholangiography (IOC)
intraoperative hippocampal cooling
intraoperative lymphatic mapping
intraoperative radiolymphoscintigraphy
intraoperative transmyocardial revascularization (ITMR)
intraoperative ultrasonography (IOUS)
intraperitoneal onlay mesh hernia repair (IPOM)
intraportal endovascular ultrasonography (IPEUS)
intravascular MRI technique
intravascular ultrasound (IVUS)
intravenous fluorescein angiography (IVFA)
intravenous pyelogram (IVP)
InVance male sling
invasive procedure
inversion-ligation appendectomy
inverted L capsulotomy

operation *(cont.)*
inverted U-pouch ileal reservoir
in vitro fertilization (IVF)
in vivo optical spectroscopy (INVOS)
iontophoresis
IR-guided pigtail catheter placement
iridectomy
iridencleisis
isolated heat perfusion of an extremity
isotopic cisternography
Isshiki thyroplasty type I
IVOX artificial lung
Jatene arterial switch (correction of transposed great arteries in neonate)
Jenckel cholecystoduodenostomy
J (jowl) lift technique
Jones first-toe repair
Joplin bunionectomy
Judd ventral hernia repair
Judkins coronary arteriography
LADARVision Custom Cornea laser treatment
Kalamchi osteotomy
Kapandji-Sauve technique for distal radial-ulnar joint repair
karate chop phaco technique
Karydakis
Kasai peritoneal venous shunt
Kech and Kelly osteotomy
keel excision
Kelikian modified Z osteotomy
Keller arthroplasty
Keller bunionectomy
Kestenbaum repair of nystagmic torticollis
keyhole resection
Kiricuta reconstructive breast
Kirsch laser welding technique
Klagsbrun harvest of chondrocytes

operation *(cont.)*
Kocher-Langenbeck ilioinguinal approach to fracture repair
Koch lens insertion
Kock modified pouch
Koenig arthroplasty
Konno patch enlargement of aorta
Kraske approach
Kreuscher bunionectomy
Kropp bladder neck reconstruction
Krupin valve with disc
krypton (red) laser photocoagulation
Kun colocolpopoiesis
kyphosis correction surgery
LABA (laser-assisted balloon angioplasty)
lacrimal scintigraphy
lacunar limbectomy
Ladd correction of malrotation of bowel
Lange tendon lengthening
laparoscopic-assisted bowel resection
laparoscopic-assisted colorectal resection
laparoscopy-assisted ileocystoplasty and ileovesicostomy
laparoscopic-assisted vaginal hysterectomy (LAVH)
laparoscopic bladder neck suture suspension
laparoscopic cholecystectomy
laparoscopic donor nephrectomy (LDN)
laparoscopic fundoplication
laparoscopic Heller myotomy
laparoscopic intracorporeal ultrasound
laparoscopic laser-assisted auto-augmentation of bladder
laparoscopic laser cholecystectomy
laparoscopic Nissen and Toupet fundoplication
laparoscopic pneumodissection

operation *(cont.)*

laparoscopic radical prostatectomy
laparoscopic sigmoid colectomy
laparoscopic total extraperitoneal (TED) hernioplasty
laparoscopic transcystic duct exploration
laparoscopic transcystic papillotomy
laparoscopic ultrasound (LUS)
laparoscopic urinary diversion
laparoscopic uterine nerve ablation (LUNA)
laparoscopic videolaseroscopy
laparoscopy-assisted abdomino-perineal pull-through
laparoscopy under local anesthesia (LULA)
Lap-Band adjustable gastric banding (LAGB)
lap Nissen (laparoscopic Nissen fundoplication)
LAR/CAA (low anterior resection in combination with coloanal anastomosis)
large loop excision of the transformation zone (LLETZ)
large particle biopsy
large-skull implant surgery
LARS (laparoscopic antireflux surgery)
laryngeal framework surgery (LFS)
laryngoplastic phonosurgery
laryngotracheal reconstruction
laser angioplasty
laser-assisted balloon angioplasty (LABA)
laser-assisted microanastomosis
laser-assisted tissue welding
laser-assisted uvulopalatoplasty (LAUP)
laser biomicroscopy of vitreoretinal structures
Laser Bra

operation *(cont.)*

laser correlational spectroscopy (LCS)
laser image custom arthroplasty (LICA)
laser in situ keratomileusis (LASIK)
laser myringotomy
laser nucleotomy
laser uterosacral nerve ablation (LUNA)
laser photoablation
laser sclerostomy
laser stapedotomy
laser thermal keratoplasty (LTK)
laser trabeculodissection (LTD)
lasertripsy
Lasertrolysis
laser welding
Lash hysterectomy
lateral acetabular shelf osteotomy
lateral crural steal (LCS) for nasal tip reconstruction
latissimus dorsi demand dynamic wrapping
Latzko vesicovaginal fistula
Lazaro da Silva technique
Lazarus-Nelson peritoneal lavage
Leadbetter-Politano ureterovesico-plasty
LeDuc-Camey ileocystoplasty
LeDuc ureteral anastomosis
LEEP (loop electrosurgical excision procedure)
LeFort I apertognathia repair
LeFort II and III fracture repairs
LeFort uterine prolapse repair
left cardiac sympathetic denervation (LCSD)
Lejour-type breast reduction, modified
Lester Martin modification of Duhamel
levatorplasty
Lewis-Tanner esophagectomy

operation *(cont.)*
LICA (laser image custom arthroplasty)
Lich-Gregoire repair
Lichtenstein hernia repair
Lichtenstein open tension-free mesh hernioplasty
Lich ureteral implantation for neobladder construction
L.I.F.T. (laser-assisted internal fabrication) technique
ligamentum teres cardiopexy fundoplication
light reflection rheography
Limberg flap closure
limb-sparing technique
Lindseth kyphectomy with posterior crisscross wires
Lindseth osteotomy
lingualplasty
lip lift
liquid crystal thermography
Linton procedure
liposuction-assisted nerve-sparing radical abdominal hysterectomy (LANS-RH)
LLETZ (large loop excision of the transformation zone)
Longo hemorrhoidectomy
loop electrosurgical excision procedure (LEEP)
loopogram (ileostogram)
loopostomy
Lortat-Jacob hepatic resection
Lovaas autism treatment program
low-dose screen-film technique
LUNA (laser uterosacral nerve ablation)
LVRS (lung volume reduction surgery)
lymphapheresis
lymphoscintigraphy
MAA lung scan
Madden incisional hernia repair
Madigan prostatectomy

operation *(cont.)*
Magerl screw placement
Magnuson-Stack shoulder arthrotomy
magnetic resonance angiography (MRA)
magnetic resonance cholangiography (MRC)
magnetic resonance elastography (MRE)
magnetic resonance mammography
magnetic resonance neurography (MRN)
magnetic resonance spectroscopy (MRS)
magnetic resonance urography
magnetic stimulation of fracture
magnetoencephalogram (MEG)
MAGPI (meatal advancement, glanduloplasty, penoscrotal junction meatotomy)
Ma-Griffith anastomosis
Malbran transscleral fixation of intraocular lens
Malone antegrade continence enema (MACE)
Malone principle of continent urinary diversion
Malone stoma (enterostomy)
mammary ptosis
mammoplasty
Mammotest breast biopsy
mandibular advancement osteotomy (MAO)
manner of Lattimer
Maquet elevation of tibial crest
Marshall-Marchetti-Krantz vesicourethral suspension
Marx osteoradionecrosis (ORN)
Masimo SET (signal extraction technology)
Masket lens insertion
masking technology
Mason abdominotranssphincteric resection

operation *(cont.)*
Mason vertical-banded gastroplasty
matricectomy
Matsner median episiotomy
Mau osteotomy, modified
maxillomandibular osteotomy
maze cut-and-sew
Mayday distal first metatarsal osteotomy for hallux valgus
Mayo culdoplasty, modified
maze procedure (ablation of refractory atrial fibrillation)
McCall posterior culdoplasty
McCraw gracilis myocutaneous flap for vaginal construction
McDonald cervical cerclage
McIndoe vaginal construction
McKee-Farrar total hip arthroplasty
McRoberts maneuver
McVay hernia repair
meatal advancement, glanduloplasty, penoscrotal junction meatotomy (MAGPI)
median sternotomy
mediastinotomy
medical holography
medulloscopy
mega-OATS (osteochondral autologous transfer system)
meloplasty
membrane stripping
Merindino GI
MESA (microepididymal sperm aspiration)
mesh plug hernioplasty
Meuli arthroplasty
MIAS (minimal incision aortic surgery)
Microdot technique
microendoscopic diskectomy (MED)
microlumbar diskectomy
microsurgical denervation of the spermatic cord

operation *(cont.)*
microsurgical epididymovasostomy (MSEV)
microsurgical tubal reanastomosis (MTR)
microvascular arterial bypass surgery for impotence
microvascular free tissue transfer for glossectomy
microwave nonsurgical treatment for benign prostatic hypertrophy
MIDCAB (minimally invasive direct coronary artery bypass)
midface sling
Millard rotation flap advancement
Millard R-A cleft lip repair
Millen retropubic prostatectomy
Millikan modified mesh-plug hernioplasty
Milligan-Morgan hemorrhoidectomy
Mimix bone replacement cranioplasty
mini-FES (functional endoscopic sinus) surgery
minilaparotomy pelvic lymph node dissection
minilaparotomy staging pelvic lymphadenectomy
minimal incision aortic surgery (MIAS)
minimally invasive video-assisted thyroidectomy (MIVAT)
Mitchell distal osteotomy
Mitchell epispadias repair technique
Mitek anchor system
Mitrofanoff appendicovesicostomy
Mitrofanoff catheterizable stoma
Mitrofanoff neourethra procedure
MIVR (minimally invasive valve repair or replacement)
M-mode echocardiogram
modified endoventricular circular-plasty

operation *(cont.)*
modified Hughes eyelid procedure
modified Isshiki type 4 thyroplasty
modified Linton procedure
modified Pereyra bladder neck suspension
Moe scoliosis
Mohs chemosurgery
Molina band
Monarc subfascial sling
Monarc transobturator tape sling
monochromatization filtering technique
Monti bladder augmentation
Monti-Malone continent urinary diversion
Moran repair
mosaicplasty
Moschowitz obliteration of cul-de-sac
Mosley anterior shoulder repair
moxibustion
moving-bed infusion-tracking MRA
MRCP (magnetic resonance cholangiopancreatography)
MRCP using HASTE with a phased-array coil
MR hydrography
MRP (magnetic resonance pancreatography)
MR peritoneography
MT (magnetization transfer) saturation
MUGA (multiple gated acquisition) scan
multi-vessel small thoracotomy (MVST)
Mumford-Gurd arthroplasty
Mustardé flap otoplasty
Mustard transposition of great vessels
myodesis
myofascial release

operation *(cont.)*
Nagahara phaco chopper and phaco chop technique
Nambudripad Allergy Elimination Technique (NAET)
nasal septal crossover flap
native tissue harmonic imaging
NDT (neuro-developmental techniques)
Nd:YAG CTLC (contact trans-scleral laser cytophotocoagulation)
near-infrared spectroscopy (NIRS)
Neer hemiarthroplasty
neoumbilicoplasty
nephroureterectomy with en bloc removal of cuff of bladder
neuroendovascular interventional procedures
New England Baptist arthroplasty
Nichols vaginal suspension
ninety-ninety intraosseous wiring
nipple-areola reconstruction (NAR)
Nissen laparoscopic fundoplication
Nissen total fundoplication
non-breath-hold MR cholangiography
Norland bone densitometry
Norwood (Fontan modification)
Norwood (Gill/Jonas modification)
Norwood (Sade modification)
no-touch technique
NovaSure endometrial ablation
nucleoplasty
Nyhus preperitoneal mesh hernioplasty
nuclectomy
Nuss repair
Ober-Barr brachioradialis transfer
Obwegeser sagittal mandibular osteotomy
oculoplethysmography-carotid phonoangiography (OPG/CPA)

operation *(cont.)*
off-center ablation
off-pump coronary artery bypass (OPCAB)
off-pump coronary revascularization with endoscopic saphenous vein harvesting (OPCRES)
OPART
open mesh-plug hernioplasty
open reduction and internal fixation (ORIF)
open-sky vitrectomy
open tension-free mesh hernioplasty
OPERA (outpatient endometrial resection/ablation) procedures
optical coherence biometry (OCB)
optical coherence tomography (OCT)
Oriental flap technique
Orr-Loygue transabdominal proctopexy
Orr rectal prolapse repair
orthotopic transplantation
osteo-odontokeratoprosthesis (OOKP)
osteoradionecrosis (ORN)
osteotomy
out-in-out technique
oxygen cisternography
PACAB (port-access CABG)
pallidal brain stimulation procedure
pallidotomy guided by microelectrode recording
Palomar EsteLux
Palva flap technique
pancreas-sparing duodenectomy (PSD)
pancreaticoduodenectomy
PANDO (primary acquired nasolacrimal duct obstruction).
pants-over-vest repair
Pap Plus speculoscopy

operation *(cont.)*
PARK (photoastigmatic refractive keratectomy)
Parker-Kerr closed end-to-end enteroenterostomy
partial encircling endocardial ventriculotomy
partial liquid ventilation
Partipilo gastrostomy
passive girdle effect (adynamic-girdling) in aortomyoplasty
patchplasty
PC-IOL (posterior chamber intraocular lens) implantation
Pearce trabeculectomy
PEARL (physiologic endometrial ablation/resection loop)
pectus excavatum repair
pedicle subtraction osteotomy
pelvic floor electrical stimulation (PFS)
Pemberton acetabuloplasty
Pemberton circumacetabular osteotomy
PEMF (pulsed electromagnetic field)
penile vein ligation
per anum intersphincteric rectal dissection with direct coloanal anastomosis
percutaneous aortic balloon valvuloplasty
percutaneous automated diskectomy
percutaneous balloon mitral valvuloplasty
percutaneous bladder neck stabilization (PBNS)
percutaneous cholecystolithotomy (PCCL)
percutaneous choledochoscopy
percutaneous coronary rotational atherectomy (PCRA)
percutaneous dilational tracheostomy (PDT)

operation *(cont.)*

percutaneous endopyeloplasty
percutaneous endoscopic gastrostomy (PEG)
percutaneous endoscopic jejunostomy (PEJ)
percutaneous endoscopic sigmoidostomy
percutaneous epididymal sperm aspiration
percutaneous epiphysiodesis using transphyseal screws (PETS)
percutaneous gastroenterostomy (PEG)
percutaneous gastrostomy (PG)
percutaneous intracoronary angioscopy
percutaneous left atrial appendage transcatheter occlusion (PLAATO)
percutaneous mitral balloon valvotomy (PMBV)
percutaneous nephrostolithotomy (PCNL)
percutaneous nephrolithotripsy (PNL)
percutaneous pinning of fractures
percutaneous radiofrequency catheter ablation
percutaneous radiofrequency facet rhizotomy
percutaneous resection of transitional cell carcinoma
percutaneous transatrial mitral commissurotomy
percutaneous transhepatic cholangiography (PTHC)
percutaneous transhepatic cholecystolithotomy (PCTCL)
percutaneous transhepatic liver biopsy with tract embolization (PBTE)
percutaneous transluminal angioplasty (PTA)

operation *(cont.)*

percutaneous transluminal myocardial (or transmyocardial) revascularization (PTMR)
percutaneous transluminal renal angioplasty (PTRA)
percutaneous transluminal septal myocardial ablation
percutaneous transperineal seed implantation
percutaneous transvenous mitral commissurotomy (PTMC)
PerFix hernioplasty
perfusion-weighted MRI imaging
periacetabular osteotomy (PAO)
perineal surgical apron technique
PerioChip
periosteal stripping
peripheral excimer laser angioplasty (PELA)
peripheral laser angioplasty (PLA)
peripheral scatter photocoagulation
peritomy
peritoneography MR
periurethral collagen injection
petaling the cast procedure
PET (positron emission tomography) scan
PET with 3-D SSP (positron emission tomography with 3-D stereotaxic surface projection)
pharyngeal flap-pushback procedure
pharaonic circumcision
Phemister-type epiphysiodesis
phonocardiography
photoangioplasty
photoastigmatic refractive keratectomy (PARK)
photocoagulation
photo epilation
photon correlation spectroscopy
photorefractive keratectomy (PRK)
phototherapeutic keratectomy (PTK)

operation *(cont.)*
photothermal sclerosis
pillar palatal restoration procedure
PIPIDA scan
PITA (powered intracapsular tonsillectomy and adenoidectomy)
plasmapheresis
platform posturography
pleural tent construction
plicectomy
plugged liver biopsy
P-MRS (phosphorus nuclear magnetic resonance spectroscopy)
pneumatic retinopexy
Politano-Leadbetter technique
polydioxanone plating procedure
Ponka herniorrhaphy
Pool cleft lip repair
Port-Access coronary artery bypass (PACAB)
Port-Access minimally invasive cardiac surgery
portoportal anastomosis
posterior capsulorrhexis with optic capture
posterior chamber intraocular lens (PC-IOL) implantation
posterior lumbar interbody fusion (PLIF)
posterior sagittal and 3-flap anoplasty
posteromedial release of clubfoot (PMR)
power Doppler sonography
Prentiss orchiopexy
pressure support ventilation
Pringle maneuver
ProDisc disk replacement surgery
Profore four-layer bandaging
profundaplasty
proliferative retinopathy photocoagulation
promontofixation
propeller flap method
ProstRcision

operation *(cont.)*
proton magnetic resonance spectroscopy
proximal row carpectomy (PRC)
psoralen inactivation technique
PTFE (polytetrafluoroethylene)
pubovaginal sling procedure
Puestow pancreaticojejunostomy
pulsatile irrigation
pulsed-dye laser (PDL) surgery
pulse oximetry
Pulvertaft anastomosis
push enteroscope/enteroscopy
push-pull wire technique
Putti-Platt arthroplasty
pylorus-preserving pancreaticoduodenectomy (PPPD)
pylorus-preserving Whipple (PPW) modification
PYP (pyrophosphate) scan
quantitative computed tomography (QCT)
quantitative coronary arteriography (QCA)
RACAB (robot-assisted coronary artery bypass)
R-A concept (in unilateral cleft lip repair)
radial keratotomy
radial thermokeratoplasty
radical prostatectomy (RP)
radiocolloid mapping
radiofrequency (RF) ablation
radiofrequency catheter ablation (RFA)
radiofrequency percutaneous myocardial revascularization (RF-PMR)
radioimmunoluminography (RILG)
radioimmunoscintimetry
radiolymphoscintigraphy
radionuclide cholescintigraphy
radionuclide scan
Raman spectroscopy
Randall-Tennison triangular flap

operation *(cont.)*
- Randall unilateral cleft lip repair
- Rashkind balloon atrial septotomy
- Rastelli cardiac
- Raz sling for urinary incontinence
- real-time ultrasonography
- rectal endoscopic ultrasonography (REU)
- rectilinear biphasic waveform for external defibrillation
- rectus abdominis myocutaneous (RAM) flap
- REDS (remote endoscopic digital spectroscopy)
- reduced liver transplant (RLT)
- reduction columelloplasty
- reflectance-guided laser selection
- remote endoscopic digital spectroscopy (REDS)
- rescue PTCA
- restorative proctocolectomy
- restorative proctocolectomy and ileal pouch anal anastomosis (RP/IPAA)
- retrocolic submesocolic gastro-enteroanastomosis
- retrograde cerebral perfusion (RCP)
- retrograde intrarenal surgery (RIRS)
- retroperitoneoscopy
- retropubic prostatectomy
- Reverdin-Green osteotomy
- Revo rotator cuff repair
- RHCT (renal helical CT) imaging
- rheography, light reflection
- rhinolaryngostroboscopy (RLS)
- rhizotomy, functional posterior
- RICE (rest, ice, compression, elevation) treatment
- Rink modification of Casale continent catheterizable vesicostomy
- Ripstein rectal prolapse repair
- robot-assisted coronary artery bypass (RACAB)

operation *(cont.)*
- robotic-assisted laparoscopic sacrocolpopexy
- Rocabado technique for manipulative (physical) therapy
- rollerball endometrial ablation
- Rosomoff cordotomy
- Ross aortic valve replacement procedure
- rotational atherectomy (RA)
- rotational scarf osteotomy
- rotationplasty
- Roux-en-Y divided gastric bypass
- ruptured abdominal aortic aneurysm (RAAA)
- Rutkow sutureless plug and patch
- sacrocolpopexy
- sacrospinous colpopexy
- sagittal approach
- saline-enhanced MR arthrography of shoulder
- saloon door approach in MIDCAB procedures
- same-day microsurgical arthroscopic lateral-approach laser-assisted (SMALL) fluoroscopic diskectomy
- Sand process
- sandwich treatment
- SASMA (skin-adipose superficial musculoaponeurotic) facelift
- Sauve-Kapandji distal radioulnar joint reconstruction
- Scanning-Beam Digital X-ray (SBDX)
- Schanz-type proximal femoral valgization osteotomy
- scaphotrapeziotrapezoid (STT) arthrodesis
- scarf osteotomy bunionectomy
- Schaubel modification of Smith-Petersen approach
- Schepens-Okamura-Brockhurst retinal detachment repair
- Schiotz tonometry

operation *(cont.)*
Schlein elbow arthroplasty
Schuknecht cochleosacculotomy
Schwartz–Pregenzer urethropexy
scintirenography
scleral buckling
sclerouvectomy, partial lamellar
Scopinaro
second-look laparotomy
sector scan echocardiography
seminal vesiculography (SVG)
Semont maneuver
serial scans
sestamibi Tc-99m SPECT with dipyridamole stress test
Sever-L'Episcopo shoulder repair
sewing machine technique
SharpShooter tissue repair
Sharrard kyphectomy
Shepherd lens insertion
Shirodkar cervical cerclage
shoelace technique for delayed fasciotomy closure
Shouldice hernia repair
SI (sensory integration)
Simonsen technique
simultaneous areolar mastopexy and breast augmentation (SAMBA)
Singapore fasciocutaneous flap
Silastic bead embolization
single photon planar scintigraphy (SPPS)
Sinu-Clear laser sinus surgery
skin-level transverse colostomy and loop ileostomy
skin-sparing mastectomy
Skoog release of Dupuytren contracture
sleeve pneumonectomy
slide-by technique
small-bowel enteroscopy (SBE)
SMALL (same-day microsurgical arthroscopic lateral approach laser-assisted) fluoroscopic diskectomy

operation *(cont.)*
smasectomy rhytidectomy technique
Smead-Jones closure
snare resection (band and snare)
Soave abdominal pull-through procedure
soft tissue shaving cannula liposhaver
Sones coronary arteriography
sonographically guided human thrombin injection
sonohysterography
sonopuncture
Southwick osteotomy
sparrow-picking technique
SPECT (single photon emission computed tomography) scan
spectral Doppler
speculoscopy
sperm aspiration technique
spinal myeloscopy
spinopelvic transiliac fixation (STIF) technique
spiral x-ray computed tomography (SXCT)
split anterior tibial tendon transfer (SPLATT)
split-liver transplantation
stacked scans
STAE (subsegmental transcatheter arterial embolization)
staged abdominal repairs (STARs)
STA-MCA (superficial temporal artery–middle cerebral artery) bypass
Stamey bladder suspension
Stamm gastrostomy
Stanmore shoulder arthroplasty
stapled hemorrhoidopexy
stapled lung reduction
stapled transanal rectal resection (STARR)
Steel osteotomy
Stenstrom otoplasty technique
step-oblique mammography

operation *(cont.)*
- stereotactic pallidotomy
- stereotactic radiosurgery (SRS)
- stereotactic tractotomy
- stereotaxic core needle biopsy (SCNB)
- stereotaxy
- STIF (spinopelvic transiliac fixation)
- stimulated graciloplasty
- STING (subureteric Teflon injection)
- Stoppa laparoscopic hernia repair
- stress cystogram
- stress-injected sestamibi-gated SPECT with echocardiography
- stress perfusion and rest function by sestamibi-gated SPECT
- stress perfusion scintigraphy
- Stretta gastroesophageal reflux procedure
- strip-biopsy
- Strother acrochordonectomy
- subclavian flap aortoplasty (SFA)
- subfascial endoscopic perforator surgery (SEPS)
- submandibular gland transfer
- submucosal saline injection technique
- subperiosteal corticotomy
- subplatysmal face-lift technique
- subpleural blanketing technique
- subsegmentectomy
- suburethral sling
- suction-assisted lipectomy (SAL)
- suction-assisted lipoplasty (SAL)
- suction-bubble technique
- Sugiura paraesophagogastric devascularization
- Sunna circumcision
- Sunrise LTK
- super-wet technique
- supraglottoplasty
- surface electromyography (sEMG)
- Swanson PIP joint arthroplasty

operation *(cont.)*
- Swenson abdominal pull-through
- Syme amputation of foot
- Syme external urethrotomy
- Synthetic Aperture Focusing Technique (SAFT)
- synthetic penetrating keratoplasty (S-PK)
- TACE (transcatheter arterial chemoembolization)
- Targis microwave catheter-based system
- TcHIDA scan
- TCP (total cavopulmonary connection)
- tease procedure
- teboroxime scan
- TECAB (totally endoscopic coronary artery bypass)
- TechneScan MAG3
- technetium scan
- tendon Z-lengthening around the knee and ankle
- Tennison-Randall cleft lip repair
- TEP (totally extraperitoneal) hernia repair
- terminal sedation (TS)
- Tesla imaging system
- T-graft configuration technique
- Thal esophageal stricture repair
- thallium stress test
- thermal quenching
- thermistor-plethysmography
- Thiersch-Duplay urethroplasty
- thin-layer chromatography
- Thom flap laryngeal reconstruction
- thoracoabdominal aortic aneurysm (TAAA) surgery
- thoracophrenolaparotomy
- thorascopic apical pleurectomy
- thorascopic talc pleurodesis
- thread-lift (same as feather-lift)
- 3-D CE (three-dimensional contrast-enhanced) MR angiography technique

operation *(cont.)*
3-D FT magnetic resonance angiography
3-D SLS (three-dimensional superficial liposculpture)
three-trocar technique of laparoscopic cholecystectomy
thromboelastograph (TEG)
ThromboScan MRU
thyroplasty type I
thyroxine radioisotope assay (T_4RIA)
Tikhoff-Linberg shoulder resection
time-resolved imaging by automatic data segmentation (TRIADS)
TIPSS (transjugular intrahepatic portosystemic shunt)
tissue engineering
tissue harmonic imaging
TKA (total knee arthroplasty)
TMR (transmyocardial revascularization)
tomodensitometric examination, abdominal
tonsillar Coblation
topodermatography
Torkildsen shunt ventriculocisternostomy
total cavopulmonary connection
total hip replacement (THR)
total lymphoid irradiation (TLI)
total mesorectal excision (TME)
Toupet hemifundoplication
Toupet partial posterior fundoplication
T-pouch technique
T-PRK (tracker-assisted photorefractive keratectomy)
trachelotomy
tracheoesophageal puncture (TEP)
tracheoplasty
tracheotomy
transabdominal preperitoneal (TAPP) hernia repair
transanal endoscopic microsurgery (TEM)

operation *(cont.)*
transarticular screw reconstruction
transbronchial biopsy (TBB)
transcarotid balloon valvuloplasty
transcatheter arterial embolization (TAE)
transcervical balloon tuboplasty (TBT)
transcoccygeal approach
transconjunctival removal of cavernous hemangioma
transcostovertebral approach
transcoronary ablation of septal hypertrophy (TASH)
transcranial color-coded sonography
transcutaneous neuromuscular electrical stimulation (TNMES)
transesophageal echocardiogram (TEE)
transfemoral liver biopsy
transferred immune response
transhepatic embolization (THE)
transient evoked otoacoustic emission (TEOAE)
transjugular intrahepatic portosystemic shunt (TIPSS)
transjugular liver biopsy
translabyrinthine removal of large acoustic neuromas
transluminal endovascular graft placement
transluminal ultrasonic angioplasty (TUA)
transmyocardial revascularization (TMR)
transnasal endoluminal ultrasonography
transpapillary endoscopic cholecystotomy
transperineal-transsphincteric approach
transplanted stamp graft
transrectal ultrasound (TRUS)
transsacral
transscrotal extratunica vaginalis

operation *(cont.)*

transthoracic echocardiogram
transthoracic needle aspiration biopsy
transtrochanteric valgus osteotomy (TVO)
transumbilical breast augmentation (TUBA)
transurethral balloon laserthermia prostatectomy
transurethral electrovaporization of the prostate (TUVP)
transurethral incision of the prostate (TUIP)
transurethral needle ablation (TUNA)
transurethral ultrasound-guided laser-induced prostatectomy (TULIP)
transvaginal sacrospinous colpopexy
transvaginal ultrasound-guided urethral reconstruction
transvenous liver biopsy
transverse retubularized sigmoidovesicostomy continent urinary diversion to the umbilicus
trapeziometacarpal silicone arthroplasty
Traverso-Longmire technique
triangular vaginal patch sling
TriVex transilluminated powered phlebectomy
TSPP (technetium stannous pyrophosphate) rectilinear bone scan
tumescent liposuction technique
Turco posteromedial release of clubfoot
Turner-Warwick urethroplasty
turn-up plasty
TVT (tension-free vaginal tape) continent procedure
2-D echocardiography
2-D IVUS (two-dimensional intravascular ultrasound)
two-incision hip replacement

operation *(cont.)*

two-layer latex and Marlex closure technique
270° Toupet fundoplication
two-stage capsulorrhexis
ultrafast CT electron beam tomography
ultrasonic aspiration
ultrasonic-assisted lipoplasty (or liposuction) (UAL)
ultrasound biomicroscopy (UBM)
ultrasonic body contouring
ultrasound-guided anterior subcostal liver biopsy
ultrasound-guided pseudoaneurysm compression
ultrasound-guided transcervical tuboplasty
umbilical artery velocimetry
under-the-skin technique
unenhanced scan
UPLIFT (uterine positioning via ligament investment fixation and truncation) procedure
ureterorenoscopy
ureteroscopy
urethrovesical suspension
urinary diversion procedure
urinary tract reconstruction augmentation cystoplasty
urocytogram
urothelial augmentation
uterine artery embolization (UAE)
uterine fibroid embolization (UFE)
uvulopalatopharyngoglossoplasty
uvulopalatopharyngoplasty (UPPP)
vaginal flap reconstruction of urethra and vesical neck
vaginal interruption of pregnancy, with dilatation and curettage (VIP-DAC)
vaginal packing
vaginal-psoas colposuspension
vaginal wall sling surgery
vagus nerve stimulation (VNS)

operation *(cont.)*
valvuloplasty
varicose vein ablation
varus derotational osteotomy (VDRO)
vascular targeting agent technology
VCAB (ventriculocoronary artery bypass)
vectorcardiography
velolaryngeal endoscopy
vertebroplasty
vertical-banded gastroplasty (VBG)
ventricular endoaneurysmorrhaphy
vertical tripod fixation (VTF)
vesicoureterogram (VCUG)
vesicourethral suspension
vestibular neurectomy
vibroacoustic stimulation
video-assisted thoracic surgery
video densitometry (VD)
videoendoscopic swallowing study (VESS)
videolaparoscopy
videolaseroscopy
Vineberg cardiac revascularization
viscosupplementation
vitrectomy
voiding cystourethrogram (VCUG)
Vollmar endarterectomy
Voxgram
V-Q (ventilation-perfusion) scan
V-to-Y advancement of the helical root
Waldhausen subclavian flap repair
Wardill palatoplasty
Warthin-Starry technique
watchband incision
Watson-Jones tenodesis
wavefront LASIK
Weir nasal alar excision
Well operation for rectal prolapse
Wheeless construction of J rectal pouch
whiplash technique
Whipple pancreaticoduodenectomy

operation *(cont.)*
Williams vulvovaginoplasty
Wirsung dilatation
Wise areola mastopexy breast augmentation (WAMBA)
Wise reduction mammoplasty
Witzel duodenostomy
Womack splenectomy
Woods screw maneuver
Woods technique of follicular relocation
wringer wrap
Wu bunionectomy
xenotransplantation
Yang-Monti
York-Mason approach
Young-Dees-Leadbetter bladder-neck reconstruction
Y stenting angioplasty
Zaidemberg technique
Zancolli clawhand deformity repair
Zavanelli maneuver
zigzag wire technique
zipper sphincterotomy
zonulolysis
Z-plasty, four-flap
zygote intrafallopian transfer (ZIFT)

operon—a chromosomal segment including one or more structural genes and associated material to regulate their function.

OPG/CPA—see *oculoplethysmography/carotid phonoangiography.*

ophthalmic *Pneumocystis*—see *AIDS-associated ophthalmic Pneumocystis.*

ophthalmodynamometry—measures the relative central retinal artery pressures and indirectly assesses carotid artery flow on each side. See *Bailliart ophthalmodynamometer.*

ophthalmoscopy—allows examination of the interior of the eye after dilation.

Opmilas CO_2 multipurpose laser.

Opmilas 144 Plus laser system—used for soft tissue applications in arthroscopic and general surgery. Uses Nd:YAG laser for gynecologic, urologic, and general surgery.

OP-1—see *Osteogenic Protein 1.*

opportunistic infection or **organism**—a microorganism that does not ordinarily cause disease but becomes pathogenic under certain circumstances (e.g., impaired immune response, or predisposing factors such as neoplasm or trauma). AIDS patients or patients who are immunocompromised are giving a new meaning to this term and to our understanding of the immune system. Opportunistic infections are responsible for approximately 90% of AIDS-related deaths.

opposed loop-pair quadrature magnetic resonance coil—MRI term.

opposition—the act of being opposite, or the state of being set in opposite manner. Usage: "The thumb and index finger could be placed in opposition." Cf. *apposition.*

OpSite—watertight polyurethane dressing that adheres to the skin around the wound, but not the wound itself.

OpSite Flexigrid—transparent adhesive film dressing.

opsonizing antibodies—antibodies that make bacteria susceptible to phagocytes.

Optibond Solo (Dentistry)—a bonding agent.

Optical Biopsy System—laser device operated through either a sigmoidoscope or a colonoscope to evaluate the benign/malignant status of a colon polyp.

optical coherence biometry (OCB).

optical coherence reflectometry (OCR).

optical coherence tomography (OCT)—a noninvasive, noncontact imaging technology capable of producing cross-sectional images of the retina in vivo with high resolution to obtain multiple cross-sectional images of the fovea, peripapillary retina, and macula.

optical pachometer—used in determining the depth of corneal pathology in an eye.

Optical Tracking System—LED wand used by neurosurgeons for image-guided intraoperative navigation (i.e., during surgical procedure).

optical trapping—see *LaserTweezers.*

optic neuritis—inflammation of that portion of the optic nerve that is not ophthalmoscopically visible.

Opti-Gard patient eye protector.

OptiHaler—a drug delivery system for use with metered dose inhalers.

optimal cutting temperature (OCT)—a synthetic water-soluble glycol and resin mounting medium; used to embed and mount tissue for cutting frozen sections.

Optimaze malleable laser tip surgical ablation system.

Optimed glaucoma pressure regulator—a tiny implant.

Option Care—a national network of home infusion and healthcare providers.

Opti-Plast XT balloon catheter—used for delivery of the SAXX renal stent.

Optipore wound-cleaning sponge.

Optisol-GS—a storage solution for human donor corneas. Usage: "The donor corneoscleral button with a 3 mm rim was preserved in Optisol."

Optistat—a power contrast injector by Mallinckrodt that introduces contrast media into the body in a controlled manner.

OptiVision—infrared laser system for treatment of presbyopia.

optokinetic nystagmus (OKN).

Opus cardiac troponin I assay—a test used to diagnose acute myocardial infarction within 22 minutes after receipt of a blood sample by the lab. A heart attack disrupts blood flow as well as delivery of oxygen to heart muscle. The result is destruction of cells and the release of cardiac troponin I into healthy tissue and the bloodstream. Measurement of cardiac troponin I and other cardiac markers permits the quick finding of heart attack. Cardiac troponin I is present in the blood from 4 to 6 hours after acute onset of myocardial infarction following heart muscle damage and remains elevated as long as 7 days.

OR, O.R. (operating room).

Oracle Focus—a line of combined ultrasound imaging and PTCA catheters.

Oracle Megasonics catheters (interventional radiology)—a line of high-pressure PTCA catheters.

Oracle Micro catheter.

Oracle Micro Plus—PTCA and ultrasound imaging catheter.

oral—pertaining to the mouth, as in oral intake, oral surgery. Cf. *aural.*

oral contraceptive—see *medications*.

OralScreen 3-panel oral fluids test—for illicit drugs, including marijuana, cocaine, and opiates. Results are available within 10 minutes.

OraQuick—HIV 1 and 2 rapid HIV test.

orascope—microfiberoptic endoscope that allows a dentist or endodontist to see inside a tooth.

OraTest—used for detection of oral cancer.

Orbasone system—noninvasive therapeutic device used to treat joints, muscles, and ligaments.

Orbis-Sigma cerebrospinal fluid shunt valve—has three pressure/flow stages, and reportedly a much lower failure rate than standard valves.

orbital rim stepoff (Oph)—an indication of fracture (and slight displacement). Usage: "Examination for fracture revealed no orbital rim stepoff."

Orbscan II—corneal diagnostic system that helps determine the best surgical ablation pattern for a patient undergoing a LASIK procedure.

OrCel bilayered cellular matrix—dressing applied to wounds to protect and promote healing. It is made from cow collagen and two types of living human skin cells.

Oreopoulos-Zellerman catheter—used for peritoneal dialysis.

Orfizip cast—a wrist cast that goes from the palm to the elbow. It closes over the forearm by means of a zipper, hence the name.

organic brain syndrome (OBS).

organ of Corti (in the cochlea)—contains hair cells, transmitting stimuli to the cochlear branch of cranial nerve VIII (acoustic, or vestibulocochlear, nerve).

organoaxial gastric volvulus—occurs when the stomach rotates along a longitudinal axis. It is rarely mesenteroaxial or vertical.

Oriental flap technique—creation of a V-Y flap.

oriented times four (oriented x 4)—oriented to person, time, place, and future plans.

oriented times three (oriented x 3)—oriented to person, time, and place.

ORIF (open reduction and internal fixation).

orifices—plural of *orifice* ("opening") and often mispronounced "or'-uh-fuh-sees."

Origin balloon, tacker, trocar—instruments for laparoscopic surgery.

origin of a vessel (Radiol)—the commencement of a vessel as it branches off from a larger vessel.

Orion anterior cervical plate—internal fixation system made of a titanium alloy, a locked screw-to-plate system used to stabilize the cervical spine after trauma, or multilevel diskectomy.

ORLAU (Orthotic Research and Locomotor Assessment Unit) **swivel walker**—orthosis for ambulation in children with cerebral palsy and myelomeningocele.

Ormond disease—idiopathic retroperitoneal fibrosis.

ORN (osteoradionecrosis).

OR1—incorporates all components of the surgical suite into a single electronic system. Developed by Karl Storz Endoscopy-America, Inc., the system includes control of endoscopic devices with options for activation by touch screen and remote control, all using PC-based architecture.

orotracheal intubation, NRSI (nonrapid sequence induction).

orphan drug—a drug used to treat a rare disease for which the manufacturer could not expect to recoup drug development and production costs due to the small number of patients who would use the drug. The Orphan Drug Act supports the development of orphan drugs by allowing tax credits to the pharmaceutical company and shortened FDA approval time.

Orr-Loygue transabdominal proctopexy—for complete rectal prolapse.

Orr rectal prolapse repair.

ortho (Oph)—a brief form for *orthophoric*, as well as *orthopedic*. See *muscle balance was ortho*.

ortho—when an ophthalmologist uses the word *ortho*, it usually refers to *orthophoric* or *orthophoria*.

Ortho Dx—an electromedical stimulator for postsurgical knee rehabilitation.

OrthoDyn—bone substitute material used to fill voids in bone as well as in multiple applications for fracture repair.

Ortho-evac—a postoperative autotransfusion system designed especially for orthopedic use, including knee, hip, and spinal surgery.

Orthofix Cervical-Stim—noninvasive cervical bone growth stimulator.

Orthofix external fixator.

Orthofix intramedullary nail.

Orthofix ISKD (intramedullary skeletal kinetic distractor)—device for leg lengthening.

OrthoGen/OsteoGen—an implantable stimulator for nonunion of fractures.

OrthoGuard AB bone pin sleeve—a sleeve on orthopedic external fixation devices, covered with Medi-Coat antimicrobial coating.

OrthoGuard AB bone pin sleeve—with

Ortho HCV 2.0 ELISA test system—a blood screening test for hepatitis C. Detects antibodies to three HCV antigens.

Ortho-Ice Multipaks—a complete system for cryotherapy (cold) or heat therapy. Special holders allow application at any joint.

Ortholav—equipment for pulsed irrigation and suction. Used with Ritter double- or single-orifice tip or Yankauer multi- or single-orifice tip.

Ortholoc Advantim knee revision system.

OrthoNail—an intramedullary fixation device.

OrthoPak II bone growth stimulator—a bone growth stimulator with electrodes. The battery-powered OrthoPak II weighs only 4 ounces and can be mounted directly on a cast or carried from a belt clip or in a pocket.

orthopedic hardware—wires, pins, screws, plates, and other devices of metal or other material implanted in or attached to bone in the course of a surgical procedure.

orthophoria—parallelism of the visual axes; the normal muscle balance.

Orthoplast jacket—a specially molded jacket used for correction of scoliosis. It is worn for 23 hours a day until skeletal maturity has taken place or until the spine has straightened and correction can be maintained out of the jacket.

orthopnea, three-pillow; **two-pillow**—difficulty breathing unless positioned in a semi-sitting position. Often measured roughly by how many pillows the patient needs in order to breathe comfortably while sleeping upright in a semi-sitting position.

Orthoset cement—radiopaque bone cement.

orthosis—an orthopedic appliance or apparatus applied externally to correct deformities, to support or improve the function of a joint. See also *prosthesis*.
- Bebax shoe
- Caligamed ankle
- CranioCap
- Gillette joint
- GunSlinger shoulder
- LSU (Louisiana State University) reciprocation-gait

orthosis *(cont.)*
- Malleoloc anatomic ankle
- MultiBoot
- Newport MC hip
- Oklahoma ankle joint
- ORLAU swivel walker
- Rebel knee
- Rochester HKAFO
- Select joint
- SportsFit thumb
- Thera-Soft hand/wrist
- TLSO (thoracolumbosacral orthosis)
- Toronto parapodium
- UCBL (University of California Berkeley Laboratory)
- Viscoheel K, Viscoheel N
- Viscoheel SofSpot

OrthoSorb absorbable pin—absorbable fixation device used to fix fractures of the phalanges or metacarpals. The pin is absorbed within six months.

orthotopic transplantation—transplantation of an organ and placing it in the recipient in its normal anatomic position. Examples: heart and liver transplantation.

Orthotrac pneumatic vest—a custom-made, physician-prescribed ambulatory device designed to reduce compressive forces on the spine by transferring upper body weight from the spine to the hips. It looks like an inflatable double belt, and it is worn around the waist for 30-60 minutes at a time, 2-3 times a day.

Ortho TriCyclen Lo (norgestimate/ethinyl estradiol)—oral contraceptive drug.

Ortolani sign—a click at the hip joint, in congenital dislocated hip.

O.S. (*oculus sinister*, left eye).

OSA (obstructive sleep apnea).

OSAS (obstructive sleep apnea syndrome).

Osborne fascia—the fascial bridge of the cubital tunnel between medial epicondyle and olecranon. Usage: "The nerve was followed into the cubital tunnel where Osborne fascia was opened."

OSCAR—an ultrasonic bone cement removal system used in hip revision procedures.

Osciflator balloon inflation syringe—used in angioplasty procedures.

oscillating saw (Ortho).

OSCM (oil-soluble contrast medium).

OS-5/Plus, OS-5/Plus 2 brace—noncustom multifunctional knee brace for postoperative and rehabilitation applications. Made by Omni Scientific (OS).

OSI arthroscopy tools—including the well-leg holder, the arthroscopic leg holder, and the extremity elevator.

Osler nodes—small tender nodules (2 to 5 mm in diameter) seen about the tips of the fingers or toes; may be found in patients with bacterial endocarditis, acute and subacute.

OSMED (otospondylomegaepiphyseal dysplasia).

OsmoCyte pillow—a highly absorptive wound dressing that cushions the wound and absorbs excess moisture/exudate over a longer period of time than a standard dressing.

osmolality—a test of concentration of a solution. It is used to determine the concentration of urine or serum, and results are expressed in milliosmoles per kilogram (mOsm/kg). Cf. *osmolarity.*

osmolarity—concentration of an osmotic solution, e.g., urine or blood serum; expressed in osmoles per liter (Osm/l). Cf. *osmolality.*

OssaTron—a noninvasive extracorporeal shock wave therapy device for treatment of chronic heel pain syndrome.

osseous—bony.

ossification of the posterior longitudinal ligament (OPLL)—one of the well-known causes of cervical radiculomyelopathy.

Ossoff-Karlan laryngoscope.

Ostase biochemical marker of bone turnover—a blood test that aids in management of postmenopausal osteoporosis. See *Access Ostase.*

osteal—bony (osseous). Cf. *ostial.*

osteoarthritis radiographic grading
- grade I, small osteophytes
- grade II, osteophytes without joint space impairment
- grade III, osteophytes with moderate loss of normal joint space
- grade IV, osteophytes with significant loss of joint space and sclerosis of subchondral bone
- grade V, grade IV with subluxation

Osteo Bi-Flex—a dietary supplement for healthy joints.

osteochondral defect (OCD) **of the glenoid fossa**—occurs most often as a result of acute trauma and has a high association with instability, labral tear, and intra-articular bodies.

osteochondral lesion of the talar dome.

osteochondral plug transfer—used for the treatment of focal chondral defects of the knee.

osteochondritis dissecans *(not* dessicans)—see *König disease.*

Osteo-Clage cable system—used in orthopedic cerclage fixation.

OsteoGen HA (hydroxyapatite)—dental implant material.

Osteogenic Protein 1 (OP-1)—Stryker patented recombinant human protein, used to initiate new bone formation in fractures.

Osteogenics BoneSource—a synthetic bone replacement material.

Osteo-Gram—a bone density test for osteoporosis used in conjunction with the OsteoView desktop hand x-ray device.

"osteointegrated" implant—mispronunciation of *osseointegrated implant*.

osteomanipulative therapy (chiropractic).

Osteomark test (NTx assay)—a simple urine test that measures the rate of bone resorption or loss.

"osteomeatal"—incorrect spelling for *ostiomeatal complex*.

osteomesopyknosis—a rare, benign osteosclerotic bone disorder limited to the axial skeleton and diagnosed from radiographs of the area. It is distinguished from superficially similar sclerosing bone conditions such as osteopetrosis, pyknodysostosis, renal osteodystrophy, and atypical axial osteomalacia.

osteoneogenesis—literally, new bone formation; also a technique being used for frontal sinus obliteration in the treatment of frontal sinusitis. Also *auto-obliteration*.

Osteonics ABC hip replacement system—surgically implanted to completely replace a diseased or dysfunctional hip joint.

Osteonics-HA coated implant (Ortho).

Osteonics Omnifit-HA hip stem.

Osteonics Total Shoulder System—for shoulder arthroplasty.

Osteonics Trident PSL acetabular shell.

osteo-odontokeratoprosthesis (OOKP) —a surgical procedure that uses the patient's own tooth root and alveolar bone as support for a corneal prosthesis. See *Falcinelli OOKP*.

Osteopatch—a transdermal patch test used in the diagnosis and management of osteoporosis. It collects sweat and checks for biochemical markers of bone loss.

osteophytes—bony excrescence or osseous outgrowth. See *bridging osteophytes*.

Osteosal—rapid office test to detect increased bone breakdown indicating the risk of osteoporosis and to monitor the adequacy of therapy.

Osteoset—bone graft substitute.

OsteoStim—implantable bone growth stimulator.

OsteoTite bone screw—made of stainless steel and coated with hydroxyapatite, a structural mineral of bone, which facilitates acceptance by the bone and the body. Used for ISKD procedures.

osteotomy (see *operations*).

OsteoView—a self-contained desktop device for taking hand x-rays. It is used in conjunction with OsteoGram bone density test in the diagnosis of osteoporosis.

OsteoView 2000—digital imaging system used to diagnose osteoporosis and arthritis.

ostial—pertaining to an ostium (an opening). Cf. *osteal*.

ostiomeatal—denoting the opening of the auditory, nasal, or urinary meatus. The word does not have anything to do with osteo (bone).

ostiomeatal complex—congenital narrowing of the middle meatus of the nasal cavity, into which the frontal, maxillary, and anterior and middle ethmoidal sinuses drain; a risk factor for recurrent and chronic sinusitis. Because the term refers to the ostia (openings) of the sinuses, and not to bone, the commonly seen spelling *osteomeatal* is incorrect.

ostiomeatal stent (ENT)—a temporary tube placed following functional endoscopic sinus surgery for the purpose of preventing adhesions and maintaining patency of a middle meatal antrostomy. In children, the stent allows postoperative suctioning, usually necessary after about three weeks, without general anesthesia.

ostium—opening into a tubular organ.

os trigonum—a separate ossicle of the lateral tubercle of the posterior aspect of the talus of the ankle. A true os trigonum forms as a secondary ossification center which does not fuse with the talus after skeletal maturation.

os trigonum syndrome (also known as *talar compression syndrome*)—produces significant pain due to inflammation of the ankle joint capsule, a fracture of the os trigonum, or pathology of the Stieda process of the talus.

OTA (oligoteratoasthenozoospermia).

OTC (over-the-counter) **drug**—generally considered safe for consumers to use (as determined by the FDA) if the label directions and warnings are properly followed. Available without a prescription.

otoacoustic emission (OAE) **testing**—a hearing test for patients who cannot (because of disability or because they are too young) give adequate feedback required in the standard hearing test.

OtoLAM—laser technology for treatment of middle ear infections in children, said to sharply reduce antibiotic utilization and help to avoid need for insertion of ventilation tubes in the operating room.

otospondylomegaepiphyseal dysplasia (OSMED)—a very rare inherited disorder of bone growth that results in skeletal abnormalities, severe hearing loss, and distinctive facial features.

otospongiosis/otosclerosis syndrome—a type of genetic deafness. Treatment with sodium fluoride in very low doses is a promising therapy where there is early detection of this syndrome.

O-to-T advancement flap—a useful technique for repair of helical rim defects of the ear that are predominantly on the posterior aspect of the helix. The flap allows for the repair of the helical contour without a significant reduction in the size of the ear or narrowing of the helix. It can be used in areas where the donor skin is insufficient for a bilobed flap.

Ototemp 3000—measures core body temperature by reading the temperature of the tympanic membrane, without actually touching the membrane, giving an accurate reading in five seconds.

ototoxic—anything harmful to the structures or process of hearing, such as some drugs causing tinnitus, or extremely loud noises (or music). Aminoglycoside antibiotics are well known for their ototoxic side effects. Usage: "She denied the use of ototoxic drugs and has no history of ear trauma or recurrent infections."

Ottawa Ankle Rules (OARs)—a decision-making process used by orthopedists to decide if an x-ray is necessary to evaluate an acute ankle injury. Currently, this assessment is validated for adult use only, but it is being tested for pediatric use. Adult statistics indicate that this simple

Ottawa *(cont.)*
assessment could safely decrease the use of x-rays by 25%.

OTW (over the wire).

O.U., OU (*oculus uterque*, each eye).

Ouchterlony double diffusion technique. Usage: "Circulating immune complexes, C3, hemolytic complement, and precipitating antibodies by Ouchterlony are pending."

Ousley insertion spatula—used in keratoplasty procedures.

Outback reentry catheter—combines with the Frontrunner XP catheter to facilitate treatment of chronic total occlusions in peripheral arteries .

OutBound—a disposable syringe infusion system used in the administration of chemotherapy.

outcomes management—use of monitored data in a way that allows individuals and healthcare systems and providers to learn from experience and make changes in the way services are provided and administered. Also called *outcomes measurement* and *outcomes monitoring*.

Outerbridge ridge (named for R. E. Outerbridge, M.D., British Columbia, Canada)—a ridge of varying height, crossing the medial femoral condyle at its osteochondral junction, described by Outerbridge in 1961. He suggested that at least one cause of patellar chondromalacia might be friction against the medial patellar facet cartilage as the patella rides this ridge in normal movement of the knee. See *Outerbridge scale.*

Outerbridge scale—for assessing joint damage or articular surface damage in chondromalacia patellae:

grade 1, softening and swelling of the cartilage.

grade 2, fragmentation and fissuring in an area half an inch or less in diameter.

grade 3, same as grade 2, but involves an area more than half an inch.

grade 4, erosion of cartilage down to bone.

outflow cannula—in laparoscopic surgery, the tube through which fluids and specimens are removed (as opposed to the inflow cannulas through which solutions are infused).

out-in-out technique—for suturing in an intraocular lens (posterior chamber) for aphakia.

outlet view (Radiol)—an x-ray showing a tangential view of the coracoacromial arch in the sagittal plane of the scapula.

outpatient endometrial resection/ablation (OPERA).

outpatient endometrial resection/ablation (OPERA) **specialized tissue aspirating resectoscope** (STAR).

outrigger splint—used following metacarpophalangeal joint arthroplasty.

oval window—see *vestibular window*.

ovarian hyperstimulation syndrome (OHSS)—a complication of hormonal therapy for in vitro fertilization. This syndrome includes massive ovarian enlargement, ascites, pleural effusions, and electrolyte and coagulation imbalances.

ovarian remnant syndrome—a condition in which remnants of ovarian cortex left behind after surgical removal of the ovaries become functional and cystic. It most often occurs in patients who have experienced a difficult oophorectomy.

OVD (ophthalmic viscosurgical device) —see *Cellugel OVD*.

oversampling—doubling the size of the field of view (FOV) in anti-aliasing techniques (MRI terms).

overshooting—failure to stop a voluntary movement when its goal or purpose has been achieved.

over-the-balloon technology—see *InfusaSleeve II catheter*.

over-the-counter (OTC) **drug**.

overtube—tube through which the EndoCinch device is advanced.

Ovès cervical cap—for use in artificial insemination procedures.

Ovès fertility cap—used by couples having difficulty conceiving as a result of low sperm counts, reduced sperm motility, or a chronically hostile vaginal environment (such as one caused by a yeast infection).

OV-1 surgical keratometer (OV, Ophthalmic Ventures).

ovotestes—gonads that can produce both sperm and eggs; found in persons diagnosed as hermaphrodites, or "intersex" babies.

OvuStick—a urinary dipstick used to detect luteinizing hormone surge in infertility patients.

Owens-type incision—a U-shaped mucosal incision used in repair of choanal atresia.

oxazolidinones—a new class of antibiotics that disrupts the initiation of bacterial protein synthesis at an earlier stage of the cycle than other antibiotics. The bacteria are then unable to manufacture proteins and are unable to reproduce. An example is the antibiotic Zyvox (linezolid).

ox cell hemolysin test.

Oxford meniscal unicompartmental knee system.

oxidized regenerated cellulose and collagen—generic term for Promogran, a wound dressing matrix that binds MMP (matrix metalloproteases) with growth factors, indicated for the treatment of exuding wounds including but not limited to diabetic, venous, and pressure ulcers.

oxidized zirconium—a new alloy used on knee and hip implants. It is said to cause fewer allergic reactions and resist scratching better than other coated prostheses.

OxiFirst—fetal oxygen monitoring system.

Oxilan-300, Oxilan-350 (ioxilan)—low-osmolar, tri-iodinated radiographic contrast agent for intra-arterial and intravenous administration.

OxiMax—pulse oximetry device.

oximeter—a photoelectric device that measures the oxygen saturation of the blood. Usage: "Oxygen saturation was monitored by ear or finger oximeter." Used in assessing sleep disorders by polysomnogram. There is no "air" oximeter.

Oxiplex—bioabsorbable product for the prevention of postsurgical adhesions and promote hemostasis during surgery.

Oxonium (oxidized zirconium)—a material used in knee systems.

oxycodone and acetaminophen capsules—a Duramed drug product that has bioequivalency and therapeutic interchangeability with Tylox.

oxygen cisternography—technique for the diagnosis of acoustic tumors. In some cases where air will not enter the internal auditory canal, Pantopaque may be introduced into the posterior fossa for cisternography.

oxygen saturation—see *SaO*$_2$ (arterial oxygen saturation).

Oxylator EM-100—emergency resuscitation device.

Oxymizer, Oxymizer Pendant—disposable oxygen-conserving devices that use lower oxygen flow rates than other devices and reduce the amount of oxygen by 50% to 75%. The devices can be used with liquid oxygen or compressed gas.

oxyphil cell.

oxytocin challenge test (OCT).

Oxytrak pulse oximeter and Dinamap blood pressure monitor—measures oxygen saturation.

P, p

p—If you can't find a word anywhere, try looking in the *p's* in a dictionary. Often an initial *p* is silent, as in *phthisis, pneumonia, psoas, psoriasis, psyllium, pterygium, pterygoid,* and *ptosis.*

P—the shorter arm of a chromosome. (Think of the French word *petit.*)

Pa (pascal).

PAAF—see *pancreatitis-associated ascitic fluid.*

PAC (papular acrodermatitis of childhood). Cf. *Gianotti-Crosti syndrome.*

PACAB (port-access CABG)—a procedure that combines the advantages of conventional CABG with MIDCAB.

Pace bipolar pacing catheter.

Pacefinder—pacemaker lead placement system that incorporates Cardima deflectable Naviport hollow-lumen guiding catheter and Vueport balloon technology.

pacemaker (cardiac)
- Activitrax
- AddVent atrioventricular
- Autima II dual chamber
- Dash
- DDD

pacemaker *(cont.)*
- Diamond II DDR
- dual chamber Medtronic Kappa 400
- Elite dual chamber rate-responsive
- Enterra
- Entity
- Ergos O_2
- escape
- Integrity AFx AutoCapture
- Jade II SSI
- Kairos
- Kappa 400 Series
- Medtronic temporary
- Micro Minix
- Microny II SR Plus (or Microny II SR+)
- Pacefinder
- Pacesetter Synchrony
- Philos DR
- Relay cardiac
- Ruby II DDD
- SAVVI synchronous
- Topaz II SSIR
- Trilogy DC+
- Trilogy SR+
- Triumph VR
- Unity-C
- Ventak AICD
- Vitatron Diamond II

pacemaker adaptive rate—the rate that the pacemaker adapts automatically to increases or decreases in the natural (intrinsic) heart rate. Also, *rate-adaptive, rate-responsive, or rate-modulated.*

pacemaker code system—a three-letter code often used to describe various types of pacemakers. The first letter represents the chamber of the heart which is stimulated to contract (i.e., paced) by an attached electrode. The second letter represents the chamber(s) in which the pacemaker can sense ongoing normal electrical activity. The third letter indicates the type of response (i.e., mode) of which the pacemaker is capable (inhibited from competing with normal heart contractions, triggered by abnormal heart activity). Example: A DDD pacemaker serves the electrical activity of both the atrium and ventricle, paces (stimulates) both the atrium and ventricle to beat, may cause (trigger) the atrium to contract while sending no signal (inhibited) to the ventricle depending on what natural electrical activity is occurring in the heart at that time.

Pacesetter APS—a portable, pocket-size pacemaker programmer.

Pacesetter Synchrony pacemaker—a permanent rate-responsive dual chamber pacemaker.

Pacesetter Trilogy DR+ pulse generator.

pachometer—instrument that measures the thickness of the cornea.

Pach-Pen—a device that measures corneal thickness in thousandths of a millimeter.

pachymetry—a measure of central corneal thickness.

Pacifico post-suture inflation technique—reduces postoperatively induced astigmatism using CU-8 bicurve needle.

pack-year smoking history—the packs per day multiplied by the number of years of smoking; the cumulative result is the important factor. Usage: "The patient has a 50-pack-year smoking history." The patient has smoked a pack a day for 50 years, or two packs a day for 25 years, or five packs a day for ten years (or ten packs a day for five years!).

PACS (Picture Archiving and Communications Systems).

PACU (postanesthesia care unit)—a newer name for the recovery room.

PAD (public access defibrillation)—a program that seeks to distribute external defibrillators at specific sites where sudden cardiac arrest may frequently occur, e.g., public places (such as airports and casinos) where large numbers of older people may be under stress.

paddle—myocutaneous paddle or skin paddle; tissue grafts anchored by a pedicle flap.

Padgett baseline pinch gauge—records thumb-finger grasp.

Padgett hydraulic hand dynamometer—measures hand strength.

Padogram device—a vascular diagnostic device used to test for peripheral diseases and coronary arterial diseases.

pad test—test for urinary incontinence, confirmed by one gram or more of urinary leakage in 60 minutes.

Paecilomyces variotii—a fungus that is an infrequent human pathogen. It has caused complications associated with prosthetic cardiac valves, synthetic lens implants, and cerebrospinal fluid shunts.

PAFD (percutaneous abscess and fluid drainage).

PAG (periaqueductal gray) **matter**. Stimulation of the PAG matter with deep brain electrodes inhibits pain. See *PVG matter.*

PAH acid (para-aminohippuric)—used in kidney function test. See *Stamey test*.

PAI (plasminogen activator inhibitor-1).

PAIgG (platelet-associated IgG).

Pain Assessment and Intervention Notation (P.A.I.N.) **tool**—a 3-step assessment process in which the nurse first observes whether the patient appears to be in pain; next, checks specific physiologic indicators delineated by the P.A.I.N. tool, and finally elicits a summary assessment based on combining the behavioral and physiologic findings.

PainBuster disposable infusion pain management kit—based on I-Flow elastomeric infusion technology, it provides continuous infusion of a non-narcotic local anesthetic (bupivacaine HCl) directly into the intraoperative site for postoperative pain management for a 24- to 48-hour period.

pain management techniques (electrically generated)
- CES (cranial electrical stimulation)
- DCS (dorsal column stimulator)
- galvanic stimulation
- HVS (high-voltage stimulation)
- interferential current therapy
- iontophoresis
- Liss CES
- LV-MS (low-voltage microampere stimulation)
- PEMT (pulsed electromagnetic therapy)
- PENS (percutaneous electrical nerve stimulation)

pain *(cont.)*
- Stryker Pain Buster
- TENS (transcutaneous electrical nerve stimulation)

painter's encephalopathy—chronic organic brain syndrome secondary to exposure to fumes from some types of paints.

PAI-1 (plasminogen activator inhibitor)—substance that inhibits the activity of tissue plasminogen activator (t-PA) and thus is felt to be associated with increased cardiovascular risk.

PAI (Preadmission Acuity Inquiry) **tool** —designed to assess functional levels of independence and acuity of applicants to long-term care facilities.

PAK (percutaneous access kit)—see *Denver PAK.*

palatal implant—for treatment of snoring. Three matchstick-sized pieces of polyester material are placed in the soft palate. The inserts support and stiffen the palate, and no tissue is removed. Implantation is done as an outpatient procedure.

palatectomy—the removal of part of all of the soft or hard palate.

palisade—a configuration created by structures lined up like the palings of a fence.

palisade screen—a barrier fashioned from wide-bore tube drains and resembling a picket fence, held in place by retention sutures for temporary abdominal closure.

palisading (Path)—a lining up of cells such that their long axis is perpendicular to some other structure. Usage: peripheral palisading.

palladium 103 (^{103}Pd) **implantation**—ultrasound-guided transperineal implantation as brachytherapy for prostate cancer.

pallidal brain stimulation—treatment for Parkinson disease. A thin wire electrode implanted in the globus pallidus of the brain is connected to a pulse generator implanted in the chest. The pulse generator sends an electric current to the brain, jamming nerve signals from the globus pallidus.

pallidotomy guided by microelectrode recording—may be more successful in treating Parkinson disease than the traditional electrical stimulation pallidotomy.

palmar beak ligament (Ortho). Usage: "It has been suggested that instability resulting from incompetence of the palmar beak ligament is responsible for initiating the progression of degenerative joint disease."

palmar erythema (erythema palmare) —redness of the palms that persists; it may be seen in patients with liver disease, rheumatoid arthritis, and a number of other diverse medical problems.

Palmaz balloon-expandable stent—for use in patients with narrowed or blocked iliac arteries after unsuccessful balloon angioplasty.

Palmaz Corinthian—transhepatic biliary stent and delivery system.

Palmaz-Schatz stent (PSS)—a balloon-expandable articulated, slotted tube stent comprised of rigid segments attached by a central articulation. The biliary stent is used to treat biliary duct stenosis. The coronary stent is used to teat focal saphenous vein graft.

Palmaz vascular stent—a cylinder of stainless steel mesh. The stent is placed over a balloon catheter and inserted into an occluded artery after angioplasty is performed. The balloon is inflated once the catheter is positioned at the site of the occlusion. The balloon is then deflated, but the stent retains its expanded shape and remains permanently at the site of the occlusion, holding the vessel walls apart and facilitating blood flow. Also, *Palmaz-Schatz stent*.

Palmer classification of cartilage tear.

palmomental—refers to the palm of the hand and the mentalis muscle. See *palmomental reflex*.

palmomental reflex—contraction of the ipsilateral mentalis and orbicularis oris muscles, with slight elevation and retraction of the angle of the mouth in response to scratching the thenar area of the hand; seen occasionally in an exaggerated form in patients with corticospinal tract lesions. Also called *palmomental reflex of Marinesco-Radovici*.

palmoplantar hyperhidrosis (PPH)—excessive or profuse sweating on the palms and soles.

Palomar EsteLux—utilizes flashlamp technology to remove skin lesions such as solar keratoses and hair removal.

Palomar SLP1000 (super long-pulse) **diode laser system**—for permanent hair reduction with all skin types.

palonosetron—see *Aloxi*.

palpation—the act of feeling with the fingers in examination of the body. Inspection, palpation, and auscultation are the three methods of examination used most. Cf. *palpitation, papillation*.

palpitation—the subjective feeling of an irregular or abnormally rapid heart beat. Cf. *palpation, papillation*.

palsy—see *tardy palsy*.

Palumbo knee brace—custom-fitted knee brace used with chondromalacia patellae.

Palva flap—operative technique used in tympanoplasty with mastoidectomy for cholesteatoma.

PAM (potential acuity meter)—used in testing vision.

PAN (periodic alternating nystagmus).

Panacryl absorbable suture—used for soft tissue approximation and/or ligation during general and orthopedic (tendon and ligament repair) procedures. It is used for extended wound support up to six months.

panallergic—allergic to everything.

pANCA (perinuclear-type autoantibody against neutrophils)—a diagnostic marker for a spectrum of diseases. Sometimes paired in laboratory studies with cANCA.

pancreas-sparing duodenectomy (PSD)—removal of the duodenum with sparing of the portion into which hepatic and pancreatic ducts drain, thereby avoiding resection of the pancreas and creation of a bilioenteric and pancreaticoenteric anastomosis.

pancreatic enzyme therapy—used in treatment of pain in chronic pancreatitis.

pancreatic islet cell transplant—surgical treatment for a patient with type 1 diabetes mellitus.

pancreaticoduodenectomy—surgical resection of the primary tumor in peripancreatic cancer.

pancreatic polypeptide (PP).

pancreatic sepsis in acute pancreatitis—treated with therapeutic concentrations of antibiotics in the pancreatic tissue in pancreatitis.

pancreatoduodenectomy, pylorus preserving (PPPD).

pancs—slang for *pancreas* in transplant surgery.

pan-cultured—used in laboratory medicine. The specimen is cultured to determine which organisms are present and to determine which antibiotics are specific for that organism. The prefix *pan* means *all, every.* Usage: "The urine was pan-cultured."

PANDAS (pediatric autoimmune neuropsychiatric disorders associated with streptococcus).

PANDO (primary acquired nasolacrimal duct obstruction).

P&K (Polaroids and Kodachromes)—photographs of specimens. Usage: "P&K were taken," or "Polaroids and Kodachromes were taken."

panel reactive antibodies (PRAs)—the formation of antibodies to human leukocyte antigen (HLA), the presence of which makes it more difficult to find a suitable donor for heart transplantation and increases the risk of rejection. This condition is associated with blood transfusion administered for post-LVAD bleeding and occurs in 30-80% of patients on left ventricular assist devices (LVADs) prior to heart transplant.

panic disorder patients—function assessed by two types of medical outcomes study: (1) the 20-item short-form survey that covers physical functioning, role functioning, social functioning, mental health, current health perception, and bodily pain; and (2) the 36-item short-form survey which covers all of the areas in the 20-item survey and also includes energy/fatigue and general health perceptions.

panic level—an abnormal test result level that may indicate a severe or life-threatening condition.

Panje ("pan-gee") **voice button**—a laryngeal prosthesis to improve esophageal speech in patients who have had laryngectomies. See also *Blom-Singer valve,* a similar prosthetic device.

panmyelosis—when erythroid, megakaryocytic, and granulocytic proliferation is present in the bone marrow. It is indicative of acute myeloid leukemia.

panniculus, hanging—see *apron.*

PanoGauze hydrogel-impregnated gauze.

PanoPlex hydrogel dressing.

Panoramic 200 nonmydriatic ophthalmoscope—combines advances in laser and optical imaging technology to digitally capture over 80% of the retina in less than 1/2 second without use of dilating drops or contact with the eye. The system is patient-activated and uses very low levels of light.

panretinal photocoagulation (PRP).

pan-sensitive—sensitive to everything.

pantaloon embolus—see *saddle embolus.*

pantaloon hernia—results when direct and indirect hernias occur simultaneously. Also called *combined hernia.*

pants-over-vest repair (Surg).

PAO (periacetabular osteotomy).

PAP (peroxidase-antiperoxidase)—see *immunoperoxidase stain.*

Papercuff—a disposable blood pressure cuff with an outer paper layer that doesn't stretch, thus transferring all of the inflation pressure to the underlying artery. The inner plastic layer does stretch, conforming closely to the patient's arm, resulting in a significantly higher pressure pulse amplitude being transmitted to cuff signal detecting devices.

papilla, optic—point at which the optic nerve fibers leave the eyeball. Also called *optic disk.*

papillation—the presence of small projections or elevations (as the papillae on the tongue). Cf. *palpation, palpitation.*

papilledema—swelling of the nerve head from increased intracranial pressure or interference with the venous return from the eye.

papilloma, inverted schneiderian—see *schneiderian papilloma.*

papillotomy—incision of a papilla, as of the duodenal papilla. See *laparoscopic transcystic papillotomy*.

PapNet—increases sensitivity of standard Pap tests by combining automated microscopy and computerized analysis to reduce screening errors.

papova—an acronym for a group of DNA viruses thought to cause warts in humans. (See *HPV.)* Comes from the first two letters of the names of the viruses:

pa papilloma virus
po polyoma virus
va vacuolate virus

PAPP A (pregnancy-associated plasma protein A).

Pap Plus HPV Screen—combines HPV Hybrid Capture 2 test with ThinPrep Pap test to enable doctors to more effectively determine whether women have, or are at risk for developing, cervical cancer.

Pap Plus speculoscopy—a visual cervical screening exam, using a small disposable blue-white light source called Speculite, as an adjunct to the traditional Pap smear.

papular acrodermatitis of childhood (PAC).

PAPVR (partial anomalous pulmonary venous return).

PAR (postanesthesia recovery). Usage: The patient was stable after the procedure and was taken to the PAR in good condition.

para—the number of times a woman has given birth. This word is frequently followed by four numbers separated by hyphens (for example, para 3-1-0-3). The first numeral refers to the number of full-term deliveries, in this case 3; the second indicates the number of premature births (1); the third numeral is the number of abortions or miscarriages (0); the fourth numeral indicates the number of living children (3). See also *GPMAL*.

para-aminohippuric (PAH).

paraconal fascia—relatively unknown fascia that is located between the lateral aspect of the perirenal fascia and the posterior parietal peritoneum. Important because it protects delicate retroperitoneal organs (duodenum, pancreas, celiac axis, and superior mesenteric artery). Locating this condensed fascia is an important step in the dissection of the high retroperitoneum in advanced videoendoscopy.

Paradigm insulin pump.

Paradigm Link—a blood glucose monitor.

paradoxical vocal cord motion (PVCM)—another name for *vocal cord dysfunction* (VCD).

paradoxus—see *pulsus paradoxus*.

paraesophageal hernia, type II—occurs when the distal esophagus is located in its normal position, anchored by the phrenoesophageal ligament, and a defect in the diaphragm allows the stomach and hernia sac to travel into the chest. Because this condition is usually asymptomatic, it may reach tremendous size with complex herniation before diagnosis is made. Surgical correction is universally advised due to the risk of sudden catastrophic gastric volvulus and death.

parafascicular thalamotomy (PFT).

paraffin block or **section**—tissue embedded in paraffin for sectioning and subsequent staining for microscopy. See *permanent section*.

ParaGard IUD—an intrauterine device that has a tiny copper wire wrapped around the plastic body and should not be used by anyone who is allergic to copper.

Paragon coronary stent.

Paragon CRT (paflufocon B), **Paragon CRT 100** (paflufocon D), **Paragon Quadra RG** (paflufocon B), and **Paragon Quadra RG 100** (paflufocon D)—rigid gas-permeable contact lenses for corneal refractive therapy.

parallel squat exercise—a rehabilitation exercise used for patients without an anterior cruciate ligament. The patient squats until the knee is at 90° and the femur is parallel to the floor.

parallel track sign (also, double stripe sign)—a radionuclide bone imaging appearance of the diaphyses and metaphyses of tubular bones in patients with primary or secondary hypertrophic osteoarthropathy. Diffuse and symmetric increase in uptake of the radionuclide agent occurs along the cortical margins.

paramagnetic artifact (MRI)—can be seen in the soft tissues after surgery.

Paramax cruciate guide system—simplifies endoscopic cruciate reconstruction, using soft tissue and bony component grafts.

parameter—one of a number of ways to test, describe, or evaluate a person or an object. Cf. *perimeter.*

paraostomy hernia—hernia occurring next to a colostomy site.

Parasmillie—double-bladed knife for patellar tendon graft harvesting.

parathormone (parathyroid hormone, PTH).

Paratrend 7 and 7+—a tiny sensor placed in the brain for monitoring blood gases of brain-injured patients.

paratrigeminal oculosympathetic syndrome (POSS). Also, known as *Raeder syndrome* or *Raeder paratrigeminal neuralgia.*

paravariceally—beside a varix.

ParCA—see *Parodi balloon catheter for angiography.*

Parental Stress Scale: PICU (PSS: PICU)—a self-reporting tool that allows parents to record perceived levels of stress in the pediatric ICU environment.

parenteral—a route of drug administration not involving the gastrointestinal tract (intravenous, intramuscular). Cf. *enteral.*

Parham bands—used to hold the fracture fragments of long bones securely in place.

Parietex—composite mesh for hernia surgery. It contains a resorbable collagen layer to prevent development of intra-abdominal adhesions, and the product can be used in either open or laparoscopic incisional and ventral hernias.

Pari LC Plus—reusable nebulizer.

Pari LC Star—reusable nebulizer.

Parinaud oculoglandular syndrome—granulomatous conjunctivitis with swelling in preauricular lymph nodes. It is caused by *Bartonella henselae* infection.

parity—a woman's reproductive history.

PARK (photoastigmatic refractive keratectomy)—a laser surgery procedure for correction of astigmatism. The cornea is reshaped using a cold-beam laser that removes corneal tissue without damaging surrounding tissue. The reshaped cornea allows light to focus directly on the retina for clearer distance vision.

Park blade septostomy (Cardio).

Parker-Kerr closed method—of end-to-end enteroenterostomy.

Parker-Kerr intestinal clamps.

Parkland formula—used to guide initial fluid resuscitation during the first 24 hours after burn trauma. The formula calls for 4 mL over the first 24 hours. Half of the fluid is administered over the first 8 hours post burn, and the remaining half is administered over the next 16 hours. The volume of fluid given is based on the time elapsed since the burn.

Parodi balloon catheter for angiography (ParCA)—gives physicians control over the flow of blood during angiography procedures. With the ParCA, physicians can take numerous images with only one volume of contrast fluid. Invented by Dr. Juan Parodi, of Argentina.

Parona space—the tissue plane over the pronator quadratus in the distal forearm that is deep to the ulnar and radial bursae.

parosteal osteosarcoma—a low-grade, well-differentiated, malignant tumor arising from the surface of the bone. Although similar in meaning, parosteal is used as the disease entity modifier, not periosteal.

paroxetine—see *Paxil.*

paroxysmal atrial tachycardia (PAT).

paroxysmal nocturnal dyspnea (PND).

paroxysmal nocturnal hemoglobinuria (PNH)—descriptive term for the clinical manifestation of red cell breakdown with release of hemoglobin into the urine, manifested most prominently by dark-colored urine in the morning. The term *nocturnal* refers to the older belief that the process took place during sleep; this was later disproved. Hemolysis is shown to occur throughout the day and is not actually paroxysmal, but the urine concentrated overnight produces the dramatic change in color. This syndrome is often seen in hemolytic anemia and large-vessel thrombosis.

paroxysmal supraventricular tachycardia (PSVT).

PARP (poly ADP-ribose polymerase) —naturally occurring enzyme, overproduction of which is believed responsible for brain cell death in stroke victims. Research is ongoing to develop a PARP inhibitor.

Parrot sign—dilation of the pupils when the skin of the neck is pinched, as in meningitis.

Parsol 1789 (avobenzone)—an ingredient commonly used in European, Canadian, and Australian sunscreens, now approved for wider use in suncare products distributed in the U.S.

Parsonage-Turner syndrome—acute brachial neuritis.

Partaject—a drug delivery system. Partaject-delivered busulfan is used as preparative treatment for pediatric bone marrow transplant.

parthenogenesis—the maturation of an unfertilized oocyte to form a new individual; occurs naturally in some insects and has been artificially induced in experimental animals. A possible means of producing embryonic stem cells without fertilization.

partial agonist—a compound that possesses both agonist and antagonist properties.

partial anomalous pulmonary venous return (PAPVR).

partial encircling endocardial ventriculotomy—see *ventriculotomy.*

partial liquid ventilation—a technique that involves introducing the chemical perflubron into a premature infant's malfunctioning lungs and then pumping oxygen into the liquid. Because it is so efficient at absorbing oxygen, perflubron allows lower ventilator pressure settings. Standard ventilator therapy with surfactants at high force can cause permanent lung injury and lead to bronchopulmonary dysplasia.

partial saturation technique—a magnetic resonance technique in which single excitation pulses are delivered to tissue at intervals equal to or shorter than T1.

party wall—a wall between two contiguous structures.

parvovirus—see *human parvovirus B19.*

parylene coating—a plastic film coating applied to medical devices to provide physical, chemical, and electrical insulation and reduction of friction.

passive girdle effect (adynamic girdling)—an aortomyoplasty technique in which the latissimus dorsi muscle is used for passive restraint of the ventricle. See *aortomyoplasty*.

PAS (periodic acid-Schiff) **stain**—a test for collagen disease and also for the presence of Whipple disease. See *Whipple disease.*

PAS (physician-assisted suicide).

PAS (pulsatile antiembolic system).

PASA (proximal articular set angle) (Ortho).

PASAT (paced auditory serial addition task)—a test in which the patient is asked to mentally add a series of numbers from 1 to 10, stating the sum as each new number is presented. Used to assess closed head trauma.

pascal (Pa)—unit of measurement of pressure in the SI system. You will be hearing about this in relation to blood gases. Blood pressures will most probably continue to be given in millimeters of mercury (mmHg). See *SI, International System*.

PASI (Psoriasis Area Severity Index).

P.A.S. (peripheral access system) **Port catheter**—implanted in the antecubital fossa for administration of chemotherapy drugs, for long-term TPN, or for administration of intravenous antibiotics. Also made with double lumens. *P.A.S. Port* is a trademark.

P.A.S. Port Fluoro-Free—implantable peripheral access system that incorporates the Cath-Finder system that tracks the catheter tip during placement without the use of fluoroscopy. Implanted in the antecubital fossa for administration of chemotherapy drugs, for long-term TPN, or for administration of intravenous antibiotics. Also made with double lumens.

Passage catheter—balloon catheter used to dilate biliary strictures. Passage is a trade name.

Passager introducing sheath.

Passy-Muir tracheostomy speaking valve—an attachment that allows ventilator-dependent patients to speak more easily.

PASTA (polarity-altered spectral selective acquisition) **imaging** (MRI).

Past Feelings and Acts of Violence (PFAV) **Scale**—assesses such indicators of violence as past history of arrests, violence against family members, violence against strangers, use of weapons.

past-pointing (*not* passed pointing)—a test used to determine the presence of incoordination in voluntary movements. When the patient is asked to touch the examiner's finger or nose, or his own nose, he goes past it. A variant of this test is used in otolaryngology to test for vestibular problems.

PASYS ("paces") and **PASYS ST**—a single chamber cardiac pacing system.

PAT (paroxysmal atrial tachycardia).

patches, Peyer—see *Peyer patches*.

patchplasty—see *endoventricular circular patchplasty*.

patella alta—a "high-riding" patella, associated with some knee problems.

patella baja—caused by abnormal shortness of the patellar tendon, a low-riding patella. See *patella alta*.

Patella disease—pyloric stenosis occurring in tuberculous patients after fibrous stenosis. Named for an Italian physician, V. Patella.

patellar apprehension test (Ortho).

pathergy—refers to the phenomenon of trivial trauma evoking new lesions or exacerbating old ones, similar to the clinical course of some keloids.

Pathfinder—a microcatheter system, manufactured by Cardima, used in the treatment of atrial fibrillation.

Pathfinder DFA (direct fluorescent antigen) **test**—detects genital *Chlamydia trachomatis*.

pathogen (including bacteria, fungi, parasites, and viruses)—a quick-reference list. See individual entries.

pathogen *(cont.)*
Acanthamoeba keratitis
Achromobacter lwoffi
Achromobacter xylosoxidans (formerly *Alcaligenes xylosoxidans*)
Acinetobacter lwoffi
Actinobacillus actinomycetem comitans
adenovirus
aeroallergen
Aeromonas sobria
Afipia felis
Alcaligenes bookeri
Alcaligenes xylosoxidans (now *Achromobacter xylosoxidans*)
Alternaria
Alteromonas putrefaciens
Andes virus
Aquaspirillum itersonii
arbovirus (arthropod-borne virus)
Arcanobacterium haemolyticum
ARV (AIDS-related virus)
Aspergillus
avian influenza A (H5N1) virus
bacillus Calmette-Guérin (BCG)
Bacillus circulans
Bacillus coagulans
bacteriophage virus
Bacteroides corrodens
baculovirus (genetically engineered)
Bartonella bacilliformis
Bartonella elizabethae
Bartonella henselae
Bartonella quintana
Basidiomycetes
Bayou (BAY) virus
Bdellovibrio
Bio-Tract
Black Creek Canal virus
Bordetella
Borrelia burgdorferi
Branhamella catarrhalis
Brevibacterium linens
Calmette-Guérin, bacillus (BCG)
Campylobacter fetus

pathogen *(cont.)*
Campylobacter jejuni
Candida albicans
Candida glabrata
Cardiobacterium hominis
Chaetomium
Chlamydia pneumoniae
Chlamydia trachomatis
Citrobacter amalonaticus
Citrobacter braakii
Citrobacter koseri
Cobactin E
Coxiella burnetii
Cryptococcus neoformans
Cryptosporidium
Curvularia
Dermatophagoides farinae
Dermatophagoides pteronyssinus
Döderlein bacillus
Ducrey bacillus
Eaton agent *(Mycoplasma pneumoniae)*
E. coli H157:H7
Eikenella corrodens
Entamoeba histolytica
Enterobacter liquefaciens
Enterobacter sakazakii
Epstein-Barr virus (EBV)
Francisella tularensis
Friedländer bacillus
Fusarium (a slime mold)
gamma-herpesvirus
Gardnerella vaginalis
GAS (group A streptococcus)
Giardia lamblia
gram-negative organism
Haemophilus aphrophilus
Haemophilus ducreyi
Haemophilus vaginalis
Hafnia alvei
Helicobacter hepaticus
Helicobacter pylori
Helminthosporium
Herellea vaginicola
herpes simplex virus (HSV)

pathogen *(cont.)*
herpes zoster virus (HZV)
H5N1 virus
HHV-8 (human herpesvirus-8)
Hib or HIB (*Haemophilus influenza* type B)
Histoplasma capsulatum
HIV (human immunodeficiency virus)
HIV-1E virus
Hormodendrum
HTLV-I retrovirus (human T-cell leukemia/lymphoma virus)
HTLV-III (human T-cell lymphotropic virus)
human immunodeficiency virus (HIV)
human herpesvirus 6 (HHV-6)
human mammary tumor virus (HMTV)
human papillomavirus (HPV)
human parvovirus B19 (HPV B19)
Iodamoeba buetschlii
Isospora parasite
Ixodes dammini
Ixodes pacificus
Juquitiba virus
Kingella kingae
Klebsiella oxytoca
Klebsiella pneumoniae
KSHV (Kaposi sarcoma-associated virus)
Lactobacillus casei
Laguna Negra virus
Legionella pneumophila
Leishmania donovani
lentivirus
leukovirus
lymphocytic choriomeningitis virus (LCMV)
MARSA (methicillin-aminoglycoside-resistant *Staphylococcus aureus)*
McKrae strain herpes simplex virus

pathogen *(cont.)*
MCV (molluscum contagiosum virus)
methicillin-resistant *Staphylococcus aureus* (MRSA)
Micrococcus sedentarius
Mima polymorpha
molluscum contagiosum virus (MCV)
monkeypox
Moraxella lwoffi
Morganella morganii
MRSA (methicillin-resistant *Staphylococcus aureus*)
Mycobacterium alvei
Mycobacterium avium
Mycobacterium avium-intracellulare complex
Mycobacterium bohemicum
Mycobacterium branderi
Mycobacterium confluentis
Mycobacterium conspicuum
Mycobacterium genavense
Mycobacterium goodii
Mycobacterium gordonae
Mycobacterium hassiacum
Mycobacterium heckeshornense
Mycobacterium heidelbergense
Mycobacterium immunogenum
Mycobacterium interjectum
Mycobacterium intermedium
Mycobacterium kubicae
Mycobacterium lentiflavum
Mycobacterium mageritense
Mycobacterium mucogenicum
Mycobacterium novocastrense
Mycobacterium palustre
Mycobacterium triplex
Mycobacterium tuberculosis
Mycobacterium tusciae
Mycobacterium wolinskyi
*Mycoplasma pneumoniae (*Eaton agent)
Neisseria

pathogen *(cont.)*
Neisseria meningitidis
Nipah virus
Nocardia
nonsyncytium-inducing (NSI) variant of the AIDS virus
oncogenic retrovirus
opportunistic infection or organism
Paecilomyces variotii
Penicillium
Penicillium marneffei
Phoma (a slime mold)
picornavirus
Pneumocystis carinii
Pneumocystis jiroveci (formerly *Pneumocystis carinii*)
porcine endogenous retrovirus (PERV)
Propionibacterium
Pseudallescheria boydii
Pseudomonas exotoxin
Pseudomonas maltophilia
Pseudomonas stutzeri
Psorospermium haeckelii
Pullularia (a slime mold)
respiratory syncytial virus (RSV)
retrovirus
Rhizopus nigricans
Rhodococcus equi
Rhodotorula
RNA virus
Rochalimaea henselae (changed to *Bartonella henselae*)
rotavirus
Rous sarcoma virus
Saccharomyces
Serratia liquefaciens
Serratia marcescens
Sin Nombre virus (SNV)
Spondylocladium
Staphylococcus aureus
Staphylococcus epidermidis
Stemphyllium
Stenotrophomonas (formerly *Xanthomonas*) *maltophilia*

pathogen *(cont.)*
Streptococcus milleri
Streptococcus mitis
togavirus
Torula histolytica
Toxoplasma gondii
Trichosporon beigelii
Ureaplasma urealyticum
vancomycin-resistant enterococci (VRE)
vancomycin-resistant *Enterococcus faecium* (VREF)
varicella zoster virus (VZV)
virus
virus-like infectious agent (VLIA)
West Nile virus
xenotropic donor organisms
Yersinia pestis
zoonotic retroviruses

pathognomonic—characteristic or diagnostic of a particular disease.

PATI (Penetrating Abdominal Trauma Index).

patient-controlled analgesia (PCA) **system**.

patient motion artifact (Radiol)—blurring on plain films; multiple bands or ghosts, mostly in the phase-encoding direction, on MRI scans.

Patient Outcomes Research Team (PORT).

Patil stereotaxic system—for biopsy, hematoma evacuation, angiographic targeting, epilepsy implants, stereotaxic craniotomy.

patty or **pattie, cottonoid**—see *cottonoid patty (pattie), Cellolite.*

paucity—deficiency, shortage. Usage: "There is a paucity of objective findings, so we will have to undertake further laboratory tests before we can make a diagnosis in this patient."

Paufique knife (Oph).

Pauwels classification of femoral neck fractures—based on the location of the fracture line. Uses roman numerals. Named for Dr. Pauwels. See *Garden classification.*

paving stone degeneration—atrophic condition in which sharply outlined, rounded lesions appear in the peripheral retina. Also, *cobblestone degeneration.*

Pavlik harness—used to correct congenital hip dysplasia in infants under six months of age. Also, *Kicker Pavlik harness.*

PAWP (pulmonary artery wedge pressure).

Paxceed (micellar paclitaxel for injection)—a medicine for the treatment of rheumatoid arthritis.

paxial, P axial (Oph)—axial power, used in measuring anterior chamber depth.

Paxil (paroxetine)—an SSRI antidepressant, now successfully used to diminish hot flashes in men who are receiving hormone therapy for prostate cancer.

"pay-ron-ee"—phonetic for *Peyronie* disease.

PBC (primary biliary cirrhosis).

PBLs (peripheral blood lymphocytes).

PBNS (percutaneous bladder neck stabilization).

PBPC (peripheral blood progenitor cell) —used in bone marrow transplants.

PBPI (penile brachial pressure index).

PBSC (peripheral blood stem cell collections)—for allogeneic bone marrow transplantation.

PBTE (percutaneous transhepatic liver biopsy with tract embolization).

PBV (percutaneous balloon valvuloplasty).

PCA (porous-coated anatomic) **knee prosthesis**—a cementless implant that permits biologic union between the implant and the bone which infiltrates into the textured surface of the prosthesis.

PCA (patient-controlled analgesia) **system**—to administer analgesics as needed. Several manufacturers are marketing a portable computerized pump with a chamber that holds a prefilled syringe. The physician programs the pump and determines the total amount of the drug that the patient can receive over a given period of time and the amount of each dose. When the patient is in pain, he can push a button on a cord attached to the pump; the pump then dispenses a small dose of the medication into the patient's I.V. line. The patient is quite likely to need less medication this way because he feels in control and therefore less anxious and less tense than when waiting for someone to dispense the medication.

PCBS (percutaneous cardiopulmonary bypass support).

PCCL (percutaneous cholecystolithotomy).

PC (phase-contrast) **technique** (MRI).

PCD (primary ciliary dyskinesia)—see *immotile cilia syndrome.*

PCD (programmable cardioverter-defibrillator)—for detection and reversal of ventricular tachycardia.

PCD Transvene implantable cardioverter-defibrillator system.

PCEEA stapler—25-mm premium circular end-to-end anastomosis instrument.

PCHA (proliferating cell nuclear antigen) (ENT, Neuro)—a technique to assess the growth rate of vestibular schwannomas.

PC-IOL (posterior chamber intraocular lens) **implantation**—performed bilaterally to correct pediatric aphakia.

PCL (posterior cruciate ligament).

PCNL (percutaneous nephrostolithotomy)—uses ultrasound waves to disintegrate kidney stones.

PCNSL (primary central nervous system lymphoma)—a brain tumor which is most common in patients with immune system deficiency. It is successfully treated with chemotherapy rather than surgical resection or radiation therapy.

PCNU—a nitrosourea-type chemotherapeutic agent. Cf. *BCNU*.

PCO (polycystic ovary).

PCO (posterior capsular opacification).

PCP (*Pneumocystis carinii* pneumonia).

PC Polygraf HR—a device that evaluates lower esophageal sphincter and esophageal motility disorders.

PCR (polymerase chain reaction).

PCRA (percutaneous coronary rotational atherectomy).

PC-7 needle—a curved needle used in intraocular lens procedures.

PCTCL (percutaneous transhepatic cholecystolithotomy).

pCT (post-stimulus peak calcitonin).

PCT (procalcitonin).

PCW (pulmonary capillary wedge).

PD (peritoneal dialysis).

PDA (patent ductus arteriosus).

PD Access with Peel-Away needle introducer—used to place central venous lines in infants and adults for long-term intravenous delivery of antibiotics, chemotherapy agents, and nutritionals.

PDB (preperitoneal distention balloon)—permits easy separation of the preperitoneal layers in laparoscopic extraperitoneal herniorrhaphy, and the transparent balloon allows for constant visualization.

PDC (peritoneal dialysis catheter).

PDE4 (phosphodiesterase 4) **inhibitor**—a class of drugs used in the treatment of chronic inflammation, including asthma and COPD.

PDN (prosthetic disk nucleus) **device**.

PDS (pancreatic duct sphincter).

PDS (pigment dispersion syndrome).

PDS (polydioxanone suture) **II Endoloop suture.**

PDT (percutaneous dilational tracheostomy).

PDT (photodynamic therapy)—a colloquial term for *laser surgery*. See *Levulan*.

PEA (pulseless electrical activity)—formerly called EMD (electromechanical dissociation). PEA covers EMD, pseudo-EMD, and idioventricular rhythms.

peak-and-trough levels—maximum and minimum blood levels of a therapeutic agent, determined by drawing blood at strategic intervals after administration. This method provides more precise information than doing random blood levels and is particularly useful with drugs having a narrow margin between effective and toxic levels. Usage: "The following studies were considered: BUN, creatinine clearance, two urinalyses, and three drug assays one peak-and-trough level each, initially, and a repeat trough level at the end of seven days."

peak flow—see *Wright peak flow.*

peak latencies of pattern electroretinogram (PERG).

Peakometer—used in testing the peak flow of the urinary bladder.

peanut—operating room term for a small sponge.

Pearce nucleus hydrodissector—used during cataract surgery.

Pearce trabeculectomy—a type of glaucoma surgery in which trabecular meshwork is excised.

Pearce Tripod—implant cataract lens.

PEARL (physiologic endometrial ablation/resection loop).

pearl chains—chains of cells or vesicles brought into alignment during electro-cell fusion, prior to electroporation. See *electroporation*.

peau d'orange ("po-do-rahnj"') (Fr., orange peel)—dimpled appearance of the skin due to interstitial edema and particularly seen in breast cancer.

pectus excavatum—depression of the sternum. *(Not* pectus recurvatum.)

pectus excavatum repair—see *funnel chest repair.*

pedestal sign—in radiology, the pedestal sign is indicative of prosthetic loosening of the femoral stem in cementless total hip arthroplasty.

pediatric autoimmune neuropsychiatric disorders associated with streptococcus (PANDAS)—believed to be caused by an autoimmune reaction to strep, in which antibodies attack healthy as well as infected cells. This leads to inflammation in the brain's basal ganglia, an area involving movement and motor control, and may result in unusual obsessions, compulsions, tics, and behaviors that mimic Tourette syndrome or Sydenham chorea. Treatment is with aggressive, extended antibiotic therapy.

pedicle subtraction osteotomy—a procedure for the treatment of dislocated hip.

pedigree (Genetics)—a diagram showing the lineal and collateral relationships of all members of a family or kindred and indicating which of them display a particular genetic trait or disorder.

Pediatric Risk of Mortality Scale (PRISM)—used to assess a child's severity of illness.

Pedi PEG tube—a percutaneous endoscopic gastrostomy tube.

Pedotti diagram—a method of analyzing gait style.

PEEP ("peep")—positive end-expiratory pressure.

PEFR (peak expiratory flow rate)—a pulmonary function test.

pegaptanib sodium injection—see *Macugen.*

Pegasus Nd:YAG—surgical laser.

Pegasys (PEG-interferon alfa-2a)—a long-acting drug form of interferon for once weekly administration in the treatment of chronic hepatitis C.

Pegasys-Copegus (peginterferon alfa-2a plus ribavirin) **protocol**—combination drug therapy used for treatment of hepatitis C.

PEG-ELS (electrolyte lavage solution) —polyethylene glycol electrolyte lavage solution. Designed to rapidly cleanse the gastrointestinal tract without disturbing patient water and electrolyte balance in preparation for a diagnostic examination such as colonoscopy. Examples: CoLyte, GoLytely. See also *SF-ELS* (sulfate-free electrolyte lavage solution).

peginterferon alfa-2a plus ribavirin —see *Pegasys-Copegus.*

PEG-Intron Redipen—a prefilled pen-type injection syringe for delivery of medication for chronic hepatitis C.

PEG-1 (prostaglandin E-1)—liposomal treatment of critical limb ischemia, which occurs when circulation in limbs becomes so inadequate that there is danger of gangrene and subsequent amputation.

PEG (percutaneous endoscopic gastrostomy) **tube**—the preferred meth-

PEG *(cont.)*
od for patients who need long-term enteral feedings. Also, *PEG-24 system.*

pegylated—referring to drug formulations containing polyethylene glycols (PEG). Usage: "This HIV-positive patient was given PEG interleukin-2."

pegylated liposomal doxorubicin—used in treatment of AIDS-associated Kaposi sarcoma.

PEH (papillary endothelial hyperplasia).

PEI (percutaneous ethanol injection).

PEJ (percutaneous endoscopic jejunostomy).

PELD (pediatric end-stage liver disease) **score**—cf. *MELD score*.

Pelger-Huët cells—seen in acute myelogenous leukemia.

pelgeroid—refers to Pelger-Huët nuclear anomaly of neutrophils and eosinophils.

peliosis hepatis—hemorrhagic cysts in the liver. (Note: *hepatis*, not *hepatitis*.)

Pelizaeus-Merzbacher disease—familial disease of the myelin sheath.

pellet artifact (Radiol)—shotgun pellets found in the GI tract of patients who have eaten wild game.

Pelorus stereotactic system.

pelvic floor electrical stimulation (PFS, *not* PFES)—to reduce urinary incontinence in women with stress urinary incontinence. May be effective in men and women with mixed and urge urinary incontinence.

pelvic floor MRI—used to identify anal sphincter anatomy and pelvic floor motion in patients with defecation disorders. The MRI records motion as the patient squeezes pelvic floor muscles and expels ultrasound gel from the rectum.

pelvic muscle rehabilitation (PMR)—one of several modalities to help incontinent patients regain control.

Pelvicol—a permanent natural collagen implant from porcine dermis tissue.

pelvic outlet syndrome—extraspinal nerve compression and lower extremity pain. Term replaces secondary piriformis syndrome.

pelviectasis—dilatation of the renal collecting system.

PelviSoft mesh—a material used in surgery for urinary incontinence.

Pemberton acetabuloplasty—procedure to correct congenital dislocation or subluxation of the hip.

PEMF (pulsed electromagnetic field) **therapy**—see *PEMT, AMT*.

PEMT (pulsed electromagnetic therapy)—used in treatment of nonunion of bone secondary to trauma.

Pencan spinal needle—reportedly allows a faster flow rate than other needles.

Penderluft syndrome—a disturbance in air exchange in which the diaphragm is out of synchronization with inhalation and expiration.

penetrance (Genetics)—the degree of frequency with which a genotype is expressed; when some persons possessing the gene do not display the relevant trait, it is said to exhibit reduced penetrance.

Penetrating Abdominal Trauma Index (PATI)—a system of scoring abdominal trauma which takes into account the number of abdominal organs injured. A low PATI correlates with less severe injuries. Patients with a PATI of less than 25 could be surgically managed by primary closure of their abdominal wounds without the need for a colostomy. Although primary clo-

Penetrating *(cont.)*
sure always carries the risk of intra-abdominal infection and possible leaks from the suture lines, a colostomy involves known psychological complications, additional surgical complications, and additional financial considerations. The PATI is used to determine which surgical course to pursue.

Penfield retractor—used in orthopedics. Usage: "A Penfield retractor could be placed behind the T11 vertebral body, as well as inferiorly along the L1 vertebra."

penicillin VK—short for *penicillin V potassium.* See *Pen-Vee K.*

Penicillium—one of the molds most prevalent in damp interior areas. See also *Aspergillus.*

Penicillium marneffei—AIDS-related illness from Southeast Asia.

penile brachial pressure index (PBPI) —Doppler study of blood flow in the penile arteries to assess cardiovascular disease. A value of 0.65 or less indicates possibility of impending myocardial infarction or stroke.

penile gangrene and penile necrosis—often occur in patients with diabetes mellitus and end-stage renal disease.

penile prosthesis—see *prosthesis.*

penile vein ligation—for impotence from venous leakage.

Pennig dynamic wrist fixator—used to treat distal radius fractures while allowing for use of the hand.

Pennig minifixator—fracture fragment fixator for use in minimally invasive surgery of the hands and feet.

Penn pouch—for continent urinary diversion. Uses terminal ileum or cecum to form pouch.

PENS (percutaneous *electrical* nerve stimulation)—not the same as percutaneous *epidural* neurostimulator. See *percutaneous electrical nerve stimulation.*

PENS (percutaneous *epidural* neurostimulator)—not the same as percutaneous *electrical* nerve stimulation.

pentagastrin stimulated analysis.

Pentax EUP-EC124 ultrasound gastroscope—a forward-viewing fiberoptic gastroscope.

Pentax FG-36UX—linear scanning echoendoscope.

Pentax-Hitachi FG32UA—endosonographic system.

penta X syndrome—a chromosomal disorder that affects females. It is caused by the presence of five X chromosomes. Major symptoms can include mental and growth deficiencies, upward slanting eyes with excess skin over the inner corners, and patent ductus arteriosus.

Pen-Vee K—a discontinued brand name; when dictated, transcribe as *penicillin V potassium.*

People-Finder—a handheld device that uses infrared to enable the deaf-blind to locate people, stoves, animals, and light sources.

PEP (progestogen-associated endometrial protein).

PepGen P-15 (peptide-enhanced bone graft)—bioengineered bone replacement graft material for the treatment of osseous defects resulting from moderate to severe periodontitis.

per anum intersphincteric rectal dissection with direct coloanal anastomosis—for lower rectal cancer.

Perative—a nutritionally complete formula for metabolically stressed patients.

Perc-DLE SpineWand—combines electrode design and Coblation technology in tools able to remove soft

Perc-DLE *(cont.)*
tissue via molecular disintegration, with minimal damage to surrounding tissue.

Perceived Stress Scale (PSS).

Perclose A-T (auto-tie)—suture-mediated vessel closure device.

Perclose closure device—from developers of the Techstar, Prostar, and Prostar Plus closure devices. In dictation, you may hear physicians use the developer's name to refer to the device rather than the brand name.

PercuCut cut-biopsy needles—used in soft tissue biopsies.

Percuflex APD all-purpose catheter with Fader Tip.

Percuflex Plus stent—flexible ureteral stent.

PercuGuide—used in diagnostic radiology for precise localization of nonpalpable lesions.

PercuPump disposable syringe and injector.

percussion—rhythmic clapping with cupped hands on the patient's chest and back to loosen pulmonary secretions so they can be coughed up or suctioned out. Also called *frappage, chest PT.*

percutaneous abscess and fluid drainage (PAFD).

percutaneous access kit (PAK).

percutaneous aortic balloon valvuloplasty—performed in patients with cardiogenic shock and critical aortic stenosis.

percutaneous automated diskectomy—a procedure which uses a 2 mm suction cutting probe into the disk under fluoroscopy; performed under local anesthesia.

percutaneous balloon mitral valvuloplasty—see *percutaneous transvenous mitral commissurotomy.*

percutaneous balloon valvuloplasty.

percutaneous bladder neck stabilization (PBNS)—procedure for treatment of women with stress urinary incontinence, using bone-anchor suspension technique.

percutaneous cardiopulmonary bypass support (PCBS)—used to support patients following cardiac arrest, or used prophylactically for high-risk patients having cardiac catheterization or PTCA.

percutaneous choledochoscopy—a nonsurgical method for diagnosing and treating biliary tree problems. Percutaneous access is via T-tubes and transhepatic drains.

percutaneous coronary rotational atherectomy (PCRA)—procedure using a high-speed rotary device to grind obstructing atheroma into fine particles.

percutaneous dilational tracheostomy (PDT)—procedure that may be performed at bedside to relieve airway obstruction and remove tracheopulmonary secretions.

percutaneous discoscope—device to visualize material removed in percutaneous lumbar diskectomy.

percutaneous electrical nerve stimulation (PENS)—only electrical impulses are administered via needles inserted through the skin into target areas for pain relief. Cf. *TENS.*

percutaneous endopyeloplasty—surgical treatment for patients with ureteropelvic junction obstruction.

percutaneous endoscopic gastrostomy (PEG).

percutaneous endoscopic jejunostomy (PEJ).

percutaneous endoscopic sigmoidostomy—surgical treatment to manage children with incontinence.

percutaneous epididymal sperm aspiration—a nonsurgical method of obtaining sperm for in vitro fertilization that involves inserting a 21-gauge butterfly needle directly into the head of the epididymis. The procedure is significantly less costly than microsurgical aspiration, but it can cause scarring.

percutaneous epiphysiodesis using transphyseal screws (PETS)—a procedure to equalize leg length.

percutaneous ethanol injection (PEI) —a promising treatment modality for small liver cancers.

percutaneous gastroenterostomy (PGE)—insertion of a tube into the small bowel, rather than just into the stomach. PG and PGE are used to permit feeding into the stomach, duodenum, or jejunum, and for decompression of a gastric outlet obstruction, or for chronic obstruction of the small bowel. PG and PGE are also used in feeding patients with strokes, with malignancies of the esophagus, and in management of patients with burns or severe trauma.

percutaneous interosseous nerve (PIN).

percutaneous intracoronary angioscopy.

percutaneous left atrial appendage transcatheter occlusion (PLAATO) —a catheter procedure in which a self-expanding nitinol cage is implanted in the mouth of the left atrial appendage so as to occlude it and thus prevent the release of stroke-causing emboli in patients with atrial fibrillation.

percutaneous mitral balloon valvotomy (PMBV).

percutaneous nephrolithotripsy (PNL) —a technique for removal of large dense stones and staghorns via a port created by puncturing the kidney through the skin and enlarging the access port to 1 cm in diameter. There is no surgical incision. The procedure is done under anesthesia and real-time live x-ray control (fluoroscopy). Because x-rays are involved, an interventional radiologist may perform this part of the procedure. The endourologist will then continue to insert instruments via this port into the kidney, break up the stone, and remove most of the stone debris.

percutaneous nephrostolithotomy (PCNL)—uses ultrasound waves to disintegrate kidney stones.

percutaneous patent ductus arteriosus closure—the insertion of occluding spring coils into the patent ductus employing cardiac catheterization techniques. Multiple techniques for patent ductus arteriosus closure exist, but this is one of the latest.

percutaneous pinning of proximal humerus fractures—circumvents extensive soft-tissue stripping. It is performed to maintain fracture alignment without ORIF (open reduction and internal fixation).

percutaneous radiofrequency catheter ablation—a potential cure for idiopathic ventricular tachycardia.

percutaneous radiofrequency facet rhizotomy—see *facet denervation.*

percutaneous resection of transitional cell carcinoma of the renal pelvis.

percutaneous sclerotherapy—a minimally invasive treatment in which radiologists inject a sclerosing agent into a low-flow vascular malformation (such as a deforming birthmark), causing the swollen veins to constrict so that they can be safely

percutaneous *(cont.)*
and effectively injected. Magnetic resonance guidance helps with needle placement, determining how much therapeutic mixture is needed to fill the malformation, and monitoring the therapeutic agent as it is injected.

percutaneous Stoller afferent nerve stimulation system (PerQ SANS)—used for treatment of urge incontinence and urinary urgency and frequency. Employs low-frequency electrical stimulation delivered through a very fine gauge needle.

percutaneous transatrial mitral commissurotomy—nonsurgical technique for patients with rheumatic mitral stenosis.

percutaneous transhepatic cholangiography (PTC).

percutaneous transhepatic liver biopsy with tract embolization (PBTE).

percutaneous transluminal angioplasty (PTA).

percutaneous transluminal myocardial (or **transmyocardial**) **revascularization** (PTMR)—procedure using a laser to create pathways for oxygenated blood to feed ischemic (oxygen-starved) heart muscle.

percutaneous transluminal renal angioplasty (PTRA).

percutaneous transluminal septal myocardial ablation—used for patients with hypertrophic cardiomyopathy. It is a primary, sometimes familial, and genetically determined form of myocardial hypertrophy with a dynamic left ventricular outflow tract obstruction.

percutaneous transperineal seed implantation—a procedure to radiate prostatic cancer locally. Small seeds of iodine 15 or palladium 103 radioactive material are inserted into prostatic tissue. The procedure is said to be cost-effective and avoid systemic radiation effects.

percutaneous transvenous mitral commissurotomy (PTMC)—an alternative to open heart surgical mitral commissurotomy that uses catheterization techniques and uses a balloon catheter to dilate the mitral valve. Bifoil and trefoil balloons used for this procedure contain two or three balloons on a single shaft, requiring one transseptal puncture and one guidewire in the left ventricle rather than the two required for a usual two-balloon method. Single balloons are not usually adequate to dilate the mitral valve sufficiently. The shaft and tip of the bifoil and trefoil balloon catheters, however, are stiffer and make the procedure somewhat more difficult, with the greater risk of left ventricular perforation.

percutaneous umbilical cord blood sampling (PUBS).

PerDUCER pericardial access device—used for delivery of therapeutic agents inside the pericardium.

Pereyra needle—a single-prong ligature carrier for use in bladder neck suspension.

perf—slang for *tympanic membrane perforation*.

Perfan I.V. (enoximone)—a medication for the treatment of acute decompensated heart failure.

Perfecta hip prosthesis—provides anatomic proximal fit with wedge-shaped cross-section in sagittal, coronal, and transverse planes.

PerFixation screws—used in tendon graft repairs

PerFix hernioplasty.

PerFix Marlex mesh plug—a preformed Marlex mesh hernia plug consisting of a fluted outside layer combined with an inside arrangement of eight mesh petals that allow it to maintain an open conelike shape.

perfluoropropane (C_3F_8) **gas**—used in pneumatic retinopexy.

perforating folliculitis—suppurative plugging of pilosebaceous follicles.

perforating verruciform collagenoma—wartlike dermal hyperplasia with epidermal perforation of collagen.

perfusion—pouring a fluid over an organ or tissue, or through vessels of an organ; used in kidney and heart perfusion surgery, and organ transplantation. Cf. *profusion.*

perfusion pressure breakthrough syndrome, normal (in giant arteriovenous malformations).

perfusion-weighted imaging—ultrafast MRI technique that shows which parts of the brain are still alive after a stroke but are still vulnerable because they are being starved of blood. Results of these scans may determine whether neuroprotective drugs will be effective.

PERG (peak latencies of pattern electroretinogram).

periacetabular osteotomy (PAO).

periaqueductal gray electrode—not a proper name; it refers to the gray matter of the brain.

periarticular heterotopic ossification (PHO)—a complication of total hip arthroplasty in which ectopic bone growth occurs in the joint, causing decreased range of motion and pain. In severe cases, the head of the femur may actually become fused to the acetabulum. The cause is unknown. The Brooker system is used to classify PHO.

peribronchial cuffing—thickening of bronchial walls by fibrosis, as seen in asthma, emphysema, and other chronic respiratory disorders.

pericardial baffle.

pericardial well (*not* wall)—the space around the heart where iced saline slush is placed in coronary artery bypass graft surgery.

pericardium—the fibrous sac surrounding the heart and roots of the great vessels. Cf. *precordium.*

Periflow peripheral balloon catheters—used for angioplasty and the infusion of solutions to the peripheral vasculature.

Peri-Guard patch—see *CV Peri-Guard patch*.

perilunate fracture dislocation (PLFD).

perilymphatic fistula (PLF).

perimeter—circumference, edge. See *Humphrey frequency-doubling perimeter*. Cf. *parameter.*

Perimount RSR pericardial bioprosthesis—see *Carpentier-Edwards Perimount*.

perineal—refers to the perineum, the area between the scrotum and the anus in the male, and between the vulva and the anus in the female. Cf. *peritoneal, peroneal.*

perineal artery fasciocutaneous flaps—used in reconstructive surgery for stenotic vagina. Cf. *peroneal artery*.

perineal surgical apron—technique used in obstetrics and surgery.

perineurium—area surrounding nerves; fibrous connective tissue.

perinuclear antineutrophil cytoplasmic antibody (pANCA)—marker for ulcerative colitis.

perinuclear-type autoantibody against neutrophils (pANCA).

PerioChip—indicated as an adjunct to scaling and root-planing procedures in patients with adult periodontitis.

periodic acid-Schiff test (PAS stain)—a test for collagen or for presence of Whipple disease.

periodic lateralized epileptiform discharges (PLEDS)—found in electroencephalograms.

Periogard oral rinse.

periorbital infantile myofibromatosis—a lesion of the eyelid and medial canthus in an infant, treated with subtotal excision.

periosteal stripping—a procedure performed in children with limb-length discrepancy to increase the length of long bones.

peripheral access system (PAS) **port**—an implantable port positioned subcutaneously in the antecubital area of the arm. See *P.A.S. Port catheter*.

Peripheral AngioJet system—used to retrieve clots.

peripheral blood lymphocytes (PBLs).

peripheral blood stem cell (PBSC) **collections**.

peripheral bulging ring—relates to position of a foldable intraocular lens implant.

peripheral excimer laser angioplasty (PELA).

peripheral laser angioplasty (PLA).

peripherally inserted catheter (PIC)—intravenous catheter for long-term venous access in patients cared for at home or in nursing homes.

peripherally inserted central catheter (PICC).

peripheral MR angiography—utilizes a combination of ultrafast high-resolution imaging sequences, a panoramic table, and a special peripheral coil to allow coverage from the renal arteries to the vessels in the feet, all in one scan.

peripheral percutaneous interventions (PPI)—the use of endovascular procedures such as percutaneous transluminal angioplasty for peripheral artery disease as opposed to surgical bypass procedures.

peripheral scatter photocoagulation—for treatment of neovascularization of the vitreous base.

peripheral vestibular deficits (PVD).

peristaltic wave—a wave of muscular contractions passing along a tubular organ (such as the esophagus or intestines), by which its contents are advanced.

Peri-Strips Dry—thin strips of bovine pericardium sutured to a backing material and used to overlap staple lines. Used in lung resection procedures and other soft tissue repairs.

peritomy—an incision of the conjunctiva and the subconjunctival tissues, going around the entire corneal circumference. Used in cataract extractions, retinal detachment procedures, and enucleation. *Not* peridimy or peridomy.

peritoneal—refers to the peritoneum, the serous membrane lining the abdominal and pelvic cavities. Cf. *perineal, peroneal.*

peritoneal dialysis (PD).

peritonealize—to cover with peritoneum. Also, see *peritonize.*

peritoneal leaves.

peritoneal melanosis—due to a ruptured ovarian dermoid cyst.

peritoneal mouse (Radiol)—a free body sometimes seen on x-ray in the peritoneal cavity.

peritoneography—magnetic resonance imaging of the peritoneal cavity. Imaging agent is instilled into the peritoneal cavity, magnetic resonance scanning is performed with the peritoneal cavity filled, and after complete drainage of the contrast

peritoneography *(cont.)* material, scan is again performed. Images are reviewed for evidence of peritoneal leaks, hernias, loculated fluid collections, and adhesions. MR peritoneography is particularly useful in patients using continuous ambulatory peritoneal dialysis.

peritoneum—serous membrane lining the abdomen.

peritonize—to cover with peritoneum. See *peritonealize.*

periurethral collagen injection—for the control of urinary incontinence in patients not responding to conservative therapy and who refuse surgery.

perivitelline space—the area around the yolk of an oocyte. Via a microinjection technique, sperm may be injected into the perivitelline space for in vitro fertilization.

Perkins Brailler—a braille embosser.

Perkins tonometer—measures intraocular pressure.

PERK (prospective evaluation of radial keratotomy) **protocol**—for correction of myopia.

Perlane (animal hyaluronic acid)—a wrinkle treatment similar to Restylane, only larger in size; therefore, it takes longer to dissipate. Perlane is usually reserved for deep facial lines in the nasolabial and glabellar regions. The treatment lasts from three months to a year.

perlèche—another term for cheilitis, or dryness and cracking around the mouth, from repeated licking or from a Candida infection.

Perlon suture (size 10-0)—a very fine (narrow) suture used in eye surgery.

PERM (Piattaforma Elettropneumatica per Riabilitazione Motoria)—developed in Italy. The English translation would be the Electropneumatic Platform for Motor Rehabilitation, but the PERM abbreviation will no doubt be used. It is a device that can be used in the treatment of the lower limbs to provide the patient with controlled and quantifiable mechanical stimuli, thus enabling the therapist to adopt a more rigorous approach to treatment even in the very early stages of rehabilitation. Alternatively, the system can be used in a different operating mode as a normal biofeedback system capable of displaying on-screen the extent to which voluntary load has been transferred to the lower limb.

Permacol injection (injectable porcine dermal collagen matrix)—a treatment composed of cryogenically milled porcine dermal collagen matrix suspended in a saline carrier for ease of injection. Permacol Injection is intended as a urethral bulking agent for urinary incontinence but is used off-label for cosmetic soft tissue augmentation. Permacol is presented in prefilled 2.5 mL syringes and is composed of 60 mg/mL of porcine collagen.

Perma-Flow coronary bypass graft —synthetic blood vessel designed to be used in place of harvesting the patient's own blood vessels for bypass grafting. This graft can be implanted and the bypass procedure completed without having to stop the beating heart and place the patient on full coronary bypass.

Perma-Hand braided silk suture.

PermaMesh—a sheet of hydroxyapatite particles woven on absorbable suture material. This material can be molded and is used to hold graft

PermaMesh *(cont.)* material in place prior to wound closure.

permanent brachytherapy—Encapsulated radioactive "seeds" are inserted directly into a tumor, through needles, during the operative procedure. The radioactive material will deliver radiation over a few months, but will not be removed; it will gradually decay until it becomes basically inert. Low-energy radionuclides such as iodine 125 (^{125}I) and palladium 135 (^{135}Pd) are used.

permanent section (*paraffin section*; *paraffin block*)—technique in which tissue removed in an operation is embedded in paraffin for microscopic examination of the pathology present. This takes more time than frozen section but has certain advantages in that the specimen is permanent and not deteriorating, as in frozen section. Cf. *frozen section.*

Perma-Seal dialysis access graft.

PermCath—double-lumen ventricular access catheter.

Perneczky aneurysm clip—has an inverted spring mechanism to facilitate visual control during clip application.

pernio, perniosis—an inflammatory disease of the skin of the arms and legs, triggered by prolonged exposure to cold temperature. The disorder is characterized by painful, itchy skin lesions on the lower legs, hands, toes, feet, ears and face. The lesions usually last for 2-3 weeks.

peroneal—refers to the fibula or to the outer side of the leg and the muscles, nerves, and vessels thereof, the peroneus longus and the peroneus brevis. Cf. *perineal, peritoneal.*

peroxidase-antiperoxidase (PAP).

per primam (*not* primum)—first intention; primary union; healing directly, without granulation; the incision closes in minimal time, with no complications and with little resulting scar tissue.

Per-Q-Cath—peripherally inserted central catheter.

PerQ SANS (percutaneous Stoller afferent nerve stimulation system).

Persantine (dipyridamole) **thallium stress test**—a chemical equivalent of the treadmill stress test. It measures EKG reading, blood pressure, and heart rate in response to exertion on people who are not able to undergo a treadmill test. A small amount of radioactive thallium is injected IV (about as much radioactivity as you would get from a chest x-ray). The thallium is carried to the heart, at which point a scanning device demonstrates which areas of the heart are not getting sufficient blood.

"per-say"—phonetic for *per se.*

per se ("per-say")—a Latin expression meaning of, in, or by itself or oneself, intrinsically. Usage: "This statement is interesting per se." "Life per se is precious."

persistent hyperplastic primary vitreous (PHPV).

persistent vegetative state (PVS).

Persona monitoring kit—a combination ovulation-prediction monitoring kit and birth control system. By testing hormones excreted in a woman's urine, the monitoring kit indicates a green light when pregnancy risk is low and a red light on the days she is at risk of becoming pregnant. It reportedly has a 95% accuracy rate, about the same as condoms.

person with AIDS (PWA)—term preferred over "AIDS victim" in AIDS self-help and awareness groups.

PERV (porcine endogenous retrovirus).

pes anserine bursitis—occurs in elderly women with osteoarthritis. It can be treated with anti-inflammatory medication and drainage if necessary. It may be associated with anserine bursitis syndrome.

petal-fugal flow. Usage: "Angiography (for esophageal varices) was performed and showed petal-fugal flow." Also, *mixed petal-fugal flow*. See *hepatopetal* and *hepatofugal flow*.

petaling the cast—taping the edge of a rough or crumbling cast with short strips of tape or moleskin in overlapping fashion so that it looks like a series of petals.

petechia (pl., petechiae)—tiny, pinpoint round red spot caused by intradermal or submucous hemorrhage.

petit pas ("petty-pah") (Fr., small step) **gait**. Usage: "His gait was petit pas, but was otherwise normal."

PETS (percutaneous epiphysiodesis using transphyseal screws).

PET (positron emission tomography) **scan**—uses deoxyglucose to distinguish tumor from necrosis.

PET with 3-D SSP—helpful in accurate assessment of Alzheimer disease.

Peutz-Jeghers ("puts-JAY-gerz") **syndrome** (PJS)—a rare autosomal dominantly inherited disorder characterized by predisposition to hamartomatous intestinal polyposis, mucocutaneous pigmentation, and various other neoplasms.

Peyer (rhymes with *flyer*) **patches**—elevated areas of closely packed lymphoid nodules on the mucosa of the small intestine.

Peyman intraocular forceps—with the functional capabilities of forceps, pick, and scissors.

Peyman vitrector—used in cataract extraction.

PFC Sigma—total knee system.

PFCI—see *permanent focal cerebral ischemia*.

PFC (press-fit component) **total hip system**—has a porous-coated stem.

Pfeiffer-Comberg method—used radiographically to locate a foreign body in the eye.

p53 adenoviral gene—mutation of which is responsible for many types of malignant tumors. See *Advexin*.

p55-IgG—p55 tumor necrosis factor receptor fusion protein.

PF (parafascicular) **nucleus** (Neuro).

PFS (pelvic floor electrical stimulation).

PFT (parafascicular thalamotomy).

PFTE (polyfluorotetraethylene)—plastic graft material; shunt.

PG (percutaneous gastrostomy)—radiologic alternative to surgical and endoscopic gastrostomy. See *PGE*.

PGD (preimplantation genetic diagnosis).

PGE (percutaneous gastroenterostomy).

PGGO—see *pure ground glass opacity*.

PGH (placental growth hormone).

PGK (Panos G. Koutrouvelis, M.D) **stereotactic device**—floor-mounted stereotactic device that allows accurate insertion of the Nucleotome aspiration probe at the L5-S1 level for percutaneous lumbar diskectomy.

P-glycoprotein (also known as *P-170 glycoprotein)*—a substance present in some types of cancer cells. When present, it enables those cells to expel chemotherapy drugs and resist their cytotoxic effects. Cancer patients with P-glycoprotein positive

P-glycoprotein *(cont.)* cells (leukemia, multiple myeloma, non-Hodgkin lymphoma, and renal cell carcinoma) respond poorly to chemotherapy regimens. The P-glycoprotein efflux mechanism has been found to be inactivated by certain calcium channel blocking drugs that allow the chemotherapy agent to enter the cancer cell and be more effectively cytotoxic. See *calcium channel blockers.*

PgR (progesterone receptor).

PGs (prostaglandins)—lipid molecules derived from fatty acids. Prostaglandins, which are technically hormones but seldom described as such, are found in virtually all tissues and have a wide variety of actions; most cause muscular contraction and mediate inflammation. Synthetic PGs are used to induce childbirth (PGE2 or PGF2, with mifepristone); to close a patent ductus arteriosus in the newborn; to prevent and treat peptic ulcer (PGE); as a vasodilator in severe Raynaud phenomenon or ischemia of a limb; and in pulmonary hypertension. Usage: "PGs at 0.1 mcg/k were prescribed."

PGX (PolyGlycopleX).

pH—the measure of the relative balance between the acids and bases in a system. It has to do with the hydrogen ions in solutions, such as urine or serum. The normal pH of arterial blood is between 7.35 and 7.45. A pH below 7.0 or greater than 7.8 is not compatible with life. See *intracellular pH* (pHi).

PHA (phytohemagglutinin antigen)—a skin test for cellular-based immunity (not antibodies).

PHA (progressive hemifacial atrophy).

PHACE syndrome—neurocutaneous syndrome consisting of:
posterior fossa brain malformations,
hemangiomas
arterial anomalies
coarctation of the aorta and cardiac defects
eye abnormalities

phacoblade.

PhacoFlex II SI-30NB—foldable intraocular lens implant. See also *Single-Stitch inserter for PhacoFlex lens.*

Phadiatop test—a system for testing the blood to more quickly diagnose the cause of cold or allergy symptoms. Results of the yes/no test are available within a few hours.

phage typing of organisms.

phage virus—a virus that infects and destroys bacteria.

phagocyte ("eating cell")—a cell which consumes other cells or foreign material.

Phalen maneuver—to determine presence of carpal tunnel syndrome. See *Phalen sign.*

Phalen sign (*not* Phelan)—in carpal tunnel syndrome. Phalen sign is present when paresthesias are produced or are exaggerated when the wrist is held in complete flexion for 30 seconds, which presses the median nerve against the upper edge of the transverse carpal ligament.

Phaneuf ("fan-oof") **clamp**.

Phantom cardiac guidewire.

phantom limb pain—pain felt by the patient in an already-amputated limb, as though the limb were still there.

Phantom nasal mask—CPAP mask with built-in exhalation port. The mask conforms to the patient's face and minimizes leaks caused by facial hair and/or body movement.

phantoms—artificial human tissue models used to test the performance of medical imaging equipment by mimicking the radiation attenuation and absorption properties of human tissue. They are also used to measure radiation dosage during therapy, for teaching purposes, and to calibrate equipment and for research.

Phantom V Plus catheter—dilating catheter used in common bile duct dilation and stone extraction.

Pharm.D. (Doctor of Pharmacy). *Not* "form D."

pharyngeal flap-pushback procedure—for repair of velopharyngeal insufficiency. The pharyngeal flap is put into the nasal pushback raw area between the hard palate and the soft palate to keep the velum from being pulled forward by scar contraction.

pharaonic circumcision—a form of female genital mutilation. See *infibulation.*

pharmacogenetics—the branch of medical genetics that studies genetically controlled variations in responses to drugs.

pharmacogenomics—the study of small genetic differences that help explain why some people respond positively to a drug, while others do not respond or experience adverse side effects.

pharmacokinetic parameters.

pharmapsychological—pertaining to psychological responses to pharmaceutical substances. Usage: "Axis IV: Pharmapsychological factors: chemical dependency."

PharmaSeed (palladium Pd 103 seeds)—radioactive ^{103}Pd seeds/implants used in brachytherapy for the treatment of prostate cancer.

PharmChek—sweat patch drug detection system.

phased-array study—inaccurate term for *phase image*, which is a form of gated blood pool study especially processed so that a little more information is obtained from it. See *gated blood (pool) cardiac.*

phase image—MRI term. See *phased array study.*

phase sensitive detector—MRI term.

pHEMA keratoprosthesis—synthetic cornea with a spongy skirt that increases the rate of cellular invasion and incorporation of the artificial cornea. The manufacturing design process creates an intimate bond between the spongy rim and the transparent central optic zone.

Phemister-type epiphysiodesis—an operative procedure for leg length discrepancy. Also, *Phemister epiphysiodesis.*

phen-fen—see *fen-phen diet.*

phenocopy (Genetics)—a phenotype, occurring accidentally as a consequence of the interaction of a given genotype and an extraneous factor, that closely resembles one normally associated with a different genotype.

Phenoptin (sapropterin hydrochloride)—a small oral molecule therapeutic for the treatment of the genetic disease phenylketonuria (PKU).

phenotype—see *Cellano phenotype, McLeod phenotype.*

phenotype (Genetics)—the sum of observable or measurable physical, biochemical, and physiologic traits or features of an individual; determined in large measure by the genotype, but distinct from it.

phenoxodiol—a broad-spectrum anticancer drug, able to stop the growth of a wide range of human cancers.

pherogram—electrophoretic pattern.

pheromones—sexual odors which play an important part in insect, mammalian, and perhaps human reproductive behavior.

PHG (portal hypertensive gastropathy).

pHi (intracellular pH).

Philadelphia (Ph1) **chromosome**—a translocation from chromosome number 22 to chromosome number 9. The Philadelphia chromosome is found in the adult form of chronic myeloid leukemia. Usage: "A bone biopsy will be done, with Philadelphia chromosome cytogenic analysis."

Philips Tomoscan SR 6000 CT scanner.

Philos DR pacemaker.

phlegm—see *Flimm Fighter*.

phlyctenule ("flick-ten'-yule")—small nodular lesion found at the edge of the cornea; thought to be a cause of neovascularization.

PHN (postherpetic neuralgia).

PHO (periarticular heterotopic ossification).

Phocas syndrome (also, Tillaux-Phocas)—see *fibrocystic breast syndrome*.

PH-1 (primary hyperoxaluria, type 1).

phonocardiography—noninvasive cardiac diagnostic procedure which tests the occurrence, timing, and duration of the various sounds in the cardiac cycle, determines the frequency (cycles per second) and intensity (amplitude), and demonstrates murmurs in low frequencies that can be missed by the ear.

PhorMax CR (computed radiography) **system**—a desktop workstation that integrates several radiology functions and that can be integrated into a picture archiving system.

Phoropter (*not* Foreopter)—American Optical Company refractor.

phosphatidylglycerol levels—present with pulmonary maturity in a premature infant; levels decrease with lung maturity.

PhotacFil (Dentistry)—a light-cured, resin-modified glass ionomer material used to fill an access cavity made for root canal surgery.

photic stimulation—flashing light stimulation, used in EEG testing.

photoablative refractive keratectomy (PRK)—alternative to radial keratotomy. Also, *phototherapeutic keratectomy*.

photoaged—premature aging process induced by overexposure to the sun, i.e., photoaged skin.

photoangioplasty—a treatment for atherosclerotic arteries that uses laser light to activate a photosensitive plaque-dissolving agent.

photoastigmatic refractive keratectomy (PARK).

photocatalytic air filtration system—uses light that reacts with a chemical catalyst to kill microbes, dust mites, and mold.

photocrosslinking oligonucleotide hybridization assay.

PhotoDerm—a computer-based machine that uses bright light similar to a camera's flashbulb to destroy spider veins by delivering controlled doses of light through a special handpiece. *PhotoDerm PL* is used to treat benign pigmented lesions (age spots, liver spots, freckles, birthmarks, melasma, hyperpigmentation, and tattoos), and *PhotoDerm VL* is used to treat noninvasive treatment of leg veins and other benign vascular lesions.

photodynamic therapy (PDT)—cancer treatment modality that utilizes light-activated drugs in combination with laser light sources to create highly reactive forms of oxygen that cause destruction of cancerous cells. Also called *light-activated therapy*. It is also used to treat age-related macular degeneration.

photo epilation—use of light energy through the surface of the skin to destroy follicles (or roots) of unwanted hair.

PhotoGenica V-Star—a pulsed-dye laser capable of treating a full range of vascular conditions, from therapeutic to cosmetic.

photometer—see *HemoCue photometer.*

photomotogram—timed Achilles tendon reflex.

Photon cataract removal system—uses ultrasonic phacoemulsification.

photon correlation spectroscopy—see *SpectRx*.

Photon DR dual-chamber implantable cardioverter-defibrillator.

photon stimulation therapy (PST)—the use of a low-energy level, cold soft-light laser on acupuncture points in the treatment of chronic pain and also to help patients quit smoking.

photonic stimulator—device that uses infrared light to penetrate the skin and promote increased blood flow and circulation. It reportedly has benefited some patients suffering from nervous system disorders such as complex regional pain syndrome, reflex dystrophy, and radiculopathy. Not to be confused with photic stimulation, used for EEG studies.

Photon Radiosurgery System (PRS)—x-ray delivery system for tumor therapy. Formerly approved only for treatment to the brain, the system is now FDA-approved for radiation therapy treatments anywhere in the body.

photopenic area—a coined word for the light area on a film or scan.

photophobia—unusual intolerance of light.

photophoresis—treatment used for cutaneous T-cell lymphoma, a rare immune system cancer. The patient is given doses of psoralen (a light-activated drug) orally. The patient is attached to a device that takes blood from one arm, separates the white cells from the red, and then exposes the white cells to a kind of ultraviolet light. The light-activated psoralen damages the cancerous white cells, which are then reinfused into the patient's other arm. After a few days, the cancerous white cells die. The treatment is repeated at intervals, and over a period of time the patient's immune system will be able to overcome the remaining infected white blood cells. See *psoralen*.

Photopic Imaging—ultrasound system that enhances visual acuity and helps clinicians more easily see signs of cancer or stroke.

PhotoPoint—laser therapy for exudative age-related macular degeneration. It seals leaking blood vessels in the macula without creating scar tissue that interferes with central vision.

photopsia—subjective sensation of sparks or flashes of light in retinal or optic diseases.

photorefractive keratectomy (PRK)—a procedure using computer-guided excimer laser ablation to reprofile the anterior corneal curvature in order to correct myopia. It is believed capable of correcting low and

photorefractive *(cont.)* moderate myopic errors with a relatively high degree of accuracy and safety. See also *LASIK* and *T-PRK.*

photostimulable luminescence intensity—the higher the intensity, the better the radiographic image.

phototherapeutic keratectomy (PTK) —removal of anterior corneal pathology with the excimer laser.

photothermal sclerosis—method of treating varicose veins that are resistant to standard medical techniques, using a laser-like photothermal device.

Photrex (rostaporfin)—drug for treatment of wet age-related macular degeneration.

PHPV (persistent hyperplastic primary vitreous).

PHT (portal hypertension).

phthalocyanine ("thay-lo-cy-a-neen") —photosensitizing agent used in laser surgery.

phthisis ("ty-sis")—a wasting of part of the body. See *ptosis.*

phthisis bulbi—shrinkage and wasting of the eyeball.

phycobiliproteins—fluorescent pigments used in immunological diagnostic products.

phycomycosis—see *mucormycosis.*

Phylax AV—dual chamber implantable cardioverter-defibrillator.

physician-assisted suicide (PAS).

Physio Partner support mechanism —a support mechanism in the nature of a boom arm used to support a device used in the treatment of lung disease.

Physios CTM 01—noninvasive cardiac transplant monitoring system. It monitors the electrophysiologic performance of a transplanted heart to assist in the detection of acute allograft rejection.

Physio-Stim Lite—a bone growth stimulator used to promote healing of non-united fractures.

phytochemicals—natural substances found in certain foods (wild blueberries, cruciferous vegetables) that are believed to have cancer-fighting and anti-aging properties.

phytohemagglutinin antigen (PHA)—a plant product used for testing human T-cell response. An absent PHA response indicates an abnormally functioning T-cell system.

phytostanol, phytosterol—plant substances found in herbal products that have been shown in clinical studies to be effective in lowering cholesterol levels by blocking absorption.

phytosterolemia—condition in patients on total parenteral nutrition (TPN), thought possibly to be a factor in the development of cholestatic liver disease, which often occurs in patients on TPN.

phytotherapy—treatment using plants.

PIC (peripherally inserted catheter).

PIC (plasmin inhibitor complex).

pica—eating of materials not usually considered edible or nourishing (e.g., starch, dirt, clay, paint), usual ly by pregnant women or malnourished children. Cf. *PICA.*

PICA (posterior inferior communicating artery). Cf. *pica.*

Picasso phone—an innovative medical teleconferencing device. Physicians can send high-quality still images of patients and their medical conditions over standard analog phone lines, while simultaneously talking to the doctors on the other end of the connection. The phone on the sending end connects to a standard camcorder and to either a TV or PC

Picasso *(cont.)* screen. Using a computer mouse, the doctor can point out areas of interest.

PICC (peripherally inserted central catheter)—inserted into the cephalic or basilic vein in the arm and threaded into the superior vena cava. Made of silicone rubber (which is soft, flexible, durable, and reduces the risk of thrombosis). Use PIC catheter, *not* PICC catheter.

Piccolo blood chemistry analyzer system.

Picker Magnascanner—scintigraphy equipment to detect skeletal metastases.

Picket Fence leg positioner.

Pick inclusion body—found in Pick disease.

picornavirus—extremely small, ether-resistant RNA virus, one of the group comprising the enteroviruses and the rhinoviruses.

Pico-ST II—low-profile balloon catheter used in percutaneous transluminal coronary angioplasty (PTCA) procedures.

Picture Archiving and Communications Systems (PACS)—an integrated information system that facilitates the practice of radiology and teleradiology. It includes, but is not limited to, picture archiving and voice reporting.

picture element (pixel)—MRI term.

PID (primary immune deficiency).

Pierre Robin ("Ro-ban") **sequence**—a combination of birth defects which usually include the lower jaw being small in size (micrognathia) or set back from the upper jaw (retrognathia), cleft palate but not cleft lip, and a tendency for the tongue to "ball up" in the back of the mouth where it can obstruct the airway. Also *Pierre Robin complex*. Based on the various features or causes of the disease, Pierre Robin sequence or complex is considered to be more appropriate than the other names applied to the same condition—Pierre Robin syndrome, Pierre Robin triad, and Robin anomalad. Cf. *micrognathia-glossoptosis syndrome*.

Pierse tip forceps.

PIE (pulmonary infiltrates with eosinophilia) **syndrome**—adverse drug reaction to nonsteroidal anti-inflammatory drug. Suspected upper respiratory infections with fever, malaise, and pulmonary infiltrates may actually be PIE syndrome.

piezo electrical stimulator—used to stimulate acupuncture sites with small electrical shock.

Piezolith-EPL (extracorporeal piezoelectric lithotriptor).

Pigg-O-Stat (Radiol)—proprietary device resembling a clear plastic high chair that enables chest x-rays to be taken of very young children. It has two clear plastic doors; the child is placed inside and the arms raised so the doors will close and the arms will be out of the field of view of the chest. Without this device, the child's parent may be exposed to radiation when trying to keep the child's arms out of the field.

piggyback, piggybacking—a method by which more than one solution, and medication, can be infused simultaneously by introducing additional intravenous lines to the main solution line. Also, *piggyback probe*.

pigment dispersion syndrome (PDS) —a common cause of glaucoma in young adults; it is most often seen in myopic Caucasian males.

pigskin graft—see *porcine xenograft.*

pigtail catheter.

PIH (pregnancy-induced hypertension).

pike-jawed forceps—see *serrated ear-vessel forceps.*

Pilates ("puh-LAH-tees") **method of exercise**—a method of physical therapy, developed originally for bedridden patients in WWI prison camps. The method restores muscular balance in the bedridden, improves posture, eliminates muscular and soft tissue pain, and builds strength and flexibility. Dancers, athletes, actors, and singers have used it to refine strength, balance, and coordination.

pillar pain—pain in the sides of the palm caused by a vertical septum of scar tissue that can result from open carpal tunnel release.

pillar palatal restoration procedure —see *palatal implant*.

pill burden—a reference to medication regimens in which the patient is on numerous different medications.

PillCam video capsule—video endoscopy imaging for detecting disease in the small bowel as well as the esophagus.

Pillet hand prosthesis.

Pilling Weck Y-stent forceps—used for bronchoscopic inset of tracheobronchial stents.

pillion fracture—a T-shaped fracture involving the distal femur, and posterior displacement of the condyles, caused by a severe blow to the knee. Usage: "The patient is now status post grade II open fracture of the left tibia, with an ipsilateral minimally displaced left pillion fracture which was treated immediately following his injury."

pill-rolling tremor—involuntary rhythmic opposing movements, or circular rolling motion, of the thumb and index finger, characteristic of Parkinson disease.

pilocarpine iontophoresis method—to measure sweat chloride levels. An elevated level of chloride in perspiration is a sign of cystic fibrosis.

pilomatrix carcinoma—a rare, low-grade malignant lesion arising from hair cortex cells, with a tendency to recur. It usually occurs as a solitary lesion on the head, neck, extremities, or trunk (in decreasing order).

pilosebaceous unit—the combination of a hair follicle with its oil gland, considered as an anatomic unit.

Pilot audiometer—used for screening of hearing disorders in preschool children.

Pilot suturing guide—used to aid in closure of laparoscopic incisions.

PIMS (programmable implantable medication system).

PIN (percutaneous interosseous nerve) (Hand Surg).

Pinard sign—in pregnancy, pain on pressure over the uterine fundus, after the sixth month. An indication of possible breech presentation.

PINC—polymer system for the delivery of gene-based products to muscle.

pincer grasp—the use of the forefinger and thumb to pick up small objects, such as beads or coins.

pinchcock mechanism—at the esophagogastric junction.

pineal apoplexy—a stroke due to a pineal cavernous hemangioma. The recommended treatment is total removal of the causative lesion to prevent repeated bleeding or life-threatening massive hemorrhage.

PINES (paracrine, immune, neural, and endocrine systems)—an acronym devised by Joseph H. Sellin, M.D. It determines how the gut responds to a specific challenge in an attempt to maintain homeostasis.

ping-pong fracture—an actual fracture or simply a concavity and depression in the skull, resembling the indentation that results from pressure by the fingers on a ping-pong ball.

ping-ponging—repeatedly reinfecting each other, when sexual partners are not treated simultaneously for a sexually transmitted infection.

pinguecula—a degenerative lesion of the conjunctiva appearing as a yellowish nodule near the limbus.

pin headrest (Neuro).

pinked up (verb) (Cardio).

pinkeye—any condition causing hyperemia of one or both eyes; usually, bacterial or viral conjunctivitis.

pink puffer—a patient with early respiratory failure, showing dyspnea but no cyanosis. Cf. *blue bloater.*

pink tetralogy of Fallot—tetralogy of Fallot with only mild cyanosis, mild pulmonary stenosis, and left-to-right shunt, and with the pulmonary pressure higher than normal. See *tetralogy of Fallot*. Cf. *Fallot trilogy, Fallot pentalogy.*

Pinky—see *Super Pinky.*

Pinn-ACL guide system—used to simplify and refine the posterior-entry ACL reconstruction.

Pinpoint stereotactic arm—used to deliver radioactive seed implants for CT-guided brachytherapy.

Pins sign—disappearance of pleuritic pain when the patient assumes a knee-chest position.

Pipelle endometrial suction catheter—used for endometrial dating, cancer screening, and monitoring the effects of hormone treatment.

pipestem sheathing—the appearance created by lipid deposition along retinal arterioles.

PIPIDA scan—a technetium ^{99m}Tc-PIPIDA hepatobiliary scan used in acute cholecystitis.

pip-tazo or **pip-taz**—slang for piperacillin and tazobactam given in combination.

Pisces spinal cord stimulation system—electrical stimulation of nerve structures, delivered by percutaneously implanted epidural electrodes.

pisotriquetral joint—in the area of the flexor carpi ulnaris.

piston stapes prosthesis—placed in the middle of the stapedectomy opening and crimped onto the long process of the incus, with the other end in an opening in the posterior-central portion of the footplate. This technique is said to bring back the normal vibratory performance of the ossicular chain.

PITA (powered intracapsular tonsillectomy and adenoidectomy) **surgery**—is said to offer significant advantages to most patients, including less postoperative pain, a faster recovery from surgery, and a faster return to normal activity.

Pit-assisted delivery—slang; transcribe as *Pitocin-assisted delivery*.

Pitié-Salpetrière saphenous vein hook—used to retract the saphenous vein while clipping and ligating branches and to provide tension during dissection.

pitting edema—on firm finger pressure, a depression lasts for several minutes; due to fluid retention.

Pittman IMA retractor system—for use in coronary artery bypass surgery.

Pittsburgh Sleep Quality Index—for evaluation of effects of obstructive sleep apnea.

Pitt talking tracheostomy tube—used in patients with ventilator-dependent quadriplegia with severe phrenic nerve damage.

pituitary (hypophyseal) **stalk distortion** (PSD)—seen on MRI scan.

PIV (primary immune deficiency).

pivot-shift sign; **test** (Ortho).

Pixie minilaparoscope—a small laparoscope that is said to adapt to any video camera system.

Pixsys FlashPoint—a 3-D digitizer used in image-guided surgery.

pizza lung—a finding on pathologic examination of a lung that has sustained damage to the point where it resembles pizza.

PJC (premature junctional contraction) (Cardio).

PLA (peripheral laser angioplasty).

PLA (pyogenic liver abscess).

PLAATO (percutaneous left atrial appendage transcatheter occlusion).

placebo ("plah-see'bo")—see *Obecalp*, which is *placebo* spelled backwards. *Placebo* is Latin for "I will please."

placental alkaline phosphatase test (PLAP)—elevated in patients with seminomas and nonseminomatous malignant germ cell tumors. PLAP may be useful as a serum marker in patients undergoing treatment for one of these tumors to determine progression or regression of the tumor. PLAP is elevated in smokers, so that must be taken into consideration in determining the usefulness of this test in those patients.

placental growth hormone (PGH)—a hormone that appears to have important implications for physiologic adjustment to gestation and in control of maternal insulin-like growth factor 1 levels. PGH is not detectable in fetal circulation.

PLAC test—a method of predicting risk for development of congestive heart disease.

plafond—the undersurface of a plateau, as in tibial plafond.

plain—simple, open, clear; used often in *plain film*, a radiographic study performed without contrast medium, as differentiated from contrast studies and tomograms. Cf. *plane*.

planar spin imaging—MRI term.

plane—a specified level, as the plane of anesthesia; also, an anatomical area between two tissue layers where an incision may be placed. Cf. *plain*.

PLA-I—a platelet antigen. This protein is sometimes lacking on the surface of platelets in patients who have received red cell transfusions from donors who are PLA-I positive, causing severe bleeding, and may also cause post-transfusion purpura.

plasma cell mastitis—see *duct ectasia*.

plasma expander—see *artificial blood*.

plasma F—another term for *cortisol*.

PlasmaGel (patient-derived plasma emulsion with vitamin C complex) —an injectable treatment for wrinkles.

plasmapheresis—removal of plasma from blood taken from the patient, with retransfusion of the solid elements (red cells, platelets) into the patient. May be used for therapeutic purposes or for laboratory studies. Note the different root words in plasma**pheresis** and electro**phoresis**. Cf. *electrophoresis*.

Plasma Scalpel—a cutting tool used in uvulopalatopharyngoplasty (UPPP) and tonsillectomy. It operates at temperatures between 40-70°C,

Plasma *(cont.)*
minimizing the thermal effect on surrounding tissue.

plasma spray stem—a titanium plasma spray-coated prosthesis used in hip replacement surgery.

plasma thromboplastin component (PTC) in bleeding diseases.

plasmids—pieces of double-stranded circular DNA outside chromosomes, thought to be responsible for bacterial resistance.

Plastibell—used in circumcising infants.

plasticity—the ability of stem cells from one adult tissue to differentiate into mature cell types of another tissue.

Plasti-Pore—porous, high-density polyethylene material employed for the fabrication of ossicular replacement prostheses in otolaryngology, and for other grafts. It is used in the same way as Proplast. Cf. *Proplast*.

Plastiport TORP (total ossicular replacement prosthesis) (ENT).

Plastizote collar (Ortho).

Plast-O-Fit thermoplastic bandage system.

plate bender (Ortho)—used to bend dynamic compression plates. See *DCP*.

platelet antigen—see *PLA-I*.

platelet-derived growth factor—may be applied topically to aid healing in chronic, nonhealing wounds.

platelet membrane fluidity, increased—a biological risk factor for Alzheimer disease.

platform posturography—used with other vestibular tests for patients with peripheral vestibular deficits, Ménière disease, benign paroxysmal positional vertigo, and central nervous system vestibular impairment. Note: *Posturography* is a word related to *posture*, not urography, which is radiography of the urinary tract.

platinum coil—used in interventional neuroradiology in a nonsurgical repair of aneurysms in inoperable areas of the brain.

platyrrhine nose—a broad or flat nose (*platy-* meaning broad, flat). This term is somewhat redundant, as *rhine* means *nose*; nevertheless, it is dictated.

platysmaplasty—see *corset platysmaplasty.*

PLC-55 stapling device.

PLD (perilunate dislocations) (Ortho).

PLE (protein-losing enteropathy).

Pleatman sac—a rigid plastic sac used in laparoscopic procedures to isolate stones, bile, suspicious or infected tissue to prevent contamination. Prevents loss of specimen and avoids contamination of abdominal wall.

pledgets—usually cotton. Cotton balls (sponges), rolled so that they have somewhat pointed ends; used to absorb blood or fluids at the operative site. In some parts of the country they are called "pollywogs."

PLEDs (periodic lateralized epileptiform discharges)—in electroencephalogram.

PlegiaGuard—safety device to prevent dangerous overpressure by inadvertent occlusion of cardioplegia line.

pleiotropy (Genetics)—the capacity of a gene or gene pair to produce more than one effect or elicit more than one trait.

plesiotherapy—the same as brachytherapy. See *brachytherapy.*

pleural—refers to the pleura, the serous membrane lining each half of the thorax: pleural cavity, pleural effusion. Cf. *plural.*

pleural effusion—an abnormal accumulation of fluid in the pleural cavity, as seen on chest x-ray.

pleural tent—constructed apically by incising the thickened parietal pleura, bluntly dissecting it from the chest wall, and allowing it to drop down to the upper surface of the remaining tissue. Used where there are diffuse air leaks or where a significant residual pleural space is present following lung surgery.

Pleur-evac suction.

PlexiPulse—postsurgical device that reduces incidence of deep vein thrombosis and postoperative edema, thereby promoting wound healing.

Plexus mattress—a brand of air mattresses used in wound management therapy.

plexus of ganglion impar—plexus interiliacus; also impar hypogastric plexus or plexus hypogastricus impar.

plexus of Santorini.

PLF (perilymphatic fistula).

PLF (posterolateral fusion).

PLFD (perilunate fracture dislocation).

plica (pl., plicae)—ridge, fold, band, or shelf of synovial tissue, as in the transverse suprapatellar, medial suprapatellar, mediopatellar, and infrapatellar plicae. These usually cause few problems, but occasionally are large enough to become symptomatic and may require surgical intervention. See *plicectomy*.

plicectomy ("ply-kek´to-me")—excision of a plica. See *plica*.

PLIF (posterior lumbar interbody fusion)—approach for surgical treatment of spondylolisthesis and segmental instability. Cf. *TLIF*.

P listening—see *A, P, T, M*.

PLK (posterior lamellar keratoplasty)—see *endothelial lamellar keratoplasty*.

PLL (posterior longitudinal ligament)—of the spine and spinal cord.

plombage ("plom-bahzh")—as in bone or chest plombage, the surgical filling of an empty space in the body with an inert material such as methylmethacrylate.

plop, tumor—heard with cardiac tumors on auscultation.

PLT (posterior lamellar transplantation)—see *endothelial lamellar keratoplasty*.

plugged liver biopsy—used in patients with impaired coagulation.

Plum-Blossom needle—used for acupuncture.

Plummer-Vinson syndrome—characterized by dysphagia, iron-deficiency anemia, and esophageal webs. Associated with an increased incidence of postcricoid carcinoma.

plural—more than one. Cf. *pleural*.

pluripotent stem cell—a stem cell with the capacity to differentiate into cells of all germ layers (endoderm, ectoderm, and mesoderm) and into most or all cell types found in the adult body. Pluripotent cells used in stem cell research are derived from the inner cell mass of a very early embryo (blastocyst) or from the gonadal ridge of a slightly more mature embryo. Pluripotent cells cannot differentiate into placenta or fetal membranes.

plus disease (Oph)—dilated, tortuous vessels exiting the optic disk, seen in retinopathy of prematurity, suggesting serious disease elsewhere in the eye.

PMBV (percutaneous mitral balloon valvotomy).

PMC (percutaneous myocardial channeling)—a minimally invasive procedure that stimulates blood flow in the heart to relieve pain from angina by creating channels in the inner wall of the heart. These channels, it is thought, promote the growth of new blood vessels to improve blood supply to heart tissues in need of nourishment.

PMC (pseudomembranous colitis).

PMDD (premenstrual dysphoric disorder)—a condition treated now with Paxil CR.

PML (progressive multifocal leukoencephalopathy).

PMMA (polymethylmethacrylate) hard **contact lens** or **intraocular lens**.

PMR (pelvic muscle rehabilitation).

PMR (posteromedial release).

P-MRS (phosphorus nuclear magnetic resonance spectroscopy)—measures energy metabolism in patients with migraine. Energy metabolism appears to be defective in migraine patients.

PMT AccuSpan tissue expander.

PMT halo system—head and neck brace, for immobilization of spine in cervical fractures.

PND (paroxysmal nocturnal dyspnea).

pneumatic retinopexy—the fixation of the retina in its proper position with the injection of a bubble of gas into the interior of the eye in the vitreous cavity. With proper postoperative positioning, the retina can be pushed back into proper position and then the gas will spontaneously disappear in a few weeks. Gases used in this procedure may be either per fluoropropane (C_3F_8) or sulfur hexafluoride (SF_6).

pneumoarthrogram sign (Radiol)—the finding of gas density within the joint, signifying that no joint effusion is present. It is a reliable sign and of great value when identified.

pneumococcal conjugate vaccine—prophylaxis against pneumococcal diseases, e.g., otitis media, pneumonia, and meningitis.

Pneumocystis carinii—species name officially changed to *Pneumocystis jiroveci.*

***Pneumocystis carinii* pneumonia** (PCP)—once a rare pneumonia, caused by a protozoan parasite, seen only in immunosuppressed patients, such as transplant patients or patients on chemotherapy. Now one of the leading causes of death in AIDS. See *AIDS, HIV, Kaposi syndrome.*

***Pneumocystis* choroidopathy**—common in AIDS patients.

Pneumocystis jiroveci—new species name for *Pneumocystis carinii.*

Pneumo-Needle—reusable instrument.

pneumoparotitis—a rare cause of enlargement of the parotid gland. Swelling results from air forced through Stensen duct; a transient or recurrent phenomenon. Recurrent parotid insufflation may predispose to sialectasis, recurrent parotitis, and even subcutaneous emphysema.

pneumophila, Legionella—*the* organism causing legionnaires' disease.

pneumoscrotum—occasionally occurs after blunt trauma and can serve as an early sign of pneumothorax.

Pneumo Sleeve—acts as an airlock during hand-assisted laparoscopic surgery (see *HALS*). It contains the CO_2 used to inflate the abdomen and provides working space.

PNH (paroxysmal nocturnal hemoglobinuria).

PNI (prognostic nutritional index).

PNK—see *P&K* ("P and K").

PNL (percutaneous nephrolithotripsy)

POAG (primary open angle glaucoma).

POAH (posterior occipitoatlantal hypermobility).

POC (point of care).

Pocket Pachymeter—measures central corneal thickness by using ultrasonic pachymetry.

podagra—gout. Usage: "She comes to the emergency department complaining of acute podagra to the right big toe for the past two days."

POEMS syndrome

P polyneuropathy
O organomegaly
E endocrinopathy
M monoclonal (M-) protein
S skin changes

This is a combination of sclerotic myeloma, polyneuropathy, and endocrinological disorder. Hepatomegaly may also be seen in these patients.

POH (presumed ocular histoplasmosis syndrome).

poikilocyte—an atypical red blood cell.

"point 8 by point 6 centimeters"—should be transcribed "0.8 x 0.6 cm." Add a zero before the decimal for values under one, and use the letter *x* for "by."

point-search instruments—identifies acupuncture points by means of electricity. Both light-band and digital instruments are available.

POLARIS (polymorphisms and risk of ischemic stroke) **study**—risk factors and genetic factors in stroke.

Polaris cage—an adjustable spinal cage implant that provides a supporting framework for bone in-growth in patients with spinal trauma, tumors, or degenerative diseases.

Polaris-Dx steerable diagnostic catheter.

Polaris 1.32 Nd:YAG laser—for tissue melding.

Polaris X steerable diagnostic catheter.

polarity—the property of having two opposite poles (physical, chemical, electrical, or conceptual) at the extremities of a longitudinal axis.

polarity-altered spectral selective acquisition (PASTA) **imaging** (MRI).

polarity on an EEG. Usage: When "zero two zero negative polarity" is dictated, it should be transcribed "0-2/0 negative."

Polar-Mate bipolar microcoagulator.

Polaroids and Kodachromes (P&K) —photographs of specimens. Usage: "Polaroids and Kodachromes were taken," or "P&K were taken."

Polarus proximal humeral fixation system.

Polar Vantage XL heart rate monitor —used by sports medicine and rehabilitation physicians to monitor patients from a distance, either at home or while in physical therapy.

Polatest vision tester—tests binocular vision.

pole of kidney—the upper or lower extremity of a kidney.

Politano-Leadbetter technique—implanting the reservoir end of the appendix in an antirefluxing fashion by bringing the amputated end of the appendix through the reservoir wall into a submucosal tunnel.

polly-beak nasal deformity—results from inadequate tissue resection from the anterior septal angle or postoperative edema and scar following rhinoplasty. The term is descriptive (like a parrot's beak), not indicative of a number (*poly*, many). It describes a bony deformity in which the nose is thin or narrowed at the

polly-beak *(cont.)* top with tip projecting down over the lips, sometimes as much as at a 90° angle. May be further designated as *cartilaginous polly-beak* or *soft tissue polly-beak.*

pollywogs—see *pledgets.*

Polo-like kinase (PLK)—a novel proliferation marker that is positive in malignant melanoma cells.

polycystic ovary (PCO).

Polydek—coated polyester suture used in plastic surgery.

Polyderm foam wound dressing.

Poly-Dial insert (Ortho)—hemispherical polyethylene cap that fits under the acetabular cup and over the metal ball of the femoral stem of S-ROM hip prosthesis to prevent excessive wear.

polydioxanone plating—a method of extraluminal laryngotracheal fixation used in the treatment of grade 2 or 3 subglottic stenosis.

polydioxanone suture (PDS).

polyethylene glycol electrolyte lavage solution (PEG-LES).

polyethylene glycol (PEG)-**hemoglobin**—a combination of PEG and specially treated blood from cows, used as a blood substitute. Because this blood has been made with a special chemical modification, the immune system does not recognize it as "foreign" and does not reject it. This is still investigational, but you could be hearing about it in the future. It should have a number of advantages, including no blood typing or cross-matching, and eliminating risk of blood-borne diseases.

PolyFlo—polyurethane peripherally inserted central catheter (PICC).

polyfluorotetraethylene (PTFE)—plastic graft material.

polygenic (Genetics)—referring to a trait or condition that is determined by the concerted action of several genes at different loci, each contributing only a small part of the total effect.

Poly GIA stapler—a stapling device which fires absorbable staples instead of the usual metal staples.

polyglactin—a suture material.

polyglecaprone 25 (Monocryl)—pliable synthetic absorbable monofilament suture material.

PolyGlycopleX (PGX)—a new fiber supplement developed in Canada that, when taken prior to high-carbohydrate meals, helps reduce postprandial serum glucose levels.

polylactide absorbable screw—alternative to stainless steel or titanium nonabsorbable implants for fixation of ankle fractures. Use of absorbable hardware has been found to create adequate syndesmosis and eliminates the necessity for a second operative procedure to remove metallic hardware.

PolyMem—foam wound dressing.

polymerase chain reaction (PCR)—a procedure used in many areas including prenatal diagnosis, human leukocyte antigen typing, paternity testing, infectious disease detection and confirmation, hematologic diagnosis, genetic disease markers, gene mapping, forensics, and screening blood supply for infectious disease. PCR uses an in vitro method of DNA replication specific for the DNA or RNA sequence targeted for amplification. That is, the targeted nucleic marker for a specific disease, virus, or other abnormal condition is identified and multiplied many times (amplification). Only a small sample

polymerase *(cont.)*
(blood, tissue, bone) is required, and that sample need contain only a single intact RNA or DNA strand with the sequence of interest (e.g. only a single cell or hair is needed). Fresh samples are not needed (making it a valuable detection technique in forensics and archaeology), and the procedure is extremely sensitive. A disadvantage is that of contamination in view of the small sample size needed to conduct the test. See also *ligase chain reaction, repair chain reaction*.

polymorphous light eruption—intense reaction to sunlight.

polypeptide—a chain of amino acids joined by bonds between the amino ($-NH_2$) group of one and the carboxyl (-COOH) group of an adjacent one. A protein is a very long polypeptide chain.

polypectomized—a coined term, meaning the patient underwent a polypectomy.

Polyphenon E—topical drug for treatment of genital warts. Polyphenon is an active ingredient in Japanese green tea.

polyploid (Genetics)—an abnormal chromosome number, that is, one that is any multiple of the haploid number (23) other than the diploid number (46).

Polyrox—Fractal active fixation lead used in cardiovascular devices.

Polyskin II—transparent, semipermeable dressing that helps prevent scab formation and dermal dryness.

polysomnogram—performed for evaluation of sleep apnea syndrome and sleep efficiency. Sleep stages are determined by EEG, EMG, and EOG recordings. Oxygen saturation is monitored by ear or finger oximeter, and EKG is used to monitor cardiac rhythm. REM and NREM sleep, slow wave sleep, number of arousals, microarousals, awakenings, respiratory events (hypoxic and apneic) are recorded. Respiratory parameters are monitored by nasal and oral thermistors.

Polysorb suture—synthetic absorbable suture made from a proprietary braiding process, which gives it strength but allows it to glide through tissue effortlessly like a monofilament material.

Polystan—perfusion cannula and venous return catheter.

polytef soft-tissue patch (ENT)—used to reconstruct postparotidectomy defects and prevent Frey syndrome.

polytene chromosomes.

polyurethane foam embolus—used in treatment of fistula of the carotid cavernous sinus. Under local anesthesia, a small compressed piece of polyurethane foam is attached to a suture, and the common carotid artery is entered and the foam embolus placed in the artery. Blood flow carries the embolus to the fistula site, and after a few minutes the foam expands and occludes the fistula site. Then the suture is attached to the arterial wall. Blood flow through the carotid artery continues unimpeded; only the fistula site is occluded.

polyvinyl alcohol splinting material—said to be easily molded, hypoallergenic, lighter than plaster of Paris, and transparent to x-rays.

PolyWic wound filling material.

Pompe glycogen storage disease, type II—an inherited form of infantile cardiomyopathy that may be treated therapeutically with secretion-reuptake of protein.

pomum adami (Adam's apple)—the prominence in the neck that is the thyroid cartilage.

PO NG or **p.o. NG** (per os nasogastric) bolus feedings. Usage: "Erythromycin 1 mg/kg PO NG 4 times daily."

Ponka technique—for local anesthesia in herniorrhaphy.

Pontén-type tubed pedicle (Plas Surg) —a fasciocutaneous flap.

Pontiac fever—nonpulmonary flu-like form of legionellosis. See *legionnaires disease.*

P-on-T pattern, P-on-T wave—ectopic P wave superimposed on the T wave of the previous QRS complex. During an electrophysiology ablation procedure, any focus producing a P-on-T wave is considered a target for ablation.

pooling of blood in extremities.

Pool technique—unilateral cleft lip repair technique.

poor R-wave progression (PRWP).

POP (plaster of Paris)—POP ("pop") bandages.

pop-off needle—used in hard-to-get-at places, such as deep in the abdomen. A pre-attached needle is used to take one stitch only; the needle is then twisted slightly, and the suture "pops" off, leaving a long suture for later tying. A series of sutures can then be tied sequentially. It is faster to use than having needles threaded by a nurse. Trade names: D-Tach and Control-Release.

Poppen Ridge Sensitometer—used for edge/depth/gap perception test.

population doubling—the doubling of the number of cells in a line of cells growing in vitro; in nonimmortal lines, differentiation potential and life expectancy decline as the number of doublings increases, while the likelihood of genetic mutations increases.

porcine endogenous retrovirus (PERV)—a zoonotic retrovirus that can be transmitted to humans through xenotransplantation.

porcine fetal lateral ganglionic eminence (LGE) **cells**—a xenotransplantation product under study for the treatment of chronic striatal and cortical strokes.

porcine xenograft—any graft of porcine, or pig, origin, including heart valves and skin grafts. When autograft material is not available in a severely burned patient, split-thickness grafts of pigskin are used to cover the burned areas. This is a temporary graft that reduces the pain, permits the wound to heal more rapidly, and helps prevent the loss of fluids through evaporation. It also helps to protect the wound from infection.

pore—small, mostly transient opening in a cell wall caused by application of a brief high electric field pulse.

pores of Kohn—communications between alveoli.

Porites coral—see *madreporic coral.*

Porocoat—a porous coating used in the interfacing surfaces of DePuy interlocking (Tri-Lock Cup) acetabular cups. See *Proplast* and *Plasti- Pore* for other porous prosthetic materials.

porous-coated anatomic (PCA) **knee prosthesis**.

porous prosthetic materials—see *Plasti-Pore, Porocoat, Proplast.*

PORP (partial ossicular replacement prosthesis).

porphyrins—biochemical compounds in hemoglobin.

port—a small rubber stopper on the side of intravenous tubing used to administer drugs by I.V. push or to insert a needle to piggyback another smaller I.V. solution. See also *I.V. push; piggyback.*

PORT—a patented electrode design for delivery of radiofrequency (RF) energy.

PORT (Patient Outcomes Research Team)—used in psychiatric care settings to address use of antipsychotic drugs, methods of therapy, psychological and family interventions, vocational rehabilitation, etc.

portable blood irradiator—a device about the size of a pencil that uses the radioactive element thulium-170 to kill white blood cells in patients being treated for such cancers as leukemia and lymphoma and for immune diseases such as AIDS and the early rejection of bone-marrow transplants.

portable film—an x-ray picture taken with movable equipment at the bedside or in the emergency department or operating room, when it is not feasible to move the patient to the radiology department.

portable volume ventilator—designed to dispense oxygen from any source in institutions, ambulances, mobile military hospitals, or the home.

Port-A-Cath—an implantable port of plastic or stainless steel with a rubber-covered entry site for inserting drugs. The port is connected to a central venous catheter which is positioned in the subclavian vein. Both the port and the catheter are implanted subcutaneously. Drugs are injected by inserting the needle through the skin and subcutaneous tissue and into the rubber-covered entry site on the port.

portacaval H graft—a decompressive side-to-side shunt used in hepatic surgery.

Port-Access coronary artery bypass (PACAB)—a coronary artery bypass graft procedure carried out without opening the bony thorax. The patient's circulation is diverted through a heart-lung machine, cardioplegia achieved, and arterial grafts placed through several small incisions.

Port-Access minimally invasive cardiac surgery—used in single- and multi-vessel bypass surgery and mitral valve repair and replacement. It allows the surgeon to operate on a stopped heart through a small incision between the ribs, thus avoiding a sternotomy.

portal azygous collaterals—in hepatic surgery.

portal embolization (PE)—uses embolization material consisting of Gelfoam powder, thrombin, Urografin, and gentamicin. Embolization is followed by extensive resection, such as extended right hepatic lobectomy combined with pancreatoduodenectomy after portal embolization.

portal hypertension—a serious complication of chronic liver disease. Techniques for assessment of portal pressure include WHVP (wedged hepatic vein pressure) measurement, umbilical vein catheterization, direct transhepatic measurement using a thin needle, and hepatic parenchymal pressure measurement.

portal hypertensive gastropathy (PHG).

Porta-Lung noninvasive extrathoracic ventilator (NEV)—often used for ventilating children.

portal venous-dominant phase (PVP) **images** (CT scan).

Porta Pulse 3—portable defibrillator.

Portex—a brand name for surgical equipment such as tracheostomy tube, etc.

port of Wilmington—a portal located 1 cm lateral and anterior to the posterior lateral tip of the acromion for arthroscopic SLAP repair.

portogram—radiographic study of portal flow through transfemoral vein and shunt cannulation.

portoportal anastomosis—an anastomosis connecting a donor portal artery to a recipient portal artery, such as might be used in transplant surgery. When dictated, it may sound like the physician is stuttering.

Porvidx—noninvasive early lung cancer screening that detects cancer and precancerous cells in a sputum specimen as early as 7 years before disease symptoms appear.

poseyed to a chair—slang for *restrained to a chair with a Posey restraint*.

Posey restraint.

POSICAM system—medical imaging device using PET (positron emission topography) technology.

position—see *view*.

positive control—a specimen that is known to be abnormal, or that should yield a positive test.

positive end-expiratory pressure (PEEP).

positive symptoms of schizophrenia—hearing voices, hallucinations, delusions of grandeur, and paranoia. Cf. *negative symptoms of schizophrenia*.

Positrol cardiac device.

positron emission tomography (PET) —a scanning technique in radiology using computers and radioactive isotopes to aid imaging and diagnosis. PET scanning depicts blood flow and measures metabolism.

POSS (paratrigeminal oculosympathetic syndrome).

POST (peritoneal oocyte and sperm transfer).

postage-stamp-type skin graft.

postanesthesia recovery (PAR).

post balloon angioplasty restenosis—a condition following angioplasty that is more likely to occur in patients with white plaque than those with yellow plaque. Restenosis is also more likely in patients with higher levels of lipoprotein-A. Knowing this, physicians may be able to predict outcomes better by noting the color of the plaque or the levels of lipoprotein-A.

posterior blue (Oph).

posterior capsular opacification (PCO).

posterior capsulorrhexis with optic capture (Oph).

posterior chamber intraocular lens (PC-IOL) **implantation**—bilateral procedure performed to correct pediatric aphakia.

posterior glottic chink—a diamond-shaped or triangle-shaped opening between the posterior ends of the vocal cords.

posterior lamellar transplantation (PLT).

posterior occipitoatlantal hypermobility (POAH)—in Down syndrome.

posterior polymorphous dystrophy (PPMD) **of the cornea**—bilateral autosomal dominant condition, usually nonprogressive, affecting the deepest layers of the cornea. Associated with this may be secondary alterations in Descemet membrane.

posterior sagittal and 3-flap anoplasty—for the repair of high and intermediate imperforate anus.

posterior subcapsular cataract (PSC).

posterior sulcus—the groove formed by the intersection of the diaphragm and thc posterior thoracic wall, as seen in a lateral chest x-ray.

posteromedial pivot shift test—demonstrates posterior cruciate ligament rupture. In order for posteromedial pivot shift to occur, the posterior collateral ligament, the medial collateral ligament, and the posterior oblique ligament all must be interrupted. If even one of these ligaments is intact, the subluxation will not occur.

posteromedial release (PMR)—a one-stage correction for talipes equinovarus (clubfoot).

postinflammatory polyps—heaped-up areas of granulation tissue occurring in patients with quiescent Crohn disease. The polyps may have a filiform configuration.

postoperative flexor tendon traction brace.

postoperative regimen for oral early feeding (PROEF)—a slushy mixture consisting of crushed ice and flavored grenadine syrup, with added electrolytes, vitamins, amino acids, trace elements, and simple sugars. It is used to prevent distention and nausea and vomiting after abdominal surgery, since it is absorbed entirely in the upper GI tract.

postpartal—refers to postpartum. It is occasionally dictated instead of postpartum and is not incorrect.

post-poliomyelitis muscular atrophy (PPMA)—found in 15% of people who have had polio in the past. It appears about 30 years later and manifests itself by extreme fatigue, often severe muscle pain, and with a muscular weakness that may be slowly progressive over a long period of time.

postprandial lipemia—a rise in blood fats, especially triglycerides, after eating. This has been found to be exaggerated in individuals with atherosclerosis, even those with normal fasting lipid levels, putting the patient at risk for a cardiac event.

post-static dyskinesia—pain in the heel with the first few steps after rest. It is used interchangeably with plantar fasciitis to refer to heel pain.

poststernotomy mediastinitis (PSM)—a dangerous complication following median sternotomy.

post-transplantation lymphoproliferative disorder (PTLD)—found in pediatric thoracic organ transplant recipients.

post-transplant diabetes mellitus (PTDM).

post-tussive (also, *posttussive*)—after coughing. Applied to rales and rhonchi that do not disappear after the patient tries to clear his trachea and bronchi by coughing.

postural drainage—positioning the body in various ways to loosen pulmonary secretions.

Posture S'port—a posture corrector worn to help patients sit up straight and eliminate back and shoulder pain.

posturing, decorticate and decerebrate—rigid involuntary positioning of unconscious patient giving evidence of brain damage.

posturography—see moving platform posturography; *platform posturography.*

postviral fatigue syndrome—see *myalgic encephalomyelitis, chronic fatigue syndrome, yuppie flu.*

potassium—see *KCl*; *SSKI.*

potassium channel openers—a new class of chemical substances possi-

potassium *(cont.)*
bly effective for the treatment of hypertension, bronchial asthma, or urinary incontinence. Also, *K channel openers*. See *aprikalim*.

potassium hydroxide (KOH)—destroys human cells and thus facilitates identification of fungus or yeast in the specimen, when added to a specimen of skin, other tissue, or vaginal secretions before microscopic examination.

potential acuity meter (PAM)—used in testing vision.

Pott puffy tumor—posttraumatic osteomyelitis of the skull, with resultant edema, but without laceration of the overlying scalp. Also, subperiosteal abscess of frontal sinus origin. (Named for P. Pott.)

Potts scissors.

pouce flottant—French term for *floating thumb or great toe*. The condition is associated with a number of congenital defects and anomalies repaired by microvascular and plastic surgeons. Associated with club hand deformity, this condition is also known as *radial ray defect* or *intercalary defect of the pollical ray.* A modified Bardenheuer bifurcation procedure is often used for correction of this problem.

pouch (see also *reservoir*)
Dennis-Brown
Duke
Florida
Fobi
hand-assisted Miami
Hunt-Lawrence
ileal pouch design
ileoanal pouch anastomosis (IPAA)
Incise
Indiana
inverted U-pouch ileal reservoir

pouch *(cont.)*
Kock modified
laparoscopic hand-assisted Miami
lateral hypopharyngeal (LHP)
Mainz pouch urinary reservoir
Marsupial pouch-like belt
Miami
neoscrotum
Penn
pouch of Douglas
Reality vaginal
rectouterine
restorative proctocolectomy
UCLA
V-Amour female condom
Wheeless construction of J rectal

pouchogram—coined word for contrast-enhanced, radiographic examination of continent urinary diversion pouch (reservoir).

poudrage ("poo-drahj")—application of a powder to a surface, as done to promote fusion of serous membranes (e.g., two layers of pericardium or pleura).

Pourcelot resistance index (Neuro).

powder—see *Karaya powder.*

powder burn spots—vesicular and hemorrhagic burnt-out lesions, resulting from untreated endometriosis, as seen at laparoscopy.

power Doppler sonography—noninvasive technique to differentiate small hepatocellular carcinoma from adenomatous hyperplasia in patients with cirrhosis of the liver. Cf. *color Doppler sonography.*

powered reciprocating cannula—for precise sculpting and contouring in plastic surgery procedures.

Powerheart—automatic external cardioverter-defibrillator device.

Powerline catheter—a low-profile rapid-exchange PTCA catheter that provides better trackability for tortu-

Powerline *(cont.)*
ous vessels and crossability for tight lesions.

PowerSculpt cosmetic surgery system—includes powered reciprocating cannulas for precise sculpting and contouring of surgical sites. It is used in multiple facial and body applications.

PP (pancreatic polypeptide)—Usage: "PP is associated with bronchogenic carcinoma and is also associated with diarrhea, possibly mediated by prostaglandins."

PP-CAP IgA enzyme immunoassay—test for detection of *H. pylori* antibodies.

PPD (purified protein derivative) **test**—a skin test for tuberculosis.

PPE—slang abbreviation for post peak exercise.

PPH (palmoplantar hyperhidrosis).

PPHN (persistent pulmonary hypertension of the newborn).

PPI (peripheral percutaneous intervention).

PPK (palmoplantar keratoderma)—see *Voerner disease.*

PPMA (post-poliomyelitis muscular atrophy).

PPMD (posterior polymorphous dystrophy) **of the cornea**.

PPPD (pylorus-preserving pancreaticoduodenectomy).

PPROM (preterm premature rupture of membranes) **in pregnancy**.

P pulmonale—an electrocardiographic syndrome of tall, narrow, peaked P-waves seen in leads II, III, and aVF, with a prominent initial positive P-wave component in V1 and V2.

Ppv (portal venous pressure).

PRA assay—see *complement-dependent cytotoxicity* (CDC) *assay*.

PRA-STAT—an enzyme-linked immunosorbent assay to detect anti-HLA class I IgG antibodies, used in cardiac transplant patients and may help to predict cardiac allograft rejection.

prasterone—see *Aslera.*

PRA test (plasma renin activity).

PRBCs (packed red blood cells).

PRC (proximal row carpectomy)—for SLAC (scapholunate arthritic collapse) deformity. See *SLAC.*

PRDPC (pooled random donor platelet concentrates).

Preadmission Acuity Inquiry (PAI) **tool**.

prebiotic (adjective); **prebiotics** (noun)—pertaining to nondigestible food substances that improve health by stimulating the growth or activity of beneficial bacteria within the colon. "The patient put herself on a prebiotic diet." Prebiotics" is often used interchangeably with probiotics.

precedence effect—used in hearing studies to determine the major stimulus events that affect ability to process sounds in reverberant spaces. It helps determine how the auditory system "ignores" echoes in reverberant environments so that the listener can distinguish the original sound as the source.

preceding (*not* preceeding)—occurring before. Cf. *proceeding.*

precessional frequency—MRI term.

Precision Osteolock—femoral component design system using LPPS (low-pressure plasma spray) hydroxyapatite for a stable cementless fixation.

Precision QID—compact handheld glucose monitoring system.

Precision SpeedTac transvaginal anchor system.

Precision Twist transvaginal anchor system.

Preclude pericardial membrane—a Gore-Tex product.

precordial honk—an abnormal heart sound.

precordium—the area over the heart and the lower part of the thorax. See *pericardium.*

preemptive analgesia—the administration of analgesic medications to a patient prior to surgery in order to lessen postoperative pain.

pregabalin capsules—see *Lyrica.*

preimplantation genetic diagnosis (PGD) **and screening**—testing of embryos that have been created by in vitro fertilization for certain genetic traits, including gender, so as to direct the choice of which one to implant. Also, a therapy-oriented embryonic screening technique using a procedure called embryo biopsy.

preinvasive urothelial neoplasia—described as generalized thickening of the urothelium, or hyperplasia; disordered arrangements of cells with nuclear atypia or dysplasia; fully developed carcinoma in situ.

Prelief (calcium glycerophosphate)—drug originally developed as a dietary supplement for people with food intolerances. Study data reportedly show it to be effective in controlling overactive bladder.

premature rupture of (amniotic) **membranes** (PROM).

premenstrual dysphoric disorder (PMDD)—characterized by severe mood and physical symptoms around the menstrual cycle.

premenstrual voice syndrome (PMVS)—characterized by vocal fatigue, decreased range, a loss of power, slight hoarseness, and loss of certain singing abilities (such as ability to hit the highest notes). The syndrome usually starts four to five days prior to menstruation and affects about one-third of women, particularly those women whose voice is important to their career. Vocal surgery (phonosurgery) is available to maintain performance level of the singing voice.

Premier type-specific HSV-1 and **Premier type-specific HSV-2 IgG ELISA tests**—used to distinguish herpes simplex virus (HSV) type 1 (oral herpes) from type 2 (genital herpes) by serological test methods.

Premium CEEA circular stapler—with a detachable anvil and stem, used in end-to-end anastomosis, as in the rectum.

Premium Plus CEEA disposable stapler—used in laparoscopic Nissen fundoplication with esophageal lengthening.

Prentice position—an optometric term used to describe the position in which a light source is calibrated perpendicular to the face of a glass prism.

Prentiss maneuver—used to lengthen the spermatic cord by taking down the floor of the canal along with the epigastric vessels in a staged laparoscopic orchiopexy. See *Fowler-Stephens orchiopexy.*

preperitoneal distention balloon (PDB).

prepped—a brief form for *prepared.* Usage: "The patient was prepped and draped in the usual sterile manner."

PREP System—thin-layer slide preparation technology for Pap smears.

PREs (progressive resistive exercises).

presbyalgos—a coined term meaning loss of pain sensibility with age.

presbyesophagus—esophageal motility disorder due to aging.

presbyopia—defect of vision in advancing age, involving loss of accommodation, or recession of near point. Onset usually occurs between 40 and 45 years of age. Synonym: farsightedness. See *SRP* (surgical reversal of presbyopia).

present (verb)—to present oneself to a physician, clinic, or hospital for treatment.

presentation—the initial overt features of an illness; also, the part of a fetus that enters the birth canal first is the presenting part.

pressured speech—a rapid, tense manner of speaking that betrays the anxiety of the speaker.

pressure-relieving cushions (as spelled by manufacturer)
AirLITE
Enhance
Isch-Dish
Quadtro
ROHO Dry Floatation
SlimLine
Stimulite
Varilite Solo
WAFFLE

PressureSense monitor—checks for compartment syndrome.

pressure sore—an alternative term for *decubitus ulcer*. The term *pressure sore* seems to be used more frequently.

pressure support ventilation (PSV) (Resp Ther)—characterized by a unique combination of simultaneous spontaneous and mechanical breathing, so that the ventilatory and flow rates and tidal volume depend on the patient's breathing pattern and the set level of pressure support. It can be used as a stand-alone ventilatory support mode and alternative to volume-controlled ventilation, and it can be used in weaning patients from mechanical ventilation.

Pressure Ulcer Scale for Healing (PUSH) **tool**.

Prestara (prasterone)—for treatment of systemic lupus erythematosus.

Prestige IQ—low-cost blood glucose monitor. It is part of the Prestige Smart System, which allows a person with diabetes to graph and upload test results for transmittal to a healthcare provider's office in real time via the Internet.

Prestige Smart System (PSS)—a reportedly lower-priced blood glucose monitoring system.

Presto cardiac device.

Preston pinch gauge—used to quantify pinch strength of the fingers.

presumed ocular histoplasmosis (POH) **syndrome**.

Prevacare—skin care products for treatment of skin conditions and decubitus ulcers.

PreVue *Borellia burgdorferi* antibody detection assay—test for Lyme disease that searches for antigens made by the *Borrelia burgdorferi* bacteria responsible for the infection. The test can be done in the physician's office and should make it easier to diagnose the infection, which sometimes goes undetected until it has caused long-lasting damage.

PREZ (posterior root entry zone)—see *DREZ*.

Prialt (ziconotide intrathecal infusion) —for patients who suffer from severe chronic pain that cannot be relieved by morphine and other potent pain drugs. It is administered

Prialt *(cont.)*
through an implanted programmable pump that releases the drug into the fluid surrounding the spinal cord.

Price and Brew staging scheme—for AIDS dementia complex.

prickle-cell layer of epidermis.

Primaderm—a semipermeable foam dressing.

Prima laser guidewire—used in angioplasty procedures. It can pass through totally occluded coronary arteries by dissolving tissue through photoablation.

Primapore absorptive wound dressing.

primary—said of a disease or condition not known to result from some other disease or abnormal condition; cf. secondary.

primary acquired melanosis (PAM).

primary angioplasty—somewhat controversial procedure in which angioplasty is the first line of treatment for a patient having symptoms of myocardial infarction.

primary biliary cirrhosis (PBC).

primary constriction—the centromere of a chromosome, where the long and short arms join.

primary hyperoxaluria, type 1 (PH-1) —presents in childhood with recurrent urolithiasis. Also the cause of idiopathic renal failure in adults.

primary immune deficiency (PID)—found in children and adolescents in whom part of the immune system is missing or not functioning properly.

primary open angle glaucoma (POAG) (Oph)—the most common form of glaucoma, occurring when pressure in the eye gradually damages the optic nerve.

primary pure teratoma—a complex tumor with a histologically benign appearance, but an unpredictable course, and believed to have metastatic potential.

primary sclerosing cholangitis (PSC) —a chronic, progressive disease that damages the biliary tract. Associated with an increased risk of colorectal cancer.

primary transcript—the first RNA copy of a gene, which contains introns as well as exons.

Primbs-Circon indirect video ophthalmoscope system—can be used with either AO (American Optical) or Keeler indirect ophthalmoscope. It uses a beam splitter; a portion of the light goes to the eyepiece used by the surgeon, and the rest of the light goes to a video camera which televises (in color) the image seen through the ophthalmoscope (the televised image of intraocular, retinal, and vitreal pathology) to members of the surgical team.

PRIME (Primary Care Evaluation of Mental Disorders).

Prime ECG (electrocardiographic) **mapping system**.

PRIME-MD (computerized version of Primary Care Evaluation of Mental Disorders)—test for dependence, hypochondriasis, conversion disorder, and eating disorders. The computer-administered version was found to diagnose double the rate of substance abuse when compared with physician interview.

primer—a short sequence of DNA or RNA that hybridizes with a complementary sequence of DNA to form the beginning of a new nucleic acid chain.

Primer—compression dressing or wrap.

primitive streak—a band of cells appearing in the third week of embryonic development, marking the

primitive *(cont.)* longitudinal axis of the body and the site of the future spinal cord.

primordial germ cell—an embryonic cell that can mature and differentiate into a gamete (oocyte or sperm).

Primovist (gadolinium EOB-DTPA)—imaging agent.

Pringle maneuver—a technique for clamping the hepatic pedicle prior to hepatectomy.

Prinzmetal angina—an angina pectoris variant in which the patient has attacks while resting, and exercise tolerance is not significantly decreased.

Prisma digital hearing aid—uses digital signal processing (DSP) and an advanced directional microphone.

PRK (photorefractive keratectomy). Also, *T-PRK*.

proarrhythmia—the appearance of a new arrhythmia or worsening of arrhythmia in the context of antiarrhythmic drug therapy in comparison with drug-free condition. Certain antiarrhythmic drugs may actually worsen a minor cardiac arrhythmia, and such drugs are given only for life-threatening arrhythmias. See *propafenone*.

proband (Genetics)—a person possessing a genetic trait or disorder who first directs attention to its presence in other family members. Usage: "A proband of this family was a 7-year-old girl with hyperextensible joints. Note: The family has several members with Ehlers-Danlos syndrome." Same as *propositus*.

probe—a synthetic DNA sequence, labeled radioactively or fluorescently, that is made to seek and hybridize with a complementary DNA or RNA sequence in a specimen.

Probe cardiac device.

probe patent—allowing the passage of a probe; said of an orifice or hollow or tubular structure.

probe toe mark—staining of the cornea by fluorescein dye after prolonged tonometry.

probiotic (adjective); **probiotics** (noun)—live microbial feed supplement which beneficially affects the host animal by improving its intestinal microbial balance. Although referring to the supplementation of animal feeds for farm animals, the definition is now being applied to the human situation, and prebiotics and probiotics are used interchangeably.

proBNP—see *NT-proBNP*.

procalcitonin (PCT)—a calcitonin precursor believed to be a serum marker of the severity of acute inflammation and infectious disease, such as systemic bacterial infection and sepsis.

procedure—see *operation* for list of procedures, including diagnostic, radiographic, nonsurgical, surgical, and therapeutic procedures and studies.

Proceed—hemostatic surgical sealant composed of collagen-derived granules, thrombin, and patient fibrinogen. It provides both chemical and physical effects to speed clotting and thus seal bleeding tissue.

proceeding—progressing. Cf. *preceding*.

Prochieve 4%, Prochieve 8% (progesterone gel)—vaginal drug in gel form for treatment of infertility and secondary amenorrhea.

Pro-Clude—transparent film wound dressing.

procrastination (delayed action). Usage: "His basic suggestions were

procrastination *(cont.)* that treatment remain conservative, and that procrastination be the procedure of choice for the time being." See also *tincture of time.*

ProCross Rely over-the-wire balloon catheter.

ProCyte—transparent adhesive film dressing.

Prodigy bone densitometer—includes DualFemur, Lateral Vertebral Assessment (LVA), and fast Total Body scanning, using standard DEXA technology.

Prodigy lens inserter—an intraocular lens inserter that requires little manipulation of the eye.

ProDisc—a spinal disk prosthesis, used for disk replacement surgery. As a surgical technique, it may replace traditional spinal fusion in the future.

PROEF (postoperative regimen for oral early feeding).

profile—see *PULSES profile.*

Profile-ER—drugs-of-abuse screening panel that produces qualitative results in 7 minutes.

Profile total hip system—has porous coating (Porocoat). Also, DePuy.

Profix component—used in joint replacements.

Pro-Flo XT catheter (Cardio).

Profore four-layer bandaging system—controls the underlying venous hypertension responsible for venous ulcers by providing effective levels of pressure and maintaining the pressure for a full week.

ProForma—double lumen papillotome.

profundaplasty, profundoplasty—surgical reconstruction of the profunda femoris, a procedure used in treatment of femoropopliteal occlusive disease.

profusion—abundance. Usage: "There was normal hair distribution and profusion." Cf. *perfusion.*

progenitor cell—a cell occurring in fetal or adult tissue that can differentiate into a more specialized cell but, unlike a stem cell, cannot renew itself indefinitely by repeated cell division.

progesterone receptor (PgR).

prognostic nutritional index—one of the better known indices to provide a quantitative estimate of surgical risk and selection criteria for preoperative nutrition support. A highly significant increase in the incidence of postoperative complications, major sepsis, and death may be observed as the PNI increases.

progressive multifocal leukoencephalopathy (PML)—catastrophic HIV-related encephalopathy for which there is, at present, no treatment.

progressive osseous heteroplasia—developmental disorder of heterotopic ossification that appears to affect only females.

progressive parenchymal restriction—see *bronchiolitis obliterans.*

progressive resistive exercises (PREs).

progressive systemic sclerosis (PSS).

Project Gargle—a data collection and analysis study on flu viruses. U.S. Air Force bases in various locations worldwide conduct active surveillance for flu viruses and submit throat swab specimens for virus isolation and characterization. The results of these laboratory analyses help determine the composition of the following year's influenza vaccine.

prokinetic agent—a drug that speeds emptying of the stomach after eating so that less acid is secreted.

Prokop intraocular lens (implant).
prolactin levels (PRL)—elevated in patients with nonsecreting adenomas or other intrasellar and parasellar diseases (pseudoprolactinomas).
prolapsing redundant arytenoids—a condition contributing to obstructive sleep apnea.
Prolene (*not* Proline)—suture material.
Prolieve—a transurethral microwave therapy (thermodilatation) system that uses microwave energy to treat benign prostatic hyperplasia (BPH). The Prolieve device treats the symptoms of BPH by compressing and heating prostatic tissue that may be blocking the flow of urine.
proliferation—expansion of a cell population by repeated cell division.
proliferative retinopathy photocoagulation (PRP).
proliferative vitreoretinopathy (PVR).
prolonged strenuous exercise (PSE)—continuous steady-state aerobic or dynamic exercise that lasts for more than 1 hour, believed to be a contributing factor in sudden death in some athletes.
PROloop—electrosurgical device for cutting, coagulation, and vaporization of tissues.
prolotherapy—injection of saline solution into a ligament or tendon at its attachment to bone. This causes localized inflammation, which then increases blood supply and flow of nutrients to the area and stimulates tissue to repair itself. Used in treatment of chronic pain.
PROM (premature rupture of membranes, amniotic) (Ob-Gyn).
Promensil—natural isoflavone-based dietary supplement derived from red clover. It is used to help women maintain estrogen levels and cardiovascular health during menopause.
Prometheus First Step—an inflammatory bowel disease screening test.
Prometheus IBD panel—a highly specific inflammatory bowel disease (IBD) serology panel that helps to confirm suspected IBD.
Promogran (oxidized regenerated cellulose and collagen).
promontofixation—fixation of a prosthetic strip to form a sling under the bladder. It is now performed laparoscopically as well.
promoter—a segment of chromosomal DNA adjacent to a gene that serves as a marker of that gene for transcription and may influence expression of the gene.
pronator sign (Radiol)—ventral bulging of the fat plane overlying the pronator quadratus muscle. Although it typically means underlying fracture is present, it may also be seen in simple soft-tissue injury of the same region.
Proneb Ultra—nebulizer compressor designed to be used with the Pari LC Plus and Pari LC Star nebulizers.
Pronova nonabsorbable suture—synthetic nonabsorbable monofilament suture. It is used for approximation and/or ligation of soft tissues during general surgical procedures.
pronucleus—the precursor or primordium of a nucleus; the chromosomal material of a gamete during fertilization but before fusion of male and female genetic material to form a zygote.
ProOsteon implant 500—a bone-void filler fabricated to resemble cancellous bone. It is made of natural coralline hydroxyapatite. Provides a matrix for bony ingrowth to improve stabilization. Replaces or augments autologous bone grafts.

Propaq Encore vital signs monitor—used to monitor neonatal and impedance respiration functions.

Propel cannulated interference screws—used in knee arthroscopy.

Pro/Pel coating (Cardio).

propeller flap method—used in lower extremity reconstruction as a refinement to the reverse flow fasciocutaneous flap.

proper lamina (L., propria)—anglicized form of *lamina propria*, the form usually dictated. Also, *proper ligament*; *proper membrane*.

prophase—the initial stage of mitosis or meiosis, in which the chromosomes condense, thicken, and shorten.

prophylactic hyperventilation—treatment for severe head injury, stroke, and cerebral edema that has come under question due to potential brain damage caused by reduced oxygen to the brain.

Propionibacterium—an anaerobic organism, one of a group of normal skin flora.

Proplast—composite of Teflon polymer and elemental carbon. It resembles a black felt sponge and is 70 to 90% porous. It is used as graft material in fashioning prostheses. The host tissue, in effect, invades the pores of this material and transforms it into a similar tissue; it is biocompatible with many tissues, such as bone, soft tissue, and dura. Used in repair of dural defects and CSF leaks. See also *Plasti-Pore.*

ProPoint—point-search instrument used to localize acupuncture points.

propositus (Genetics)—a person possessing a genetic trait or disorder who first directs attention to its presence in other family members. Same as *proband*.

proprietary medicine—the name given to trademarked, brand name medications, both prescription and over-the-counter drugs.

proprioception—relates to the sensory system mechanism that has to do with movement of the body, its posture, balance, and coordination.

proptosis—a forward displacement of the eyeball in exophthalmic goiter or in an inflammatory condition of the orbit. Cf. *ptosis.*

Prosorba column—an apheresis device that works much like dialysis to treat severe joint swelling and pain in rheumatoid arthritis patients who have not been helped by other therapies. The patient's blood is removed, the plasma separated and treated by the Prosorba machine, and the blood then remixed and transfused back into the body. The machine is a column filled with silica and "protein A" from the cell wall of a bacterium that clings to human antibodies. As plasma runs through the column, the "protein A" separates out a small amount of antibodies before the plasma is retransfused.

PROST (pronuclear-stage embryo transfer).

ProstaCoil—self-expanding stent used in treatment of urethral obstruction caused by enlargement of the prostate gland.

prostaglandins (Pgs).

prostaglandin E-1—liposome-encapsulated form of PEG-1.

Prostalase laser system—an investigational Nd:YAG laser system used for TURP. See *transurethral balloon laserthermia prostatectomy.*

ProstaLund CoreTherm system—a medical device that uses microwave energy to treat benign prostatic

ProstaLund *(cont.)* hyperplasia. The CoreTherm device shrinks the prostatic tissue that may be blocking the flow of urine.

ProstaLund feedback treatment (PLFT)—feedback microwave thermotherapy.

Prostar, Prostar Plus, and **Prostar XL percutaneous closure devices**. See *Perclose closure device.*

ProstaSeed ^{125}I—radiation drug treatment for prostate cancer.

prostate—the prostate gland, which surrounds the beginning of the urethra in the male. Cf. *prostrate.*

prostate cancer detection test—using retrieval of prostate cells from ejaculate rather than needle biopsy, making it a more precise and less invasive procedure for prostate cancer detection.

prostate-specific antigen (PSA)—a protease produced by prostatic epithelium, found elevated in primary and metastatic adenocarcinoma of the prostate as well as in some cases of prostatitis and benign prostatic hyperplasia.

ProstRcision ("PROS-ter-si-shun")—a treatment for prostate cancer in which the prostate cells, normal and cancerous, are destroyed (excised) with irradiation. All prostate cells are "cut out" with ProstRcision, which leaves intact the sex nerves and muscles that control urination.

prostate-specific antigen bound to alpha-1-antichymotrypsin—see *PSA-ACT.*

prostate-specific antigen (PSA) **free/total index**—see *free/total PSA index.*

prostate-specific membrane antigen (PSMA)—a substance often expressed in the most aggressive clones of prostate cancer cells. Using a prostate cancer monoclonal antibody conjugate, a team of researchers targeted PSMA in an effort to detect circulating prostate cancer cells. With this test, much higher rates were found than with using prostate-specific antigen alone. Researchers believe this test may provide physicians with a method of identifying patients at high risk of advanced disease at the time of initial diagnosis or following therapy.

Prostatron—a mobile device that uses microwave energy to provide long-term relief from symptomatic benign prostatic hypertrophy. The procedure takes approximately one hour and can be done on an outpatient basis with local anesthesia. See *TUMT.*

prosthesis—an artificial substitute or internal device to replace a body part, such as a hip, knee, joint, or cardiac valve; joint replacement material; and breast and penile implants. Also, an external device such as an arm, hand, leg, or foot, or an orthopedic appliance or device. May also be called *appliance, fixation device, implant, orthosis,* or *valve.*

Prostheses in this book include:
Acticon Neosphincter
AcuMatch A Series acetabular
Airprene hinged knee
alumina-alumina total hip replacement
AMS (American Medical Systems) 700 CX inflatable penile
AMS Sphincter 800 urinary
Angelchik antireflux
Applebaum incudostapedial joint
Apollo hip
Apollo knee
Atkinson endoprosthesis
Atlas shoulder

prosthesis *(cont.)*
attic defect plate implant of ear
Austin Moore hip
Bateman UPF II bipolar endoprosthesis
Becker tissue expander/breast
Bigliani-Flatow shoulder
Bio-Chromatic hand
Black ossiculoplasty spanner strut
bladder neck support continent
Blom-Singer indwelling low pressure voice
Buechel-Pappas total ankle
Caffinière
Calnan-Nicolle synthetic joint
CardioFix Pericardium patch
Carpentier-Edwards Perimount RSR pericardial bioprosthesis
CPHV OptiForm mitral valve
crutched-stick type endoprosthesis
DANA (designed after natural anatomy) shoulder
Deon hip
DHS (dynamic hip screw)
Dilamezinsert penile
DoubleStent biliary endoprosthesis
Duraphase
Dynaflex penile
endoprosthesis
Excluder bifurcated cardiac endoprosthesis
Finney Flexi-Rod penile
Finn hinged knee replacement
Flatow/Bigliani shoulder
Flatt finger/thumb
Flowers mandibular glove
Foundation shoulder
Freedom prosthetic foot
Freestyle aortic root bioprosthesis
GFS Mark II inflatable penile
Gianturco expandable (self-expanding) metallic biliary stent
Groningen voice
Guepar II hinged knee
Hancock M.O. bioprosthesis

prosthesis *(cont.)*
Hanger ComfortFlex knee
HD II (or 2) total hip
Hemobahn endovascular
incontinence ring
Inter-Op acetabular
IntraStent DoubleStrut biliary endoprosthesis
Introl bladder neck support
J-FX bipolar head
Judet hip
Kaster mitral valve
Kinematic rotating hinge
Kirschner Modular IIC shoulder
Lap-Band rigid silicone band
Leeds-Keio ligament
Link cementless reconstruction hip
Link Endo-Model rotational knee
Lord total hip
lunate
madreporic hip
McCutchen SLT hip
McNaught keel laryngeal
Mentor Alpha 1 inflatable penile
Mentor saline-filled testicular
Metasul metal-on-metal hip
Microknit vascular graft
Monostrut cardiac valve
Mosaic porcine
Natural-Hip
NCP (NeuroCybernetic Prosthesis)
NeuroCybernetic Prosthesis (NCP)
Neville tracheal and tracheobronchial
Niebauer
Noiles posterior stabilized knee
Noiles rotating hinge total knee
Omnifit HA hip stem
Omniscience single leaflet cardiac valve
On-X prosthetic heart valve
Osteonics Total Shoulder system
oxidized zirconium
Panje voice button laryngeal
Passy-Muir tracheostomy speaking valve

prosthesis *(cont.)*
PCA (porous-coated anatomic) knee
Perfecta hip
Perimount RSR pericardial bioprosthesis
pHEMA keratoprosthesis
Pillet hand
piston stapes
Pitt talking tracheostomy tube
plasma spray stem
porous-coated anatomic (PCA) knee
ProDisc
Provox speaking valve
Richards hydroxyapatite PORP and TORP
Ring hip
Sense-of-Feel
Singer-Blom speech valve
Sivash
Small-Carrion penile
Souter-Strathclyde elbow
St. George total elbow
supradescemetic keratoprosthesis
TARA (total articular replacement arthroplasty)
titanium rib
TMJ fossa-eminence
TORP (total ossicular replacement)
Townley TARA
UroLume endoprosthesis
Utah artificial arm
vertical expandable titanium rib (VEPTR)
Vibrant D and Vibrant P soundbridge
Vitallium alloy cobalt chrome
Wallstent iliac endoprosthesis
Wayfarer
Weavenit (no *k*) vascular
Wehrs incus
Zweymuller

prosthetic disk nucleus (PDN) **device**—spinal implant for the treatment of low back pain, designed as an alternative treatment to spinal fusion.

prostrate—lying prone. Cf. *prostate.*

ProstRcision—an outpatient procedure that treats prostate cancer with a combination of seed implants followed by conformal beam irradiation.

protean—said of a disease having various symptoms in different patients.

ProtectaCap—a shock-absorbent foam whole-head protective cap which fastens under the chin. Designed for children under age 6, it has a colorful vinyl cover and none of the bulk or weight of commonly used helmets. Used to protect the skull following cranial surgery.

Protectaid contraceptive sponge.

Protect-a-Pass suture passer—used in percutaneous bladder neck stabilization for women with stress urinary incontinence. The passer utilizes a thumb lever that opens the suture channel and releases the suture, preventing entrapment of vaginal tissue in the open slot, and places a Z-stitch.

Protector suturing system—used in arthroscopic surgery for meniscal repair.

Protect Point needle—tapered tip reduces risk of glove puncture.

PROTECT trial of oral heparin.

Protege GPS nitinol self-expanding long stent—cardiac device used during a minimally invasive procedure to open strictures and blockages.

protein
ALZ-50
anti-Tamm-Horsfall
aquaporin-1
A68
autocrine motility factor (AMF)
bone morphogenic
BPI (bactericidal/permeability-increasing

protein *(cont.)*
C
CHUK (conserved helix-loop-helix ubiquitous kinase)
COUP-TF thyroid hormone receptor auxiliary
C-reactive (CRP)
CREB (cAMP response element binding)
cytokeratin
endostatin
epidermal growth factor
ESAT-6
estramustine binding (EMBP)
glial fibrillary acidic
GLQ223 (compound Q)
glycated
human Complement Factor H-related
ICAM-1 marker
IL-4R immune system
lactoferrin
leukemia inhibitory factor
Lp(a)
microtubule-associated
M-protein
M spike monoclonal
neuronal apoptosis inhibitory (NAIP)
Nogo nerve regeneration
Novel erythropoiesis stimulating (NESP)
nuclear matrix (NMP)
Osteogenic Protein 1 (OP-1)
P-glycoprotein
p24 antigen
p55-IgG tumor necrosis factor receptor fusion
phycobiliproteins
Raf-1 human
rhBMP-2 (recombinant human bone morphogenetic)
rhBMP-2/ACS (recombinant human bone morphogenetic protein-2/absorbable collagen sponge)

protein *(cont.)*
ribonuclear (RNP)
S
SCA (single-chain antigen-binding)
single-chain antigen-binding (SCA)
solder
Sonic Hedgehog (Shh)
ST2
surface marker
TGF-B (transforming growth factor-beta)
TpP (thrombus precursor)
transcription

protein C—a naturally occurring anticoagulant protein that inhibits the coagulating activity of blood factors V and VIII. The protein C levels are of concern in patients with renal disease. See *protein S.*

ProteinChip—evaluates protein biomarkers that are present in various cancers to predict the presence and extent of the disease. It is presently being used to evaluate the presence and degree of ovarian cancer.

protein-losing enteropathy (PLE).

protein S—a naturally occurring anticoagulant that is necessary for the activity of protein C in treating patients with renal disease. See *protein C.*

protein solder—human albumin preparation used for tissue welding, e.g., in urologic surgery, used in place of staples or sutures or clips, which have an inherent lithogenic reaction. It decreases operative time, promotes healing, and provides immediate intraoperative watertight seal in such procedures as arterial anastomoses, nerve coaptation, bowel anastomoses, and ureteral reconstruction. Also, *tissue solder, tissue glue.*

Protek joint implant.

Proteque SPS—steroid-sparing topical treatment for eczema and dermatitis.

pro time—brief form used in dictation for *prothrombin time* (PT), a test for defects in blood clotting. (*Pro time* should be written as two words.)

protocol—see *medications* for chemotherapy protocols. Other protocols include:
CeQUAL protocol
CIWA (Clinical Institute Withdrawal Assessment) detox
CT PE (computed tomography pulmonary embolus)
CVEMC protocol
maze cut-and-sew protocol
Raskin DHE-45 protocol
TG-60 dosimetry parameters

Protocult—stool sampling device that reduces the chance of contamination.

protodiastolic gallop—prominent fourth heart sound.

proton density images—MRI term.

proton magnetic resonance spectroscopy—performed on the fetus via MRI. May serve as a noninvasive approach to monitoring the fetus.

proto-oncogene
c-fms (growth factor receptor gene)
c-myc/myb/fos (nuclear proteins)
c-sis (growth factor gene)
c-src (cytoplasmic protein tyrosine kinase)

Protouch—synthetic orthopedic padding.

Pro-Trac—cruciate reconstruction measurement device.

Protractor—a combination retractor and wound protector indicated for use during both laparoscopic and open surgical procedures.

protruding atheromas—cause embolic disease. Can be seen on transesophageal echocardiography.

PRO 2000 Gel—drug used for the prevention of HIV-1 infection and other sexually transmitted diseases.

proud flesh—exuberant granulation tissue of skin or mucous membrane.

Provenge—therapeutic vaccine for treatment of prostate cancer.

proverbs, Benjamin (Psych).

Providencia rettgeri—newer name for the former *Proteus rettgeri;* commonly found in stool.

provocative maneuvers—on physical exam, diagnostic manipulations that reproduce the patient's symptoms in certain conditions, e.g., thoracic outlet syndrome.

Provox speaking valve—a type of laryngeal prosthesis implanted following laryngectomy. Air exhaled from the lungs is redirected through a surgical fistula in which the prosthetic speaking valve has been implanted. Advantages include more natural speech which is synchronized with breathing rather than speech using regurgitated air or the use of an external vibrator applied to the neck (which creates a mechanical, monotone-like speech). The name of the implant comes from the Latin *pro* 'for' and *vox* 'voice.'

proximal articular set angle (PASA).

Proximate flexible linear stapler.

Proximate linear cutter—a surgical stapler.

PRP (panretinal photocoagulation).

PRP (proliferative retinopathy photocoagulation).

Pruitt-Inahara carotid shunt—a long polyvinyl tube with an inflatable balloon at each end. The inflated balloon keeps the shunt tube within the vessel; thus no clamps are utilized, resulting in less trauma to the blood vessel. This shunt may also be used

Pruitt *(cont.)*
in some patients undergoing vascular reconstruction of the leg.

prune-belly syndrome—see *Eagle-Barrett syndrome.*

PRWP—slang abbreviation for *poor R-wave progression.*

PS (pulmonary sequestration).

PSA (prostate-specific antigen).

PSA-ACT (prostate-specific antigen bound to alpha-1-antichymotrypsin) —the ratio of PSA-ACT to "free" PSA in serum is indicative of prostate cancer risk. High levels, as revealed by sensitive PSA tests, indicate higher risk for prostate cancer.

PSA4—home blood test to screen for prostate cancer.

PSA (prostate-specific antigen) **index**—see *free/total PSA index.*

psammoma ("sah-mo´mah")—a tumor, especially a meningioma, that contains psammoma bodies.

psammoma bodies—microscopic laminated calcified bodies commonly seen in thyroid and ovarian cancer.

PSC (posterior semicircular canal).

PSC (posterior subcapsular cataract).

PSC (primary sclerosing cholangitis).

PSC fertility monitor—ovulation prediction device which is housed in a wristwatch-like device with an LCD readout and is worn at night during sleeping hours. It predicts ovulation by measuring ion changes on the surface of the skin.

PSD (pancreas-sparing duodenectomy).

PSD (pituitary stalk distortion).

PSE (prolonged strenuous exercise).

Pseudallescheria boydii—fungus originally identified as one of the agents thought responsible for Madura foot. *P. boydii* is an opportunistic pathogen and has been recognized with increasing frequency as a cause of pulmonary, central nervous system, prostatic, osteomyelitic, ophthalmologic, otitic, and disseminated infections, particularly in patients who are immunocompromised.

pseudoaccommodation amplitude—accommodation in the presence of an intraocular lens (IOL) implant. Usage: "We assessed the degree of pseudoaccommodation amplitude correlated with shifts along the anteroposterior axis of the BioComFold foldable IOL."

pseudo-Billroth I sign—continuous tubular narrowing of the pyloric antrum and adjacent duodenum as a result of scarring from Crohn disease. So-called because of the resemblance on barium studies to the postsurgical stomach after a Billroth I procedure.

pseudodermachalasis—slackening of the skin below the eyebrow, giving the upper eyelid a redundant appearance. Usage: "Gravitation of the eyebrow downward caused pseudodermachalasis of the upper eyelids."

pseudoendoleak—contrast medium trapped in the aneurysm sac during endovascular aneurysm repair. It may be misinterpreted as an endoleak on postprocedural CT scans. Pseudoendoleaks can be distinguished from true endoleaks by examination of prebolus noncontrast CT images as well as by duplex ultrasound scanning.

pseudofracture—see *kink artifact.*

pseudo-Hurler deformity—see *mucolipidosis III.*

pseudolaminar necrosis—cell death of layers of cortical neurons, typical of a patient in a persistent vegetative state who is on life-support systems.

pseudomallet finger—exostosis around the distal interphalangeal joint that resembles mallet finger.

pseudomembranous colitis (PMC).

pseudomeningitis—recovery of microorganism on CSF culture or smear that does not clinically correlate with clinical meningitis.

***Pseudomonas* exotoxin**—a natural poison from a common bacterium used in the treatment of malignant brain tumors. It is delivered to the tumor site in combination with interleukin 4, a substance to which cancer cells have a receptor. The *Pseudomonas* exotoxin destroys the cancer cell's ability to produce protein and stay alive. Since healthy brain cells do not have interleukin-4 receptors, they are not exposed to the bacterium's toxin.

Pseudomonas maltophilia *(Alcaligenes bookeri)*—an opportunistic pathogen found in soil, plants, water, sewage, animals, and raw milk. Seen in meningitis, septicemia, pleuritis, infected wounds.

Pseudomonas stutzeri—opportunistic pathogen found in soil but occasionally in sputum specimens, in wounds, ear drainage, and infected eyes; found also on aerosol equipment.

pseudomyotonia—a rare neuromuscular disorder with onset usually in late childhood or early adulthood, characterized by intermittent or continuous widespread involuntary muscle contractions, fasciculation, hyporeflexia, muscle cramps and weakness, hyperhidrosis, tachycardia, and myokymia. Involvement of pharyngeal or laryngeal muscles may interfere with speech and breathing. The continuous motor activity persists during sleep and general anesthesia, distinguishing this condition from stiff-person syndrome. Cf. *stiff-person syndrome*.

pseudoseizure—an attack resembling an epileptic seizure but having purely psychological causes. It lacks the electroencephalographic characteristics of epilepsy and the patient may be able to stop it by an act of will. Also called *pseudoepilepsy* and *hysterical epilepsy*.

PSF (posterior spine fusion)—spine surgery.

p.s.i., psi ("sigh") (pounds per square inch)—unit of measurement used in procedures involving pressure. See *Brown-McHardy pneumatic dilator.*

PSIL (percentage signal intensity loss) —MRI term.

P6—acupressure point. See *Neiguan point*.

PSM (poststernotomy mediastinitis).

PSMA (prostate-specific membrane antigen).

psomophagia ("somophagia")—swallowing food without chewing it thoroughly.

psoralen inactivation technique—used to inactivate a variety of infectious agents including some that are considered more difficult to inactivate than HIV. Involves exposing an active infectious agent to psoralen or one of its derivatives, and thereafter exposing it to ultraviolet light, by which process the psoralen forms chemical bonds with the nucleic acids (DNA or RNA) in the infectious agents.

Psoriasis Area Severity Index (PASI) —a standard measure of severity of psoriasis.

psoriasis of the penis—can develop from prolonged use of fluorinated steroid creams.

psoriatic onychopachydermoperiostitis—psoriasis condition of the nails consisting of onychopathy, soft tissue thickening, and x-ray evidence of bone erosion and periosteal reaction of the terminal phalanx.

Psorospermium haeckelii—may be confused with helminth eggs in laboratory analysis of feces of individuals who have recently eaten crayfish.

PSP (progressive supranuclear palsy).

PSS (progressive systemic sclerosis). Scleroderma is a form of this disease.

PST (photon stimulation therapy [or treatment]).

PSV (pressure support ventilation).

PSVT (paroxysmal supraventricular tachycardia).

psychedelic drugs (*not* psychodelic)—refers to certain types of drugs that act on the central nervous system, e.g., LSD, mescaline, etc., producing heightened perception, visual hallucinations, delusions.

PSY Inventory—for assessment of six behavioral characteristics (Sense of Responsibility, Energy and Competitiveness, Obsessive Behavior, Anger and Hostility, Stress-related Disturbances, Time Urgency) in patients who have suffered an acute myocardial infarction.

PTA (percutaneous transluminal angioplasty). Cf. *PTCA*, *Dotter-Judkins technique.*

PTAH (phosphotungstic acid-hematoxylin)—a histochemical diagnostic stain. See *Mallory PTAH.*

PTBD (percutaneous transhepatic biliary drainage).

PTC (percutaneous transhepatic cholangiography).

PTC (plasma thromboplastin component)—in bleeding diseases.

PTCA (percutaneous transluminal coronary angioplasty). See *Grüntzig.*

PTDM (post-transplant diabetes mellitus).

PTEN gene—recent findings suggest up to 50% of all endometrial cancers may contain a mutation in this gene.

PTFE (polytetrafluoroethylene)—suburethral sling material used to treat stress urinary incontinence. PTFE does not need pre-clotting, as Dacron does. It is also used as vascular access in hemodialysis.

PTH (parathormone, parathyroid hormone).

P-thal—slang for *Persantine-thallium stress test.*

PTHC (percutaneous transhepatic cholangiogram).

PTHi (intact parathyroid hormone).

P-32—a chromic phosphate suspension given via intraperitoneal administration to patients with ovarian cancer. It is used only after a second-look laparotomy has yielded negative findings and its purpose is to attempt to improve survival time. Also, phosphorus-32 or ^{32}P.

PTK (phototherapeutic keratectomy).

PTL (pharyngeal lumen airways).

PTLD (post-transplantation lymphoproliferative disorder).

PTMC (percutaneous transvenous mitral commissurotomy).

PTMR (percutaneous transluminal myocardial revascularization).

ptosis ("toe´sis") (noun)—a prolapse or drooping of an anatomic structure, such as the upper eyelid. Cf. *proptosis, phthisis.*

ptotic ("tot´tic") (adj.)—see *ptosis.*

PTPE (percutaneous transhepatic portal vein embolization).

PTRA (percutaneous transluminal renal angioplasty).

PTVA (percutaneous transseptal ventricular assist)—see *TandemHeart PTVA.*

p22 phox gene—a gene that appears to provide protection against coronary artery disease by affecting the production of free radicals that oxidize low-density lipoproteins (LDL), the bad form of cholesterol that increases risk of heart diseases.

p24 antigen—an HIV core protein that can be detected in HIV-infected blood several weeks before HIV antibodies first appear.

p24 protein—found in the core of the HIV virus and seems to be a relatively stable part of this quickly changing virus.

P300—a test for dementia.

public access defibrillation (PAD).

pubovaginal sling—constructed as part of a one-stage repair of urethral damage.

PUBS (percutaneous umbilical cord blood sampling).

PUD (peptic ulcer disease).

puddle sign—a quick, if unsophisticated, method of differentiating minimal ascites from edema. The patient lies prone for five minutes and then assumes the knee-chest position; dullness on percussion in the periumbilical region indicates ascites rather than edema.

pudendal neurogram (Peds)—used in treating spasticity in plantar flexors in children with cerebral palsy. It is an indirect approach to the assessment of bladder and bowel reflex pathways using sensory evoked potentials from dorsal nerve of the penis or clitoris (a branch of the pudendal).

puerperal abscess—may be caused by *Salmonella bredeney* and group B Streptococcus.

Puestow pancreaticojejunostomy—a procedure performed on patients with obstruction of the pancreatic ductal system resulting in dilated duct, with points of stenosis and distal calculi.

puffer, pink—a patient with early respiratory failure, showing dyspnea but no cyanosis. Cf. *blue bloater.*

puff of smoke (moyamoya)—angiographic diagnosis of bilateral stenosis or occlusion of the internal carotid arteries above the clinoids.

Puig Massana anuloplasty ring—allows for precise final adjustments to ensure atrioventricular competence.

Pulec and Freedman—classification of congenital aural atresia.

Pulmicort Turbuhaler (budesonide) (*not* pulmo, *not* turbo)—unusual spelling.

Pulmios inhaler—for treatment of pulmonary hypertension.

Pulmo-Aide nebulizer—used to permit easier breathing in patients with allergies, asthma, chronic obstructive pulmonary disease, cystic fibrosis.

pulmonary alveolar proteinosis (PAP) —a rare disease characterized by accumulation of surfactant-like phospholipid within the alveolar spaces; untreated, it causes progressive respiratory failure.

pulmonary artery wedge pressure (PAWP).

pulmonary autograft (PA)—the patient's own pulmonary valve used in aortic valve replacement. In the Ross procedure the patient's own pulmonary valve is essentially used as a "spare part" to replace the diseased aortic valve.

pulmonary parenchymal window—a CT setting for examining lung tissue. See also *bone window; brain window; soft tissue window; subdural window.*

pulmonary sequestration—a mass of abnormal lung parenchyma with an anomalous systemic blood supply not communicating with the normal tracheobronchial tree. An intralobar sequestration is contained within the visceral pleura of a lower lobe receiving its blood supply from the abdominal aorta or other thoracic vessel; an extralobar sequestration is a congenital malformation with variable ectopic blood supply.

pulmonary sling syndrome—aberrant left pulmonary artery causing tracheal stenosis and a variety of unilateral aeration disturbances. On x-rays, the left pulmonary artery appears as a small rounded mass between the trachea and esophagus. The left pulmonary artery, as it arises from the right pulmonary artery and hooks around the trachea, can cause compression of the right bronchus with resulting underinflated right lung, but overexpansion of the right lung, or even the left lung, can occur.

pulmonary toilet—postural drainage, percussion, hydration, and other means of clearing the respiratory tract.

pulmonary vascular markings—as seen on chest x-ray, the normal radiographic appearance of the branches of the pulmonary arteries and veins about the hila of the lungs.

pulmonary vascular redistribution—on chest x-ray, increased prominence of upper pulmonary vessels and reduced prominence of lower pulmonary vessels at the lung hila in left ventricular failure and other disturbances of circulatory dynamics.

PulmoSphere—particle-processing technology that doubles the quantity of a drug delivered to deep lung using a metered-dose inhaler.

Pulsar Max II pacemaker system—incorporates separate, simultaneous dual-chamber electrocardiograms, which provide a record of both atrial and ventricular heart rhythms to help physicians make therapy decisions.

pulsatile catheter (PUCA) **pump**—a transarterial, transvalvular blood pump that can be used as a vascular assist device. The catheter position is verified by pressure readings rather than by x-ray.

pulsatile irrigation—used with an enhanced nasal moisturizing formula to relieve the symptoms of empty nose syndrome, which includes the loss of function of nasal cilia. The pulsation mimics the cilia action and can act as a partial replacement of this action. Pulsatile irrigation also removes crusts, bacteria and pollen which healthy turbinates would normally deal with.

Pulsavac III wound debridement system—used to clear excess cement from a surgical site, to wash debris from open trauma fractures, to clear the intramedullary canal for rod or prosthesis placement, or to clean wounds before closure.

pulsed dose therapy—the opposite of a continuous dosing regimen. Medication or treatment is administered in several sessions with longer intervals between. Chemotherapy is an example of pulsed dose therapy. Also called pulse dose therapy, pulse therapy, pulsed therapy.

pulsed-dye laser (PDL) **surgery**—a technology used in dermatologic and cosmetic surgery, and also to treat voice disorders. The laser fires at and destroys abnormal tissue while ignoring healthy tissue. It is also used for ureteral stone lithotripsy. Cf. *ESWL*. It is said to be effective in selectively destroying warts without damaging the surrounding skin.

pulse deficit—the arithmetical difference between the apical pulse and the radial or other peripheral pulse. Generally it indicates the number of cardiac contractions per minute that are not sufficiently strong to generate a peripheral pulse.

pulsed electromagnetic therapy—electrically generated magnetic fields for pain relief.

pulsed-field gel electrophoresis—lab test for neurological diseases.

pulsed gradient—MRI term.

pulsed lavage—used in surgery reports. Usage: "The wound was thoroughly irrigated with pulsed lavage and then closed as follows."

PulseDose technology—delivers oxygen in a precise dose with every breath, rather than continuously. Used in DeVilbiss Walkabout portable series.

pulsed ultrasound—said to decrease healing time in fractures by accelerating callus formation.

pulse inversion harmonic imaging—ultrasound technique.

pulseless electrical activity (PEA)—formerly called *EMD* (electromechanical dissociation). PEA covers EMD, pseudo-EMD, and idioventricular rhythms.

PulseMaster laser—used for laser curettage, or removal of diseased or inflamed soft tissue in the periodontal pocket.

pulse-ox—slang for *pulse oximetry devices*.

pulse oximetry—a noninvasive method for determining blood oxygenation, usually dictated as "pulse ox."

pulse oximetry devices—used extensively in the intensive care unit and operating room to continuously monitor the patient's arterial blood oxygen saturation. They are composed of a sensor which emits two types of light (red and infrared) and a photodetector. The red and infrared light beams are transmitted through the patient's tissue and through arterial blood vessels. When they reach the photodetector on the other side, a computer calculates how much of each type of light was transmitted. Oxygenated hemoglobin within the arteries absorbs more infrared light, while deoxygenated blood absorbs more red light. These devices can be placed around the patient's finger or over the bridge of the nose, and around the foot or even around the great toe of neonates. Also called *finger oximetry*.

pulse pressure—the difference of the two blood pressure measurements: systolic (the higher number) and diastolic (the lower number). Increased pulse pressure is a predictor of coronary heart disease.

Pulse Pro—heart rate monitor that displays functions on a wristwatch that has most of the features of a normal sport watch. Pulse Pro does not require a chest strap transmitter and is said to be extremely accurate even during vigorous exercise.

PulseSpray—a pulsed infusion system consisting of a syringe and catheter,

PulseSpray *(cont.)*
used to inject thrombolytic agents into a vessel.

PULSES profile—a disability profile:
P physical condition
U upper extremity function
L lower extremity function
S sensory and communication abilities
E excretory control
S social support
Scored from 1 (total independence) to 4 (total dependence). A score of 2 represents symptomatology, but no impairment in activities of daily living. A score of 3 means impairment and need for assistance from others.

pulsing current (electrostimulation)—used in nonunion of fractures. When bone is placed in an electromagnetic field, and the field switched on and off, a current in the microampere range is generated in the bone, causing changes in the environment of the cells in the gap region. This leads to bone healing.

Pulsolith laser lithotripter—for nonsurgical removal of gallstones and urinary tract stones.

pulsus bisferiens (biferious pulse)—a pulse with two beats, sometimes palpable in combined aortic stenosis and aortic regurgitation.

pulsus paradoxus (*not* paradoxicus). Also, *paradoxical pulse.*

Pulvertaft anastomosis—a technique used for proximal tenorrhaphy for the correction of wrist flexor contracture. Also called *Pulvertaft weave technique.*

Pulvertaft weave—a method used in microsurgical tendon transfer.

pulvinar—(1) the expanded posterior extremity of the thalamus; (2) fibrofatty debris found in the hip joint in developmental dysplasia of the hip. You will hear the term dictated in orthopedic surgery and also in radiology, as pulvinars can be seen on x-ray.

PumpMate system—a device for pumping, storing, and feeding breast milk.

punctum plug (Oph). See *Freeman punctum plug.*

puncture site complications
arteriovenous fistula
dissection
hematoma
pseudoaneurysm
thrombosis

Punctur-Guard needle—self-blunting needles which reduce the risk of accidental needlesticks.

Puntenney forceps (Oph).

PuraPly wound dressing—indicated for the management of acute and chronic partial- and full-thickness wounds.

pure ground glass opacity (PGGO)—a finding in the lungs on high-resolution CT scanning, possibly indicative of lung cancer.

Puri-Clens wound cleanser.

pursed-lipped breathing—a breathing technique spontaneously adopted by patients with chronic obstructive pulmonary disease and others in various kinds of respiratory distress; pursing (near closure) of the lips delays expulsion of air during expiration and thus helps to maintain blood oxygen level. Not "first-lipped."

purse-string mouth—fissures or scarring left by syphilitic lesions around the mouth of neonates with congenital syphilis. Also called *rhagades.*

pursestring or **purse-string suture**—a continuous running suture placed about an opening, and then drawn tight, like a drawstring purse.

Pursuer CBD Helical or Mini-Helical stone basket—an instrument used to trap small stones remaining in the common bile duct (CBD) during laparoscopic cholecystectomy.

pursuit mechanism—the slow, involuntary movement of both eyes as they follow a moving object.

push (Surg)—(1) A term used to refer to maneuvering objects or tools into an area. (2) Aggressive or high-dose administration of drugs. "We will push corticosteroids and await developments." (3) Bolus intravenous administration of a drug.

push enteroscope/enteroscopy—diagnostic instrument and treatment procedure for jejunal angiodysplasias and small intestine bleeding sites and lesions. A child-size colonoscope is introduced via the mouth into the upper gastrointestinal tract and advanced to distances beyond the ligament of Treitz.

Pushita—blood glucose monitoring device that measures biological markers present in interstitial fluid rather than glucose concentrations. It does not require a finger stick.

push-pull wire technique—a technique used in cardiac catheterization for advancing the delivery sheath over the guidewire.

PUSH (Pressure Ulcer Scale for Healing) **tool**—developed by National Pressure Ulcer Advisory Panel to replace reverse staging of pressure ulcers.

"puts-YAY-gerz"—phonetic for *Peutz-Jeghers syndrome.*

Putti-Platt arthroplasty—for acromioclavicular separation. Subscapularis muscle and capsular repair, for chronic shoulder separation.

PUVA (psoralens, ultraviolet A) **regimen, therapy** ("poo-vah")—used for psoriasis. Ultraviolet A is a long-wave ray.

PVAC—a therapeutic vaccine used to treat psoriasis.

PVA (polyvinyl alcohol) **particles**—an embolic material used in embolization of the potential blood supply to a cranial nerve in interventional radiology procedures of the extracranial head and neck.

PVE (prosthetic valve endocarditis).

PVG (periventricular gray) **matter**—stimulated with deep brain electrodes to inhibit pain. Cf. *PAG matter.*

PVP (percutaneous vertebroplasty).

PVP (portal venous-dominant phase) **images** (CT scan).

PVR (postvoiding residual).

PVR (proliferative vitreoretinopathy).

PVS (persistent vegetative state).

PWA (person with AIDS).

pyknosis—phenomenon where the cell becomes opaque and darkly stained under the microscope, as seen in cell death.

Pylon intramedullary nail system—consists of intramedullary rods and screws for internal fixation of tibial or femoral fractures.

pyloric string sign—an elongated, narrowed pyloric canal; a sign of pyloric hypertrophy which does not change on administration of antispasmodics.

Pylori-G Fiax—objective quantitative IFA (indirect fluorescent antibody) serology assay for *Helicobacter pylori.*

Pylori Stat—rapid EIA (enzyme-linked immunoassay) serology assay for *Helicobacter pylori.*

PyloriTek—test for *Helicobacter pylori.*

pylorus preserving pancreaticoduodenectomy (PPPD)—a procedure that is said to improve upon the standard Whipple procedure. Leaving the pylorus intact results in improved eating habits in postoperative patients and ability to gain weight; no marginal ulceration as is seen in standard Whipple procedure. Transit time is preserved; no dumping, no change in glucose metabolism. After the new procedure, patients are said to have better food intake, increased body weight, no development of gastric or jejunal ulcers, and no clinical signs of digestive disorders such as dumping. Nutrition and digestion are not impeded by the preserved opening mechanism of the pylorus. See *dumping syndrome.*

pylorus-preserving Whipple (PPW) **modification**—used to treat patients with malignant periampullary disease.

pyogenic granuloma—benign polypoid growth containing proliferating capillaries. It may result from trauma and often becomes infected. Also, *granuloma pyogenicum.*

pyogenic liver abscess (PLA).

PYP scan (technetium pyrophosphate)—for myocardial infarct imaging.

pyramidal signs (or symptoms)—weakness and spasticity secondary to antipsychotic drugs or chemical imbalances in the brain. When an affected extremity is moved passively, it shows a gradual increase in resistance, then a sudden letting go, resulting in a classic "lengthening and shortening" or "clasp-knife phenomenon." Cf. *extrapyramidal signs, akathisia, tardive dyskinesia.*

pyranocarboxylic acid—a class of drugs chemically different from nonsteroidal anti-inflammatory drugs such as ibuprofen, but exert the same effects in treating inflammation, pain, and fever. Examples: Lodine, Ultradol (etodolac).

pyridostigmine—see *Mestinon.*

pyridoxylated stroma-free hemoglobin (SFHb)—artificial blood capable of carrying oxygen, can sustain life at a hematocrit of zero, and is nontoxic to the kidneys.

Pyrilinks-D—a screening urine test that detects bone loss by measuring the rate of bone resorption.

pyrophosphate scan (PYP).

pyrosis—heartburn.

Pyrost—bone replacement material used as a complement to homologous or heterologous bone grafts.

PYtest—urea breath test for *Helicobacter pylori.*

PZT (plumbeous zirconate titanate) **tip**—used with Bovie ultrasonic aspirator.

Q, q

q—the longer arm of a chromosome.

QALY (quality-adjusted life-year).

Q bands—light and dark transverse bands seen under fluorescent light in chromosomes after quinacrine staining.

Q-beta replicase—uses an enzyme replicase that makes cRNA from the DNA sequence of interest at a constant temperature detected by ethidium bromide staining of a specimen. See *polymerase chain reaction.*

QCA (quantitative coronary arteriography).

QCT (quantitative computed tomography).

q deletion syndrome—see *13q deletion syndrome* (in the *T*'s).

QDR-1500 or **QDR-2000 Bone Densitometer** (Nuclear Med)—devices that can assess the hip, lumbar spine, and total skeleton. The QDR-2000 includes 5-second scanning capability.

QEEG (quantitative EEG).

Q fever—disease endemic to sheep in the western part of the U.S. It causes flu-like symptoms in humans who are exposed to diseased sheep. These symptoms can be mild, occasionally severe, and can prove fatal. The organism causing Q fever is *Coxiella burnetii,* a rickettsia.

QFT (QuantiFERON-TB) **test**.

QHS (quantitative hepatobiliary scintigraphy).

Q-LAS 10—Q-switched YAG laser fully integrated into the arm of a slit lamp, allowing the ophthalmic surgeon to utilize the lamp for laser capsulotomy treatments and also as a standard examination unit.

QMST (quantitative muscle strength testing).

q.n.—every night.

QNS—quantity not sufficient, usually indicating that the specimen submitted is inadequate for the performance of the test requested.

q.o.d., QOD—every other day. An abbreviation that should be expanded when dictated.

QOL, QoL (Quality of Life) **assessment**.

QPD (quadrature phase detector)—MRI term.

QSART (quantitative sudomotor axon reflex test)—a test that measures the autonomic nerves that control sweating and is used to assess autonomic nervous system disorders, peripheral neuropathies, and some types of pain disorders.

Q sign—slang for a moribund patient, with gaping mouth and lolling tongue.

Qsma (superior mesenteric artery blood flow). Cf. *Rsma*.

Q-switched Nd:YAG laser—used to perform irradiation for postinflammatory hyperpigmentation secondary to granuloma faciale. Also, *Q-switched ruby laser.*

Q-Tc interval—corrected Q-T interval.

QTR (quadriceps tendon rupture)—in the knee.

Q-TWiST (quality-adjusted time without symptoms or toxicity)—a quality-of-life statistical model that discounts survival by time with side effects and symptoms. Originally developed for breast cancer therapies and now applied to AIDS and rectal cancer.

Quad-Lumen drain—perforated drain with a radiopaque stripe, used to monitor closed wound drainage postoperatively.

quadrature detector—MRI term.

quadrature phase detector (QPD)—MRI term.

quadrature surface coil system for MR imaging—MRI term.

quadriceps boot (DeLorme boot)—a metal plate that fits over the sole of a shoe and can be fitted with weights of various sizes for therapeutic exercise of the quadriceps muscles.

quadriceps muscle (*not* quadricep)—as in the quadriceps and hamstring muscles. It is one muscle with four heads.

quadriceps tendon rupture (QTR)—results in inability to extend the knee, which is essential in walking.

quadriplegia—*not* quadraplegia.

Quadripolar cutting forceps—an instrument that limits thermal spread without compromising hemostasis. The forceps is able to dissect, grasp, coagulate, transect, and retract for precise laparoscopic surgery.

quad sets—an exercise to strengthen the quadriceps muscles (for knee pain, as in chondromalacia patellae). Standing, with the legs straight, tighten the thigh muscles for three seconds, and relax. Do ten of these, and repeat a set of ten about 20 times a day.

QUAD 12000 and **QUAD 7000**—high-field, whole-body, open MRI scanners. The QUAD 12000 does not require the patient to be placed in the traditional tunnel-type MRI scanner and utilizes a magnet with a field strength of 0.6 tesla.

QualiCode *Borrelia burgdorferi* IgG and **IgM Western blot kits**—in vitro diagnostic tests for the detection of *Borrelia burgdorferi* antibodies for diagnosis of Lyme disease. It is used for patients who have positive or indeterminate ELISA tests.

quality factor—MRI term.

Quality of Life (QOL, QoL) **Assessment.**

quality of life, health-related (HRQoL, HRQL).

quant—slang for beta hCG quantitative.

Quanticyt (quantitative cytology)—urine test for transitional cell carcinoma.

QuantiFERON-TB test (QFT)—a whole-blood test for diagnosing latent tuberculosis (TB) infection

QuantiFERON-TB *(cont.)*
(LTBI). If not detected and treated, LTBI may later develop into TB disease. The QFT measures the patient's immune reactivity to *Mycobacterium tuberculosis*, the bacterium that causes TB.

Quantiplex HIV RNA assay—directly quantifies the amount of HIV in the plasma of people infected with the AIDS virus.

Quantiplex HCV-RNA 2.0 quantification assay—a branched DNA assay for HCV.

quantitative computed tomography (QCT)—using single photon absorptiometry, a noninvasive test for assessment of the skeleton with regard to bone mineral density in osteoporosis, hyperparathyroidism, Cushing syndrome, and other metabolic diseases known to affect the bones.

quantitative hepatobiliary scintigraphy (QHS).

quantitative muscle strength testing (QMST)—an objective standardized method of testing the strength of various muscles and muscle groups and of comparing the results with predicted or normal values based on age, gender, and body mass index.

Quantitative Sudomotor Axon Reflex Test (QSART)—to assess both pre- and post-synaptic activity of the sympathetic sudomotor system. The test is useful in evaluation for reflex sympathetic dystrophy.

quantity not sufficient (QNS).

Quantum Maverick catheter—a coronary balloon dilatation catheter.

Quantum pacemaker.

QuantX color quantification tools—used for transesophageal echocardiography (TEE) imaging on the V5M Multiplane and V510B Biplane TEE transducers. These tools provide numeric and graphic display of color data generated from two user-selectable regions of interest.

QUART (quadrantectomy, axillary dissection, and radiotherapy)—used in treatment of carcinoma of the breast.

Quartet system—used in the diagnosis and treatment of obstructive sleep apnea.

quartz fiberoptic probe.

quaternary ammonium chloride—skin cleansing compound, used in skin preparation prior to surgery.

Quattro mitral valve.

Queckenstedt sign—failure of cerebrospinal fluid pressure to rise and then fall when neck veins are compressed; indicative of a vertebral CSF canal block.

quellung reaction (*not* quelling)—technique for demonstrating the presence of capsular polysaccharide antigen. It is used to diagnose pneumococcal pneumonia.

quench, quenching—a term used when the magnet of the MRI equipment fails or goes down.

Quervain abdominal retractor.

Quervain disease—see *de Quervain disease.*

Quervain fracture.

QuestDirect—offers diagnostic screening tests for cholesterol, osteoporosis risk, allergies, and more, in a convenient location for an average of $20–25.

QuesTests—trademarked name of the diagnostic screening tests offered by QuestDirect. See *QuestDirect.*

questionnaire—see *test.*

Questionnaire for Identifying Children with Chronic Conditions (QuICCC).

Quest medical tape and hard pledget—used in beating heart surgery.

Questus Leading Edge—arthroscopic grasper-cutter.

Quetelet BMI index—body mass index to assess nutritional status. The formula for BMI is weight divided by height x 705. See *body mass index*.

Queyrat—see *erythroplasia of Queyrat*.

Quick Confusion Scale—a 6-item, 15-point instrument for testing for impaired mental status in an emergency department setting.

QuickDraw venous cannula—can be placed percutaneously to provide venous drainage in open-chest cardiac procedures, thus eliminating another cannula from the operative field.

QuickSeal arterial closure system—a device to stop femoral artery bleeding after cardiac catheterization.

QuickSilver—hydrophilic-coated guidewire.

Quick Tack periosteal fixation system—designed to replace the use of sutures during a Carticel implant procedure in the knee.

QuickVue Chlamydia test.

QuickVue influenza test—rapid point-of-care test for detection of influenza A and B.

QuickVue one-step *H. pylori* test—uses a smaller blood sample and provides faster results than the original test. *H. pylori* is believed to be associated with over 80% of the cases of peptic ulcer disease.

QuickVue UrinChek 10+ urine test strips.

Quiet interference screw—biodegradable screw that lessens the likelihood of an inflammatory response.

QuikHeel lancet—device for obtaining blood sample from the heel of an infant.

Quill self-anchoring suture—barbed polydioxanone suture, for wound closure of dermal tissue.

Quinaband—wound dressing used in the management of venous and gravitational ulcers as an adjunct to compression therapy.

Quincke spinal needle.

Quintessence—formulation of essential amino acids which can be used to supplement protein needs (as in low-protein diets used by kidney failure patients) or to enhance nutritional status in individuals with normal protein intake.

Quinton Mahurkar dual lumen catheter—for hemodialysis and peritoneal use. It comes in femoral and subclavian sizes. Also, *Mahurkar dual lumen catheter.*

Quinton PermCath (*not* PermaCath)—a large-bore, double-lumen silicone catheter placed in the internal jugular vein and used for long-term vascular access for hemodialysis.

Quinton-Scribner shunt—a vascular shunt used in dialysis patients.

Quinton suction biopsy instrument (Rubin tube)—used in esophageal biopsies.

Quinton tube—used for small bowel biopsy.

Quire mechanical finger forceps—for removal of foreign bodies from the ear.

Quixil (concentrated cryoprecipitated clottable proteins) **spray**—tissue adhesive.

R, r

r—when a lowercase *r* (and sometimes lowercase *rh*) appears before abbreviations or numbers, it often stands for *recombinant*.

RA (rhinocerebral aspergillosis).

RA (rotational atherectomy)—see *high-speed rotational atherectomy.*

RAAA (ruptured abdominal aortic aneurysm).

rAAT (recombinant alpha-1 antitrypsin).

RAB (remote afterloading brachytherapy).

rabbit nose—habitual repeated wrinkling of the nose by a person with itching of the nares due to allergic rhinitis.

rabbit stools—stools expelled as small pellets. Cf. *ribbon stools*.

RACAB (robot-assisted coronary artery bypass).

raccoon eyes—discoloration below or around the eyes due to subcutaneous hemorrhage, sometimes seen in basal skull fracture. Same as *raccoon sign*.

raccoon sign—periorbital ecchymoses, a possible indication of a number of different conditions including basilar skull fracture, other trauma, immunoglobulin amyloidosis, and even severe allergies. See *raccoon eyes*.

racemic fluoxetine, S-fluoxetine—drug used in an attempt to prevent migraine headache attacks.

rachitic—pertaining to rickets.

rachitic rosary—seen in patients with rickets. So-called because the enlargement of the cartilages at the costochondral junctions has the appearance of a string of beads.

R-A concept (in unilateral cleft lip repair)—see *Millard R-A cleft lip repair.*

Racz epidural catheter—see *epidural neuroplasty.*

rad (radiation absorbed dose)—see *centigray, gray, joule.*

RAD (renal tubule assist device).

RAD55 self-irrigating suction bur—for ENT surgery.

RAD40 sinus blade—for ENT surgery.

radial artery graft—tried and abandoned in the 1970s as a coronary artery bypass graft, but recently reinvestigated for the same purpose.

radial head subluxation (RHS) (also called *nursemaid's elbow*)—occurs when the radial head slides under the annular ligament and becomes entrapped. Reduction is achieved through a combination of supination, flexion, and extension, usually with prompt return of function. Recurrent RHS occurs in nearly one-fourth of patients.

radial keratotomy—a procedure for improving vision in myopic patients. Developed by Dr. Fydorov in the Soviet Union. Radial cuts (8 or 16) are made in the cornea, not quite all the way through. This flattens the shape of the eye, and changes myopia to more normal vision.

Radial Jaw—single-use biopsy forceps.

radial ray defect—see *pouce flottant.*

radial thermokeratoplasty—for correction of hyperopia.

Radiance (calcium hydroxylapatite, [CaHA] microspheres suspended in polysaccharide gel)—not yet FDA approved for cosmetic applications, but is approved for radiographic tissue marking.

radiation dosages—may be given as rads in a tissue dose, and in roentgens as an air dose. See *centigray; gray; joule.*

radiation-related optic neuropathy (RON).

radical—going to the root or source of a morbid process; directed to the cause, as in "radical excision of a tumor." Also, a fundamental constituent of a molecule; "free radical." Cf. *radicle.*

radical prostatectomy (RP).

radicle—one of the smallest branches of a nerve or a vessel, as in "intra-hepatic biliary radicles." Cf. *radical.*

radiculopathy—see *salon sink.*

Radiesse—an injectable implant used for plastic and reconstructive surgery including subdermal soft tissue augmentation and restoration of the facial area. It provides a matrix into which the body's own tissue can grow and maintain the implant in place.

radioactive iodinated serum albumin study (RISA).

radioactive seed implants—drug used to treat early-stage prostate cancer. The implants are tiny radioactive seeds, each one the size of a grain of rice. Each grain is placed at a precise location around the prostate gland and delivers a high dose of radiation to the prostate, while minimizing radiation to nearby organs such as the bladder and the rectum. The procedure is done on an outpatient basis and only takes about an hour to complete. There are said to be few side effects, and the majority of men return to work within five days of treatment. Examples:

BrachySeed
BrachySeed Pd-103
Cs131 (Cesium-131) Seed
I-Plant brachytherapy seeds
low-dose radiation (LDR) seeds
percutaneous transperineal seed implantation
PharmaSeed (palladium Pd 103 seeds
radioactive seeds
Symmetra I-125 brachytherapy seeds
Ultraseed

radioallergosorbent test (RAST).

radiocolloid mapping—see *intraoperative lymphatic mapping.*

radiodermatitis emulsion (RE)

Radiofocus Glidewire *(not* guidewire) —trade name for an angiographic

Radiofocus *(cont.)*
polymer-coated guidewire. It reduces friction and the risk of thrombus formation. The tip of the wire is flexible, to minimize trauma to the vessel.

radiofrequency (RF) **catheter ablation** —a treatment in paroxysmal supraventricular tachycardia when other forms of therapy have not proved effective. Radiofrequency, an electrical current, is delivered via a special type of intracardiac electrode catheter, to the area that is the source of the tachyarrhythmia, e.g., an area of abnormal conduction or impulse formation. This energy heats a tiny bit of tissue, only a few millimeters in diameter and depth, which produces coagulation necrosis. If, on testing, the doctor can reproduce the tachyarrhythmia, further RF current is applied to the tachyarrhythmic focus. The ablation is considered to be satisfactory if the tachyarrhythmia can no longer be induced. Also, *radiofrequency ablation* (RFA).

radiofrequency (RF) **coil; pulse**—MRI term.

radiofrequency percutaneous myocardial revascularization (RF-PMR)—a process that delivers radiofrequency (RF) energy to the oxygen-deprived heart muscle through a catheter, creating small crater-like injuries in the endocardium. It is believed to stimulate the body's healing response and initiate angiogenesis (creation of new vessels).

radiofrequency (RF) **spatial distribution problem**—MRI term.

Radiogardase (insoluble Prussian blue) —an agent given to people with known or suspected exposure to radioactive cesium-137 or radioactive or nonradioactive thallium.

radioimmunodetection (RAID)—an invaluable method in the management of patients with malignant melanoma, for the entire body can be surveyed with one test.

radioimmunoluminography (RILG)—a system for direct measurement of quantity and distribution of protein in histological specimens.

radioimmunoscintimetry—a means by which surgeons can more readily localize abdominal tumors. A week to ten days prior to surgery, the patient is injected with a monoclonal antibody that is specific to the tumor, and a radioactive substance (marker) attached to the antibody. This enables identification of the tumor intraoperatively with the use of a Geiger counter. Also, *immunoscintimetry*.

radioisotope (see also *technetium*)
- Cardiolite (^{99m}Tc sestamibi)
- CardioTec (^{99m}Tc teboroxime)
- CEAker
- Choletec (^{99m}Tc mebrofenin)
- fluorodeoxyglucose (FDG)
- Hedspa
- ImmuRAID (CEA-Tc99m)
- indium-111-labeled human nonspecific immunoglobulin G (^{111}In-IgG)
- iodine 131 MIBG (^{131}I)
- iridium 192 (Iriditope) (^{192}Ir)
- Macrotec (^{99m}Tc albumin)
- nitrogen 13 ammonia (^{13}N)
- OncoScint CR103 MOAB labeled with indium 111 (^{111}In)
- palladium 103 (^{103}Pd)
- ProstaScint (CYT-356 radiolabeled with 111 indium chloride)
- Renotec (^{99m}Tc iron-ascorbate DTPA)
- rubidium 82 (^{82}Rb)
- selenium 75 (^{75}Se)
- specific immunoglobulin G (^{111}In-IgG)

radioisotope *(cont.)*
TcHIDA (technetium-HIDA)
Techneplex (^{99m}Tc pentetate)
TechneScan MAG3 (^{99m}Tc mertiatide)
technetium ^{99m}Tc albumin
technetium ^{99m}Tc albumin aggregated
technetium ^{99m}Tc albumin colloid
technetium ^{99m}Tc bicisate
technetium ^{99m}Tc colloid
technetium ^{99m}Tc disofenin
technetium ^{99m}Tc etidronate
technetium ^{99m}Tc ferpentetate
technetium ^{99m}Tc furifosmin
technetium ^{99m}Tc gluceptate
technetium ^{99m}Tc glucarate
technetium ^{99m}Tc-GSA (diethylenetriaminepentaacetic acid-galactosyl-human serum-albumin)
technetium ^{99m}Tc iron-ascorbate-DTPA (Renotec)
technetium ^{99m}Tc lidofenin
technetium ^{99m}Tc macroaggregated albumin (^{99m}TcMAA)
technetium ^{99m}Tc albumin (Macrotec)
technetium ^{99m}Tc mertiatide (TechneScan MAG3)
technetium ^{99m}Tc oxidronate
technetium ^{99m}Tc pentetate (Techneplex)
technetium ^{99m}Tc pertechnetate sodium
technetium ^{99m}Tc PIPIDA
technetium ^{99m}Tc pyrophosphate
technetium ^{99m}Tc sestamibi (Cardiolite)
technetium ^{99m}Tc siboroxime
technetium ^{99m}Tc sodium
technetium ^{99m}Tc succimer
technetium ^{99m}Tc sulfur colloid (^{99m}Tc-SC) (Tesuloid)
technetium ^{99m}Tc teboroxime (CardioTec)

radioisotope *(cont.)*
technetium ^{99m}Tc tetrofosmin
technetium stannous pyrophosphate (TSPP)
Tesuloid (^{99m}Tc-SC, sulfur colloid)
thallium 201 (^{201}Tl)
xenon 133 (^{133}Xe)

radioisotope stent—a very low-dose radiation-emitting stent implant designed to prevent or reduce the re-stenosis of blood vessels following treatment for coronary artery disease.

radiolabeled peptide alpha-M2—imaging agent used in breast cancer imaging and possible therapy.

radiolucent—offering relatively little resistance to x-rays (by analogy with *translucent*).

radiolucent spine frame—a modification of the Relton-Hall spine frame. Made of strong radiolucent plastic compounds that achieve x-rays without metallic shadows that are common to metal frames. Used in intraoperative radiography to assess spinal alignment to prevent overcorrection of the spinal curve and decompensation. Recommended to assist in assessment of hook placement and spine alignment.

radiolymphoscintigraphy, intraoperative—combined with blue dye mapping during lymphadenectomy for melanoma.

radionuclide—radioactive isotope; a species of atom that spontaneously emits radioactivity. Often mispronounced as "radio-nucl-ee-ide" and misspelled "radionucleide."

radionuclide esophageal transit test (RETT)—a procedure used to assess esophageal motility, including esophageal mean transit time (MTT), residual fraction (RF), and retrograde index (RI).

radionuclide scan—the introduction into the body of a radioactive substance whose distribution in tissues, vessels, or cavities can be detected and recorded by a device that senses radiation. The choice of radioactive substances (radionuclides, isotopes) is governed by the tendency of certain organs or tissues to take up (absorb, concentrate) certain elements or compounds. Radionuclides may be swallowed, inhaled, or injected into a body cavity or into the circulation. Scanning may be performed immediately after the material is administered (as in studies of blood flow) or after an interval (as when absorption or concentration of a substance in an organ must occur first). The standard lung scan procedure includes two separate scans of the lungs, one after inhalation of a radionuclide and the other after injection of a second radionuclide into the circulation. Scanning is done with a scintillation camera (scintiscanner, gamma camera) which creates a picture on film representing the distribution and intensity of gamma radiation emitted by the patient.

radiopaque—resisting penetration by x-rays.

radiotherapy
- Beta-Cath radiation therapy
- CHART (continuous hyperfractionated accelerated radiotherapy)
- coronary radiation therapy (CRT)
- crossfire radiation therapy
- CyberKnife stereotactic radiosurgery/radiotherapy system
- EBIORT (electron beam intraoperative radiotherapy) procedure
- EBRT (external beam radiation therapy)
- fractionated stereotaxic radiation therapy

radiotherapy *(cont.)*
- Galileo intravascular radiotherapy
- gamma-ribbon radiation therapy
- Generation 6 integrated radiotherapy
- GliaSite radiation therapy
- image-guided radiation therapy (IGRT)
- Intrabeam intraoperative radiotherapy (IORT)
- intraoperative radiotherapy (IORT)
- IMRT (intensity-modulated radiation therapy or radiotherapy)
- lens-sparing external beam radiation therapy
- LINAC radiosurgery
- MammoSite RTS (radiation therapy system)
- microwave thermoradiotherapy
- Mobetron intraoperative radiation therapy (IORT)
- Nucletron radiotherapy
- Photon Radiosurgery System (PRS)
- QUART (quadrantectomy, axillary dissection, and radiotherapy)
- single-field hyperthermia combined with radiation therapy
- skeletal targeted radiotherapy (STR)
- SmartBeam high-resolution, intensity-modulated radiotherapy
- telecurietherapy
- TMS 3-dimensional radiation therapy
- vascular brachytherapy

RadiStop radial compression system—for prolonged controlled mechanical compression of the radial artery, which is becoming an alternative to the femoral approach for angiography and angioplasty.

Radius enteral feeding tubes.

RADIUS program—see *Rheumatoid Arthritis DMARD.*

Radstat—a device and its accompanying wrist splint that allows selective compression of the radial artery following catheterization through the wrist.

RAE endotracheal tubes—both oral and nasal tubes can be bent to keep them out of the respective surgical fields.

RA (rheumatoid arthritis) **factor**—protein in the blood of most patients with rheumatoid arthritis. It is detected by a blood test. Cf. *Rh factor.*

Raf-1—a human protein found to be an autoantigen in Ménière disease.

Ragnell handheld retractor.

RAI (radioimmunoassay)—used to measure various hormone levels in the blood.

Rai classification of chronic lymphocytic leukemia—classifies progression of the disease from stages 0 through 4.

Stage 0 patients are low risk and have lymphocytosis.

Stage 1 patients are intermediate risk and have lymphocytosis plus lymphadenopathy.

Stage 2 patients are also intermediate risk but have lymphocytosis plus hepatomegaly or splenomegaly, with or without lymphadenopathy.

Stage 3 patients are high risk and have lymphocytosis plus anemia (hemoglobin < 11 g/dL), with or without lymphadenopathy, hepatomegaly, or splenomegaly.

Stage 4 patients are also high risk but have lymphocytosis plus thrombocytopenia.

RAID (radioimmunodetection)—used in combination with a monoclonal antibody against carcinoembryonic antigen. See *ImmuRAID.*

rainbow coverage—sliding scale insulin coverage for inpatient glucose control, an unphysiologic and now obsolete method of basing insulin dosage on urine sugar, as measured by color changes in test tablets or strips (hence "rainbow"); since the urine sugar can only reflect an elevation of blood sugar one to six hours earlier and can never indicate low blood sugar, this way of calculating insulin dosage produced erratic responses, with the blood sugar bouncing from one extreme to the other ("roller coaster control").

rainbow passage—a term used to refer to the glottic space between the vocal cords on visual examination.

Raji cell assay test—for immune complexes.

rake—a bent-tine, forklike retractor.

rale—a fine crackling, static-like sound heard through the stethoscope, indicating a pathologic condition. Take a lock of hair and roll it between your thumb and index finger near your ear; you've just heard what a crackling rale sounds like. Also, *Velcro rales.*

rale indux—a crepitant rale that is heard in patients with pneumonia at the stage when consolidation begins. Cf. *rale redux.*

rale redux—an unequal subcrepitant sound caused by the passage of air through the fluid in bronchial tubes. This rale is heard when pneumonia is resolving. Also, *rale de retour* (rattle of return).

RAM (rapid alternating movements).

Raman spectroscopy—method of detecting plaque or remote sensing of diseased artery wall in laser angioplasty. Cf. *spectrofluorometry.*

ram's horn sign—a tubular funnel-shaped antrum caused by fibrosis and scarring associated with Crohn disease of the stomach.

Ramirez shunt—a vascular access shunt, used in performing dialysis.

RAMP Reader—provides a quantitative measurement of cardiac enzymes in a whole blood sample.

Ramsay Hunt (no hyphen) **syndrome** —herpetic eruption of the external ear and ipsilateral facial paralysis, usually with additional symptoms of pain in the affected ear (occasionally with auditory symptoms), oral lesions, reduced tearing, and reduced taste on the anterior two-thirds of the tongue.

Ranawat/Burstein total hip system—porous femoral components for noncemented hip replacement.

Rancho cube—part of an orthopedic apparatus used with the Ilizarov method for leg lengthening. The cube is actually a rectangular pin gripper made from titanium. The cubes come with one to five holes through them to hold the pins and connecting rods of the Ilizarov apparatus. The cubes replace the steel transfixion wires usually used. The advantage of the Rancho cube is that it does not work its way through to the skin surface as the wire can.

Rancho los Amigos cognitive scale in rating posttraumatic amnesia, levels I to VIII.

Level I—no response to any stimulus.

Level II—generalized response, often only to pain, but limited, and inconsistent, nonpurposeful.

Level III—localized response, withdrawal from painful stimuli, and can make purposeful responses. May follow simple commands, but only inconsistently and hesitantly.

Level IV—alert, but may be agitated, confused, aggressive, and disoriented. Cannot perform self care.

Level V—confused, with inappropriate response.

Level VI—confused, but with appropriate response.

Level VII—automatic, but appropriate response.

Level VIII—purposeful and appropriate response. Alert, oriented, and can recall past events. Can learn new activities and can perform activities of daily living. Judgment and abstract reasoning are impaired, and there is reduced tolerance to stress; may function at less than optimal level.

Rancho fixation system—modification of the Ilizarov external fixation system that allows the surgeon to build hybrid frames using half-pins or pins and wires.

Randall-Tennison triangular flap—see *Randall unilateral cleft lip repair.*

Randall unilateral cleft lip repair—a modification of an older technique, the Tennison triangular flap operation, for repair of unilateral cleft lip.

Rand microballoon—used in microballoon embolization of cerebral aneurysms, arteriovenous malformations, and carotid cavernous fistula occlusion.

randomize—a term used in testing new medications or chemotherapy protocols. Patients are selected at random, rather than in any predetermined manner, to test responses.

Randot ("ran-dot") **test**—not a physician's name; it is a coined word for the random dots that become recognizable as geometric figures when the patient wears a certain kind of eyeglasses. This is a test of binocular depth perception.

Raney clip—used in repair of facial fractures requiring bicoronal incision, to obtain hemostasis of the galea and skin.

Ranfac cholangiographic catheters—LAP-13 for insertion through the lateral port; ORC-B for open procedure, XL-11 for percutaneous or three-puncture technique. Also, *Ranfac laparoscopic instruments.*

range of motion (ROM).

Ranke complex—calcified node, or mass, or granuloma in the chest, from old tuberculosis.

Ranson criteria—a predictor of mortality in acute pancreatitis. The Ranson variables, however, are not specific for pancreatitis but rather general markers of organ system dysfunction.

RAP cannula—see *remote access perfusion (RAP) cannula.*

Rapicide—high-level disinfectant and sterilant for disinfection of flexible endoscopes in automated endoscope reprocessors.

rapid acquisition with relaxation enhancement (RARE)—a version of STIR. See *STIR.*

rapid alternating movements (RAM).

Rapid Drug Screen (trademark)—drugs-of-abuse urine test kit that can be used at home or by businesses.

Rapide suture.

rapid eye movement (REM).

RapidFlap—a cranial fixation device that affixes the bone flap from both sides of the bone.

Rapidgraft—an arterial vessel substitute.

rapid HIV test—provides preliminary results in 20 minutes.

Rapid Susceptibility Assay (RSA)—a laboratory test for fungal susceptibility to antifungal agents.

Rapid Syndrome Validation Project—early disease detection computer network for physicians. The doctor enters the patient's symptoms into the database to find out if similar cases have been reported elsewhere and what malady might be associated with the symptoms.

rapid urease test (RUT)—a rapid and accurate test to detect *Helicobacter pylori* in gastric lesions. The test produces a color change in one minute with a specimen of gastric mucosa obtained via endoscopic biopsy. Other tests for *H. pylori* take much longer: Gram stain (1 to 3 hours); culture (4 to 7 days). The RUT allows appropriate treatment to be initiated immediately.

RapiSeal patch—collagen-based biodegradable patch used to control surgical bleeding in solid organs such as liver and spleen.

RAPP (Routine Assessment of Patient Progress)—an assessment instrument for psychiatric inpatients that allows nurses to incorporate both interview and observational data into a comprehensive assessment.

Rapp-Hodgkin syndrome—congenital multisystem disorder characterized by cleft palate and/or cleft lip, partial or complete, and/or absence of teeth, impaired ability to sweat, dysplastic nails, and occasionally other physical abnormalities.

Raptor over-the-wire delivery system—used with Bx Velocity stent. It reduces the risk of edge dissection and prevents *dog-boning*. See *dog-boning*.

Raptor PTCA balloon—see *Raptor over-the-wire delivery system.*

RARE (rapid acquisition with relaxation enhancement) **technique**—MRI term.

Rashkind balloon atrial septotomy—a procedure in which a cardiac catheter with a balloon is inserted; the balloon is inflated, thus enlarging the aperture.

Rashkind cardiac device.

Rashkind double umbrella device—used in reopening a previously occluded ductus arteriosus.

Raskin DHE-45 protocol—a combination of metoclopramide and dihydroergotamine IV scheduled round the clock for two to three days with doxepin or amitriptyline as prophylaxis for the treatment of chronic daily headache.

Rasmussen syndrome—chronic idiopathic progressive unilateral hemisphere inflammation.

Rasor blood pumping system (RBPS)—disposable device used in circulatory support and cardiopulmonary bypass. Also an alternative to intraaortic balloons for acute postoperative cardiac support.

RAST (radioallergosorbent test)
- RAST class 0, no likelihood of atopy.
- RAST 0/I—borderline.
- RAST class I response is thought by some to have some significance.
- RAST class II and above represents the presence of atopy.
- RAST results are reported in units per milliliter (U/ml).

ratbite fever—see *Haverhill fever.*

rating of perceived exertion (RPE)—self-assessment scale to rate breathlessness and fatigue during exercise.

ratio
- bone and limb growth velocity
- C/N (contrast-to-noise)
- CT (cardiothoracic)
- cup-to-disk

ratio *(cont.)*
- FPSA vs. TPSA
- gyromagnetic
- helper/suppressor cell
- high nuclear-to-cytoplasmic
- I-E ratio ("I to E ratio") (inspiratory-expiratory)
- I/E (inspiration/expiration)
- international normalized (INR)
- L/S (lecithin/sphingomyelin) (in amniocentesis)
- M/E (myeloid/erythroid)
- RV/TLC (residual volume/ total lung capacity)
- S/N (signal-to-noise)
- T-lymphocyte subset
- ventilation-perfusion (V-P)
- waist-to-hip (WHR)

"rat"—phonetic for *WRAT* (Wide Range Achievement Test).

rational drug design—use of x-ray crystallography, molecular modeling, or MRI scanning to determine the target molecule of a pathogen, and then use of computers to design an effective drug.

ratty—a descriptive term meaning shabby, unkempt, but more likely ragged in a medical context, used to describe many findings at surgery or in the pathology laboratory. Usage: "A ratty placenta was sent to pathology."

ratty changes—slang for damaged tendons and muscles in the orthopedic exam.

Raulerson syringe—used with guidewire insertion in the Seldinger technique.

Rayleigh scattering law (Neuro).

ray resection—resection of a finger or toe, a ray of the hand or foot.

Ray-Tec sponge—x-ray detectable surgical sponge. Cf. *Vistec.*

Ray threaded fusion cage (TFC)—used in lumbar fusion surgery, this titanium stabilization device is placed between the vertebrae to maintain the height of the disc space. It has hollow threaded cylinders that are packed with fragments of the patient's bone. The bone then grows through tiny openings in the cylinders to fuse the vertebrae.

Raz double-prong ligature carrier—for performing bladder and bladder neck suspensions.

Razi cannula introducer—used to simplify the procedure and diminish postoperative strokes and memory loss following aortic cannulation.

RazorVac ArthroWand—device used to remove torn knee joint tissue by dissolving the problem areas in a field of ionized gas about the width of a strand of human hair.

Raz sling operation—for urinary incontinence. See *vaginal wall sling procedure.*

RCA (rotational coronary atherectomy)—see *directional coronary atherectomy* and *radiofrequency catheter ablation.*

rCBF (regional cerebral blood flow)—PET (positron emission tomography) term. See also *rCBV.*

rCBV (regional cerebral blood volume)—PET (positron emission tomography) term. See also *rCBF.*

RCC (renal cell carcinoma).

RCMD (refractory cytopenia with multilineage dysplasia)

RCP (retrograde cerebral perfusion)—used in cardiac surgery. Usage: "The Dacron graft was de-aired using RCP, which filled the conduit with dark blood, displacing luminal air."

rCPP (regional cerebral perfusion pressure).

rd (rutherford)—unit of radioactivity.

RDI (respiratory disturbance index).

RDRV (adsorbed)—Rhesus diploid cell strain rabies vaccine. See *HDRV.*

RDS (respiratory distress syndrome).

RDW (red cell diameter width)—a term used in hematology.

RDX coronary radiation catheter delivery system—designed to prevent restenosis in patients who have implanted coronary stents.

RE (radiodermatitis emulsion).

reactive airways disease (RAD)—bronchial asthma.

reactive perforating collagenosis (RPC)—an uncommon disorder in which altered collagen bundles are eliminated through the skin, presenting as cup-shaped epidermal depressions and umbilicated papules or nodules with a central adherent keratotic plug. Both childhood and adult forms are believed to be a cutaneous response to superficial trauma, the adult form always associated with pruritus.

reactive, reparative atypia (Ob-Gyn)—presence of immature cells formed in the process of healing or regrowth of the squamous epithelium. A common finding that often follows treatment of dysplasia and other conditions such as cervical or vaginal infections.

ReAct NMES (neuromuscular electrical stimulation) **device**—used in physical therapy to treat disuse atrophy and other neuromuscular disorders. The system uses Multi-Ply or Soft-EZ reusable electrodes.

reagent—substance involved in a chemical reaction; also a substance used to detect the presence of another substance by chemical means. See *Millon reagent.* Cf. *reagin.*

reagin—a type of antibody. See *RPR, reagent.*

REAL (Revised European American Lymphoma) **classification of lymphoma**—considers lymphoma in terms of "real" diseases rather than pathologic entities. The major entities are diffuse large B-cell lymphoma, follicular lymphomas, mucosa-associated lymphoid tissue (MALT) lymphoma, peripheral T-cell, small lymphocytic, and mantle cell. Less common are mediastinal large B-cell, anaplastic large T-cell, Burkitt marginal zone, and peripheral T-cell.

Reality vaginal pouch—reservoir (similar to a diaphragm) placed in the vagina for several hours to collect amniotic fluid. Used to diagnose PPROM (preterm premature rupture of membranes).

real-time color flow Doppler—permits two-dimensional color-coded imaging of blood flow.

real-time 4-D ultrasound—four-dimensional color images in real time.

real-time position management (REAL) **tracking system**.

real-time ultrasonography—intraoperative scanning technique (frequency around 30 cycles per second [cps]) which permits physiological movement to be observed while it is happening, e.g., it is possible to see a cyst collapsing as its wall is entered. It is used for determining the precise location of tumors of the brain, beneath the cerebral cortex, for removal through very small and accurately placed incisions. It also permits the accurate guiding of biopsy needles, localizing of intracranial cysts, aneurysms or abscesses, or foreign bodies, and makes it possible to position catheters in the ventricles for draining fluids or to measure pressure. In a laminectomy, the spinal cord can be visualized without opening the dura. It is also used for noninvasive exploration of the pelvis and abdomen. It is particularly useful in that the examination can be taped on magnetic tape and individual frames can be placed in the patient's record. There is no radiation hazard associated with the use of real-time ultrasonography or examination. See *ultrasound.*

Rebar microcatheters—used for both neurologic and peripheral vascular procedures.

Rebel knee orthosis—a pre-sized knee brace designed not to migrate.

Rebif in a thin-needle (29-gauge) **prefilled syringe**—ready-to-use for subcutaneous administration in the treatment of multiple sclerosis. Rebif (interferon beta-1a) is a disease-modifying drug used to treat relapsing forms of multiple sclerosis and is similar to the interferon beta protein produced by the human body.

rebound tenderness—test for rebound tenderness; the fingers are pushed into an area far from the area of suspected inflammation and then quickly removed. The rebound of the indented structures causes pain in the area of inflammation.

recanalization—see *transcervical balloon tuboplasty.*

recession—the moving of the end of an eye muscle (usually the medial rectus or lateral rectus, that adducts or abducts, respectively, the eyeball) and reimplanting it in a slightly different position, for correction of strabismus. Cf. *resection.*

recessive—said of a trait or gene that is expressed only in homozygotes. See *autosomal.*

reciprocating cannula, powered—for precise sculpting and contouring in plastic surgery procedures.

reciprocating saw.

recombinant (Genetics)—referring to an individual who has a combination of genes not found together in either parent.

recombinant DNA—an artificial gene; a strand of genetically active DNA that has been synthesized in a laboratory by combining segments of DNA from various sources. If a recombinant gene that codes for the synthesis of human insulin or hepatitis B vaccine is introduced into a strain of nonpathogenic bacteria, a large culture of such bacteria can be induced to make the hormone or vaccine in sufficient quantity to meet therapeutic demands.

recombinant enzyme replacement therapy—used to treat Pompe disease, an inherited and usually lethal glycogen storage disease that often afflicts children. In the disease, glycogen accumulates and destroys skeletal, heart, and lung muscle.

recombinant human granulocyte colony stimulating factor (r-HuG-CSF).

recombinant human neutral endopeptidase (rNEP).

recombinant immunoblot assay (RIBA)—used to detect the hepatitis C virus.

recombinant novel plasminogen activator (rNPA).

recombinant platelet-derived growth factor (rPDGF-BB)—stimulates migration and proliferation of fibroblasts and smooth muscle cells and induces the rapid development of granulation tissue.

recombination (Genetics)—the formation of new combinations of linked genes by crossing over between their loci.

recons—slang for CT reconstructed images.

reconstitution—a term used in angiography for maintenance of flow in an artery beyond an area of narrowing or obstruction by establishment of collateral circulation.

reconstruction artifact (Radiol)—error in CT imaging.

reconstruction study—generation of an image by computer processing of scan data. Used in computed tomography scan.

recording electrode—that one of an array of ECG or EEG electrodes whose input is balanced against the input of one or more indifferent electrodes. Cf. *indifferent electrode.*

recovery—a term that seems to be replacing "harvest" in the literature in reference to obtaining donor organs for transplantation. See *harvest.*

recruitment—when, in testing hearing, a slight increase in decibel level causes a disproportionate increase in loudness perceived.

rectal endoscopic ultrasonography (REU)—a sonographic transducer is inserted endoscopically to evaluate for possible tumors in the rectum.

rectal linitis plastica (RLP)—a rare colorectal carcinoma with a long delay between onset of symptoms and diagnosis.

rectilinear biphasic waveform for external defibrillation—provides successful defibrillation with less delivered current than conventional monophasic waveform.

Rector-Gordon-Healey-Mendoza-Spitzer type IV renal tubular acidosis—a rare type named for five physicians in different cities who first found and identified it.

rectus abdominis myocutaneous (RAM) **flap**—used in vaginal reconstructive procedures.

recurred (*not* reoccurred). Usage: "The symptoms recurred with the advent of cold weather."

recurrence risk (Genetics)—the probability that a genetic trait or disorder that is present in one or more members of a family will recur in another member of that family in the same or a later generation.

recurrent abdominal pain (RAP).

recurrent respiratory papillomatosis (RRP)—recurrent benign growths in the respiratory tract, most common in the larynx in children. Caused by HPV (human papillomavirus).

recurrent spontaneous abortions (RSA).

red cell diameter width (RDW).

red clot—composed of a mesh of cross-linked fibrin molecules and entrapped red cells. It is superimposed over a white clot, the result of coagulation cascade in myocardial infarction with associated ST-segment elevation.

Reddick cystic duct cholangiogram catheter—used during laparoscopic cholecystectomy.

Reddick-Saye screw—inserted through trocar to provide fixation and traction during laparoscopic cholecystectomy.

red flag—a condition or laboratory value ("panic level") indicating severe or urgent condition.

red herring—a misleading diagnostic clue.

Redifurl TaperSeal IAB catheter—for percutaneous insertion in the femoral artery.

Redipen—see *PEG-Intron Redipen.*

red reflex—an ophthalmologic finding. When the light from the ophthalmoscope is flashed on the patient's pupil at a slight angle lateral to the patient's line of vision and at about a distance of 12 inches, a bright orange glow will be noted.

REDS (remote endoscopic digital spectroscopy).

reduced liver transplant (RLT) or **reduced-size liver transplant** (RSLT) —a segmental liver transplant, reduced from a larger liver to fit a smaller recipient, such as a child. Such transplants can be taken from a parent or other compatible living relative. Also called *cut-down liver*.

reduced signal intensity in the center of the blood vessels on MR angiograms that can mimic intraluminal thrombus.

reducing substances—positive in stools of premature infants who are not properly digesting formula, consists of various sugars tested by making a mixture of stool and water and Clinitest tablet.

reduction columelloplasty—a procedure for refinement of the nasal bone or narrowing splayed medial crura, increasing the nasolabial angle, modifying the shape of the nares, and for increasing tip projection.

reduction division—meiosis; more specifically, the first meiotic division, during which the chromosome number in each cell is reduced from diploid (23 pairs) to haploid (23 unpaired chromosomes).

reefing—folding or tucking of skin or other tissue: Usage: "We then performed arthrotomy, lateral release, and medial reefing of the right patella for lateral subluxation."

Reese dermatome—a drum-type dermatome that makes grafts from .008 to .034 inch.

Reese-Ellsworth classification of retinoblastoma—groups I through V.

Reese retinal telangiectasia.

Reese stimulator—used in sectioning of recurrent nerve for spastic dysphonia.

Reeve rests—rests of thyroid tissue entirely separate from the thyroid or extending from it into the thyrothymic area. They may be mistaken for lymph nodes or parathyroids and may be clinically significant during thyroid surgery. Also *thyrothymic thyroid rests.*

refer, referred—also, *referring, referral,* but *referable.*

reference, ideas of—delusions that strangers such as radio or television broadcasters are referring to the patient.

Refinity—brand-name skin products, including an in-office skin peel treatment.

Refinity Coblation system—wrinkle reduction procedure.

reflectance-guided laser selection—used for removal of tattoos. It uses skin reflectance measurements to determine the optimum laser wavelength to remove various colors in the tattoo.

reflectant spectral photometer—an endoscope with a probe in the biopsy port that reflects light off mucosa and back into the instrument, and then into a processor. An index of mucosal blood flow is then obtained.

reflex—reflected action or movement. Cf. *reflux.*

re-flex (verb)—a hyphen is needed to distinguish *re-flex* (to flex again) from the noun *reflex* (an involuntary action).

reflexes, deep tendon
- 0 absent
- 1+ decreased
- 2+ normal
- 3+ hyperactive
- 4+ clonus

reflex sympathetic dystrophy (RSD) —a response to an injury consisting of vasomotor instability, trophic skin changes, swelling, and pain.

ReFlex Wand—disposable surgical device used in the office environment to debulk tonsils without removing them. Also for the treatment of snoring by creating channels in the soft palate for tissue removal and stiffening in a matter of seconds.

reflux—backward or return flow. Cf. *reflex.*
- gastroesophageal
- hepatojugular
- intrarenal
- vesicoureteral

reflux esophagitis, classification—written as grades, with roman numerals:
- E-I erythema, edema
- E-II erosions
- E-III localized deformity
- E-IV stricture

refraction—determination of the refractive errors of the eye for distance and near vision.

refractory cytopenia with multilineage dysplasia (RCMD)—a myelodysplastic syndrome.

regenerative (or reparative) **medicine** —a mode of treatment in which stem cells are induced to differentiate into

regenerative *(cont.)*
the specific cell type required to repair damaged or depleted adult cell populations or tissues.

Regency SR+ single-chamber, rate-responsive pulse generator.

Regen flexion exercises (Ortho)—pronounced like "region."

Regent aortic heart valve—mechanical heart valve implant.

regimen (*not* regime)—a systematic course of therapy, diet, or exercise meant to achieve certain ends. Also, *protocol*.

regime—government or social system; mode of rule or management. Often misused in medicine for *regimen*. Cf. *regimen*.

regional cerebral blood flow (rCBF).

regional cerebral blood volume (rCBV).

regional cerebral perfusion pressure (rCPP).

Registered Health Information Administrator (RHIA)—formerly RRA (Registered Record Administrator).

Registered Health Information Technician (RHIT)—formerly ART (Accredited Record Technician).

Regnauld-type degeneration—results in first metatarsophalangeal joint space narrowing, loss of joint cartilage, bony spurring, and painful range of motion of the great toe.

Regulus frameless stereotactic system.

Reifenstein syndrome—partial androgen insensitivity, familial incomplete male pseudohermaphroditism.

Reil, island of—in the brain.

Reimer migration index—a radiographic method of determining the percentage of hip subluxation.

Reinke crystals—crystals contained in interstitial cells (Leydig cells) of human testes. See *Leydig cell*.

Rein rib-cutting knife—autopsy instrument for severing the costosternal joints.

Reis-Bückler corneal dystrophy.

Reitan CatheterPump—a left ventricular assist device. (No space in CatheterPump.)

rejection
acute cellular xenograft
cellular xenograft
delayed xenograft (DXR)
hyperacute (HAR)
transplant

relaxation rate; relaxation time—MRI terms.

relaxin (recombinant human relaxin)—drug used for the treatment of scleroderma.

relaxing (or **relief**) **incision**—an incision made to relieve tension in tissue.

Relay cardiac pacemaker—dual chamber rate-adaptive pacemaker.

Relia-Flow device—a surgically implanted device for hemodialysis access or vascular bypass.

Reliance CM femoral component.

Reliance urinary control insert—a disposable balloon-tipped device that is placed in the urethra and expanded, to prevent urine loss.

ReliefBand NST (nerve stimulation therapy)—watchlike electronic device for drug-free treatment of nausea and vomiting due to motion sickness, chemotherapy, and pregnancy.

Relton-Hall spine frame.

Relume system—used to treat stretch marks and acne scars. The device uses a fiberoptic light source to darken the scar tissue until it matches the healthy normal skin.

rem (roentgen-equivalent-man)—unit of measurement of maximum toler-

rem *(cont.)*
ance dose of radiation (for hospital personnel). A permissible dose is 0.1 rem/week, or 5 rems per year. See *gray.*

remote afterloading brachytherapy (RAB)—remote-controlled implantation of a radioactive source in a patient for brief treatment without exposing the physician or nurse to radioactivity. The applicator is placed manually, and the radioisotope is administered under computer control by machine, after the physician or nurse has left the treatment room. The most commonly used radioisotopes for this procedure are iridium 192 (^{192}Ir) and cesium 137 (^{137}Cs). Iodine 125 (^{125}I), a low-energy radionuclide, may also be used. Cf. *brachytherapy.*

remnant-like particle (RLP) **lipoprotein**—form of cholesterol that results from metabolism of very low density lipoproteins and chylomicrons, the major triglycerides that carry lipids in the blood. These cholesterol-rich particles are believed to promote plaque formation, which leads to arterial disease and sets the stage for a heart attack.

remote access perfusion (RAP) **cannula**—multifunction catheter used to stop the heart and provide arterial blood flow for the body without need to open the chest. This minimally invasive cardiac surgery is performed through small incisions, or "windows," between the ribs.

remote endoscopic digital spectroscopy (REDS).

REM (rapid eye movement) **sleep**—that period of sleep when the heart rate and respiration are irregular, brain waves are rapid and of low voltage, and dreaming occurs. Cf. *NREM sleep.*

renal cell carcinoma (RCC)—solid renal tumor.

renal helical CT (RHCT)—imaging modality in the evaluation of potential renal donors.

renal transit time (RTT)—used to identify obstructive uropathy in children. It is used in contrast-enhanced MR urography to indicate the time it takes for a contrast agent to go through the kidney and collecting system.

renal tubule assist device (RAD)—for use with the bioartificial kidney.

renin levels, serum—elevated in cardiac patients. In addition to cholesterol and triglyceride levels in cardiac patients, you will be hearing about serum renin levels. Studies have shown that elevated cholesterol and triglycerides are not the only factors responsible for an increased risk of heart attacks. It has been found that the risk of heart attack is seven times higher in patients with elevated renin levels. In addition, elevated renin levels may provide the key to the question of why more than half the patients experiencing a myocardial infarction have normal cholesterol levels.

repair—see *operation.*

repair chain reaction—involves the use of a polymerase and ligase that is highly specific to detect a known DNA or RNA sequence in a specimen. See *polymerase chain reaction.*

repeated FID (free induction decay)—MRI term.

Repel—bioresorbable barrier film used to prevent postoperative adhesions.

Repela surgical glove—resistant to tear and puncture. Made of Kevlar and Lycra.

reperfusion edema after lung transplantation (Radiol)—appears as air-space disease in the middle and/or lower lung zones and is a form of noncardiogenic pulmonary edema.

repetition time (TR)—given in seconds—MRI term.

repetitive strain injury (RSI)—see *carpal tunnel syndrome.*

repetitive transcranial magnetic stimulation (rTMS)—uses an electromagnet placed on the scalp to generate brief magnetic pulses, about the strength of an MRI scan, which stimulate the cerebral cortex. It is being used to treat individuals with partial spinal cord injury.

rephasing gradient—MRI term.

RepHresh ("re-fresh") **vaginal gel**—a feminine hygiene product.

Repicci II unicondylar knee system.

re-place (verb)—a hyphen is needed to distinguish *re-place* (to place again) from *replace* (to take the place of).

replant splint—designed to treat metacarpal, wrist, and forearm replants. A high-profile crane has constant tension designed for protective extrinsic muscle mobilization.

RepliCare hydrocolloid dressing material.

Repliderm—a collagen-based dressing for wounds, decubitus or diabetic ulcers, and first- and second-degree burns.

Replogle tube.

Repose—a surgical system for treating obstructive sleep apnea and snoring. It is a minimally invasive procedure that stabilizes and prevents the tongue from collapsing back and obstructing the airway passage. The procedure does not require incisions and can typically be performed in less than 30 minutes. Recovery time is expected to be much shorter relative to other surgical methods.

repressor (Genetics)—a substance produced by a regulator gene that inhibits the action of another gene, chiefly by preventing synthesis of the protein for which the second gene codes.

reproductive cloning—cloning of an embryo for transplantation into a uterus in order to produce a mature organism that is genetically identical to the nuclear donor.

rescue PTCA—PTCA to the infarct-related artery after failed thrombolysis.

research cloning—see *therapeutic cloning*.

resection—excision of a portion of an organ or of a structure. Cf. *recession.*

reservoir (see also *pouch)*
- Camey ileocystoplasty
- Camey
- continent supravesical bowel urinary diversion
- continent urinary diversion
- double bubble flushing
- Florida pouch
- heparin lock
- Hunt-Lawrence pouch
- ileal conduit
- ileal neobladder
- Indiana pouch
- inverted U-pouch ileal
- J-Vac suction
- Kock pouch
- Le Bag
- Mainz pouch urinary
- Mitrofanoff
- Ommaya
- Reality vaginal pouch
- reservoir ileostomy
- retubularized ileum
- Rickham

reservoir *(cont.)*
Rowland pouch
Salmon-Rickham ventriculostomy
sigmoid colon
W-stapled urinary (or ileal neobladder)

residual—lasting effect of disease or injury.

residual volume/total lung capacity (RV/TLC) **ratio.**

resigned person (Psych)—a possible precursor to borderline personality disorder.

resipump—reservoir/pump component of inflatable penile prosthesis.

resolution—the ability of an optical, radiographic, or other image-forming device to distinguish or separate two closely adjacent points in the subject. In computed tomography, resolution is measured in lines per millimeter; the higher the resolution, the sharper and more faithful the image.

Resolve Quickanchor—used for intraosseous screw fixation.

resonators (Plas Surg)—cavities (mouth, nose, throat) that can be used to change the nature of sound produced by the larynx.

ReSound Digital 2000 hearing device—uses digital signal processing circuit technology made by Philips.

RESOURCE Beneprotein instant protein powder—see *Beneprotein*.

RESPeRATE apparatus—a device that interactively coaches the user in performing therapeutic breathing exercises to lower blood pressure. Although the registered trademark is spelled as presented here, it can also be transcribed as *Resperate*.

Respiradyne—an electronic instrument that measures pulmonary function.

respirator—see *ventilator.*

respiratory distress syndrome (RDS)—formerly *hyaline membrane disease*. Occurs in the lungs of premature infants due to the lack of surfactant (lubricant). It is this lubricant which helps keep the air sacs in the lungs open on exhalation. Without surfactant, the walls of the air sacs collapse and stick together, making it difficult or impossible to inhale. See *Exosurf, Survanta, lamellar body number density.*

respiratory disturbance index (RDI)—the number of sleep disordered breathing events per hour of sleep.

respiratory symptoms (RS)—associated with GERD (gastroesophageal reflux disease).

respiratory syncytial virus (RSV).

respiratory syncytial virus, immunoglobulin (RSV-IG).

respiratory triggering—MRI term.

Respironics CPAP (continuous positive airway pressure) **machine**—device for treatment of sleep apnea and in all-night polysomnogram.

Respironics nasal mask—used in respiratory therapy.

respirophasic—a term meaning associated with respiratory activities (inspiration and expiration), as in pleuritic chest pain.

Respitrace machine—used in sleep studies to measure nasal and oral airflow, as well as chest and abdominal respiratory effort.

Response CV catheter system—electrophysiology catheter that is used to evaluate cardiac conditions and electrically restore the heart's normal rhythm when the upper chambers of the heart (the atria) are beating rapidly or irregularly.

Response GM—a handheld device allowing patients to test their own granulocyte count using a drop of blood.

Res-Q ACD (arrhythmia control device)—a 40-joule implantable cardioverter-defibrillator. Also, *Res-Q AICD* (automatic implantable cardioverter-defibrillator).

Res-Q Micron—an implantable cardioverter-defibrillator used in the management of arrhythmia to prevent sudden cardiac death.

Restenosis in Intervened Coronaries with Hyperhomocysteinemia (RICH) **study**.

Resting Heart system—a complete intuitive system designed to address the traditional challenges of arrested-heart surgery.

Reston—foam wound dressing; also hydrocolloid dressing material.

restorative proctocolectomy—an ileal pouch procedure used as surgical treatment for ulcerative colitis. The procedure involves removal of the colon and either all or most of the rectum with preservation of the anal sphincters.

restorative proctocolectomy and ileal pouch anal anastomosis (RP/IPAA)—surgical therapy for patients with mucosal ulcerative colitis and familial adenomatous polyposis.

Restore—a close tolerance dental implant system that uses an external hex-based screw system. The term *close tolerance* means that the oral surgeon is able to select an implant that matches the space almost exactly, allowing for a stable fit.

Restore ACL guide system—used in total knee replacement. It includes a tibial guide, a StraightShot graft passer, and an Advantage screw.

Restore alginate wound dressing.

restriction enzyme (restriction endonuclease)—any of various enzymes that cleave DNA strands at the site of specific sequences. Restriction enzymes of bacterial origin are used in recombinant DNA technology.

restriction fragment length polymorphism (RFLP)—a variant DNA sequence that can be isolated and detected by application of an enzyme that cleaves at a specific site.

restriction map—a graphic display of DNA sites that are cleaved by various restriction enzymes.

Restylane and Restylane Fine Lines injectable gel—transparent hyaluronic acid (a substance produced naturally by the body) gel that is injected into facial tissue to smooth wrinkles and folds, especially around the nose and mouth. The smoothing effect lasts about six months.

Resuscitaire radiant warmer (Peds)—a warmer designed for use in the nursery and in labor and delivery.

retained bladder syndrome—a condition resulting from the urinary bladder being left in, even when a supravesical urinary diversion is done, e.g., in cases of neurogenic bladder or interstitial cystitis.

RetCam 120—a digital camera that takes pictures of the back of the eye. It is used to follow up premature infants for possible retinopathy of prematurity, which usually strikes in the fourth to tenth week of life and can be treated with laser surgery if diagnosed early.

rete ("ree-tee") **ridges** (Path)—epidermal projections into dermal tissue.

retention sutures (also, *stay sutures)*—heavy nonabsorbable sutures to rein-

retention *(cont.)*
force wound closure where there is likely to be unusual postoperative stress.

RET gene test for familial medullary thyroid carcinoma.

Rethi incision (Plas Surg)—a surgical incision in the nose. Usage: "Correction was achieved by inserting a columella strut and a tip graft through a Rethi incision."

reticent—reserved, quiet, not inclined to speak out. Dictators use it *incorrectly* thus: "We discussed having an upper GI and barium enema, which she was reticent to get." Of course, what is meant is *reluctant.*

reticular—pertaining to or resembling a net. Do not confuse with *Roticulator.*

reticulation artifact (Radiol)—a cobweb pattern sometimes seen if film emulsion shrinks because of variation in processing temperature.

retina—innermost, or third tunic, of the eye, that receives the image formed by the lens, and is the immediate instrument of vision.

retinal commotio (concussion)—usually a result of trauma to the eyeball.

retinal detachment—pathological condition where the retina, or part of it, becomes separated from the choroid. Surgical correction includes cryotherapy (cold), diathermy (heat), photocoagulation (laser), and scleral buckling. These therapies induce a sterile inflammatory reaction that causes retinal re-adherence. See *pneumatic retinopexy; rhegmatogenous retinal detachment; Schepens-Okamura-Brockhurst technique for retinal detachment repair.*

retinal nerve fiber layer (RNFL) **thickness**—a factor related to visual function in glaucomatous eyes.

retinal pigment epithelial (RPE) **depigmentation**.

retinal tear; **retinal hole**—injuries, disease, or degeneration may cause small holes or tears in the retina, allowing the vitreous humor from the large chamber in the back of the eye to seep in between the retina and the choroid, causing the two layers to separate, reducing the blood supply to the retina, and resulting in retinal detachment.

retinopathy—any disorder of the retina.
arteriosclerotic
central serous
chloroquine
circinate
diabetic
hypertensive

retinopathy of prematurity (ROP), **posterior**—treated by argon laser photocoagulation.

retinopexy—see *pneumatic retinopexy.*

retinoschisis—splitting of the sensory layers of the retina, usually due to aging.

Retisert—intravitreal drug implant that releases fluocinolone acetonide into the eye for the treatment of diabetic macular edema.

RET proto-oncogene—its presence predicts multiple endocrine neoplasia type 2A syndrome (MEN-2A) and medullary thyroid carcinoma. Its discovery has led to prophylactic thyroidectomy to prevent the occurrence of the neoplasia.

retractor
Airlift balloon
Alm self-retaining
Assistant Free self-retaining soft tissue
Bennett bone
bent malleable
Berkeley-Bonney

retractor *(cont.)*
Bookwalter
Breisky-Navratil
Brewster
Buck-Gramcko
Eccentric Y
Echols
Elite Farley
EndoRetract
eXpose
Favaloro-Morris
FlexPosure endoscopic
Fujita snake
Fukushima cranial
Gazayerli endoscopic
Gilvernet
Goligher
Greenwald
Harrington
Hawkins-Bell
Hays
Henning meniscal
Hohmann
Jarit P.E.E.R.
Laparolift Airlift balloon
Lapro-Flex self-forming laparoscopic
Lone Star
Magrina-Bookwalter vaginal
malleable
Mark II Chandler
Mediflex-Gazayerli
MicroFrance Angot-Vanecloo
Mini-Hohmann
Miskimon cerebellum
Nathanson liver
Navratil
Nevyas drape
Octopus
Omni
Omni-Tract adjustable wishbone
Penfield
Pitie-Salpetriere saphenous vein hook
Protractor

retractor *(cont.)*
Quervain abdominal
Ragnell handheld
R-Med miniretractor
Rosenkranz pediatric
SaphLITE/SaphLITE II
Scoville
Sewell
Shadow-Line
Spacekeeper
RETT (radionuclide esophageal transit test)
Space-OR flexible internal
TLC
Tupper hand-holder and retractor
Upper Hands
Weitlaner
wishbone

retrobulbar neuritis—inflammation of the orbital portion of the optic nerve, usually unilateral.

retrocolic submesocolic gastroentero-anastomosis—an approach in laparoscopic biliopancreatic diversion for obesity.

retrograde cerebral perfusion (RCP).

retrograde intrarenal surgery (RIRS)—a procedure in which a fiberoptic endoscope is placed through the urethra into the bladder and into the ureter and kidney. The stone is seen through this optical instrument and can be manipulated, crushed by ultrasound probe, evaporated by laser probe, grabbed by small forceps, or pushed back into the kidney (for subsequent ESWL).

retrolisthesis—the displacement posteriorly of a vertebra on the one below.

retromammary space view (mammography)—for patients with breast implants, the retromammary space view allows for visualization of the posterior border of the implant and the tissue posterior to the implant,

retromammary *(cont.)* not visible with conventional views. A limitation is that the posterior aspect of a retropectoral implant is more difficult to visualize than in prepectoral implants.

retroperitoneoscopy—laparoscopy of retroperitoneal area.

retropharyngeal implant—for correction of velopharyngeal incompetence using a rib cartilage graft.

retropubic prostatectomy.

retrospectoscope—a physician's coined term for 20/20 hindsight.

retrovirus—any of several RNA viruses, including HIV, that produce reverse transcriptase; this enzyme reverses the normal pattern of nucleic acid transcription, so that DNA is synthesized on an RNA template. Genetically altered retroviruses are used to import alien genes into cells for research and therapy; many are carcinogenic. See *HIV*.

Retrox fractal active fixation lead—consisting of bipolar pre-formed J and bipolar straight lead configurations, allowing atrial and ventricular applications.

RetroX hearing system.

RETT (radionuclide esophageal transit test).

retubularized ileum—option for creating a continent vesicostomy in the absence of the appendix. A segment of small bowel is harvested, retubularized, and reimplanted in the reservoir in a submucosal or seromuscular tunnel.

REU (rectal endoscopic ultrasonography).

Reuter bobbin tube (ENT)—a tube that looks like a sewing machine bobbin (the round kind).

Reuter suprapubic trocar and cannula system—used in transurethral resection of the prostate.

Revatio (sildenafil citrate)—an erectile dysfunction drug which is now used in the treatment of pulmonary arterial hypertension (PAH) related to connective tissue disease.

Reveal insertable loop recorder—an implantable heart monitor manufactured by Medtronic. It is inserted under the skin in the chest area, allowing patients to bathe, swim, and engage in other activities that may be difficult or impossible with an external monitoring device.

Reveal Plus—an implantable loop recorder that helps to establish symptom-rhythm correlation during syncope, near-syncope, palpitations, and acute life-threatening events.

Reveal Plus insertable loop recorder—implantable heart monitor with autoactivation capabilities. The recorder continuously monitors the heart's electrical activity and records ECG information in up to a 12-minute "loop," replacing old ECG data with new data.

Reveal XVI—a PET/CT imaging system that can perform high-speed cardiac procedures and tests for cancer detection in about 13 minutes.

Revelation microcatheters—for temperature-guided radiofrequency ablation procedures, including the Helix, T-Flex, and Tx.

Reverdin-Green osteotomy—of the metatarsal head.

reverse anorexia syndrome (Psych)—a condition seen in male bodybuilders who feel they are too small, often resulting in (or sometimes a result of) anabolic steroid abuse. The opposite

reverse *(cont.)*
of anorexia nervosa in women, this condition may be due in large part to sociocultural factors evidenced in the gym subculture, bodybuilding magazines and movies starring bodybuilders.

reverse transcriptase—an enzyme that promotes the synthesis of DNA on a template of RNA.

reverse transcription-polymerase chain reaction (RT-PCR)—used to detect CEA (carcinoembryonic antigen) to help determine cancer staging.

reversible ischemic neurological deficit (RIND)—an episode that may last several hours, longer than a transient ischemic attack.

reversible obstructive airway disease (ROAD)—used synonymously with *asthma*.

reversible posterior leukoencephalopathy syndrome (RPLS)—an acute reversible neurologic dysfunction characterized by headache, decreased alertness, transient visual loss, with subsequent development of seizures. Common precipitants include acute elevations of blood pressure, acute renal decompensation, eclampsia, and treatment with immunosuppressive drugs such as cyclosporine, tacrolimus, or mycophenolate derivatives.

Reviderm—a hyaluronic acid in which dextran beads are suspended, used as a wrinkle treatment that lasts as long as nine months.

Revised European American Lymphoma classification of lymphoma —see *REAL*.

Revitalase erbium cosmetic laser.

Revo retrievable cancellous screw—acts as a suture anchor in rotator cuff repair.

Revo rotator cuff repair system—used for arthroscopic and open rotator cuff repair.

Rey and Taylor Complex Figure Test —a neurological test.

Rey Auditory Verbal Learning Test.

Reye syndrome—a rare, but often fatal, disease in children, marked by edema of the brain, fatty infiltration of the liver, unconsciousness, and seizures. Seen after viral illnesses such as chickenpox and influenza. Thought possibly related to the administration of aspirin during these illnesses.

RF (radiofrequency) **coil**; **pulse**—MRI terms.

RFA (radiofrequency catheter ablation) —used for recurrent tachyarrhythmias.

RFLP (restriction fragment length polymorphism).

RF-PMR (radiofrequency energy in percutaneous myocardial revascularization).

RGO (reciprocating gait orthosis).

RGP (rigid gas permeable) **contact lens** (Oph).

rgp120—a protein associated with HIV, *rgp120* stands for recombinant gp120 protein. See also *MN rgp120*.

rhabdomyolysis (disintegration or dissolution of muscle)—newly recognized as a complication following cocaine use.

rhagades (rag'-ah-dez)—fissures or scarring in the skin around the mouth or anus. White linear scars at the corners of the mouth can be a sign of congenital syphilis. See *purse-string mouth*.

rhBMP-2 (recombinant human bone morphogenetic protein)—used in conjunction with a lordotic threaded interbody fusion cage.

rhBMP-2/ACS (recombinant human bone morphogenetic protein-2/absorbable collagen sponge)—a novel protein device that enhances bone healing, now approved for use in the treatment of acute open tibia shaft fractures in adults.

RHCT (renal helical CT) **imaging**.

rhegmatogenous retinal detachment—caused by a retinal tear.

rheography, light reflection—imaging procedure that detects deep vein thrombosis using near-infrared light. The light is beamed from diodes to a depth of 1-2 mm into the skin. In the absence of disease, dorsiflexion of the foot will empty the venous plexus of the calf, reduce the amount of light absorbed, and result in an increase in signal. In chronic venous insufficiency, light absorption is reduced to 10-15 seconds. In deep vein thrombosis, light absorption is reduced to less than 10 seconds, showing significantly reduced venous emptying.

Rheolog—a toaster-sized device with tubing that accurately and quickly measures blood viscosity. It improves doctors' ability to assess the efficacy of blood-thinning drugs and could shed light on the role thicker blood plays in heart disease and stroke. The device needs less than a teaspoonful of blood.

Rhesus diploid cell strain rabies vaccine (RDRV) (adsorbed).

rheumatic fever diagnosis—see *Jones criteria, revised.*

Rheumatoid Arthritis DMARD Intervention and Utilization Study (RADIUS)—a clinical trial to evaluate the impact of a tumor necrosis factor inhibitor in patients with rheumatoid arthritis in the U.S.

rheumatoid factor (RH factor, *not* Rh)—an abnormal protein in the blood of most patients with rheumatoid arthritis. Testing for RH factor helps to diagnose this disease.

Rh factor (Rhesus)—an antigen, genetically determined, which is found on the surface of erythrocytes. Incompatibility of the antigens in a mother and fetus is the cause of *erythroblastosis fetalis.* See *RhoGam.*

RH factor (rheumatoid)—see *rheumatoid factor.* Not to be confused with *Rh* (Rhesus) *factor.*

RHIA (Registered Health Information Administrator)—formerly RRA (Registered Record Administrator).

RhinoBur rhinoplasty bur—part of the XPS 2000 microresector system instrument set, used in plastic surgery.

rhinocerebral aspergillosis (RA)—fatal complication common in bone marrow transplantation patients.

rhinolaryngostroboscopy (RLS)—used in the diagnosis of laryngeal disorders.

Rhinoline endoscopic system.

Rhino Rocket—nasal packing designed for mucosal compression after nasal surgery or for tamponade of anterior or middle segment epistaxis. The compressed foam is in a plastic syringe to protect it from moisture and to aid in insertion. When in place and in contact with moisture, the material swells to six times its compressed diameter.

Rhinotherm—treats nasal congestion and rhinorrhea with hyperthermia, using water-saturated pressured air at 110°F directly to the nasal passages.

Rhino Triangle—polypropylene hip abduction brace for treating hip dysplasia in toddlers up to 2½ years of age.

RHIT (Registered Health Information Technician)—formerly ART (Accredited Record Technician).

Rhizopus nigricans—an allergen.

rhizotomy, functional posterior (including the S2 dorsal rootlet)—procedure for treatment of spasticity in children with cerebral palsy.

Rhodes Inventory of Nausea and Vomiting—an eight-item pencil and paper form that measures the prevalence and amount of distress caused by nausea with or without vomiting.

Rhodococcus equi—aerobic, gram-positive coccobacillus infecting horses, swine, and cows that has also been reported in immunocompromised human patients, such as those having undergone organ transplantation or who have HIV disease.

RHS (radial head subluxation).

rhuFab—see *Lucentis (ranibizumab).*

Rhythm Catheter, The—a disposable electrical catheter for use in diagnosing and correcting arrhythmias of the heart.

RIBA (recombinant immunoblot assay)—an FDA-mandated laboratory test to rule out HCV in blood donors.

ribbon stools—stools of greatly narrowed diameter, often due to partial obstruction of the lower bowel by a tumor. Cf. *rabbit stools.*

rib cartilage graft—with arrow flap, used in nipple-areola reconstruction for long-lasting nipple projection.

ribonuclear protein (RNP)—results of ENA testing.

ribonucleic acid—see *RNA.*

ribosomes—cytoplasmic organelles containing ribosomal RNA and protein, the site of polypeptide synthesis by messenger RNA.

RICE (rest, ice, compression, elevation)—an acronym for basic treatment of most sprains, strains, and other closed soft-tissue injuries, particularly of the extremities. Also used in instructions to patients who have undergone orthopedic surgery or arthroscopy.

RIC fluid exchange resuscitation catheter—a catheter for emergency fluid exchange resuscitation sold as a component part of a rapid infusion exchange set.

RICH (Restenosis in Intervened Coronaries with Hyperhomocysteinemia) **study.**

Richards hydroxyapatite PORP and TORP prostheses—made of a biocompatible material for ossicular reconstruction.

Richards Solcotrans Plus—see *Solcotrans Plus.*

Richmond Agitation-Sedation Scale (RASS)—a 10-level scale (from +4 to -5) for the assessment of sedated and agitated patients.

Richter hernia—a type of hernia in which only part of the circumference of the bowel passes through the defect; may develop in a trocar site following laparoscopy.

Rickham reservoir—used in obtaining serum methotrexate levels.

ridges, rete ("ree-tee") (Path)—epidermal projections into dermal tissue.

Rid Mousse (pyrethrum extract)—for treatment of head and body lice.

Riechert/Mundinger stereotactic device—used in the treatment of post-traumatic tremor.

Riedel struma (*not* stroma)—thyroiditis in which the gland is slowly replaced by hard, dense, fibrous tissue which is difficult to distinguish from cancer. Surgery may be necessary to relieve tracheal compression.

Riester otoscope (*not* Reister).

Right Angle ArthroWand.

Right Clip—applier used for minimally invasive surgery. It has a right angle that allows for better visualization and manipulation of vessels.

Rigiflex TTS balloon catheter—a through-the-scope catheter with a balloon at the tip that is inserted through the patient's mouth, into the GI tract. Dilates a stenosis in the ileum or colon resulting from Crohn disease.

RigiScan—device for real-time evaluation of penile tumescence and rigidity in erectile dysfunction.

Rigler sign (Radiol)—detection of pneumoperitoneum on supine radiographs of the abdomen. With visualization of both sides of the intestinal wall on radiography, the bowel wall is outlined very clearly as if etched by a pencil because the gas in the peritoneal space outlines the outside wall. Rigler sign is symptomatic of bowel obstruction with pneumoperitoneum.

rigor—rigidity, stiffness (as in *rigor mortis*). Cf. *rigors*.

rigors—chills. Cf. *rigor.*

RIGS/ACT (adaptive cellular therapy) —products for treating patients with advanced carcinoma.

RIGScan and **RIGScan CR49**—used with Neoprobe RIGS technology for surgical detection of metastatic colorectal cancer.

RIGS system—consists of cancer-specific targeting agents, such as RIGScan CR49, handheld gamma detectors, and methods for their use. A cancer patient is injected before surgery with a low-level radioactive cancer-specific targeting agent. During the operation the surgeon uses the RIGS gamma radiation-detecting probe to locate tissue that contains a significant amount of the radioactive targeting agent.

Riley-Day syndrome (familial dysautonomia)—symptoms include abnormal gastrointestinal motility, ataxia, extremely labile blood pressure, insensitivity to pain, and spinal deformity.

RILG (radioimmunoluminography).

rim sign (Radiol)—(1) Enhancement or widening of a normal rim, margin, or edge as seen on x-ray; e.g., widening of the space between the anterior rim of the glenoid fossa and the humeral head in posterior shoulder dislocation. (2) Appearance of a rim, outline, or halo in a radiographic or sonographic image of soft tissues representing an abnormal zone of different density; e.g., a rim appearing around a ureteral calculus, due to ureteral distention and edema, helps to distinguish it from a phlebolith.

RIND (reversible ischemic neurological deficit).

ring chromosome (Genetics)—a structurally abnormal chromosome in which the end of each arm has been deleted and the broken ends have united to form a ring.

ring curet (curette).

Ringer lactate—see *lactated Ringer solution*.

"ringer rap"—phonetic for *wringer wrap*.

Ringer solution—a physiologic salt solution used for irrigation in surgery. See *lactated Ringer solution*.

ring forceps *(not* Ring forceps)—also called *sponge forceps*.

ring fracture—encircles the foramen magnum; may be considered a basilar or occipital fracture.

Ring hip prosthesis.

Ring–McLean sump tube—Usage: "The tract was dilated to 12 French, and a 12 French Ring–McLean sump tube was placed."

ring scalpel.

ring stand—a device used to hold surgical equipment during surgical procedures.

Rink modification of Casale continent catheterizable vesicostomy—a procedure done for continent urinary diversion without bladder augmentation.

Rinne ("rin-nay") **test**—a test for conductive hearing loss, using air and bone conduction. A tuning fork is stroked or tapped and held close to the external auditory meatus until it is no longer heard. Then the base of the tuning fork is placed near the mastoid bone. If the patient cannot hear it on the mastoid bone, the test is considered normal (positive). If the patient can hear it better by bone conduction, the Rinne is negative, and the patient has a conductive hearing loss.

RinoFlow—micronized nasal irrigation system for treatment of rhinosinusitis.

rippling muscle disease—a rare disease that is usually inherited. May be triggered by an autoimmune phenomenon.

Ripstein procedure—for rectal prolapse.

RIRS (retrograde intrarenal surgery).

RIS (Radiology Information System).

RISA (radioactive iodinated serum albumin) **study**.

Risser localizer cast—used in treatment of scoliosis.

Risser sign—indication of skeletal immaturity.

Risser table—used in making an orthosis or body brace. It is a tubular steel frame that supports the shoulders and hips of the patient but permits the technologist ready access to the rest of the torso.

Rituxan (rituximab)—intravenous infusion monoclonal antibody for non-Hodgkin B-cell lymphoma. It is investigational for rheumatoid arthritis and chronic lymphocytic leukemia.

Rivas vascular catheter—long-term implantable catheter.

Rivetti-Levinson intraluminal shunt—designed for use during beating-heart bypass procedures.

Riza-Ribe needle—used with R-Med plug to effect laparoscopic closure of trocar defects.

RLP (rectal linitis plastica) **colorectal carcinoma**.

RLP (remnant-like particle) **lipoprotein**.

RLS (rhinolaryngostroboscopy) **system**.

RLT (reduced liver transplant).

R-Med mini-retractor—used for evaluation of lateral pelvic fossa and posterior surface of the ovaries during diagnostic and operative laparoscopy and mini-laparoscopy.

R-Med Plug—used with Riza-Ribe needle for closure of laparoscopic trocar defects.

RM (Riechert-Mundinger) **stereotaxic system**—used in performing stereotaxic craniotomy as well as 3-D stereotaxic treatment planning for convergent beam irradiation and radioactive seed implantation.

RNA (ribonucleic acid)—a nucleic acid consisting of molecules of ribose (a 5-carbon sugar) joined in a long helically coiled chain by phosphate bonds with side-chains consisting of pyrimidines (cytosine and uracil) and

RNA *(cont.)*
purines (adenine and guanine). A molecule of RNA is formed on a template of DNA. In turn, polypeptides are synthesized on a template of messenger RNA (mRNA). Transfer RNA (tRNA) assists in the alignment of amino acids along the mRNA template. Ribosomal RNA (rRNA), a component of the ribosomes, functions as a nonspecific site of polypeptide synthesis.

rNEP (recombinant human neutral endopeptidase).

RNFL (retinal nerve fiber layer) thickness.

RNP (ribonuclear protein)—result of ENA testing.

ROAD (reversible obstructive airway disease)—another term for *asthma*.

Road Interview—psychiatric assessment tool. The patient is led along an imaginary road and asked to describe obstacles encountered during the walk. Named obstacles are said to be a key indicator of a person's mental state and may be a warning signal about suicidal intentions.

Robert G. Edwards catheter—a device used for the introduction of an embryo into the uterine cavity after fertilization in vitro.

Robert Jones bulky soft dressing with Hemovac drainage.

robertsonian translocation (Genetics) —a translocation in which two acrocentric chromosomes fuse at the centromere and the short arms are lost.

Robicsek vascular probe (RVP)—intravascular flexible surgical probe. Has different sizes of bulbs at the end of the probe and has a flexible one-piece construction without a metal stylet to be removed.

Robin ("ro-ban") **syndrome**—see *Pierre Robin syndrome, micrognathia-glossoptosis syndrome.*

robin's egg–blue gallbladder—the color of a normal gallbladder, as seen on laparoscopy. An alternative finding when cholecystitis is suspected.

Robin McKenzie exercises—see *McKenzie extension exercises*.

Robodoc—a computerized "surgical assistant" developed in Sacramento, California. It is used to drill the femur cavity for hip replacement surgeries.

robot—see *ZEUSS robot*.

robot-assisted coronary artery bypass (RACAB)—see *beating heart surgery.*

robotic-assisted laparoscopic sacrocolpopexy—procedure to repair vaginal prolapse. It pins back in place the vault of a vagina that has fallen down within the vaginal canal or even outside the vaginal opening. In the new robotic approach, the surgeon operates remotely from a computer terminal, guiding the robotic hand that performs the surgery, rather than standing over the patient. This technique also offers 3-D vision, better ability to maneuver, and reduction of any tremor that might be present in the human hand.

Robotrac passive retraction system—mounted on the operating room table, this apparatus holds all types of retractors in a fixed position until repositioned, thus allowing surgical assistants to perform other duties.

ROC (receiver operating characteristic) —MRI term.

ROC and **ROC XS suture fasteners**—used in treatment of female urinary incontinence. These polymer-based devices are used to attach the sag-

ROC *(cont.)*
ging bladder neck or uterus to the pubic bone.

Rocabado technique—for manipulative (physical) therapy.

Roche-Microwell Plate Hybridization Method—a test useful in diagnosing *Mycobacterium tuberculosis*.

Rochester bone trephine—a long tube with jagged cutting edges at the distal end; used to remove a dowel of cancellous bone from the iliac crest and insert it into the foot during arthrodesis to correct hallux valgus.

Rochester HKAFO—a hip-knee-ankle-foot orthosis which has separate hip and knee joint locks. For ambulation in children with cerebral palsy and myelomeningocele.

rockerbottom foot—congenital vertical talus foot deformity.

Rockey-Davis incision *(not* Rocky).

RODEO (rotating delivery of excitation off-resonance)—3-D MRI technique.

rod-sleeve instrumentation—for treatment of thoracolumbar burst fractures.

Roeder loop—the most commonly used slipknot in laparoscopic surgery. Originally developed for tonsillectomy but modified by Semm for use in laparoscopic surgery.

roentgen-equivalent-man—see *rem*.

roentgen knife—not a knife, but a type of stereotaxic radiosurgical device used in surgery to reach deep-seated tumors or arteriovenous malformations in the brain. See *Gamma Knife*.

roentgen stereophotogrammetric analysis (RSA) (Ortho)—allows 3-D measurement of relative implant movement and sometimes measurement of wear. Now being used to assess aseptic prosthetic loosening.

rofecoxib—oral drug said to be as effective in relieving pain and inflammation as the maximum doses of nonsteroidal anti-inflammatory drugs (such as aspirin and ibuprofen), without GI side effects.

Roger ("ro-zhay") **disease**—see *maladie de Roger.*

Rogozinski spinal fixation system—system of rods, hooks, and screws used to provide sacral fixation. Provides two points of spinal fixation combined with cross-linking to create strong, stable fixation. Also called *Richards Rogozinski spinal fixation system.*

Roho mattress—air-filled device that helps prevent pressure sores (decubitus ulcers).

ROI (region of interest).

Rokitansky-Aschoff sinuses—small outpouchings of the gallbladder mucosa extending through the lamina propria and muscular layer.

Rokitansky disease—see *Budd-Chiari syndrome.*

rolandic epilepsy (also *jacksonian)*—see *jacksonian seizure.* Note: The adjective *rolandic* is not capitalized.

rolfing—a type of massage therapy.

rollerball endometrial ablation—an alternative to hysterectomy in a select group of patients with menorrhagia. It uses a rollerball electrode to coagulate the endometrium during a brief outpatient procedure with a short recovery.

roller coaster glucose control—see *rainbow coverage*.

Rolyan Firm D-Ring wrist support—see *Firm D-Ring*.

Rolyan Gel Shell splint—a hand splint with a gel pad that applies gentle pressure on the incision site of a carpal tunnel release to help de-

Rolyan *(cont.)*
sensitize the area and prevent hypertrophic scar formation.

ROM (range of motion).

Romano surgical curved drilling system—used to drill curved holes, particularly in the bones of the foot and ankle.

roman sandal fashion, tied in—a suture technique.

Romberg test—for differentiating between peripheral and cerebellar ataxia. The patient stands with feet together, first with the eyes closed, then with the eyes open. The examiner evaluates the amount of body swaying. Some swaying is normal. If the Romberg is positive or equivocal, the patient may be asked to hop in place on one foot and then the other.

Rome I and **Rome II criteria**—for irritable bowel syndrome.

ROMI (rule out myocardial infarction)—medical slang used as a verb, as in "The patient was romied." It means a myocardial infarction was ruled out.

RON (radiation-related optic neuropathy).

R1 Rapid Exchange balloon catheter—for PTCA.

R on T phenomenon—premature ventricular contractions coming so closely together that ventricles are stimulated in their resting period, which can lead to fatal ventricular tachycardia or fibrillation. The name reflects the appearance on the electrocardiogram.

Roos test—a maneuver performed to detect thoracic outlet syndrome.

rooting reflex—the turning of an infant's mouth toward the stimulus when its cheek is gently touched (as if it is searching for food).

root signs—signs of compression or injury of spinal nerve roots, such as absence of deep tendon reflexes in a patient with a slipped intervertebral disk.

ROP (retinopathy of prematurity).

ROPA (Regional Organ Procurement Agency)—matches potential donors and recipients for organ transplants.

ROPE (respiratory ordered phase encoding)—a respiratory compensation technique—MRI term.

Rorschach test (Psych)—ink blot test.

ROS '95—wheat flour that has been modified to remove starch and replaced with enriched wheat proteins and fibers. It is available in different formulations, with sugar modulation ranging from zero percent (sugar-free) to 25 percent.

Rosai Dorfman disease—sinus histiocytosis of uncertain origin, characterized by massive lymphadenopathy, increased erythrocyte sedimentation rates, and elevated serum immunoglobulins.

Rosch-Uchida—transjugular liver access needle-catheter.

Rosedale psychiatric home care scale—a 10-item rating scale that identifies essential elements for psychiatric nursing care within the home.

Rosenkranz pediatric retractor system—for use in open heart surgery.

Rosen needle—used in ear surgery. Usage: "The tube was positioned in place with a Rosen needle."

Rosenthal fibers—seen in pilocytic astrocytoma.

Rosenthal needle—used for bone marrow biopsy and aspiration.

rose thorn sign—radiologic finding on arthrogram of inverted labrum between femoral head and acetabulum in developmental dysplasia of the hip.

rosettes, Homer-Wright—sometimes seen on histologic examination of medulloblastomas.

rosiglitazone—a medication taken to help improve blood sugar levels. It also helps to boost the effectiveness of a treatment for opening clogged arteries. Marketed under brand name Avandamet.

Rosomoff cordotomy—a percutaneous radiofrequency cervical cordotomy.

Ross aortic valve replacement procedure—combines use of the patient's own pulmonary valve in the aortic position with use of a homograft to replace the pulmonary valve and right ventricular outflow tract. The patient's own pulmonary valve is essentially used as a "spare part" to replace the diseased aortic valve.

Rossavik growth equation (or model)—equation using fetal growth curves to compare a fetus's growth in the third trimester with its own pattern in the first and second trimesters. Helps to differentiate between fetuses that achieve their growth potential and those with growth failure who are at a greater risk for fetal compromise or postnatal complications.

Rossiter system—unique, inexpensive stretching program that reduces pain in individuals in such diverse occupations as assembly-line worker, computer operator, and musician—any job or activity that requires repetitive tasks. Employees undergo training in powerful two-person stretches, done at the job site, to relieve chronic pain, tingling, stiffness, and numbness.

Ross procedure—uses the pulmonary valve from the right side of the heart to replace a defective aortic valve on the left side. To replace the relocated pulmonary valve, surgeons implant a pulmonary valve taken from the hospital's tissue bank of donated human valves. The native pulmonary valve is an ideal substitute because it is about the same size and shape as the aortic valve and is able to close tightly even under high pressure.

Ross pulmonary porcine valve—stentless pulmonary heart valve designed by Dr. Donald N. Ross for pediatric patients. Because it is stentless, it does not require any artificial material, such as a sewing ring, to immobilize tissue.

Ross syndrome—an uncommon disorder characterized by segmental anhidrosis, hyporeflexia, and tonic pupils. It is a dysautonomic condition of varying expression resulting from a generalized injury to ganglion cells or their projections.

rostaporfin—see *Photrex*.

Rotablator—a high-speed, elliptical, rotating abrasive bur used in percutaneous coronary rotational atherectomy. Resulting particles that are small or smaller than red blood cells wash out downstream from the site of the lesion.

ROTACS guidewire—used to prevent restenosis, or occlusion, of an artery post angioplasty.

RotaLink (and **RotaLink Plus**) **rotational atherectomy device**—for removal of plaque from a coronary artery using a high-speed diamond-tipped burr.

Rotalok cup—uncemented acetabular component.

rotating frame of reference—MRI term.

rotational coronary atherectomy—see *directional coronary atherectomy*.

rotationplasty—limb-sparing technique used to remove the diseased portion of bone, turn the shortened portion of the leg bone in a half-circle, and reattach it, with the ankle joint functioning as a knee. It has been used in very young children to treat Ewing sarcoma behind the knee, for example.

rotavirus—a group of viruses involved in acute gastroenteritis in infants.

RotaWire Floppy Gold guidewire.

Rotazyme diagnostic procedure—an enzyme immunology kit from Abbott Labs for rotavirus antigen in stool and liver aspirates.

Roth-Bernhardt disease—see *meralgia paresthetica*.

Roth Grip-Tip suture guide (Urol).

Rothman Gilbard corneal punch.

Rothmund-Thomson syndrome—oculocutaneous disorder seen with linitis plastica (a gastric carcinoma), and characterized by skin changes including atrophy, telangiectasias, alterations in pigmentation, and sparse or absent eyelashes and eyebrows. Some patients are also found to have cataracts, bone defects, dystrophic nails, and small stature.

Roth retrieval net—gauze-covered net for polyp retrieval.

Roth spots—small hemorrhages, round or oval lesions with small white centers. May be seen in the ocular fundi in cases of subacute bacterial endocarditis.

roticulating endograsper—a surgical instrument used in minimally invasive surgeries.

Roticulator stapler—*not* reticulator, as sometimes dictated.

Rotograph Plus—panoramic dental tomography imaging system.

Roto-Rest bed.

Rotunda perineum needle.

Rous sarcoma virus—oncogenic retrovirus.

Routine Assessment of Patient Progress (RAPP).

Rouviere ligament—fibulocalcaneal ligament.

Rouviere, node of.

Roux-en-Y divided gastric bypass—procedure to treat massive obesity. The stomach is divided into two sections, reducing the size of the new pouch from about 2 quarts to 2 ounces. This drastic reduction in size limits the stomach's capacity to hold food. It may be performed as either an open or laparoscopic procedure, depending on the patient's condition and the existence of previous scars. The laparoscopic surgery uses only a few small incisions in the abdominal wall.

Roux stasis syndrome—a syndrome of nausea, vomiting, abdominal pain, and postprandial fullness following Roux-en-Y gastrojejunostomy. It is thought to result from the jejunal transection performed during the construction of a conventional Roux limb. Construction of Roux-Y limbs greater than about 40 cm in length may increase the incidence of the Roux-Y stasis syndrome.

Roux-Y ("roo-Y") **chimney**—surgical technique. Usage: "Transjejunal approaches have been used to examine patients following Kasai procedures, to dilate stenotic hepaticojejunostomies in a retrograde manner, to place a U tube percutaneously, to perform percutaneous hepaticojejunostomy, and to accomplish intermittent biliary access in patients with Roux-Y chimneys brought up to the skin." Also, *Roux-en-Y anastomosis*.

Rovsing sign—indicative of acute appendicitis. Pain elicited in the lower right abdomen at McBurney point when the corresponding point in the lower left is pressed.

Rowe disimpaction forceps (Oral Surg).

Roy-Camille plates—used in screw placement in lower cervical spine.

RP (radical prostatectomy).

RPC (reactive perforating collagenosis).

rPDGF (recombinant platelet-derived growth factor).

RPE (rating of perceived exertion).

RPE (retinal pigment epithelium) **dropout**; **clumping**.

RP/IPAA (restorative proctocolectomy and ileal pouch anal anastomosis).

RPM (real-time position management) **tracking system**—used in electrophysiologic procedures for real-time visualization of catheters. It assists physicians in precisely manipulating catheters within the heart during procedures.

RPR (rapid plasma reagin)—a test for syphilis, faster than the VDRL, and macroscopic rather than microscopic. See *reagin*.

RPR-CT (rapid plasma reagin circle-card test)—for syphilis. Cf. *RPR*.

RRA (registered record administrator)—see *RHIA*.

RRFs (ragged-red fibers)—a hallmark of mitochondrial encephalopathies.

RRI (recurrent respiratory infections).

RRP (recurrent respiratory papillomatosis).

RS (respiratory symptoms).

RSA (recurrent spontaneous abortions).

RSA (roentgen stereophotogrammetric analysis).

RSI (rapid sequence induction) **orotracheal intubation**—said to have a higher success rate, fewer complications, and produce better patient outcome than noninduced orotracheal intubation and blind nasotracheal intubation. Emergency medicine physicians prefer RSI orotracheal intubation as the method of choice for trauma airway management in the helicopter.

RSI (repetitive strain injury).

RSLT (reduced-size liver transplant).

Rsma (superior mesenteric artery resistance). Cf. *Qsma*.

RSR (reduced sewing ring)—see *Carpentier-Edwards Perimount RSR pericardial bioprosthesis.*

RSV (respiratory syncytial virus).

rTMS (repetitive transcranial magnetic stimulation).

RTT (renal transit time).

Rubens flap—used for breast reconstruction after mastectomy. It is a modification of the deep circumflex iliac artery-iliac crest flap in that there is no bony transfer. The name of the flap is derived from the appearance of the female form in paintings by Peter Paul Rubens, which shows an area of particular fullness at or just above the iliac crest. This technique is used in patients who have had a previous abdominoplasty and have few other tissues available for an autologous graft except a fullness above the iliac crest region as a result of the abdominoplasty. See *breast reconstruction donor sites.*

ruboxistaurin—a medication that may reduce vision loss from diabetes-induced eye disease.

RU-486—former name of *Mifeprex* (mifepristone).

Rufus and Ruby, The Bears With Diabetes—teddy bears used to educate children with type 1 diabetes mellitus. They have patches sewn onto

Rufus *(cont.)* them to help children learn about the spots on their bodies that are best for insulin injections and blood glucose testing (tummy, thighs, arms, bottom, and fingers). You may hear Rufus and Ruby mentioned in pediatric dictation.

rugger-jersey spine—increased density in the upper and lower zones of the vertebral body in a striated appearance (sclerotic banded vertebrae). The pattern is similar to the alternating colors of the rugby player's jersey at the time of the description of this entity. Rugger jersey spine is typically observed only in secondary hyperparathyroidism.

Ruiz-Cohen round expander—a device used for acute intraoperative arterial elongation, which is a reliable method of repairing a small arterial defect as opposed to using an interposition vein graft. The interposition vein graft has been shown to have a higher incidence of thrombosis than the Ruiz-Cohen round expander. However, a vein graft is still the technique of choice for large arterial defects.

Ruiz microkeratome—disposable instrument used to create the corneal flap during a LASIK procedure for vision correction.

Rule of Nines—formula by which the percentage of body surface which has been burned is determined. The head is figured at 9%, as is each arm. Each leg is 18% (2 x 9), as are the anterior trunk and the posterior trunk. This all adds up to 99%. The perineum is figured at 1%. See also *Berkow formula*.

rule of 100—an accurate way to assess sports on-the-field trauma. Simply stated, if the systolic blood pressure is greater than 100 and the pulse and temperature are less than 100, significant sports trauma is unlikely. On the other hand, if an elevated heart rate or temperature above 100 is detected, or the systolic blood pressure is under 100, serious trauma may have occurred and the patient needs immediate transport to a trauma facility.

RUMI uterine manipulator and injector.

runoff—the flow of blood (and contrast medium) through the branches of an artery into which the medium has been injected.

ruptured abdominal aortic aneurysm (RAAA).

rush immunotherapy—consists of a number of injections given over a short time to desensitize a person to certain allergens, such as dust mites, cat dander, or certain plants.

Russel (one *L*) **gastrostomy kit**.

Russell-Taylor (R-T) **nail**.

Russell traction—used as a temporary measure to stabilize femoral fractures until the patient can be taken to surgery.

Russell viper venom time, dilute (dRVVT)—a modified prothrombin time that has been made sensitive to the lupus anticoagulant (LA). This may be heard in rheumatology dictation.

Russian forceps.

RUT (rapid urease test).

rutherford (rd) **unit**—a unit of radioactivity; abbreviated *rd*.

Rutkow sutureless plug and patch—repair for inguinal hernia using a simple mesh plug made of preformed polypropylene mesh that maintains a permanent open cone-like shape. It requires no suturing.

Rutzen ileostomy bag.

RVCD—slang abbreviation for *right ventricular conduction delay.*

RVH (right ventricular hypertrophy).

RV/TLC (residual volume/total lung capacity) **ratio**.

RWECochG (round window electrocochleography)—a test for assessing children with cochlear implants for residual hearing in low frequencies.

Rx5000 cardiac pacing system.

RX Herculink 14—pre-mounted stent system for treatment of malignant obstructions of the biliary duct.

RX Herculink Plus—biliary stent system.

RX stent delivery system—a rapid exchange technology that allows cardiologists and catheter lab personnel to decrease their radiation exposure due to the reduced need for fluoroscopy during placement and catheter exchanges.

"rye"—phonetic rendering of Reye syndrome, acquired encephalopathy in children following a febrile illness, believed to be associated with aspirin use.

Rye histopathologic classification—used in Hodgkin disease.

Ryna-12 S (phenylephrine tannate/pyrilamine tannate) **suspension**—for symptomatic relief of the coryza and nasal congestion associated with the common cold, sinusitis, allergic rhinitis, and other upper respiratory tract conditions.

Rythmol—see *propafenone.* Note the spelling of this drug is *Ry,* not *Rhy,* although it affects the rhythm of the heart.

S, s

SAA (slotted acetabular augmentation).

SAANDs (selective apoptotic antineoplastic drugs).

SAARD (slow-acting antirheumatic drug)—utilized to slow the progression of rheumatoid arthritis. Examples: antimalarial agent, gold salts, penicillamine, sulfasalazine, methotrexate.

SAB (*Staphylococcus aureus* bacteremia).

SAB (stereotactic aspiration biopsy).

Saber Bisector ArthroWand—an arthroscopic instrument that slices through soft tissues and is used for lateral retinacular release during patellar realignment or in management of severe ligament tears. Also used to release frozen shoulders.

Sable—balloon catheter used in angioplasty procedures.

"Sabo"—phonetic for *Szabo-Berci*.

Sabouraud medium—culture medium for growing fungi.

Sabreloc spatula needle.

sabre shin deformity—in congenital syphilis, the leading edge of the tibia bows forward.

saccade—series of involuntary, abrupt, rapid small movements or jerks of both eyes simultaneously in changing the point of fixation.

saccadic pursuit—following movements of the eyes.

saccadic slowing (Oph, Neuro).

Saccomanno collection fluid and fixative—a premixed, ready-to-use fixative used for the collection of sputum and other mucoid fluids prior to processing and staining.

sacculotomy—see *Fick sacculotomy.*

SACH (solid-ankle, cushioned heel) **heels**—for orthopedic appliances.

Sacks-Vine PEG (percutaneous endoscopic gastrostomy) **tube**, or *Sacks-Vine feeding gastrostomy tube.*

sacral insufficiency fracture (SIF)—usually present as nonspecific pelvic or low back pain, often overlooked in the elderly.

sacralization—abnormal bony fusion between the fifth lumbar vertebra and the sacrum.

sacral nerve stimulation (SNS) **therapy**—implantable device for patients with urge incontinence, resulting

sacral *(cont.)*
from neurological conditions such as spinal cord injury, stroke, spina bifida, or multiple sclerosis. The pulse generator is implanted in the abdominal wall, and a wire lead is attached to a nerve near the sacrum.

sacrococcygeal pilonidal sinus—surgically treated by rhomboid excision and Limberg flap closure.

sacrocolpopexy—see *abdominal sacrocolpopexy.*

sacrospinous colpopexy—gynecologic procedure for restoring vaginal support in women with vault prolapse, massive vaginal eversion, or procidentia.

saddle anesthesia—a term often dictated by neurologists when reporting a patient's sensation to light touch and pin prick in areas where the body would touch a saddle if mounted on a horse. Not to be confused with *saddle block anesthesia*.

saddle coil—MRI term.

saddle embolus—a blood clot lodged at the bifurcation of an artery, thus blocking both branches. Also called *pantaloon embolus* or *straddling embolus*. "Significant past history includes a history of saddle embolus."

saddle leather friction rub—observed on heart examination.

Sade modification of Norwood procedure—for hypoplastic left-sided heart syndrome. See *Fontan, Gill/Jonas.*

Sadowsky hook wire—used in breast surgery.

SAE (subcortical atherosclerotic encephalopathy).

SAECG (or SAEKG) (signal-averaged electrocardiogram).

Saethre-Chotzen ("say-ther-cho-tzen") **syndrome**—form of familial craniofacial anomaly in which there may be cranial synostoses and other anomalies.

safari
scalpel
surgery

SAFER (saphenous [vein graft] angioplasty free of emboli randomized).

SafeTap tapered spinal needle.

Safety AV fistula needle—for use in hemodialysis.

SAF-Gel hydrogel dressing—for wound hydration.

SafetyGlide needle—has a shield that covers the needle tip to help protect the healthcare practitioner from an accidental needle stick. Also called *BD SafetyGlide needle*.

SAF (self-articulating femoral) **hip replacement**.

SAFHS (sonic-accelerated fracture-healing system) **therapy**—ultrasound therapy which accelerates healing of Colles fractures and tibial diaphysis fractures.

SAFT (Synthetic Aperture Focusing Technique).

Saf-T E-Z set—translucent needle shield to protect against accidental needlesticks.

SAF-T shield—postoperative eye protection.

sagging brain—spontaneous intracranial hypotension, the result of a hole or tear in the sac around the spinal cord that causes fluid to leak into surrounding tissues. Such tears are not uncommon following spinal taps and other forms of neurosurgery and can also occur with rupture of a benign cyst at the juncture of the sac and a surrounding nerve.

sagging rope sign—a radiodense curvilinear shadow at the base of the femoral neck indicative of Legg-Calvé-Perthes disease.

sagittal orientation (Radiol).

sagittal roll spondylolisthesis (Ortho).

sagittal T1-weighted image—MRI term.

SAH (subarachnoid hemorrhage).

Sahara Clinical Bone Sonometer—portable device for estimating bone strength using ultrasound measurements; it transmits high-frequency sound waves through the patient's heel for about 10 seconds and automatically analyzes results.

Sahli needle—used for bone marrow biopsy and aspiration.

SA-IGIV (*Staphylococcus aureus* immune globulin intravenous [human]).

SAIL protocol—for reducing polypharmacy in physician practice. Protocol for each patient should consist of:

Simplicity: Prescribe as few medications as possible, adjusting dosages and individual medications so that fewer meds need to be taken per day and cost to the patient is as low as possible.

Adverse effects: Be constantly aware of possible reaction to or interaction between prescribed medications.

Indications: Be certain that indications for any medication are clear.

Lists: Maintain a precise and current list of all drugs taken by the patient, making sure that the patient and all treating physicians are aware of all meds being taken.

sail sign—anterior and superior elevation of the fat pad in the elbow joint. The sail sign is highly suggestive of intra-articular fracture.

SAL (suction-assisted lipectomy).

SAL (suction-assisted lipoplasty).

salaam activity—a form of seizures.

SalEst system—a test that identifies pregnant women at risk for preterm labor. A saliva sample is checked for estriol level. An elevated estriol level could be a warning sign that preterm labor and delivery may occur within 2-3 weeks.

salient—pertinent, noticeable, outstanding; said of diagnostic findings, findings at surgery, etc.

saline-enhanced MR arthrography of shoulder—used as an inexpensive alternative to gadopentetate dimeglumine.

saliva ovulation test—an over-the-counter ovulation tester available for women who are trying to get pregnant or trying to prevent pregnancy. The device is a lipstick-sized portable microscope that a woman can use to determine if she is, or will soon be, ovulating. She simply licks the slide contained in the device and allows it to dry. She attaches a small eyepiece, focuses the lens, and checks what pattern appears. If she sees short random hair-like patterns, that means she'll be ovulating in 1-3 days. During ovulation, a distinct fern-like pattern appears. It is said to be about 98% accurate.

Salmon law—a method of locating the internal opening of an anal fistula.

salmon-patch hemorrhages (Oph)—usually found in patients with sickle cell disease, occurring in the mid-peripheral part of the fundus of the eye. They are initially red but often turn a salmon color after several days.

Salmon-Rickham ventriculostomy reservoir (Neuro).

Salonpas—over-the-counter pain-relieving patch containing herbal and

Salonpas *(cont.)* other ingredients that are absorbed through the skin.

salon sink radiculopathy—a neurologic condition, presenting as pain, tingling, and weakness radiating from the neck to the upper extremities, caused by compression of a nerve root in the cervical spine when leaning the head back (hyperextension) for shampooing in hair salons. People most at risk are those suffering from preexisting injuries or arthritis of the cervical spine.

saloon door approach—in MIDCAB (minimally invasive direct coronary artery bypass) procedures, a technique in which the intercostal muscles are incised laterally and the adjacent cartilages folded back. It disconnects rather than removes the fourth and fifth costal cartilages and thus helps prevent skeletal defects that occur with complete removal.

SALT (skin-associated lymphoid tissue).

Salter fracture

- I fracture through the plate only
- II fracture through the growth plate and through a portion of the metaphysis
- III fracture through the growth plate and through the epiphysis
- IV fracture through the growth plate, the metaphysis, and the epiphysis
- V a crushing fracture injury of the growth plate
- VI fracture of the perichondrial ring surrounding the epiphysis

Salter osteotomy.

Salt II candidate—a patient who is a candidate for the Salt II-hyponatremia study that compares a vasopressin antagonist with a placebo.

Salt II hyponatremia study—see *Salt II candidate.*

saluresis—excretion of sodium and chloride ions in the urine.

saluting—repeated rubbing of the nose upward to scratch an itchy nose and open the obstructed airway (seen in patients with allergies). Also called *allergic salute.*

salvia rubus—see *Avlimil.*

Salyer modification—of Obwegeser mandibular osteotomy.

Salzmann nodules—in the cornea.

Salz nuclear splitter—used to fracture the nucleus in phacoemulsification (refers to vitreous loss in an extracapsular cataract extraction).

SAM (scanning acoustic microscope).

SAM (subcutaneous augmentation material).

SAM (systolic anterior motion)—as seen on 2-D echocardiogram.

SAMBA—automated image analysis system (Système d'Analyse Microphotométrique à Balayage Automatique).

SAMBA (simultaneous areolar mastopexy and breast augmentation). Cf. *WAMBA*.

same-day microsurgical arthroscopic lateral-approach laser-assisted (SMALL) **fluoroscopic diskectomy**.

"sammoma"—see *psammoma.*

Sampaolesi line (Oph).

SampleMaster biopsy needle—used with INRAD HiLiter ultrasound-enhanced stylet.

Samsoon modification of Mallampati airway classes I through IV—see *Mallampati classification*.

Sam splint—foam pad with aluminum center which is invisible on x-ray, waterproof, and reusable.

Samter triad—asthma, aspirin sensitivity, and nasal polyps. Also, *ASA triad* and *triad asthma.*

Samuels Micro-Scler catheter—used in treating spider veins.

sand, brain—gritty material found in the pineal body, the choroid plexus, and other structures within the brain.

Sandia Decon Foam—an anti-anthrax foam spray used to decontaminate rooms infected with anthrax spores. Named for the Department of Energy Sandia Laboratory, where it was developed.

Sandifer syndrome—rare manifestation of gastroesophageal reflux in children that is associated with abnormal movements and postures of the head, neck, and trunk; treated with Nissen fundoplication and a Heineke-Mikulicz pyloroplasty.

Sandman—a line of sleep disorder diagnostic systems.

Sandoz Clinical Assessment Geriatric Scale (SCAG)—a 97-point scale which assesses 18 different symptoms as well as global performance.

Sandoz suction/feeding tube.

Sand process (Dr. Bruce Sand)—uses a holmium laser-based system for collagen shrinkage to correct ophthalmic conditions.

S&S—slang for *seated and supine*; expand when it is dictated. Usage: "Straight leg raise negative S&S."

sandwich—see *Marlex methylmethacrylate.*

sandwich nucleic acid hybridization assay—a method of assaying hepatitis C virus in which an oligonucleotide probe hybridizes to (binds) viral RNA in a serum specimen and is in turn bound by a probe integrated into the test plate. The capture probe thus forms the "filling" of a "sandwich." Use of various probes permits detection of various HCV genotypes.

sandwich sign—in radiology, refers to the appearance of a contrast-filled stomach which has herniated into the chest and folded upon itself.

sandwich treatment—combination of two or more therapies.

Sanger-Brown syndrome.

sanguineous—bloody.

S-A (sinoatrial) **node**.

SANS (Stoller afferent nerve stimulation)—used for the treatment of urge incontinence syndrome. It stimulates the sacral region of the spine that controls bladder function. This reconditions the nerves, suppressing overactivity and restoring normal reflex control.

Santorini plexus—a network of veins in the region of the prostate gland.

Sanvar IR (vapreotide)—a somatostatin analog for acute treatment of esophageal variceal bleeding to stop hemorrhage prior to endoscopic intervention and to prevent recurring bleeding during the critical five days following treatment. Also, for the management of life-long symptoms of carcinoid tumors and acromegaly, for which it was granted orphan-drug designation by the FDA.

SaO_2 (arterial oxygen saturation)—the percentage of hemoglobin in the arterial blood that is saturated with oxygen. Normal values are 95% to 100%.

SAP (superabsorbent polymer).

SAPHFinder surgical balloon dissector—used with EndoSaph in saphenous vein harvesting for CABG procedures.

SaphLITE/SaphLITE II retractor system—stainless steel device for retraction of subcutaneous tissue to afford

SaphLITE *(cont.)*
exposure and visualization of the saphenous vein during saphenous vein harvesting procedures.

SAPHtrak balloon dissector—used to remove the saphenous vein in a minimally invasive procedure. The balloon is inserted through a 1 to 3 cm incision and then inflated, separating the natural tissue planes to create a subcutaneous space along the length of the saphenous vein. Upon removal of the balloon, this “dissected” space can be insufflated with gas to create a surgical working space.

SAPPHIRE (study of angioplasty with protection in patients at high risk for endarterectomy).

sapropterin hydrochloride—see *Phenoptin*.

SAPS (simplified applied physiology score).

sarcoglycanopathy—a form of dystrophy caused by a mutation of any one of the four sarcoglycan genes, formerly referred to as severe childhood autosomal recessive muscular dystrophy (SCARMD).

sarcoma—derived from a Greek word meaning ‘to become fleshy’. It is a cancerous tumor arising from connective tissue (muscle, bone). Cf. *cancer* and *carcinoma*.

Sarns aortic arch cannula.

SARS (severe acute respiratory syndrome)—a viral respiratory illness, first recognized as a global threat in March 2003, after first appearing in Southern China in November 2002. The illness usually begins with a high fever, sometimes associated with chills or other symptoms including headache, general feeling of discomfort, and body aches. Some people also experience mild respiratory symptoms at the outset. Diarrhea is seen in approximately 10-20% of patients. After two to seven days, SARS patients may develop a nonproductive cough that might be accompanied by or progress to a condition in which the oxygen levels in the blood are low (hypoxia). In 10-20% of cases, patients require mechanical ventilation. Most patients develop pneumonia. SARS is caused by a previously unrecognized coronavirus, called SARS-CoV (SARS-associated coronavirus). It is possible that other infectious agents might have a role in some cases of SARS. SARS appears to be spread by close person-to-person contact (droplet spread). In addition, it is possible that it might be spread more broadly through the air or by other ways that are not now known.

SAS (sleep apnea syndrome).

SASMA (skin-adipose superficial musculoaponeurotic) **system**—a face-lift technique said to achieve more lasting results than other techniques.

Sassone score—a system of scoring the appearance (in transvaginal ultrasonography) of ovarian and adnexal masses to distinguish between malignant and benign masses. The score is based on characteristics of the mass: wall structure, presence of septa, loss of echo behind the structure on ultrasound, and echogenicity.

satellite DNA—a strand of DNA containing many tandem repeats of a short basic repeating unit.

satellite lesion—a smaller lesion, near the primary lesion; accompanying, nearby, subordinate lesions. Usage: “There was an indurated, excoriated

satellite *(cont.)*
rash which had no satellite lesions or any appearance of tinea." "Examination reveals an erosive vaginal lesion at 6 o'clock, consistent with herpes, and several satellite lesions which are also erosive, ulcerative lesions."

Saticon vacuum chamber pickup tube—for video camera used in arthroscopy. Cf. *Circon, Newvicon, Vidicon.*

Satietrol Complete—one of a new generation of weight-loss products that works by activating cholecystokinin, an important satiety signal in humans. Can be taken as a premeal beverage to reduce hunger or as a meal replacement. Studies have shown that it significantly reduces hunger for up to 5 hours.

SatinCrescent tunneler, SatinShortcut, SatinSlit keratome—ophthalmic products, satin finish.

sats—(oxygen) saturation.

satting—slang for saturating.

Sattler veil—see *bedewing of cornea.*

saturation—see SaO_2 (arterial oxygen saturation).

saturation recovery technique—MRI term.

Saturn splint—splinting device for noninvasive treatment of carpal tunnel syndrome.

saucerize—to create a saucer-shaped excavation surgically.

Sauflon PW (lidofilcon B)—soft extended-use hydrophilic contact lens for aphakia in children.

sausage digits—erythematous fingers resembling link sausages. It refers to fusiform soft-tissue swelling involving an entire single digit within the hand. It is classically associated with the single-ray pattern of involvement seen in some patients with psoriatic arthritis and may be the initial manifestation of the disease.

sausaging of a vein—refers to a narrowing of the vein so that it looks like a string of sausages.

Sauvage graft—filamentous velour Dacron arterial graft material.

Sauve-Kapandji procedure—for reconstruction of distal radioulnar joint. Also called *Kapandji-Sauve procedure.*

SAVANT (Surgical Anatomy Visualization and Navigation Tools)—provides anatomical positioning and true 3-D visualization for minimally invasive surgeries of the brain, spine, and other locations.

Savary dilator (*not* savory).

Save-A-Tooth—tooth preserving system that can keep a knocked-out tooth alive for up to 24 hours.

save for—a colloquial expression meaning *except*. Usage: "Save for some platelike atelectasis at the right base, chest film is normal."

SAVVI (not an acronym)—synchronous pacemaker that needs only a single lead. It is used for patients with acquired, congenital, or postoperative atrioventricular block.

SAXX renal stent.

SB Charité III intervertebral dynamic disc spacer—vertebral disk prosthesis for patients with single-level degenerative disk disease for whom back pain, rather than leg pain, is the major complaint.

SBE (small bowel enteroscopy).

SBE (subacute bacterial endocarditis).

SBE p-lax—slang for *subacute bacterial endocarditis prophylaxis*.

SBGM (self blood glucose monitoring).

SBP (spontaneous bacterial peritonitis).

SBSP (simultaneous bilateral spontaneous pneumothorax).

SBRN (sensory branch of the radial nerve).

SCAD (spontaneous coronary artery dissection).

SCA-EX and **SCA-EX ShortCutter catheters with rotating blades**—used for directional coronary atherectomy.

SCAG (Sandoz Clinical Assessment-Geriatric) scale.

scale (see *classification, score, test)*
- Abbreviated Injury
- ADAS (Alzheimer Disease Assessment)
- Adolescent and Pediatric Pain Tool (APPT)
- AIMS (Abnormal Involuntary Movement)
- ALS (amyotrophic lateral sclerosis) Functional Rating (ALS-FRS)
- Alzheimer Disease Assessment Scale cognitive subscale (ADAS-cog)
- ASIA impairment
- Bayley Scales of Infant Development
- Behavioral Pathology in Alzheimer Disease Rating
- Bethesda rating (for Pap smears)
- Brazelton Neonatal Assessment
- Cattell Infant Intelligence
- CES-D (Center for Epidemiological Studies–Depression)
- Child Pugh
- CINA (Clinical Institute Narcotic Assessment)
- CIWA–A (Clinical Institute Withdrawal Assessment–Alcohol)
- Daumas-Duport glioma pathology grading
- Dementia Rating (DRS)
- Dubowitz scale for infant maturity
- ECOG (Zubrod) performance status

scale *(cont.)*
- Edinburgh Postnatal Depression Scale (EPDS)
- Epworth Sleepiness
- Exercise Self-efficacy
- FACT (Functional Assessment of Cancer Therapy)
- FLACC pain
- Flint Colon Injury (FCIS)
- French (sizing)
- Gastroesophageal Reflux Disease–Health-Related Quality of Life (GERD-HRQL)
- Geriatric Depression (GDS)
- Global Deterioration (GDS)
- Glasgow Coma
- Glasgow Outcome (GOS)
- Harris hip
- Health Failure Self-Care Behavior, revised
- Hospital Anxiety and Depression (HAD)
- House-Brackmann facial weakness
- HSC (Hospital for Sick Children) pain
- Karnofsky rating
- Kurtzke Disability Status (KDSS)
- Mitsuo
- Montefiore Organic Brain
- National Institutes of Health Stroke Scale (NIHSS)
- nomogram
- Numeric Rating Scale (NRS, NRS-101)
- Obsessive Compulsive Drinking (OCDS)
- Outerbridge
- Parental Stress Scale: PICU (PSS: PICU)
- Past Feelings and Acts of Violence (PFAV)
- Pediatric Risk of Mortality (PRISM)
- Pressure Ulcer Scale for Healing (PUSH) Tool

scale *(cont.)*
Q-TWiST (time without symptoms or toxicity)
Quick Confusion
Ranchos los Amigos cognitive
Rating of Perceived Exertion (RPE)
Richmond Agitation-Sedation (RASS)
Sandoz Clinical Assessment Geriatric (SCAG)
Self-perceived Dyspnea
Self-Regard Questionnaire
sense of coherence (SOC)
SHRS (St. Hans Rating Scale for extrapyramidal syndromes)
Stanford Sleepiness
Suicide Risk (SRS)
Tanner Developmental
Unified Parkinson Disease Rating (UPDRS)
Vineland Social Maturity
Visual Analog Scale (VAS)
WAIS (Wechsler Adult Intelligence)
Wechsler Memory
Woodson and Hamilton Motor Activity (MAS)
Zung Depression
Zung Self-rating Anxiety (SAS)

scalloping of vertebrae (Radiol)—sometimes seen on x-ray of patient with sickle cell anemia.

scalp electrode—EKG lead attached to scalp of infant about to be delivered to evaluate intrauterine heart rate.

scalpel safari—surgery jargon for a trip to a third-world country for cosmetic surgery (such as liposuction) at a much lower price than in the U.S. The patient is on "safari" (away from scrutiny) while the wounds heal. Also called *surgery safari*.

scalp pH—blood sample taken from scalp of infant about to be delivered to evaluate intrauterine oxygenation.

scan, scanner—see also *operation*.
Aloka scanner
ATL real-time Neurosector scanner
biphasic helical CT
BladderScan
B-scan
Bruel-Kjaer ultrasound scanner
Cardiolite
CardioTek
cine CT scanner
contrast material enhanced
coronary artery (CAS)
CT (computed tomography)
CT/T 8800 scanner
Denver Developmental Screening
Dermascan
DEXA (dual energy x-ray absorptiometry)
EMI scanner
Evolution XP scanner
FiberScan laser system scanner
Fonar-360 MRI
four-slice coronal CT scan of sinuses
F-scan
gallium
General Electric CT-T scanner
Gyroscan ACS NT MRI
HeartView CT
HIDA or TcHIDA
Imatron ultrafast CT scanner
indium 111 scintigraphy
Lumiscan 150 scanner
MAA lung
medronate
milk
mPower PET
MUGA (multiple gated acquisition)
open sky MRI
PET (positron emission tomography)
PIPIDA, or Tc-PIPIDA
PYP (pyrophosphate)
QUAD 12000 and QUAD 7000 MRI scanner
radionuclide

scan *(cont.)*
sector echocardiography
sector scanner
serial scans
sestamibi stress scan
SkinScan
SLUScan for Your Heart
SoftScan
Somatom DR 1 (2, 3) CT scanner
SPECT (single photon emission CT)
spiral XCT (x-ray computed tomography) scanner
stacked scans
tagged red blood cell nuclear
teboroxime scan
TechneScan MAG3 scan
technetium
3-Scape real-time 3-D imaging
ThromboScan
TransScan TS2000 electrical impedance breast scanning
T-Scan 2000
TSPP rectilinear bone
unenhanced scan
Vision 1.5-T Siemens MRI
V-P (ventilation-perfusion)
V-Q (ventilation-perfusion)
xenon 133 (^{133}Xe)

Scanmaster DX x-ray film digitizer—digitizes x-ray film, allowing the image to be viewed on a computer monitor. This permits radiologists to make clinical diagnoses directly from the monitor, bypassing the need to examine the original film.

scanning acoustic microscope (SAM).

Scanning-Beam Digital X-ray (SBDX)—a low-radiation fluoroscopy system used in the diagnosis and treatment of cardiovascular disease.

scanning laser polarimetry—a laser for measuring the angle of rotation in polarization.

Scan-O-Grams of lower extremities.

scaphocephaly (sagittal synostosis)—an abnormally long and narrow skull in a newborn, as a result of premature closure of the sagittal suture. It is treated with sagittal craniectomy and biparietal morcellation. See also *craniosynostosis*, *endoscopic strip craniectomy*, and *helmet-molding therapy*.

Scaphoid-Microstaple system—a simple staple device used for osteosynthesis.

scapholunate arthritic collapse—see *SLAC wrist*.

scarf osteotomy bunionectomy—used for correction of hallux valgus deformity of the great toe.

SCARMD (severe childhood autosomal recessive muscular dystrophy). See *sarcoglycanopathy*.

scatoma—stercoroma; tumorlike mass in the rectum formed by an accumulation of fecal material. Cf. *scotoma*.

SCC (small cell carcinoma) **of the lung**. Also, *squamous cell carcinoma*.

SCD (sequential compression device).

Schanz screw (Ortho)—used in performing a proximal femoral valgization osteotomy. Usage: "Good exposure was obtained by inserting a large Schanz screw in the greater trochanter region and retracting the trochanter bone with a T-handled universal chuck."

Schanz-type proximal femoral valgization osteotomy. See *Schanz screw*.

Schaubel modification of Smith-Petersen approach. Instead of dividing the fascia lata at the iliac crest, an osteotomy of the iliac crest between the attachments of the external oblique muscle medially and the fascia lata laterally is performed. Tensor fasciae latae, gluteus medius,

Schaubel *(cont.)* and gluteus minimus attachments are subperiosteally dissected distally to expose hip joint capsule.

Schepens-Okamura-Brockhurst technique—for retinal detachment repair.

Scheuermann disease—osteochondrosis of vertebral epiphyses in the young.

Scheuermann juvenile kyphosis.

Schiek back support—a belt that assists in maintaining proper alignment of the lower back.

Schiller test—when iodine is painted on the cervix, healthy tissue is stained but cancerous tissue is not.

Schinzel acrocallosal syndrome—rare disorder inherited as an autosomal recessive genetic trait and characterized by craniofacial abnormalities, absence or underdevelopment of the mass of white matter that unites the two halves of the brain, additional fingers and/or toes, loss of muscle tone, and mental retardation.

Schiötz tonometry—measures intraocular pressure. See *applanation tonometry*.

Schirmer test—a strip of filter paper or soft tissue paper (called *tear strips*) placed between the eyelids to determine the quantity of tear production. Used in the diagnosis of Sjögren syndrome and one of its elements, keratoconjunctivitis sicca, also known as *dry eye*.

schizencephaly—a developmental disorder of cortical migration often associated with epilepsy. Patients with this disorder have significant neurological impairment and often paresis and subnormal intelligence.

schizophrenia—see *negative symptoms of schizophrenia*, *positive symptoms of schizophrenia*.

Schlemm canal—in the inner scleral sulcus, against the sclera, a large vessel filled with aqueous humor, closely resembling a large lymphatic channel.

Schlesinger solution—a morphine and scopolamine solution used for palliative purposes in patients with advanced carcinoma.

Schmidt elastic–Giemsa stain.

schneiderian papilloma, inverted—an epithelial neoplasm of the nasal wall of uncertain etiology. It has a tendency to recur and has a propensity to be associated with malignancy. Another attribute is its destructive capacity. It appears in men more often than in women, whites more than blacks, and in the sixth and seventh decades of life.

schneiderian respiratory membrane—lines the lateral nasal wall, turbinates, and paranasal sinuses. (Victor Conrad Schneider, late 1600's.)

Schneider Wallstent—see *Wallstent*.

Schober test—measures lumbar flexion for evaluation of spondylitis. Measurements are given in degrees, with normal being 20° or more.

Scholten endomyocardial bioptome and biopsy forceps—used in heart transplantations.

Schon hemodialysis catheter (also SchonCath).

Schönlein-Henoch purpura—a kidney disease with urticaria, erythema, arthritis, arthropathy. Also, *Henoch-Schönlein purpura*.

Schuco nebulizer—used in pediatric settings to produce moist nebulized air as an adjunct to therapy for respiratory problems.

Schuco 2000—a self-contained, portable nebulizer for aerosolization therapy at home or elsewhere.

Schüffner dots—cytoplasmic stippling.

Schuknecht classification of congenital aural atresia—type A, atresia limited to the fibrocartilaginous part of the external auditory canal; type B, narrowing and sometimes tortuosity of both fibrocartilaginous and bony parts of the external auditory canal; type C, totally atretic canal but well-developed pneumatization of the temporal bone; and type D, total atresia with reduced pneumatization of the temporal bone.

Schuknecht cochleosacculotomy—for treatment of progressive endolymphatic hydrops (Ménière disease). Involves the placement of an endolymphatic shunt to control a chronic state of excessive accumulation of endolymph.

Schulman syndrome—seen in a list of conditions that may respond to pentoxifylline therapy; no description given.

schwannoma—see *neurilemmoma.*

Schwartz-Pregenzer urethropexy—developed and named after Drs. Marlan K. Schwartz and Gerard J. Pregenzer. The procedure is performed laparoscopically with three small incisions that allow insertion of a microscopic camera through the abdominal wall. A nonreactive mesh graft is then used to attach the neck of the bladder to a ligament on the pubic arch, returning the bladder to its normal position and alleviating the stress that causes incontinence.

Schwartz test—for patency of the deep saphenous veins.

SCID (severe combined immunodeficiency disease). See *bare lymphocyte syndrome, Swiss-type SCID, x-linked SCID.*

scintigraphy, quantitative hepatobiliary (QHS).

scintillating scotoma—flashing lights and expanding circles of light, seen in migraine headache and in disorders of the occipital lobe of the brain. See *fortification spectrum.*

scintimammography (SMM)—screening technique for detection of carcinoma of the breast, using technetium ^{99m}Tc sestamibi (Cardiolite). Is said to be more sensitive than conventional mammography for detecting carcinoma and may reduce the number of mammographically indicated biopsies of the breast that yield negative results for carcinoma.

scintirenography (Urol).

scirrhous ("skir-us")—refers to a hard cancer, e.g., scirrhous carcinoma of the breast. Cf. *serous.*

scissors—see *device.*

scissors gait (Ortho, Neuro).

SciTojet—needle-free injector for use with human growth hormone.

SCIWORA (spinal cord injury without radiographic abnormality) **syndrome**—occurs when the elastic ligaments of a child's neck stretch during trauma. As a result, the spinal cord also undergoes stretching, leading to neuronal injury or, in some cases, complete severing of the cord.

SCJ (squamocolumnar junction).

SCLC (small cell lung carcinoma, or cancer)—see *NSCLC.*

sclera (pl., sclerae)—the tough white tissue that covers the so-called white of the eye.

scleral buckling procedure—used as treatment for primary retinal detachment. Silicone sponge, solid silicone, or fascia lata are attached to the sclera or buried in it. The sclera indents (or buckles) toward the cen-

scleral *(cont.)*
ter of the eye. Subretinal fluid is drained, and the retina is reattached (after the fluid has been drained or resorbed) and is in contact with the pigment epithelium. The buckling element can be applied locally or can encircle the eye, as appropriate. Cf. *pneumatic retinopexy,* a newer procedure.

scleral expansion band (SEB)—device used to correct presbyopia. It consists of four segments that are implanted just below the surface of the sclera.

scleroderma (*n*ot scler*a*derma)—a form of progressive systemic sclerosis, a disease of no known cause, no means of treatment, and no cure. It can be manifested by a small area of dry, hard skin or it can be what is called a *diffuse systemic sclerosis*, usually affecting the arms and hands. The skin becomes hard and thickened, making it difficult to use the hands. This process can also affect internal organs—lungs, GI tract, kidneys. This disease is not what one would call an equal opportunity disease; 80% of its victims are women.

scleroderma sine scleroderma—a category of scleroderma in which the characteristic features of internal organ involvement are present without the usual detectable skin features.

ScleroLaser—a laser system used for photothermolysis of leg telangiectasias. It avoids laser exposure to surrounding tissue.

ScleroPLUS HP—a laser system used to treat leg veins plus other vascular conditions such as facial spider veins, port wine stains, hemangiomas, rosacea, stretch marks, angiomas, scars, and warts.

sclerosing encapsulating peritonitis—occurring in a cirrhotic patient with *Listeria* peritonitis and an indwelling peritoneovenous shunt. Treated by repeated operative interventions for removal of the fibrinopurulent exudate encasing the small bowel.

sclerotherapy—see *EVS.*

sclerotome—see *Lundsgaard.*

sclerouvectomy, partial lamellar (Oph)—used to remove a uveal tumor and leave intact outer sclera and sensory retina.

SCL-90-R (Symptom Checklist-90 Revised).

SCNB (stereotaxic core needle biopsy)—for breast microcalcifications.

SCNT (somatic cell nuclear transfer)

SC-1 needle—used to reposition a subluxated lens in intraocular surgery.

SCOOP 1—a transtracheal oxygen catheter with an opening at the distal tip for oxygen flow. Also, *SCOOP 2*—a catheter with distal and side openings.

scope—see *endoscope.*

scoped—slang for examined by endoscope (bronchoscope, cystoscope, colonoscope).

Scopette device—used to reduce genital prolapse during urodynamic evaluation.

Scopinaro procedure—biliopancreatic diversion, a bariatric surgery technique.

scorbutic white line—radiologic finding in scurvy.

score (see also *classification, index, scale, test)*

Agatston
APACHE II, APACHE III
Apgar
AUA BPH
Ballard
Ballard gestational assessment

score *(cont.)*
Banff
Baylor bleeding
bother
Braden
cardiac morbidity
Champion Trauma Score
Cockcroft-Gault equation
Cooperman event probability
coronary artery scoring
Detsky modified risk index
Dripps-American Surgical Association
Duke treadmill exercise
Eagle equation for cardiac morbidity
Esterman visual function
Euler-Byrne (EB)
Glasgow Coma
Gleason
Goldman cardiac risk index
Green and O'Brien wrist function
Harris hip
Hughston knee
Inappropriate Sleep Composite Score
Injury Severity Score
International Prostate Symptom Score (IPSS)
Knee Society Score
Kurtzke disability
LAP (leukocyte alkaline phosphatase)
Lysholm knee
Mallampati
McGill pain
MELD (Model for End-Stage Liver Disease)
metology score summarizing cervical rotation
Mississippi 3-class scoring system
modified Rodnan total skin-thickness
PELD (pediatric end-stage liver disease)

score *(cont.)*
Penetrating Abdominal Trauma Index (PATI)
PULSES profile
SAPS (simplified applied physiology score)
Sassone
Selvester QRS
sepsis-related organ failure assessment (SOFA)
SmartScore
Tegner activity
treadmill duration (TDS)

scoring incision—in surgery. Usage: "This allowed a vertical scoring incision posteriorly, as well as another scoring incision along the bone ridge, permitting swiveling of the cartilage to a more midline position."

Scorpio total knee system.

Scotchcast 2 casting tape (Ortho).

scotoma—an area of depressed vision in the visual field surrounded by an area of more normal vision. Examples: Bjerrum, scintillating, Seidel. Cf. *scatoma*.

scotopic sensitivity screening, whole-field (Oph)—may be of value in field-based screening for glaucoma.

scotty dog sign—diagnostic of spondylolysis on x-ray. On oblique view of the lumbar spine, the outline of a dog can be seen. The parts of the dog are as follows: the transverse process is the nose; the pedicle is the eye; the pars interarticularis is the neck; the superior articular facet is the ear; the inferior articular facet is the front leg. A break in the neck of the dog, or a dog collar, corresponds to a fracture in the region of the pars interarticularis, which is specific for spondylolysis.

Scoville retractor—double-hinged for spinal surgery retraction.

screen craze (Radiol)—a filigree pattern or cobweb appearance on the radiograph, produced by cracked old intensity screens.

screw—see *device*.

scrim—ENT slang for speech or auditory discrimination.

Scully Hip S'port—a functional hip support that can be applied in multiple configurations to treat a wide range of hip injuries.

Sculptor anuloplasty ring—combines the features of flexible, rigid, and adjustable rings to adapt to the natural geometry of the anulus.

Sculptra wrinkle filler—soft tissue filler to surgically treat wrinkles, furrows, and folds in the skin.

scurf—flaky material seen usually around the eyelashes but also other parts of the body.

scybalous ("sib-uh-lus") **stool**—hard, dry fecal matter. Usage: "He was taking laxatives and enemas, with production of scant, scybalous stools." Cf. *sibilant*.

scyphoid ("si´foid")—cup-shaped. Cf. *xiphoid*.

SD (serologically determined) **antigens**.

SDAP (single donor apheresis platelets).

SDAT (senile dementia of Alzheimer type).

SDB (sleep-disordered breathing).

SD Plasma—designed to climinate the risk of viral transmission during blood plasma transfusion. While screening of donor transfusions has improved the safety of blood transfusions, SD Plasma reduces the risk of blood-borne viruses from donors who test negative but have been recently infected.

Sea-Band acupressure wristband—said to control nausea and vomiting in some pregnant women.

seabather's eruption (Derm)—itching and rashes appearing on protected and unprotected skin within hours of exposure, believed to be due to contact with larvae of the thimble jellyfish. May also be accompanied by headaches, fever, chills, nausea, and fatigue. Symptoms usually subside within 12 days.

sea-blue histiocyte syndrome—one of the reasons for liver transplant in children.

seabuckthorn seed oil—extracted from the seabuckthorn plant and used for centuries by Tibetan and Mongolian physicians to treat diseases of the GI system. This nutritional supplement is said to work by providing damaged cells in the GI tract the necessary nutrients to repair themselves, including vitamins, fatty acids, flavonoids, and carotenoids.

Sea-Clens wound cleanser.

sea fan—in patients with sickle cell retinopathy. Major nutrient arterioles and draining venules grow in neovascular patches or channels, which develop slightly dilated aneurysmal tips resembling the typical fan shape of *Gorgonia flabellum* (sea fan).

sea fronds—description of neovascularization seen on eye examination.

seagull bruit.

SEA (side entry access) **port**.

Seasonale—oral contraceptive drug, referred to as the "four-month pill." As opposed to women taking an oral contraceptive 21 consecutive days and having 13 menstrual periods a year, the Seasonale regimen involves taking "the pill" for 84 consecutive days and having four menstrual periods a year.

SeaSorb alginate wound dressing.

seat belt fracture—see *Chance fracture.*

seat belt sign—abrasion across the abdomen following trauma in an automobile accident in which the lumbar vertebrae are fractured from extreme forward flexion. See *Chance fracture.*

sebaceous miliaria—nonfollicular pustulosis of the newborn caused by *Malassezia furfur* yeasts. Cf. *Malassezia furfur pustulosis*.

Sebastian syndrome (SBS)—autosomal dominant platelet disorder with macrothrombocytopenia and characteristic leukocyte inclusions. See also *MYHIIA syndrome*.

"seb kers" ("sub cares")—slang for *seborrheic keratoses*.

secondary intention—an old term referring to a healing process in a surgical or traumatic wound that is delayed. A wound in which the reapposed surfaces healed promptly back together without becoming infected was said to heal by primary intention. A wound that didn't heal that way but remained open because of drainage, retained foreign material, tissue defects, or other reasons, finally closing and filling in as the open surfaces cicatrized, was said to heal by secondary intention. In the days before antisepsis, asepsis, and antibiotics, the main reason for failure of primary closure was wound infection (often not recognized as such). Nowadays healing by secondary intention occurs in wounds that are intentionally left open because of extensive tissue damage or contamination (e.g., facial bite wounds), mechanical difficulties in effecting primary closure, or other reasons.

second impact syndrome—seen in sports medicine. This syndrome affects patients with a previous head injury who are not fully recovered when they experience a second head trauma. Thought to be caused by a temporary inability of the brain to control vascular constriction following head injury, even a slight second injury can cause brain swelling and possible death.

second-look laparotomy—reoperation, for further investigation.

secretin—a human polypeptide hormone secreted by the mucosa of the duodenum and upper jejunum. Secretin has recently been approved for use in the treatment of autism, but its effectiveness is questionable.

secreting the infant—jargon for *suctioning secretions from the infant*. Usage: "As the nurse was secreting the infant, I entered the room, clamped the cord, cut same, and handed the infant to the mother." Edit "secreting" to "suctioning secretions."

secretory phase endometrium, early—the second half of the menstrual cycle, after ovulation, in which the corpus luteum secretes progesterone, preparing the endometrium for implantation of the embryo. Menstruation takes place if fertilization does not occur. Note spelling of *secretory*.

sector scan echocardiography—see *two-dimensional echocardiography.*

Secu clip ("C-Q")—clip used in tubal ligation.

secundum atrial septal defect (ASD).

Secur-Fit HA (hydroxyapatite) **hip system**.

sedentary death syndrome (SeDS)—a condition which is linked to syndrome X, dysmetabolic syndrome,

sedentary *(cont.)*
obesity, increased rates of type 2 diabetes mellitus, and childhood obesity.

sediment—see *spun urine sediment.*

Sedlackova syndrome—also known as velofacial hypoplasia. Sedlackova syndrome and velocardiofacial (Shprintzen) syndrome have a corresponding phenotype and are both associated with chromosome deletion of 22q11.2.

sed rate (sedimentation rate)—a good indicator of the possible presence (or absence) of generalized systemic illness. When the brief form *sed rate* is dictated in a report, it may be typed as dictated or written out. One would certainly never type *sed rate* if *sedimentation rate* were dictated.

SeDS (sedentary death syndrome).

seeds—see *radioactive seed implants.*

"see-ess-eye-eye"—phonetic for *CS/II* (continuous subcutaneous insulin infusion).

SeedNet system—minimally invasive cryotherapy that permits controlled coverage of a target area in the prostate with IceSeeds, using ultrathin needles, effecting rapid destruction of cancerous tissue.

SEE IT substernal epicardial echocardiography—imaging technology utilizing an insertion port/pathway for an ultrasound transducer probe, combined with a mediastinal drain lumen. Placed in lieu of a mediastinal drain prior to closure of the sternum. The SEE IT sleeve allows the surgeon to pass a standard adult or pediatric echoprobe into the patient's chest overlying the epicardium. This permits visualization of virtually all the structures of the heart, providing real-time information that allows immediate assessment and treatment of the patient.

"see-pap"—see *CPAP.*

SeeQuence II—disposable contact lens.

Segard (afelimomab)—for the treatment of sepsis and septic shock.

SEG-CES (segmented cement extraction system)—removes cement in a femoral revision procedure.

segmentally demineralized bone technology—allows bone to be softened in portions, combining flexible and inflexible bone sections in one implant. The flexible section of a graft, composed of the same collagen protein as tendons and ligaments, remodels in the body into natural ligament and tendon; the hard bone section can be machined and threaded for anchoring into the patient's bone and will remodel as bone.

segmental mediolytic arteriopathy—a variant of fibromuscular dysplasia, it is a noninflammatory disease of small and medium arteries characterized by focal segmental disruption of the medial smooth muscle cells. This leads to dissection, intramural hemorrhage, and aneurysm formation.

segmental misty mesentery (SSM)—an imaging term describing a segment of increased density in the mesenteric fat. See *misty mesentery.*

segmental range of motion (SROM).

segments, middle cerebral artery
M_1 sphenoidal
M_2 insular
M_3 opercular
M_4 cortical

Segond fracture—bony avulsion of the rim of the lateral tibial plateau indicating an injury to the anterior cruciate ligament.

segregation (Genetics)—the normal separation of allelic genes during meiosis, one going to each of the two gametes formed.

Seguin sign—involuntary contracture of muscles just prior to an epileptic seizure.

Segura CBD (common bile duct) **basket**—for use in retrieving gallstones from the common bile duct. See *In-Surg laparoscopic instrumentation.*

Seidel humeral locking nail.

Seidel intramedullary fixation.

Seidel test—used with fluorescein dye to locate wound leaks.

seizure threshold—refers to the relative likelihood that a seizure will occur. For example, it might be said that sleep deprivation lowers the seizure threshold—that is, makes a seizure more likely.

SE (spin-echo) **image**—a magnetic resonance image obtained by the spin-echo technique; with this technique, T2 is determined indirectly, as a function of TE, the echo time.

Seitzinger tripolar cutting forceps—a multiple-function endoscopic instrument; it permits the surgeon to grasp, coagulate, and transect tissue with a single insertion of the instrument. These forceps can be used in a variety of laparoscopic procedures, e.g., colectomy, laparoscopically assisted vaginal hysterectomy (LAVH), oophorectomy, myomectomy, lysis of adhesions, uterosacral nerve ablation, and Nissen fundoplication.

SELCA (smooth excimer laser coronary angioplasty).

Selecta 7000 laser—for the performance of selective laser trabeculotherapy as a new treatment option for open-angle glaucoma in patients who have not improved with medical and argon laser therapy.

selective apoptotic antineoplastic drugs (SAANDs).

selective estrogen receptor modulator (SERM) class of drugs.

selective tubal assessment to refine reproductive therapy (STARRT) **falloposcopy system**.

selective tubal occlusion procedure (STOP) **contraceptive device**.

Seldinger gastrostomy needle.

selection (Genetics)—the operation of forces that determine the relative fitness of a particular genotype, thus affecting the frequency of the relevant genes in a population.

selective excitation; **irradiation**—MRI terms.

Select joint—orthosis for ambulation in children with cerebral palsy and myelomeningocele.

Select Specialty Hospital—a facility for patients who need a longer acute stay than a traditional hospital usually offers.

Selenia—a full-field digital mammography system.

selenium-75 (^{75}Se)—radioisotope used in pancreatic scan.

self-aspirating cut-biopsy needle—see *PercuCut cut-biopsy needle.*

self-blood glucose monitoring (SBGM)—a more precise method than urine tests in keeping blood glucose levels under control. The blood glucose meter has a lancing device and is used together with reagent strips. One such meter is the Accu-Chek III. It uses a Chemstrip bG reagent, so the color reading can be checked against the digital reading. It also has a memory that holds the last 20 test values with the date and time of each test so they can be compared. Other such meters are *Medisense Pen 2* and *Companion 2*.

self-limiting (or **self-limited**)—said of a disease such as the common cold that typically runs its course and resolves spontaneously without complications or sequelae, even when left untreated.

Self-perceived Dyspnea Scale—records patient's perception of degree of dyspnea while performing daily activities.

Self-Regard Questionnaire—a quantitative rating scale to measure stress-personality interactions, expected to be used by clinicians.

self-selected gait speed—a predictor of overall function.

Sellick maneuver—pressure on the cricoid during anesthesia induction/intubation. Used to prevent aspiration of stomach contents. Pressure is maintained until the anesthesiologist inflates the cuff on the endotracheal or nasoendotracheal tube.

Sellin test—a test done to evaluate diarrhea to determine its type or cause.

Selverstone clamp (*not* Silverstone).

Selvester QRS scoring system—a method of measuring the ischemic risk region and infarct size as calculated from the standard 12-lead EKG.

SEM (scanning electron microscope).

sEMG (surface electromyography)—measures the electrical activity of muscles and uses computerized biofeedback therapy to treat patients with chronic pain or injuries. A computer translates information from surface electrodes placed on the muscles into a display on a computer screen. Through the display people learn to identify tensed muscles and learn to relax them.

semidisposable monocrystant antimony pH electrodes—a device for ambulatory pH monitoring in patients with gastroesophageal reflux.

seminal vesiculography (SVG)—evaluation of the distal male reproductive tract.

Semmes-Weinstein nylon monofilaments—used in determining cutaneous pressure thresholds. Color-coded filaments of different weights are placed, with enough pressure to just bend the fibers, on each phalanx of the fingers, radial and ulnar side, and along the nerve distributions. The patient is not allowed to watch the application of the fibers. A delayed response of more than three seconds is abnormal. The report is coded with colored pencils corresponding to the color-coded, weighted fibers.

Semm hysterectomy—see *CASH*.

Semont maneuver—used in the treatment of benign paroxysmal positional vertigo. This is a procedure whereby the patient is rapidly moved from lying on one side to the other. Also called the *liberatory maneuver.*

SEMRUSB—slang for *systolic ejection murmur, right upper sternal border.*

Senning intra-atrial baffle—for repair of transposition of the great vessels.

Senographe 2000D—digital mammography imaging system.

SenoScan full-field digital mammography system—for use in the detection of breast cancer and other abnormalities.

Sensability—lubricated plastic sheet that a woman holds over her breast to more easily feel for lumps during self-examination.

Sensar—foldable acrylic posterior chamber intraocular lens. The Sensar is delivered into the eye through the Unfolder. See *Unfolder.*

Sens-A-Ray—digital dental imaging system that utilizes existing x-ray source and replaces traditional x-ray film with a sensor unit that digitizes and transfers images to a computer, providing instant images on a monitor.

sense of coherence (SOC) **scale**—measures overall orientation toward demanding life situations.

Sense-of-Feel prosthesis—an artificial foot which uses a pager-sized pressure transducer to send signals to the residual leg, enhancing balance and a more natural gait and possibly helping to reduce "phantom" pain.

SensiCath optical sensor—used with the OnLineABG blood gas monitoring system.

Sensipar (cinacalcet HCl)—a medication for the treatment of secondary hyperparathyroidism associated with chronic kidney disease and hypercalcemia in patients with parathyroid carcinoma.

sensitize—to introduce radioactive material into a fluid, tissue, or space for purposes of performing a radioactive scan; essentially the same as *label*. Cf. *label*.

Sensi-Touch anesthesia delivery system. Also called *Sensi-Touch anesthesia needle*.

sensorimotor skills—alertness, responsiveness, interest in surroundings. *Not* sensory-motor.

sensorineural (*not* sensory neural).

Sensor PTFE-nitinol guidewire with hydrophilic tip.

sensory branch of the radial nerve (SBRN).

sensory integration (SI)—a method of treatment in physical and occupational therapy, often in conjunction with NDT (neuro-developmental techniques) and myofascial release.

sensory nerve action potential (SNAP).

Sensory Organization Test (SOT)—used in conjunction with computerized dynamic posturography.

Sentinel implantable cardioverter-defibrillator—used for treatment of cardiac arrhythmia.

sentinel bleed—the initial show of blood in a threatened abortion.

sentinel clot—a mesenteric hematoma or a focal area of higher density clotted blood seen on CT, suggestive of vascular injury.

sentinel loop—an isolated, gas-filled, distended loop of small bowel that represents paralytic ileus.

sentinel lymph node (SLN)—the node identified as most likely among the 25 or 30 nodes in the axillary basin to contain metastatic disease. Also defined as an enlarged lymph node in the left supraclavicular fossa containing cancer metastatic from the stomach; called *Virchow* or *Troisier node.*

sentinel pile—a hemorrhoid or hemorrhoid-like nodule of tissue that forms below an anal fissure.

sentinel skin paddle—a small portion of skin placed over a muscle pedicle graft to facilitate postoperative monitoring by capillary refill.

SEP (somatosensory evoked potential) —used to monitor spinal cord function in spinal injury, and in spinal cord monitoring in surgery. See also *SSEP,* which is synonymous.

SEPA—a dermal absorption enhancer that can accelerate the passage of pharmaceutical agents through the skin.

Sepacell RZ-2000—device for removing white blood cells from a unit of whole blood (leukoreduction).

Seprafilm tissue barrier—used in wound closure.

Sepramesh—a prosthetic surgical mesh designed to be sutured in place along the abdominal wall to support and strengthen hernia repairs, especially incisional hernias. It contains a bioresorbable barrier that separates the mesh from underlying tissue and organ surfaces to minimize tissue attachment to the mesh.

SEPS (subfascial endoscopic perforator surgery).

sepsis-related organ failure assessment (SOFA) **score**—measurement of PCT (procalcitonin) concentrations during multiple organ dysfunction syndrome provides more information about the severity and the course of the disease than that of CRP (C-reactive protein).

sepsis syndrome—an acute systemic illness characterized by hypotension, coagulopathies, and multiorgan failure. The term includes a broad group of patients with systemic inflammatory response syndrome (SIRS), sepsis, septic shock, and/or multiorgan dysfunction syndrome (MODS).

Septopal implant—gentamicin-impregnated PMMA beads on surgical wire.

sequela (pl., *sequelae;* usually used in the plural)—a persistent effect of an illness or injury, such as paralysis after a stroke.

sequence—a technique for noninvasive exploration of the biliary tract.

sequential compression device (SCD) —for the treatment of leg edema and lymphedema. Usage: "SCDs were used to prevent deep vein thrombosis."

Sequential Multiple Analyzer (SMA).

Sequestra 1000—a blood processing system used to conserve blood during major surgery and perform autotransfusion. It separates blood components such as platelets and plasma prior to surgery for use during the operation. Separated platelets may be used to make "platelet gel," which reduces bleeding and facilitates healing when applied to surgical wounds.

sequestration of medication—gradual withdrawal.

Sequoia ultrasound system—from Acuson.

SER (somatosensory evoked response).

"serb"—see *Srb syndrome.*

SER-IV (supination, external rotation-type IV fracture).

serial scans—a series of scans made at regular intervals along one dimension of a body region.

SERM (selective estrogen receptor modulator)—a class of drugs including tamoxifen and raloxifene and used in the treatment of cancer and osteoporosis, respectively.

seroconversion symptoms—response to a viral illness, including HIV. The symptoms feel like a case of the flu and occur approximately three weeks after exposure.

Seroma-Cath—wound drainage system used to treat postoperative seromas which can be a complication of mastectomy, axillary dissection, abdominoplasty, and some other procedures.

seromuscular intestinal patch graft—used in repair of radiation-induced vesicovaginal and rectovaginal fistulas. A segment of intestine is removed and repaired by end-to-end anastomosis. The removed segment is opened, the muscular surface denuded, and

seromuscular *(cont.)* the patch applied over the debrided fistulous tract of bladder or rectum.

seromyectomy—see *duodenal seromyectomy.*

serotonin type-3 receptor antagonists—a class of drugs used to treat chemotherapy-induced nausea and vomiting. See *ondansetron.*

serous ("se´rus")—pertaining to serum, resembling serum, or containing serum (as in serous cystadenoma). Cf. *scirrhous.*

SERPACWA ("sir-pack'-wuh") (skin exposure reduction paste against chemical warfare agents)—developed by the U.S. military to reduce absorption of chemical warfare agents through the skin.

serpiginous—snake-like.

serrated ear-vessel forceps—a forceps used in tendon anastomosis of the Pulvertaft type. Also called *pike-jawed forceps.*

Serratia liquefaciens—formerly classified as *Enterobacter liquefaciens.* It has been isolated from the intestinal tract, respiratory tract, blood, and urine.

Serratia marcescens—an organism that frequently figures in nosocomial infections, mainly in immunocompromised individuals. It causes infections in much the same areas as *E. coli* and is the cause of gram-negative ulcers in infectious keratitis.

Sertoli-cell-only syndrome—characterized clinically by aspermia and histologically by complete loss of the epithelium in the testicular tubules.

serum cidal—see *cidal.*

serum pepsinogen test—uses a fasting blood sample in screening for gastric cancer.

serum p24 antigen concentration—a marker used to monitor HIV serum levels.

Servo pump—used in cases of hydrocephalus to control intracranial pressure at desired levels.

sestamibi stress test—using radioactive imaging agent ^{99m}Tc sestamibi (Cardiolite) to show areas of myocardial infarction in a stress test.

sestamibi Tc-99m SPECT with dipyridamole stress test—used to predict the extent of perfusion abnormalities that occur during coronary occlusion and may facilitate estimation of the total myocardium in jeopardy from a stenotic lesion.

SET three-lumen thrombectomy catheter—Its tip delivers a high-pressure saline stream that microfragments clots. The clot fragments then move through the outflow lumen into a collection bag.

setting sun sign—with increased intracranial pressure or irritation of the brain stem, deviation of the eyes downward so that white sclera is seen above the iris.

sevelamer hydrochloride—see *Renagel.*

7C Gold test—proprietary urine test that measures neuronal thread protein, which is selectively increased in the brain and spinal fluid of an individual with Alzheimer disease. The test provides rapid results and is easy to read.

17-beta-Estradiol—seven-day transdermal hormone replacement therapy patch.

severe acute respiratory syndrome—see *SARS.*

severe childhood autosomal recessive muscular dystrophy (SCARMD)—may be caused by a deficiency of the adhalin gene, which has been isolated and found on chromosome 17. When adhalin is absent, muscle cells are more prone to damage, and as

severe *(cont.)*
the cells break down, the muscles begin to waste away. SCARMD is rare in the U.S. but more common in some Middle Eastern countries.

Sewell retractor (ENT).

sewing capsule—part of EndoCinch device.

sewing machine technique—see *endoscopic sewing machine technique.*

Sex After MI Knowledge Test—measures knowledge about resumption of sexual activity after a myocardial infarction.

sex chromatin—a mass of chromatin visible near the periphery of cell nuclei in genetic females; it represents the inactive X chromosome of the XX pair that determines femaleness. Synonym: Barr body.

sex chromosome—either of the two chromosomes (X and Y) that determine gender and sex-linked traits. Genetic females have two X chromosomes; genetic males, one X and one Y.

sex-influenced—referring to a genetic trait that, although it is not X-linked, is expressed differently, in either degree or frequency, in the two sexes.

sex-limited—referring to a genetic trait that, although it is not X-linked, is expressed in only one sex.

sex-linked—in genetics, referring to a trait, disease, or pattern of transmission involving one of the sex chromosomes, that is, either the X (female) or the Y (male) chromosome. In actual usage, virtually synonymous with *X-linked.* See *X-linked.*

Sextant Medtronic Sofamor Danek spinal system.

Sextant system—a minimally invasive pedicle screw instrumentation technique for spinal stabilization.

sexually transmitted disease (STD).

Sézary syndrome—exfoliative erythroderma, manifested by hyperkeratosis, edema, alopecia, and pigment and nail changes.

SF_6 (sulfur hexafluoride)—a gas used in pneumatic retinopexy.

SFA (subclavian flap aortoplasty).

SF-ELS (sulfate-free electrolyte lavage solution)—used to treat constipation. Designed to rapidly cleanse the gastrointestinal tract without disturbing patient water and electrolyte balance, in preparation for diagnostic examination such as colonoscopy. Example, NuLytely. See also *PEG-ELS.*

S-fluoxetine, racemic fluoxetine—drug used in an attempt to prevent migraine headache attacks.

SFS (small fragment system)—see *Alphatec.*

SGA (small for gestational age).

Sgambati reaction or **test** ("zgahm-bah-tee")—a lab test for peritonitis. When the patient's urine is combined with nitric acid and chloroform, a resulting red tint is a positive sign of peritonitis.

SGAP (superior gluteal artery perforator) **flap**.

SGOT—see *AST.*

SGPT—see *ALT.*

SGRO (St. George Respiratory Questionnaire).

Shade UVAGuard—a broad-spectrum sunscreen lotion containing Parsol 1789. See *Parsol 1789.*

Shadow-Line retractors.

SHAFT (sad, hostile, anxious, frustrating, tenacious) **syndrome**—factitious disorder in which a patient manipulates the surgeon to perform operations to fulfill his or her psychological needs.

SHAFT (shopping, housework, accounting [bills], food preparation, and transportation [driving]—a mnemonic for instrumental activities of daily living (ADLs). Cf. *DEATH*.

shagreen lesions of the optic lens.

Shah permanent tube—a middle ear ventilating tube used in patients with otitis media.

shaken baby syndrome—see *shaken impact syndrome.*

shaken impact syndrome—the newer name for *shaken baby syndrome*. Caregivers, by violently shaking an infant, cause permanent neurological damage by the abrupt acceleration and deceleration of the brain against the cranium, resulting in intracranial hemorrhage.

shake test—tests the maturity of fetal lungs. See *foam stability test.*

Shaldon catheter.

sham feeding—the use of something like chewing gum to aid in the restoration of bowel function and prevent postoperative ileus after colon surgery.

sham therapy—in which the main treatment or ingredient is inactive. Placebos are a form of sham therapy.

ShanStar Cranberry—an over-the-counter concentrated herbal extract, given to maintain correct pH balance of urine.

Shapshay-Healy—20 cm phonatory and operating laryngoscope.

Shark disposable biopsy forceps—used to obtain endoscopic mucosal tissue biopsies for microscopic examination and foreign body retrieval.

sharp and blunt dissection—a surgical term referring to separating or cutting apart tissues with sharp instruments (scalpel, scissors) where necessary and with blunt instruments or fingers where possible. Separation of structures and development of tissue planes by blunt dissection is less traumatic and causes less bleeding.

Sharpey fibers—collagenous fibers of a tendon, ligament, or periosteum buried in the subperiosteal bone.

Sharplan SilkTouch flashscan surgical laser—now approved for use in hair transplantation.

sharps—operating room slang for suture needles, scalpel blades, hypodermic needles, cautery blades, and safety pins, all of which require special handling to avoid injury to healthcare personnel and to reduce their risk of acquiring bloodborne infections. Sometimes a *sharps count* is dictated at the end of an operative report.

SharpShooter—used for "inside-out" tissue repair technique of meniscus suturing.

Sharrard-type kyphectomy (Ortho).

Shaw I and **Shaw II scalpel**—a Teflon-coated hemostatic scalpel used in hot conization of the cervix.

Shaw scalpel—an electrical scalpel. A dictator mentioning this instrument will usually give settings in degrees of temperature.

Sheehy syndrome—rapidly advancing sensorineural hearing loss in younger age groups.

sheet sign—psychological despair in AIDS patients shown by their hiding under bedcovers and refusing human contact.

Sheffield pedobarograph—a floor-mounted system for measuring pressure underneath the foot.

shepherd's crook area of the right coronary artery.

Shepherd internal screw fixation—for sagittal split ramus osteotomy.

Shepherd technique—for intraocular lens insertion using a 3-4 mm incision and closure with suture knots covered with conjunctiva.

Sherpa guiding catheter—directs balloon catheters rapidly into coronary arteries or other sites where obstructions are treated.

Sherwood intrascopic suction/irrigation system for laparoscopic procedures—allows surgeon to use suction/irrigation and electrocautery without removing the irrigator from the cannula during the cauterization.

Shiatsu therapeutic massage—see also *Ohashiatsu massage.*

shifting dullness on percussion—indicates the presence of ascites. The abdomen is percussed with the patient lying in the supine position, then with the patient lying on each side. If the area of dullness shifts, this indicates the presence of ascitic fluid, rather than edema or cyst.

shift to the left (white blood cells)—means there are increased numbers of immature neutrophils which may indicate presence of infection. The term refers to a white blood cell differential counted manually; the technician uses a diagram which places the younger, developing cells on the left side of the page. A rise in the number of these cells, a shift to the left, is a sign of the body's reaction to an infection, or of leukemia. See *shift to the right.*

shift to the right—means that there are increased numbers of older neutrophils present in the blood. Cf. *shift to the left.*

Shikani middle meatal antrostomy stent—a temporary stent to be placed following endoscopic sinus surgery. May be removed after mucosal layer heals in 10 to 14 days.

shim coil; shimming—MRI terms.

shin splints—painful spasm of shin muscles due to strain, usually as a result of running.

Shirley wound drain.

Shirodkar cervical cerclage procedure.

shock blocks—blocks placed under the foot of a bed to elevate it manually for a patient in shock.

shock on T-wave induction capability—programming of an implanted cardioverter-defibrillator to deliver a rhythm-converting shock during the ventricular repolarization phase of the cardiac cycle, represented by the T wave of the electrocardiogram.

shocky—in shock, or showing signs (tachycardia, pallor, diaphoresis, restlessness) suggestive of shock.

shoelace technique—a surgical technique for delayed primary closure of fasciotomy. Skin staples spaced approximately 2 cm apart function as eyelets for a Silastic vessel loop that serves as the lace. The shoelace technique involves running a Silastic vessel loop through skin staples placed at the skin edge along the initial fasciotomy incision. Daily tightening of the shoelace permits gradual reapproximation of the skin edges while compartment edema resolves. Closure using a simple suture or Steri-Strip is then possible after 5-10 days. This allows for gradual closure of open fasciotomy wounds, avoiding the morbidity and cost associated with skin graft or secondary closure.

shoe, WACH (wedge adjustable cushioned heel)—a cast shoe used in orthopedics.

short arc progressive resistive exercises.

short-bore magnet—MRI term.

ShortCut knife—an ophthalmic knife with a unique rounded tip and short length for intraocular incisions. Also, *A-OK ShortCut knife.*

Short-Form Health Survey, 36-item (SF-36) and **12-item** (SF-12)—self-reported quality-of-life surveys with 36 questions (long form) and 12 questions (short form).

shorthand vertical mattress stitch—rapid skin everting suture technique.

short inversion time inversion recovery (STIR) (MRI term)—a pulse sequence sensitive enough to detect a broad range of pathologic conditions.

short-limb dwarfism—form of dwarfism in which the extremities are abnormally short, as differentiated from the true, or normal, dwarf, in which the only abnormality is the small size.

short-rod/two-claw technique—spinal instrumentation used to treat thoracic or lumbar spine wedge compression or burst fractures. Although not indicated in every situation, advantages include decreased pain and stiffness and elimination of the need for instrumentation removal.

short tandem repeats (STRs)—genetically inactive nucleotide sequences that appear between active sequences of a chromosome; they are highly distinctive of an individual and are useful in DNA fingerprinting. See also *variable number tandem repeats.*

short TR/TE (or T1-weighted)—MRI terms. TR (repetition time); TE (echo time).

short wavelength autoperimetry (SWAP)—a test for glaucoma. Different intensities of blue light are flashed across a screen, and the patient presses a button every time a blue light is seen. It is hard for a patient with glaucoma to see the blue light since nerve fibers most sensitive to the color blue are the first to be affected by glaucoma. SWAP test is able to spot glaucoma three to four years before white-light testing, allowing stabilization with eye drops or surgery. This test is usually advised for anyone in a high-risk category: over 40; African-American; family history of glaucoma. It is typically given in conjunction with white-on-white testing.

shotty nodes—as in B-B shot. Not to be confused with "shoddy," as in "shoddy merchandise."

shoulder pad sign—an appearance of the shoulders caused by amyloid infiltration of periarticular tissues, pathognomonic for immunoglobulin amyloidosis.

Shouldice hernia repair—used for either direct or indirect hernias; a variation of the Halsted-Bassini repair.

shower of infarcts—minor infarcts in the brain leading to vascular dementia.

"shrom"—phonetic for *SROM* (spontaneous rupture of membranes).

SHRS (St. Hans Rating Scale for extrapyramidal syndromes)—a scale for rating tardive dyskinesia.

shuck—a term used in orthopedic surgery. Usage: "This trial component had good stability with inferior, posterior, and anterior shuck and excellent range of motion." It refers to the relative amount of motion observed when applying a longitudinal distraction force to the hip or to the test for motion.

Shuffors internal screw fixation—used in sagittal split ramus osteotomy.

shunt
- Allen-Brown vascular access
- Anastaflo intervascular
- Buselmeier
- Cordis-Hakim
- coronary anastomotic
- Denver pleuroperitoneal
- endolymphatic mastoid (EMS)
- Flo-Thru intraluminal
- Gibson inner ear
- Gott
- Holter
- House and Pulec otic-periotic
- Kasai peritoneal venous
- LeVeen peritoneal
- Mason
- MBTS (modified Blalock-Taussig)
- mesocaval (MCS)
- Orbis-Sigma cerebrospinal fluid
- PFTE (polyfluorotetraethylene)
- Pruitt-Inahara carotid
- Quinton-Scribner
- Ramirez
- Rivetti-Levinson intraluminal
- Thomas vascular access
- TIPSS (transjugular intrahepatic portosystemic)
- Torkildsen
- transjugular intrahepatic portosystemic
- ventriculoperitoneal (VP)
- ventriculosubarachnoid (VS)
- Vitagraft arteriovenous
- Warren splenorenal
- Winters

Shur-Clens wound cleanser.

Shur-Strip (Deknatel)—a sterile wound closure tape.

Shutt Mantis retrograde forceps—used in ipsilateral approach to anterior horn of meniscus in arthroscopic knee surgery.

Shwachman syndrome—pancreatic exocrine insufficiency and cyclical neutropenia with growth retardation, steatorrhea, and abnormalities in bones and joints, often giving rise to profound short-stature deformities and sometimes fatal infections and visceral hemorrhages.

SI—see *International System*.

SI (sensory integration).

SIADH (syndrome of inappropriate antidiuretic hormone secretion).

SI (sacroiliac) **belt**—see *SI-LOC*.

sib, sibling—brother or sister.

sibilant—having a shrill or whistling sound. Cf. *scybalous*.

Sibley-Lehninger—test for serum aldolase.

SIBS (social interaction between siblings) **interview**—a new instrument to assess sibling relationships in antisocial youth.

SIBS (surgical isolation bubble system).

sick building syndrome—nausea, headache, and some other symptoms experienced by people who work in some new buildings in which windows cannot be opened. Apparently caused by many of the chemicals found in carpeting and furniture.

Sickledex—a screening test for sickle cell disease.

sickle knife (ENT). Usage: "The periorbita was opened with a sickle knife in a posterior-to-anterior direction" (in an endoscopic orbital decompression for Graves disease).

sick sinus syndrome—referring to the sinoatrial node.

SICOR—a computer-assisted cardiac catheterization recording system that automatically calculates, displays, and reports all hemodynamic parameters, valve areas and shunts, and then prints a report immediately after catheterization.

side-biting clamp.

Side Branch Occlusion system—minimally invasive procedure used in treatment of peripheral vascular disease. Fiberoptic visualization allows the vascular surgeon to work inside of saphenous vein, removing vein valves and sealing off the side branches.

side-cutting spatulated needle—comes in one-fifth circle and one-third circle and is threaded with 4-0 cable-type Supramid Extra suture material.

side-cutting Swanson bur—used in revision of total wrist arthroplasty and other procedures.

side entry access (SEA) **port**.

Side-Fire reflecting dish—used with Surgilase Nd:YAG laser to perform prostate resection in benign prostatic hypertrophy. It consists of a Teflon-coated light guide with a solid gold reflecting dish crimped to the end of a light guide. The gold reflecting dish enables a more precise energy delivery system to the prostatic tissue by deflecting energy at right angles. Solid gold is used because of its high reflectivity and low absorption of laser energy. The device has a venturi aperture that helps to prevent debris adherence on the dish with resultant distortion of the reflecting surface during lasing. Continuous irrigant keeps the reflecting gold dish cool during lasing and prevents distortion and melting of the delivery system.

siderotic nodules in the spleen (Radiol)—seen on x-rays; also called *Gamna-Gandy nodules* or *bodies*. See *Gamna-Gandy bodies.*

SIEP (superior epigastric [artery] perforator) **flap**—used in autologous breast reconstruction surgery.

SieScape imaging—ultrasound imaging technology that provides panoramic views of ultrasound images in real time. Radiologists are able to view one image rather than having to piece together a series of separate smaller pictures.

sievert (Sv) ("see´vert")—the SI unit of radiation absorbed dose equal to 1 gray (Gy) or 1 joule (J) per kilogram, or 100 rem.

sieving coefficient (SC)—the mathematical expression of the ability of a solute to cross a membrane (such as Bowman capsule in the kidney) or a filter, based on the ratio of the concentrations of the substance on both sides of the membrane or filter.

SIF10 Olympus enteroscope.

"sigh"—phonetic for *p.s.i.*

"sigh-ee-sis"—phonetic for *cyesis*.

Sigma—method used in testing serum CPK. See also *Oliver-Rosalki*.

sigmaS—a serum tumor marker used to distinguish between early and advanced stages of breast cancer. (No space in sigmaS.)

sigmodontine rodents—vectors of hantaviruses associated with hantavirus pulmonary syndrome.

sign
- absent bow-tie
- Aaron
- accordion
- alien hand
- Allis
- Apley
- Aufrecht
- Babinski
- banana
- Bard
- Battle
- bite (avascular necrosis)
- blade of grass
- blue dot

sign *(cont.)*
Blumberg
Boas
bone bruise
bone in bone
bounce home
bow-tie
Branham
brim
Brockenbrough-Braunwald
Brudzinski
C
Carabello
Chadwick
chandelier
Clarke
cobblestone appearance
cockade image
Collier
comb
cortical ring
cotton-wool
Courvoisier
crescent
crowded carpal
Cullen
Cupid's bow contour
dagger
Dalrymple
Dance
David Letterman
deep lateral femoral notch
de Musset
doll's eye
Dorendorf
double anterior horn
double-bubble
double halo
double PCL (posterior cruciate ligament)
double stripe
double-wall
drawer
drooping shoulder
dural tail

sign *(cont.)*
Earle
echo
elbow fat pad
empty can
Ewart
extrapyramidal
fabere
fadir
Fajersztajn crossed sciatic
fat-blood interface (FBI)
fat pad
Federici
Finkelstein
Fischer (obsolete)
fissure
Fleischner
flipped meniscus
Fodéré
football
formication
fragment-in-notch
Froment
frontal release
Galeazzi
Gauss
Goodell
Gowers
Griesinger
hair-on-end
Hamman
heel pad
Hill-Sachs
Hitzelberger
Hoehne
Homans
Hoover
impingement
inverted Napoleon hat
ivory phalanx
ivory vertebra
J
Jackson
Jacquemier
Joffroy

sign *(cont.)*
Lasègue
lateral femoral notch
lemon
linguine
long tract
Macewen
main d'accoucheur
McCort
McMurray
Moebius
Moses
Mulder
mute toe
navel
Nicoladoni-Branham
obturator
oil drop change
Ortolani
parallel track
parrot's
pedestal
Phalen
Pinard
Pins
pivot-shift
pneumoarthrogram
pronator
pseudo-Billroth I
puddle
pyloric string
pyramidal
Q
Queckenstedt
raccoon
ram's horn
Rigler
rim
root
rose thorn
Rovsing
rugger-jersey spine
sagging rope
sail
sandwich

sign *(cont.)*
scotty dog
seat belt
Seguin
setting sun
sheet
shoulder pad
signet-ring
soft neurologic
soft tissue rim
Spurling
steeple
Stellwag
string
target
teardrop
tenting
Terry fingernail
Terry-Thomas
Tinel
too many toes
tooth
track
tram-track
trolley-track
trough line
Trousseau
tumbling bullet
turtle
Unschuld
vacuum disk
Valleix
vital
von Graefe
Weill

SignaDress—hydrocolloid dressing material.

Signa I.S.T. MRI **scanner**.

signal amplification technique—amplifies a secondary probe attached to the sample via a synthetic DNA probe to isolate a particular DNA or RNA sequence in a specimen. See *polymerase chain reaction*.

signal-averaged electrocardiogram (SAECG)—device that allows non-invasive recording of low-amplitude cardiac signals such as ventricular late potentials. It has been used to predict life-threatening cardiac events.

signaling, myocardial adrenergic.

signal intensity—in magnetic resonance imaging, the strength of the signal or stream of radiofrequency energy emitted by tissue after an excitation pulse.

signal-to-noise ratio (S/N)—MRI term.

Signa SP/i 0.5T MR imaging unit—an MRI machine.

signet-ring pattern—a cellular change wherein the cell has a ring-like configuration, as seen in gastric carcinoma.

signet-ring sign—caused by abnormal orientation of the scaphoid on x-ray (rotary subluxation). Also called the *cortical ring sign* and not to be confused with *signet-ring pattern*.

Sigvaris compression stockings—for treatment of venous disease in ambulatory patients.

SIHC (surgically implanted hemodialysis catheter).

SIL (squamous intraepithelial lesions).

Silastic bead embolization—used as therapy for some types of arteriovenous fistulae fed by several small arteries in areas not amenable to surgical repair, or if the vessel is not a critical artery which may be obliterated without fear of causing distal ischemia. See *Gianturco coil,* used for the same purpose.

Silastic silo reduction of gastroschisis—see *Silon tent*.

sildenafil citrate—see *Revatio, Viagra*.

silent (disease)—asymptomatic; the lack of apparent symptoms in the presence of disease. Usage: silent heart attack, silent gastroesophageal reflux disease, silent migraine.

silent areas of the brain—seizures starting from a focus in these areas produce no aura. See *eloquent areas*.

silent, EKG—see *dipyridamole*.

silent epidemic—predicted by epidemiologists when, around the year 2030, 20 percent of the population will be over 65. The epidemic referred to is Alzheimer and other dementing diseases.

silent gene—a mutant gene that has no detectable effect on the phenotype of the individual possessing it.

silent infarction—refers to a myocardial infarction that is undiagnosed because symptoms are absent or are attributed to some other cause.

silent prostatism—a condition in which progressive obstruction occurs slowly, without symptoms, and the patient presents without urinary complaints. The presence of benign prostatic hypertrophy may be suspected if there is azotemia and if ultrasound shows bilateral hydronephrosis.

Silhouette—therapeutic massage system.

silicon—a chemical element present in sand and various types of rock. Cf. *silicone*.

silicone—an organic compound used in the manufacture of various medical devices such as breast implants, catheters, drains. Cf. *silicon*.

silicone flexor rod—placed in the sheath of the flexor tendon for reconstruction of a finger.

silicone ring.

silicone synovitis—a condition induced by particles of silicone debris that come loose from a silicone implant.

Silipos Distal Dip—prosthetic sheath/liner which reduces friction and pistoning of an extremity prosthesis.

silk free ties—free ties performed with silk.

Silk guidewire (Cardio).

Silk Laser—aesthetic carbon dioxide laser system for laser skin resurfacing. See *2040 erbium laser*.

SilkTouch laser—used for hair transplantation. It creates holes in the skin that are small enough to transplant a single hair.

SI-LOC—a type of sacroiliac belt designed to stabilize the SI joint and pubic symphysis after fractures of the pelvic ring. The belt prevents the innominates from being pushed away from each other, pressing the joint surfaces firmly together.

Silon tent—used in an operative procedure for gastroschisis. The tent is placed over the abdominal opening and the intestines are gradually reduced back into the abdomen by ligating the top of the tent progressively. See also *Silastic silo*.

Silon wound dressing—transparent, nonadherent dressing used for partial-thickness wounds such as donor sites and second-degree burns.

Silsoft extended wear contact lenses—used in treating pediatric aphakia.

Silverlon wound packing strips—sterile, nonadherent wound dressing with silver for protection against microbial contamination. It is used to control local wound bleeding and nasal hemorrhage; to encourage draining and wicking of fluids from a body cavity, infected area, or abscess; and to remove necrotic tissue from ulcers or other infected wounds when used as a wet-to-dry packing.

Silverstein facial nerve monitor.

Silverstein stimulator probe—used to determine nerve stimulation.

Silverstone—see *Selverston clamp*.

silver wire effect—effect created by narrowing of arterioles in the retina.

Simal cervical stabilization system.

Similac Alimentum Advance protein hydrolysate formula with iron.

simkin analysis—**sim**ulation **kin**etics analysis to determine serum acetaminophen levels. It is not named for a person.

Simonsen technique—for large rectovaginal fistula repair. It is based on the creation of a neovagina associated with an established abdominal pull-through operation.

simplex (Genetics)—referring to a family pedigree containing only one member affected by a given trait or disorder.

Simplex P—a radiopaque bone cement.

Simplicity spirometer—for measuring lung capacity and performance.

SimpliCT—an interventional guidance system that uses a laser beam to significantly improve the accuracy of computed tomography-guided puncture procedures.

simplified applied physiology score (SAPS).

Simpson atherectomy catheter—used for atherectomy in atherosclerotic peripheral vascular disease (removal and retrieval of atheroma).

Simpson Coronary AtheroCath (SCA) **system**—a catheter system with a small rotating blade inside used for directional coronary atherectomy.

Simpson peripheral AtheroCath—see *Simpson atherectomy catheter.*

Simpulse system—high-pressure, high-volume pulsed lavage used in joint replacement procedures.

simultaneous areolar mastopexy and breast augmentation (SAMBA). Cf. *WAMBA*.

simultaneous Malone antegrade continent enema (MACE) **and Mitrofanoff procedure using the divided appendix**—formation of both a Malone continent enema and a Mitrofanoff channel from separate segments of the appendix, feasible only with an appendix of 9 cm or more. When the appendix is shorter, it is used for the Mitrofanoff channel, and a pedicled tube flap is created from the cecum for the MACE.

simultaneous volume imaging—MRI term.

Sinding Larsen–Johannson disease—of the patella. (Sinding Larsen *and* Johannson.)

Sine-U-View nasal endoscope—provides optically precise images when doing sinus surgery.

sine-wave pattern—indicative of hyperkalemia, seen on electrocardiogram. (Pronounced like *sign-wave*.)

Singapore fasciocutaneous flap—a pedicled graft used in vaginal reconstruction.

Singer-Blom valve—used for esophageal speech in patients who have had laryngectomies.

singer's node—not an eponym, but a small white nodule which is often seen on the vocal cords of singers, or others who use their voices excessively.

Singh–Vaughn–Williams classification of arrhythmias.

single breath-hold sequence—on CT scan.

single-chain antigen-binding (SCA) **proteins**.

single-contrast arthrography—for evaluation of ligamentous injuries of the knee.

Single-Day Baxter infuser—used for postoperative pain control in forefoot operations. It functions by continuous infusion of anesthetic into the malleolar internal space.

single donor apheresis platelets (SDAP).

single-field hyperthermia combined with radiation therapy (radiation oncology)—a technique used for recurrent or advanced carcinoma of the breast. Using ultrasound technology, the tumor is superheated to the point of cell destruction. It can be used for local or regional control of recurrent, previously treated breast cancers.

single-lung transplant (SLT) **recipient**.

single photon emission computed tomography (SPECT).

single shot fast spin echo (SSFSE)—magnetic resonance imaging of fetal anatomy.

single slice fast dynamic in vivo sequence—MRI term.

Single-Stitch inserter for PhacoFlex lens—a silicone intraocular lens which folds for easy insertion through the small incision used for cataract surgery. The tiny opening can then be closed with one stitch (hence, Single-Stitch).

single-stripe colitis (SSC)—a single stripe of ulcerated mucosa seen on colonoscopy is diagnostic of colitis.

Singleton–Merten syndrome—a rare disorder characterized by abnormalities of the teeth, accumulation of calcium deposits in the aorta and other heart valves, and/or osteoporosis. Its cause is unknown.

singultus—hiccups. Usage: "The patient was observed to have multiple episodes of singultus during his emergency room stay."

sinking redundant arytenoids—synonym for prolapsing redundant arytenoids.

sink test—referring to a sham lab test, in which the unexamined specimen is discarded "down the sink."

sink-trap malformation—a condition resulting in redundancy and obstruction of an interposed colon segment used to replace an esophagus that has been rendered unusable by the ingestion of a caustic substance.

Sin Nombre virus (SNV)—the cause of Hantavirus pulmonary syndrome.

sinoatrial node (SA or S-A node)—the pacemaker of the heart and what is referred to in "sinus rhythm." See *Flack node* and *Koch node* (which are synonymous).

Sinskey hook (Oph).

Sinu-Clear laser sinus surgery—outpatient procedure using a patented laser delivery system in combination with warmed irrigating fluid to safely remove nasal polyps and diseased sinus tissue.

sinuscope—a rigid-rod lens optics system for ENT diagnosis and procedures.

sinus rhythm—normal rhythm generated by the sinoatrial node.

sinus tarsi syndrome—a frequently misdiagnosed condition in which patients have pain over the lateral aspect of the ankle (the sinus tarsi region) and the sensation of hindfoot instability. Patients often have a history of an inversion ankle injury that results in chronic pain.

SiPAP—a device for the delivery of intermittently increased and constant positive airway pressure to the lungs of infants or neonates. Note lowercase *i*.

Sippy diet—named for Dr. Bertram Welton Sippy, who wrote on gastric and duodenal ulcers.

SIRS (systemic inflammatory response syndrome).

SIR-Spheres—treatment for liver tumors. The physician injects the small spheres into the liver tumor through the common hepatic artery or through the right or left hepatic artery. The spheres lodge in the area of the tumor where the radiation helps slow the growth of the cancer cells. The radioactivity disappears within 11 days, but the spheres remain in the liver permanently.

SIRS/sepsis (systemic inflammatory response syndrome)—sepsis as a result of confirmed infectious process.

SISCOM (Subtraction Ictal SPECT coregistered to MRI)—imaging approach used to pinpoint location of seizure onset by electronically superimposing SPECT images over an MRI of the patient's brain. Surgeons can utilize the new approach in the operating room, in conjunction with other tools, to further confirm location of a seizure prior to removal.

SISI (short increment sensitivity index) —used in hearing test.

SIS technology—an acellular biomaterial that supports tissue repair with a scaffold-like matrix having an all-natural structure and composition. A new biomaterial that does not encapsulate when surgically implanted, but is gradually remodeled, leaving behind organized tissue. See various Oasis and Surgisis products.

Sister Mary Joseph node—lymph node near the umbilicus. Named for the nurse who first observed that when she found such a node, the patient always had pancreatic carcinoma.

sitaxsentan sodium—see *Thelin*.

site—place or position. Usage: "The site of the abscess was located quickly." Cf. *cite*.

SiteGuard MVP—transparent adhesive film dressing.

Site-Rite and Site-Rite II ultrasound systems—for vascular imaging.

SiteSelect—percutaneous breast biopsy system from Imagyn Medical Technologies.

sitostanol ester margarine—a margarine that contains sitostanol ester, a cholesterol blocker.

situ—see *in situ*.

SI (syncytium-inducing) **variant of HIV**—see *nonsyncytium-inducing*.

Sitzmark study--to determine bowel transit time.

Sivash prosthesis—total hip prosthesis that does not require use of cement.

SIVD (subcortical ischemic vascular dementia)—a type of vascular cognitive impairment (VCI).

sivelestat—neutrophil elastase inhibitor drug for treatment of acute lung injury and respiratory distress syndrome.

6-minute walk distance, 6-minute walking test (6MWT)—used to evaluate patients with heart disease. Patients are asked to walk for 6 minutes as far as they can at a brisk pace but may rest as needed. The distance completed correlates with the functional status of the individual.

6-22 ureteral stent or 6, 22 ureteral stent—a 6-French, 22-cm ureteral stent.

-sized—commonly dictated as an adjective, as in 1.5-cm-sized polyp. Also, pint-sized, Olympic-sized, adult-sized, medium-sized, 50-mL-sized.

SJM-Seguin anuloplasty ring—a ring with variable flexibility. It is sufficiently rigid in its anterior region to maintain intercommissural distance, yet sufficiently flexible in its posterior region so as not to interfere with left ventricular function and to permit the natural three-dimensional anular mobility, thereby remodeling the mitral valve, correcting dilatation, and preserving physiologic anular function.

Sjögren ("sho-grenz") **syndrome**—symptom complex marked by keratoconjunctivitis sicca.

SjO_2 (oxygen saturation in the internal jugular vein)—measured by an intravenous catheter in the internal jugular vein. Used to assess cerebral perfusion in head-injury patients.

skeletal targeted radiotherapy (STR)—a radionuclide, holmium-166, linked to a drug that targets the bone in patients with Ewing sarcoma. By injecting STR into the blood, the radiation can localize in tumors in the bone, thus delivering more radiation to the areas of bone that are directly affected by tumor than the rest of the skeleton.

skeletonize—in Webster's, meaning "to produce in or reduce to skeleton form." Rarely found in medical dictionaries, although doctors use the word in dictation.

SKF (skilled nursing facility).

skier's tear—a rupture of the ulnar collateral ligament of the thumb.

skier's thumb—rupture of the adductor pollicis tendon after forced abduction, an injury from ski poles during falls.

Skil saw—an electric saw you will run into (figuratively speaking) in orthopedic surgery transcription in reference to the etiology of an injury.

Skimmer RRP laryngeal shaver—used to reduce an exophytic mass in the larynx.

skin depth—MRI term.

Skindex, revised—a 29-item quality-of-life questionnaire administered to dermatology patients.

skin exposure reduction paste against chemical warfare agents (SERPACWA, pronounced "sir-pack'-wuh")—to reduce absorption of chemical warfare agents through the skin.

skin fold (skin crease) artifact (Radiol)—a common finding on x-rays of patients with a large body habitus. Skin folds can mimic the streaks of atelectasis on a chest film. Prior studies, follow-up examination with repositioning, and/or clinical correlation may be required to make the differentiation.

skin graft—see *graft, skin*.

skin lesion artifact (Radiol). Occasionally an astute radiologist will recognize that the pattern of an artifact could be caused by a skin lesion such as a melanoma in the worst possible case. Radiologists usually rule out artifacts with other views, but if they remain, in a case like this they would say "clinical correlation recommended."

skin-level transverse colostomy and loop ileostomy—an emergency treatment for toxic megacolon (in the absence of perforation) because the colon's friability precludes the standard surgical approach of colectomy. The skin-level transverse colostomy and loop ileostomy compress the colon and diverts intestinal contents. After recovery, a subsequent colectomy can be performed safely.

Skinlight erbium:YAG laser—used for skin resurfacing, reportedly more gentle than the CO_2 laser, causing less thermal damage and a shorter recovery time.

Skinny dilatation catheter—used in cardiac catheterization. *Skinny* is a trade name.

Skinny needle with Chiba tip—a 22-gauge needle used in percutaneous biopsy or aspiration cytology. See *Chiba*.

Skinny Pill—over-the-counter "thermic and herbal formula" that purports to be a weight-loss remedy.

Skinny Pill for Kids—controversial over-the-counter "thermic and herbal formula" for obese children ages 6-12.

SkinScan—microprocessor-driven device used for aesthetic laser surgery. It ensures consistent, precise treatment for soft tissue applications, particularly on face.

Skin Skribe—a skin marker used in surgery.

skin slip—abnormal mobility of the skin over subcutaneous structures due to early putrefactive changes in a dead body.

skin-sparing mastectomy—designed to remove only cancerous breast tissue, thereby maintaining much of the overlying skin, resulting in a better cosmetic outcome, a small scar, and excellent symmetry of the native and reconstructed breast.

SkinTegrity hydrogel dressing.

Skinvisible—hypoallergenic hand lotion provides a skin barrier that protects against the transmission of nosocomial infections and absorption of noxious chemicals.

skip metastasis—development of recurrent nodal disease in the regional

skin-sparing *(cont.)* axillary basin when no sentinel nodes have been previously identified.

"skir-us"—phonetic rendering of scirrhous.

Skoog release—of Dupuytren contracture.

SK-SD, SKSD (streptokinase-streptodornase)—skin test for immune function.

"SKUD-HEFT"—phonetic for the acronym *SCD-HeFT*.

SKY—epidural pain control system.

Skylight—gantry-free nuclear medicine gamma camera.

skyline view of patella (Radiol)—study of the knee region in which the patella is visualized above the distal femur and appears like a rising (or setting) sun.

SLAC (scapholunate arthritic collapse) **wrist**—in which a fracture/deformity has healed in a rotated position and eroded the radioscaphoid joint.

Slant lens—a single-piece intraocular lens with a design which incorporates slanted haptics and a low profile for easy insertion through the longer scleral tunnel and more acute angle of entry now used in intraocular lens surgery. *Slant* is a trademark. Also, *Cilco Slant haptics lens*.

SLAP (superior labrum [or labral] anterior posterior) **lesion**—a specific type of labral tear of the shoulder joint. It occurs at the point where the tendon of the biceps muscle inserts on the labrum of the shoulder joint. A fall onto an outstretched arm is usually the cause of this injury. Usage: "He has a SLAP lesion where the labrum is detached superiorly. We used a bur in order to get down to good bloody bone in that area, in an attempt to get the SLAP lesion to heal down to bloody bone."

Slattery-McGrouther dynamic flexion splint.

sleep apnea—disorder associated with snoring, irregular heartbeat, and wakefulness in which soft tissues in the throat can obstruct breathing. In severe cases, this can cause death.

sleep deprivation—lack of total sleep, rapid eye movement (REM) sleep, or nonrapid eye movement (NREM) sleep. Fatigue, irritability, difficulty remembering, difficulty in concentrating, and problems with muscle coordination may be manifestations of sleep deprivation. On the average, adults require from 6 to 9 hours of sleep per night, with older people thought to require less than younger ones.

sleep-disordered breathing (SDB).

sleeve pneumonectomy—an operative procedure to treat proximal tumors of the lung.

SLHA (syringolymphoid hyperplasia) **with alopecia and anhidrosis**.

slice fracture—a spinal fracture that goes through the disk or through the vertebral body.

slice profile—MRI term.

slide-by technique—a technique that involves inserting the colonoscope by pushing its tip along the colon wall. This technique involves some risk. By pressing the scope against the colon wall, tears and bleeding can occur in the mesentery supporting the colon. Perforations may be more common when the slide-by technique is used. Many experts strongly recommend insertion of the scope only when the lumen can be visualized.

Slider GDS (graft deployment system).

slide tracheoplasty.

slim disease—the term used for AIDS in some countries in Africa because of the great loss of weight seen in this disease. Cf. *wasting syndrome.*

sling
cardiac
esophageal
fascia lata suburethral
Gynecare TVT urethral
Hemi Sling shoulder
InVance male sling
ligamentum teres cardiopexy
Martius flap and fascial
midface
Monarc subfascial
pubovaginal
pulmonary
Raz urinary incontinence
Straight-In male
Stratasis TF (tension free) urethral
Stratasis urethral
suburethral
SurgiSis sling/mesh
Suspend
transvaginal Cooper ligament
Triangle gelatin-sealed
triangular vaginal patch
UltraSling
vaginal wall

sling and swathe—used for immobilization of fractured humerus if comminution is not extensive.

sling ring complex—used to describe tracheal stenosis caused by a combination of a fixed, complete cartilaginous ring and pulmonary sling syndrome. See *pulmonary sling syndrome*.

Slinky catheter—PTCA (percutaneous transluminal coronary angioplasty) catheter for use in invasive catheterization procedures.

slipped rib syndrome—a condition caused by an increased mobility of the 8th to 10th ribs (which are not attached to the sternum like ribs 1 to 7), a result of ligament laxity of the costovertebral joints.

slipped upper femoral epiphysis (SUFE)—the most common hip disorder in adolescents.

slip-ring CT technology.

slit-lamp biomicroscopy—allows well-illuminated microscopic examination of eyelids and anterior segment of the eyeball in a three-dimensional cross-section view. See *Haag-Streit slit lamp*.

SLK-View stent.

slotted acetabular augmentation (SAA)—a procedure that provides a congruous extension of the acetabulum to establish the normal load-bearing area of the acetabulum. An acetabular slot is created to control the level and anteroposterior extent of the augmentation and to secure the medial portion of the graft.

sloughed urethra syndrome.

slow-channel blocking drugs—another name for calcium channel blockers.

slow code—CPR efforts carried out perfunctorily and with little expectation of success.

SLRT ("slert") (straight leg raising test) (or tenderness).

SLS (Spectranetics laser sheath).

SLS (Spectranetics laser sheath) **laser**.

SLT (single-lung transplant) **recipient**.

Sly disease—a form of mucopolysaccharidosis, with onset at the age of one to two years, manifested by cardiac anomalies, mental retardation, short stature, pectus carinatum, and facies seen in Hurler syndrome.

slump test—assesses the mobility of the pain-sensitive structures in the vertebral canal. It tests cervical/trunk flexion, straight leg raising, and ankle

slump *(cont.)*
dorsiflexion. When all components are in place, with the nervous system at full stretch, the cervical flexion is released. Response is deemed positive or negative based on this release.

SLUScan for Your Heart—a noninvasive test that uses an ultra-fast computed tomography (CT) scanner to look inside the heart and its arteries for calcium buildup. It's a way to check for heart disease before there are symptoms. This test is safe, quick, and painless. It takes only 30 minutes and uses no needles, dyes, or shots. Exercise is not required, and clothing does not have to be removed.

SMA (superior mesenteric artery).

SMAC (Sequential Multiple Analyzer plus Computer) ("smack")—automated serum chemistry panels (profiles) comprising multiple tests.

small-bore feeding tube.

SmartBeam—high-resolution, intensity-modulated radiotherapy treatment (IMRT).

SmartCath esophageal balloon catheter—a device used to measure physiologic parameters in the esophagus such as temperature and pressure.

SmartNail—see *Bionx SmartNail.*

Smart Scalpel—a closed-loop surgical system for efficient excision of diseased tissue, leaving adjacent healthy tissue intact.

SmartScore—uses high-speed CT images to provide evaluation of heart disease risk.

SMA-6 (Sequential Multiple Analyzer) —test for sodium, potassium, chloride, bicarbonate (CO_2), BUN, and creatinine.

SMA-12 (Sequential Multiple Analyzer) —test for calcium, phosphorus, glucose, BUN, uric acid, cholesterol, total protein, albumin, total bilirubin, alkaline phosphatase, LDH, and AST (SGOT).

SMA-20 (Sequential Multiple Analyzer) —automated serum chemistry panels (profiles) of 20 tests: glucose, BUN, creatinine, sodium, potassium, chloride, calcium, phosphorus, uric acid, cholesterol, total protein, bilirubin, alkaline phosphatase, LDH, AST (SGOT), ALT (SGPT), direct bilirubin, triglycerides, albumin, iron.

small bowel enteroscopy (SBE)—a technique used to visualize the small bowel in patients with idiopathic gastrointestinal bleeding.

small bowel transit time (Radiol)—on upper GI series, the time required for swallowed contrast medium to pass through the small bowel and appear in the colon.

Small-Carrion penile prosthesis—*Small* is an eponym, not a size.

small cell lung carcinoma (or **cancer)** (SCLC).

SMALL (same-day microsurgical arthroscopic lateral-approach laser-assisted) **fluoroscopic diskectomy**—a surgical alternative to open surgical diskectomy.

small for gestational age (SGA).

small patella syndrome—a rare autosomal dominant disorder. Characterized by patellar aplasia or hypoplasia and abnormalities of the pelvic girdle.

SmallPort needle—a phacoemulsification needle used in cataract extraction to remove the nucleus and polish the capsule. It has a smaller opening at the tip than other phacoemulsification needles.

Sm (Smith) **antigen**—in systemic lupus erythematous.

SMAP (systemic mean arterial pressure).

SMART (sperm microaspiration retrieval technique)—infertility procedure.

SMART (surgical myomectomy as reproductive therapy).

SmartBrace—a brace used to treat repetitive stress injuries of the wrist.

smart defibrillator—a semiautomatic defibrillator that can be used by emergency medical technicians. It automatically checks impedance to determine loose leads and analyzes the rhythm. If ventricular fibrillation or ventricular tachycardia is detected, the system recommends a shock. This may be repeated as often as necessary. The system will not charge if ventricular fibrillation or ventricular tachycardia are not detected.

SmartFlow—a device that provides real-time blood flow information during cardiac catheterization procedures.

SmartKard digital Holter system—directly outputs ECG data from Holter recorder to any Hewlett-Packard laser printer, saving time and eliminating expense of a computer system.

SmartMist—asthma management system designed to improve the effectiveness of metered-dose inhalers.

SmartNeedle—hooked to a Doppler that emits an audio signal that helps locate femoral, subclavian, or internal jugular vessels for catheterization.

SmartWrap elbow brace—used to treat repetitive stress injuries of the elbow, often referred to as epicondylitis or tennis elbow.

SMAS ("smass") (superficial musculoaponeurotic system)—a term referring to a layer of the face, used in plastic surgery in rhytidectomies.

smasectomy—rhytidectomy technique, coined from SMAS (superficial musculoaponeurotic system).

smile (or smiling) **incision**.

SMIP (sustained maximal inspiratory pressure).

Smith-Lemli-Opitz syndrome—autosomal recessive disorder characterized by multiple congenital anomalies, including microcephaly, mental retardation, unusual facies, and genital abnormalities.

Smithwick hook.

SMM (scintimammography).

SMM (segmental misty mesentery).

SMo (stainless steel with molybdenum) —used in orthopedic appliances. It causes minimal tissue reaction.

SMO (supramalleolar orthosis)—allows for plantar flexion and dorsiflexion in orthosis for ambulation in children with cerebral palsy and myelomeningocele.

SmokEvac electrosurgical probe—see *Nezhat-Dorsey Trumpet Valve.*

SmokEvac—trumpet-valve smoke evacuator for laparoscopic surgery.

Smoothbeam—nonablative diode laser technology for skin renewal. It works by heating the upper dermis of the skin to induce a mild thermal injury. The body's natural healing response initiates collagen remodeling and the deposition of new, organized collagen.

smooth brain (lissencephaly)—syndrome in which the organized "layered" structure of normal brains is lost, resulting in severe neurological dysfunction. All humans born with type 1 lissencephaly suffer from severe mental retardation, and most experience recurrent seizures.

SMP (sympathetically maintained [pelvic] pain).

SMPV (superior mesenteric-portal vein).

SMV (superior mesenteric vein).

SNA, SNB—measurements in orthodontics. S stands for sella, N for nasion (nasal point), A and B are reference points.

SNAP (sensory nerve action potential) (Neuro).

snap gauge band (Urol)—a band made of elastic fabric and Velcro. It has three snaps, designed to open at progressively higher degrees of penile rigidity. Used to test for organic vs. psychogenic impotence. See *Dacomed snap gauge.*

Snarecoil—see *Goldenberg Snarecoil.*

snare resection (band and snare)—technique for cutting tissue in the esophagus.

Sneddon syndrome—livedo reticularis and cerebrovascular lesions involving all the extremities and the trunk, worsening in cold weather and during the acute phase of neurological complications.

Snellen chart—a test for visual acuity, using progressively smaller letters or symbols.

SNHL (sensorineural hearing loss). Note: *Not* sensory neural.

snapping triceps syndrome—characterized by medial elbow pain, snapping, neuropathy, or a combination of symptoms. Two palpable "snaps" may be detected clinically, with the first representing dislocation of the ulnar nerve and the second representing dislocation of the medial head of the triceps muscle.

SND (spontaneous nipple discharge).

"snick or sniff or snick unit"—phonetic for *SNF* (skilled nursing facility [or floor]).

sniff test—forced rapid inspiration under fluoroscopic visualization to detect paralysis of one or both diaphragms. (*Not* an eponym.)

SNIP (Strategic National Implementation Process)—a group that works with WEDI in identifying industry best practices for implementation of HIPAA standards.

"S, N, N"—slang abbreviation for abdomen: *soft, nontender, nondistended.*

SNOCAMP—acronym for report format required by some managed care entities to justify reimbursement:

S Subjective
N Nature of presenting problem
O Objective
C Counseling and coordination of care
A Assessment
M Medical decision making
P Plan

"snoos"—phonetic for *snus*, a Swedish smokeless tobacco.

Snorenz—snore relief throat spray.

snowball opacities (Oph).

snowbanks (Oph)—aggregation of inflammatory cells seen on the anterior inferior retina, characteristic of pars planitis.

snowstorm shadow—on chest x-ray, one of the indications for diagnosis of neurogenic pulmonary edema.

S/N ratio (signal-to-noise)—used in MRI scans.

SN60AT AcrySof soft foldable lens—intraocular lens implant.

snuffbox—see *anatomical snuffbox.*

snuffles—*not* a mispronunciation of *sniffles*, but actually a medical term for a hemorrhagic nasal discharge, generally associated with congenital syphilis in infants.

snus—Swedish smokeless tobacco. "[The patient exhibits] focal epithelial hyperplasia (FEH) from possible snus use.

SOAE (spontaneous otoacoustic emission).

soaker catheter—used for pain management of large surgical incisions. The catheter distributes fluid in the same way a soaker hose saturates a lawn, allowing delivery of local anesthetic without the undesirable effects of narcotic pain relievers.

SOAP (Subjective, Objective, Assessment, Plan) **note**—refers to a format setup of clinic, hospital, and physician chart notes or progress notes. Paragraph headings of the report are usually presented vertically:
SUBJECTIVE:
OBJECTIVE:
ASSESSMENT:
PLAN:
or may be abbreviated vertically:
S:
O:
A:
P:

Soave abdominal pull-through procedure—surgery for Hirschsprung disease. This procedure does not require pelvic dissection. The aganglionic rectal musculature is not removed; instead, the rectal mucosa is removed, and the normal ganglionic segment is then brought down through the rectal muscular cuff.

Social Adjustment Scale—assessment inventory used to evaluate patients with traumatic brain injury. Evaluates function in categories of work, social and leisure, extended family, marital, parental, and family unit roles.

SODAS (spheroidal oral drug absorption system)—trademark system that controls release and absorption rate of a drug.

SOD (sphincter of Oddi) **dysfunction**.

Soehendra dilator—used to dilate the cystic duct.

Soehendra stent retriever—for use in removing biliary stents.

Soemmering area or **ring**—an oval yellowish spot located exactly in the center of the posterior part of the retina.

Sofamor spinal instrumentation device—allows 3-D correction of the spine to treat spinal deformity, trauma, or degenerative disease.

SOFA score—see *sepsis-related organ failure assessment score*.

Sof-Gel palm shield—a soft splint with a self-contained gel that prevents skin breakdown associated with neuromuscular and skeletal tightness of the hands.

SofPulse—a device that uses pulsed magnetic energy to treat pain and edema in soft tissue injuries and to accelerate and improve revascularization following injury or grafting.

Sofsorb absorptive dressing.

Sof-Tact glucose monitor—automated "alternate-site" glucose monitoring system, which allows a blood sample to be taken from much less sensitive areas of the body (as opposed to fingers) for blood sugar testing.

SoftCloth absorptive dressing.

SoftForm facial implant—constructed of ePTFE (expanded polytetrafluoroethylene) and similar to Gore-Tex but shaped in tubes rather than solid strips.

Softgut—a surgical chromic suture.

SoftLight—laser hair removal system, combining a low-energy laser with

SoftLight *(cont.)* carbon-based activating lotion to prevent hair growth without affecting the surrounding tissue.

Soft N Dry Merocel sponge—a fiber-free material that is used in wound dressings to keep the patient dry.

soft neurological signs—nonlocalizable (focal) signs. Cf. *localizing or focal neurological signs*.

soft-passed—medical jargon for pass without encountering resistance. Usage in neurosurgery: "A ventricular catheter was then passed into the right occipital horn, and subsequently it soft-passed a total of 12.5 cm."

Softscan—laser scanner used in superficial skin resurfacing.

SoftScan laser mammography system—radiation-free system that can be used without painful breast compression. This technology is particularly useful in younger women, whose breast tissue is more dense and therefore more difficult to assess radiographically.

Soft Shield collagen corneal shield—used for lubrication and protection.

soft tissue rim sign (Radiol)—see *rim sign*.

soft tissue shaving cannula (liposhaver)—an alternative to conventional liposuction.

soft tissue window—CT setting for best visualization of nonosseous anatomy. See *bone window, brain window, pulmonary parenchymal window,* and *subdural window*.

Soft Torque uterine catheter—radiopaque tip for fluoroscopic visualization for accurate placement of the catheter and injection of contrast, dye, or washed sperm.

Soft Touch cup (Ob-Gyn)—a disposable, truncated cone-shaped plastic cup constructed of semirigid polyethylene, used for vacuum-assisted deliveries.

Soft-Vu Omni flush catheter—for improved abdominal aortography and studies of iliac arteries and arteries of lower extremities.

Sof-Wick dressings; drain sponges.

SolarGen 2100s—an advanced laser console for performing transmyocardial revascularization and percutaneous myocardial channeling procedures.

solar keratosis—horny skin growth in some individuals, caused by overexposure to sunlight.

Solcotrans closed vacuum-drainage system—for postoperative use following total hip replacement.

Solcotrans drainage/reinfusion system—used as a blood-saving system, especially in spinal fusion procedures.

SoLight—device that attaches to forceps to illuminate the surgical area.

Solitaire needle—slightly curved needle used for closure following small-incision cataract surgery.

Solo catheter with Pro/Pel coating (Cardio).

SoloPass—a combination stent and catheter used in endoscopic bile duct procedures.

SoloSite—a nonsterile hydrogel that provides moist wound healing.

SoloSite wound gel—clear wound gel that is noncytotoxic and appropriate for use with chronic wounds.

soluble CD4—a drug used to treat AIDS.

Soluset—a volume control device for administering intravenous solutions.

solution—see *medication*.

Solvang graft—a tip graft to the nose.

SomaSensor—a rectangular plastic pad placed across the patient's forehead. This sensor uses an infrared light source directed through the patient's scalp, skull, and brain to continuously measure cerebral oxygen content. The sensor is attached to the Somanetics INVOS cerebral oximeter, which provides a computerized output of the O_2 saturation in both numerical and graphic form. This device is used during anesthesia and in the critical care unit. It has an advantage over pulse oximetry in that it provides accurate readings during periods of hypotension and even cardiac arrest.

somatic cell—all cells of a developing or mature organism except germline cells.

somatic cell genetics—the study of the genetics of somatic cells cultured in vitro.

somatic cell nuclear transfer (SCNT) —transplantation of the diploid nucleus of a somatic cell into an unfertilized oocyte from which the haploid nucleus has been removed. The resulting chimera has the genetic makeup of the donor cell but the developmental potential of a primitive germ cell. Cell division of the chimera yields a clone of totipotent stem cells that are genetically identical with the donor of the nucleus.

somatic genetic transfer (also called somatic genetic modification)—a process in which desired genes are introduced into the somatic cells of the body by means of a viral vector.

somatic mutation—any mutation occurring in a somatic cell rather than in the germline.

somatic stem cell—see *adult stem cell.*

somato-emotional release (SER)—use of therapeutic visualization and dialogue techniques to treat posttraumatic stress disorder. Often used in conjunction with CST (craniosacral therapy).

somatomedin levels—drawn for growth hormone testing.

Somatom Plus-S CT Scanner.

SOMATOM Volume Zoom—computed tomography system that aids physicians in monitoring progression of coronary artery disease and evaluating graft patency following bypass surgery.

somatosensory evoked potential (SEP).

somatosensory evoked response (SER).

Somavert (pegvisomant)—injectable drug that treats acromegaly by blocking the effects of excessive growth hormone production by a pituitary tumor.

Somersize diet—actress Suzanne Somers' eating regimen, which allows all food groups but forbids combining carbohydrates and fats/proteins at the same meal. No sugar, processed foods, or white flour allowed.

Somer uterine elevator.

Somjee-Crabtree temporal bone support clamp—for holding temporal bones during dissection. It is structurally very different, more practical, and effective for securing the bone than the temporal bone-holding bowl which has been in use.

Somnoplasty system—minimally invasive radiofrequency-based devices used for ablation of excess tissue in the upper airway in order to reduce or eliminate habitual snoring.

Somogyi effect—a swing to a high level of glucose in the blood from extremely low level.

Somogyi units—results of serum amylase testing expressed in Somogyi units.

"somophagia"—see *psomophagia*.

Sonablate 200 system—for the treatment of benign prostatic hyperplasia utilizing high-intensity focused ultrasound technology.

"sonameter"—see *centimeter.*

Sonde enteroscope—used in intraoperative enteroscopy in localizing small-intestinal bleeding sites, providing complete visualization of the small-bowel mucosa without enterotomy, while avoiding the trauma that can be caused by push endoscopy.

Sondergaard cleft—the interatrial groove.

S-100 antibody test—a test for melanomas and other tumors.

Sones catheter.

Sones selective coronary arteriography.

Songbird disposable hearing aid—delivers 40 days of life when used 12 hours per day, at a cost of $39 plus professional fees; a major advantage for those who cannot afford the cost of traditional hearing aids.

sonic-accelerated fracture healing system (SAFHS).

sonicator (Cardio)—a device that uses sound waves to create a disruption. Usage: "A sonicator was used to produce microbubbles in the contrast medium that was injected into both coronary arteries."

Sonic hedgehog (Shh)—protein that is active in promoting the survival of specific neurons from the midbrain, striatum, and spinal cord in vitro. It has implications for treatment of certain neurologic diseases.

Sonksen-Silver visual acuity cards—to test visual acuity in children ages 3 and up or those with communication problems.

SonoCT (real-time spatial compound imaging)—an ultrasound technique using electronic beam steering of a transducer array to rapidly acquire 3-9 overlapping scans of an object from different view angles. It compiles up to 9 times the information of conventional ultrasound. It offers multiple lines of sight and has the ability to visualize pathologies such as breast lesions. Also, *HDI 5000 SonoCT*.

Sonocur Basic system—extracorporeal shock wave therapy system for treating tennis elbow.

sonographically guided human thrombin injection—a procedure to treat false aneurysms. Thrombin is injected into the hematoma under ultrasound guidance.

SonoHeart—handheld digital echocardiography system that provides two-dimensional and PowerMap directional color Doppler images on demand. Allows trained clinicians to instantly assess and document left ventricular function, chamber size, source of murmurs, wall thickness, valve regurgitation, and cardiomyopathies.

sonohysterography—a technique in which the uterus and endometrial cavity are examined by vaginal ultrasound after instillation of fluid into the uterine cavity. Can be performed in the office without need for anesthesia.

SONOLINE Sierra—ultrasound imaging system.

Sonolith Praktis—portable lithotriptor used to treat stones in the kidney and ureters.

sonolucent—offering relatively little resistance to ultrasound waves (as air or fluid) and hence generating few or no echoes. Cf. *radiolucent; translucent.*

Sonoprobe SP-501 system for endoscopic procedures.

sonopuncture—stimulation of acupuncture points with sound waves.

SonoSite 180 portable ultrasound—hand-carried ultrasound system designed to augment routine bimanual pelvic exams, assess pelvic pain or abnormal bleeding, and aid in basic fetal assessment, using either transabdominal or intravaginal imaging, all at point of care.

Sonotron—a pulsed radiofrequency therapeutic device used in treating carpal tunnel syndrome and other repetitive stress conditions.

Soothe-N-Seal—a cyanoacrylate adhesive product for the treatment of canker sores. It provides immediate pain relief with a protective barrier against irritation from ingestion of food and liquids.

Soothies—glycerin gel pads used by nursing mothers to relieve nipple pain and promote natural healing of sore nipples.

Sophy programmable pressure valve—used in neurosurgery in the management of hydrocephalus.

Soprano—a cryoablation system.

SorbaView—composite wound dressing.

Sorbie Questor elbow system—for reconstruction of the elbow joint damaged by rheumatoid, degenerative, or post-traumatic joint diseases.

Sorbsan topical wound dressing—used to treat decubitus ulcers.

"sore-a-len"—see *psoralen.*

SOT (Sensory Organization Test).

souffle ("soo´flay")—a soft blowing sound heard on auscultation.

Soundtec hearing aid—a partially implanted hearing aid. A neodymium-iron-boron magnet is implanted at the incudostapedial joint and driven by a magnetic coil placed within an ear canal mold.

Souter-Strathclyde elbow prosthesis—used in arthroplasty.

southern access—posterior access in operative therapy of fracture dislocation of the hip, appropriate for certain fractures, depending on where the fracture line is.

Southwick osteotomy.

SPA (sperm penetration assay).

Spacekeeper retractor—used in saphenous vein harvesting procedures.

Spacemaker balloon dissector—used in subfascial endoscopic perforator surgery (SEPS). It is a nondistensible balloon filled with saline used to create large laparoscopic working space within the extraperitoneal pelvic region, eliminating risks associated with entry into and closure of the peritoneum.

Space-OR flexible internal retractor—used for retraction of organs and tissues in abdominal surgery.

Space-Saver volumetric pump—infusion pump for delivery of total parenteral nutrition.

sparrow-picking technique—an acupuncture technique where an herb is placed on the tip of the acupuncture needle or used in a stick form and passed over a tender joint. See *moxa* and *moxibustion*.

SpaTouch PhotoEpilation system—laser/light hair removal device.

spatulated half-circle needle (Oph).

SPE (streptococcal pyrogenic exotoxin).

specialized tissue aspirating resectoscope (STAR). See *OPERA STAR*.

SPECT (single photon emission computed tomography)—a cardiac imaging technique using thallium and a single gamma camera or scintillation camera which moves in a series of positions around the chest of the patient, receiving radionuclide signals from many angles. This provides a three-dimensional image and helps to localize regions of poorly perfused myocardium by eliminating image overlap. Also useful in neurologic diagnosis, especially in assessing stroke prognosis.

spectacular shrinking deficit syndrome (Neuro)—profound hemispheric ischemia that resolves rapidly over hours to days, usually leaving patients with minimal residual effects.

SPECT/MRI—imaging system that is helpful in diagnosing patients with fibromyalgia syndrome, chronic fatigue syndrome, and major depressive disorder.

spectral Doppler (Radiol).

Spectranetics laser sheath (SLS)—an excimer laser device to assist in removal of larger-sized pacemaker and implantable cardioverter-defibrillator leads.

Spectraprobe-Max probe (Cardio).

spectrofluorometry—an investigational method to detect and identify bacteria using fluorescence spectroscopy. Expected to provide rapid identification of bacteria without the need for culturing with antigens. Compared with the nonresonance Raman spectroscopy, it is a very sensitive technique. This process is expected to have great impact on the diagnosis and treatment of otitis media, where the often empiric choice of an antibiotic to which the bacteria is resistant can mean prolonged disease and increased morbidity. The only method currently available for accurate identification of bacteria is tympanocentesis, which requires the insertion of a needle through the tympanic membrane and is mildly painful. Tympanocentesis may not be readily available in the primary care office, but spectrofluorometry can be used in a physician's office and is noninvasive.

Spectrum tissue repair system—used for arthroscopic or open suturing of knee and shoulder soft tissue.

SpectRx (capital R)—test to measure LDL and HDL cholesterol levels. This will likely replace fingerstick and blood drawing. It works by shining a low-power red light beam into the eye. The light beam "scatters" the LDL and HDL particles in the aqueous, and, by a technique called photon correlation spectroscopy, it is possible to count these particles.

Speculite—a tiny bar light attached to a speculum and used in speculoscopy as an adjunct to a Pap smear.

speculoscopy—a visual cervical screening exam used as an adjunct to a traditional Pap smear. The procedure combines 4-6 times magnification, an acetic acid wash of the cervical area, and a small disposable blue-white light source called Speculite. This aids in exposing potentially abnormal cervical areas. Studies have shown that Pap smear alone detected 31% of early precancerous changes, but Pap and speculoscopy together found 83%.

speech mapping of the brain.

speech reception threshold (SRT).

Speedicath intermittent catheter—prepacked in sterile saline solution and in an easy-to-open foil container. It is especially easy to use by individuals with limited dexterity.

Speed test (J. Spencer Speed)—used to assess biceps tendon for inflammation, SLAP lesion, and avulsion. Resistance is applied to the arm with the shoulder at 90° of forward elevation and forearm in full supination. The test is positive when pain in the shoulder is experienced.

Speedy balloon catheter—used in percutaneous transluminal coronary angioplasty.

Spence, tail of—also called *tail of the breast*. It is the tail-like segment of mammary gland tissue that extends to the axillary region.

SPEP ("ess-pep") (serum protein electrophoresis).

sperm—a male gamete; this abridged term is now preferred to spermatozoon; plural sperm or sperms.

sperm aspiration—technique for obtaining sperm directly from the testicle of a man who has no sperm in his ejaculate.

Sperma-Tex preshaped mesh—knitted polypropylene monofilament mesh used for the repair of inguinal hernia defects.

SpermCheck test—to check for sperm antibodies.

SP-501 Sonoprobe endoscopy system.

SpF Spinal Fusion Stimulator (trademark)—an adjunct to spinal fusion to increase probability of fusion success and to increase the rate of healing after spinal fusion. Implanted cathodes produce a direct current which initiates an electrochemical reaction and stimulates osteogenesis. This process is called *osteoinduction* by the manufacturers.

SPGR (spoiled gradient-recalled) (echo sequences)—MRI term.

sphincter of Oddi dysfunction (SOD).

sphincterotome, Wilson-Cook (modified) **wire-guided**.

sphincter-saving procedure—used in resection of rectal cancer. Sphincter preservation is the goal of preoperative irradiation of locally advanced rectal cancer in combination with chemotherapy.

Sphrintzen syndrome—velocardiofacial syndrome, caused by a deletion on chromosome 22.

Sphygmocorder—consists of a mercury sphygmomanometer, an occluding cuff, an inflation source, a stethoscope, a microphone capable of detecting Korotkoff sounds, a camcorder, and a display screen, used for recording blood pressure without the intervention of a human observer.

SPI-Argent II—peritoneal dialysis catheter designed to exit site infections.

spica bandage.

spica cast.

spicules of periosteal new bone, **irregular perpendicular**.

SPIDER (steady-state projection imaging with dynamic echo-train readout).

Spiessel lag screws, position screws, internal screw fixation—used in sagittal split ramus osteotomy.

spiking fever—a fever characterized by recurrent, sudden brief elevations that look like a row of spikes on a temperature graph.

spill—excrete inappropriately in urine, as glucose or protein.

spinal cord injury without radiographic abnormality (SCIWORA) **syndrome**.

spinal cord stimulation—see *dorsal column stimulator*.

spinal epidural hematoma—diagnosed on MRI and treated with surgical decompression and treatment of the underlying disorder.

spinal Galant reflex—alternative name for Galant reflex, in which the stroking of a baby's back from the neck to the paravertebral area, with baby in the prone position, causes the back to curve toward the side that is stroked. It is present at birth and normally disappears by 3-6 months of age.

spinal myeloscopy—fiberoptic endoscopic examination of the epidural space for examination and treatment of pain due to inflamed lower back nerves and/or pain after lower back surgery. By applying fluid under pressure, along with manipulation of the myeloscope, nerves can be released from scar tissue, and local anesthetic and steroid can be injected directly onto damaged nerve roots to reduce inflammation and speed the healing process.

SpinaLogic 1000—a bone growth stimulator used for nonoperative treatment for failed spinal fusion surgery, nine months post-surgery. It is a noninvasive, portable, battery-operated, low-energy magnetic field bone growth stimulator.

spin density; **spin echo**—MRI terms.

spindle—a system of microtubules within a cell that direct the organization of chromosomes during mitosis.

SpineAssist—a miniature robot that offers surgeons improved accuracy during complicated back surgery while minimizing risks associated with spinal surgical procedures. The size of a soda can, SpineAssist is attached directly to the patient's body, pointing surgeons to the exact positioning needed for tools and implants.

SpineCATH—for use in intradiscal electrothermal therapy.

spin-echo image (SE)—an MRI image obtained by the spin-echo technique. With this technique, T2 is determined indirectly, as a function of TE (echo time).

SpineWand—see *Perc-DLE SpineWand.*

spin-lattice relaxation time—MRI term.

spinopelvic transiliac fixation (STIF) **technique**—for lumbosacral fusion. It facilitates compression across the sacroiliac joints, which promotes sacroiliac joint fusion and can provide a stable base for curvature correction and lumbosacral fusion.

spin-warp imaging—MRI term.

SPIR (selective partial inversion-recovery)—prepared T2-weighted fast spin-echo acquisition on MR imaging; fat suppression images.

spiral band of Gosset—the second palmar layer in the hand. Sometimes referred to in dictation of operative procedures for Dupuytren contracture.

spiral CT—reportedly shows better resolution of tumors and anatomic structures than conventional angiograms. Also called *helical CT*.

spiral vein grafts—used for vascular conduits in irradiated and contaminated tissue beds. A greater saphenous vein is harvested, split longitudinally, and wrapped in a spiral around a chest tube and then stitched to form a tube itself.

spiral XCT (x-ray computed tomography) **scanner**.

spiral x-ray computed tomography (SXCT).

SpiraStent—a ureteral stent designed to facilitate urine flow and relieve obstruction of the ureter.

Spira-Valve—an implantable device for chronic obstructive pulmonary disease.

SpiroFlo—bioabsorbable prostate stent for treatment of temporary urethral obstruction.

spirometer—see *incentive spirometer.*

spirometric gating (or guidance)—in helical CT technology.

Spirulina Pacifica—a nutritional supplement made from microalgae.

Spitz-Holter valve—an old type of valve for ventriculoatrial shunting in hydrocephalus.

Spivack valve—a technique used in performing a Depage-Janeway gastrostomy.

S-PK (synthetic penetrating keratoplasty).

SPLATT (split anterior tibial tendon transfer)—a surgical technique used to correct equinovarus deformity due to cerebral palsy or brain injury. The anterior tibial tendon is split and the lateral part is transferred through the cuboid and then sutured on itself, with the foot in an everted and dorsiflexed position.

splenic perfusion measurement by dynamic CT scan—used in evaluation of portal hypertension.

spline—see *Calcitek spline*.

splint
- Accuform nasal
- acrylic wafer TMJ (temporomandibular joint)
- air (also inflatable)
- AirFlex carpal tunnel

splint *(cont.)*
- AirFlex Plus
- birdcage
- Breathe-Easy nasal
- Brooke Army Hospital
- buddy
- Budin toe
- Bunnell active hand and finger
- Bunnell finger extension
- Bunnell knuckle-bender with outrigger
- Carpal Lock cock-up
- Cool Comfort D-ring thumb and wrist
- Delbet
- Denis Browne clubfoot
- Denver nasal
- DonJoy knee
- Doyle Shark nasal
- eZY WRAP
- Firm D-Ring wrist support (Rolyan)
- Flexisplint
- Friedman Splint brace
- HIPciser abduction
- HVO (hallux valgus orthosis)
- Hydro-Splint II
- inflatable
- Joint-Jack finger
- Kennedy sinus
- Liberty One
- Link Stack Split
- MindSet toe
- outrigger
- plaster
- polyvinyl-alcohol
- Radstat wrist
- replant
- Rolyan Gel Shell
- Sam
- Saturn
- shin
- Slattery-McGrouther dynamic flexion
- Sof-Gel palm shield

splint *(cont.)*
Stader
sugar-tong plaster
synergistic wrist motion
talipes hobble
Thomas
Thumz'Up functional thumb
turnbuckle functional position
Versi-Splint

splinter hemorrhage—a short linear hemorrhage under a fingernail or toenail, longitudinally oriented and looking somewhat like a splinter; often due to trauma but sometimes a sign of infective endocarditis.

splinting—stiffening of muscles to avoid pain in a part or extremity. Usage: "She is splinting rather markedly, and on this basis appears to be short of breath." "This may be associated with a certain amount of splinting and a reluctance to take deep inspirations."

splinting therapy—used not only to facilitate activities of daily living, such as maintaining function in the hand or elbow, but also to correct orthopedic problems and assist in postoperative rehabilitation after replant, flexor tendon, and rheumatoid arthritis reconstruction surgery.

Splintrex—instrument used for rapid removal of wood or metal splinters; consists of forceps and a loupe.

split-flap technique—in vaginal surgery.

split-liver transplantation (SLT)—division of donor liver for transplantation into two recipients.

split renal function (SRF)—a finding on MR urography.

split sheath catheter.

split spinal cord malformation (SSCM)—identified in infants by a screening MR imaging study, with type I or II defined by CT myelography. It should be surgically treated when diagnosed.

SP (stump pressure) **measurement**.

spondy—slang for *spondylolisthesis* by radiologists.

spondylodiskitis—inflammation of the vertebra and disk, the etiology of which is not well understood but believed to be an expression of the inflammatory disease encountered in ankylosing spondylitis.

spondylophyte impaction set—used for correction of bony impingements of neural structures.

sponge
Helistat absorbable collagen
hemostatic
K-sponge
Lapwall laparotomy
Merocel
peanut
pledgets
Protectaid
Ray-Tec x-ray detectable surgical
Sof-Wick
Taka microneurosurgical
Vistec x-ray detectable
Weck-cel

sponge and needle counts—a phrase used in operative reports to indicate that no foreign material or object has been inadvertently left inside the patient in the surgery. It is standard practice for sponges, needles, and certain other articles to be counted before the beginning of surgery and again just before the surgeon begins to close the wound. Usually two persons perform the counts together for greater security. The surgeon does not begin closure of the wound until the sponge and needle counts are reported correct.

sponge dissector (dissecting sponge)—used in surgery. Also called *peanut* or *cherry*. Cf. *spud dissector*.

spontaneous bacterial peritonitis (SBP).

spontaneous coronary artery dissection (SCAD).

spontaneous nipple discharge (SND), **nonbloody**—an indication of breast cancer and the need for surgical intervention. Breast cancer can present as unilateral nonbloody SND, indicating the importance of surgical intervention. Papilloma is more common in women with SND than without and most often presents as bloody SND.

spontaneous otoacoustic emission (SOAE)—used in studies of comparative hearing.

spoon forceps.

sporadic (nonfamilial) **clear cell carcinoma**—the most common type of kidney cancer. The gene responsible is the same as the cause of the inherited cancer syndrome called von Hippel-Lindau (VHL) disease.

Sporicidin—a glutaraldehyde-phenate cold sterilizing solution for disinfecting surgical instruments, endoscopes, respiratory therapy equipment.

SportsFit thumb orthosis—low-profile orthosis used to protect a thumb joint from sudden forceful motions that could cause injury.

SportsRAC—a PC-based shoulder training and injury rehabilitation system that enables the patient to perform a series of exercises designed to assess and train neuromuscular control.

SPOT—a prepackaged sterile FDA-approved formulation of pure carbon particles in suspension, used for tattooing of colonic neoplasms.

spotting—scanty vaginal bleeding, menstrual or otherwise.

spot urine—a random urine collection, not the first urine of the morning. Usage: "Spot urine for albumin-to-creatinine ratio . . ."

SPPS (single photon planar scintigraphy).

SprayGel absorbable adhesion barrier system—an adhesion barrier that can be delivered laparoscopically or via laparotomy to form a strongly adherent hydrogel film to prevent adhesions in gynecological surgery.

SprayGel adhesion barrier system—reduces or eliminates adhesions following gynecological surgery.

spray-on skin—see CellSpray.

spreader graft—insertion of a piece of cartilage, as between the anterior margin of the nasal septum and the upper lateral cartilage, to reestablish appropriate width (in this case, of the middle third of the nose). May also be called *batten graft*.

spring fixation—the use of springs after lumbosacral fusion to hold graft material in place.

spring-loaded silo—used in staged closing of gastroschisis deformity.

Sprint catheter with Pro/Pel coating (Cardio).

S protein—see *protein S*.

sprung pelvis—traumatic dislocation of the pubic symphysis.

SPTL-1b vascular lesion laser—used for selective photothermolysis of port wine stains, hemangiomas, facial spider veins, scars, angiomas, warts, stretch marks, rosacea, and other vascular abnormalities.

SPTTL (superficial posterior talotibial ligament).

spud dissector—used in surgery.

spun urine sediment—urine specimen centrifuged to concentrate sediment (cells, casts, crystals, and other formed elements) before microscopic examination. Usage: "Spun urine sediment demonstrated 15-20 white cells."

Spurling sign or **test**—for nerve root compression. To conduct this test, the examiner approaches the seated patient from above and, with both hands, presses down on the patient's head, with added pressure on the spinal nerve roots. Pain indicates impingement on the nerve root by a herniated disk.

spurring (Radiol)—formation of one or more jagged osteophytes, as in osteoarthritis.

Spyglass angiography catheter.

SpyroDerm—a water-absorbent wound and burn dressing.

SQS-20 subcuticular skin stapler—uses absorbable staples that result in less scarring. Places staples just below the epidermis for better cosmetic result.

squamous cell carcinoma (SCC).

squamous intraepithelial lesion (SIL)—squamous intraepithelial lesions on Pap smear, reported as low grade or high grade.

square knot—an easy and reliable knot used for tying most suture materials, including surgical gut, collagen, silk, cotton, and stainless steel sutures. May also be indicated in Ethilon (nylon), Ethibond (polyester), and Prolene (polypropylene) sutures.

squeeze test—to diagnose sprain of the syndesmotic ligaments of the ankle.

Squirt wound irrigation system—for large-volume irrigation of a wound site.

Srb ("serb") **syndrome**—costosternal malformation present from birth; named for Srb J. Ueber (no vowel in *Srb*).

SRF (split renal function)—a finding on MR urography.

SRMD (stress-related mucosal disease).

SROM (segmental range of motion).

SROM ("shrom") (spontaneous rupture of membranes).

S-ROM femoral stem prosthesis.

SRP—see *surgical reversal of presbyopia.*

SRS (stereotactic radiosurgery).

SRT (speech reception threshold).

SRT (smoke removal tube) **vaginal speculum**—used in laser surgery.

SSBE (short-segment Barrett esophagus).

SSC (single-stripe colitis).

SSCM (split spinal cord malformation).

SSD (shaded surface display)—MRI term.

SSD (Social Security Disability).

SSEP (somatosensory evoked potential). See also *SEP,* which is synonymous.

S7 coronary stent—for use in percutaneous transluminal coronary angioplasty (PTCA).

SSFP (steady state free precession)—MRI term.

SSFSE (single shot fast spin echo)—MRI term.

S660 small vessel stent—coronary stent system specifically developed for stenting of vessels that are 2.2 to 2.9 mm in diameter.

S670 coronary stent—over-the-wire stent for maintaining patency of coronary vessels after angioplasty procedures.

SSI (Social Security Income).

SSKI (saturated solution of potassium iodide).

S-sleep (synchronized sleep).

SSM (segmental misty mesentery).

SSP (stereotaxic surface projection).

SSR (sweat secretion rate).

SSRO (sagittal split ramus osteotomy).

SST (stainless steel rod).

S-Stent—a new-generation smaller stainless steel corrugated ring stent with a proprietary Quadrature Link system allowing for easier maneuvering in smaller, more tortuous vessels.

S.S.T. small bone locking nail—used as an intramedullary nailing device for the forearm or fibula.

STAAR implantable contact lens (ICL)—a permanently implanted contact lens that is inserted through a microincision in the eye and placed behind the iris and in front of the patient's natural lens to correct mild to severe myopia and hyperopia.

STAAR Toric—implantable contact lens.

Stability total hip system—made of titanium Porocoat in one piece to reduce fretting.

Stableyes capsular tension ring—intraocular lens.

Stableloc—external wrist fixation system.

stabs—another name for band cells in the differential count.

Staccato—a pharmaceutical delivery device for administering drugs and diagnostic agents via inhalation.

stacked scans—in computed tomography, a series of scans without intervals of unexamined tissue between them. Same as *contiguous images*.

Stacker 2—an OTC diet supplement.

Stacker 3 with Chitosan—an OTC diet supplement and metabolism booster.

Stader splint—a metal bar with pins at right angles to the bar; the pins are driven into the fragments of the fractured bone, and the bar holds the pieces in alignment.

STAE (subsegmental transcatheter arterial embolization).

staged abdominal repairs (STARs)—closure of serious abdominal wounds in stages, perhaps with the use of devices such as the STAR system.

stages of labor—first stage, dilatation of the cervix until it is fully dilated and flush with the vagina; second stage, expulsion of infant; third stage, expulsion of placenta and membranes and contraction of the uterus.

staging—see *classification*.

stagnation—a term used in the report of a thrombin injection for pseudoaneurysm: "The neck of the pseudoaneurysm was occluded during the injection to promote stagnation and prevent thrombin leakage."

Stahl classification of Kienböck disease—see *modified Stahl classification*.

Stahl ("stall") **ophthalmic calipers**—used in measuring orbital implants.

stain—see *tests*.

Stalevo—a medication for the treatment of idiopathic Parkinson disease.

stalk-section effect (Neuro).

STA-MCA (superficial temporal artery–middle cerebral artery) **bypass procedure**.

Stamey needle—a single-prong ligature carrier used in the Stamey bladder suspension procedure.

Stamey-Malecot catheter (Urol).

Stamey test—used in evaluating patients thought to have renovascular hypertension. The prognosis after corrective surgery is better in patients with a positive Stamey test. In the

Stamey *(cont.)*
test a differential ureteral catheterization is done in which urinary flow rate and creatinine or PAH (para-aminohippuric acid) concentrations are measured from each kidney on diuresis. Patients with renal hypertension caused by obstruction of the renal artery will have a significantly decreased flow rate and a significantly increased creatinine or PAH concentration on the same side, as compared with the normal kidney on the other side.

Stamm gastrostomy.

Stammberger antrum punch (ENT).

Stammberger circular punch.

stamp graft, transplanted—a technique that makes endoscopic mucosal grafting possible and offers a potential breakthrough in the management of laryngotracheal stenosis.

standard deviations from the mean, as in "DEXA scores are *x* "standard deviations from the mean." The standard deviation is a mathematical expression, used by statisticians, for the extent to which a given value varies from the average or expected value. When a measurement (such as bone densitometry) yields a particularly abstract result, it is often more meaningful to express the patient's reading in standard deviations from the average, or normal, than in raw numbers.

Stanford Dependency Index (SDI)—derived from the Fagerstrom Tolerance Questionnaire and classifies addiction on the basis of five questions: how soon after waking the patient has a first cigarette; does patient smoke when ill in bed; does patient smoke more in the morning than the rest of the day; does patient have difficulty refraining in places where smoking is prohibited; how deeply does the patient inhale.

Stanford Sleepiness Scale—for evaluating effects of obstructive sleep apnea.

Stanmore shoulder arthroplasty.

stapedectomy—see *laser stapedectomy.*

Staphylococcus aureus **bacteremia** (SAB).

Staphylococcus aureus **Immune Globulin Intravenous (Human)** (SA-IGIV)—purified immune globulin G (IgG) derived from pooled adult human plasma used to treat *S. aureus* infections. See *Altastaph*.

Staphylococcus aureus **septicemia**—seen in AIDS patients.

Staphylococcus epidermidis—skin flora (formerly *Staph. albus*).

stapled hemorrhoidopexy—a surgical procedure for prolapse and hemorrhoids, believed to be less painful and have fewer adverse events than traditional hemorrhoidectomy.

stapled lung reduction—procedure for treatment of diffuse emphysema.

stapler
- Auto Suture Multifire Endo GIA 30
- Auto Suture Premium CEEA
- EEA
- Endo-GIA suture
- Endo-Hernia
- Endopath EMS hernia
- ILA
- Multifire Endo GIA
- Multifire GIA
- Poly GIA
- Premium CEEA circular
- Proximate flexible linear
- Proximate linear cutter
- Roticulator
- SQS-20 subcuticular skin
- Surgeons Choice
- TL-90 (Ethicon)

STAR (specialized tissue aspirating resectoscope)—used in endometrial resection/ablation procedures. See *OPERA STAR*.

STARs (staged abdominal repairs).

STAR (suture tension adjustment reel) **system**—originally developed for delayed closure of calf wounds but now used for staged closure of abdominal wounds.

stare, thyroid—see *Collier sign*.

star figure—a star-shaped folding or pleating of the retina due to edema.

Starfish NS (nonsternotomy) **heart positioner**.

Stargardt dystrophy—prolongation in dark adaptation, possibly a result of vitamin A deficiency.

STARR (stapled transanal rectal resection).

STARRT (selective tubal assessment to refine reproductive therapy) **falloposcopy system**—used for diagnosis of proximal tubal occlusion.

starry-sky pattern—as dictated in pathology reports. Usage: "There was a starry-sky pattern with phagocytosis of tumor cells."

START SMART Program—for patients about to begin assisted reproductive technology techniques. It emphasizes the A, R, and T of Assisted Reproductive Technology: **A**sking questions of doctors and nurses, **R**eading and **R**esearching the course of treatment prescribed, and **T**alking to doctors and nurses throughout the treatment process.

stat or **STAT** (L., *statim*)—immediately. Often used in a request for an emergency lab report or x-ray, or a rush report from Transcription, in which case it means "I need it yesterday." Dictionaries show a period after *stat* because it is an abbreviation, but most medical personnel do not treat *stat* like an abbreviation and do not place a period after it. Often it appears in all caps.

Statak—soft tissue attachment device for use as alternative to conventional transosseous techniques.

State-Trait Anxiety Inventory—consists of two subscales to measure anxiety state (subjective feelings of tension, nervousness, and worry) and trait anxiety (relatively stable individual differences in disposition to anxiety).

Statham electromagnetic flow meter—flow measurements in blood vessels.

statin drugs—a class of cholesterol-lowering drugs that have also been found to protect against stroke and death from cardiovascular disease. Statin drugs are also called *reductase inhibitors* (e.g., simvastatin).

STATLase-SDL diode laser—for use in endoscopic surgery.

StatLock hemodialysis catheter—fastening device that replaces suture for securement of central venous catheters used in renal dialysis.

StatLock Universal Plus—used for suture-free anchoring of percutaneous drainage catheters.

Stat 2 Pumpette—disposable I.V. pump that maintains flow rate under changing conditions.

status post—the condition or fact of having sustained an injury or illness or having undergone a surgical procedure, as in *status post appendectomy*.

Stayoden 9000F TENS—see *TENS*.

stay sutures—see *retention sutures*.

STD (sexually transmitted disease).

steady state free precession (SSFP)—MRI term.

steal, stealing—see *coronary-subclavian steal syndrome; crural steal procedure; lateral crural steal (LCS) for nasal tip reconstruction; subclavian steal syndrome.*

STEAM (stimulated echo acquisition mode) **sequence**—on MR spectroscopy.

Steell—in Graham Steell murmur.

steel-winged butterfly needle.

Steeper Powered Gripper—electric terminal prosthetic device that allows grasping, picking up, and holding a wide variety of objects.

steeple sign—on chest x-ray.

steerable guidewire system—used in invasive radiological vascular procedures.

Steerocath-A ablation catheter.

Steerocath-Dx octapolar and valve mapping catheters.

Steerocath-T ablation catheter.

STE MI (ST-segment elevation in myocardial infarction).

Steffee plates and screws—used in lumbar fusion.

Steinhauser lag screws, position screws, or internal screw fixation—used in sagittal split ramus osteotomy.

Steinmann pin—threaded and nonthreaded.

steinstrasse (Ger., stone street or rocky road)—urinary sand and stone fragments which result from extracorporeal shock wave lithotripsy of kidney stone.

Steis needle—used for bone marrow biopsy and aspiration.

Stela electrode leads—vitreous carbon-tip pacing electrodes.

Stellwag sign—infrequent blinking in patients with Graves disease.

stem cell—an undifferentiated multipotent precursor cell that is capable both of perpetuating itself as a continuing line of stem cells and of undergoing differentiation into one or more specialized types of cells. See *hMSCs* and *HSC*. Examples:

adult stem cell
bone marrow stromal stem cell
hematopoietic stem cell
human embryonic stem cell
mesenchymal (MSC) stem cell
multipotent stem cell
neural stem cell
pluripotent stem cell
somatic stem cell
totipotent stem cell
umbilical cord stem cell
undifferentiated stem cell
unipotent stem cell

stem cell autograft—used to create new skin around cornea scarred by chemical burns or congenital defect of the iris. Damaged skin can lead to rejection of a corneal transplant. Once the stem cells are growing and creating new skin, a routine corneal transplant can be carried out.

stem-cell marrow harvesting—for autologous frozen stem-cell marrow storage. This is done in patients with acute lymphoblastic leukemia while in relative remission, for use in relapse when an HLA-matched compatible donor is not available.

Stemgen—stem cell factor.

STEMI (ST-segment elevation myocardial infarction). Usage: "Treatment was instituted following the new STEMI guidelines."

Stenotrophomonas (formerly ***Xanthomonas***) ***maltophilia***—a cause of urinary tract infection.

Stensen duct.

Stenstrom otoplasty technique—surgical correction of lop ears. A small postauricular incision is made and

Stenstrom *(cont.)*
an otoabrader used to rasp the anterior surface of the antihelix to weaken the cartilage and to recreate the antihelical fold.

stent (see also *tube)*
Acculink self-expanding
ACS OTW HP coronary
ACS RX Multi-Link coronary
Advanta V12
AneuRx
AngioStent cardiovascular
Atkinson tube
balloon-expandable
Bard Memotherm colorectal
Bard XT coronary
Beamer injection
BeStent
BeStent2 laser-cut
BiodivYsio coronary
BioSorb resorbable urology
Bridge Assurant biliary
Bridge extra support over-the-wire renal
Bx Sonic
Bx Velocity coronary
CardioCoil coronary
Contour closed end
Contour stent with HydroPlus coating
Contour VL Percuflex
Cragg Endopro System I
CrossFlex LC coronary
crutched-stick-type biliary duct
Cypher sirolimus-eluting coronary
Dexamet
digestive-respiratory fistula (DRF)
DISA S-Flex coronary
Double J indwelling catheter
Double J ureteral
drug-eluting (DES)
Dua antireflux
Dumon tracheobronchial
Dynalink self-expanding biliary
Elastalloy Ultraflex Strecker nitinol

stent *(cont.)*
Endocare Horizon prostatic
EndoCoil biliary
endoscopic biliary endoprosthesis
EsophaCoil self-expanding esophageal
esophageal Z-Stent with Dua antireflux valve
Excluder bifurcated endoprosthesis
expandable esophageal (EES)
expandable metallic
Fader Tip ureteral
Focustent coronary
GFX coronary
Gianturco expandable (self-expanding) metallic biliary
Gianturco-Rösch Z-stent
Gianturco-Roubin flexible coil
Gianturco-Roubin (GRS)
Guidant Multi-Link Tetra coronary
Harrell Y
Hepamed-coated Wiktor
Hood stoma
Horizon prostatic
HydroPlus
InStent Carotid Coil
IntraCoil nitinol
IntraStent DoubleStrut biliary endoprosthesis
IntraStent DoubleStrut LD
INX stainless steel
IRIS coronary
Jostent coronary stent-graft
KISS (kidney internal splint/stent)
Lubri-Flex
Magic Wallstent
Mardis firm stent with HydroPlus coating
Megalink biliary
Memotherm nitinol
MeroGel nasal dressing and sinus
metallic
MINI Crown
MPD (main pancreatic duct)
Multi-Flex

stent *(cont.)*
Multi-Link Duet coronary
Multi-Link Penta coronary
Multi-Link Tetra coronary
Multi-Link Vision RX and OTW (over-the-wire) coronary
Neuroform microdelivery
NexStent carotid
NIRflex coronary
Niroyal Elite Monorail
NIR Primo Monorail coronary
NIR with SOX coronary
nitinol mesh
Omni–Link .018 and .035 biliary
OmniStent
ostiomeatal
Palmaz balloon-expandable
Palmaz Corinthian biliary
Palmaz-Schatz coronary and biliary
Palmaz-Schatz (PSS)
Paragon coronary
Percuflex Plus ureteral
ProstaCoil
Protege GPS nitinol self-expanding long
radioisotope
RX Herculink 14
RX Herculink Plus
SAXX renal
Schneider Wallstent
self-expanding
Shikani middle meatal antrostomy
6-22 ureteral stent or 6, 22 ureteral
SLK-View
SoloPass
SpiraStent ureteral
SpiroFlo prostate
S7 coronary
S660 small vessel coronary
S670 coronary
SLK-View
S-Stent
Strecker
Stretch VL Flexima
Stryker

stent *(cont.)*
Symbiot
Symphony
tacrolimus-eluting
Talent LPS endoluminal stent-graft
Taxus Express2 paclitaxel-eluting coronary
T–Y
Ultraflex
UroCoil
UroLume urethral
UroLume Wallstent
VascuCoil peripheral vascular
Vistaflex
Wallstent
Wiktor balloon expandable coronary
Wiktor GX
XT radiopaque coronary
Z
Zeta coronary

Stenvers views (Radiol).

step-oblique mammography—involves obtaining additional images at stepped increments in obliquity, usually 15° increments, beginning from the view in which a radiographic density is seen and proceeding toward the view in which the density is not seen.

step-off—a gap between bone fracture fragments.

stepping of vessels—abrupt change in the direction of retinal vessels passing over the brim of an abnormally deep optic cup.

Step trocar—a trademarked product from a line of minimally invasive surgical access devices, including radially expanding dilation technology for surgical access.

stereognosis—relates to the ability to perceive, recognize, and understand the form of objects only by touching and manipulating them; a test of the function of the parietal lobes of the cerebral cortex.

stereognosis tests—Seddon coin, Moberg pick-up, Downey object recognition, Ayres tactile discrimination tests.

StereoGuide—stereotactic needle core biopsy.

stereolithography—for assessment and surgical planning in treating congenital aural atresia. Fabricates a precision model of the temporal bone from CT imaging and 3-D image reconstruction.

StereoPlan—stereotactic surgery planning software used in neurosurgery.

stereotactic aspiration biopsy—used to biopsy nonpalpable nodules of the breast.

stereotactic core needle biopsy (SCNB) —minimally invasive procedure for tissue diagnosis of nonpalpable breast lesions.

stereotactic needle biopsy—a nonsurgical breast biopsy.

stereotactic pallidotomy—performed for treatment of Parkinson disease. The neurosurgeon destroys a portion of the globus pallidus, thereby decreasing a patient's muscle rigidity from Parkinson disease.

stereotactic percutaneous lumbar discectomy (Neuro)—use of stereotactic equipment for precise insertion of the Nucleotome probe and aspiration of the herniated disk.

stereotactic radiosurgery (SRS)—uses a noninvasive (no pins in the scalp) relocatable system for precise localization of a tumor during radiosurgery. See *fractionated stereotaxic radiation therapy; LINAC radiosurgery.*

stereotactic tractotomy—a psychosurgical technique to relieve intractable depression, anxiety, or obsessional states.

stereotactic vacuum-assisted biopsy (SVAB) **device**—used for breast biopsy and other tissue biopsies.

stereotactic vs. stereotaxis—often used interchangeably, although *stereotactic* is preferred. *Stereotaxis* is the general term referring to the field. Etymology: Greek *stereos*, solid or three-dimensional; *taxis*, an arrangement; Latin *tactus*, to touch.

stereotaxically guided interstitial laser therapy—to perform in situ ablation of a tumor. A potential alternative to surgical lumpectomy for treatment of breast cancer.

stereotaxic core needle biopsy (SCNB).

stereotaxic surface projection (SSP).

stereotaxy—the use of the Leksell stereotaxic device, modified for use with the CT scanner, for localizing areas of the brain for implanting radioactive sources, or implanting brain electrodes.

Steri-Drape—a plastic incise drape.

sterilely *(not* sterilly or sterily)—performed in a sterile manner.

sterile talc powder—a powder placed within the chest cavity to decrease the recurrence of malignant pleural effusions in symptomatic patients.

Steri-Oss dental implant device—for use with threaded and cylindrical implants. Also, *Steri-Oss type 2210 endosteal dental implant*.

steroid—adrenocortical steroid.

steroid-eluting electrode—pacemaker electrode that reportedly increases electrical efficiency when delivering impulses in the pacing range, allowing more of each electrical impulse to reach the inner heart wall.

stethodynia—chest pain.

Stevens-Johnson syndrome (SJS)—characterized by a severe adverse drug reaction. The sometimes fatal

Stevens *(cont.)*
condition is characterized by a blistering rash that can lead to detachment of the skin and inflammation of the gastrointestinal and respiratory lining. More than 100 drugs—including antibiotics, NSAIDS, anticonvulsants, and the gout drug allopurinol—are known to cause SJS in rare cases. Researchers have recently directly linked a gene of the immune system to the syndrome.

Stewart-Treves syndrome—lymphangiosarcoma.

St. George Respiratory Questionnaire (SGRO)—a disease-specific instrument that measures symptoms, activity, and impact.

St. George total elbow prosthesis.

St. Hans Rating Scale (SHRS)—for extrapyramidal syndromes.

Stickler syndrome (Oph).

stick tie—in some operating rooms a suture ligature (or transfixion suture), in others a long strand of suture clamped on a hemostat.

Stieda process—the lateral bony process which is an extension of the talus of the ankle.

STIF (spinopelvic transiliac fixation).

Stifcore aspiration needle—used to obtain gastric or bronchial biopsies.

stiff-heart syndrome—see hyperreflectile granular sparkling appearance of the myocardium.

stiff-person syndrome—a progressive neurological disorder characterized by constant painful contractions and spasms of voluntary muscles, particularly the muscles of the back and upper legs, in response to stimuli such as loud noises. Also known as *stiff-man syndrome* and *Moersch-Woltmann syndrome.*

STIF (spinopelvic transiliac fixation) **technique.**

Stilling–Türk–Duane syndrome—see *Duane syndrome.*

Still disease—juvenile rheumatoid arthritis.

Stiman test—a test for meniscal tear. With the patient's foot hanging off the edge of the table and the thigh stabilized on the table, the knee is forcefully internally and externally rotated. Pain is positive for meniscal tear.

Stim Plus—a battery-operated, handheld microcurrent stimulator designed to detect and treat areas of injury. It can also be used to locate and stimulate traditional acupuncture trigger points.

stimulated echo artifact (MRI)—produced by inadequate tuning of fast imaging sequences.

stimulated graciloplasty—see *DePalma staple procedure.*

Stimuplex Dig RC (remote control) **peripheral nerve stimulator**.

STING (subureteric Teflon injection)—used for treatment of vesicoureteral reflux in children.

Stinger ablation catheter—used to create focal "lesions" inside the heart to treat cardiac arrhythmia.

stippled salt-and-pepper nuclei—description of a finding in a biopsy diagnosed as oat cell carcinoma.

STIR (short inversion time inversion-recovery) **sequence**—MRI term.

St. Jude 4F Supreme—fixed-curve electrophysiology catheters.

St. Jude Medical Port-Access—a mechanical heart valve system used to perform a minimally invasive mitral valve repair and replacement using small incisions ("ports") between the ribs instead of opening the thoracic cavity.

St. Jude Pacesetter Atlas DR ICD (implantable cardioverter-defibrillator.

STN (subthalamic nucleus).

stockinette (stockinet)—a knitted, elastic material, used for wrapping over dressings.

stockings or **hose**
- Activskin
- Jobst
- Juzo knee-high compression hosiery
- Sigvaris compression
- T.E.D. (thromboembolic disease) thigh-high antiembolic

Stoller afferent nerve stimulation (SANS).

Stomeasure—part of the Montgomery tracheal cannula system. Allows accurate measurement of the patient's tracheostomy stoma.

stone-age scalpel—for applications where extremely fine cutting action is required, or for studies where trace metals from ordinary scalpel blades cannot be tolerated. They are so fine that they are used in human surgical procedures where objectionable scar tissue might result from the use of a coarser scalpel. The blade is made from obsidian—a type of volcanic glass—which allows a much finer blade than is possible with the conventional steel blade, and much less expensive than a diamond knife.

Stone Cone nitinol stone retrieval device.

StoneRisk profile—diagnostic tests that measure risk factors for the five major classifications of kidney stones. The StoneRisk test analyzes the composition of a kidney stone.

STOO Series Ten Thousand Ocutome—a probe and vitreous cutter.

stooling—defecation. Used generally of infants not yet toilet-trained.

STOP (selective tubal occlusion procedure)—nonsurgical permanent contraception device for women. The implantable device is a small metal coil that is placed through a hysteroscope and deployed into each fallopian tube. The nonsurgical procedure may be performed in the physician's office under local anesthesia (cervical block).

Stoppa operation—preperitoneal prosthetic mesh repair of hernia via laparoscopy.

Stormer balloon catheter—over-the-wire balloon dilatation catheter system for the treatment of coronary artery disease.

Storz Calcutript—see *Karl Storz Calcutript.*

Storz cholangiograsper—a cholangiocatheter grasper.

Storz infant bronchoscope.

Storz radial incision marker—used in cataract surgery.

STR (skeletal targeted radiotherapy).

strabismus—the deviation of one eye from parallelism with the other. Types: A-pattern, concomitant, incomitant, nonconcomitant.

straddling embolus—same as *saddle embolus.*

Straight-In male sling system—minimally invasive surgery that uses a transperineal approach to bolster the urethra by placing a sling below it. The sling is held in place with bone screws attached to the descending rami of the pubic bone. It replicates lost natural support and helps restore voiding function.

Straight-In surgical system—used for performing open or laparoscopic bladder neck fixation procedures to

Straight-In *(cont.)*
treat stress urinary incontinence in women.

straight last shoe—see *last*.

StraightShot arterial cannula—allows surgeon to incise and cannulate the aorta in one easy step.

StraightShot Magnum handpiece—used with a variety of powered plastic surgery instruments in the XPS 2000 Microresector System.

strandy infiltrate (Radiol)—pulmonic infiltrate that appears as strands or streaks of increased density on chest x-ray.

strangury—slow, painful urination, caused by spasm of the urinary bladder and urethra. Usage: "He has no dysuria, but does have some chronic urinary urgency and frequency. There is no strangury."

Strata hip system.

Stratasis TF (tension-free) urethral sling—a minimally invasive tension-free sling specifically designed to treat stress urinary incontinence resulting from urethral hypermobility type 2 and/or intrinsic sphincter deficiency.

Stratasis urethral sling—surgically implanted to provide pubourethral support in the treatment of stress urinary incontinence.

Stratasorb composite wound dressing.

Strategic National Implementation Process (SNIP).

Stratus cardiac troponin I test—provides stat assessment of myocardial damage.

Strecker stent—a tantalum-metal mesh, self-expanding stent that may be used in biliary tract or coronary arteries. It is placed on a balloon catheter and inserted and positioned endoscopically. Covered with a gelatinous layer which dissolves in one to two minutes, the stent then expands and remains expanded due to special memory metal fibers in the stent.

strep throat—streptococcal infection of throat. *(Not* strept throat.)

streptococcal pyrogenic exotoxin (SPE).

streptococcus A infection—not a new infection, but much in the news because of heavy media coverage of a few severe cases of flesh-eating bacteria or necrotizing fasciitis. Group A strep can be spread by foods, surgical instruments, coughs, or handshakes. The infection is virulent in the victim and spreads through the body with astonishing speed, resulting in severe toxic shock syndrome or necrotizing fasciitis. Infection may enter the body via a bruise, chickenpox blister, sore, surgical wound, or other injury. The bacteria multiply rapidly, with the patient exhibiting swollen lymph nodes, rising fever, and excruciating pain at the site of infection. Readily cured with penicillin in its early stages, the infection may be irreversible in as little as four days. In the U.S., the infection affects about 10,000 to 15,000 people each year and leads to 2,000 to 3,000 deaths. In about 5 to 10% of those affected, it leads to necrotizing fasciitis, a gangrenous-type condition in which muscle and fat are broken down by the infection, necessitating surgery and even amputation. Approximately 20 to 30% of those with necrotizing fasciitis die. According to the CDC, the infection affects mostly adults and usually those with other medical or surgical problems. See *flesh-eating*

streptococcus *(cont.)* *bacteria*; *necrotizing fasciitis*; and *toxic shock syndrome.*

Streptococcus milleri—a recently identified microaerophilic gram-positive organism; thought to be a significant pathogen in childhood appendicitis.

Streptococcus mitis—an organism seen in subacute bacterial endocarditis, in the upper respiratory tract, and in the eye. Usage: "Culture of the anterior chamber, vitreous, and the intraocular lens revealed no growth, but culture of the en bloc lens capsule revealed coalescent growth of *Streptococcus mitis* on chocolate agar."

streptogramin—class of bacteriostatics.

streptokinase-streptodornase (SK-SD) —skin test for immune function.

stress cystogram (Radiol)—study of the bladder to demonstrate stress incontinence. Contrast medium is instilled into the bladder and films are taken while the patient coughs and bears down.

stress-injected—sestamibi-gated SPECT with echocardiography.

stress Myoview—noninvasive nuclear imaging technique for patients unable to undergo traditional stress testing.

stress perfusion and rest function—by sestamibi-gated SPECT.

stress perfusion scintigraphy.

stress-related mucosal disease (SRMD)—caused by diminished blood flow to the gastrointestinal tract with a secondary irritant, usually gastric acid, and not related to the presence of *Helicobacter pylori*. Gastrointestinal hypoperfusion may occur in up to 50% of critically ill patients.

stress riser—the concentration of mechanical forces that results in weakness, such as the junction between two orthopedic rods.

STRETCH cardiac device.

Stretch VL Flexima stents—variable length stents.

Stretta procedure—for treatment of gastroesophageal reflux disease. The procedure employs a balloon from which rows of needles are passed into the area to be treated. Radiofrequency energy is produced at the needle tips using a processor that controls the rate and degree of the resultant injury.

striatal nigral degeneration—a form of atypical parkinsonism. The name comes from the corpus striatum adjacent to the foramen of Monro.

string of beads appearance (Radiol)—sometimes seen on angiography of patients whose renovascular hypertension is secondary to fibromuscular dysplasia.

string phlebitis—a variant of Mondor disease occurring in pregnancy and which may appear in the axillary area, antecubital fossa, and groin.

string sign—long, severe stenosis of the distal segment of the internal carotid artery. See *myositis ossificans*. Also, *string sign* refers to marked narrowing of the terminal ileum or neoterminal ileum as a result of severe edema, inflammation, and spasm without actual fibrosis. It is found in Crohn disease patients. See also *pyloric string sign*.

strip-biopsy—used in obtaining large particle biopsies in the GI tract.

stripe of salmon red mucosa (GI)—the description of an endoscopic finding.

StriVectin-SD—marketed as a stretch-mark reducing cream. It is gaining popularity as an anti-aging, anti-wrinkle product.

Strobel formula—a method of accurately positioning pH probes for evaluation of gastroesophageal reflux in preterm infants.

Strobel method—a rapid, accurate, and precise method of determining the amount of vitamin A in breast milk.

stroked out—slang for *had a stroke*.

stroma-free hemoglobin (SFHb) **solution**—for blood transfusions.

stromal—pertaining to the stroma or connective tissue framework of an organ rather than to its functioning cells or tissues.

Strong-Campbell Vocational Interest Inventory (SCVII).

Strother acrochordonectomy—a procedure for removing acrochordons (flesh-toned skin tags) without anesthesia or cryosurgery. A surgical clamp is applied to the base of the lesion and left in place for approximately 15 minutes, following which the clamp is removed and the lesion is excised using fine, delicate scissors.

structural gene—a gene that codes for an RNA or protein product other than a regulator.

struma—see *Riedel struma*.

Stryker compartment pressure monitor. Also, Stryker manometer; Stryker intracompartmental pressure monitor system. May be erroneously referred to as Stryker "compartmental checker."

Stryker drain (Ortho).

Stryker leg exerciser—device that provides continuing passive motion to the leg to help restore a patient's range of motion postoperatively.

Stryker microdebrider—see *Hummer*.

Stryker Pain Buster pain management system.

Stryker stent.

ST-segment elevation in myocardial infarction (STE MI).

STT (scaphotrapeziotrapezoid) **arthrodesis**—used in treatment of Kienböck disease. See *Kienböck disease*.

ST-T wave changes—commonly dictated, although the dictator actually means *ST segment and T wave changes*. There is no *ST-T wave* or *ST wave*.

ST2 protein—an inflammatory biomarker (heart cell "stress" protein) found in increased blood levels, indicating a higher risk of death and congestive heart failure in the 30 days after a heart attack. A blood test for ST2 may help predict the prognosis of patients after a heart attack, but measuring ST2 will not help in diagnosing heart attacks because patients with asthma can also have increased levels of ST2 in their blood.

Stuart factor—see *blood coagulation factors*.

study or trial

- ACCLAIM (Advanced Chronic Heart Failure Clinical Assessment of Immune Modulation Therapy) trial
- ADEPT (Advanced Elements of Pacing Trial)
- AFFIRM (Atrial Fibrillation Follow-up Investigation of Rhythm Management study
- ALLHAT (Antihypertensive and Lipid-Lowering Treatment to Prevent Heart Attack Trial)
- ARIES I and II trials
- carperitide

study *(cont.)*
CREST (Cilostazol for Restenosis) study
EarlyBird
EMERALD (Enhanced Myocardial Efficacy and Recovery by Aspiration of Liberalized Debris) study
FOLFOX4 colorectal cancer trial (oxaliplatin)
Folstein MMSE (mini mental status exam)
HIDA-CCK scintigraphy
HIFI (High-Frequency Ventilation in Premature Infants)
JNC 7 report of the Joint National Committee on the Detection, Evaluation, and Treatment of High Blood Pressure
MRCP (abdominal MRI/magnetic resonance cholangiopancreatography)
multi-slab and cine techniques for single breath-hold cardiac-synchronized angiography
OPALS (Ontario Prehospital Advanced Life Support Study)
pelvic floor MRI
pharmacogenomics
POLARIS stroke
PROTECT trial of oral heparin
RICH (Restenosis in Intervened Coronaries with Hyperhomocysteinemia)
RADIUS (Rheumatoid Arthritis DMARD Intervention and Utilization Study)
Salt II hyponatremia
SAPPHIRE (study of angioplasty with protection in patients at high risk for endarterectomy)
Thrive Treatment Study
VALIANT (VALsartan in acute myocardial infarction) study
VEPARAF study

study *(cont.)*
Z-FAST trial of Femara and Zometa
ZODIAC (Ziprasidone Observational Study of Cardiac Outcomes) study

Stulberg hip positioner—attaches directly to operating table to convert for hip replacement surgery.

STUMP (spindle tumor of uncertain malignant potential).

stump pressure—pressures measuring retrograde flow.

stump-related neovascularity—resulting from hypoxia-induced proliferation of endothelial cells distal to the stump ligature in vascular surgery.

sty, stye—see *hordeolum.* Some might think that there is a differentiation—that *stye* is a hordeolum and that *sty* is an enclosure for pigs, but dictionaries list both spellings for *hordeolum.*

Stylet—internal esophageal MRI coil; used to image health conditions related to the esophagus and aorta from inside the body.

Stylus cardiovascular sutures—stainless steel needles used during coronary artery bypass grafting, peripheral graft implantation, and valve replacement procedures.

subarachnoid hemorrhage (SAH).

subbacterial endocarditis prophylaxis (SBE p-lax).

subclavian flap aortoplasty (SFA)—a technique used to correct aortic coarctation in children.

subclavian steal syndrome (Radiol)—cerebrovascular insufficiency caused by obstruction of the subclavian artery proximal to the vertebral artery, reversing the blood flow through the vertebral artery. The subclavian artery thus, in effect, "steals" cerebral

subclavian *(cont.)* blood, causing cerebral or brain stem ischemia.

sub-Coblation—nonablative Coblation technique that shrinks tissue by reducing the level of radiofrequency applied.

subcortical atherosclerotic encephalopathy (SAE).

subcortical dementia—any of a group of dementias thought to be caused by lesions affecting subcortical brain structures more than cortical ones, and characterized by memory loss with slowness in processing information or making intellectual responses. Included are multi-infarct dementia and dementias that accompany Huntington chorea, Wilson disease, and paralysis agitans.

subcortical ischemic vascular dementia (SIVD)—the main type of vascular cognitive impairment.

subcu—could mean either *subcutaneous* or *subcuticular. Subcutaneous* is the deeper layer, and *subcuticular* the more superficial layer. This may help in determining which is meant. When "subcu" is dictated and you are unsure which term is intended, spell *subcu*. Do not use the abbreviation *subQ* or *sub q* because the *Q or q* can be mistaken for a medication dosage. Usage: "The wound was closed with running subcu stitches of 5-0 Prolene."

subcutaneous augmentation material (SAM)—facial implant material made of expanded polytetrafluoroethylene and used in plastic and reconstructive maxillofacial surgery. See also *Gore-Tex SAM facial implants.*

subcutaneous emphysema (Radiol)—air or gas in subcutaneous tissues as evidenced on an x-ray.

subcutaneous fat lines (Radiol)—the edges or borders of the subcutaneous fat layer as seen on an x-ray.

subcutaneous injection artifact (Radiol)—occurs in a study such as an intravenous pyelogram, if the contrast agent is accidentally injected subcutaneously instead of intravenously. The arm will opacify instead of the kidneys. This is a very rare error.

subcutaneous polytef patch (Gore-Tex)—used in minimally invasive percutaneous facelift procedure, to suspend the midface and efface the melolabial fold.

subdiaphragm—used in dictation as a noun but not found in dictionaries. It is a back-formation from *subdiaphragmatic.* Usage: "Pelvic washings were then obtained from the right paracolic gutter, right subdiaphragm, left subdiaphragm, and cul-de-sac of Douglas."

subdural window—CT setting used when a subdural hematoma is suspected.

subependymal heterotopia—a hereditary disease, probably linked to the X chromosome, in which collections of normal neurons are found in an unusual location in the brain (ectopic gray matter.) Patients with subependymal heterotopia tend to have mild clinical symptoms, consisting of mixed partial-complex and tonic-clonic seizures, usually starting in late childhood or in the second decade of life.

subepithelial hematoma of the renal pelvis (Antopol-Goldman lesion).

suberosis—extrinsic allergic alveolitis caused by exposure to oak bark or cork dust.

subfascial endoscopic perforator surgery (SEPS)—treatment for chronic venous insufficiency.

Subjective, Objective, Assessment, and Plan—see *SOAP.*

sublux (verb)—brief form. *Subluxate* (verb) is the proper term. Usage: "I could not subluxate the patella."

submandibular gland transfer—done prior to radiation therapy for cancer, to preserve the submandibular gland.

submental SAL—see *SAL.*

Sub-Microinfusion catheter—low-profile catheter with ability to navigate within the cerebral vasculature for precise delivery of agents. It has radial infusion ports which provide mixing of blood and contrast media, an important key to excellent visualization.

submucosal saline injection technique—for treatment of early duodenal cancers and adenomas.

suboptimal films—not as good as might have been expected; usually referring to technical factors in an x-ray study, such as positioning, film quality, and patient cooperation.

subperiosteal corticotomy.

subplatysmal face-lift technique—a deep plane rhytidectomy using tissue mobilization, advancement, and repair.

subpleural blanketing technique—a technique in which the esophagogastric anastomosis is slipped under the upper mediastinal pleura, which is kept intact, after the azygos vein has been ligated and divided. This pleural "blanket" may act as an efficient barrier against potential digestive spillage into the mediastinum.

Sub-Q-Set—see *CSQI.*

subsegmental transcatheter arterial embolization (STAE).

subsegmentectomy—excision of a subsegment of the liver.

subset—as in "T-cell subset studies," a group within a group (T-4 cells, T-8 cells).

subthalamic nucleus (STN)—area of the brain that contributes to movement. An electrical lead is implanted into this area to effect deep brain stimulation to block abnormal nerve signals that cause tremors and other symptoms of Parkinson disease. See also *globus pallidus internal segment* (GPi).

subtraction films (Radiol)—a method to visualize the arteries and veins on x-ray. A scout film is taken first, before the dye is injected. The scout negative is made into a positive (darkens it). Then the angiogram is taken (this is a negative). Then a scout positive is taken and put under the dye-injected negative (the patient, not the film, has had the dye injection), which screens out the bone, so that all that is then visible are the arteries and veins.

Subtraction Ictal SPECT Co-registered to MRI (SISCOM) **imaging system**.

subureteric Teflon injection (STING).

suburethral sling procedure—made of PTFE (polytetrafluoroethylene) and used to treat stress urinary incontinence.

subwakefulness syndrome—daytime drowsiness and daytime sleep episodes that are always composed of non-REM sleep stages 1 or 2. The naps occur repetitively.

succus entericus—a term meaning secretions from the intestinal mucous membrane (Latin, "intestinal juice").

succussion splash—a splashing sound heard when a patient's body is

succussion *(cont.)* shaken. It indicates the presence of fluid and air in a body cavity, usually the stomach or chest.

suction-assisted lipectomy (SAL)—a procedure in which fat is removed by a suction device, rather than by sharp dissection.

suction-assisted lipoplasty (SAL).

suction-bubble technique—an easily visualized movement of air bubbles in attached tubing caused by the vacuum created by hip-joint distraction, thereby verifying intra-articular needle placement for hip aspiration and arthrography.

Suction Buster catheter—a combination duodenal decompression tube and feeding tube with multiple holes down the side of the tube. Also called *Moss Suction Buster tube.*

suction test—used during laparoscopic procedures. See *drip test*.

Sudan stain—an iodine compound used as a test for stool fat. It colors the droplets of fat, thus making them visible under the microscope. If there is excessive fat in the stool (steatorrhea), it may indicate liver disease, small bowel malabsorption problems, or pancreatic problems. If, on the other hand, the stool fat is extremely low, that may mean a vitamin D deficiency (since vitamin D is fat soluble).

Sudeck atrophy—acute osteoporosis.

SUDS HIV-1 (single-use diagnostic system for HIV screening)—can be performed in a healthcare setting without special equipment.

SUFE (slipped upper femoral epiphysis).

sugar-tong plaster splint—used for immobilization in Colles fracture.

sugar to pack a wound—see *brown sugar.*

Sugita right angle aneurysm clip.

Sugiura esophageal varices procedure—esophageal transection with paraesophagogastric devascularization.

Suh ventilation tube (ENT).

SUI (stress urinary incontinence).

suicide gene—a synthetic nucleic acid sequence, introduced into tumor cells by a viral vector, that renders those cells vulnerable to chemotherapeutic agents that are nontoxic to normal cells.

Suicide Risk Scale (SRS)—assesses past history of suicide attempts, present suicidal ideation, and feelings of hopelessness or depression.

sulfur hexafluoride (SF_6)—a gas used in pneumatic retinopexy.

summation gallop (S3 and S4)—in cardiac examination.

summation shadow artifact (Radiol) (also called *superimposition* or *construction artifact*)—superimposition of pulmonary vessels on end and/or bony shadows, which may mimic a lesion. Different views can resolve the issue. This artifact occurs frequently.

Summit LoDose collimator.

sump syndrome—cholestasis in patients who have undergone choledochoduodenostomy (CDS). It occurs when ingested food particles lodge between the CDS and ampulla of Vater.

sundown syndrome—complex of symptoms such as disorientation, agitation, and emotional stress which appear in elderly patients about the time of sunset. The hypothesized causes include decreasing light levels which increase disorientation in patients whose sight is already impaired, dehydration, or

sundown *(cont.)* progressive fatigue. The patient afflicted with this syndrome is termed a *sundowner*, a pejorative term.

Sundt-Kees clip—for clipping aneurysms.

Sunna circumcision—female genital mutilation consisting of removal of prepuce and/or tip of clitoris. (*Sunna* in Arabic means "tradition.") See also *clitoridectomy* and *infibulation*.

Sunrise LTK procedure—laser thermokeratoplasty procedure for farsightedness, expected to provide relief for 10 years or more.

sunrise view of the patella (Radiol).

sunset eyes—an abnormal appearance of the eyes in which the pupils lie at or below the level of the lower lids; seen in infantile hydrocephalus and due to retraction of the upper lids.

sunset legislation—a type of legislation that incorporates an expiration date so that it must be reevaluated at a later time; this allows for changes in policy as public opinion and perceived needs change.

superabsorbent polymer (SAP)—a promising embolic material that may be used in place of the other particle embolic materials.

Superblade—a small blade used in ophthalmology.

supercharged TRAM flap—see *TRAM flap*, used in breast reconstruction. When the blood supply provided by the intact vascular pedicle of the transplanted muscle is supplemented by microsurgical augmentation of arterial or venous supply (or both), it is said to be "supercharged."

superconducting magnet—MRI term.

superficial musculoaponeurotic system (SMAS).

superficial posterior talotibial ligament (SPTTL).

Superglue (cyanoacrylate)—a tissue adhesive.

superimposition artifact (Radiol)—see *summation shadow artifact*.

superior epigastric [artery] **perforator** (SIEP) **flap**.

superior gluteal artery perforator (SGAP) **flap**—used in simultaneous bilateral breast reconstruction after mastectomy. Dissection of the flap is performed with complete preservation of gluteus maximus muscle function. The resulting vascular pedicle obtained via dissection through the muscle is longer than that of gluteal musculocutaneous flap and affords the surgeon the luxury of avoiding vein grafts in the anastomotic phase of surgery.

superior mesenteric vein (SMV).

superior vena cava (SVC) **syndrome**.

supernate—the liquid material that rises to the top, after the solid material, or sediment, has settled to the bottom. Also, *supernatant*. Cf. *infranate*.

Super-9 guiding cardiac device.

supernumerary—more than the usual number, as of digits, or parathyroid glands.

superparamagnetic iron oxide (SPIO) contrast medium.

Super PEG tube—percutaneous endoscopic gastrostomy tube. *Super* is a trade name.

Super Pinky—a pink rubber ball with attached elastic headband. The ball is applied over the closed eyelids to lower intraocular pressure prior to surgery on the eye.

SuperQuad assistive device—a walking cane with a quad base and a lower hand grip designed to reduce the amount of effort and strength required to stand up.

Super Quant—see *HCV Super Quant RT-PCR assay.*

SuperStitch—for use in suturing vascular puncture sites.

super stress test—cardiac test used to detect T-wave alternans in order to identify patients at high risk for sudden cardiac death. Similar to an exercise stress test.

super-wet technique—plastic surgery liposuction technique that uses fluid to aid in the liposuction process. Uses less fluid than the tumescent technique.

Supple Peri-Guard patch—see *CV Peri-Guard patch.*

suppressor cell, or **T-8 suppressor cell**—lymphocytes, part of the immune system. These are different from the T-4 lymphocytes attacked by the virus, but they need to interact with T-4 cells for the immune system to function correctly. Also called *cytotoxic cells.*

supradescemetic keratoprosthesis—an artificial cornea placed above the level of the Descemet membrane.

supraglottoplasty—a procedure to treat severe laryngomalacia.

supramalleolar orthosis (SMO).

Supramid suture—a multiple monofilament nylon stranded suture in a nylon sheath, used for intestinal anastomoses.

suprasellar—above the sella turcica.

supratentorial symptoms—a way for physicians to indicate confidentially that there might bc a functional overlay to an illness. The tentorium lies at the base of the cerebrum in the brain; hence, by definition, activity the patient can control is above this point. It can also be used in a somewhat pejorative sense or whenever physicians want to indicate among themselves, without being understood by laymen reading the record or overhearing, that the patient might have an element of hypochondriasis to his complaints.

supratip nasal tip deformity—the characteristic rounded shape of a baby's nose; also called the *universal nose of childhood.*

supraventricular tachycardia (SVT) or **tachyarrhythmia**.

Supreme electrophysiology catheter.

surcingle ("sur-single")—a girdle; also a band, belt, or girth passing over a horse's back or saddle. See *Von Lackum surcingle.*

SureBite biopsy forceps—a flexible tube with a cup biopsy tip for gastrointestinal biopsies.

SureCell Chlamydia test kit.

SureCell herpes (SC-HSV) **test kit**.

"sure-clens"—phonetic for *Shur-Clens.*

Sure-Closure—a skin-stretching system used to approximate wounds or incisions that might normally require grafting or that have a high probability of separating. Currently used in podiatric surgery, particularly on the bottom of the foot.

SureCuff—tissue in-growth cuff that provides catheter fixation.

SurePress compression dressing or **wrap**.

SureSight—a hand-held, child-friendly vision screening device.

Suresite—transparent adhesive film dressing.

Suretac, Suretac IXC—bioabsorbable shoulder fixation device.

SureTrans—autotransfusion system for orthopedics.

surface coil—in magnetic resonance imaging, a simple flat coil placed on the surface of the body and used as a receiver.

surface electromyography (sEMG).

surface marker—a surface protein unique to certain types of cell, used by antibodies and other substances to identify cells.

surfactant—a combination of the phospholipids, lecithin and sphingomyelin, which coat the alveoli. In premature infants, surfactant levels are so low and the resulting surface tension of the alveoli so high that the lungs collapse with each breath. Surfactant derived from amniotic fluid or from cows' lungs can be used to correct the deficit.

surfactant, heterologous—surfactant derived from sources other than human, including bovine or porcine sources. Surfactants reduce surface tension of pulmonary fluids and contribute to the elasticity of the lung and are important in treatment of conditions such as cystic fibrosis.

surfactant, homologous—surfactants derived from human sources, the only source at this time being amniotic fluid collected from uncomplicated term pregnancies. It is the only surfactant replacement that contains all the surfactant proteins. Disadvantages of human-derived surfactants are the limited supply and the risk of transmission of viral agents.

Surfit ("sure-fit") adhesive.

surf test—medical slang for surfactant test of amniotic fluid.

Surgeons Choice—the trade name of the ILA surgical stapling system. (Note that there is no apostrophe used.) See *ILA stapler*.

surgeon's knot (also *friction knot)*—used in tying Vicryl and Mersilene sutures.

surgery safari—surgery jargon for a trip to a third-world country for cosmetic surgery (such as liposuction) at a much lower price than in the U.S. The patient is on "safari" (away from scrutiny) while the wounds heal. Also called *scalpel safari*.

surgical gut—catgut, an absorbable suture. May be made from the serosal layer of beef intestine or the submucosal layer of sheep intestine.

surgical isolation bubble system (SIBS) —used to maintain sterile operative field.

surgically implanted hemodialysis catheter (SIHC)—a dual lumen central venous catheter.

Surgical Navigation Network—Windows NT image-guided surgery software platform.

Surgical No Bounce Mallet—designed to allow easier orthopedic prosthesis installation, resulting in less trauma to the patient and less fatigue to the surgeons. (Note: *not* Surgicel.)

Surgical Nu-Knit—absorbable hemostatic material (like a loosely knitted fabric, but thicker and more closely woven than Surgicel), oxidized regenerated cellulose.

surgical reversal of presbyopia (SRP) —a procedure using the scleral expansion bands. It allows a patient to focus and read by expanding the diameter of the eye overlying the ciliary muscle, increasing the distance between the ciliary muscle and the edge of the crystalline lens, thus allowing the ciliary muscle to exert more force on the lens. Four polymethylmethacrylate segments are inserted around the circumference of the eye and expand the area around the lens, allowing the muscles more room in which to work and enabling the eye to once again focus on small objects such as words on a page.

Surgical Simplex P—radiopaque bone cement.

Surgicel—an oxidized regenerated cellulose product that will be absorbed by body tissues; used for hemostasis. Cf. *Surgical Nu-knit*.

Surgicel Fibrillar—absorbable hemostat.

Surgicel Nu-Knit—absorbable hemostatic agent.

Surgidac—braided polyester suture material.

Surgidyne—closed wound drainage devices, namely, drainage tubes, bulb evacuators, and collection bags; vacuum controllers for drainage devices.

Surgifoam absorbable gelatin sponge—sponge for obtaining hemostasis during surgical procedures when control of bleeding by other means is ineffective or impractical.

Surgilase CO_2 laser—a laser using gold as an additional catalyst, allowing more controlled tissue effects and a higher peak power.

Surgilase 150—high-powered CO_2 laser with three operating waveforms: SurgiPulse, PowerPulse, and continuous wave.

Surgilav machine—used in washing the acetabulum or other operative area in orthopedic surgery.

SurgiLav Plus—hydrodebridement portable system for cleaning debris and necrotic tissue from chronic wounds.

Surgilene—a monofilament polypropylene suture material.

Surgilon—braided nylon suture material.

Surg-I-Loop—silicone loops, available in a variety of widths and colors, used during surgery to provide retraction, occlusion, and identification of veins, arteries, and nerves.

Surgiport—disposable surgical trocar and sleeve to be used during endoscopic procedures and laparoscopic surgery.

Surgi-Prep—see **Betadine Surgi-Prep** (povidone-iodine) **Sponge Brush**.

Surgipro—a prolene mesh used in hernia repairs.

SurgiScope—uses robotic arm with MR and CT interactive guidance to plan and perform brain surgery, allowing smaller incisions and reducing risk to patient.

Surgisis Gold hernia repair graft—mesh graft used for implantation to reinforce soft tissue in the repair of a hernia or body wall defect. Used in colorectal, plastic, general, thoracic, and trauma surgery.

Surgisis IHM (inguinal hernia matrix)—used to reinforce soft tissues in the inguinal floor to repair inguinal hernias in both open and laparoscopic surgery.

SurgiSis sling/mesh—for reinforcement of soft tissues where weakness exists. It is intended for colon and rectal prolapse repair, reconstruction of the pelvic floor, bladder support, tissue repair, and sacrocolposuspension. Also used for pubourethral support for the treatment of urinary incontinence due to hypermobility and intrinsic sphincter deficiency.

Surgitron—portable radiosurgical unit; it has four therapeutic currents, as well as bipolar capabilities for microsurgical procedures.

Surgiview—multiuse disposable laparoscope.

Surgi-Vision Intercept urethral coil—enables high-resolution MRI images of the urethral wall to be made from inside the body.

Surlyn molding helmet—a helmet applied on an infant after surgery for craniosynostosis, designed to minimize growth in the anteroposterior direction while allowing for expansion of the skull in the lateral dimensions.

sursumduction—upward movement of only one eye in testing for vertical divergence. Also, *supraduction, superduction, supravergence, sursumvergence.* Cf. *circumduction*.

survivor's guilt—a phenomenon that afflicts those who live through devastating circumstances, such as epidemics, or who simply outlive peers or spouses. If the spouse became demented and had to be institutionalized, the guilt is especially intense and a cause of depression.

Susac syndrome—microangiopathy of the brain, branch retinal artery occlusions, and hearing loss in young women between the ages of 21 and 41. It is self-limiting, most often one to two years in duration, but about half of the patients will have residua, including total deafness.

Suspend sling—surgical implant device for the treatment of stress incontinence in women.

Sustain—HA (hydroxyapatite) biointegrated dental implant system.

sustained maximal inspiratory pressure (SMIP).

sustention (postural) **tremor**—a tremor of a limb that increases when the limb is stretched.

Sutralon—nonabsorbable synthetic polyamide suture used in general soft tissue approximation and/or ligation, including use in cardiovascular, ophthalmic, and neurological procedures.

SutraSilk—nonabsorbable silk suture used in general soft tissue approximation and/or ligation, including cardiovascular, ophthalmic, and neurological procedures.

Suturamid suture material.

suture—a quick-reference list of suture material, technique, and type. The burgeoning field of laparoscopic and other minimally invasive surgeries may bring with it a number of new suture and knot techniques, as surgeons develop intracorporeal suturing methods. Tying sutures long distance by means of instruments viewed through a scope or video camera is a skill in itself and far removed from the suturing of open procedures. Examples:

Aberdeen knot
Acier stainless steel
Ailee
Arthrosew
barbed
baseball stitch
Biosyn
Bondek absorbable
braided Mersilene
braided Nurolon
bridle
Brolin antiobstruction stitch
bunching
Caprosyn
catgut
collagen
convertible slip knot
coupled
crossed-swords technique
Dacron
Dafilon surgical
Deklene
Deknatel
Dermalene
Dermalon
Dexon Plus
Dexon II
DG Softgut

suture *(cont.)*
double-armed
Endoknot
Endoloop
Ethibond
Ethiflex
Ethilon monofilament nylon
free tie
funicular
Gambee
gift wrap technique
Gillies horizontal dermal
guy
Heaney
Herculon
interrupted near-far, far-near
Krackow
Maxon polyglyconate monofilament
Mersilene
Mersilk braided silk
Monocryl (polyglecaprone 25)
Novafil (*not* Novofil)
Nurolon
out-in-out technique
Panacryl absorbable
PDS (polydioxanone) II Endoloop
Perma-Hand braided silk
Pilot
Polydek
polyglactin
Polysorb
Prolene
Pronova nonabsorbable
pursestring or purse-string
Quill self-anchoring
Rapide
retention
roman sandal fashion
Roth Grip-Tip
Sabreloc (spatula needle)
Sepramesh
shorthand vertical mattress
Softgut
stay
stick tie (suture ligature or transfixion suture)

suture *(cont.)*
Stylus cardiovascular
SuperStitch
Supramid
Suretac
surgical gut
Surgidac braided polyester
Surgilene
Surgilon
Sutralon
SutraSilk
Suturamid
Sutureloop colposuspension
swaged-on
Synthofil
Teflon
Tevdek
Thiersch
Ti-Cron
transfixion
T12
undyed braided polyglycolic acid
Vicryl Rapide
wing
Z-stitch

sutured in place, shield-shaped tip graft (ENT)—sounds poetic? At least alliterative. Included because it's the kind of expression, dictated rapidly, that can become unintelligible unless one knows it. The tip referred to is the tip of the nose.

SutureGroove gold eye weights—weights of 99.9% pure gold used for the treatment of lagophthalmos. A small incision is made in the eyelid, just above the lashes, and a small pocket created. The weights are secured to the lid with sutures placed through small channels or grooves in the weight, and the incision closed. Placement of the eyelid implant may be septal, mid pretarsal or low pretarsal.

suture ligature—see *stick tie* and *transfixion suture.*

Sutureloop—ready-to-use needle/colposuspension suture suitable for use with various procedures and needles. It consists of two Novafil sutures with prethreaded Teflon pledgets. A radiopaque clip is applied to each pledget to enable postoperative x-ray visualization of buttress position.

Suture Strip Plus—a stretch wound closure strip.

Suture/VesiBand organizer—attaches to drape or skin within the sterile field to eliminate entanglement of multiple sutures and silicone bands.

SVAB (stereotactic vacuum-assisted biopsy) **device**.

SVC (superior vena cava) **syndrome**—caused by obstruction of the SVC due to a variety of malignant and benign entities.

SVG (seminal vesiculography).

SVR (surgical ventricular restoration).

SVR (systemic vascular resistance).

SVT (supraventricular tachycardia, or supraventricular tachyarrhythmia).

swaged-on (rhymes with "wedged") suture. The suture and needle are fused together. Also called *atraumatic suture.*

swamp-static artifact—see *tree artifact*.

Swan-Ganz catheter—used to monitor pulmonary capillary wedge pressure.

swan-neck catheter.

Swanson PIP joint arthroplasty. Usage: "A Swanson PIP joint arthroplasty of the right ring finger and extensor pulley reconstruction, for boutonnière deformity, was performed, using a Swanson prosthesis."

Swanson Silastic implant (Ortho).

SWAP (short wavelength autoperimetry).

Swartz SL Series Fast-Cath introducer.

sweat chloride levels—an elevated level of chloride in perspiration is a sign of cystic fibrosis. One method of measurement is the pilocarpine iontophoresis method.

sweat secretion rate (SSR).

Swede-O-Universal braces (Ortho).

sweetheart—operating room slang for Harrington retractor, so-called because the tip of the blade is somewhat heart-shaped. See *Harrington retractor.*

sweet oil—an old-fashioned remedy for earache; can refer to any refined vegetable oil (e.g., olive oil), particularly one with a pleasant fragrance (e.g., almond oil).

Sweet Tip pacing lead—with screw-in tip for permanent implantation. It is used for either atrial or ventricular applications. Also, *Sweet Tip Rx pacing lead.*

Swenson papillotome—used to perform a papillotomy during an endoscopic transpapillary catheterization of the gallbladder in patients with symptomatic gallstones.

Swenson pull-through procedure—for Hirschsprung disease.

swimmer's view (Radiol)—an oblique view of the thoracic spine in which the arm nearer to the x-ray source hangs at the patient's side and the opposite arm is upraised.

SwingAlong walker caddy—attachment to a walker to hold additional objects such as trays, hooks, and dinnerware.

swing test—measures heart rate variability in patients with congestive heart failure.

Swiss lithoclast—intracorporeal lithotripter for endoscopic stone disintegration.

Swiss-type SCID (severe combined immunodeficiency disease)—caused by lymphoid stem-cell defect.

Swivel-Strap brace (Ortho)—wraps anatomically and allows counter-rotation.

Swiss ball therapy—therapeutic exercises using a heavy-duty vinyl ball. It helps to increase range of motion, strength, endurance, motor skills, and balance and is useful in treating upper body ailments.

SWJ (square-wave jerks) (Neuro).

sword-fighting—refers to the placing of laparoscopic or thoracoscopic ports too close together, which interferes with maneuverability of the instruments. Also called *fencing-in.*

SXCT (spiral x-ray computed tomography).

Syed-Neblett brachytherapy method.

Syed template—an interstitial gynecologic brachytherapy. Previously, the technique required blind insertion of the interstitial needles, risking inaccurate placement of the radioactive sources and viscus perforation.

Symbion J-7-70-mL-ventricle—total artificial heart.

Symbiot stent—an ePTFE-covered self-expanding stent intended to reduce plaque embolization during stenting and post-stenting restenosis.

Syme amputation—ankle disarticulation. Usage: "The patient should consider talking with other amputees about the likelihood of a below-knee amputation prosthesis, as I don't feel that a Syme amputation would be indicated in this patient."

Symmetra ^{125}I brachytherapy seed—for treatment of prostate cancer.

symmetrical phased array—term used in B-scan, Doppler, and color Doppler imaging. See *B-scan*.

Symmetry endobipolar generator.

sympathetically maintained (pelvic) **pain** (SMP).

Symphony stent—a self-expanding nitinol stent used in diseased arteries of the legs, usually in conjunction with balloon angioplasty.

Symptom Checklist-90 Revised (SCL-90-R)—measures degree of parental stress symptoms.

SynchroMed infusion system—an implanted programmable pump and catheter used to deliver morphine into the epidural space. It is used to treat cancer patients with unrelieved pain. This pump can also deliver chemotherapy drugs, clindamycin (to treat osteomyelitis), and baclofen (to treat chronic muscle spasticity).

synchronized sleep (S-sleep, or non-REM [NREM] sleep)—precedes desynchronized sleep and is the time when the muscles begin to relax, when fatigue is relieved. There are also changes in electrical activity on EEG. Cf. *REM* and *desynchronized sleep*. See *polysomnogram*.

synchronous airway lesions (SALs)—associated with laryngomalacia, requiring epiglottoplasty.

synchronous cancer—cancer occurring at two primary sites.

Synchrony system—records the breathing movements of a patient's chest and combines that information with sequential x-ray pictures of tiny markers inserted inside a tumor, to enable precise delivery of radiation during any point in the respiration cycle.

syncytial ("sin-sish-al") **knot formation**—a placental layer which proliferates and folds on itself, producing tangles of tissue.

syncytium-inducing (SI) **variant of HIV**—causes a more rapid decline in CD4 cells and progression to AIDS than does the nonsyncytium-inducing variant. See *nonsyncytium-inducing*.

syndactyly—a congenital anomaly in which the webbing between two (or more) digits extends to fusing the fingers to each other.

syndrome
- Aarskog
- abdominal compartment (ACS)
- abdominal cutaneous nerve entrapment
- ablepharon macrostomia (AMS)
- acquired long QT (aLQTS)
- acute compartment
- acute tumor lysis (ATL)
- adult respiratory distress (ARDS)
- AFP (acute flaccid paralysis)
- ALCAPA (anomalous origin of left coronary artery from the pulmonary artery)
- alien hand
- anosognostic
- anserine bursitis
- anticonvulsant hypersensitivity
- antiphospholipid
- antiphospholipid antibody (APS)
- apallic
- apple peel
- Arndt-Gottron
- atypical mole
- Baastrup
- Baller-Gerold
- bare lymphocyte
- Bartter
- Bazex
- Beare-Stevenson cutis gyrata
- beat knee
- Beckwith-Wiedemann
- beer drinker's hyponatremia
- Behçet
- Blackfan-Diamond
- Bland-Garland-White

syndrome *(cont.)*
- Bloodgood
- Bloom
- Blue Angel
- blue diaper
- blue rubber-bleb nevus
- blue toe
- blue velvet
- Boerhaave
- Bowen Hutterite
- BPTI (brachial plexus traction injury)
- brain death
- Brett
- bronchio-oto-renal (BOR)
- Brown
- Brown tendon sheath
- Brueghel
- Brugada
- Budd-Chiari
- buried bumper
- burning mouth (BMS)
- burning vulvar
- calciphylaxis
- capillary leak
- Carney complex
- carpal tunnel (CTS)
- cast
- cat's cry
- cauda equina
- cerebral salt-wasting (CSW)
- Cheatle
- Chilaiditi
- chronic fatigue
- chronic fatigue immune dysfunction
- chronic intestinal pseudo-obstruction
- Churg-Strauss
- Cobb
- Coffin-Lowry
- compartment
- complex regional pain (CRPS)
- constipation-dominant irritable bowel (C-IBS)
- Cooper
- corneal exhaustion

syndrome *(cont.)*
Cotton-Berg
CPD (chorioretinopathy and pituitary dysfunction)
CREST
cri du chat
Crigler-Najjar
CRST
CTS (carpal tunnel)
cubital tunnel
Cushing
cyclic vomiting
Dandy-Walker
de Clérambault
delayed pulmonary toxicity (DPTS)
de Morsier
de Morsier-Gauthier
Denys-Drash
diarrhea-predominant vs. constipation-predominant irritable bowel
DiGeorge
DIMOAD
DOOR (deafness, onychodystrophy, osteodystrophy, retardation)
double whammy
drug reaction with eosinophilia and systemic symptoms (DRESS)
Duane retraction
dumping
dysplastic nevus
Eagle-Barrett
economy class
EEC
Ehlers-Danlos
empty nest
empty nose (ENS)
empty sella
eosinophilia-myalgia (EMS)
failed back surgery (FBSS)
false memory
familial visceral neuropathy
FAMMM (familial atypical multiple mole melanoma)
fat embolism (FES)

syndrome *(cont.)*
Fechtner
fetal hydantoin
fibrocystic breast
fish-odor (primary trimethylaminuria)
Fitz-Hugh and Curtis
Floating-Harbor
Fournier
fragile X
Funston
GALOP
Garcin
Garin-Bujadoux-Bannwarth
gas-bloat
Gastaut
gastroduodenal intussusception due to Peutz-Jeghers syndrome in infancy
GEMSS (glaucoma, lens ectopia, microspherophakia, stiffness of the joints, and shortness)
Gerstmann
Gianotti-Crosti
Gilles de la Tourette
Gitelman
Goldenhar
Greig cephalopolysyndactyly
Guillain-Barré
half base
Halbrecht
Hamman-Rich
Hantavirus pulmonary (HPS)
Harada
heart and hand (heart-hand)
HEE (hemiconvulsion, hemiplegia, epilepsy)
HELLP
hemolytic uremic (HUS)
Henoch-Schönlein
hepato-renal (HRS)
HPRC (hereditary papillary renal cancer)
HVS (hyperventilation)
hyperlexia

syndrome *(cont.)*
hypersensitivity
hypothenar hammer
ICE (iridocorneal-endothelial)
immotile cilia
impaired regeneration (IRS)
insulin resistance
Ivemark
Jackson-Weiss
Jaffe-Campanacci
Janus (Brett syndrome)
Jerusalem
Josephs-Blackfan-Diamond
Joubert
Juberg-Marsidi
Kasabach-Merritt
Kaznelson
Kearns-Sayre-Shy
Klinefelter (XXY)
Klippel-Feil
Koerber-Salus-Elschnig
Kousseff
LADD (lacrimoauriculodentodigital)
LAMB
Landry-Guillain-Barré-Strohl
laparoscopic surgeon's thumb
large vestibular aqueduct
late luteal phase dysphoric disorder (LLPDD)
Laurence-Moon-Biedl
lazy leukocyte (LLS)
Lejeune
Lennox-Gastaut
LEOPARD
Leriche
Lesch-Nyhan
Lewy body dementia
Li-Fraumeni (LFS)
locked-in
locker-room
Löffler (Loeffler)
loin pain hematuria
lottery fantasy
Louis-Bar
Lowe

syndrome *(cont.)*
Lown-Ganong-Levine
lymphadenopathy (LAS)
Lynch, Lynch I, Lynch II
Maffucci
Marcus Gunn jaw-winking
Marshall
MAS (meconium aspiration)
Mayer-Rokitansky-Kuster-Hauser (MRKH)
McCune-Albright
medial tibial stress (MTSS)
Meige
Meigs
MELAS
MEN (multiple endocrine neoplasia)
MEN 1 (type 1)
meningococcal supraglottitis
Menke steely hair
metabolic
minor vestibular adenitis
micrognathia-glossoptosis
Mirizzi
Moersch-Woltmann syndrome
mole
monosomy 7
Mouchet
MRKH (Mayer-Rokitansky-Kuster-Hauser)
mucocutaneous lymph node (MLNS)
multiple endocrine neoplasia type 2b
multiple evanescent white dot
multiple organ dysfunction (MODS)
multiple organ failure (MOF)
Munchausen
myalgic encephalomyelitis (ME)
myelodysplastic (MDS)
MYHIIA
Myhre
nephrotic
nerve root compression
Nezelof

syndrome *(cont.)*
normal perfusion pressure breakthrough (in giant arteriovenous malformations)
Norrie neurodevelopmental disorder
NSTE acute coronary
obstructive sleep apnea (OSAS)
Ogilvie
oligoteratoasthenozoospermia
organic brain
os trigonum
otospongiosis/otosclerosis
ovarian hyperstimulation (OHSS)
ovarian remnant
painter's encephalopathy
pallid infantile
paratrigeminal oculosympathetic
Parinaud oculoglandular
Parsonage-Turner
pelvic outlet
Penderluft
penta X
perfusion pressure breakthrough
Peutz-Jeghers (PJS)
PHACE
Phocas
Pierre Robin
pigment dispersion (PDS)
Plummer-Vinson
POEMS
Poland
postviral fatigue
P pulmonale
premenstrual voice (PMVS)
presumed ocular histoplasmosis (POH)
primary ciliary dyskinesia (PCD)
prune-belly
pulmonary sling
Ramsay Hunt
Rapp-Hodgkin
refractory cytopenia with multilineage dysplasia (RCMD)
Reifenstein
respiratory distress (RDS)

syndrome *(cont.)*
retained bladder
reverse anorexia
reversible posterior leukoencephalopathy (RPLS)
Reye
Riley-Day
Robin
Ross
Rothmund-Thomson
Roux stasis
Saethre-Chotzen
Sandifer
Sanger-Brown
SAS (sleep apnea)
Schinzel-type acrocallosal
Schwachman
SCIWORA (spinal cord injury without radiographic abnormality)
sea-blue histiocyte
Sebastian
second impact
sedentary death (SeDS)
Sedlackova
sepsis
Sertoli-cell-only
severe acute respiratory (SARS)
Sézary
SHAFT (sad, hostile, anxious, frustrating, tenacious)
Sheehy
SIADH
sick building
sick sinus
Singleton–Merten
sinus tarsi
SIRS/sepsis (systemic inflammatory response)
Sjögren
slipped rib
sloughed urethra
small-patella
Smith-Lemli-Opitz
smooth brain (lissencephaly)

syndrome *(cont.)*
snapping triceps
Sneddon
spectacular shrinking deficit
Sphrintzen
Srb
Stevens-Johnson (SJS)
Stewart-Treves
Stickler
stiff-heart
stiff-person
Stilling-Türk-Duane
subclavian steal
subwakefulness
sump
sundown
sundowner
superior vena cava (SVC)
Susac
systemic capillary leak (SCLS)
systemic inflammatory response (SIRS)
Takatsuki
talar compression
tarsal tunnel
Terson
tethered cord
13q deletion
thoracic endometriosis (TES)
3-M (Miller, McKusick, and Malvaux)
Tillaux-Phocas
Tolosa-Hunt
tooth and nail
Tourette
transient bone marrow edema
translocation Down
triad asthma
triad of Rigler
trisomy-D
tumor lysis (TLS)
Turner
UGH+
ulnocarpal abutment (UAS)
Unverricht-Lundborg
Usher
VACTERL
vanishing lung
VATER
venous leak
vestibular adenitis
Vogt-Koyanagi-Harada
vulvar vestibulitis
wasting
white clot
white dot
Winchester
Wiskott-Aldrich
WPW (Wolff-Parkinson-White)
XXY (Klinefelter)
Yentl
yo-yo
Yunis-Varon
Zollinger-Ellison (ZES)

syndrome X—refers to typical angina pectoris in a patient with normal blood flow in coronary arteries, as shown by imaging studies. It is presumed to be due to vascular spasm. Not to be confused with *metabolic syndrome X*.

synechialysis (Oph).

SynerG detachable coil system.

synergism—a positive interaction between two or more drugs in which each boosts the effect of the others.

synergistic wrist motion splint.

Synergraft—tissue-engineered replacement heart valves.

Synergy neurostimulation system—implantable dual channel therapy designed to aid in management of chronic intractable pain in trunk or limbs.

syngamy—the fusion of sperm and oocyte at fertilization.

synovial frost (Ortho).

Syntel latex-free embolectomy catheter—balloon embolectomy catheter used on patients with latex allergies.

synteny—the presence of two or more loci on the same gene.

Synthaderm—synthetic (polyurethane) occlusive wound dressing used on ulcerations, usually on the lower extremities.

Synthes CerviFix system—used for stabilization and promotion of fusion of the cervical spine and occipital-cervical junction.

Synthes compression hip screw—American version of the German AO hip compression screw.

Synthes dorsal distal radius plate—for fixation of fractures, osteotomies, and carpal fusions involving the distal radius; applied to the dorsal aspect.

Synthes drill.

Synthes mini L-plate (Hand Surg).

Synthes transbuccal trocar (Oral Surg).

Synthetic Aperture Focusing Technique (SAFT)—used in intravascular ultrasound imaging, uses a limited number of A-scan signals. and requires far less computation time.

synthetic cornea—a soft, flexible plastic disk with a central optical element. It has a specially treated skirt that fits in a hollow cut into the damaged cornea and allows the surrounding cells to grow into it. Implanting is less invasive than current corneal transplantation and does not penetrate the innermost epithelial and Descemet membrane layers of the cornea. It is for patients unsuitable for standard penetrating keratoplasty (PK) or who have had a prior unsuccessful PK.

synthetic penetrating keratoplasty (S-PK).

Synthofil suture—nonabsorbable polyester braided and coated suture for skin closure and cardiovascular and arterial surgery.

syntonic—characterized by normal emotional response. Usage: "His affect was generally appropriate, and mood syntonic."

Syringe Avitene—an endoscopic delivery system for Avitene, a collagen hemostat. Note that *Syringe* is part of the trade name.

syringolymphoid hyperplasia with alopecia and anhidrosis (SLHA)—a syringotropic variant of mucinosis follicularis and a precursor lesion of mycosis fungoides. It may manifest as a slowly but continuously progressing single lesion as on the ankle.

system (see also *device*; *imaging system*)
- ABBI
- Access AFP immunoassay
- Access MV
- Accu-Chek InstantPlus
- Accu-Chek II Freedom blood glucose
- AccuLength arthroplasty measuring
- Accura hemofiltration
- AccuSway balance measurement
- Achieve off-pump
- Acolysis ultrasound intravascular thrombolysis
- Acusyst Xcell monoclonal antibody culturing
- Acutrak fusion
- Add-On Bucky digital
- Advanta V12 stent graft
- Advantim revision knee
- Advia 120 Hematology
- AFFINITY cage
- Affymetrix GeneChip
- Agee carpal tunnel release
- Agee-WristJack fracture reduction
- AFFINITY cage
- Allegretto Wave excimer laser
- Aloka color Doppler
- Alphatec mini lag-screw (MLS)
- Altaire MRI

system *(cont.)*
AMK (Anatomic Modular Knee) total knee
AML (Anatomic Medullary Locking) total hip
Amset ALPS (anterior locking plate system)
AnCore anuloplasty
AngeCool RF (radiofrequency) catheter ablation
AngioJet Rheolytic thrombectomy
AnuloFlex anuloplasty ring
Anscore health management
aortic connector
Apex irrigation
APR total hip
AquariusNET
Argyle Turkel safety thoracentesis
arrhythmia mapping
Arthro-Flo
Arthro-Lok
Asnis 2 guided screw
Aston cartilage reduction
Atavi atraumatic spine fusion
AtLast blood glucose monitoring
Aurora dedicated breast MRI
automated cellular imaging (ACIS)
automated lamellar therapeutic keratoplasty (ALTK)
BAK/C (cervical) and BAK/T (thoracic) interbody fusion
BACTEC blood culture
Baculovirus Expression Vector (BEVS)
BAK Vista interbody fusion
Bard EndoCinch endoscopic suturing
BAROS (Bariatric Analysis and Reporting Outcome System)
beating-heart bypass
BiliBed phototherapy
BiliCheck handheld battery-powered
BIO-INTRAFIX soft tissue tibial fixation

system *(cont.)*
BioZ
BladderScan
Brackmann II EMG
Brava breast enhancement
Bravo pH monitoring
Breast Cancer System 2100
breast imaging and reporting data system of the American College of Radiology (BI-RADS)
Bremer Halo Crown
Bridge Assurant biliary stent delivery
Bridge extra support over-the-wire renal stent
Brown-Roberts-Wells (BRW) stereotactic
CADD-Prizm pain control (PCS)
CADstream
Calcitek drill
Canal Finder
Cardiofreezer cryosurgical
cardiopulmonary support (CPS)
CathTrack catheter locator
C-bloc continuous nerve block
C-CAP (custom contoured ablation pattern) method
CD Horizon Eclipse spinal
CD Horizon Sextant spinal
cell recovery (CRS)
Cell Saver Haemolite
CG Future anuloplasty
Checkmate intravascular brachytherapy
Cheng-Ferkel grading
Concentric retriever
Concise compression hip screw
Continuum MR-compatible infusion
Cormet hip resurfacing
CorRestore
CPT hip
CRTD (cardiac resynchronization therapy defibrillation)
CS-5 cryosurgical

system *(cont.)*

C-Tek anterior cervical plate
CustomCornea Wavefront
C-VEST radionuclide monitoring
Dall-Miles cable grip
DentiPatch lidocaine transoral delivery
DePuy total hip system with porous coating
DeWrap three-layer compression
Diascan glucose monitoring
digital holography
Doc-U-Dose drug delivery
Dodick Laser Photolysis
Drake-Willock automatic delivery
Duran AnCore anuloplasty
Dyna-Lok plating
Dynasplint shoulder
Easi-Lav gastric lavage
EBI bone healing
Eccovision acoustic rhinometry
Ectra
Electronic HouseCall
electronic portal imaging
EnAbl thermal ablation
Encompass Cardiac Network
End-Flo laparoscopic irrigating
EndoCinch suturing
Endomed LSS laparoscopic
EndoSaph vein harvest
Endotak lead defibrillation
En Garde spring coil fixation
Entree Plus and Entree II trocar and cannula
EntSol nasal wash
Envoy middle ear implantable
EpiStar Diode Laser
ErecAid
Essure sterilization
Exactech total knee
Explorer X 70 intraoral radiography
EX-FI-RE external fixation
E-Z Flap
Expedium MIS spine
Express2 coronary stent

system *(cont.)*

F.A.S.T. (First Access for Shock and Trauma) 1 intraosseous infusion
FASTak suture anchor
FasT-Fix
FastPack
Flo-Stat fluid management
Flowtron DVT pump
FluoroNav virtual fluoroscopy
FluoroTrak
Freehand neuroprosthetic
Free-standing Tissue Retraction Bridge
Frontier biventricular cardiac pacing
Frostline
Fujinon Sonoprobe
functional MRI (fMRI)
Gamma locking nail
Gatekeeper reflux repair
GDC SynerG Detachment
GeneChip
GenESA
Giraffe Spot PT Lite phototherapy
Given diagnostic imaging
GlucoWatch G2 Biographer
Grosse and Kempf locking nail
GTS great toe
Guidant TRIAD three-electrode energy defibrillation
Haid Universal bone plate
HBS (headless bone screw) bone screw
HDI 1000 ultrasound
HDI 5000 ultrasound
Halifax interlaminar clamp
HeartMate vented electric LVAS (left ventricular assist system)
HeartMate SNAP-VE LVAS (sutures not applied-vented electric left ventricular assist system)
Heartport Port-Access

system *(cont.)*
HEARTS (healthy early alarm recognition and telemonitoring system) project
Heartstring proximal seal
Hepcon
Hexcel total condylar knee
HomMed monitor
Horizon AutoAdjust CPAP
Hot and Cold Sensory
House-Brackman facial nerve grading
HydroFlex arthroscopy irrigating
HY-TEC automated diagnostic
IDXrad
IGS (implantable gastric stimulation)
Ilizarov
Illumina PROSeries laparoscopy
Imagecast
ImageChecker detection for mammography
Indiana Tome
Infant Flow nasal CPAP
In-Fast bone screw
InnerVision transillumination
Innova home therapy
Innovator Holter
Insall/Burstein II
Intelect laser
Intercept platelet
International Association of Enterostomal Therapists stages
international normalized ratio (INR)
Intrel 3 spinal cord stimulation
IRIS (intensified radiographic imaging system)
Isola spinal instrumentation
Isolex
i-STAT
Jay seating
Kaneda spine stabilizing
Keramos ceramic total hip
Knee Signature (KSS)

system *(cont.)*
K2 hemi toe implant system
Lactosorb plating
LADARWave Custom Cornea Wavefront System
Laitinen CT guidance system and stereotactic head frame
Lap-Band rigid silicone band
Lapro-Clip ligating clip
Leibinger miniplate
Leibinger Profyle
less invasive stabilization (LISS)
LifeCare PCA Plus II infusion
LIFE-Lung fluorescence endoscopy
LiteNest portable seating
LORAD StereoGuide stereotactic breast biopsy
Luhr fixation
Luxtec fiberoptic
Magnetic Surgery
Magnetom MRI
Mallinckrodt sensor
Mammomat Novation digital mammography
Mammex TR mammography
MammoSite RTS (radiation therapy system)
Mammotest breast biopsy
Marx bridging plate
Maxilift Combi patient lifting
Maxim modular knee
McCain TMJ arthroscopic
MDS
Medi-Ject needle-free insulin injection
Medi-Jector Vision needle free insulin injection
Medisorb drug delivery
MedNext bone dissecting
Metrix implantable atrial defibrillation
METRx
Micro-Aire pulse lavage
MicroLap and MicroLap Gold microlaparoscopy

system *(cont.)*
MicroLysus drug delivery
MicroSpan microhysteroscopy
microvascular anastomotic coupler
MicroVas vascular treatment
microwave cardiac ablation
microwave endometrial ablation (MEA)
mini Hoffmann external fixation
Mirage nasal ventilation mask
MKM AutoPilot stereotactic
Mobetron intraoperative radiation therapy (IORT) treatment
Monticelli-Spinelli
Moss Miami load-sharing spinal implant
MOST options rotating hinge revision knee
MRSI (magnetic resonance spectroscopic)
Multi-Link Vision RX and OTW (over-the-wire) coronary stent
Musgrave pedobarograph
Navitrack
National Notifiable Disease Surveillance (NNDSS)
NC-Stat
Neotrend
NeuroCybernetic Prosthesis (NCP)
Neuroform microdelivery stent
Neuroshield cerebral protection device
Neurotrend
Nomos pin-free attachment stereotactic
NovaSure endometrial ablation
Octopus 2+ tissue stabilization
Ocutech vision enhancing
Omnifit Plus hip
ON-Q anesthesia delivery
Operating Arm
Optical Biopsy
Optical Tracking
Orbscan II

system *(cont.)*
Ortholoc Advantim knee revision
osteochondral autologous transfer (OATS)
Osteo-Clage cable
Osteonics ABC hip replacement
Osteonics total shoulder
Oxford meniscal unicompartmental knee system
Palomar EsteLux
Partaject drug delivery
Patil stereotaxic
Pelorus stereotactic
percutaneous Stoller afferent nerve stimulation (PerQ SANS)
peripheral access (PAS) port
PFC Sigma total knee
PhorMax CR (computed radiography)
photocatalytic air filtration
Photon Radiosurgery (PRS)
Piccolo blood chemistry analyzer
Polarus proximal humeral fixation
PowerSculpt cosmetic surgery
Precision SpeedTac transvaginal anchor
Precision Twist transvaginal anchor
Prestige Smart system (PSS)
Profile total hip system with porous coating
ProstaLund CoreTherm
Protector suturing
Pulsar Max II pacemaker
Pulsavac III wound debridement
PumpMate
Quartet
QuickSeal arterial closure system
Quick Tack periosteal fixation
Ranawat/Burstein total hip
Rancho fixation
Raptor over-the-wire delivery
Rasor blood pumping (RBPS)
RDX coronary radiation delivery
Regulus frameless stereotactic
Relume

system *(cont.)*
Repicci II unicondylar knee
Resting Heart
Restore ACL guide
Reuter suprapubic trocar and cannula
Reveal XVI PET/CT
Rhinoline endoscopic
RIGS
RLS (rhinolaryngostroboscopy)
RM (Riechert-Mundinger) stereotaxic
Robotrac passive retraction
Rogozinski spinal fixation
Romano surgical curved drilling
Rx5000 cardiac pacing
RX stent delivery
SB Charité III intervertebral dynamic disc
Scaphoid-Microstaple
Sensi-Touch anesthesia delivery
Sextant
Sextant Medtronic Sofamor Danek spinal
Sherwood intrascopic suction/irrigation
Side Branch Occlusion
Silhouette therapeutic massage
SiteSelect percutaneous breast biopsy
SKY epidural pain control
Sleep-In Bone Screw
Slider GDS (graft deployment system)
SmartKard digital Holter
SODAS (spheroidal oral drug absorption system)
Somnoplasty
sonic-accelerated fracture healing (SAFHS)
Sonocur Basic
Soprano cryoablation
SpaTouch PhotoEpilation
SP-501 Sonoprobe endoscopy
SportsRAC shoulder rehabilitation

system *(cont.)*
SprayGel absorbable adhesion barrier
Stability total hip
Stableloc external wrist fixation
STARRT (selective tubal assessment to refine reproductive therapy) falloposcopy
STAR (suture tension adjustment reel)
Straight-In surgical
Stryker Pain Buster pain management
SureTrans autotransfusion
SynchroMed infusion
Synchrony
SynerG detachable coil
TAG (tissue anchor guide)
TandemHeart PTVA
Targis
TCPM pneumatic tourniquet
TD Glucose monitoring
Tetrax interactive balance
ThermaCool TC
ThermoChem
Thoraseal
THORP (titanium hollow-screw osseointegrating reconstruction plate)
thrombolytic assessment (TAS)
TMS 3-dimensional radiation therapy treatment planning
TOTAL O_2
TRANSCEND articulation hip
transesophageal pacing
Trellis infusion catheter
TriActiv
Trident hip replacement
TriGen intramedullary nail
TwinFix Ti Quick-T fixation
Trilogy acetabular
Trinica
Tru-Close wound drainage
T3
Tylok cerclage cabling

system *(cont.)*
Ulson fixator
Unilink
Universal2 (no space) total wrist implant
UPlink
V.A.C. Freedom system
VAPR-3
VasoView balloon dissection
Vectra Genisys laser system
Versalok fixation
Versaport trocar
VersaPoint
Vertetrac ambulatory traction
ViewPoint CK (Conductive Keratoplasty)
Vicon
Visica cryoablation
VISX WaveScan Wavefront
VNUS Restore catheter
Wallaby phototherapy
WarmTouch patient warming
Wartner wart removal
WCD 2000
Welch Allyn ear wash
WNM
Wurzburg plating
X-PRESS vascular closure
Zest Anchor Advanced Generation (ZAAG) bone anchoring
Zeus robotic
Zimmer CPT (collarless polished taper) hip
ZMS intramedullary fixation

systemic and topical hypothermia.

systemic capillary leak syndrome (SCLS)—a rare condition characterized by unexplained episodic capillary hyperpermeability due to a shift of fluid and protein from the intravascular to the interstitial space. This results in diffuse swelling, weight gain, and renal shut-down. The disease evolves into multiple myeloma in some patients.

systemic lupus erythematosus (SLE)—an inflammatory disorder of the connective tissues, characterized by a "butterfly" erythema over the malar area and the bridge of the nose, arthralgias. It may include renal involvement, recurrent pleurisy, splenomegaly, and involvement of other body systems. It is thought to be an autoimmune disorder. It is seen predominantly in young women but is also seen in children. Also called *disseminated lupus erythematosus*. See also *Farr test*.

systemic mean arterial pressure (SMAP).

systemic vascular resistance (SVR).

System-S soft skeletal implant—used in hand arthroplasty.

systolic anterior motion (SAM) **on 2-D echocardiogram.**

Szabo-Berci needle drivers—designed for use with Karl Storz endoscopes for advanced suturing techniques.

T, t

T (tesla)—SI unit of magnetic strength (used in MRI). The term *gauss* was formerly used.

TAAA (thoracoabdominal aortic aneurysm) **surgery**.

TAB (tumescent absorbent bandage)—a post-tumescent wound dressing to keep the patient dry.

TAC (tetracaine, adrenaline, cocaine) —slang for topical analgesia for superficial lacerations. TAC is used especially for repair of open wounds in small children to avoid needle infiltration. Do not confuse with TAC (triamcinolone cream) used to treat dermatologic conditions.

TAC (transient aplastic crisis).

TAC ("tack") (triamcinolone cream)—used in the treatment of psoriasis and other dermatological conditions.

TACE (transcatheter arterial chemoembolization)—the most common nonsurgical treatment for hepatocellular carcinoma.

Tachyarrhythmia Detection Software —provides fully automatic detection and treatment of life-threatening arrhythmias.

tacrolimus-eluting stent.

Tactilaze angioplasty laser catheter—vaporizes atherosclerotic plaque by means of an angioplasty catheter threaded through the artery.

tactoid bodies—fibrillary aggregates which can be seen in neurofibromas representing rounded aggregates of collagen and cell processes, and probably represents a degenerative change.

TAE (transcatheter arterial embolization).

tag (Nuclear Med)—to label, i.e., to render a substance radioactive by incorporating a radionuclide in it; also, to cause a tissue or organ to take up radioactive material. Cf. *label, sensitize*.

Tagarno 3SD cine projector—for angiography.

tagged red blood cell nuclear scan—a magnetic resonance imaging scan in which the red blood cells have been "tagged" with a radioactive element.

tag image file format (TIFF).

TAG (tissue anchor guide) **system**.

tail—slender appendage, as in tail of Spence, tail of the breast. Cf. *cauda*.

tail of breast—in mammography, a wedge-shaped zone of breast tissue extending toward the axilla. Also known as the *axillary tail of Spence*.

tail of Spence—also called *tail of the breast*. It is the tail-like segment of mammary gland tissue that extends to the axillary region.

tailor's bunion—a name from the distant past when tailors sat cross-legged on the floor to do their sewing, and thus developed bunions on the fifth metatarsal (rather than the first metatarsal where they usually occur).

tailor tacking, **tailor tacked**—terms used in breast surgery.

Taka microneurosurgical sponge—developed by Dr. Takanori Fukushima.

Takatsuki syndrome (Neuro).

Takayasu arteritis—arteritis involving the aortic arch and its branches.

Take-apart scissors and forceps.

takeoff of a vessel (Radiol)—in angiography, the commencement (or origin) of a vessel as it branches off from a larger vessel.

talar tilt test—assesses the integrity of the calcaneofibular ligament (CFL) and the inversion and eversion range of motion of the ankle mortise.

talcosis—intravascular, perivascular, and alveolar granulomatous inflammation in which foreign bodies (talc and sometimes starch) can be identified. This talcosis is found in almost all I.V. drug abusers. It may cause abnormalities in pulmonary function.

talc poudrage—used to perform pleurodesis.

talc powder, sterile.

talc slurry—used to perform pleurodesis.

Talent LPS endoluminal stent-graft system—used for the treatment of abdominal aortic aneurysms.

talipes hobble splint—see *Denis Browne clubfoot splint*.

TAM (total active motion).

T&B or **T and B cells**—an abbreviation for helper T cells and B cells, important immune system markers.

T and C—slang for Tylenol and codeine. When a physician dictates, "The patient was given T and C for pain," one should transcribe, "The patient was given Tylenol and codeine for pain."

Tandem cardiac device.

TandemHeart—small 8-ounce centrifugal pump/ventricular assist device that can be implanted percutaneously and provides a steady flow of blood throughout the body, allowing the heart to rest and begin the healing process.

TandemHeart PTVA—a minimally invasive percutaneous transseptal ventricular assist system.

tandem mass spectrometry—screening blood test for newborns that scans for over 25 genetic diseases.

tandem repeats—many copies of the same DNA sequence occurring in succession along a chromosome without intervening DNA sequences of different configuration.

tangent screen—used in visual field testing.

tangential cut—a cut which is slightly off center, or glancing.

tangential speech—rambling, tending to go off on tangents.

Tanne corneal punch.

tanned red cells (TRC) **test**.

Tanner Developmental Scale—stages secondary sexual characteristics on a scale of I to V, I indicating no de-

Tanner *(cont.)*
velopment, V indicating full development; "breasts Tanner stage II," for example. Also, *Marshall and Tanner pubertal staging*.

Tanner mesher—a device used to mesh skin in preparation for grafting; permits the skin to stretch, thus covering a greater area. See also *Tanner-Vandeput mesh dermatome*.

Tanner-Vandeput mesh dermatome—an instrument that cuts small parallel slits in split thickness skin grafts, permitting the graft to expand two to three times its original size. When the graft is applied, the slits expand and become diamond-shaped areas which then epithelialize from the surrounding skin edges.

Tanner-Whitehouse bone age reference values for North American children.

Tannihist-12—prescription product containing antihistamine, decongestant, and antitussive, indicated for symptomatic relief of congestion, rhinorrhea, and cough associated with viral upper respiratory infection.

tantalum bronchogram (using powdered tantalum).

tantalum mesh, plate, ring, wire. Tantalum is not an alloy; it is biologically inert, having great tissue acceptability and high tensile strength. In plate form it is used for skull plates.

tap—see *glabellar tap*.

TAP (Thornton adjustable positioner).

TAP (tumor-activated prodrug)—technology used with proprietary antibodies for drug research.

tape
Cath-Secure hypoallergenic
Dacron
Elastikon elastic
Hy-Tape
lap
MaxCast
Microfoam surgical
Scotchcast 2 casting
Shur-Strip
Transpore surgical

taper—to reduce the dose of a medicine gradually; to change size gradually.

TAPET (tumor amplified protein expression therapy)—drug delivery that uses genetically altered strains of *Salmonella* as a vehicle for the delivery of antineoplastic drugs to tumor sites with minimal effect on healthy tissue.

TAPP (transabdominal preperitoneal) hernia repair.

TARA (total articular replacement arthroplasty) **prosthesis**—see *Townley TARA prosthesis*.

tardive dyskinesia (Psych)—involuntary tics, which may consist of continuous chewing motions or darting movements of the tongue, jerky dancing motions, or slow writhing motions of the hands or arms, secondary to long-term administration of antipsychotic drugs. Symptoms usually resolve on discontinuing the drug or reducing the dosage. See *extrapyramidal signs*. Cf. *pyramidal signs, akathisia*.

Tardy MicroBur—part of the XPS 2000 Microresector System instrument set, used in plastic surgery.

tardy palsy—referred to in electromyograph reports and nerve conduction velocities, with reference to carpal tunnel syndrome. Usage: "Impression: Slowing of ulnar nerve, slowing across the elbow, consistent with a tardy palsy."

tardy posterolateral rotatory instability of elbow—a condition developing 2-3 decades after the occurrence of either congenital or postinjury cubitus varus.

targeted cryoablation devices—used to treat liver and other cancers.

target lesion—a skin lesion consisting of concentric rings of erythema. For example, target lesion (of Lyme disease). See *erythema migrans*.

target sign—a test for cerebrospinal fluid leak. If a cerebrospinal fluid leak is suspected, examination of the bloody fluid placed on porous paper will show a clear halo around the inner bloody residue if positive. See *double halo sign*.

Target Tissue Cooling System (TTCS) —allows for the use of a cooling medium (such as water) on human tissue during the application of laser energy. The cooling of the target tissue prevents thermal damage, and the coolant facilitates the establishment of a photo-acoustic effect which aids in the removal of tissue.

Targis microwave catheter-based system—nonsurgical, catheter-based transurethral thermoablation system to treat benign prostatic hypertrophy.

Tarlov ("tar-loff") **perineurial cyst**.

tarsal cyst—see *chalazion*.

tarsal tunnel syndrome—a group of symptoms caused by compression of the posterior tibial nerve, or the plantar nerves, in the tarsal tunnel, resulting in pain, numbness and paresthesias of the plantar aspect of the foot. Usage: "The left medial great toe pain was suggestive of tarsal tunnel syndrome." Cf. *carpal tunnel syndrome*.

Tart cells—named for the patient in whom the cells were discovered. They can be seen in some cases of rheumatoid arthritis or serum sickness.

TASH (transcoronary ablation of septal hypertrophy).

TAT (thrombin-antithrombin III complex) **inhibitor**—a drug to treat HIV-positive patients.

tattooing of colonic neoplasms—endoscopic marking of intestinal lesions, most commonly with India ink, for subsequent localization during surgical resection or polypectomy surveillance.

Taussig-Bing anomaly—a congenital defect of the heart, characterized by complete transposition of the pulmonary artery in association with a ventricular septal defect. Symptoms may include cyanosis, dyspnea on exertion, severe pulmonary hypertension, systolic murmur, loud pulmonic second sound, and polycythemia. Incomplete bundle branch block or right ventricular hypertrophy may also be present.

Taut cystic duct catheters—several different types of catheters utilized for intraoperative cholangiography.

Taxus Express2—paclitaxel-eluting coronary stent system.

Taylor pinwheel—used in sensory examination in neurologic testing.

TBB (transbronchial biopsy).

TBNA (transbronchial needle aspiration).

TBP (total body pain)—a slang term referring to a patient with many severe but largely subjective complaints.

TBSA (total body surface area).

TBT (transcervical balloon tuboplasty).

TCA (trichloroacetic acid)—a topical treatment for human papillomavirus (genital warts).

TCA (tricyclic antidepressant).

TCCB (transitional cell carcinoma of the bladder).

TCCO (transcranial cerebral oximetry).

TCCS—see *transcranial color-coded sonography*.

TCD/CBDE (transcystic duct/common bile duct exploration)—performed via laparoscopy.

TCD (transcranial Doppler) **measurements**.

TCD (transcranial Doppler) **velocities**.

T-cell—thymus-derived lymphocyte, a part of the immune system. See *B-cell, T-4, T-8*.

T-cell function test—can detect lack of T4-helper (CD4) cell activity in fighting infection before counts actually start to diminish. It gives clinicians more information on their patients' actual immune status and aids in making the timing of antiviral treatment more effective.

TcHIDA ("tek-high-dah")—see *HIDA, PIPIDA*.

Tc 99m or **^{99m}Tc** (technetium). See *medications* and *technetium*.

TCN-P (triciribine phosphate)—chemotherapy drug.

TCP (total cavopulmonary connection) —the Fontan procedure preferred over atriopulmonary (AP) connection in recent studies. Patients having TCP are shown to recover with less exercise intolerance, perfusions, arrhythmia, thrombus, and protein-losing enteropathy (PLE) than patients having AP.

TCP/IP (transmission control protocol/ Internet protocol)—computer telecommunications term, also used in teleradiology.

TCPM pneumatic tourniquet system—for orthopedic procedures.

TCR (tear clearance rate) (Oph).

TCR (T-cell receptor) **peptide vaccine** —used in treatment of multiple sclerosis. It works by reducing specific T-cell populations in cerebrospinal fluid.

TCu380A IUD (intrauterine device).

T-cuts—for corneal astigmatism.

T'd ("teed")—a brief form used in operative procedures as a verb, referring to the extension of an incision in a T shape. Usage: "The pericardium was opened vertically and T'd horizontally, superiorly, and inferiorly."

TDD (thoracic duct drainage).

TD Glucose monitoring system—incorporates a small skin patch and electronic meter to monitor glucose levels. After the patch has been placed on the forearm for 5 minutes, a small electronic meter is held up to the patch and produces a glucose reading. The single-use patch is then removed and discarded.

t-dimer (thrombin dimer). It is very unlikely that what you hear is "t-dimer." See *D-dimer*.

TDOG (tissue Doppler gated) **dynamic three-dimensional ultrasound imaging**.

TDP (torsades de pointes).

TDS—slang abbreviation for a *technically difficult study* in radiology when the radiologist is unable to see all structures clearly.

TDS (treadmill duration score).

TE (echo time)—in magnetic resonance imaging, the interval between the first pulse in a spin-echo examination and the appearance of the resulting echo.

TEA (transluminal extraction atherectomy).

TEA (transepicondylar axis).

tear—see *Mallory-Weiss tear, retinal tear.*

tear clearance rate (TCR) (Oph).

teardrop sign—(1) a classic radiographic finding in blowout fractures of the orbit; the teardrop represents the herniated orbital contents, periorbital fat, and inferior rectus muscle; (2) a teardrop-shaped density, seen on x-ray, extending anteriorly from the ankle joint along the neck of the talus. It is diagnostic of ankle effusion.

Tearisol—artificial tears.

tear strips—see *Schirmer test.*

Tear-Trough implants—two varieties of Implantech facial implants.

tease—to separate tissues gently with a probe or other blunt instrument instead of cutting. Usage: "The adhesions were teased free (or teased off) the uterus."

Tebbetts rhinoplasty set—designed for open and closed rhinoplasty procedures. Includes an osteotome, alar stabilizing jig, speculums, and retractors.

teboroxime scan—a cardiac scan using radioactive imaging agent CardioTec (^{99m}Tc teboroxime) to show areas of myocardial infarction. Used for emergency scans, it clears rapidly from the blood to allow subsequent scans, if necessary.

TEC (transluminal extraction catheter).

TECAB (totally endoscopic coronary artery bypass).

tecadenoson—selective A1-adenosine receptor agonist drug, used to convert paroxysmal supraventricular tachycardia to normal sinus rhythm.

TECA (technetium albumin) **study.**

TechneScan MAG3—renal diagnostic imaging agent that uses technetium ^{99m}Tc mertiatide to determine kidney function.

technetium—an element, an isotope of which Tc 99m (^{99m}Tc) is used as a diagnostic aid in liver, brain, lung, and kidney scans. See *medications; radioisotopes.*

technetium pertechnetate (Tc 99m)—a tracer used in radionuclide studies for active gastrointestinal bleeding; this material labels red blood cells. If bleeding occurs in a period of up to 24 hours that the labeled red blood cells remain in the circulating blood, the tracer will extravasate and accumulate at or near the site. It is also used to demonstrate the presence of a Meckel diverticulum.

Techni-Care surgical scrub.

technique—see *operation.*

Techstar and **Techstar XL**—percutaneous vascular surgery system.

Techstar percutaneous closure device—also referred to as *Perclose closure device* (the manufacturer).

T.E.D. (thromboembolic disease) **stockings** or **hose**—antiembolism stockings. Trademark *T.E.D.* has periods.

TEE (transesophageal echocardiography)—see *Acuson V5M.*

"teed"—see *T'd.*

TEF (tracheoesophageal fistula).

Teflon-coated hollow-bore needle (ENT)—used in ear surgery.

Teflon paste injection for incontinence—a procedure in which injection of a Teflon paste (Polytef, Ethicon) into the periurethral tissues at the bladder neck is done on an outpatient basis to restore urinary control in incontinent women, particularly the elderly. The injection works by adding bulk to these tissues, compressing the urethral lumen and increasing the resistance to the outflow of urine.

Tegaderm transparent dressing—a waterproof dressing for wound and I.V. site coverage. Made by 3M.

Tegagel—hydrogel dressing and sheet.

Tegagen HG—alginate wound dressing.

Tegagen HI—alginate wound dressing.

Tegapore—contact-layer wound dressing.

tegaserod maleate ("te-GAS-a-rod") —see *Zelmac*; *Zelnorm*.

Tegasorb dressing—a hydrocolloid wafer dressing used in treatment of wounds, e.g., pressure ulcers (decubitus ulcers). These dressings are permeable to moisture vapor and to oxygen, so they permit oxygen exchange; but they are impermeable to bacteria, so they prevent contamination. These dressings are contraindicated in the presence of infection.

Tegner activity score—done pre- and postoperatively for knee reconstruction surgery.

Teichholz ejection fraction—used in echocardiogram.

T-8 cell—also called suppressor/cytotoxic cell. See *suppressor cell*.

Tekna mechanical heart valve.

Telangitron—a device used in the removal of telangiectases, cherry angiomas, and other small vascular blemishes and lesions.

TeleCaption decoder—allows hearing-impaired or deaf persons to read program captions on television.

telecurietherapy—radiotherapy.

telemedicine—a live, two-way audio/video exchange of medical information, education, and surgery procedures.

telepathology—transmission and interpretation of tissue specimens via remote telecommunication, generally for the purpose of diagnosis or consultation but also for continuing education.

teleradiology—the transmission of images from a local (transmitting) site to a remote (receiving) site for interpretation at the remote site.

Telescopic Plate Spacer (TPS)—expandable titanium spacer intended to replace one or two vertebral bodies that must be removed due to cancer, thus avoiding the destabilization of the spine that occurs due to corpectomy.

telesensor—Star Trek technology today, consisting of miniature computerized devices the size of a computer chip which attach to the body to sense vital signs and electrical conductivity of the skin and transmit the information to geographically distant receiving stations. Telesensors are developed for applications in medicine as well as the military.

Teletrast—an absorbable surgical gauze which contains a plastic thread that has been impregnated with barium sulfide, thus making it radiopaque. Among other applications, it is used in microvascular decompression to displace a vessel that is compressing the trigeminal nerve.

Teller acuity card (TAC)—used for acuity measurement in examination for macular heterotopia and for macular fold.

telogen—the resting phase of hair growth. See *anagen*.

telomerase—an enzyme produced by germ cells, bonc marrow stem cells, and tumor cells. It helps to prevent the attrition of telomeres (terminal sequences of chromosomes) during mitosis and confers immortality on a cell line.

telomerase reverse transcriptase, human (hTERT)—correlates with the development of adenoma and dysplasia of the esophagus.

telomere—a repeating sequence of double-stranded DNA at either end of a chromosome. As cells divide and differentiate throughout the lifespan of an organism or cell line, the occasional failure of a telomere sequence to be replicated during mitosis leads to gradual shortening of chromosomes. This genetic erosion plays an important part in normal aging and sets a natural limit on the number of times that such cells can undergo mitosis.

telophase—the final stage of cell division, beginning when the daughter chromosomes reach the poles of the dividing nucleus and continuing until cell division is complete.

TEM (transanal endoscopic microsurgery).

temporal arcade.

temporal instability—MRI term.

temporal squamosa (pars squamosa of the temporal bone)—the thin, flat anterior and superior part of the temporal bone.

temporomandibular joint (TMJ).

Tenckhoff—peritoneal dialysis catheter.

Tender Touch Ultra cup (Ob-Gyn)—a disposable, truncated, cone-shaped plastic cup constructed of silicone elastomer (a soft, pliable plastic), for vacuum-assisted deliveries.

tendinitis—*not* tendonitis.

tendo Achillis (or Achilles tendon).

tendon—the fibrous cord by which a muscle is attached. Cf. *tenon*.

10-EDAM—see *EDAM*.

Tendril DX—implantable pacing lead with a tip electrode that releases steroid upon entering the heart tissue. The steroid reduces inflammation, allowing for a lower voltage stimulation threshold.

Tendril SDX—steroid-eluting, active fixation pacing lead with a diameter of 6.2 French (less than 1/10 inch), allowing a less traumatic insertion procedure.

tenecteplase—see *TNKase*.

Tennant nuclear ball rotator (Oph).

Tennessee slider knot—used in arthroscopic repairs.

Tennison-Randall repair—for cleft lip.

Tennis Racquet catheter—used in angiography. This is a trade name, and the catheter does look like a tennis racquet.

tenofovir disoproxil fumarate and emtricitabine—see *Truvada*.

tenon (not tendon)—a projecting member in a piece of wood or other material for insertion into a mortise to make a joint. See *mortise*. Cf. *tendon*.

TENS (transcutaneous electrical nerve stimulation)—a nondrug, noninvasive, nonaddictive alternative for control of pain. It appears to enhance the concentration of beta-endorphins significantly. The TENS system consists of a small battery-powered stimulator with lead wires that attach to two or more surface electrodes. See *AdvanTeq II TENS, Eclipse TENS, Maxima II TENS, Stayoden 9000F TENS*, and *PENS*.

Tensilon test—for myasthenia gravis.

tension-free vaginal tape (TVT) **procedure**.

tensor fasciae latae—note the proper spelling of this muscle. The tensor fasciae latae lies on the lateral side of the thigh, enclosed between two layers of the fascia lata (note change in spelling with different usage) which form its sheath.

"ten-ten"—phonetic rendering of specific gravity value, 1.010. Specific gravity is always written as 1 followed by a decimal and three additional digits. Normal values range from 1.001 to 1.030.

tenting of hemidiaphragm—on chest x-ray, a distortion of the diaphragm by scarring, in which an upward-pointing angular configuration (like a tent) replaces all or part of the normal curved contour of a hemidiaphragm.

tenting sign—a simple test for severe dehydration; a pinched fold of skin will stay tented up.

10-20 System—see *International 10-20 System.*

Tenzel calipers—modification of Jameson calipers. Used to measure the eyelid crease.

TEOAE (transient evoked otoacoustic emission).

TEP (tracheoesophageal puncture).

TEP (totally extraperitoneal) **hernia repair**—identical to the TAPP (transabdominal preperitoneal) technique, but takes place in the preperitoneal space.

terahertz waves—new imaging technology that can peer inside living and inanimate objects and provide 3-D images.

teratogen—any agent or factor that causes, or increases the likelihood, of congenital malformations.

teratoma—a tumor containing tissues from all three embryonic germ layers, usually arising in a gonad (ovary or testis). Can be artificially induced by injection of stem cells into immunodeficient laboratory animals, in order to assess the pluripotency of the cells.

terb—slang for *terbutaline*.

Terlux—a plastic based on methylmethacrylate and other substances.

terminal sedation (TS)—palliative option for the terminally ill, along with VSED (voluntarily stopping eating and drinking), undertaken at the request of a mentally competent patient who is suffering consistent intolerable pain. See also *PAS*, *VAE*, and *VSED*.

termination codon—a codon (UAG, UAA, or UGA) that terminates the synthesis of a peptide or protein by preventing the addition of further amino acids.

terrible triad of the shoulder—concomitant presentation of rotator cuff tear, brachial plexus injury, and anterior shoulder dislocation. This combination of injuries most often occurs in patients over age 40.

Terrien degeneration—marginal thinning and degeneration of the upper nasal quadrants of the cornea.

Terry fingernail sign—see *Terry nails*.

Terry keratometer—enables surgeons to measure astigmatism while the patient is still on the operating table after surgery, and while the final wound closure is being accomplished.

Terry-Mayo needle (Urol)—a heavy, small Mayo needle.

Terry nails—white opaque ground-glass appearance of the nails proximally, with a normal pink area distally. Seen in cirrhosis of the liver and certain other liver diseases. Usage: "Terry nails are present, and he has some clubbing."

Terry-Thomas sign—see *David Letterman sign*.

Terry trephine—used in keratoplasty procedures.

Terson syndrome—characterized by vitreous hemorrhage with intracranial hemorrhage. Can include perimacular retinal folds. Previously described only in association with *shaken baby syndrome*.

tertiary contractions—on upper GI series, aberrant contractions of the esophagus, occurring after the primary and secondary waves of normal swallowing.

tertipara—a woman who has given birth three times (para 3).

Terumo dialyzer—for hemodialysis.

Terumo guidewire—used to pass strictures encountered during ERCP.

Terumo SteriCell processor trypan blue—dye exclusion test to measure bone marrow viability.

TES (thoracic endometriosis syndrome).

tesaglitazar—see *Galida*.

TES (*Toxocara* excretory secretory) **antigen**.

tesla (T)—SI unit of magnetic strength (used in MRI). The term *gauss* was formerly used.

Tesla system—imaging technique that facilitates brain scans on small babies, visualizing structures of the brain that were previously indiscernible.

test or **assay**—a quick-reference list of laboratory, neurologic, orthopedic, and other specialty tests. See also *classification, index, scale, scan, score*.

ACB (albumin cobalt binding)
Access AFP immunoassay system
Access Ostase serum-based
AccuPoint hCG Pregnancy Test Disk
acetowhite
acoustic stimulation
Actalyke activated clotting time (ACT)

test *(cont.)*

Adams
adenovirus
Ad7C cerebrospinal fluid
Advanced Care cholesterol
Affirm one-step pregnancy
Affymetrix GeneChip lab analysis
agarose gel electrophoresis (AGE)
agglutination
air conduction
Alamar Blue
AlaSTAT latex allergy
Alatest latex-specific IgE allergen
Albert Famous Faces Test
Albumin Cobalt Binding myocardial infarction screening
AMI panel
Alexagram breast lesion diagnostic
alkaline phosphatase antialkaline phosphatase (APAAP) antibody
Allen circulatory
Allen picture visual acuity
alpha-fetoprotein (AFP)
alpha-2 antiplasmin functional assay
alternans noninvasive cardiac diagnostic
AlzheimAlert
Amplicor *Chlamydia* Assay
Amplicor CT/NG
Amplicor *Mycobacterium tuberculosis*
Amplified *Mycobacterium tuberculosis* Direct (MTD)
amplified restriction fragment length polymorphisms (ARFLP)
Amsler grid
Ana-Sal saliva-based HIV
ANCA (antineutrophil cytoplasmic antibody)
androgen receptor mutation assay
anticytoplasmic antibody
antiendomysial antibody IgA
antigen enzyme immunoassay
Anti-MPO (p-ANCA) ELISA autoimmune

test *(cont.)*
Apo E
applanation tonometry
apprehension
Apt-Downey alkali denaturation
Aptima Combo 2
Aptima CT
arginine tolerance (ATT)
ASTY colorimetric microdilution panel
AtLast blood glucose monitoring
AUA symptom index
auramine-stained buffy coat smear
Autoclix blood glucose
Autolet blood glucose
AutoPap
Aware AccuMeter rapid HIV
AxSYM antibody to hepatitis C virus
AxSYM Free PSA
BAEP (brain stem auditory evoked potential)
BAER (brain stem auditory evoked response)
Bang horseshoe-crab blood
Bard BTA
Barlow hip dysplasia
Bates-Jensen pressure ulcer status tool
bcr/abl protein
BDProbeTec ET system
Bender Gestalt
bentonite flocculation
benzalkonium chloride patch
Berens 3-character (eye)
Berkson-Gage breast cancer survival rates
Berryhill functional capacity
Bielschowsky head tilt
BiliCheck
Bing auditory acuity
Biocept-5 pregnancy
Biocept-G pregnancy
Bioclot protein S assay
Biosafe PSA4

test *(cont.)*
BioStar strep A OIA Max
Bladder Tumor assay
Blessed Information Memory Concentration
bone conduction
Bonney
bounce home
BRACAnalysis comprehensive gene
brachial plexus tension (BPTT)
brain natriuretic peptide (BNP)
branched chain DNA assay
breath hydrogen excretion
breath pentane
Brief Neuropsychological Mental
Brief Pain Inventory (BPI)
bronchoprovocation
Brown-Brenn stain
Brown-Hopps stain
Bruininks-Oseretsky test of motor proficiency
BTA stat
BTA Trak urine assay
buccal smear
buffy coat smear
B-VAT (Baylor Visual Acuity test)
CA15-3 RIA
cake mix kit for hematopoietic progenitor assay
caloric test of vestibular function
Cambridge Biotech HIV-1 urine Western blot
c-ANCA (cytoplasmic antineutrophil cytoplasmic antibody)
capillary blood sugar
capillary electrophoresis
carbolfuchsin stain, Tilden
Cardiac STATus
Cardiac T rapid assay
Caring Behavior Assessment (CBA) tool
carotid sinus massage
carpal compression
C-cholyl-glycine breath excretion
cell assay

test *(cont.)*

Chemstrip bG
ChemTrak *Helicobacter pylori*
Cherry-Crandall serum lipase
Cholestech LDX system with the TC and glucose panel
Cholesterol Manager
Cholesterol 1,2,3
CholesTrak home cholesterol
chromopertubation
Chronic Pain Coping Inventory (CPCI)
CHST6 (carbohydrate sulfotransferase-6) gene assay
CIE (countercurrent immunoelectrophoresis)
CIWA-A (Clinical Institute Withdrawal Assessment–Alcohol)
Clancy circumduction-adduction shoulder maneuver
Clarke
Clinical Triage Instrument
clock-drawing
clonogenic assay
CLOtest (*Campylobacter*-like organism)
Coat-A-Count Free PSA IRMA
Coat-A-Count PSA IRMA
COBAS Amplicor HBV monitor
COBAS Amplicor HCV assay (or test)
coin
Colaris
cold water calorics
ColoCARE
colorectal cancer screening
Colorgene DNA hybridization
complement-dependent cytotoxicity (CDC) assay
complement fixation
complex tone
concealed straight leg raising
C1q assay
Confide HIV

test *(cont.)*

Copalis (coupled particle light scattering)
Copalis ToRC total antibody assay
Copalis treponemal antigen total antibody assay
copper-binding protein (CBP)
Core-Assure biopsy kit
corneal impression (CIT)
cotinine
Coulter HIV-1 p24 antigen assay
cover-uncover
cracker
cribogram
cross-chest adduction
cross-cover
cryocrit
C-terminal assay
CTFC (corrected TIMI frame count)
C-urea breath excretion
C-urinary excretion
Cybex
CYP2D6 drug screening
dark-field microscopy
D blood typing and antibody screening
DDT ([fluorescein] dye disappearance test)
Denver Developmental Screening
dermoscopy (dermatoscopy) using epiluminescent microscopy
DFA (direct fluorescent antibody)
Diagnex Blue
Diatest
Diff-Quick stain
Digene HIV RNA
digital movement analysis (DMA)
Dimension Free Prostate Specific Antigen (FPSA) Flex reagent cartridge
dipyridamole thallium stress
direct fluorescent antibody (DFA)
Directigen latex agglutination
Dix-Hallpike

test *(cont.)*
DNA ploidy analysis
DNA sequencing
Doppler perfusion index (DPI)
Downey texture discrimination
Draw-a-Bicycle (DAB)
Draw-a-Flower (DAF)
Draw-a-House (DAH)
Draw-a-Person (DAP)
drip and suction
DR-70 blood
duck waddle
duction
Dunlop synoptophore
Durkan CTS (carpal tunnel syndrome) gauge
dye exclusion
EAST
EDR (extreme drug resistance) assay
Efficacy Sources Inventory
EIA, EIA-2 (enzyme-linked immunoassay)
Elecsys Anti-HBs immunoassay
Elecsys PreciControl Anti-HBs
Elecsys proBNP immunoassay
electrochemiluminescence immunoassay (ECLIA)
electrotransfer
ELISA (enzyme-linked immunosorbent assay)
Ellestad treadmill stress
EMIT (enzyme-multiplication immunoassay)
empty can sign
endotoxin activity assay
Enfant pediatric vision testing
Entero-Test
Envacor
EP (evoked potential)
epiluminescence light microscopy (ELM)
Equate Legionella water
ER (evoked response)
ergonovine maleate

test *(cont.)*
estrogen receptor
$ETCO_2$
EUCAST
ExacTech blood glucose meter
exercise tolerance
extreme drug resistance (EDR) assay
EZ Detect
EZ-Screen Profile
Eysenck Personality Inventory
fabere
Factor III multimer
factor V Leiden mutation
fadir
Fagan
Family Assessment Measure III (FAM III)
Farr
Fastex proprioceptive and agility
FastPack System
FDT (fluorescein disappearance)
fecal occult blood (FOBT)
F_ECO_2
FEF_{25-75}
FemCard
FemExam TestCard
fern
Ferrans and Powers Quality of Life Index, Cardiac Version
fetal fibronectin (fFN)
Fick cardiac output
FILE (Family Inventory of Life Events and Changes)
finger-to-nose (F to N)
Finkelstein
First Check Ecstasy
Fisher exact
5'nucleotidase
FlexSure HP (*Helicobacter pylori*)
flocculation flow cytometry
flow cytometry crossmatch (FCXM)
Flu-Glow
FLU-OIA rapid

test *(cont.)*
Fluor-i-Strip
fluorescein dye disappearance (DDT)
fluorescein uptake
fluorescent cytoprint assay
foam stability
Folstein Mini-Mental Status Exam (MMSE)
FoodSCAN
foraminal compression (FCT)
forced oscillation technique (FOT)
14-3-3 assay
free beta
free PSA (prostate-specific antigen)
free/total PSA (prostate-specific antigen) index
Frick
FTA-ABS (fluorescent treponemal antibody absorption test for syphilis)
Fukuda
Functional Capacity Evaluation (FCE)
functional intact fibrinogen (FiF)
Gaenslen
gait and station
galactose-1-phosphate uridyl transferase
galvanic body sway (GBST)
Galveston Orientation and Amnesia Test (GOAT)
Gastroccult
GeneAmp PCR
GenESA System pharmacological stress
get-up-and-go
GGTP liver function
glabellar tap
glial fibrillary acidic protein (GFAP)
glove-juice technique
Glucatell test kit
Gluco-Protein
glycosylated hemoglobin

test *(cont.)*
Gomori (or Grocott) methenamine silver (GMS)
gonioscopy
Goodenough
GRASS
Gravindex pregnancy
guaiac
Gungor
Gurd criteria
Guthrie LEAP assay
Hallpike caloric stimulation
Hallpike-Dix maneuver
halo
Halstead-Wepman Aphasia Screening Test
HBV
HC II
HCV 3.0 Strip Recombinant Immunoblot Assay
HCV Super Quant RT-PCR assay
Heart Failure Knowledge Test
Heartsbreath
Heartscan heart attack prediction
heavy metal screening
heel-to-shin
heelstick hematocrit
Heinz body
Helisal rapid blood
HemaStrip-HIV 1 and 2
hematopoietic progenitor clonogenic assay
Hemoccult Sensa system
Hemoccult II
Hemochron high-dose thrombin time (HiTT)
HemoCue
heparin anti-XA assay
Heprofile ELISA
HercepTest
Heritage Panel
Herp-Check
hexagonal phospholipid
HI (hypopnea index)
High-Risk Hybrid Capture II HPV

test *(cont.)*
histoculture drug response assay (HDRA)
Histoplasma capsulatum polysaccharide antigen
HIV phenotype
HIVAGEN
HMB-435 melanosome
homocysteine
homogeneous gene assay system
horizontal adduction
Hot Sampler
Hpfast agar gel
H reflex electrodiagnostic
HRL color vision
H-SLAP (human stromelysin aggregated proteoglycan)
Humphrey frequency-doubling perimeter
Hybrid Capture II HBV
Hybrid Capture II *Neisseria gonorrhoeae*
Hybritech Tandem PSA ratio (free PSA/total PSA)
Hycor rheumatoid factor (RF) IgA ELISA autoimmune
HY-TEC automated diagnostic
HZA (hemizona)
ice water calorics
IDIF (indirect immunofluorescent assay)
^{125}I iothalamate GFRtest, intraoperative hourglass
IDI-Strep B
I-HAST (In-Home Alzheimer Screening Test)
iliopsoas
Illness Severity Instrument
Immulite assays and confirmatory kits for hepatitis
Immulite PSA assays
immunobead assay
ImmunoCard STAT! Rotavirus
ImmunoCyt
Immuno 1 complex PSA (cPSA)

test *(cont.)*
Impact assays
Incomplete Sentence Blank Test (ISB)
indirect fluorescent antibody (IFA)
Infant Distraction Test
Inform HER-2/neu gene-based
ink potassium hydroxide
InPath cervical cancer screening
!nSure fecal occult blood
Intercept oral fluid drug
intracavernous injection
intraoperative endoscopic Congo red
INVOS 2100 breast cancer
Ishihara color vision
islet cell antibodies screening (ICA)
Isletest and Isletest-ICA
Jaeger
Jamar grip
k82 ImmunoCap blood
KetoSite
Kleihauer
Kleihauer-Betke
Krimsky
Kruskal-Wallis
Kveim
Lachman
lamellar body number density
Landolt ring
LAP (leukocyte alkaline phosphatase)
latex agglutination
LDL Direct
Legionella Urinary Antigen (LUA) ELISA
leucine aminopeptidase
leukocyte esterase
Lezak Malingering Test
LifePoint Impact
Lifestream personal cholesterol monitor
lift-off
ligase chain reaction

test *(cont.)*
Limulus amoebocyte lysate (LAL)
lipid-laden macrophage index (LLMI)
litmus
liver function (LFT)
liver panel plus 9
Lp(a)
LRUT (locally made rapid urease)
Ludington
lung diffusion
Maddox rod
MAIPA (monoclonal-antibody-specific immobilization of platelet antigens) assay
Mallampati
Mancini plates
Mantoux tuberculosis
Master two-step
maternal serum alpha-fetoprotein (MSAFP)
Matles
Matritech NMP22 test for bladder cancer
Mayo Clinic system test for primary biliary cirrhosis
McNemar
MCT (motor control test)
Medical Outcomes Study–Social Support Network
Melastatin
mental status
Mentor BVAT
MEP (multimodality evoked potential)
MHA-TP (microhemagglutination test for *Treponema pallidum*)
Micral chemstrip
Micral urine dipstick
Microflo test strip for glucose monitoring
Micro-monitor
microsomal TRC (tanned red cells)
Mini-Mental State Examination (MMSE)

test *(cont.)*
Miniquant assay
Minnesota Multiphasic Personality Inventory (MMPI)
Minnesota Test for Differential Diagnosis of Aphasia
Miraluma
Mississippi Scale for Combat-Related Posttraumatic Stress Disorder (PSD)
Miyazaki-Bonney
modified rapid urease (RUT)
Moire topographic assessment
monoclonal antibody-based enzyme immunoassay
Monojector blood glucose
motor control (MCT)
multiple sleep latency (MSLT)
MultiVysion PB assay
MycoAKT latex bead agglutination for *Mycobacterium* detection
Myers-Briggs Personality Inventory
nail fold capillaroscopy
Nardi (morphine-Prostigmin)
NAT (nucleic acid testing)
Naughton cardiac exercise treadmill
Neo-EpCAM cancer detection kit
Neurobehavioral Cognitive Status
N-geneous HDL cholesterol
N High Sensitivity CRP (C-reactive protein) assay
NicCheck-I
Nirschl scratch
N-MID osteocalcin ELISA
NMP22 urinary marker
NT-proBNP immunoassay
nuclear contour index (NCI) on blood lymphocytes
nucleic acid-based crosslinking assay
nucleic acid sequence-based amplification assay
nucleic acid testing (NAT)
Nuremberg Activities Inventory (NAI)

test *(cont.)*
Nymox urinary
O&P (ova and parasites)
octopus peripheral vision
octopus visual field
OligoDetect
Oliver-Rosalki serum CPK
ophthalmodynamometry
ophthalmoscopy
Opus cardiac troponin I assay
OralScreen 3-panel oral fluids
OraQuick HIV-1 antibody
OraSure
OraTest
Ortho HCV 2.0 ELISA
osmolality
Ostase biochemical marker of bone turnover
Osteo-Gram
Osteomark
Osteomark NTx assay
Osteopatch transdermal patch
otoacoustic emission (OAE)
Ouchterlony double diffuse
ox cell hemolysin
oxytocin challenge (OCT)
pad urinary incontinence
Pain Assessment and Intervention Notation (P.A.I.N.) tool
PainBuster disposable infusion pain management kit
pANCA (perinuclear antineutrophil cytoplasmic antibody)
PapNet
Pap Plus HPV Screen
Paragon immunofixation electrophoresis
PASAT (paced auditory serial addition task)
past-pointing
patellar apprehension
Pathfinder DFA
Patrick (fabere)
PCR (polymerase chain reaction)
peak expiratory flow rate (PEFR)

test *(cont.)*
PEFR (peak expiratory flow rate)
pentagastrin stimulated analysis
periodic acid-Schiff (PAS)
Persantine thallium stress
Phadiatop
PharmChek
PHA skin
Phalen
photocrosslinking oligonucleotide hybridization assay
pilocarpine iontophoresis
pivot-shift
PLAC
Polateset vision
polymerase chain reaction (PCR)
Porvidx
posteromedial pivot shift
PP-CAP IgA enzyme immunoassay
PPD skin
PPL skin
PRA (plasma renin activity)
PRA-STAT
Preadmission Acuity Inquiry (PAI) tool
preimplantation genetic diagnosis (PGD) and screening
Premier type-specific HSV-1 ELISA
Premier type-specific HSV-2 IgG ELISA
PreVue *Borellia burgdorferi* antibody detection assay
PRIME-MD (computerized version of Primary Care Evaluation of Mental Disorders)
Profile–ER
Prometheus First Step
prostate cancer detection
prostate-specific antigen (PSA) free/total index
Protocult
PSA (prostate-specific antigen) index
PSA4 home blood

test *(cont.)*
PSY Inventory
P300 dementia
Pylori Fiax assay
Pylori Stat assay
PyloriTek
Pyrilinks-D urinary assay
PYtest
Q-beta replicase
QSART (quantitative Sudomotor Axon Reflex Test)
QualiCode *Borrelia burgdorferi* IgG and IgM Western blot kits
Quanticyt (quantitative cytology)
QuantiFERON-TB (QFT)
quantitative muscle strength testing (QMST)
quantitative sudomotor axon reflex (QSART)
Quantiplex HBV-DNA quantification assay
Quantiplex HIV RNA assay
Quantiplex HIV-RNA quantification assay
Queckenstedt
quellung reaction
QuestDirect
QuesTests
Quetelet BMI index
QuICCC (Questionnaire for Identifying Children with Chronic Conditions)
QuickVue *Chlamydia*
QuickVue influenza
QuickVue one-step *H. pylori*
radioallergosorbent (RAST)
radionuclide esophageal transit (RETT)
Raji cell assay
RAMP Reader
Randot
Rapid Drug Screen
rapid HIV
Rapid Susceptibility Assay
recombinant immunoblot assay (RIBA)

test *(cont.)*
rapid plasma reagin (RPR)
RAPP (Routine Assessment of Patient Progress)
RAST test for measuring atopy
recombinant immunoblot assay
refraction
Reitman-Frankel SGOT and SGPT
renin
repair chain reaction
RET gene
reverse transcription-polymerase
Rey and Taylor Complex Figure
Rey Auditory Verbal Learning
Rheolog
Rhodes Inventory of Nausea and Vomiting
RIBA (recombinant immunoblot assay)
RIGScan CR49 test for colorectal cancer detection
Rinne
RISA (radioactive iodinated serum albumin)
Road Interview
Roche-Microwell Plate Hybridization Method
roentgen stereophotogrammetric analysis (RSA)
Romberg
Roos
Rorschach
Rotazyme diagnostic
RPR (rapid plasma reagin)
RPR-CT (rapid plasma reagin circle card test)
rule of 100
RUT (rapid urease test)
SalEst system
saliva ovulation
sandwich nucleic acid hybridization assay
Schiller
Schirmer
Schwartz

test *(cont.)*
- scotopic sensitivity screening, whole-field
- sed rate (sedimentation rate)
- Seidel
- self-blood glucose monitoring (SBGM)
- Sellin
- Sensory Organization Test (SOT)
- SEP (somatosensory evoked potential)
- SER (somatosensory evoked response)
- serum pepsinogen
- serum protein electrophoresis
- 7C Gold urine
- Sex After MI Knowledge Test
- Sgambati test for peritonitis
- shake
- Short-Form Health Survey, 36-item (SF-36) and 12-item
- short wavelength autoperimetry
- Sibley-Lehninger serum aldolase
- SIBS (social interaction between siblings) interview
- Sickledex
- Sigma CPK
- signal amplification technique
- simkin analysis
- sink
- Sitzmark study
- 6-minute walk distance, 6-minute walking (6MWT)
- Skindex questionnaire, revised
- slit-lamp
- slump
- SLUScan for Your Heart
- SMAC
- SMA-6
- SMA-12
- SMA-18
- SMA-20
- Snellen chart
- sniff
- S-100 antibody

test *(cont.)*
- Sonksen-Silver acuity cards
- SpectRx
- Speed
- squeeze
- Stamey
- State-Trait Anxiety Inventory
- St. George Respiratory
- Stiman
- StoneRisk profile
- straight leg raising (SLRT)
- Stratus cardiac troponin I
- streptokinase-streptodornase (SK-SD)
- Strobel formula for evaluation of gastroesophageal reflux
- Strobel method of detecting vitamin A in breast milk
- Strong-Campbell Vocational Interest Inventory (SCVII)
- suction
- Super Quant assay
- super stress
- surf (surfactant)
- sweat chloride
- Symptom Checklist-90 Revised (SCL-90-R)
- talar tilt
- tandem mass spectrometry
- tanned red cells (TRC)
- T-cell function
- Teller acuity cards
- Tensilon
- tenting
- Tes-Tape urine glucose
- Test of Incremental Respiratory Endurance (TIRE)
- TestPackChlamydia
- thallium stress
- Thayer-Martin gonorrhea
- Thematic Apperception Test (TAT)
- ThinPrep and ThinPrep 2000
- ThinPrep Pap
- 36-Item Short Form Health Survey
- Thompson

test *(cont.)*
- Thorn
- three-tube stool set
- Thrombus Precursor Protein (TpP)
- thyrocalcitonin for pheochromocytoma
- thyroperoxidase antibody
- thyroxine radioisotope assay (T_4RIA)
- ThyroTest for hypothyroidism
- tilt
- tine
- tiptoe
- tissue pO_2 diagnostic study
- Titmus
- T-lymphocyte subset ratio
- Toronto Hospital Alertness Test
- touch prep analysis
- TOVA ("toe-vah") (Test of Variables of Attention)
- *Toxocara* ELISA
- TPMT (thiopurine methyltransferase) level
- TpP (thrombus precursor protein)
- Tracer Blood Glucose
- Trail Making Test
- TRAx ELISA assay
- treadmill
- Triage BNP
- Triage cardiac system
- T.R.U.E. (thin-layer rapid use epicutaneous) allergen patch
- T water fructose intolerance
- tyramine test for pheochromocytoma
- tyrosine tolerance
- Tzanck
- UBT breath
- Uni-Gold *H. pylori*
- Unterberger
- Unterberger-Fukuda stepping
- uPM3 urine
- upper limb tension (ULTT)
- Uricult dipslide
- Uriscreen

test *(cont.)*
- Urocyte diagnostic cytometry
- van den Bergh
- VAP cholesterol
- VDRL
- Velogene rapid MRSA assay
- Velogene rapid TB assay
- Velogene rapid VRE assay
- VEP (visual evoked potential)
- VER (visual evoked response)
- Verdict-II
- Versant HCV RNA 3.0 assay (bDNA)
- vertebral artery
- VEX (vasodilator plus exercise) treadmill
- ViraPap
- ViraSTAT immunofluorescence assay
- Virgo Anti-Cardiolipin screening kit
- Visidex, Visidex II
- visual field
- Visual Neglect
- Vitros immunodiagnostic
- von Kossa calcium
- Vysis PathVysion
- Vysis UroVysion DNA probe assay
- Wada
- WAST (Woman Abuse Screening Tool)
- WAST-Short form
- Watts Sexual Function Questionnaire
- Weber
- Wellcogen latex agglutination
- WEST (Weinstein Enhanced Sensory Test)
- Westergren sedimentation rate
- Western blot electrotransfer
- Wide Range Achievement Test (WRAT)
- wing
- Wirt stereo
- Wisconsin Card Sorting
- Wood light

test *(cont.)*
Worth four-dot (W4D)
Wroblewski serum LDH
YeastOne colorimetric antifungal panel
Yergason
zona hamster egg
ZstatFlu

testicular interstitial fluid (TIF).

Testim—testosterone drug replacement gel.

testisin—a novel serine protease expressed by premiotic testicular germ cells, a cancer target.

Test of Incremental Respiratory Endurance (TIRE)—software used in conjunction with equipment to test a spontaneously breathing patient's respiratory endurance.

TestPackChlamydia—a quick office test for *Chlamydia* based on enzyme-linked immunosorbent assay. No spaces in trademark.

testosterone—see *Testim.*

testosterone gel—see *Fortigel.*

TET (tubal embryo transfer).

tethered cord syndrome—seen when an area of the spinal cord is firmly caught up in scar tissue or between vertebrae.

tetracaine, adrenaline (epinephrine), and cocaine (TAC). See *TAC.*

tetralogy of Fallot ("fal-lo")—complex of four congenital cardiac anomalies: pulmonary stenosis, ventricular septal defect, dextroposition of the aorta, and right ventricular hypertrophy. Cf. *Fallot pentalogy, Fallot trilogy*. See also *pink tetralogy of Fallot*.

Tetrax interactive balance system—used for posturography evaluation of central and peripheral neurologic disturbances.

tet spell—medical slang for a "spell typical of tetralogy of Fallot."

TEVs (tissue-engineered blood vessels)—a new source for replacement blood vessels in vascular surgery. It is a matrix of vascular smooth muscle embedded in fibrin gels.

Texas Scottish Rite Hospital (TSRH).

TFC (threaded fusion cage)—see *Ray threaded fusion cage.*

TFC (triangular fibrocartilage).

TFCC (triangular fibrocartilaginous complex)—a structure in the wrist that may exhibit thinning in patients with gymnast's wrist.

TFCI (transient focal cerebral ischemia).

TFD—see *tight fingertip dilated.*

TFL (tensor fasciae latae).

T-4 cell—the cell specifically attacked by the HIV virus. Called helper/ inducer T-cell.

TFPI (tissue factor pathway inhibitor).

TGA (transposition of the great arteries).

The Female Condom—*see Female Condom, The.*

TGF-B (transforming growth factor-beta)—a protein found to promote bone healing and now used in treatment of nonunion of fractures, as a bone graft material, and to promote ingrowth of tissue into a hip prosthesis.

T-graft configuration technique—a new technique in coronary artery bypass graft surgery using arteries from both the arm and chest to form a T-shaped conduit around the diseased portions of the heart. It is said to offer patients hope for longer-lasting bypasses with reduced chances for postoperative infections.

TG-60 dosimetry parameters—dosing protocol for Novoste Beta-Cath 90Sr/Y source trains for intravascular brachytherapy.

THA (total hip arthroplasty).

ThAIRapy Vest—portable device that utilizes high-frequency chest wall oscillation (HFCWO) to provide airway clearance. The vest is linked to an air pulse generator which inflates and deflates the vest from 5 to 25 times per second, gently squeezing the thorax and creating high expiratory air flow within the lungs, moving mucus toward the larger airways for clearance by coughing. See also *ABI Vest airway clearance system.*

thallium SPECT (thallium 201 single-photon emission computed tomographic) **imaging**—evaluates the presence and extent of myocardial perfusion defect. Also used in stroke and other neurological assessment.

thallium stress test—used to reveal the presence and extent of coronary artery disease by comparing blood flow in the heart during treadmill exercise with the blood flow at rest. Thallium is taken up by the heart in direct proportion to the blood flow, and images of areas of the heart showing thallium retention delineate the areas of arterial blockage. The radioisotope used is thallium 201 (Tl-201).

Thal repair of esophageal stricture.

Thayer-Martin culture medium—used in testing for *Neisseria gonorrhoeae*.

THC:YAG laser (thulium, holmium, chromium: YAG crystal)—performs a sclerostomy to reduce intraocular pressure in uncontrolled glaucoma.

THE (transhepatic embolization).

theca cell—found in the ovary after ovulation, derived from nurse cells surrounding the developing egg.

theca lutein cyst (of the ovary)—caused by high HCG (human chorionic gonadotropin) levels in molar pregnancies.

The Closer—see *Closer, The.*

thelarche—the beginning of breast development.

Thelin (sitaxsentan sodium)—investigational drug used in the treatment of pulmonary arterial hypertension.

Thematic Apperception Test (TAT)—mental status examination.

Therabite jaw motion rehabilitation system—a device designed for patients with reduced jaw movement or jaw hypomobility following surgery and/or radiation treatment. It helps patients open their mouths, encourages healing, improves speech, and promotes better oral hygiene.

Thera-Boot compression dressing or wrap.

TheraCLEC-Total—a treatment for pancreatic insufficiency, a condition that affects most people with cystic fibrosis.

Thera Cool cold therapy—used to treat postoperative pain and swelling as well as during rehabilitation.

TheraGym exercise balls—used for improving gross motor control, range of motion, muscle tone, and balance by both pediatric and adult orthopedic patients.

Theralux—ex vivo photodynamic therapy, currently being evaluated in three therapeutic areas: the prevention of acute graft-versus-host disease (aGvHD), the purge of cancerous cells from bone marrow transplants in non-Hodgkin lymphoma, and the treatment of chronic GvHD and other autoimmune diseases by extracorporeal photochemotherapy.

therapeutic cloning—creation by somatic cell nuclear transfer of a

therapeutic *(cont.)*
clonal embryo, which is induced to divide until the blastocyst stage, during which embryonic stem cells are harvested from the inner cell mass.

therapeutic lifestyle changes (TLC)—a combination of changes including diet, exercise, stress control, etc., recommended by the ATP I, II, and III guidelines for patients with obesity and elevated cholesterol.

therapy
ablative therapy with bone marrow rescue
ActiPatch
Activa dystonia stimulation
active specific immunotherapy (ASI)
adaptive cellular (RIGS/ACT)
Advanced Chronic Heart Failure Clinical Assessment of Immune Modulation Therapy (ACCLAIM)
antegrade scrotal sclerotherapy
aversion
balloon brachytherapy
balloon photodynamic
Bead Block
Blinkeze external lid weights treatment for lagophthalmos
brachytherapy
breast-conserving (BCT)
cardiac shock wave (CSWT)
cell-based
CeQUAL protocol
cervical nerve root block (CNRB)
chelation
circulator boot
ClearLight
cognitive behavior (CBT)
continuous renal replacement (CCRT)
coronary radiation (CRT)
craniosacral (CST)
crossfire radiation
CVEMC chemotherapy protocol

therapy *(cont.)*
CyberKnife radiosurgery
Cyriax physiotherapy
cytoablative
therapy, deep brain stimulation
Dornier Epos Ultra
D-Prevent circulatory
dynamic conformal
electrochemotherapy
electron beam intraoperative radiotherapy (EBIORT)
electroporation
embolotherapy
endolaser venous (ELVT)
endoscopic cryotherapy
endoscopic injection (EIT)
endoscopic variceal sclerotherapy (EVS)
episcleral plaque brachytherapy
external beam radiation (EBRT)
Enterra therapy
Enteryx procedure
extracorporeal photochemotherapy (ECP)
ex vivo liver-directed gene
feedback microwave thermotherapy
Flutter chest percussion
Foscan (temoporfin) mediated photodynamic
fractionated stereotaxic radiation
Galileo intravascular radiotherapy
gamma-ribbon radiation
gastric electrical stimulation
gene
gene-silencing (GST)
Gerson
Giraffe Spot PT Lite phototherapy
GliaSite radiation
HAART (highly active antiretroviral)
HDR (high-dose-rate) brachytherapy
helmet-molding
HHH or triple-H (hypertensive hypervolemic hemodilution)
home ambulatory inotropic

therapy *(cont.)*
HS-tk gene
hyperbaric oxygen
IGRT (image-guided radiation therapy)
IMRT (intensity modulated radiation)
inotropic
intralesional laser
intraoperative high-dose-rate (IOHDR) brachytherapy
intraoperative radiation (IORT)
intraoperative radiotherapy (IORT)
intraperitoneal hyperthermic chemotherapy (IPHC)
intravascular red light (IRLT)
lens-sparing external beam radiation (LSRT)
LITT (laser-induced thermotherapy)
liver-directed ex vivo gene
maternal blood clot patch
McKenzie extension exercises
meridian
microvascular (MVT)
microwave thermoradiotherapy
monodrug
neoadjuvant hormonal (NHT)
Novoste Beta-Cath brachytherapy
osteomanipulative (chiropractic)
palladium 103 brachytherapy
pancreatic enzyme
panretinal photocoagulation (PRP) and focal laser
percutaneous sclerotherapy
permanent brachytherapy
photodynamic (PDT)
photon stimulation (PST)
phytotherapy
Prolieve transurethral microwave
prolotherapy
ProstaLund feedback treatment (PLFT)
ProstRcision treatment
pulsed dose
pulsed dye laser

therapy *(cont.)*
pulsed electromagnetic field (PEMF)
QUART (quadrantectomy, axillary dissection, and radiotherapy)
recombinant enzyme replacement
remote afterloading brachytherapy (RAB)
remote brachytherapy
RIGS/ACT (adaptive cellular therapy)
rush immunotherapy
sacral nerve stimulation (SNS) therapy
SAFHS (sonic-accelerated fracture healing system)
SeedNet cryotherapy
sham
single-field hyperthermia combined with radiation
skeletal targeted radiotherapy (STR)
SMART (surgical myomectomy as reproductive)
SmartBeam radiotherapy
somato-emotional release (SER)
sonic-accelerated fracture healing system (SAFHS)
Sonocur Basic system
stereotaxically guided interstitial laser
Swiss ball
TAPET (tumor amplified protein expression)
Thera Cool cold
Theralux
Theralux ex vivo photodynamic
ThermaChoice uterine balloon
Thermoflex water-induced thermotherapy (WIT)
tracheal toilet
Trager
transpupillary thermotherapy
transurethral microwave thermotherapy (TUMT)
triple-H therapy (hypertensive hypervolemic hemodilution)

therapy *(cont.)*
- Trojan horse technique
- ultrasound-guided compression
- Urowave thermotherapy
- uterine balloon
- vacuum-assisted negative pressure wound
- vascular brachytherapy
- VAX-D (vertebral axial decompression)
- ventricular resynchronization
- water-induced thermotherapy (WIT)

TheraSeed—an alternative permanent implant with a 17-day half-life. A palladium 103 (Pd-103) active isotope in a titanium capsule, it is used in the treatment of rapidly growing tumors.

Thera-Soft hand/wrist orthosis—used for wrist drop and finger contraction.

TheraSphere—nonsurgical outpatient therapy that uses microscopic glass beads to deliver radiation therapy treatment for inoperable hepatocellular carcinoma.

ThermaChoice uterine balloon therapy—treatment for excessive menstrual bleeding. It can be performed on an outpatient basis under local anesthesia. A balloon catheter is inserted vaginally and inflated with a small amount of sterile fluid, after which a heating element inside the balloon raises the temperature to approximately 87° Celsius for a total of 8 minutes. The result is thermal ablation of the uterine lining. Also, Thermachoice III uterine balloon.

ThermaCool system—a nonlaser radiofrequency device used in facial rejuvenation without invasive surgery. It heats the lower layers of the skin and may tighten the skin and improve skin texture. In addition, it may dramatically improve the skin of patients with acute cystic acne.

Therma Jaw (or Thermajaw) **hot urologic forceps**—allows simultaneous tissue sampling and electrocoagulation of a biopsy site, eliminating the need for exchange of instruments through a flexible cystoscope.

Thermal Angel—a blood and IV fluid infusion warming device, portable and disposable.

Thermaline—malleable multielectrode surgical ablation system with fluid-cooled and bipolar options.

thermal quenching—a cooling technique that protects the skin during laser treatments for hair removal or vascular lesions.

thermistor—a type of thermometer that registers very small changes in temperature. Usage: "Respiratory parameters were monitored by nasal and oral thermistor and abdominal and chest wall strain gauges."

thermistor-plethysmography (Cardio).

ThermoChem-HT system—used in intraperitoneal hyperthermic chemotherapy (IPHC). It heats fluids (chemotherapy agents) and recirculates them into the peritoneal cavity to treat GI and other cancers within the peritoneal cavity.

thermodilution catheter—specially designed, triple-lumen Swan-Ganz catheter. One lumen is used to inject a cold solution to measure cardiac output. See *thermodilution technique*.

thermodilution technique—to obtain numerical values to calculate cardiac output. Following injection of a cold solution (saline, 5% dextrose in water, or autologous blood) into the right atrium, a change in temperature of the circulating blood can be detected by a temperature-sensitive catheter in the pulmonary artery.

Thermoflex system—a water-induced thermotherapy (WIT) system for the treatment of benign prostatic hyperplasia and associated urinary obstruction.

Thermo Fuel—ready-to-drink energy beverage.

Thermophore—moist heat pads for external application of heat, to relieve pain.

Thermoscan Pro-1-Instant thermometer—able to obtain a reading in just two seconds using infrared technology. Using a special speculum which fits into the ear canal, the thermometer accurately reflects the body core temperature because of its closeness to the tympanic membrane. An aural temperature reading is unlike oral readings which can be affected by eating, drinking, or smoking.

Thermoskin arthritic knee wrap—a heat retainer with a Trioxon lining used to help ease the pain and discomfort of arthritis sufferers. The heat retainers are also available for the back, hand/wrist, ankle, and elbow areas.

Thermo-STAT—a new arm-cuff device that speeds delivery of heat to the heart and internal organs of patients who develop hypothermia during surgery.

TherOx 0.014 infusion guidewire—used primarily in percutaneous transluminal coronary angioplasty (PTCA). It also provides site-specific delivery of drugs or fluids into the coronary arteries.

The Sensar—see *Sensar.*

The Unfolder—see *Unfolder.*

THI needle—used in cardiac surgery to express air from the ventricle.

Thiersch-Duplay urethroplasty.

Thiersch graft—a delayed pedicle skin graft.

Thiersch suture.

thigh-high antiembolic stockings—see *stockings*.

thin-layer chromatography screen—an analytic technique used to screen serum or urine samples for poisons or drugs of abuse.

ThinLine EZ—a bipolar cardiac pacing lead.

ThinPrep, **ThinPrep Pap**, **ThinPrep 2000**—screening tests for cervical cancer, which may replace the conventional Pap smear. The FDA supports the claim that ThinPrep improves the detection of low-grade lesions by 65% and reduces the number of inadequate specimens by more than 50%. It assures uniformity of slide samples.

ThinProfile eyelid implants—see *SutureGroove gold eye weights*.

THINSite dressing—multilayer dressing that has an extremely low profile and will conform to almost any body contour.

THINSite with Biofilm—hydrogel topical wound dressing used to treat pressure ulcers, arterial and venous stasis ulcers, and dermal wounds.

thiopurine methyltransferase (TPMT).

third intercondylar tubercle of Parsons (TITP)—frequent and prominent in patients with osteoarthritis of the medial FTJ (femorotibial joints) and prominent tibial spines. TITP is also known as *Parsons knob* or *Parsons tubercle*, depending on size.

third spacing—movement of fluids in the body into the third space (not the vascular space, in the blood vessels, and not inside cells, in the intracellular space). This interstitial fluid can be in one organ or systemic, and can

third *(cont.)*
be caused by lymphatic blockage, increased capillary permeability, or lowered plasma proteins.

13-cis retinoic acid, 13cRA.

13q deletion syndrome (46 Dr or 46 Dq)—due to a deletion of the long arms of chromosome 13 (one of the group D chromosomes). The syndrome may include mental retardation and physical retardation, broad nasal bridge, large and prominent low-set ears, facial asymmetry, hypertelorism, ptosis, epicanthus, microcephaly, microphthalmia, imperforate anus, and a number of other anomalies.

34-day supply—the standard amount of prescription medicine allowed by many health insurance programs is 34 days' worth. Apparently the idea is that it gives the patient enough for every day of a 31-day month plus 3 days to allow for weekends and other obstacles to prompt refilling of the prescription.

36-Item Short Form Health Survey (SF-36)—used to measure personal evaluation of health and levels of well-being.

Thomas needle—used for bone marrow biopsy and aspiration.

Thomas shunt—vascular access shunt used in performing dialysis.

Thomas splint.

Thom flap—laryngeal reconstruction.

Thompson test—Achilles tendon test. With the foot at rest, compression of the calf (gastrocnemius) muscle causes ankle flexion if the Achilles tendon is intact. Usage: "The Achilles tendon is intact by Thompson test."

thoracic duct drainage (TDD)—being evaluated as an adjunct to classical immunosuppression (preoperatively) in the prevention of early rejection of organ transplants.

thoracic endometriosis syndrome (TES)—deposition of endometrial tissue in the pleuropulmonary organs. There is a significant association between the presence of pelvic endometriosis and TES. Chest pain is the presenting symptom, and pneumothorax is the most common manifestation.

thoracic OPLL (ossification of the posterior longitudinal ligament)—a rare entity causing thoracic myelopathy. One of the well-known causes of cervical radiculomyelopathy.

thoracic Schober test—term used in assessing ankylosing spondylitis.

thoracic splenosis—a rarely encountered condition, consisting of multiple pleural-based nodules that are most often identified accidentally on routine chest x-rays. The splenic nodules may mimic neoplasms radiographically.

thoracolumbar burst fractures (Ortho).

thoracolumbosacral (TLSO) **brace**.

thoracophrenolaparotomy—minimally invasive surgery involving entry into the thorax and abdomen around the diaphragm.

thoracoscopic apical pleurectomy—for treatment of SBSP (simultaneous bilateral spontaneous pneumothorax). Also, thorascopic.

thoracoscopic microwave epicardial AF (atrial fibrillation) **ablation**.

thoracoscopic talc pleurodesis—performed under local anesthesia for treatment of SBSP (simultaneous bilateral spontaneous pneumothorax). Also, thorascopic.

Thoralon—biomaterial used in Aria coronary artery bypass graft for patients with few or no suitable native vessels.

Thora-Port—used for safe insertion of thoracoscopic instruments.

Thoraseal—a drainage system for the chest cavity.

Thoratec ventricular assist device (VAD)—provides mechanical circulatory support via left or right ventricle or both. The patient's blood is diverted from the failing ventricle into the assist device, which pumps the blood back to the body, simulating the function of the heart. Two blood-pumping sacs, one for each side of the heart, are attached to the body and tethered to a machine the size of a ventilator. This is not a permanent solution; what it does is "buy time" until the heart recovers (if it can) or until a suitable donor heart becomes available.

Thorel bundle—a bundle of muscle fibers in the heart that connects the sinoatrial and atrioventricular nodes.

Thorn test—a test of uric acid excretion, and also a test to help in the diagnosis of Addison disease.

Thornton adjustable positioner (TAP) —simple and apparently effective oral appliance for the treatment of snoring and obstructive sleep apnea. Custom molded from each patient's dental impressions, the TAP is a small plastic device similar to an orthodontic retainer that is worn in the mouth during sleep. By adjusting the appliance to reposition the jaw, soft throat tissue is prevented from obstructing the airway, eliminating snoring and improving breathing.

Thornton double corneal ruler (Oph).

Thornton 360° arcuate marker—used during corneal surgery and during keratotomy for astigmatism.

Thornwaldt cyst (also, *Tornwaldt*)—can be seen on CT scan as a mass high in the nasopharynx, midline between the longus capitis muscles, or just off midline. It may contain only fluid, but sometimes there is a calcification within it.

THORP (titanium hollow-screw osseointegrating reconstruction plate) **system**—screws and plates for alloplastic mandibular reconstruction.

THR (total hip replacement).

threaded interbody fusion cage—hollow cylinder packed with bone graft material and implanted between the vertebrae to facilitate spinal fusion.

thread lift (Derm)—minimally invasive lifting procedure of the face that entails smaller incisions and can be performed by a dermatologic surgeon using local anesthesia. It uses specially designed threads to support the soft tissue upwards. The procedure is achieved by placing Aptos or anti-drooping suturing threads underneath the skin surface. These serve as a truss to elevate a drooping jowl, brow, or cheek pad. The thread has bidirectional knotlike barbs that hook tissue and lift it into place with more stability than conventional sutures. The thread can be gently tightened for added support. Also called *feather lift*.

threadwire saw—a new device for cutting bone.

3-D CEMRA (three-dimensional contrast-enhanced magnetic resonance angiography) **technique** using MR fluoroscopy and 3-D spiral recording of data acquisition—MRI term.

3-D FT (three-dimensional Fourier transform)—a less frequently used image reconstruction process in MRI than 2DFT.

3-D FT magnetic resonance angiography—noninvasive vascular imaging technique.

3-D gadolinium-enhanced MR angiography—for aortoiliac inflow assessment plus renal artery screening.

three-dimensional superficial liposculpture (3-D SLS)—liposuction of fat in the superficial and intermediate layers. It is associated with a more contoured look and greater skin retraction.

3-D IVUS (three-dimensional intravascular ultrasound).

3DKnee—artificial knee implant designed to provide increased knee strength, a higher and more consistent range of motion, and longer-term performance for total knee replacement patients.

3-D-MSI (magnetic source imaging).

3-Dscope—three-dimensional laparoscope said to cut operative time for complicated laparoscopic procedures by adding the third dimension of depth perception.

3-D SLS—see *three-dimensional superficial liposculpture*.

3-D SSP (3-D stereotaxic surface projection).

3-D time of flight magnetic resonance angiographic sequences (3-D TOF MR angiographic sequences).

3-D Turbo FLAIR (fluid-attenuated inversion recovery)—MRI technique that allows for better visualization of tissue structures because the imaging passes are actually interleaved rather than stacked.

3M Clean Seals—a waterproof protection bandage.

3-M syndrome—named for last initials of three researchers (J.D. Miller, V.A. McKusick, P. Malvaux) who were among the first to identify the disorder, characterized by low birth weight, dwarfism, abnormalities of the craniofacial area, distinctive skeletal malformations, and/or other physical abnormalities. It is thought to be inherited as an autosomal recessive genetic trait.

three-pillow or **two-pillow orthopnea**—refers to the number of pillows a patient must use to prop up in bed in order to sleep comfortably without difficulty breathing.

3-prong (or three-prong) **rake blade**—a self-retaining retractor blade.

3-Scape real-time 3-D imaging—used with Sonoline Elegra ultrasound platform to improve detection and characterization of organ tumors.

three-trocar technique of laparoscopic cholecystectomy—uses suture retraction of the gallbladder instead of a fourth trocar. Usage: "Monofilament nylon with a straight needle was inserted through the right seventh intercostal space in the anterior axillary line, and the seromuscular layer of the gallbladder fundus was punctured and retracted toward the anterior abdominal wall."

three-tube stool set—a laboratory screening procedure for *Salmonella* consisting of a triple sugar iron agar slant, lysine-iron agar slant, and a Christensen urea agar slant.

3 vag deliveries and 1 tab—slang for 3 vaginal deliveries and 1 therapeutic abortion.

THRIVE (T1 high resolution isotropic volume examination) **technique**—a

THRIVE *(cont.)* powerful new imaging sequence that combines a 3-D T1-weighted TFE sequence with SPIR fat suppression and SENSE, enabling fast, high-resolution imaging with large FOV coverage and excellent fat suppression in as short as a single 20-second breath hold.

Thrive Treatment Study—a study investigating ximelagatran or enoxaparin followed by warfarin.

thrombocidins—another term for human antimicrobial peptides.

thromboelastograph (TEG)—used to confirm coagulopathy such as that which occurs during liver resection. This allows for rapid diagnosis and institution of proper hemostatic treatment for platelet and coagulation factor abnormalities.

thromboembolic disease (TED).

thrombolytic assessment system (TAS) —a system about the size of a desktop calculator. It uses a disposable cord with a test well for a single drop of blood to perform coagulation studies. The card is encoded with the patient's ID number and the coagulation study results. It can also be linked to printers and computers for archiving and future retrieval.

ThromboScan MRU (molecular recognition units)—imaging agent combined with molecular recognition units to produce better scans.

thrombosis—formation or presence of thrombus. See *central splanchnic venous thrombosis* (CSVT); *deep venous thrombosis* (DVT)

ThromboSol—extends the shelf-life of transfusable platelets.

thrombotic thrombocytopenic purpura (TTP)—complication in AIDS patients.

thromboxanes (TxA_1 and TxB_2)—stimulators of platelet aggregation.

thrombus—a clot in the cardiovascular system. See also *thrombosis*.

Thrombus Precursor Protein (TpP)—test for early diagnosis of preeclampsia. Women with preeclampsia have lower levels of TpP in the second trimester, prior to onset of clinical manifestations.

thulium-holmium-chromium:YAG laser (THC:YAG laser).

thumb, gamekeeper's.

thumbprinting (Radiol)—indentations that look like thumbprints, seen radiographically on the surface of the colon in a barium enema. They are indicative of ischemic colitis or of hematoma formation on the bowel wall.

ThumZ'Up—a functional thumb splint consisting of a clear plastic shield over the base of the thumb and an elastic bandage that encircles the wrist and base of thumb. The splint holds the thumb in an upright position, such as when you give the "thumbs up" sign, hence the name. (Note apostrophe in trade name.)

thunderclap headache—a sudden, extremely painful, high-intensity headache (not migraine, tension, or cluster headache). The name is very descriptive. May indicate a brain aneurysm and impending rupture.

thymidylate synthase—expression of this substance might be useful in determining tumor response to 5-fluorouracil.

thymine—a pyrimidine (symbol T), one of the four bases found in DNA; in the formation of a double-stranded nucleic acid, it always pairs with the pyrimidine cytosine (C).

thyrocalcitonin—test for pheochromocytoma.

thyroid stare—see *Collier sign*.

thyroid storm—episode of heightened thyroid hormone activity due to sudden release of an abnormal amount of hormone into the circulation. A thyroid storm may be induced by stress or infection, or it may occur spontaneously. Symptoms are anxiety, rapid pulse, fear, high fever, restlessness, breathing problems, exhaustion. In severe cases, which may prove fatal, the patient may be delirious and then become comatose. Also, *thyroid crisis*.

thyroperoxidase (TPO)—a thyroid enzyme, present in over 95% of patients with malignant thyroid tumors.

thyroperoxidase antibody test—for thyroid disease.

thyroplasty type I (also called laryngoplasty)—used in treatment of unilateral vocal cord paralysis with resulting hoarseness or inaudibility. It involves placing a silicone implant through a "window" made in the thyroid cartilage. The implant pushes the paralyzed vocal cord medially to meet the functioning (moving) cord. The operation is performed under local anesthesia so the patient can phonate during the course of the procedure, and the surgeon can evaluate the quality of the patient's voice and assess the movement of the vocal cords. Thyroplasty types II and III are used to change tension of the vocal cord and the pitch of the voice. These are new procedures. The procedure previously in general use, the injection of Teflon into the vocal cord, is said to still be the treatment of choice for some debilitated or elderly people, but one of its disadvantages is that Teflon has been known to "migrate" and cannot easily be removed.

ThyroTest—a rapid assay for the detection of hypothyroidism. Results are available in 10 minutes from a whole-blood sample.

thyrothymic thyroid rests—rests of thyroid tissue entirely separate from the thyroid or extending from it in the area between the thymus and the thyroid. They may be mistaken for lymph nodes or parathyroids and may be clinically significant during thyroid surgery. Also *Reeve rests*.

thyrotoxicosis factitia—thyroid disease caused by the intake of excess thyroid medication. Also called *thyrotoxicosis medicamentosa*.

thyrotoxicosis medicamentosa—thyroid disease caused by the intake of excess thyroid medication. Also called thyrotoxicosis factitia.

thyroxine radioisotope assay (T_4RIA).

TI (inversion time)—MRI term.

TIA (transient ischemic attack)—cerebrovascular occlusion, in which the symptoms resolve within 24 hours. Cf. *CVA*.

tibial plateau—a flattened surface at the upper end of the anterior aspect of the tibia.

tic—involuntary repetitive muscle movement. See *Tourette syndrome and Gilles de la Tourette syndrome*. Cf. *tick*.

tick—a small bloodsucking arthropod; the lesion produced by its bite may cause anything from a small papule to a large ulcerating wound, with acute pain and swelling. See *Lyme disease*, which is transmitted by the deer tick. Cf. *tic*.

TICL—trademarked abbreviation for Toric implantable contact lens.

Ti-Cron (also TI-CRON)—surgical suture. Correct U.S. spelling is not *Tycron*, which appears to be a European spelling.

tidal volume—the amount of air exchanged with each breath. A respiratory response to exercise.

Tielle absorptive dressing.

Tiemann Meals tenolysis knife.

tiered-therapy programmable cardioverter-defibrillator (PCD).

"tie-sis"—see *phthisis*.

TIF (testicular interstitial fluid).

TIFF (tag image file format)—computer graphics format used in teleradiology.

tight asthmatic—an asthmatic with extreme difficulty breathing, that is, with extreme bronchospasm. Usage: "Examination revealed a very tight asthmatic, using accessory muscles, and breathing at 28. He had tight inspiratory and expiratory wheezing."

tight fingertip dilated (TFD)—refers to measurement of dilation of the cervical os at the beginning of the delivery process. Usage: "The cervical os was TFD."

Tikhoff-Linberg shoulder resection—used in bone and soft tissue sarcomas of proximal upper limb that do not involve nearby neurovascular structures. Resection includes distal clavicle, proximal humerus, and part or all of scapula, as well as adjacent muscles, while preserving the function of the forearm and hand. A skeletal prosthesis is used to preserve limb length and stabilize the arm to the chest. A TRAM (transverse rectus abdominis myocutaneous) flap may be used to ensure wound healing.

TIL (tumor-infiltrating lymphocytes).

Tillaux-Phocas syndrome—see *fibrocystic breast syndrome.*

tilt-table test (Cardio)—a test to identify and counsel patients who are likely to experience recurrent syncope. The patient is restrained on an electric tilt table. The table is tilted to a head-up position, an I.V. infusion of isoproterenol given, and the test is concluded at the end of a 10-minute head-up tilt or when the patient faints.

tilt test—a commonly used clinical tool for assessment of volume status with orthostatic change in pulse and blood pressure. It is particularly valuable in evaluating patients with hemorrhage, diarrhea, vomiting, and increased insensible fluid losses.

time
- acquisition
- activated coagulation (ACT)
- dilute Russell viper venom (dRVVT)
- Duke bleeding
- echo (TE)
- interpulse
- inversion (TI)
- Ivy bleeding
- relaxation
- renal transit (RTT)
- repetition (TR)
- Russell viper venom, dilute (dRVVT)
- tincture of (TOT)

time-of-flight echoplanar imaging (MRI term)—venous occlusion of the structure in question is carried out and released to augment blood flow and enhance visualization.

time-resolved imaging by automatic data segmentation (TRIADS).

TiMesh—titanium mesh bone-plate and screw system used for rigid fixation of bone fractures.

TIMI (thrombolysis in myocardial infarction).

timolol formulation—see *Istalol*.

Timoptic Ocumeter—single-dose eye drops for glaucoma.

tincture of time (TOT)—physician jargon. It's a physician's way of saying, "Let's just wait a bit and see if it doesn't clear up on its own." Physicians say that aggressive treatment may cure only a small number of illnesses, and that tincture of time (watchful waiting) cures a large proportion of curable illnesses. Usage: "Given tincture of time, we may soon see a resolution of his symptoms."

tinea ("TIN-ee-uh") **vs. tenia** ("TEH-nee-uh")—similar terms frequently confused. Tinea is a fungal infection (tinea versicolor), and tenia or taenia is a bandlike structure (tenia coli, longitudinal bands of the colon) or a tapeworm (*Taenia solium*, the pork tapeworm).

Tinel sign—positive if there is tingling and numbness at the distal end of a limb when percussion is performed over the site of a divided nerve. The fact that there is some sensation indicates that the nerve has not been completely divided, or that there is some regeneration of the nerve.

tine test—a tuberculin skin test in which a multiple-puncture device is used. The blades resemble the tines of a fork, hence the name. Not as reliable as the Mantoux test, but a good mass screening test.

tin-mesoporphyrin—see *SnMP*.

TIPS (transjugular intrahepatic portosystemic) **shunt**—a procedure for treatment of gastric antral vascular ectasia with portal hypertension.

tiptoe test—a simple method developed at Mayo Clinic to determine if arterial narrowing is present in the legs. Blood pressure is first taken in the arms and at the ankles. The patient is then asked to stand against a wall and raise up onto tiptoes 50 times. Afterward, blood pressure is taken again at the arms and ankles. If pressure is lower at the ankles than arms, significant arterial disease is strongly suspected.

TIRE (Test of Incremental Respiratory Endurance).

Tischler cervical biopsy punch forceps.

Tis disease—carcinoma (tumor) in situ of the bladder.

Tisseel—"surgical glue" made from two naturally occurring compounds derived from human blood: fibrinogen (a human blood protein) and thrombin (an enzyme). The product works by forming a flexible material that can stop oozing from small, sometimes inaccessible blood vessels during surgery when conventional surgical techniques are not feasible.

Tissucol—biological adhesive used in surgery.

tissue Doppler gated (TDoG) **dynamic three-dimensional ultrasound imaging**—a technique, in fetal imaging, in which tissue Doppler data are used to calculate a gating signal, in the absence of an ECG signal, for synchronization between loops.

tissue engineering—creation of tissues that can be used to augment a normal tissue, replace abnormal tissue, or stimulate the development of normal tissue. New tissue engineering technologies are utilizing live cells to help heal chronic wounds.

tissue-engineered blood vessels (TEVs).

tissue factor pathway inhibitor—important in the coagulation process.

tissue glue or solder—see *protein solder*.

tissue harmonic imaging—an ultrasound technique. The notion incorporated in the term is that the imaging technique depends on harmonics (wave patterns) that are characteristic of the tissue in question.

TissueLink Monopolar Floating Ball—combines radiofrequency energy with conductive fluid for hemostasis and coagulation of tissue during surgery.

tissue morcellator—instrument used to reduce large organs or tissue masses (enclosed in a specially designed bag) to small pieces for removal through the small incisions created for minimally invasive surgery, such as laparoscopy. Cf. *morselize*.

tissue plasminogen activator (t-PA).

tissue pO_2—a diagnostic study done on a wound to determine the oxygen content of the tissues, a factor important in healing.

tissue regeneration barrier—see *Atrisorb FreeFlow*.

tissue-selective estrogens (Ob-Gyn)—show promise as treatment of osteoporosis in postmenopausal women.

titanium rib—an expandable prosthesis made of titanium implanted into patients with chest wall and spine deformities that impair lung function and bone growth. The titanium rib is implanted onto a patient's rib and spine during the initial surgery. Follow-up surgeries are performed every four to six months to expand the device, which facilitates growth of the chest wall. The device exerts pressure on the spine without fusion and allows growth to continue while also helping to control the scoliosis. Also known as *vertical expandable titanium rib* (VEPTR).

Titanium VasPort (Cardio)—implantable vascular access device.

titer
- anti-RHO-D
- antistreptolysin (AST)
- anti-teichoic acid
- HI (hemagglutination inhibition)
- microsomal TRC antibody
- TRC (tanned red cells) antibody

Titmus test—for stereo acuity. The test pattern can be seen in three dimensions only when both eyes are working together. Cf. *litmus test*.

titrate—to make fine adjustments in the dose of a medicine by observing its effects.

TITP (third intercondylar tubercle of Parsons).

t.i.w.—three times a week.

TJF-100 Olympus endoscope with reusable biopsy channel caps.

TKA (total knee arthroplasty).

TKO-type I.V. (to keep open [the vein])—intravenous infusion given as slowly as possible to keep the blood from clotting in the needle, but not to give the patient significant fluid volume. Also, *KVO-type I.V.* (keep vein open).

TLC (therapeutic lifestyle changes). Do not confuse with *TLC* (tender loving care.)

TLC (total lymphocyte count).

TLC (triple-lumen catheter).

TLC (brand name) **retractor**.

T-lens—therapeutic contact lens.

TLI (total lymphoid irradiation)—used previously for cancer, now used with organ transplant patients to suppress

TLI *(cont.)*
T cells and decrease organ rejection. It may even allow transplant patients to avoid taking immunosuppressive drugs.

TLIF (transforaminal lumbar interbody fusion)—minimally invasive approach for surgical treatment of spondylolisthesis and segmental instability. The TLIF approach is a unilateral PLIF (posterior lumbar interbody fusion), which provides 360-degree fusion, avoids anterior access and associated complications, decreases manipulation of neural structures, reduces damage to ligamentous elements, minimizes excessive bone removal, enhances biomechanical stability, and provides early mobilization. Cf. *ALIF, PLIF.*

T listening—see *A, P, T, M.*

TL-90 (Ethicon) **stapler**—used in hepatic resection to minimize the blood loss from the cut surface of the liver as well as time consumed for the procedure. Livers from adults (parents, for example) must be cut down to fit children.

TLSO (thoracolumbosacral orthosis)—a semirigid plastic jacket (brace) used to treat scoliosis in children. The jacket is worn during the years of growth to prevent or slow further progression of the curve beyond 30°.

T-lymphocyte subset ratio—used to measure an AIDS drug's ability to improve immune function.

TMA (transmetatarsal amputation).

TMA (trimethylamine).

t-mastoid—slang for *temporal mastoid.*

T-max—slang for temperature maximum, the highest recorded temperature.

T-min—slang for minimum temperature.

TMJ (temporomandibular joint).

TMJ fossa-eminence prosthesis—used to treat internal derangement, adhesions, perforations, and ankylosis of the temporomandibular joint.

TMR (transmyocardial revascularization)—a holmium laser procedure performed on the beating heart to create pathways within the heart muscle.

TMST (treadmill stress test).

TMS 3-dimensional radiation therapy treatment planning system—provides extremely accurate information allowing for precise delivery of the radiation treatment plan.

TMZF femoral component—see *Accolade.*

TNB (transthoracic needle biopsy).

TNB (Tru-Cut needle biopsy).

TNDM (transient neonatal diabetes mellitus).

TNF (tumor necrosis factor)—a chemical toxin released from a gene (introduced by genetic engineering into human white blood cells) and toxic to malignant tumors. Therapy currently used to treat patients with malignant melanoma. Certain white blood cells known as tumor-infiltrating lymphocytes (TIL), which the body naturally produces to fight malignancies, are removed from the patient's body and genetically altered to include the gene that produces tumor necrosis factor. These cells are then given back to the patient. They migrate to the tumor site and begin manufacturing TNF.

TNK (tenecteplase). Do not confuse with *TNKase*, which is a specific brand name, or *TNK-tPA*, a genetically engineered tissue plasminogen activator.

TNKase (tenecteplase)—single-bolus "clot buster" drug that can be administered over 5 seconds when treating a heart attack.

TNK-tPA—a second-generation tissue plasminogen activator (t-PA). Note: While *t-PA* (with the hyphen) is preferred, Genentech, the manufacturer, specifically left out the hyphen in the drug name, perhaps to avoid a double hyphen.

TNM classification of malignant tumors: *T* represents the size of the tumor, *N* the clinical status of the nodes, and *M* metastasis.

T1 Direct extension of primary tumor.
T2 Direct extension of primary tumor to specific organs.
T3 Direct advanced extension of tumor, unresectable.
TX Direct extension of tumor not assessed.
N0 Regional lymph nodes not involved.
N1 Regional lymph nodes involved.
NX Regional lymph nodes not assessed.
M0 No distant metastases.
M1 Distant metastases present.
MX Distant metastases not assessed.

Stage I, T1-2, N0, M0—No extension or node involvement.
Stage II, T3, N0, M0—Advanced extension, unresectable.
Stage III, T1-3, N1, M0—Node involvement.
Stage IV, T1-3, N0-1, M1—Distant metastases present.

TNMES (transcutaneous neuromuscular electrical stimulation).

tNOX (quinol oxidase)—an overactive form of an enzyme known as *NOX*. The NOX enzyme is found on the surface of cells and plays a key role in growth of both normal and cancerous cells. Green tea has been found to inhibit the activity of this enzyme.

"to be to a"—phonetic for IIb/IIa (platelet inhibitor).

Todd-Wells guide—used in stereotaxic procedures. Cf. *BRW CT stereotaxic guide*.

toe-in gait—in ambulatory children with congenital clubfeet.

toeing in, toeing out—turning the forefoot in or out in walking.

toe-out gait.

toe-to-hand transfer and **foot-to-hand transfer**—the transplantation of toes to the hand to replace traumatically amputated or congenitally absent digits (e.g., great toe may be transplanted to thumb position).

toe web infection—no hyphen needed.

Toffel angled thru-cutting forceps.

TOF (time-of-flight) **MR angiography**.

togavirus—a subgroup of arboviruses (arthropod-borne viruses) that includes viruses carried by mosquitoes and ticks. The togavirus is so-called because it wears a covering (or toga) and is the cause of hemorrhagic fever.

toileting—using bathroom facilities without assistance; said in connection with partially disabled persons.

tokos or **tocos**—slang terms for tocodynamometer, a uterine contraction monitoring device. Cf. *Tokos*.

Tokos—former name of Matria, a company that provides remote electronic uterine contraction monitoring services. Cf. *tokos*.

Toldt ligament; **line of Toldt**—see *white line of Toldt*.

tolerogen—a substance that the immune system recognizes as "self," and not

tolerogen *(cont.)*
a foreign substance. Tolerogens are made by chemically linking fragments of DNA with specific protein molecules which the body already recognizes as "self." Tolerogens have potential in the control of autoimmune diseases such as systemic lupus erythematosus, rheumatoid arthritis, myasthenia gravis, etc.

Tolosa-Hunt syndrome—painful ophthalmoplegia.

toluidine blue stain.

Tom Jones closure—heavy retention suture closing all layers together (instead of in separate layers) except for the skin.

tomodensitometric examination, abdominal—to measure tissue densities. A technique that might be used to diagnose pheochromocytoma (in an unusual location).

tomography
ACAT (automated computerized axial tomography)
Cardiac Protect
cine CT (computed tomography)
computed (CT)
computed tomographic angiography (CTA)
computed tomography laser mammography (CTLM)
computed tomography angiographic portography (CTAP)
computed tomography colonography
computed tomography laser mammography (CTLM)
computerized axial (CAT)
digital tomosynthesis
dynamic computerized
electron beam computed
electron beam (EBT)
endoscopic optical coherence (EOCT)
FDG (18-fluorodeoxyglucose) positron emission

tomography *(cont.)*
magnetic resonance (MRT)
multidetector computed (MDCT)
optical coherence (OCT)
PET with 3-D SSP (positron emission tomography with 3-D stereotaxic surface projection)
positron emission (PET)
quantitative computed (QCT)
single photon emission computed (SPECT)
SOMATOM Volume Zoom
spiral x-ray computed (SXCT)
tomosynthesis
tuned aperture computed (Delta 32 TACT)
ultrafast CT electron beam
ultrasonic

tomosynthesis—a derivative of conventional geometric tomography, but it has the advantage that a full volume of data can be produced at radiation dosages less than with conventional tomography. See *digital tomosynthesis.*

Tonalin (conjugated linoleic acid)—an over-the-counter natural supplement that has been shown in double-blind randomized placebo studies to reduce body fat in obese people.

T1—the time it takes for protons to return to their orientation to a static magnetic field after an excitation pulse (MRI term).

T1FS (T1-weighted fat-suppressed) **images** (MRI term).

T1 high resolution isotropic volume examination (THRIVE) **technique**

T1-weighted fat-suppressed gadolinium-enhanced SE images—MRI term.

T1-weighted gadolinium-enhanced SE images—MRI term.

T1-weighted image—a spin-echo image generated by a pulse sequence

T1-weighted *(cont.)*
using a short repetition time (0.6 seconds or less) (MRI term). Also called *"short TR/TE."*

tongue display unit (TDU)—allows blind people to "see with their tongue." It can activate areas that are normally reserved for visual information and are unused when someone suffers from congenital blindness.

tongue-retaining device (TRD).

tonic-clonic seizure—the newer name for *grand mal seizure.*

tonometry (*not* tenometry)—measurement of intraocular pressure in the diagnosis of glaucoma. See *applanation tonometry; Goldmann applanation (GAT); Schiötz tonometry*.

Tono-Pen tonometer (Oph)—used in measuring intraocular pressure.

tonsil channeling—creation of channels in the tonsils using Coblation Channeling technique as a debulking procedure.

tonsils kissing bilaterally (ENT).

too many toes sign—visibility of four or even all five toes when the walking subject is observed from behind, an indication of splayfoot, flatfoot, or both.

Toomey syringe kit—designed to reduce cross-contamination in office aspiration procedures.

tooth and nail syndrome—ectodermal disorder in which certain primary teeth and/or several secondary teeth may either be absent or widely spaced and misshapen. Certain nails may be absent at birth and then grow extremely slowly, particularly during the first two to three years of life. The toenails are usually more severely affected than the fingernails. It is inherited as an autosomal dominant genetic trait.

tooth sign (Radiol)—a jagged superior pole of the patella, indicating chronic recurrent tendinopathy.

Topaz CO_2 laser—used in skin rejuvenation procedures.

Topel knot—a twist knot designed for laparoscopic procedures. See also *Aberdeen knot, convertible slip knot.*

tophaceous gout—one of the causes of carpal tunnel syndrome, especially in older males.

Top-Hat supra-anular aortic valve.

topodermatography—an imaging technique used to identify and evaluate changes of cutaneous lesions in melanoma screening or followup of cancer patients.

topography—see *Humphrey Systems ablation planner topography*.

TORCH screening (titer)—acronym
T toxoplasmosis
O other
R rubella
C cytomegalic inclusion disease
H herpes
Also:
TO toxoplasmosis
R rubella
C cytomegalovirus infections
H congenital herpes

Toric intraocular lens—a foldable lens used in cataract surgery that corrects preexisting astigmatism.

Toriumi curved rasp—has a reduced cutting surface and a lower profile to allow a targeted reduction of the dorsal hump of the nose.

Toriumi sharp and dull suction elevators—allow elevation of delicate mucosal structures while maintaining optimal visibility.

Toriumi 2.5 mm osteotome—rhinoplasty instrument shaped to steer the instrument along the lateral surface of the bone during lateral osteotomy

Toriumi *(cont.)*
without traumatizing superficial tissues.

Torkildsen shunt procedure—ventriculocisternostomy.

Tornwaldt bursitis.

Tornwaldt (Thornwaldt) **cyst** (ENT)—can be seen on CT scan as a mass high in the nasopharynx, midline between the longus capitis muscles, or just off midline. It may contain only fluid, but sometimes there is a calcification within it.

Toronto Hospital Alertness Test—for evaluating effects of obstructive sleep apnea.

Toronto parapodium—has one lock for both hip and knee joints. Orthosis for ambulation in children with cerebral palsy and myelomeningocele.

Toronto SPV valve—a stentless porcine heart valve entirely supported by the patient's aorta. Without a stent apparatus to occupy space, larger heart valves can be implanted, thus improving blood flow.

TORP (total ossicular replacement prosthesis)—in otological surgery.

torque tube catheter.

torr—a unit of measurement that relates to pressure in the patient in neurosurgery, when hypothermia and hypotension are used. Usage: "The pressure was kept at 70 torr and then dropped to 60 torr."

torsades de pointes ("tor-sahd´duh pwahnt") (Fr., fringe of pointed tips)—very rapid ventricular tachycardia in which there is waxing and waning of amplitudes in the QRS complexes as seen on the electrocardiogram. It could be self-limiting or go on to ventricular fibrillation. *Torsades de pointes* refers to the twisting, torsion, or waving of points in the appearance of the ECG tracing.

Torula histolytica—the cause of torulosis, the old name for cryptococcosis.

TOT (tincture of time).

total abdominal evisceration (TAE)—a technique for harvesting transplant organs from a dead donor. The kidneys, liver, pancreas, duodenum, and spleen are removed en bloc rather than individually. This harvesting technique is faster, and preliminary reports suggest that there is a lower incidence of loss of function in donor organs removed by this method.

total cavopulmonary connection (TCP)—used in a modified Fontan procedure for surgical correction of a double-inlet left ventricle. Venous blood from the inferior vena cava is channeled directly into the main pulmonary artery via an intra-atrial baffle created with autologous pericardium. Blood from the distal superior vena cava is diverted directly into the right pulmonary artery, and the single ventricular chamber is thus dedicated to systemic circulation. This procedure avoids the prosthetic conduits used in other types of repairs.

total knee arthroplasty (TKA).

Total-Lo—see *Cholesterol Manager.*

totally extraperitoneal (TEP) **hernia repair**.

total lymphocyte count—a quick and inexpensive test that may be a useful indicator of nutritional status and outcome.

total lymphoid irradiation (TLI).

total mesorectal excision (TME)—meticulous surgical dissection of the mesorectal tissues to improve the results of surgery for rectal cancer.

Total O_2 system—a supplementary oxygen system. It provides home oxygen patients with stationary

Total *(cont.)*
oxygen as well as the ability to fill portable oxygen cylinders for ambulation.

totipotent stem cell—a zygote or any cell of the very early (3 to 4-day) embryo, which has the capacity to differentiate into all cell types that are found in an embryo, fetus, newborn, or adult, including the embryonic components of the trophoblast and placenta required to support development and birth. No artificially created stem cell line to date has been shown to have these properties.

touch prep analysis—a fast method for pathologic diagnosis of tumor margins.

Toupet (partial posterior) **fundoplication**—a posterior, 270° wrap of the esophagus as surgical treatment of severe gastroesophageal reflux disease. It replaces the 360° wrap of the Nissen fundoplication. Results are said to be excellent with fewer complications than the Nissen procedure.

Tourette syndrome (maladie des tics) —a disorder of tics, throat sounds, generalized jerking movements, and the uncontrollable use of obscene language. Also, *Gilles de la Tourette syndrome*.

Tourguide guiding catheters—a line of French guiding catheters (sizes 6 through 10) to be used in interventional cardiac procedures, including PTCA, atherectomy, and stenting.

TOVA ("toe-vah") (Test of Variables of Attention) testing.

Towne projection in x-rays (Radiol)—occipital view of the skull.

Townley TARA prosthesis (Ortho)—see *TARA prosthesis*.

Townsend knee brace—made of lightweight titanium and graphite.

toxic—showing signs of toxemia or septicemia, such as fever, tachycardia, flushing, and mental confusion.

toxic shock syndrome—not a new infection, but mentioned often in the news in connection with group A streptococcal infections. It was big news during the tampon scare of the 1980s. See *streptococcus A infection; necrotizing fasciitis;* and *flesh-eating bacteria*.

toxic colitis—diffuse abdominal tenderness and systemic signs of toxicity, such as tachycardia, fever, leukocytosis, anemia, and hypoalbuminemia. Initially it is treated medically with fluid replacement, nasogastric decompression, high-dose intravenous steroids, and broad-spectrum antibiotics. For a patient who does not improve quickly with medical therapy or patients who develop peritonitis or perforation, a subtotal colectomy with ileostomy and either a Hartman stump or mucous fistula is the preferred operation.

***Toxocara* ELISA**—test for endophthalmitis.

***Toxocara* excretory secretory antigen** (TES antigen)—indicative of *Toxocara* nematodes (on ELISA test).

Toxoplasma gondii—can cause central nervous system toxoplasmosis in patients with AIDS.

t-PA (tissue plasminogen activator) (Activase)—given intravenously to dissolve a thrombus.

TP-53 mutation—found in non-small-cell lung tumors.

T-piece oxygen—administration of humidified oxygen through a tube connected to a T-shaped connector attached to an endotracheal tube.

TPM (total passive motion).

TPMT (thiopurine methyltransferase) **level**—a lab test performed before starting azathioprine (Imuran). If TPMT is very low, azathioprine is best avoided; if somewhat low, dosage of azathioprine should be reduced; and if high, a standard dosage may undertreat.

TPN (total parenteral nutrition) **line**.

T-pouch technique—a bladder augmentation technique for continent urinary diversion.

TpP (thrombus precursor protein)—an in vitro diagnostic test for the risk assessment of blood clot formation.

TPPN (total peripheral parenteral nutrition).

T-PRK (tracker-assisted photorefractive keratectomy).

TQa—transcutaneous access flow device.

TR (repetition time)—in magnetic resonance imaging, the interval between one spin echo pulse sequence and the next.

TRA (all-trans-retinoic acid)—a form of vitamin A given orally to patients with malignant solid tumors unresponsive to other chemotherapy.

trabecula (pl., trabeculae)—thin fibrous band of tissue.

trabecular metal—a material used in orthopedic implants.

trabeculoplasty—brief laser treatment which produces tightening of the outflow mechanism in glaucoma patients by placing a number of pinpoint lesions directly over the drain. Usually performed under topical anesthesia on an outpatient basis. Also, *argon laser trabeculoplasty.*

Tracer Blood Glucose Micro-monitor for self-testing by diabetics.

TracerCAD—a computer program used to create better-fitting limb prostheses.

Tracer—hybrid wire guide for endoscopic surgery.

trach—slang for *tracheostomy*.

trache 'go bag'—a bag of supplies for tracheostomy patients when traveling, including De Lee suction catheter, bulb syringe, disposable suction catheters, tracheostomy tube with tie (same size and size smaller), scissors, water-soluble lubricant (sterile single use packets), saline (two or three 5-cc vials), 4 x 4's or trach sponges, portable suction machine, emergency phone numbers, HME (heat moisture exchanger) devices, Ambu bag, portable oxygen, and hospital, insurance, and pharmacy cards available in baby's own "wallet."

tracheal toilet—routine care of a curved metal tracheal tube, including passage of a suction catheter into the trachea for removal of mucus.

tracheal tug—downward impulse imparted to the trachea by aortic aneurysm, synchronous with heartbeat.

trachelotomy—incision into, or excision of, the neck of the uterus (cervix uteri); also called *cervicectomy*. Cf. *tracheotomy*.

tracheoesophageal puncture (TEP)—a promising option for post total laryngectomy patients (other than esophageal speech or an artificial larynx). TEP can be performed at the same time as the laryngectomy (primary TEP) or at a later time (secondary TEP). Delaying the procedure would be for poor tissue quality, poor clinical status, or the need for planned postoperative radiation treatment.

tracheostomy—see *percutaneous dilational* (PDT).

tracheotomy—incision of the trachea. Cf. *trachelotomy*.

Trachlight—lighted stylet used in intubation of surgical patients.

track—the path along which something has moved and left a mark, e.g., needle track. This word is not often used in medical dictation. Cf. *tract*.

tracker-assisted photorefractive keratectomy (T-PRK).

Tracker-18 Soft Stream catheter—a microcatheter used to deliver drugs to lyse intracoronary thrombi. The holes in the sides of the catheter deliver a soft stream which does not injure the blood vessel.

track sign—see *parallel track sign*, *double stripe sign*, *trolley-track sign*.

tract—a collection of nerve fibers that have a common origin, function, and termination—as in *spinal tract*; or a group of organs that are arranged serially and together perform a common function—as in *gastrointestinal tract*; or an abnormal passage through tissue—as *sinus tract*, *fistulous tract*. Usage: "In further dissection around the right lateral aspect of the pancreas graft, we came across a *tract* from a previous Jackson-Pratt drain. Once this was taken down, there was gross pus in this *tract*, and this *tracked* all the way supraperitoneally into the oblique muscles." Do not confuse with *track,* which is often used as a verb in medical dictation, meaning to follow a path or course.

traction
- Bryant
- Buck
- Cotrel
- Crutchfield skeletal
- halo
- halter
- Russell

traction artifact—abnormal appearances created in tissue by suction or stretching during the obtaining of a biopsy specimen.

tract of Lissauer—a white matter tract immediately posterior to the dorsal horn of the spinal cord gray matter through which small nociceptive nerve fibers pass.

Trager therapy—gentle rocking movements used to ease pain and tension in conditions such as Parkinson disease, irritable bowel syndrome, chronic back pain, and multiple sclerosis.

tragus-to-wall distance—term used in assessing lateral cervical mobility in ankylosing spondylitis.

TRAIDS (transfusion related AIDS, acquired immunodeficiency syndrome).

Trail Making Test—neurological test.

Trak Back—disposable pullback device that provides steady and precise pullback of intravascular ultrasound catheters, facilitating viewing of 3-D-like images, in addition to conventional cross-sectional displays.

TRAM (transverse rectus abdominis myocutaneous) **flap**.

tram-track sign—as seen in cortical calcifications of optic nerve or perineural orbital lesion.

transabdominal preperitoneal (TAPP) **hernia repair**—an approach to laparoscopic inguinal hernia repair using balloon distention to permit better exposure and reduce risk of preperitoneal adhesions.

transabdominal thin-gauge embryofetoscopy (TGEF)—fiberoptic endoscope inserted into the uterus to obtain information (in addition to that already provided by transvaginal ultrasound) to aid in diagnosing fetal anomalies.

transanal endoscopic microsurgery (TEM)—a minimally invasive technique for resection of sessile adenomas and some rectal carcinomas.

transarticular screw reconstruction —for management of C1-2 fracture instability.

transaxial fat-saturated 3-D images —MRI term.

transbronchial biopsy (TBB)—histopathological findings of specimens graded on the International Society for Heart and Lung Transplantation system.

transbronchial needle aspiration (TBNA).

transcarotid balloon valvuloplasty—used in infants with congenital aortic valve stenosis. The neck artery is used because it is larger and can be directly repaired, and surgeons are able to avoid losing a leg artery. The procedure is monitored by transesophageal echocardiogram.

transcatheter ablation—used to describe interventional electrophysiology procedures in which direct current or radiofrequency energy is used to ablate (remove) arrhythmogenic areas in the myocardium.

transcatheter arterial chemoembolization (TACE).

transcatheter arterial embolization (TAE)—used to deliver chemotherapeutic agents through the common hepatic artery to liver neoplasms.

Transcend articulation hip system—a ceramic-on-ceramic total hip replacement system, surgically implanted to completely replace a diseased hip joint.

Transcend implantable gastric stimulator (IGS)—a pacemaker-like device implanted laparoscopically to induce and maintain weight loss. The IGS consists of a stimulation lead implanted in the gastric wall connected to an electric programming unit implanted under the skin of the abdomen. The operative technique is relatively simple, and the system does not alter gastrointestinal anatomy.

transcervical balloon tuboplasty (TBT) —procedure to open blocked fallopian tubes that are the cause of infertility. Anesthesia is obtained with a paracervical block and a catheter is inserted into the blocked fallopian tube under fluoroscopic guidance. Less expensive than standard surgery for blocked tubes or in vitro fertilization. Also called *recanalization*.

transconjunctival approach to orbital tumors.

transcoronary ablation of septal hypertrophy (TASH)—believed to be an effective way to relieve resting left ventricular outflow tract obstruction in hypertrophic cardiomyopathy.

transcostovertebral approach—for the excision of herniated thoracic disks.

transcranial color-coded sonography (TCCS)—bedside procedure using ultrasound that traces the cerebral blood flow to ascertain the presence and location of an arteriovenous malformation.

transcranial Doppler (TCD) **velocities**.

transcription—the synthesis of a strand of RNA on a complementary template of DNA.

transcription factor—any of various proteins that bind to specific sites on DNA and turn the expression of different sets of genes on or off.

transcutaneous electrical nerve stimulation (TENS).

transcutaneous neuromuscular electrical stimulation (TNMES).

transcutaneous oxygen level ($TcPO_2$).

TransCyte—a human-based, bioengineered temporary skin substitute for the treatment of burns.

transdermal patch for glucose monitoring—a disposable transdermal patch applied to the skin for 5 minutes; a pocket-sized monitor then reads the patch and indicates the patient's blood glucose level.

transdermal testosterone gel—has been approved for use in men and is currently in clinical trials for women.

transdifferentiation—the ability of a stem cell from one type of tissue to differentiate into a cell type characteristic of another tissue.

Transeal transparent adhesive film dressing.

transepicondylar axis (TEA).

transesophageal echocardiography (TEE)—a semi-invasive procedure that provides views of the posterior structure of the heart and is the investigation of choice for diagnosis of acute dissection of the aorta, assessment of aortic graft dehiscence, and in search for a potential cardiac source for thromboembolism.

transesophageal pacing system—eliminates the use of drugs in nonexercise stress testing for patients with congestive heart failure and other late-stage cardiovascular diseases.

transfemoral liver biopsy.

transferred immune response—technique of transferring antibodies from cancer cells of one cancer patient to a healthy patient, and then transplanting healthy bone marrow back into the cancer patient.

transferrin (as in ferrous)—a glycoprotein. Also, *iron binding protein*.

transfixion suture—suture ligature; used to suture a large blood vessel closed; secures against slippage of the knot; sometimes called stick tie.

TransFix pin—used in arthroscopically assisted anterior and posterior cruciate ligament reconstruction. It provides a single and strong tibial attachment point for the 4-stranded semitendinosus and gracilis tendons, and it provides adequate graft length for secure fixation.

transforaminal lumbar interbody fusion (TLIF)—a variation of the posterior lumbar interbody fusion (PLIF) approach for surgical treatment of spondylolisthesis and segmental instability. The TLIF approach is a unilateral PLIF, which provides 360-degree fusion, avoids anterior access and associated complications, decreases manipulation of neural structures, reduces damage to ligamentous elements, minimizes excessive bone removal, enhances biomechanical stability, and provides early mobilization.

transgenic—referring to laboratory transfer of genetic material from one genome to another.

transhepatic embolization (THE).

transhepatic gallbladder litholysis—contact dissolution (also known as direct solvent dissolution or litholysis) for the treatment of gallstones.

transhiatal esophagectomy.

transient aplastic crisis (TAC)—an illness in which red cell production virtually stops, and the red blood cell count falls rapidly; a complication of parvovirus B19 infection.

transient bone marrow edema syndrome—a self-resolving condition related to the bone marrow edema pattern seen on MR imaging.

transient evoked otoacoustic emission (TEOAE)—frequently used to determine the physiological condition of the cochlea in studies of comparative hearing.

transient ischemic attack (TIA).

transient neonatal diabetes mellitus (TNDM)—a condition affecting babies who initially cannot produce insulin. Symptoms disappear after about three months; however, two-thirds of those affected will develop diabetes later in life, usually in their teens.

TransiGel—hydrogel-impregnated gauze.

transitional cell carcinoma of the bladder (TCCB).

transient focal cerebral ischemia (TFCI)

transjugular intrahepatic portosystemic shunt (TIPS or TIPSS)—a treatment modality for portal hypertension-induced variceal hemorrhage unresponsive to sclerotherapy. Although the procedure has been improved with the use of an expandable Wallstent for better shunt patency, stenosis may still occur in about half of the patients, necessitating shunt revision by stent replacement or angiographic dilation of the shunt or addition of a second one.

transjugular liver biopsy.

translabyrinthine removal of large acoustic neuromas.

translation—the synthesis of a polypeptide having an amino acid sequence complementary to, and derived from, the codon sequence of a corresponding strand of messenger RNA.

translocation (Genetics)—an accidental interchange of fragments between two chromosomes. Chronic myelogenous leukemia results from a translocation between chromosomes 9 and 22, resulting in the so-called Philadelphia chromosome.

translocation Down syndrome—a variation of Down syndrome, caused by an extra 21st chromosome that moves from the 21st chromosome pair to either the 13th or 15th pair, resulting in 13/21 or 15/21 translocation Down syndrome. Cf. *trisomy-D syndrome.*

transluminal endovascular graft placement—a procedure in which a compactly folded graft is delivered through a sheath, deployed, and pressed against the vessel by balloon inflation. It is performed to reduce an aortic aneurysm.

transluminal extraction catheter (TEC)—cone-shaped rotating device with suction that cuts plaque from the lumen and sucks out the pieces.

transluminal ultrasonic angioplasty (TUA)—the use of high-energy and low-frequency ultrasound to recanalize obstructed veins in deep venous thrombosis.

transmission control protocol/Internet protocol (TCP/IP).

transmyocardial revascularization (TMR).

transnasal endoluminal ultrasonography—a method to study the anatomy of the GI tract.

Transorbent—multilayer dressing that includes an extra soft foam layer to protect and cushion a wound.

transpapillary endoscopic cholecystotomy—drains the gallbladder in acute acalculous cholecystitis. It is done in place of more aggressive percutaneous, laparoscopic, or open cholecystotomy, primarily in patients at high surgical risk.

transparent adhesive film—semi-permeable membrane dressings that are waterproof yet permeable to oxygen and water vapor. These dressings help prevent bacterial contamination and maintain a moist wound environment. They also facilitate cellular migration and promote autolysis of necrotic tissue by trapping moisture at the wound surface. Some newer transparent films are designed simply to keep I.V. sites dry; these have a higher moisture vapor permeability (MVP) and are not used on wounds. See *dressing*.

transperineal-transsphincteric approach—for repair of rectourethral fistula.

transperineal ultrasonography—technique that enables imaging of anal sphincters and anal canal structures.

transplant, transplantation
AuBMT (autologous bone marrow transplantation)
amniotic membrane transplantation
arthroscopic autologous chondrocyte transplantation
autologous ovarian transplantation
auxiliary transplant
BMT (bone marrow)
cellular xenotransplantation
fetal neuron allotransplantation
fetal pig cell transplantation
fetal tissue
fetal ventral mesencephalic tissue
foot-to-hand transfer
hematopoietic stem cell (HSCT)
LRT (living related transplant)
orthotopic
pancreatic islet cell
posterior lamellar (PLT)
reduced liver transplant (RLT)
reduced-size liver transplant (RSLT)
single-lung transplant (SLT) recipient

transplant *(cont.)*
split-liver transplantation
stamp graft
toe–to–hand transfer
UD-BMT (unrelated donor, bone marrow transplantation)
xenotransplantation

transplant rejection classification—The classification system of the International Society for Heart and Lung Transplantation divides acute rejection (AR) into grades: grade AO, none; grade A_{2a}, minimal, mild, with evidence of bronchiolar inflammation; grade intermediate, and severe acute rejection. It also recognizes four categories of chronic rejection (CR) and inflammation in describing airways and vessels.

transposition of the great arteries (TGA).

transpupillary thermotherapy—ophthalmological treatment of occult wet age-related macular degeneration.

transrectal ultrasound (TRUS)—used in assessing and characterizing the degree of pathology of prostatic abscess.

TransScan TS2000 electrical impedance breast scanning system—real-time noninvasive radiation-free imaging device that maps local electrical impedance properties of breast tissue, using inherent differences between neoplastic and normal tissues.

transscrotal extratunica vaginalis procedure—a technique for bilateral varicocele repair using a single scrotal incision that can be performed on an outpatient basis.

transthoracic echocardiography (TTE)—evaluates the structure, function, and size of pulmonary and aortic valves.

transthoracic needle aspiration biopsy of benign and malignant lesions.

transthoracic needle biopsy (TNB)—used to diagnose thoracic lesions.

transtracheal oxygen catheter—can replace a nasal cannula for better patient comfort and aesthetics. Inserted at the base of the neck through a small, permanent, surgically created tract into the trachea. The catheter is connected to tubing to a portable oxygen tank.

transtrochanteric valgus osteotomy (TVO)—orthopedic procedure that utilizes a wedge bone fragment between the greater trochanter and the proximal femoral fragment.

transtympanic steroid administration—steroids administered directly to the middle ear effective in treating sudden-onset sensorineural hearing loss in patients who have failed to respond to systemic steroid therapy.

transumbilical breast augmentation (TUBA)—an innovative technique using a small incision in the navel as an access point for insertion of saline-filled breast implants.

transurethral balloon laserthermia prostatectomy—investigational procedure in which the prostate is irradiated with a Prostalase (Nd: YAG) laser system inserted transurethrally through a balloon device. The balloon can be monitored via transrectal ultrasound. See *Prostalase laser system.*

transurethral electrovaporization of the prostate (TUVP)—a procedure similar to TURP, but TUVP uses a roller electrode to vaporize superficial layers of prostate tissue while coagulating deeper layers. TUVP may result in fewer bleeding complications.

transurethral incision of the prostate (TUIP)—an alternative to transurethral resection of the prostate (TURP). TUIP is nearly as effective in reducing symptoms of benign prostatic hypertrophy and can be done on an outpatient basis. It is limited to patients who have 30 g or less of prostatic tissue to be resected.

transurethral microwave thermotherapy (TUMT)—heats the prostate via a transurethral application. It houses a microwave antenna in a water-cooled sheath, thus protecting prostatic mucosa while delivering deeper heating to obstructing parenchyma. When tissues are heated to greater than 45°C, necrosis occurs, resulting in ablation or resorption of overgrown prostatic tissue.

transurethral needle ablation (TUNA)—procedure for treatment of benign prostatic hypertrophy. Radiofrequency is delivered through side-deploying needles to create coagulative necrotic lesions within the prostate. The prostate then retracts, opening the prostatic urethra.

transurethral ultrasound-guided laser-induced prostatectomy (TULIP) (Urol)—a surgical treatment for benign prostatic hypertrophy. Ultrasound is used to visualize the enlarged prostate, and a 90° angle side-firing laser is used to destroy the obstructing prostatic tissue. Postoperative complications such as hemorrhage are minimal, and most patients go home the next day. See also *transurethral balloon laserthermia prostatectomy*.

Transvac transdermal patch—a patch sold without medication for delivering bioactive agents through enhanced permeability of the skin.

transvaginal Cooper ligament sling—see *Capio CL.*

transvaginal sacrospinous colpopexy—a modification of the sacrospinous colpopexy for women with vaginal vault prolapse. See *sacrospinous colpopexy.*

transvaginal suturing (TVS) **system**—a surgical device to correct female stress urinary incontinence.

transvaginal ultrasound (TVS)—may replace endometrial biopsy as the standard diagnostic procedure for vaginal bleeding among postmenopausal women.

transvenous liver biopsy—a faster (takes about 10 minutes to perform), simpler method for obtaining liver tissue that is used when percutaneous liver sampling is contraindicated by bleeding tendency, ascites, pulmonary emphysema, peliosis hepatis, or liver amyloidosis. Under fluoroscopy, a sheathed needle is inserted via the jugular vein down to the hepatic vein, which is pierced to obtain a specimen of liver parenchyma. The procedure produces a smaller specimen but is safer because liver capsule is not pierced and any bleeding is confined to venous bleeding.

transverse magnetization; **orientation**—MRI term.

transverse rectus abdominis myocutaneous (TRAM) **flap**—used in breast reconstruction. In this technique to reconstruct the breast, tissue is transferred from the central portion of the abdomen onto the chest wall, or tunneled beneath the skin to the breast. Also called *tummy tuck flap*.

transverse retubularized sigmoidovesicostomy continent urinary diversion to the umbilicus—a procedure used to create a catheterizable sigmoidovesicostomy to the umbilicus for continent urinary diversion. The procedure avoids having to anastomose two segments of ileum together, which is necessary in larger patients.

TRAP (tartrate resistant acid phosphatase)—osteoclast marker enzyme used in the diagnosis of histological aspects of heterotopic bone.

trapeziometacarpal silicone arthroplasty—joint replacement for severe degenerative arthritis.

Traube space—the gastric bubble, which causes a different tympanitic note from percussion over the lungs.

TraumaJet—wound debridement system capable of removing contamination, as well as damaged tissue, from a traumatic wound.

traumatic aortic injuries in children—diagnosed by helical CT scan and transesophageal echocardiography. Injuries may include left apical cap, pulmonary contusion, aortic obscuration, and mediastinal widening.

Travenol infuser—a disposable device for the delivery of continuous parenteral drug therapy to patients who can be ambulatory.

Traverso-Longmire technique—for resection of a malignant tumor of the pancreas.

TRAx ELISA assay—technology system with application to a broad range of diagnostic assays.

TRC (tanned red cells) (microsomal TRC antibody titer)—a test used in the study of thyroid antibodies.

TRD (tongue-retaining device).

treadmill testing—stress testing of cardiac response, in which the patient progressively increases walking speed, and the incline of the tread-

treadmill *(cont.)*
mill is also increased. The test is continued until signs of ischemia are noted, or when the target heart rate is reached. The test is discontinued when the patient becomes fatigued, short of breath, or notes claudication or vertigo.

treatment—see *medications*, *operation*.

tree artifact (Radiol)—a tree-shaped spot on a radiograph caused by exposure of undeveloped film to visible light including sparks of static electricity. Also, *crown artifact* and *swamp-static artifact* (the same phenomenon).

trefoil balloon catheter—see *percutaneous transvenous mitral commissurotomy*.

Trelex mesh—used for reinforcement of repair during inguinal herniorrhaphy.

Trellis infusion catheter and system—minimally invasive thrombolytic catheter system, designed to facilitate the delivery of clot-dissolving drugs into the arteries and veins in the upper and lower limbs and evacuate the treated area.

tremor, pill-rolling.

trepopnea ("tree-pop-nee´uh")—preference for the recumbent position, because breathing is easier in that position.

T_4RIA—thyroxine radioisotope assay.

TriActiv system—a device designed to treat saphenous vein graft disease in patients who have previously had coronary artery bypass surgery and now have blockages in the grafts. It consists of a protection balloon guidewire which creates a protected space, a flush catheter which washes the graft, and an extraction system which removes the debris found in the grafts. These three features work in combination to prevent the debris found in the graft from going downstream and potentially causing a heart attack.

triad asthma—aspirin sensitivity, asthma, and nasal polyps. Also known as *ASA triad* and *Samter triad*.

triad of Rigler—air in the bile ducts, small bowel ileus, and a visible gallstone in the small bowel, all diagnostic of gallstone ileus.

TRIADS (time-resolved imaging by automatic data segmentation) (MRI) — provides variable resolution of an individual's respiratory cycle.

Triage BNP test—a blood test for B-type natriuretic peptide, a protein released when the left ventricle is overloaded or stretched, for the rapid diagnosis of heart attacks.

Triage cardiac system—rapid diagnostic test designed to aid in detection of heart attacks.

trial—see *study*.

triamcinolone cream (TAC, pronounced "tack").

Triangle gelatin-sealed sling material—designed for a less invasive transvaginal procedure to treat female stress incontinence. Triangle material is sealed with an absorbable bovine gelatin that is crosslinked to control the rate of its resorption in the body. This may help to reduce inflammation during the healing process.

triangle of doom—see *triangle of pain*.

triangle of pain (also, electric zone; "triangle of doom")—used to describe the triangular area between the gonadal vessels medially and the iliopubic tract laterally. May be dictated in hernioplasty or laparoscopic herniorrhaphy reports. The truly

triangle *(cont.)*
dangerous region is deep to the iliopubic tract where position of nerves cannot be seen or predicted with certainty.

triangular vaginal patch sling—a sling created from the anterior vaginal wall. A procedure for stress urinary incontinence and hypermobile urethra.

Triano digital hearing aid—a behind-the-ear hearing aid that claims to be able to help the patient distinguish between speech and background noise.

Tricep hooked-prong grasping forceps—used in kidney stone extraction.

triceps skin fold—useful in nutritional status analysis.

trichiasis—inversion of the eyelashes so that they rub against the cornea, causing continual irritation of the eyeball.

trichinosis—infection with trichinae; caused by eating undercooked pork and some other meats containing *Trichinella spiralis*. Cf. *trichocyst, trichosis*.

trichloroacetic acid (TCA)—a topical treatment for human papillomavirus (genital warts).

trichocyst—a cell structure which is derived from the cytoplasm. Cf. *trichinosis, trichosis*.

trichosis—a disease of, or abnormal growth of, the hair. Cf. *trichinosis, trichocyst*.

Trichosporon beigelii—seen in post-surgical soft tissue infections.

trichotillomania—compulsive tugging at one's hair. Usage: "Her symptoms included rather depressive features and trichotillomania."

Tricodur Epi (elbow) compression support bandage.

Tricodur Omos (shoulder) compression support bandage.

Tricodur Talus (ankle) compression support bandage.

tricorrectional bunionectomy—bunion repair procedure also used to repair juvenile hallux valgus deformity. The bunion deformity is corrected in all three planes with a distal metatarsal osteotomy involving a transverse V-osteotomy with a long plantar hinge using cannulated bone screws for fixation. Does not interfere with the epiphyseal growth center of the first metatarsal.

tricyclic antidepressant (TCA).

Trident ceramic acetabular insert.

Trident hip replacement system—surgically implanted to completely replace a diseased or dysfunctional hip joint.

TriFix spinal instrumentation system—pedicle screw fixation system used for stabilization of the spine.

triflange acetabular cup—a hemispherical uncemented device with flanges used in acetabular surgery.

TriGen FAN nail—a femoral antegrade nail.

TriGen intramedullary nail system.

triggering mechanism—a precipitous event or process causing onset of acute disease, e.g., acute cardiovascular disease or sudden death.

trigger point—a localized zone of tenderness, especially in a muscle.

Trillium T2T—heparin biocompatible surfaces on cannulas used in arrested heart surgery.

Trilogy acetabular cup—comes in non-holed, cluster-holed, or multi-holed models.

Trilogy acetabular system—acetabular component designed for use in minimally invasive hip replacement surgery.

Trilogy DC+—pacemaker used in patients with sick sinus syndrome and intermittent heart block.

Trilogy SR+—single-chamber pacemaker that "learns" the patient's lifestyle and adapts to changes during activity and rest.

Trilucent breast implants—breast implants filled with vegetable oil.

trimodal injury pattern—injury to the lower body, thorax, and head and/or upper extremities in pedestrians hit by automobiles.

trimodal spectroscopy—used for the detection and characterization of cervical precancers in vivo. It uses three techniques (intrinsic fluorescence, diffuse reflectance, and light scattering) in combination.

trimsulfa—slang for *trimethoprim-sulfamethoxazole.*

Trinica—a select anterior cervical plate system and spinal fixation system.

Trinovin—dietary supplement made from red-clover-based isoflavones said to reduce symptoms of benign prostatic hypertrophy.

Triosyn resin—an iodine formulation proven effective against a broad spectrum of microorganisms; it is versatile and equally effective in fluid, air, surface, and dermatological applications.

Triosyn T-1000 respirator—a disposable personal facemask designed to provide protection against airborne SARS virus.

tripe palm—cutaneous marker for internal malignancy which produces a rugose or corrugated thickening of the skin of the palm. It often precedes the diagnosis of a new or recurrent tumor. Malignant acanthosis nigricans is most commonly associated with intra-abdominal malignancies. Also, tripe palms can be associated with endometrial carcinoma and may be the first sign of malignancy.

triple A (AAA)—medical slang for *abdominal aortic aneurysm.*

triple-antibiotic therapy.

triple-dose gadolinium-enhanced MR imaging without MT (magnetization transfer).

triple-H therapy (hypertensive hypervolemic hemodilution) **after subarachnoid hemorrhage**.

triplet—a codon; a unit of three DNA or RNA bases, coding for a specific amino acid.

triploid (Genetics)—pertaining to a cell with three of each chromosome instead of the usual pair.

tripoding—Gowers sign, classical sign of Duchenne muscular dystrophy.

Trippi-Wells tongs—used for traction.

triptorelin pamoate, injectable—see *Trelstar Depot*.

triquetrum—the triquetral bone in the wrist, between the pisiform and lunate bones; os triquetrum, also called *triangular bone*.

Triseptin (ethyl alcohol, skin conditioning emollients, surfactants and preservatives)—a waterless surgical scrub.

trisomy (Genetics)—a condition in which three copies of a given chromosome occur instead of the usual two, as in trisomy 21 (Down syndrome).

trisomy-D syndrome—manifested by the following clinical features: apneic spells, apparent deafness, capillary hemangioma, cardiac defects, char-

trisomy-D *(cont.)* acteristic dermal pattern, cleft lip and palate, death in early infancy, ear malformation, polydactyly, scalp defects, and severe central nervous system defects. Cf. *translocation Down syndrome, trisomy-G.*

trisomy-G—genetically determined disorder; one of a group of such disorders associated with increased risk of leukemia.

Triumph VR pacemaker—a single chamber adaptive rate pacemaker.

TriVex transilluminated powered phlebectomy procedure—for varicose vein removal. In this procedure, the surgeon removes the vein using a small powered surgical device while viewing the vein using a transilluminating light.

TroCam—endoscopic system placing the camera and lighting directly into the surgical field for computerized imaging.

Trocan disposable CO_2 trocar and cannula.

trochanteric Gamma locking nail—used in repair of complex femoral fractures.

troika of consciousness cycle—a model for determining sleep debt and sleepiness.

Troisier node—see *sentinel node*.

Trojan horse technique—an investigational therapeutic approach to Alzheimer disease. It protects brain cells in culture by drastically reducing the neurotoxic amyloid protein aggregates that are critical to the development of the disease. The treatment involves dispatching a small molecule into the cell to enlist the aid of a larger "chaperone" protein to block the accumulation of the brain-clogging protein.

trolley-track sign—an appearance on frontal radiographs of the spine in some patients with ankylosing spondylitis. This abnormality is characterized by the presence of three vertical radiodense lines resulting from ossification of supraspinous and interspinous ligaments and apophyseal joint capsules.

trophectoderm—the outer cellular envelope of the blastocyst, which will develop into the placenta and fetal membranes.

trophoblast—the outer envelope of the blastocyst, containing cells that will differentiate to form the placenta and fetal membranes.

troponin T—see *cardiac troponin T lab test*.

trospium hydrochloride—a drug for treatment of overactive bladder.

trough line—seen in posterior shoulder dislocation on x-ray.

"trouser" balloon delivery system—see *Bard XT coronary stent*.

Trousseau sign—the occurrence of carpal spasm, in latent tetany, when the upper arm is compressed (as with the use of a tourniquet).

troxacitabine—anticancer compound for the treatment of leukemia and a variety of solid tumors.

TR/TE, long—see *T2-weighted image*.

TR/TE, short—see *T1-weighted image*.

Tru-Area Determination—wound-measuring device.

Tru-Close wound drainage system—a completely closed wound drainage system with a unique splittable design providing two drains through one exit site. Because the evacuator is never opened or emptied, patients and healthcare personnel are protected from exposure to contaminated body fluids.

Tru-Cut needle—used for liver biopsy.

T.R.U.E. (thin-layer rapid use epicutaneous) **allergen patch test**—a ready-to-apply allergen patch test that can be used for 24 allergens and allergen mixes, capable of detecting up to 85 of the most common substances that cause allergic contact dermatitis.

trueFISP (true fast imaging with steady-state precession) (MRI).

True-Flex intramedullary nail—fluted titanium nail for fixation of upper extremity fractures.

true vertigo—a feeling that everything is revolving around the patient, or that he himself is revolving. Differentiated from mere dizziness.

Trufill—a brand name of n-butyl cyanoacrylate (n-BCA).

Trufill n-BCA—liquid embolic system for presurgical embolization of cerebral arteriovenous malformations.

TruJect—self-administered autoinjector drug delivery system. Approximately the size of a pen, it is spring-activated and pre-filled to deliver subcutaneous or intramuscular injection of medication with the touch of a button.

Trumpet Valve hydrodissector—see *Nezhat-Dorsey Trumpet Valve hydrodissector*.

truncation band artifact—see *edge ringing artifact, Gibbs phenomenon*.

TruPulse CO_2 laser system—used for skin resurfacing.

Truquant BR—an in vitro test kit for the detection of recurrent breast cancer in women with stage I or stage II disease. The test detects the presence of the CA27.29 antigen, a breast cancer tumor marker, in the blood.

TRUS (transrectal ultrasonography)—to evaluate prostate carcinoma.

Truvada (tenofovir disoproxil fumarate 300 mg and emtricitabine 200 mg) —a fixed-dose combination of the antiretroviral drugs for treatment of HIV infection.

TruWave pressure transducer—disposable transducer in a closed, needleless blood sampling system.

TruZone PFM (peak flow meter)—for asthma and emphysema in both children and adults.

trypsin, balsam, castor oil—see *Xenaderm*.

TS (terminal sedation).

T-Scan 2000—transpectral impedance scanner that performs electrical mapping of breast lesions in patients who have had ambiguous mammogram results. The device is designed to improve diagnostic accuracy and lower the number of unnecessary biopsies.

TSF (triceps skin fold).

TSH-01—a transdermal tape with natural estrogen and 17 beta-estradiol. Used as treatment for climacteric disturbances and postmenopausal osteoporosis. The base material of the tape is polymer technology that mitigates skin irritation.

T-Span tissue expander.

TSPP rectilinear bone scan (technetium stannous pyrophosphate).

TSRH (Texas Scottish Rite Hospital) **Crosslink**—a spinal instrumentation system used to stabilize the rods used in correction of scoliosis. Also, *Cotrel-Dubousset*.

T-TAC (transcervical tubal access catheter).

TTB-USA (through-the-balloon ultrasound ablation).

TTE (transthoracic echocardiography).

T3 system—a targeted transurethral thermoablation system for treatment

T3 *(cont.)*
of benign prostatic hyperplasia. The system is catheter-based to provide a "nonsurgical," anesthesia-free procedure.

TTP (thrombotic thrombocytopenic purpura).

TTP (time to peak).

T12 needle.

T12 suture.

T2 (MRI term)—the time it takes for protons to go out of phase after having been shifted in their orientation by an excitation pulse.

T-2 protocol—for treatment of Ewing sarcoma.

T2-weighted fast SE images (MRI).

T2-weighted image (MRI term)—a spin-echo image generated by a pulse sequence using a long repetition time (2 seconds or more). Also called *long TR/TE*.

T2-weighted turbo SE images (MRI).

TUA (transluminal ultrasonic angioplasty).

TUBA (transumbilical breast augmentation).

tube (see also *stent*)
Abbott-Rawson
Activent antimicrobial ventilation tubes for myringotomy
Baldwin ventilation
Bard Genie button
Bivona TTS (tight-to-shaft) tracheostomy
Blakemore-Sengstaken
Broncho-Cath endobronchial
Caluso PEG
Cantor
Celestin latex rubber
Combitube
Corflo enteral feeding
Entristar skin-level gastrostomy
Ewald
fenestrated tracheostomy

tube *(cont.)*
fil d'Arion silicone
Flexiflo Stomate low-profile gastrostomy
germination
Guibor Silastic
Keofeed feeding
K-Tube
Kurz ventilation
Lanz low-pressure cuff endotracheal
Luki
Mark IV
MIC gastroenteric
MIC-Key G gastrostomy
MIC-Key J gastrostomy
Micron bobbin ventilation
MIC-TJ (transgastric jejunal)
Miller-Abbott
Miser
Molteno seton
Montgomery Safe-T-Tube
Moretz Tab ventilation
Moss G-tube PEG kit
Moss nasal
Moss Suction Buster
nasogastric (NG) feeding
nasojejunal (NJ) feeding
Newvicon vacuum chamber pickup
NG (nasogastric) feeding
Nuport PEG
Nyhus-Nelson
Olympus One-Step Button
ostiomeatal stent
overtube
Pedi PEG
PEG (percutaneous endoscopic gastrostomy)
Pitt talking tracheostomy
Radius enteral feeding
RAE endotracheal
Replogle
Reuter bobbin
Ring–McLean sump
Sacks-Vine PEG (percutaneous endoscopic gastrostomy)

tube *(cont.)*
Sandoz suction/feeding
Saticon vacuum chamber pickup
Shah permanent
small-bore feeding
Suh ventilation
Super PEG
Ultrasil tube
Versatome laser fiber
Vidicon vacuum chamber pickup

Tubegauz—see *tube gauze*.

tube gauze vs. Tubegauz (brand name). Use the generic name for a product when it is not known if the generic or trade name is dictated and the products are pronounced the same. "The digit was then dressed with Neosporin and tube gauze."

tube harvester—used in harvesting osteochondral plugs and occasionally bone for grafting.

tubercle of Zuckerkandl—embryonic thyroid appendage.

tuberculosis, classification of:
TB0—no exposure, no infection.
TB1—exposed to tuberculosis, infection status unknown.
TB2—latent infection, no disease (positive PPD).
TB3—active tuberculosis
pulmonary—receiving no chemotherapy
pleural—receiving chemotherapy (date).
lymphatic—chemotherapy terminated (date).
bone and/or joint—completed prescribed chemotherapy course.
genitourinary—incomplete chemotherapy course.
other locations: disseminated (miliary), meningeal, peritoneal.
TB4—inactive tuberculosis, healed or adequately treated.
TB5—possible tuberculosis, status unknown (rule out TB).

tuberculosis tests—see *Amplified Mycobacterium tuberculosis direct test*, *Roche-Microwell plate hybridization method,* and *tine test*.

Tubex injector—a closed injection system to protect doctors and nurses against needle-stick injuries.

tubing forceps—used in glaucoma patients for trimming, handling, and insertion of drainage tube into scleral entry site.

tuboplasty—see *transcervical balloon tuboplasty*.

tubularized cecal flap—used in continent urinary diversion procedures.

TUIP (transurethral incision of the prostate).

tularemia—a febrile illness, first described in Tulare, California. The vector (carrier) is thought to be *Ixodes pacificus*, a common deer and cattle tick.

TULIP (transurethral ultrasound-guided laser-induced prostatectomy).

tulip probe.

tulip tip—on end of PEG feeding tube.

tumbling bullet sign—on radiographs, a bullet which changes its location and orientation within a solitary bone cyst.

tumescent absorbent bandage (TAB) **dressing**.

tumescent technique—a liposuction technique where high-volume, pressurized fluid formula is infiltrated, distending, anesthetizing and exsanguinating the region, allowing for almost bloodless and painless surgical removal of excess fatty tissues during liposuction.

Tum-E-Vac—gastric lavage kit for use in emergency situations.

tummy tuck flap—method of breast reconstruction in which the transverse rectus abdominis muscle (TRAM) flap is used to create a myocutaneous

tummy *(cont.)*
flap which is tunneled beneath the skin to the breast. Similar in procedure to an abdominoplasty, hence the name *tummy tuck flap*. Also called *TRAM flap*.

tumor—see *disease.*

tumor-activated prodrug (TAP).

tumoral calcinosis—a rare systemic disorder characterized by ectopic soft tissue calcification near the joints.

tumor amplified protein expression therapy (TAPET).

tumor blush—vascularization seen on angiography. Increased vascularization is a clue to the presence of a tumor and may represent a malignancy rather than hypertrophy.

tumor-infiltrating lymphocytes (TIL).

tumor lysis syndrome (TLS)—a rare complication following chemotherapy in which massive lysis of malignant cells releasing their intracellular components causes an acute episode of hyperuricemia, hyperkalemia, and hypocalcemia. TLS can lead to renal failure and even death.

tumor marker—a biochemical indicator (CA 15-3, CA 19-9, CA27.29, CA 72-4, DR-70, for example) that, when found in the blood, urine, or serum, indicates the presence of a tumor. Examples of these markers are *carcinoembryonic antigen* (CEA) as a marker for carcinomas of the lung, digestive tract, and pancreas; *prostate-specific antigen* (PSA) for cancer of the prostate; *alpha-fetoprotein* (AFP) for hepatomas and teratomas, Paget disease of the bone, and Hodgkin disease. Examples:
alpha-fetoprotein (AFP)
antigen
Bcl-2 oncogene
BRCA1 oncogene

tumor *(cont.)*
BRCA2 oncogene
carcinoembryonic antigen (CEA)
chromosome 14q tumor
CYFRA 21-1
gene
neuron specific enolase
oncogene
prostate-specific antigen (PSA)
thymidylate synthase

tumor necrosis factor—see *TNF*.

tumor plop—the sound made by a pedunculated myxoma in a cardiac chamber when the patient is rolled over.

tumor suppressor gene—a gene that suppresses cellular proliferation; when damaged or deleted it may permit development of malignant tumors. Examples:
APC (adenomatous polyposis coli)
DCC (deleted in colon carcinoma)
NF1 (neurofibromatosis)
NF2 (neurofibromatosis)
RB1 (retinoblastoma)
TP53 (p53)
VHL (von Hippel-Lindau)
WT1 (Wilms tumor)

TUMT—see *transurethral microwave thermotherapy*.

TUNA—see *transurethral needle ablation.*

TUNEL stain—terminal deoxynucleotidyl transferase-mediated deoxyuridine triphosphate used to stain the placenta to identify apoptosis (programmed cell death).

Tun-L-Kath epidural catheter—used for epidural neuroplasty.

tunnel views (Radiol).

Tuohy needle—used to insert a lumbar subarachnoid catheter.

Tupper hand-holder and retractor—provides total accessibility and stability required for meticulous hand surgery.

turbo spin-echo sequences (MRI)—superior to gradient-echo sequences in visualizing the biliary tree.

turbo spin-echo T_2-weighted sequence (MRI).

turbo STIR images—MRI term.

TurboVac 90—suction ArthroWand.

Turbo Whisker—an arthroscopic surgical blade.

Turco posteromedial release of clubfoot.

turgor pressure—pressure in capillaries.

turnbuckle functional position splint—designed to reduce wrist flexion contractures. The splint controls wrist-hand angle with a turnbuckle, which can be adjusted in fine increments.

Turner mosaicism (syndrome).

Turner needle—a biopsy needle for aspiration and cutting of solid tissue specimens.

Turner-Warwick method—uses the right gastroepiploic artery as the vascular supply for a pedicle graft in a bowel reconstruction procedure.

Turner-Warwick urethroplasty.

turn-up plasty—a seldom-used procedure that provides a stump for an above-the-knee prosthesis by removing the infected femur, foot amputation, knee disarticulation, and then turning the lower leg up, using the tibia to support the femoral component of a joint replacement.

turtle sign—(1) In shoulder dystocia, the baby's head emerges but then recedes into the birth canal. (2) In an obstetrical ultrasound image of a male fetus, the genitalia resemble the head and forelimbs of a turtle.

Turvy internal screw fixation—used in sagittal split ramus osteotomy.

Tutofix—cortical pin for fixation of small and medium fractures. Tutofix pins are produced from bovine compact bone.

Tutoplast—brand name for tissues which have been treated through a process of preservation and viral inactivation and then implanted or reimplanted into the patient. Reportedly shows great promise for bone tumors.

TUVP (transurethral electrovaporization of the prostate).

Tuwave—programmed TENS waveform treatment mode used to reduce edema and pain following surgery or trauma. See *TENS*.

TVO (transtrochanteric valgus osteotomy).

TVS (transvaginal ultrasound).

TVT (tension-free vaginal tape) **procedure**—for treatment of female stress urinary incontinence. Prolene mesh tape is woven through pelvic tissue and positioned underneath the urethra, creating a supportive sling. The procedure is performed under local anesthesia, and results of surgery can be assessed before the patient leaves the operating room.

T water test—for fructose intolerance.

twenty-nail involvement (or *20-nail*)—psoriatic involvement of all 20 fingernails and toenails.

2040 erbium SilkLaser—computerized erbium laser used for plastic and dermatological surgery, including incision, excision, ablation, vaporization, and/or coagulation of soft tissue.

2010 Plus Holter system—computerized digital systems for analysis of data collected from Holter monitoring; used for monitoring, analysis, and diagnosis of possible cardiac abnormalities.

20/30 Indeflator inflation device—for inflating and maintaining consistent pressure during surgical procedures.

21-channel EEG (electroencephalogram).

twig—smaller than a branch, e.g., in a vessel or nerve. Usage: "There is a possibility that a neural branch or twig was injured, and should the sensory symptoms persist, she was advised to return."

TwinFix Ti Quick-T fixation system—a device used in rotator cuff and glenohumeral instability repair in the shoulder.

Twin Jet nebulizer—for administration of aerosolized drugs such as pentamidine.

twinning—naturally occurring division of a blastocyst into two identical parts, each of which develops into a fetus; the result is a pair of monozygotic (identical) twins (twin offspring from one zygote).

Twisk needle holder, forceps, scissors—a combination instrument used in microsurgery.

IIb/IIa ("to be to a") **platelet inhibitor**—a term that may be hard to decipher when encountered in dictation if not completely clear.

2C3—anti-VEGF (vascular endothelial growth factor) antibody with the ability to block the binding of a growth factor to receptors found on tumor vasculature, with the effect of inhibiting tumor vessel growth.

TwinFix—suture anchor with needles for orthopedic surgical procedures.

two-dimensional echocardiography (sector scan)—noninvasive technique for diagnosis, making catheterization unnecessary for some cardiac lesions.

2-D FT (two-dimensional Fourier transform)—a mathematical process that creates MRI images from raw data; 3-D FT also exists but is used less.

2-D IVUS (two-dimensional intravascular ultrasound).

two-flight dyspnea—difficulty breathing that occurs on climbing two flights of stairs. (But what is a flight? Ten steps? Twenty steps?)

two-incision hip replacement—minimally invasive hip replacement using the Zimmer VerSys femoral hip stem and the Trilogy acetabular system. It affords all the benefits of other minimally invasive procedures; patients generally walk out of the hospital on crutches the day after the operation.

two-layer latex and Marlex closure technique—a simplified wound management technique consisting of a temporary two-layer sandwich of synthetic materials (Esmarch latex rubber bandage and Marlex nonabsorbable synthetic mesh). Effects temporary abdominal wall closure and thus protects the intestine, prevents adhesions, and can be easily revised at bedside.

Two-Photon Excitation (TPE)—light-based technology that uses short pulsed bursts of long-wavelength light for destruction of cancerous and diseased tissues.

270° Toupet fundoplication—surgical procedure used to treat gastroesophageal reflux disease.

two-stage capsulorrhexis—for endocapsular phacoemulsification (Oph).

two-stick or **three-stick technique**—colloquial term for two or three ports (incisions) used during thoracoscopy or other minimally invasive procedure.

Tyco #3—medical slang for Tylenol No. 3 (Tylenol with codeine).

Tycron suture—nonabsorbable polyester fiber surgical suture. *Tycron* and *Ti-Cron* are sold by different manufacturers but appear to be the same material.

Tygon tubing—used in venovenous bypass for transplantation of the liver, and for other uses.

Tylenol No. 3—edit to correct name, Tylenol with Codeine No. 3.

Tylok cerclage cabling system.

tylosis—callosities. See *hypertylosis*.

tympanocentesis—see *spectrofluorometry*.

tympanoplasty—see *crowncork tympanoplasty*.

Tyndall effect—see *aqueous flare*.

typhlitis—inflammation of the cecum; also, *cecitis*.

Typhoon microdebrider blade—self-irrigating, disposable cutter blade used in endoscopic sinus surgery.

tyramine test—for pheochromocytoma.

tyrosine tolerance test.

T–Y stent—a tracheobronchial stent which has both T-shaped and Y-shaped sections. Used to maintain a patent airway after burns or trauma.

TZ (transition zone).

Tzanck ("zank") **preparation**.

U, u

UAC (umbilical artery catheter).
UAD (upper airway dysfunction).
UAE (uterine artery embolization).
UAL (ultrasonic-assisted lipoplasty [or liposuction]).
UAS (ulnocarpal abutment syndrome).
UBC (University of British Columbia) **brace**.
UBIS 5000 ultrasound bone sonometer—a portable medical device that uses ultrasound to measure the strength of the heel bone. Since the heel bone is similar to the bones in the hip and spine, this measurement can indicate the strength of those bones as well.
UBM (Ultrasonic Biomicroscope).
UBOs (unidentified bright objects)—used in MRI dictation on the breast.
UBT breath test—noninvasive procedure for diagnosis of *Helicobacter pylori*.
UCBL (University of California Berkeley Laboratory) **orthosis**.
UCLA pouch—for continent urinary diversion, formed from colon.
UC strip—catheter tubing fastener.
UD-BMT (unrelated donor, bone marrow transplantation).
UDS (urine dipstick).
UES (upper esophageal sphincter).
UFE (uterine fibroid embolization).
UFT (Uracil and ftorafur)—chemotherapeutic agent.
UGH+ syndrome—symptoms of uveitis, glaucoma, hyphema, plus vitreous hemorrhage.
UHMWPe (ultra-high molecular weight polyethylene) **ball liner**—Enduron acetabular liner.
Uhthoff ("oot'-hoff") **phenomenon**; **sign**—nystagmus in patients with multiple cerebrospinal sclerosis.
Uldall *(not* Udall) subclavian hemodialysis catheter.
ulegyria—destruction of the cortex in a deep sulcus of a gyrus.
ulnocarpal abutment syndrome (UAS).
Ulson fixator system—orthopedic device used for percutaneous pinning and external fixation techniques. It is used to repair Colles wrist fractures, requiring the insertion of two percutaneous pins into the intramed-

Ulson *(cont.)*
ullary canal followed by application of an external Ulson fixator with a clamp assembly.

Ultec—hydrocolloid dressing.

Ultima C femoral component. Usage: "The femoral canal was then reamed up to a #2 Ultima C size femoral component."

Ultrabrace—a custom-fitted, postop knee orthosis in which patients can ambulate with adjustable dynamic assistance or resistance.

Ultracal HN Plus—a nutritional supplement used for tube feeding.

UltraCision ultrasonic knife—ultrasonically activated scalpel used to dissect tissue with simultaneous hemostasis in minimally invasive surgery. Improved healing and reduced tissue injury are the result of minimal thermal injury produced by this instrument compared to the heat-generating electrocautery or laser. In addition, there is no smoke, char, or odor. Its use requires no protective eye gear or special safety equipment. See *Harmonic Scalpel*.

Ultra-Drive bone cement removal system—used in total hip revision to remove old cement without damage to the cortical wall. Ultrasonically tuned tool tips to provide audible and tactile feedback in order to differentiate between cement and bone.

Ultra 8 balloon catheter.

ultrafast CT—see *cine CT*.

ultrafast CT electron beam tomography—computed tomography that is more accurate and rapid than digital fluoroscopy.

UltraFine erbium laser system—used for skin resurfacing.

UltraFix RC—implant that provides fixation strength for rotator cuff repair.

Ultraflex stent—a self-expanding stent made of an elastic metal, nitinol, which is encased in gelatin and an outer plastic sheath. It is implanted endoscopically over a guidewire. Once in place, the plastic sheath is removed and the stent expands as the gelatin dissolves. It is used to treat esophageal stenosis in patients with unresectable esophageal carcinoma.

Ultraject—contrast media in prefilled plastic syringe, providing accurate dosing and protection against accidental needle-stick injuries.

UltraKlenz wound cleanser.

UltraLite—flow-directed microcatheter.

Ultramark 4 ultrasound.

Ultramax coated knitted velour vascular graft.

UltraPulse CO_2 laser—used for laser resurfacing treatment of wrinkled, scarred, or sun-damaged skin of the face.

Ultraseed system—ultrasound-guided brachytherapy system for treatment planning of transperineal prostate implantation of radioactive seeds in prostate cancer.

Ultrasil tube—ventilation tube for myringotomy.

UltraSling—supports the glenohumeral joint in neutral position with 10° of abduction. It is used for postoperative rehabilitation following arthroscopic repair of SLAP (superior labrum anterior posterior) lesions.

ultrasmall superparamagnetic iron oxide (USPIO)—a class of imaging agents.

ultrasonic aspiration—a safe and effective method for obtaining local control of large neuroblastomas.

ultrasonic-assisted lipoplasty (or **liposuction**) (UAL)—liposuction technique that removes fat only from the

ultrasonic *(cont.)*
deeper layers rather than the superficial layers.

Ultrasonic Biomicroscope (UBM)—a device used for viewing structures in the front half of the eye.

ultrasonic body contouring—uses ultrasound to disrupt, destroy, and disperse targeted fat cells, giving patients the benefits of liposuction without the pain and recovery time.

ultrasonic dissection coagulator—the generic name for devices such as Harmonic scalpel, now used for tonsillectomy.

ultrasonic pachymetry—can be used intraoperatively to measure corneal thickness.

ultrasonography—a means of visualizing internal structures by observing the effects they have on a beam of sound waves. The sound used for this procedure is at a higher frequency (pitch) than the human ear can detect. Ultrasound waves pass through air, gas, and fluid without being reflected; however, they bounce back from rigid structures such as bone and gallstones, creating an "echo" that can be detected by a receiver. Solid organs such as the liver and kidney partially reflect ultrasound waves in predictable patterns. Waves are also reflected from the interface between two structures. Ultrasonography might be compared to taking a flash photograph. Light from the flashbulb bounces off the patient and comes back to create an image on film of the surface contours of the patient; however, the echo must be converted electronically to a visible image before it can be interpreted. Sophisticated electronic equipment permits ultrasound scanning of a body region with generation of a two-dimensional picture of internal structures. In practice, the same device that generates the sound waves (called a transducer) also acts as the receiver. Although it emits signals at a rate of 1000 per second, the transducer is actually functioning as a receiver 99.9% of the time.

ultrasound (US) (see also *imaging*)
ADR
Aloka
ATL real-time
BladderScan
B-mode
contrast echocardiography
diathermy
duplex
endoscopic (EUS)
endovaginal (EVUS)
four-dimensional (4-D)
frequency domain imaging (FDI)
gray scale
high-intensity focused (HFU)
laparoscopic ultrasonography (LUS)
NeuroSector
Nicolet Elite Doppler
Olympus EU-M30S endoscopic ultrasonography receiver
Photopic Imaging
real-time
real-time 4-D
SonoSite portable
TDOG (tissue Doppler gated) dynamic three-dimensional ultrasound imaging
transcervical tuboplasty
transnasal endoluminal
transrectal
TRUS (transrectal ultrasound)
Ultramark 4

ultrasound biomicroscopy (UBM).

ultrasound diathermy—heats to a tissue depth of 5 to 6 cm and is used to

ultrasound *(cont.)*
warm areas around tissue interfaces such as joints.

ultrasound-guided anterior subcostal liver biopsy.

ultrasound-guided compression—a noninvasive treatment for persisting false aneurysms using direct compression on the point of communication between the artery and the hematoma. It is thought to be an improvement over surgical repair but is in less favor than the newer sonographically guided human thrombin injection.

ultrasound-guided pseudoaneurysm compression—treatment for catheter-related femoral injuries.

ultrasound transcervical tuboplasty—unblocks obstructed fallopian tubes, without exposing the patient to abdominal surgery, x-rays, or x-ray dyes. A cervical cannula is positioned, and Doppler ultrasound is used (instead of fluoroscopy) to thread a catheter into the blocked tube, where normal saline is injected to check catheter position. Then a flexible wire is threaded through the catheter to break up the obstruction.

Ultrasure DTU-one (yes, the "one" is lower case)—imaging ultrasound system for assessment of osteoporotic fracture risk.

Ultrathon—highly effective insect repellant originally developed for use by the U.S. military, now being released to the public in response to serious mosquito and tick-borne diseases in the northeast part of the country. It has a 33% DEET (diethyltoluamide) content in a controlled-release polymer-based cream.

Ultratome—small sphincterotome manufactured by Microvasive.

ULTT (upper limb tension test).

umami (pronounced "you-mommy")—a newly discovered human taste receptor that responds to glutamate, a savory tasting molecule found in a variety of meats, cheeses, and vegetables.

umbilical artery velocimetry—used to determine the gestational age of a fetus. This technique uses a Doppler ultrasound to compare systolic and diastolic blood flow in the umbilical artery. Other techniques used to determine fetal gestational age include mean amniotic fluid index and biophysical profile.

umbilical coiling index—a reference point for diagnosing fetal problems. The normal umbilical cord consists of three intertwining blood vessels in Wharton jelly, which fall into fixed coils. The average umbilical cord has 11 such coils. However, 5% of umbilical cords are completely straight. This phenomenon has been associated with fetal anomalies, fetal heart rate decelerations, passing meconium, premature labor, and even fetal death. The umbilical coiling index (expressed as coils/cm) is determined by dividing the number of coils by the length of the umbilical cord. An index of less than 0.1 coils/cm is associated with the above-mentioned fetal problems. A normal value (the mean index) is 0.21 coils/cm.

umbilical cord stem cell—a hematopoietic stem cell that is present in umbilical cord blood during the immediate postpartum period; similar to bone marrow stem cells.

umbilicated—having a central pit or dimple.

umbrella cell—found on the surface of the urothelium.

uncooperative—often used euphemistically for a negative, disobedient, defiant patient.

under-the-skin technique—a technique of skin closure in which there are only two stitch holes, one at each end of the incision, and no knots are required. A button or pearl is simply attached to each end instead of a knot.

undifferentiated—said of a stem cell that has not undergone differentiation into a specific cell type.

undyed braided polyglycolic acid suture.

unenhanced scan—a scan made without the use of a contrast material.

Unfolder—intraocular lens (IOL) implantation system used to deliver The Sensar foldable acrylic posterior chamber IOL. See also *Sensar*.

ungual tuft—tip of the nail.

UNHS (Universal Neonatal Hearing Screening).

unicornuate uterus—often found in women with urinary tract anomalies, such as renal agenesis contralateral to the hemi-uterus and ectopic kidney. A rare malformation that is difficult to recognize without invasive procedures. Thus, it is diagnosed only by the presence of gynecological symptoms such as pelvic pain, infertility, or repeated abortion.

Unified Parkinson Disease Rating Scale (UPDRS)—a rating tool to follow the longitudinal course of Parkinson disease. It is made up of three main sections: (1) mentation, behavior, and mood, (2) activities of daily living, and (3) motor. A total of 199 points is possible; 199 represents the worst (total) disability, and 0 is no disability.

Uniflex intramedullary femoral nail system.

Uniflex polyurethane adhesive surgical dressing.

Uni-Gold—*H. pylori* one-step test using only one drop of whole blood, serum, or plasma to test for the presence of IgG antibodies to the bacterium.

Unigraft bone graft material—synthetic bioactive glass material used in the repair of oral defects, including periodontal defects, extraction sites, and augmentation of the alveolar ridge.

Unilab Surgibone—nonantigenic, sterile, specially processed mature bovine bone used instead of autologous or homologous bone for implantation into humans to fill cavities from which tumors or cysts have been removed. There are also specially prepared onlay grafts that have cancellous bone on one side and cortical bone on the other, and also load-bearing cancellous bone blocks and dowels.

UNILINK system—a mechanical anastomotic device, designed for work under the operating microscope, to anastomose small blood vessels.

Unimar J-Needle—a suturing needle for closing deep tissue layers in a small opening into a body cavity.

unipotent stem cell—a stem cell that is capable of sustaining a self-renewing line or of differentiating into a single mature cell type.

UniPuls electro-stimulation instrument—provides full TENS application along with stimulation of acupuncture sites.

UniShaper—a single-use keratome.

uni-tip deformity—often the result of nasal tip surgery in which the domes

uni-tip *(cont.)*
of the lower lateral cartilages become pinched or over-narrowed and take on a uni-tip shape. The tip of the nose has a normal bidomal shape.

Unitron Esteem CIC (completely-in-the-canal) **hearing aid**.

Unity-C pacemaker—single-pass, rate-adaptive cardiac pacing system.

universal donor cells—cells of genetically engineered transgenic animals, such as pigs, the organs of which may be used for xenotransplantation.

Universal fixation screws.

Universal Neonatal Hearing Screening (UNHS)—new screening test that utilizes otoacoustic emissions to test neonatal hearing. It can be carried out in the first few days of life and is said to be much more sensitive than the Infant Distraction Test which was normally performed at 7 to 8 months.

Universal Spine Classification—in which fractures are categorized as type A, B, or C. Type A fractures involve only one column, have no translation or angulation, and are managed conservatively. Type B fractures involve two columns, with insignificant translation and angulation, and may be managed either conservatively or surgically. Type C fractures either involve all three columns, have significant translation, or have significant angulation, and are generally managed surgically.

Universal2 (no space) **total wrist implant system**.

universal vacuum release (UVR).

University of Akron artificial heart—fully implantable artificial heart that does not need to be connected to a machine outside the patient. Contains batteries to provide power and electromagnets to move the blood through its chambers.

University of Wisconsin solution—for donor heart preservation.

Unna boot (Ortho)—see *Unna paste.*

Unna-Flex compression dressing and wrap.

Unna-Pak compression dressing and wrap.

Unna paste—a moist paste impregnated with zinc oxide, calamine lotion, and glycerin. It is applied as a "cast" (Unna boot) and provides topical treatment and compression for venous stasis ulcers.

unreamed femoral nail (UFN)—an intramedullary nail used for repair of pathologic, epiphyseal, subtrochanteric, and ipsilateral fractures of the femoral neck. There is less iatrogenic damage to the vascularization of the bone (than with a reamed femoral nail), the risk of fat embolism syndrome and ARDS is reduced, and the operation is a less time-consuming procedure, associated with less blood loss.

Unschuld sign—a tendency to have cramps in the calves, an early indication of diabetes mellitus.

Unterberger test—see *Fukuda test.*

Unterberger-Fukuda stepping test—see *Fukuda test.*

Unverricht-Lundborg syndrome—progressive myoclonus epilepsy, a genetic syndrome. The malignant form, associated with progressive dementia may be called *Lafora body disease*, the benign form *Baltic myoclonus.*

upbiting forceps.

UPDRS (Unified Parkinson Disease Rating Scale).

UPEP ("yoo-pep") (urine protein electrophoresis).

UPF prosthesis (Universal proximal femur)—see *Bateman UPF prosthesis*.

upgoing toes—abnormal response to the Babinski test, in which the great toe curls upward when the sole of the foot is stroked. Diagnostic of disorders of the central nervous system.

UPLIFT (uterine **p**ositioning via **li**gament **i**nvestment **f**ixation and **t**runcation) **procedure**—a laparoscopic procedure that shortens and strengthens the round ligaments to perform uterine suspension.

UPlink—a highly sensitive drug monitoring system, capable of performing up to 10 drugs-of-abuse tests on one sample in less than 10 minutes.

uPM3 urine test—found to be 80% correct in detecting a gene marker of prostate cancer. The test may eliminate the need for painful prostate biopsy in many cases.

upper airway dysfunction (UAD)—similar to vocal cord dysfunction and has similar treatment but is not a surgical condition. See *vocal cord dysfunction*.

Upper Hands—a self-retaining retractor used in liver transplantation.

upper limb tension test (ULTT)—considered an analog to the straight leg raising test for the lower limb, it assesses pain responses consequent to passive movements of the upper limb and neck.

UPPP (uvulopalatopharyngoplasty).

uptake—in radionuclide scans, the absorption or concentration of a radionuclide by an organ or tissue. Also, *fluorescein uptake*.

urachus, patent—in a neonate, incomplete closure of the umbilicus through which urine escapes; a urachal cyst may form and require surgical treatment.

uracil—a pyrimidine (symbol U), one of the four bases found in RNA; in the formation of a double-stranded nucleic acid, it always pairs with the pyrimidine cytosine (C).

uracil mustard—chemotherapy drug.

Ureaplasma urealyticum—organism suspected of creating a higher incidence of infertility in women. It is also a risk factor for respiratory disease in the first three years of life.

Ureflex ureteral catheter—for intravenous pyelogram.

ureter vs. urethral—refers to two totally different anatomical structures. (Spelling hint: There are two *e*'s in ureter and there are two ureters; there's one *e* in urethra, and there is only one urethra.)

ureteral calculi in pregnancy—may be diagnosed with small instruments and treated without resorting to ionizing radiation, but using only ultrasound monitoring and rigid ureteroscopy.

ureteropelvic junction (UPJ).

ureterorenoscopy—rigid or flexible retrograde, combined with percutaneous resection, used as treatment for transitional cell carcinoma of renal pelvis.

ureteroscopy—with small rigid instruments, such as the Gautier ureteroscope, may be performed on the entire urinary tract even during advanced pregnancy. Stones may be fragmented, extracted, or displaced, and double pigtail ureteral catheters may be applied with only sonographic guidance, at times without use of anesthesia.

urethral and vesical neck damage to women—caused by aggressive trans-

urethral *(cont.)*
urethral resection of the bladder neck; incontinence procedures (including anterior plication, anterior colporrhaphy, and needle urethropexy); injudicious use of indwelling urethral catheters in neurologically impaired or debilitated patients; invasive tumors (e.g., cervical carcinoma); obstructed obstetrical delivery; pelvic trauma; radiation; and urethral diverticulectomy.

urethral reconstruction complications
detrusor muscle instability
fistula formation
hydronephrosis
ischemia or sloughing of the flap
urinary incontinence
urinary retention
vesical neck stenosis

urethral surgical reconstruction—used to fashion an unobstructed neourethra and maintain continence.

URF-P2 choledochoscope.

Uricult dipslides—used in testing urine for bacteria.

uridine rescue—a drug regimen which allows larger than usual doses of fluorouracil to be given to patients with metastatic colorectal carcinoma.

urinary diversion procedure—for intestinal urinary conduit.

urinary tract anomalies—often associated with unicornuate uterus in women.

urinary tract reconstruction augmentation cystoplasty—technique for continent urinary diversion.

urine analysis—transcribe urinalysis when "urine analysis" is dictated.

urine protein electrophoresis (UPEP).

urines—urine specimens.

urines are cooking—medical slang for "reports of urine cultures and sensitivity studies are pending."

Uriscreen—a urine specimen test to detect bacteriuria, especially in pregnancy. It is said to be a reliable alternative to culture screening of all pregnant patients and is estimated to save as much as 80% of all unnecessary cultures.

UroCoil—self-expanding stent used to treat strictures of the male urethra.

Urocyte diagnostic cytometry system—noninvasive test for carcinoma of the urothelium.

urocytogram—study of estrogen effect on desquamated cells from the urogenital tract (used in investigation of precocious puberty).

Urolase fiber—for visual laser ablation of prostate.

Urologic Targis—a targeted transurethral thermoablation system.

Uroloop—a surgical device that cuts and vaporizes tissue simultaneously.

UroLume endoprosthesis—tiny, expandable wire stent used to open and keep the urethra patent as treatment for benign prostatic hyperplasia.

UroLume urethral stent—used for recurrent bulbomembranous urethral strictures.

Urolume Wallstent—a metallic stent placed in the urinary tract.

UroMax II catheter—a high pressure ureteral balloon catheter.

urothelium—epithelium of the urinary bladder.

urothelial augmentation—an alternative to gastrointestinal segments in augmentation cystoplasty. Also *autoaugmentation*.

UroVive—a self-detachable balloon system for treating urinary stress incontinence. It is a urethral bulking agent consisting of a micro-balloon permanently implanted in a minimally invasive fashion into the urinary

UroVive *(cont.)*
sphincter muscle. It is a one-time treatment performed on an outpatient basis.

Urowave—uses microwave thermotherapy to reduce the size and symptoms associated with an enlarged prostate.

ursodeoxycholic acid (ursodiol)—drug used to dissolve stones. Usage: "To consider use of ursodeoxycholic acid in a person this young would not be appropriate, as he has a high possibility of recurrence, even after dissolution of the stones."

urushiol ("oo-roo-she-all")—that component in poison oak, poison sumac, and poison ivy that causes the contact dermatitis in people who are sensitive to these plants.

USCI cannula.

USCI Goetz bipolar electrodes.

USCI NBIH bipolar electrodes.

Usher syndrome type 1—congenital nerve deafness and retinitis pigmentosa.

USPIO (ultrasmall superparamagnetic iron oxide)—a class of imaging agents.

Utah artificial arm—a myoelectric prosthesis for amputations above the elbow; it comes with either a hook or an artificial Myobock hand.

uterine artery embolization (UAE)—a procedure in which a bolus is injected and remains permanently in the uterine arteries in order to block the flow of blood through those vessels; attempts to shrink fibroids by cutting off their blood supply.

uterine balloon therapy—a procedure using a catheter and balloon to heat the inside of the uterus and destroy its lining to stop excessive menstrual bleeding. An alternative procedure to hysterectomy.

uterine cry—see *cry, uterine*.

uterine fibroid embolization (UFE)—treatment for uterine fibroids. A less-invasive procedure than hysterectomy, UFE is performed under local anesthetic, using a catheter passed through a small incision in the groin into the uterine artery. When the catheter reaches the uterine artery, tiny particles are released into the artery which flow to the fibroids, blocking the blood flow, thereby starving the fibroid. See *uterine artery embolization*.

uterine positioning via ligament investment fixation and truncation (UPLIFT) procedure.

uterus didelphys—double uterus.

"u-thymic"—see *euthymic*.

"u-thyroid"—see *euthyroid*.

U-Titer—a computer-based assessment technique used in nearly all clinical domains.

Utrata capsulorrhexis forceps—used in small-incision eye surgery. Cf. *Kraff-Utrata tear capsulotomy forceps*.

uveitides—plural form of uveitis.

UVR (universal vacuum release) (Ob-Gyn)—used in vacuum deliveries.

uvulopalatopharyngoplasty (UPPP)—a surgical treatment for sleep apnea in patients who cannot tolerate or do not respond to medical therapies, such as wearing a CPAP (continuous positive airway pressure) or BiPAP (bi-level positive airway pressure) mask during sleep. UPPP involves the removal of the tonsils, adenoids, posterior soft palate, and extra mucosal tissue in the pharynx. Note the similarity to *uvulopalatopharyngoplasty*.

V, v

V (ventricular).

Vabra aspirator—disposable system for endometrial screening.

V.A.C. (vacuum-assisted closure)—trademarked with periods and without hyphen.

V.A.C. Freedom system—a lightweight model of the vacuum-assisted [wound] closure device.

vaccine (see also *medications*)
- ActHIB (*H. influenzae* type B)
- bacillus Calmette-Guérin (BCG)
- Dryvax
- edible
- Helivax
- Hemophilus B conjugate
- HIV AC-le
- human diploid cell strain rabies (HDRV)
- Hib polysaccharide
- HspBcor
- influenza
- MN rgp120
- MPL (monophosphoryl lipid A)
- pneumococcal conjugate
- Provenge
- PVAC therapeutic
- RDRV (Rhesus diploid cell strain rabies)

vaccine *(cont.)*
- TCR (T-cell receptor) peptide
- zoster immune globulin

Vac-Lok—a patient immobilization cushion that creates a precise, rigid mold to hold the patient's body in place during imaging procedures. The cushion is radiotranslucent and artifact-free.

Vac-Pak Pad—a pad used for immobilization in total hip surgery.

VACTERL syndrome
- V vertebral or vascular defects
- A anorectal malformation (imperforate anus)
- C cardiac anomaly
- TE tracheoesophageal fistula
- R renal anomaly
- L limb anomaly

Vacurette—suction curet (Ob-Gyn).

Vacutainer—rubber-stoppered vacuum tube to draw blood.

vacuum-assisted closure (V.A.C.)—assists in wound closure by applying localized negative pressure to draw edges of the wound toward the center. Applied to a special dressing positioned in the wound cavity or over

vacuum-assisted *(cont.)*
a flap graft, this pressure-distributing wound packing helps remove fluids from the wound and increase blood perfusion.

vacuum-assisted negative pressure wound therapy—in which an open-cell foam sponge is fitted into the wound, the wound sealed with an adhesive drape, and subatmospheric pressure applied through an evacuation tube by a computerized pump. This method evacuates wound fluid, reduces localized edema, stimulates granulation tissue formation, and reduces bacterial colonization.

vacuum disk (or vacuum phenomenon)—the presence of a linear radiolucency in the disk space, a typical finding of degenerative disk disease on radiography.

vacuum phenomenon, spontaneous —(1) A finding on x-ray of the lateral compartment of the knee, possibly related to traction on a joint or the absence of an effusion. The presence of this finding on a plain radiograph, or of artifacts associated with it on magnetic resonance imaging, is said by some to create the false impression of a meniscal tear, especially in the medial compartment. Others consider it a true indication of meniscal degeneration with tearing. (2) Linear radiolucency in the disk space (vacuum phenomenon), which is a typical finding of degenerative disk disease. It is often associated to other findings of degenerative disk disease such as disk space narrowing and endplate sclerosis.

VAD (ventricular assist device)—see *Thoratec ventricular assist device*.

VAE (voluntary active euthanasia). See also *PAS*, *TS*, and *VSED*.

vagal nerve implant—given to a patient with epilepsy that cannot be controlled by drugs or surgery. The implant is placed subcutaneously under the collarbone, and two electrodes from it are placed on the vagal nerve. When patients sense the onset of a seizure, they activate the implant to stimulate the vagal nerve. This appears to interrupt epileptic activity in the brain.

vagal paraganglioma—see *glomus vagale*.

vaginal birth after (previous) **cesarean section** (VBAC).

vaginal candle (Oncol)—used in radium insertion.

vaginal construction techniques—see *operations*.

vaginal contraceptive film (VCF)—spermicidal contraceptive drug in film formulation that begins to dissolve instantly and washes away with the body's natural fluids, thereby not having to be removed.

vaginal flap reconstruction of urethra and vesical neck in women—approaches are (1) anterior bladder flap (Tanagho procedure); (2) posterior bladder flap (Young-Dees-Leadbetter procedure); (3) vaginal flap. Vaginal flap reconstruction is said to be more successful than bladder flap operations.

vaginal flap reconstruction and pubovaginal sling procedure—used to treat women with extensive vesical neck and/or urethral damage.

vaginal interruption of pregnancy, with dilatation and curettage (VIP-DAC).

vaginal packing—used in beating heart surgery. A technique using the

vaginal *(cont.)*
Medtronic Octopus 2+ tissue stabilization system forms a 'heart sling,' and the two arms of the vaginal packing cradle the heart and allow it to be manipulated to access all walls of the heart. Usage: "A two-inch sterile vaginal packing was then snared with a rummel at its midpoint with the deep pericardial suture and cinched down into the pericardial well."

vaginal-psoas colposuspension—modification of the psoas hitch procedure used for ureterovesicostomy, for repair of uterovaginal prolapse.

vaginal wall sling procedure—for recurrent stress urinary incontinence in elderly women due to severe genital prolapse. Similar to the Raz procedure, this procedure uses a vaginal wall graft to provide increased urethral compression and stability of the bladder base. Because it results in vaginal shortening, it is not recommended for sexually active women. See also *abdominal sacral colpoperineopexy*, *Raz procedure*, *sacrospinous colpopexy*, and *triangular vaginal patch sling*.

vagus nerve stimulation (VNS)—provided by implanted pulse generator in patients with epilepsy and other neurological disorders.

Vairox high compression vascular stocking.

Valchev uterine manipulator.

VALIANT (valsartan in acute myocardial infarction) **study**.

Validyne manometer.

Valle hysteroscope.

Valleix sign—an uncomfortable burning pain that radiates proximally toward the calf upon palpation of the course of the posterior tibial nerve from the proximal aspect of the medial malleolus distally toward the anterior aspect of the calcaneus.

ValleyLab—laparoscopic and electrosurgical instruments.

ValleyLab Ligasure.

valley-to-peak dose rate—lowest dose to highest dose.

Valtrac BAR (biofragmentable anastomotic ring).

valve (see also *prosthesis*)
antireflux flap
ATS Open Pivot bileaflet heart
Bauhin ileocecal
Benchekroun ileohydraulic
Biocor porcine stented aortic and mitral
Biocor stentless porcine aortic
Capetown aortic prosthetic
Contegra pulmonary valved conduit
CPHV OptiForm mitral
CryoLife-O'Brien
CryoValve-SG
dual switch (DSV)
flap (*not* flat)
Freestyle aortic root bioprosthesis
glutaraldehyde-tanned porcine heart
Hall prosthetic heart
Hancock M.O. II Bioprosthesis porcine
Heister
Ionescu tri-leaflet
Kock nipple
Krupin-Denver eye
Medtronic Hancock II tissue
mitral valve homograft
Mosaic heart
Mosaic porcine bioprosthesis
On-X prosthetic heart
Orbis-Sigma cerebrospinal fluid
Quattro mitral
Regent aortic heart
Ross pulmonary porcine
Spitz-Holter
Synergraft

valve *(cont.)*
Tekna mechanical heart
Top-Hat supra-anular aortic
Toronto SPV
Xenomedica prosthetic
Xenotech prosthetic

valvotomy—see *percutaneous mitral balloon valvotomy* (PMBV).

V-Amour female condom—a soft latex pouch attached to a flexible V-shaped frame. A polyurethane sponge is inside the pouch.

Van Bogaert disease—a rare familial disease, resulting in hepatomegaly secondary to very high concentrations of cholesterol esters.

vanc—slang for *vancomycin*.

vancomycin-resistant enterococci (VRE).

vancomycin-resistant *Enterococcus faecium* (VREF) **infection**.

van den Bergh test—of the concentration of bilirubin in the blood. Normal range: direct bilirubin 0.0 to 0.1 mg per 100 ml of serum; total bilirubin 0.2 to 1.4 mg per 100 ml of serum.

Van Herick grading system (Oph)—a method for estimating anterior chamber depth. Usage: "Anterior chambers were deep by Van Herick."

van Heuven anatomic classification—diabetic retinopathy.

vanishing lung syndrome—a progressive disorder characterized by presence of large upper lobe bullae occupying at least one-third of the hemithorax and compressing surrounding normal lung. Also called "type 1 bullous disease" and "primary bullous disease of the lung."

van Loenen operating keratoscope.

Vannas capsulotomy scissors.

VANS (video-assisted neck surgery).

vanSonnenberg sump—for percutaneous abscess and fluid drainage. (Note: There is no space in *vanSonnenberg*.) See also *vanSonnenberg-Wittich catheter.*

VAP (ventilator-assisted pneumonia).

VAP cholesterol test—breaks the HDL fraction down into HDL2 and HDL3, HDL2 being thought to be the "protective" fraction. It also breaks the LDL down into LDL-R (real), Lp(a) (lipoprotein A), considered the highest risk factor, and IDL (intermediate density lipoprotein). The VLDL (very low-density lipoprotein) is also broken down into VLDL1 and VLDL2. This test has shown that patients with normal traditional cholesterol tests may be at risk for heart disease and stroke. The manufacturer recommends specific treatment regimens for different combinations of test results.

VaporTrode—roller electrode specially designed for electrovaporization of prostate tissue.

VAPR-3—a radiofrequency system for arthroscopic surgery.

variable number tandem repeats (VNTRs)—genetically inactive nucleotide sequences that appear between active sequences of a chromosome; they are highly distinctive of an individual and are useful in DNA fingerprinting. See also *short tandem repeats*.

variable screw placement (VSP)—used along with slotted plates with transpedicular screws to correct spondylolisthesis.

variable stiffness endoscope—instrument that allows passage through the sigmoid loops with a flexible setting. Stiffness can then be increased to allow passage through

variable *(cont.)* the transverse colon and around the hepatic flexure to the cecum.

variable threshold angina—see *mixed angina.*

varicella zoster virus—see *VZV.*

varicoses—a widely used term meaning "varicosities." The term has come into use in this sense only in recent years. This is a case in which an abstract noun, *varicosis* (the condition of having varices, or varicosities, or varicose veins) has been "concretized" to *varicosis* (a varix, varicosity, or varicose vein), and then used in the plural, *varicoses.*

varicose vein ablation—a minimally invasive alternative to saphenous vein stripping. It is done on an outpatient basis, and there is often no need for sedation.

Varidyne drain (ENT).

Variflex—cardiac device.

VariLift spinal cage—implantable device used for vertebral fusion in the treatment of degenerative disk disease.

Vari/Moist wound dressing—has nonadherent moisture vapor characteristics.

Varivas R—denatured homologous vein harvested after saphenous vein stripping and used in various lengths for vascular access and bypass surgeries.

varus derotational osteotomy (VDRO).

vasa deferentia—plural of *vas deferens.*

Vas-Cath—acute and chronic catheters for insertion in subclavian or jugular veins. Usage: "An 11.5 French Vas-Cath was then passed through the peel-away sheath and into the inferior vena cava."

VascuCoil peripheral vascular stent—a self-expanding nitinol stent used in smaller blood vessels, such as femoral arteries of the thigh, whereas conventional peripheral vascular stents are used only in the large iliac arteries of the pelvic region.

Vascu-Guard—a peripheral vascular patch derived from bovine pericardium. Used in carotid endarterectomy.

vascular and airway modeling—a finding on CT scan.

vascular brachytherapy—used to apply gamma radiation therapy to help prevent reblockage of arteries. It uses a closed-end catheter containing radioactive seeds of IR-192 that can deliver a therapeutic dose up to a diameter of several millimeters.

vascular cognitive impairment (VCI)—ranges from mild cognitive impairment to severe dementia. May be caused by stroke or transitory ischemic attacks. The main type of VCI is *SIVD* (subcortical ischemic vascular dementia).

vascular endothelial growth factor (VEGF) (Ob-Gyn; Oph)—known to be particularly responsible for promoting neovascularization in human breast cancer. Also, an angiogenic protein and vasopermeability factor whose intraocular concentrations are closely correlated with active neovascularization in patients with diabetes mellitus, central retinal vein occlusion, retinopathy of prematurity, and rubeosis iridis.

vascular flasks—term used to describe pathologic appearance after pancreaticoduodenectomy and other procedures. Usage: "Endoscopic

vascular *(cont.)*
ultrasonogram revealed a well-circumscribed hyperechoic pancreatic tumor, with anechoic areas corresponding to vascular flasks."

vascularized fibula graft—insertion of a portion of fibula into an osteonecrotic hip. With blood vessels attached, the fibular bone grows and strengthens the hip, thereby obviating the need for hip replacement.

vascular Parkinson disease—characterized by sudden onset and rapid progression of clinical symptoms, absent or poor response to dopamine, and postural instability with shuffling gait and absence of tremor. These symptoms make it clinically distinct from Parkinson disease.

vascular targeting agent—technology for treatment of solid tumors based on targeting components that deliver a variety of therapeutic agents to the blood vessels supplying tumors. These localized agents then specifically destroy or occlude the tumor vessels.

VascuLink—vascular access graft.

vasculopath—a coined term referring to a patient with vasculopathy.

Vascutek Gelseal—knitted and woven vascular grafts. Also, Vascutek Gelsoft.

vasoactive intestinal peptides—see *VIP*.

vasomotor rhinitis—enlargement of the inferior turbinate due to increase in circulation. There may be huge pools of blood in the turbinate, or there may be a physical swelling due to this enlargement that blocks breathing. See *empty nose syndrome*.

VasoSeal VHD (vascular hemostatic device)—designed to provide an immediate hemostatic seal at the area of arterial puncture site wound by delivering highly purified collagen directly to the surface of the artery. Used during coronary angiography and angioplasty procedures as well as radiologic procedures.

Vasotrax—small 4-inch monitor/sensor that is placed over the radial artery at the wrist and registers accurate systolic and diastolic blood pressures as well as heart rate, all without the necessity for removal of clothing or even rolling up the sleeve. Said to be more accurate at measuring BP than a standard cuff.

VasoView balloon dissection system.

VasoView Uniport—endoscopic saphenous vein harvesting system requiring only a single 2-cm incision. All instruments operate through a single multilumen catheter.

VAT (volume as tolerated). Usage: VAT feeds (pediatrics).

VATER syndrome
V vertebral and/or vascular defects
A anorectal malformation
TE tracheoesophageal fistula
R radial, ray, or renal anomaly

VATS (video-assisted thoracic surgery)

Vaughn-Williams antiarrhythmic effect.

VAX-D (vertebral axial decompression) **therapy**—for treatment of herniated or slipped disks, sciatica, and degenerative disk disease not responding to standard medical therapy. A special decompression table is used in 30-minute sessions over a period of two months; the procedure stretches the spine and slowly decompresses the injured disk.

VBAC (vaginal birth after [previous] cesarean section).

Vbeam—a pulsed dye laser system used to treat cutaneous vascular lesions.

VBG (vertical-banded gastroplasty).

VBMCP (vincristine, BCNU, melphalan, cyclophosphamide, prednisone) —chemotherapy protocol.

VCAB (ventriculocoronary artery bypass) revascularization procedure.

VCD (vocal cord dysfunction).

VCDF (volume-cycled decelerating-flow ventilation).

VCF (vaginal contraceptive film).

VCI (vascular cognitive impairment).

VCS clip adapter—tiny metal clips used to join vascular structures without penetrating the lumen.

VCUG (vesicoureterogram).

VCUG (voiding cystourethrogram).

VDRL (Venereal Disease Research Laboratory) **test**—diagnostic test for syphilis. Do not translate *VDRL* in reports.

VDRO (varus derotational osteotomy).

vectis—a curved lever used for traction on the fetal head during delivery.

vector—in cloning, the plasmid or phage used to carry the cloned DNA segment.

vectorcardiography—noninvasive cardiac diagnostic procedure that presents the same diagnostic information as that given by electrocardiography, but in a different form. It gives a three-dimensional picture of the conduction of electrical impulses from the sinoatrial node, across the right atrium to the atrioventricular node, down the bundle of His, through the bundle branches to the apex, and upward into the Purkinje fibers, stimulating the myocardial muscle.

Vector intertrochanteric nail.

Vector and **VectorX large-lumen guiding catheters**—used with interventional technologies such as stents and atherectomy devices.

Vectra Genisys laser system—orthopedic/physical therapy device that provides topical heating for temporary increase in local blood circulation, temporary relief of minor muscle and joint aches, pain and stiffness, and muscle spasm.

Vectra vascular access graft (VAG)—for use in renal dialysis patients, primarily as a shunt between an artery and a vein to gain access to the circulatory system in order to remove toxins from patients' blood during hemodialysis.

VED (vacuum erection device)—vacuum constriction device used to treat erectile dysfunction.

VEGF (vascular endothelial growth factor).

vein contrast enhancer (VCE)—a device used to enhance subcutaneous veins in order to pinpoint a suitable vein for an injection or a drip. Patients walk out of the procedure with supportive leg stockings, which they wear for one week.

Veingard—transparent dressing which is moisture-permeable, waterproof, and sterile. Used over an intravenous site, so the site can be monitored.

vein of Galen—vena cerebri magna, the great cerebral vein, formed by the two internal cerebral veins; named after a second century A.D. Greek physician.

vein of Labbé ("lab-bay").

Velcade (bortezomid)—anticancer drug that may have broad application in the treatment of cancer.

Velcro rales.

Veletri (tezosentan)—endothelin receptor antagonist drug for the treatment of acute heart failure.

Veley headrest—Light-Veley headrest used in neurosurgical procedures.

Velocity—a digital x-ray system that is meant to replace regular plain film systems.

velocity encoding—on brain magnetic resonance angiography.

Velogene rapid MRSA assay—gene-based diagnostic assay for rapid identification of methicillin-resistant *Staphylococcus aureus*.

Velogene rapid TB assay—gene-based diagnostic assay for the rapid identification of *Mycobacterium tuberculosis*.

Velogene rapid VRE assay—gene-based diagnostic assay for the rapid identification of vancomycin-resistant *Enterococcus faecalis* and *Enterococcus faecium*.

velolaryngeal endoscopy—endoscopy of the soft palate (velum palatinum) and laryngeal mechanisms.

velopharyngeal insufficiency (VPI).

Velpeau dressing or bandage—used for treatment of dislocation of the shoulder or other shoulder girdle injuries. It consists of bandaging the arm in such a manner that the injured arm is bent at the elbow over the patient's chest, with the palm of the hand at the uninjured shoulder, taking the weight off the injured shoulder.

VenaFlow compression system—intermittent pneumatic compression system indicated for deep vein thrombosis prophylaxis. Not to be confused with *Venaflo needle*.

Venaflow vascular graft—used to reduce the incidence of hyperplasia.

Venaport guiding catheter—for venous mapping.

Vena Tech LGM filter—an inferior vena cava filter used to prevent recurrent pulmonary embolism. Can be placed in the jugular or femoral artery. *LGM* is for *Lehman, Gerofliea,* and *Metais*—the French engineers who developed the filter.

venetian blind artifacts—secondary to interleaving of magnetic resonance images.

venipuncture (*not* veno- or vena-).

Venodyne compression system—for deep venous thrombosis (DVT).

venogram (*not* venagram).

veno-occlusive disease (VOD).

venous leak syndrome (Urol)—disorder that interferes with veno-occlusive mechanism of the corpora cavernosa, resulting in failure to trap blood within the penis. It prevents storage of blood so that an erection cannot be maintained.

venous web disease (hepatic)—see *hepatic venous web disease*.

Ventak AICD pacemaker.

Ventak AV III DR—automatic implantable cardioverter-defibrillator system.

Ventak Mini II (and **III**) **AICD** (automatic implantable cardioverter-defibrillator)—a small implantable defibrillator that, with the incorporation of Guidant TRIAD defibrillation energy delivery system, is used for treating patients with life-threatening rapid heart arrhythmias.

Ventak Prizm—dual chamber physiologically shaped implantable defibrillator.

Ventavis (iloprost)—an inhalation treatment for pulmonary hypertension.

VentCheck—handheld monitor that verifies and confirms ventilator settings.

venter (noun)—belly, or belly-shaped part. See *ventral.*

Ventex dressing—a two-level wound dressing system for deep wounds, such as those associated with venous ulcers, donor sites, stage II and III pressure ulcers, and abrasions. It controls moderate to heavy exudative drainage. The first layer closest to the skin is a vented transparent film that allows for wound inspection without disturbing new granulation or epithelial tissue. Centrally located vents allow controlled escape of excess exudate. Over this, an outer absorbent dressing is placed, which can absorb more than 15 times its weight in exudate. Its polyurethane backing forms a barrier against bacteria and fluids and seals out the external environment on all four sides. Cf. *Aquasorb*, *Curasorb*, and *ClearSite*.

ventilate (verb)—to express verbally, especially as a release for pent-up emotions. Also, to breathe for a patient either by means of a hand-held bag or mechanical respirator.

ventilation—high-frequency jet and high-frequency oscillation assisted respiration for premature infants. See *noninvasive extrathoracic ventilation* (NEV).

ventilation-exchange bougie—an airway device that can be mounted on a fiberoptic laryngoscope for passage through the larynx into the trachea via a laryngeal mask airway. Subsequent removal of the fiberoptic laryngoscope and laryngeal mask airway allows a tracheal tube to be railroaded into position over the ventilation-exchange bougie.

ventilation-perfusion (V-P) **ratio**. Use a hyphen, not a virgule (slash), between these terms.

ventilation-perfusion (V-P) **scan**.

ventilator or **respirator**
- ACD (active compression-decompression) resuscitator
- BABYbird respirator
- BagEasy respirator
- Bennett PR-2 ventilator
- Bird respirator
- Bourns-Bear ventilator
- Bourns infant ventilator
- cuirass respirator
- high-frequency jet ventilator
- high-frequency oscillation ventilator
- Inspiration
- KinetiX ventilation monitor
- Monaghan 300 ventilator
- MVV (maximal voluntary ventilation)
- Porta-Lung noninvasive extrathoracic ventilator (NEV)
- portable volume ventilator
- Triosyn T-1000 respirator

ventilator-associated pneumonia (VAP).

Ventra catheter—used for percutaneous thromboendarterectomy.

ventral (adj.)—toward the belly, anterior. See *venter*.

Ventralex mesh, Ventralex patch—materials used in hernia repairs.

ventricular assistance device—see *DMVA*.

ventricular assist device (VAD).

ventricular containment device—see *Acorn cardiac support device*.

ventricular ejection fraction—portion of the total volume of a ventricle that is ejected during ventricular contraction (systole); usually expressed as a percent rather than a fraction. Determined in multiple gated acquisition scan, or MUGA.

ventricular endoaneurysmorrhaphy—a procedure for the repair of ventricular aneurysm using an elliptical

ventricular *(cont.)*
patch graft that both restores normal shape, internal contours, and volume of the ventricle and preserves its external anatomy, permitting revascularization of the anterior descending or other coronary arteries when indicated.

ventricular fibrillation—ineffectual twitching of damaged heart muscle instead of normal contractions.

ventricular geometry change—a new concept in the treatment of heart failure that reduces left ventricular (LV) wall stress and improves cardiac function by reducing effective LV radius.

ventricular resynchronization therapy—uses a battery-powered pulse generator implanted in the upper chest to deliver electrical impulses simultaneously to both sides of the heart in order to improve its ability to pump oxygenated blood to the body. See *Frontier 3 x 2*.

ventriculocisternostomy—Torkildsen shunt procedure.

ventriculocoronary arterial fistula—communication between the left ventricular cavity and the left coronary artery in the fetus.

ventriculoperitoneal (VP) **shunt**—used in the treatment of normal pressure hydrocephalus. A small catheter is passed into a ventricle of the brain. A pump is attached to keep fluid away from the brain. Another catheter is attached to the pump and tunneled under the skin, behind the ear, down the neck and chest and into the peritoneal cavity.

ventriculotomy, partial encircling endocardial—to relieve ventricular tachycardia in patients with ischemic heart disease.

Ventritex Angstrom MD implantable cardioverter-defibrillator.

Ventrix catheter—the only advanced intracranial pressure (ICP) monitoring and drainage catheter designed to tunnel away from the brain.

ventroposterolateral thalamic electrode—see *VPL thalamic electrode*.

Ventureyra ventricular catheter—a process for the prevention and treatment of proximal obstruction in CSF shunts.

venturi mask—used in the administration of oxygen.

VEP (visual evoked potential)—see *brain tests, noninvasive*.

VEPARAF study—a study to evaluate the use of verapamil plus antiarrhythmic drugs to reduce atrial fibrillation recurrences after electrical cardioversion.

VER (visual evoked response) (Neuro).

Verbatim balloon catheter—so named because the balloon expands precisely to preprogrammed sizes. Used in coronary angioplasty.

Verbrugge bone clamp (Ortho)—used in acetabular fracture repair.

Verdict-II—drugs-of-abuse screening panel.

Veress needle (*not* Verres)—used in laparoscopy for insufflation of carbon dioxide.

Veripath peripheral guiding catheter—single-lumen guiding catheter used to provide a pathway through which therapeutic and diagnostic devices are introduced into the peripheral vasculature.

vermian veins—veins of the cerebellar vermis.

Vernier calipers—used to measure the amount of intervertebral disk protrusion present, or for any other fine measurement.

VERP (ventricular effective refractory period).

VerreScope—microlaparoscopic entry and instrument system designed for laparoscopy under local anesthesia (LULA).

VersaBond—a medium-viscosity bone cement.

Versadopp 10 probe—pen-size ultrasonic Doppler probe.

Versa-Fx—femoral fixation system which requires removal of less bone.

Versalab ultrasonic medical device—a device to aid in the diagnosis of peripheral vascular disease.

VersaLight laser—for skin resurfacing.

Versalok—a low-back fixation system that uses polyaxial screws rather than set screws or locking nuts.

Versant HCV RNA 3.0 assay (bDNA)—a transcription-mediated amplification method of detecting hepatitis C virus RNA. Also *Versant HCV RNA Qualitative TMA assay*.

VersaPoint system—a minimally invasive hysteroscopic fibroid removal device. It utilizes bipolar electrovaporization technology to instantly vaporize tissue upon contact.

Versaport—trocar system requiring a smaller incision site, reducing risk of herniation and improving cosmetic results.

VersaPulse holmium laser (Neuro)—for use in laser nucleotomy. See *laser nucleotomy*.

Versatome laser fiber—a specialized fiberoptic tube used to deliver laser energy.

versions—in ophthalmology, binocular voluntary movement of the eyes in conjugate gaze (in the same direction). See also *ductions*.

Versi-Splint—a carry bag with ABS plastic components of splints which can be used to stabilize any joint in an emergency.

vertebral artery testing—performed to assess the relationship between cervical spine movement and symptoms which may be vertebrobasilar in origin. Tests include sustained rotation, left and right; sustained extension; sustained rotation and extension, left and right; and any position that is described by the patient to elicit dizziness.

vertebral body impactor—an instrument used in the management of thoracic and lumbar spine fractures, after first performing hemilaminectomy and resection of the pedicle on the side where there is most compression of the spinal canal. Usage: "With the impactor, the bone graft was securely seated."

vertebroplasty—the injection of polymethylmethacrylate to stabilize and strengthen a collapsing vertebral body.

Vertetrac ambulatory traction system—noninvasive device for relief of low back pain.

vertex—top, generally used alone to refer to the top of the head, as in "vertex presentation," but also used in referring to the top or apex of other organs. Cf. *vortex*.

vertical-banded gastroplasty (VBG).

vertical expandable titanium rib (VEPTR)—originally developed in San Antonio. See *titanium rib*.

vertical tripod fixation (VTF)—for transscleral fixation of intraocular lens.

vertigo—see *true vertigo*.

Vesica—percutaneous bladder neck stabilization kit used in treating stress urinary incontinence.

vesical (adj.)—pertaining to the bladder. Cf. *vesicle*.

vesicant—a drug or agent that causes blistering. Usage: "Serious tissue damage can result if vesicants leak from a previously punctured site."

vesicle (noun)—a small blister, a small bladder or sac containing liquid. Cf. *vesical*.

vesicoureterogram (VCUG).

vesicourethral suspension—Marshall-Marchetti-Krantz procedure.

vesicular breathing—the sound of normal breathing, as heard on auscultation of the lungs; sometimes likened to the sound of a breeze blowing through trees.

vessel-sizing catheters—used to determine size of a stent to be placed or a vena cava filter to be used. They are also used to measure and size stent-grafts for procedures involving abdominal aortic aneurysms. The catheters are marked with 2, 11, or 20 platinum bands, depending on need and area to be measured, and dictators may refer to them as 2-band catheters, 11-band catheters, etc.

Vest, the—see *ABI Vest airway clearance system*.

vestibular adenitis—see *vulvar vestibulitis syndrome*.

vestibular neurectomy—surgical treatment for vertigo in patients with Ménière disease.

vestibular window—opening between the tympanic cavity and the scala vestibuli of the cochlea, into which the footplate of the stapes fits. Also called *oval window*, *fenestra ovalis*, *fenestra vestibuli*.

vestibulodynia—combination of constant vulvar pain of vestibular origin and dyspareunia, affecting women who are older than those with vestibulitis alone. It is associated with human papillomavirus DNA and dysuria. Also called *vulvar vestibulitis syndrome*.

V.E.T. (vacuum erection technologies) —a manual vacuum device used to produce penile erections in patients with erectile dysfunction. The trademark spelling includes periods.

VEX (vasodilator plus exercise) **treadmill test**.

VFA (vocal fold atrophy).

V fib (ventricular fibrillation).

V5M Multiplane transducer—delivers superior image quality by combining higher frequency image quality with penetration appropriate for a complete TEE exam. See *QuantX* and *Doppler tissue imaging*.

V510B Biplane TEE transducers—see *QuantX* and *Doppler tissue imaging*.

VFSS (videofluoroscopy swallowing study).

VHL (von Hippel-Lindau) **disease**.

VHL (von Hippel-Lindau) **gene**.

VHL (von Hippel-Lindau) **syndrome**.

VHS variable-angle hip fixation system.

Viagra (sildenafil citrate)—a possible new use for treatment of pulmonary arterial hypertension related to connective tissue disease.

Viasorb wound dressing.

Vibracare—percussor machine for patients with cystic fibrosis. Provides optimal postural drainage. See also *Flimm Fighter*.

Vibram—soled rockerbottom shoe used after foot surgery.

Vibrant D and **Vibrant P Soundbridges**—implantable medical prostheses indicated for the treatment of hearing impairment due to sensorineural deafness. The devices convert acoustic sounds to amplified vibrations inside the middle ear.

vibrational medicine—a category of alternative medical practices that encompass homeopathic remedies, flower essences, crystal healing, therapeutic touch, acupuncture, radionics, electrotherapy, herbal medicine, psychic healing, and therapeutic radiology.

vibration-assisted CRP (canalith repositioning procedure). See *CRP*.

vibrissae ("vi-bris´ee")—the hairs that grow in the nostrils.

vibroacoustic stimulation (Ob-Gyn)—application of vibrations against a mother's stomach to help rouse a fetus and aid in external cephalic version. It is performed to reposition the fetus to avoid vaginal breech delivery or cesarean section.

Vickers ring tip forceps.

Vicks VapoRub—an over-the-counter product used, but not approved for, the treatment of fungal nail infections.

Vicon system—commercial gait analysis system that combines both kinetic and kinematic analysis. The system employs a force plate and goniometer system as well as four cameras. In addition, electromyographic equipment may be used.

Vicotuss (guaifenesin with hydrocodone)—a medication used for treatment of intractable cough.

Vicryl Rapide—a synthetic absorbable suture (polyglactin 910) for short-term wound closure. It is said to have a rapid absorption rate—about seven to ten days.

victim impact panel (VIP)—a panel which offenders, such as domestic abuse offenders or DUI offenders , are required to attend to hear victims talk about how they've been affected by domestic violence or drunk driving. The first of these was instituted by the Mothers Against Drunk Driving (MADD), and various other types of VIPs have been established across the country.

VID (vitello-intestinal duct)—a patent (clear) VID in neonates can produce a T-shaped prolapse of intestine through the umbilicus.

vidarabine (adenine arabinoside, Ara-A, Vira-A)—an antiviral drug for herpes simplex and herpes zoster infections.

video-assisted thoracic surgery (videothoracoscopy)—minimally invasive surgery of the chest, using techniques similar to laparoscopy.

video densitometry (VD).

videoendoscopic surgical equipment—for minimally invasive surgical approaches, such as removal of a mediastinal cyst between right lower lung vein and right atrium.

videoendoscopic swallowing study (VESS)—used for evaluation of pharyngeal dysphagia, particularly in elderly patients.

videofluoroscopy swallowing study (VFSS).

video Hydrolaparoscope—contains a port for viewing and one for irrigation and removal of fluid.

videokeratography (Oph)—provides mapping of the corneal structure with a high degree of efficiency.

videolaparoscopy—allows full and meticulous explorations of the small bowel to be performed. It allows direct observation of lesions of the bowel or digestive hemorrhages of obscure origin.

videolaseroscopy—see *laparoscopic laser cholecystectomy*.

videomicroscopy—used in examining skin lesions of patients with solar lentigines.

video-stroboscopic laryngoscopy—study used in evaluation of abnormalities of vocal cord vibrations in patients with vocal cord dysfunction (VCD). The studies are done between VCD attacks and are more revealing than regular laryngoscopy.

Vidicon vacuum chamber pickup tube—for video camera used in arthroscopy.

view
Arcelin
Caldwell
Chausse
coned-down
dens
Hughston
Laurin x-ray
Law
Low-Beer
Mayer
outlet
Owen
retromammary space
Schuller
Stenvers
sunrise
Towne
tunnel
Waters

Viewing Wand—a combination of a medical imaging workstation and a probe that allows the surgeon to see the trajectory of the probe relative to the location of a tumor, cyst, or other lesion, as well as the surrounding anatomy.

ViewPoint CK (conductive keratoplasty) **system**—device used to perform conductive keratoplasty, a nonlaser radiofrequency procedure that reshapes the cornea for correction of hyperopia.

Vigilance CCO/SvO$_2$/CEDV monitor—provides automatic continuous measurement of end-diastolic volume, cardiac output, and mixed venous oxygen saturation to provide optimal therapy for critically ill and injured patients.

Vigilon dressing—a synthetic (polyethylene) occlusive dressing, for use on ulcerations. The dressings relieve pain, cause debridement, and stimulate the formation of granulation tissue. Usage: "The recipient sites were protected with Vigilon dressing material, then covered with wet Kerlix gauze, and then dry Kerlix gauze."

villose (adj.)—variant spelling of *villous.*

villous—shaggy with soft hairs; covered with villi; "villous adenoma." Also spelled *villose.* Cf. *villus.*

villus (pl., villi)—small vascular protrusion, particularly a protrusion from the surface of a membrane, commonly seen in small bowel. Cf. *villous.*

Vilmann-Hancke biopsy handle instrument—consisting of a steel needle with stylet, metal spiral sheath, and an aluminum biopsy handle. Used for gastrointestinal endoscopy.

Vincent infection—necrotizing ulcerative gingivitis.

Vineland Social Maturity Scale—used in psychiatry/psychology evaluation.

violaceous ("vi-o-lay´shus")—violet-colored. Usually refers to lesions on the skin.

VIP (vasoactive intestinal peptides). Usage: "Elevations of VIP are associated with bronchogenic carcinoma."

VIP-DAC (vaginal interruption of pregnancy, with dilatation and curettage).

vipoma—an endocrine tumor that produces VIP. See *VIP* (vasoactive intestinal peptides).

vipoma syndrome—also known as *WDHA* (watery, secretory diarrhea, hypokalemia, and achlorhydria) *syndrome*.

viral hepatitides—hepatitis A, B, C.

viral vector—an engineered virus that is used in gene therapy to introduce a foreign gene into a cell.

ViraPap—human papillomavirus detection test used along with the standard Pap smear.

ViraSTAT—immunofluorescence assay for viral culture of parainfluenza, using fluorescently labeled monoclonal antibodies which are type-specific.

Viratrol—a handheld battery-operated device that delivers a minute charge to prevent oral and genital herpes lesions from forming or to speed the healing process.

Virchow node—enlarged supraclavicular lymph node; often the first sign of a malignant abdominal tumor. Also called *sentinel* or *signal node*.

Virend—used to treat herpes simplex virus.

virgin—a term used to refer to previously unoperated anatomy, stenosis, or herniation, such as virgin lumbar anatomy, virgin lumbar spinal stenosis, virgin disk herniation.

Virgo anti-cardiolipin screening kit—ELISA test kit used in screening patient serum for the presence of autoantibodies that are typically observed in patients with systemic lupus erythematosus and other connective tissue diseases.

Viringe—a prefilled, needleless, vascular access flush device for both saline and heparin applications.

viroid—a virus-like unenveloped infective RNA particle.

virtual colonoscopy—noninvasive CT procedure used to detect small colorectal polyps by rendering a 3-D view of the interior of the colon; however, for polyp removal and biopsy, standard colonoscopy is still necessary.

virtual cystoscopy—use of pelvic helical CT scanning after distention of the bladder for diagnosing and monitoring of transitional cell carcinoma.

Virtual Hospital Room Communicator—a hardware communications module located at the point of patient care, storing data from a variety of monitoring devices. Captured data is valuable to both providers and payors for clinical, utilization management, and reimbursement purposes.

virtual labor monitor (VLM)—one receiver is attached to the laboring mother's torso; another is fastened to the fetal presenting part, thus allowing the recording of the movement of the fetus down the birth canal. Under development is a VLM with 3-D computer graphics simulation.

Virtuoso—a portable three-dimensional imaging system.

virus—not a living organism, but a very small segment of genetic material (DNA or RNA) encased in a protective protein shell. Upon entering a living cell, the virus assumes control of that cell's function and reproduction. The normal operations of the cell are suspended and it becomes a factory for the synthesis of more virus. Finally the cell disintegrates, releasing hundreds of new virus particles, which can then invade other cells. Viral

virus *(cont.)*
infection typically elicits an acute, self-limited inflammatory response, without suppuration or fibrotic reaction. Viruses show a predilection for skin and mucous membranes, and even those that cause systemic disease often produce eruptions of papules or vesicles (as in measles and chickenpox). Viruses cause the common cold, influenza, measles, mumps, chickenpox, warts, herpes simplex, hepatitis, poliomyelitis, AIDS, and rabies. For quick-reference list, see *pathogen* and individual entries:
adenovirus
AIDS-related
Andes
arbovirus
ARV
avian influenza A (H5N1)
baculovirus (genetically engineered)
Bayou
Black Creek Canal
Epstein-Barr (EBV)
gamma-herpesvirus
hepatitis B (HBV)
herpes simplex virus (HSV)
herpesvirus
herpes whitlow
herpes zoster (HZV)
H5N1
HHV-8 (human herpesvirus-8)
HIV (human immunodeficiency)
HIV-1E
KSHV (Kaposi sarcoma-associated)
HTLV-I retrovirus (human T-cell leukemia/lymphoma)
HTLV-III (human T-cell lymphotropic)
human herpesvirus 6 (HHV-6)
human mammary tumor (HMTV)
human papillomavirus (HPV)
human parvovirus B19 (HPV B19)

virus *(cont.)*
Laguna Negra
Juquitiba
lentivirus
leukovirus
lymphocytic choriomeningitis (LCMV)
McKrae strain of herpesvirus
MCV (molluscum contagiosum)
Nipah
nonsyncytium-inducing (NSI) variant of the AIDS
oncogenic retrovirus
phage
picornavirus
porcine endogenous retrovirus (PERV)
respiratory syncytial (RSV)
retrovirus
RNA
rotavirus
Rous sarcoma
Sin Nombre (SNV)
togavirus
varicella zoster (VZV)
West Nile
zoonotic retrovirus

virus-like infectious agent (VLIA)—a microbacterium.

virus-like particle—see *VLP*.

Visage Cosmetic Surgery System—wrinkle reduction procedure using Coblation.

Visa II PTCA catheter.

VISC (vitreous infusion suction cutter).

viscera—plural form of *viscus*.

Viscoheel K, Viscoheel N—orthosis used to reduce shock load to joints and spine, as well as to correct varus and valgus position of the heel and leg axis.

Viscoheel SofSpot—orthosis used to reduce heel spur pain and plantar fascial pain.

viscosupplementation—injection of a special viscous fluid into a joint to decrease pain and improve function in patients with osteoarthritis. It is thought that the addition of such material in the joint may help make the joint lining manufacture more normal synovial fluid.

viscous—thick, not readily flowing. Cf. *viscus*.

viscus (pl., viscera)—an internal organ, particularly one in the abdominal or thoracic cavities. Cf. *viscous*.

Visi-Black surgical needle—a needle with a nonshiny finish and a slim, tapered point. The black finish is intended to provide greater visibility within the operative field.

Visica cryoablation system—a minimally invasive treatment for breast fibroadenoma for women who do not want to undergo open surgery. It is performed in a doctor's office, conserves breast tissue, and visibly reduces scarring of the patient's breast. The fibroadenoma is "quick-frozen," killing the tumor cells and causing the tumor to progressively shrink and disappear.

Visicath—a small endoscopic instrument, which may be used for bedside examination of the airway.

Visick (grades I-IV)—grading system for postgastrectomy recurrence of carcinoma.

Visidex, Visidex II—blood glucose testing strips.

Visijet Hydrokeratome—high-energy, supersonic waterjet beam used to cut the cornea, specifically developed to create a LASIK flap in refractive surgery. See *LASIK*.

Visilex—polypropylene mesh specifically designed for laparoscopic hernia repair.

Vision 1.5-T Siemens MRI scanner.

Vision PTCA catheter.

Visipaque (iodixanol) **intravascular injection**—radiographic nonionic isosmolar contrast medium (IOCM).

Visitec circular knife.

Visitec crescent knife.

Visitec EdgeAhead phaco slit knife (Oph).

Visitec stiletto knife (Oph)—used in vitreoretinal surgery. Also, *cannula, cystitome, needle, nucleus hydrodissector.*

Vistaflex—balloon expandable, platinum alloy biliary stent.

Vistec x-ray detectable sponge—a surgical sponge with radiopaque strands running through it for x-ray visualization (just in case the sponge count is incorrect!).

Visual Analog Scale (VAS)—instrument for patient measurement of pain, consisting of a 10-cm line with "no pain at all" at one end and "worst pain imaginable" at the other.

visual evoked potential (VEP).

visual field testing—to test the function of retina, optic nerve, and optic pathways when both central and peripheral visual fields are examined.

Visual Neglect Test—to assess neurological deficit following an incident such as a subarachnoid hemorrhage. The patient is shown a page with 32 lines scattered randomly across it and is asked to cross out each line. If the patient fails to cross out more lines on one side of the page than the other, the side with the most errors corresponds to the side of visual neglect.

Visuflo—a device that blows a stream of filtered, humidified air onto a suture site to remove unwanted blood flow.

Visulas Nd:YAG laser.

visuscope—an instrument for testing the amblyopic eye.

VISX excimer laser—used in laser vision correction procedures to correct astigmatism.

VISX Star S2 excimer laser system—considered safe and effective for treatment of up to 14 diopters of myopia and up to 5 diopters of astigmatism.

VISX Star 3 excimer laser system—for ophthalmologic surgeries.

VISX WaveScan Wavefront System (Oph)—allows instant measurement of refractive aberrations using highly advanced optics that project light into the eye and analyze the returning wavefront. The system produces a WavePrint, much like a "fingerprint" of the eye.

Vitacor Plus—a dietary supplement.

VitaCuff antimicrobial cuff—a subcutaneous attachable cuff containing silver, for use with central venous catheters, to decrease bacterial infections at the site of entry.

Vita-Gummies—a popular brand name of vitamins for children.

Vitallium—trademark for an alloy used in prostheses and in skull plates. See *McKeever Vitallium cap prosthesis*.

Vitalograph spirometer.

vital signs—pulse, respiration, temperature. Sometimes a physician dictates, "Four vital signs are normal." In that case, blood pressure is the fourth sign.

Vitatron catheter electrode (Cardio).

Vitatron Diamond pacemaker—responds to circulatory needs caused by a patient's emotional state as well as level of physical activity.

Vitatron Diamond II—a dual sensor, dual chamber pacemaker that is designed to improve a patient's exercise tolerance and provide a steady, stable ventricular beat.

Vitatron pacing systems—include the QT sensor and the Activity (ACT) sensor, as well as the Diamond II DDR, the Ruby II DDD, the Topaz II SSIR, and the Jade II SSI.

Vitatron Selection AFm—atrial fibrillation monitor.

vitelliform macular degeneration.

Vitesse Cos—laser catheter by Spectranetics containing optical fibers that are "optimally spaced" to improve debulking efficiency (the dissolving of tissue blocking an artery).

Vitesse E-II—eccentric, rapid-exchange coronary catheter.

Vitex (equal amounts of human thrombin and fibrinogen)—a tissue adhesive.

Vitrasert intraocular implant—a form of Cytovene (ganciclovir) available in a timed-release delivery form implanted in the eye to treat cytomegalovirus.

vitrectomy—surgical procedure used for bleeding inside the eye, usually caused by diabetic retinopathy. The blood-filled vitreous is removed and replaced with a clear solution. See *open-sky vitrectomy*.

vitrector probe—used during cataract surgery to simultaneously aspirate, cut, and irrigate with balanced salt solution.

vitreoretinopathy—vitreoretinal membrane shrinkage or contraction of the eye.

vitreous base—attachment to the ciliary epithelium (near the ora serrata).

vitreous body—a transparent jelly-like mass that fills the cavity of the eyeball.

vitreous cutter—instrument used in eye surgery such as vitrectomy.

vitreous face—anterior surface, that which is behind the lens.

vitreous space—vitreous body or the cavity it occupies.

vitro—see *in vitro*.

Vitros immunodiagnostic test—a laboratory test that detects early antibodies associated with hepatitis B virus (HBV) infection.

vivo—see *in vivo*.

VLAP (visual laser ablation of prostate).

VLCD (very low-calorie diet)—a specific diet of nonfat milk with vitamins and mineral supplements.

VLDL (very low-density lipoprotein).

VLIA (virus-like infectious agent)—a microbacterium.

VLM (virtual labor monitor).

VLP—a virus-like particle believed to be the etiologic agent of enterically transmitted non-A, non-B hepatitis.

V-MAX—virtual reality device that magnifies and makes things clearer for individuals with low vision.

VMO strengthening and "short arc" quads.

VNS (vagus nerve stimulation).

VNUS Closure catheter; **radiofrequency generator**—a device for shrinking varicose veins to occlusion. Used as an alternative to vein-stripping surgery.

VNUS Restore catheter—partially shrinks over-dilated varicose veins to restore competency of vein valves as a possible treatment for deep vein reflux.

vocal cord—*not* vocal chord.

vocal cord dysfunction (VCD)—adduction of the vocal cords on inspiration, a cause of inspiratory dyspnea. Related terms: episodic laryngeal dyskinesia (ELD), paradoxical vocal cord motion (PVCM), upper airway dysfunction (UAD), among others.

Vocare bladder system—designed for patients with spinal cord injuries that cause loss of bowel and bladder control. Sensory nerves are severed and electrodes connected directly to nerve roots. The electrodes are also attached to a receiver implanted under the skin. The patient places the stimulator over the receiver, and the bladder is emptied.

VOD (veno-occlusive disease).

Voerner disease—rare form of hereditary epidermolytic palmoplantar keratoderma, which includes hyperkeratosis of the skin of the palms and soles, with fissuring and marked hyperhidrosis.

Vogt-Koyanagi-Harada disease.

Vogt lines—seen on the cornea in keratoconus.

voiceprints—acoustic spectrographic methods to detect abnormalities in the cries of infants.

Volkmann contracture—neurovascular contracture of an extremity due to arterial occlusion.

Volkmann spoon—a small spoon used in removal of pancreatic calculi.

Volk Pan Retinal Lens—for binocular indirect ophthalmoscopy.

Volk Quadraspheric fundus lens—a diagnostic/therapeutic contact lens with four aspheric surfaces.

Volk SuperPupil XL lens—for indirect ophthalmoscopy to view small pupils.

Vollmar endarterectomy—an alternative surgical treatment for occlusive superficial femoral artery in the absence of a greater saphenous vein or in young smoking patients.

volume acquisition—MRI term.
volume analysis—MRI term.
volume as tolerated (VAT). Usage: VAT feeds (pediatrics).
volume element (voxel)—MRI term.
volume rendering of helical CT data.
volumetric segmentation—allows for quantifying the tumor burden in patients with cancer.
voluming artifact (Radiol).
voluntarily stopping eating and drinking (VSED)—undertaken at the request of a mentally competent patient, along with terminal sedation, a palliative option for the terminally ill. See also *PAS*, *terminal sedation (TS),* and *VAE*.
voluntary active euthanasia (VAE).
Voluson ultrasound system—provides three-dimensional images in real time, including clear color real-time video of fetus in utero.
Volutrol—control apparatus for intravenous infusion.
volvulated Meckel diverticulum—a term coined from "volvulus."
Volz total wrist arthroplasty.
Von Frey test—test of cutaneous sensibility performed with a Semmes-Weinstein pressure anesthesiometer.
von Graefe sign—in exophthalmos, the upper lid lags behind the lower, exposing the eyeball.
von Hippel-Lindau (VHL) **disease**—an inherited disease in which affected persons are predisposed to develop multiple tumors, including cancers of the kidney, eye, brain, spinal cord, and adrenal gland. The identification of the VHL gene in affected families has led to better management of the disease.
von Hippel-Lindau (VHL) **gene**—identified by researchers at the National Cancer Institute in Bethesda, Maryland, as the gene for von Hippel-Lindau disease. The gene is also involved in clear cell skin cancer, which is not hereditary.
von Hippel-Lindau (VHL) **tumor suppression gene**—leads to identification of proteins that seem to interact with this gene product.
von Kossa staining—demonstrates the presence of calcium in tissues.
Von Lackum surcingle—a traction device using straps that apply contralateral pressure; for correction of scoliosis. See also *surcingle*.
von Recklinghausen disease—neurofibromatosis.
von Rokitansky disease—see *Budd-Chiari syndrome*.
von Willebrand factor (vWF)—antigen levels most elevated in giant cell arteritis, but also found in Sjögren syndrome, choroiditis, and polymyalgia rheumatica. Elevation of the vWF antigen levels may help in the differential diagnosis of giant cell arteritis. Cf. *giant cell arteritis*; *von Willebrand knee*.
von Willebrand knee—nothing to do with the knee, but is a group of optic nerve fibers, located in the anterior optic chiasm, that loop forward into the contralateral optic nerve and then back into the appropriate optic tract. Cf. *von Willebrand factor*.
Voorhees needle (Ob-Gyn). *Not* to be confused with *Veress needle*.
Voptix—a computer program that stores and displays corneal thickness data taken from a variable array of corneal positions.
VOR (vestibulo-ocular reflex).
vortex—a whorled pattern or arrangement, such as is found in fingerprints or the pattern of hair growth at the crown of the head. Cf. *vertex*.

Vortex (guaifenesin with hydrocodone) —a medication used for treatment of intractable cough.

Vortex router (ENT).

Vortex stabilization system—utilizes vacuum-assist technology, enabling physician to immobilize the artery while performing beating-heart bypass.

Voxgram—multiple-exposure hologram of CT image. See *digital holography system.*

Voyager aortic device—for use in stopped-heart procedures that include CABG, mitral valve replacement, and valve repair; allows performance of four critical functions through a single incision.

Vozzle Vacu-Irrigator—used for controlled irrigation and evacuation of body tissue and fluids in surgery.

VPAP (variable positive airway pressure).

VPI (velopharyngeal insufficiency).

VPL thalamic electrode (ventroposterolateral)—used to alleviate intractable pain by deep brain stimulation, and is internalized in much the same way as a pacemaker. See also *electrode*.

V-Q (ventilation-perfusion) **scan** or **ratio**. Also, *VQ*. (The *Q* stands for *quotient*.) Use a hyphen, not a virgule (slash), between *ventilation* and *perfusion*.

VQ or VQQ technique—in continent urinary diversion procedures, a stomal construction technique that is a combination of separate triangular (V) and single quadrilateral (Q) or double quadrilateral (QQ) skin flaps for prevention of complications at the stomal level.

VRE (vancomycin-resistant enterococci).

VRE (vancomycin-resistant *Enterococcus faecium*).

VREF (vancomycin-resistant *Enterococcus faecium*) **infection**.

VScore with AutoGate—high-quality cardiac imaging that uses existing helical CT scanners without EKG recording devices to detect coronary heart disease.

VSED (voluntarily stopping eating and drinking). Also, *TS (terminal sedation)*.

VSP (variable screw placement).

VS (ventriculosubarachnoid) **shunt**—used in spine surgery.

V tach ("vee-tack")—medical slang for ventricular tachycardia or ventricular tachyarrhythmia.

VTED (venous thromboembolic disease).

V3 loop—part of the envelope surrounding the HIV virus. V3 loop vaccines are in the process of development.

V-to-Y advancement of the helical root—see *Antia-Buch chondrocutaneous advancement flap procedure.*

VT/VF (ventricular tachycardia/ventricular fibrillation).

Vueport balloon-occlusion guiding catheter—for intravascular electrophysiologic mapping.

vulnerable myocardium—heart wall at risk for injury from infarction.

vulsellum clamp (Ob/Gyn).

vulsellum forceps (Ob/Gyn).

vulvae—see *kraurosis vulvae*.

vulvar vestibulitis syndrome—a symptom complex associated with a significant long-term history of moderate to severe chronic introital dyspareunia and tenderness of the vulvar vestibule. A treatment program consisting of electromyographic biofeedback-assisted pelvic floor muscle rehabilitation exercises

vulvar *(cont.)*
is reported to produce significant decreases in subjective pain. See *vestibulodynia*.

vWF (von Willebrand factor).

Vysis PathVysion—a genomic disease management test that detects HER-1 neu gene status in women with metastatic breast cancer and accurately identifies patients who are possible candidates for treatment with Herceptin.

Vysis UroVysion DNA probe assay—to detect bladder cancer recurrence.

Vytorin (ezetimibe/simvastatin)—for the treatment of high LDL cholesterol (LDL-C) in patients with primary hypercholesterolemia or mixed hyperlipidemia as adjunctive therapy to diet when diet alone is not enough. Approved to treat the two sources of cholesterol by inhibiting the production of cholesterol in the liver and blocking the absorption of cholesterol in the intestine, including cholesterol from food.

VZV (varicella zoster virus)—a virus often found in patients who have had bone marrow transplants.

W, w

WACH ("watch) **shoe** (wedge adjustable cushioned heel)—a cast shoe used in orthopedics.

Wada test—a test to determine hemispheric dominance.

Wagner distraction device (Ortho)—increases the length of the femur or tibia.

WAIS (Wechsler Adult Intelligence Scale).

waist-to-hip ratio (WHR)—used in calculating the distribution of fat. A high waist-to-hip ratio, indicating a relative excess of fat in the abdomen as contrasted with the hips and buttocks, may indicate a more serious risk of cardiovascular disease and type 2 diabetes mellitus.

Waldhausen subclavian flap technique—used in repair of coarctation of the aorta.

walkaway—an instrument used to measure timing of foot contact and/or the position of the foot on the ground.

Wallaby phototherapy system (Peds)—illuminator (light source) box and fiberoptic cable with a panel on the end that can be wrapped around or placed under the baby.

Wallace Flexihub—central venous pressure cannula.

Wallace pipette—a one-step procedure to collect cells from the ectocervix and endocervix without the trauma of an endocervical brush or swab and spatula.

Wallach Endocell—a sterile, disposable endometrial cell sampler.

Wallach pencil—a cryosurgery instrument, used for treatment of retinal tears and trichiasis.

wallerian degeneration—reaction resulting from a cut or injury to distal nerve fragments.

Wallstent—a self-expanding arterial stent placed in percutaneous transluminal angioplasty to prevent mural thrombus formation. The Wallstent biliary endoprosthesis is a self-expanding metal stent that may be used in esophageal, biliary tract, or coronary artery stenosis or obstruction. See *Schneider Wallstent; transjugular intrahepatic portosystemic shunt.*

Wallstent with Unistep—a Wallstent endoprosthesis with a Unistep catheter delivery system. It is designed to improve central venous luminal diameter following unsuccessful angioplasty in patients on chronic hemodialysis with stenosis of the venous outflow tract.

Walsham forceps—used in repair of facial fractures.

WAMBA (Wise areola mastopexy breast augmentation)—plastic surgery technique based on the Wise pattern mammoplasty. The procedure lifts and enlarges breasts that have fallen after pregnancy, with weight loss, or just as part of their natural development. It results in an anchor-shaped scar with a purse-string closure around the areola. The procedure is named for Dr. R. J. Wise, and the acronym WAMBA is trademarked. Cf. *SAMBA*.

wandering spleen—a rare condition in which the spleen has a long vascular pedicle that allows the organ to move freely in the abdomen. Pedicle may become torsed.

WAP (wandering atrial pacemaker).

Wardill palatoplasty.

Warheads—a sour candy for salivary gland stimulation.

Warm 'n Form—lumbosacral corset.

WarmTouch patient warming system—manages patient body temperatures intraoperatively to prevent postoperative hypothermia.

Warren splenorenal shunt.

Wartenberg pinwheel—used in sensory examinations.

Warthin-Starry technique—silver stain used to identify *Helicobacter pylori*.

Warthin tumor—adenolymphoma. (Alfred S. Warthin, M.D., U.S. pathologist.) Cf. *Wharton tumor*.

Wartner wart removal system—an over-the-counter wart removal device that uses cryotherapy.

Was-Cath—catheter for percutaneous thromboendarterectomy.

washerwoman's skin—the macerated appearance of the skin after long immersion in water. Used in autopsy dictation.

Washington regimen—postoperative care following tendon repair.

washout phase—in radionuclide scans, scintiscanning of the lungs at the conclusion of the inhalation phase of a lung scan, after an interval during which all inhaled radionuclide has been exhaled.

WAST (Woman Abuse Screening Tool). Also, **WAST-Short** form.

wastebasket diagnosis—a vague or general diagnosis, such as chronic fatigue or nonspecific back pain.

wasting syndrome—a life-threatening weight loss, often seen in AIDS.

watchband incision—for endoscopic radial artery harvesting. The incision averages 3 cm in length.

water brash—regurgitation of excessive saliva from the esophagus, often combined with some gastric juice; heartburn; pyrosis.

Waterfield needle—used for bone marrow biopsy and aspiration.

water hammer pulse—a very rapid upstroke and falloff, indicative of a number of cardiac problems, the common denominator being a low resistance of the runoff of blood.

water-induced thermotherapy (WIT)—treatment of benign prostatic hyperplasia by introducing heated (60°C) water into the prostatic urethra by means of a special heat-transmitting balloon catheter. The precisely controlled heated water de-

water-induced *(cont.)* stroys a predictable amount of tissue, which is reabsorbed into the body, and the obstructed urethra is reopened. WIT is an outpatient procedure requiring only topical anesthesia. See *Thermoflex system.*

watering can perineum—descriptive term for a perineal deformity caused by fistulae.

watermelon stomach—gastric antral vascular ectasia (GAVE). It is associated with cirrhosis, scleroderma, and atrophic gastritis. The stomach exhibits prominent erythematous stripes running from the pylorus to the antrum that resemble the stripes on a watermelon. The "stripes" exhibit ectasias and intravascular thrombi, and can cause GI bleeding and anemia. Treatment includes laser or bipolar coagulation to control bleeding.

Water-Pik irrigator—may be used as a verb. Usage: "The canal was Water-Piked, packed with epinephrine-soaked sponges, and then packed with a dry sponge and sucked dry."

watershed region—in anatomy a "continental divide" from which vascular supply (or ascites) can go in either of two directions. Strokes in watershed regions of the brain are more devastating. There is an abdominal watershed and one in the upper pulmonary area which divides tracheal blood supply from retrograde lung supply. Lung transplants usually have the anastomosis in this region, and bronchial dehiscence can result from airway ischemia following disruption of the vascular supply in the watershed area.

water-soluble contrast medium (WSCM).

Waterston method—uses a portion of the transverse and descending colon as an interposition graft to replace an esophagus destroyed by caustic substance ingestion.

Waters view (Radiol)—occipital film for view of the maxillary sinuses. Named for Charles Alexander Waters, M.D., U.S. radiologist.

Watson-Jones tenodesis—corrects instability arising from injury of both the anterior talofibular ligament and calcaneofibular ligament.

Watts Sexual Function Questionnaire—measures self-reports of sexual function and concerns about sexual interest and satisfaction.

Watzke Silicone sleeve—used in scleral buckling procedures.

wavefront LASIK procedure—an enhanced version of LASIK that allows eye surgeons to customize the procedure for each eye, providing the possibility of even better vision.

wavefront mapping (Oph)—a means of identifying problems with vision by passing a narrow beam of light through the eye and analyzing the behavior of the light as it passes through all the optical media, not just the cornea and lens.

wavefront measurement—measures unique optical aberrations in a patient's eye by projecting light into the eye and analyzing the returning wavefront. This allows treatment with a wavefront-guided ablation pattern to reshape the cornea for indications such as myopia, hyperopia, astigmatism, and ocular abnormalities.

wavelet scalar quantization (WSQ).

WaveWire—high-performance angioplasty guidewire used to measure blood pressure in the coronary arte-

WaveWire *(cont.)*
ries. By taking blood pressure measurements on both sides of a lesion, the cardiologist can determine whether the lesion is significantly affecting blood flow. It may be used in combination with the FloWire Doppler guidewire if a patient has more than one blockage or lesion in an artery.

Wayfarer prosthesis—modifiable foot prosthesis.

WBAT (weightbearing as tolerated).

WBCL (Wenckebach cycle length).

WCD (wearable cardioverter-defibrillator)—a combination of two different devices. As a cardioverter, it uses low-energy electrical shocks to return an abnormally fast heart beat to a normal rhythm. As a defibrillator, it uses high-energy shocks to return a very fast, disordered heart beat to a normal rhythm. The patient wears a vest-like garment that holds the WCD parts—a monitor, electrodes, and small alarm module. Thus, the WCD is noninvasive, requires no surgery, implantation, or entry into the body. Cf. *ICD* (implantable cardioverter-defibrillator).

WCD 2000 system—a wearable defibrillator, indicated for adult patients who are at risk for sudden cardiac arrest and either are not candidates for or refuse an implantable defibrillator.

WCST (Wisconsin Card Sorting Test).

WDE (wound dressing emulsion).

WDHA (watery, secretory diarrhea, hypokalemia, and achlorhydria) **syndrome**. See *vipoma syndrome*.

wean—to slowly decrease a person's dependence on something—a ventilator, for example; to discontinue a medicine by gradually reducing the dose.

weapon (ENT)—an otologic instrument; an angled, round canal knife.

weave—see *Pulvertaft weave*.

Weavenit (no *k*) **vascular prosthesis**—see *Microknit vascular prosthesis*.

weave technique, Pulvertaft—see *Pulvertaft anastomosis*.

Weber test—for conducting hearing loss. The Weber test uses bone conduction. The base of the activated (tapped or stroked) tuning fork is placed against the forehead, the vertex of the skull, or the front teeth, and the patient is asked in which ear he hears the sound best. In conductive hearing loss, the sound is referred to the deafer ear. In perceptive hearing loss, the sound is referred to the better ear. See *air conduction, bone conduction*, and *Rinne test*.

Wechsler Adult Intelligence Scale—mental status examination.

Wechsler Memory Scale or **Test**—mental status examination.

Wedeen wire passers—designed with S-curve to pass around bone in orthopedic procedures.

Wedge—electrosurgical resection device used in transurethral resection of the prostate.

Wedge, The—bioresorbable interference-fit implant used to attach a graft during cruciate ligament reconstruction.

wedged hepatic vein pressure (WHVP) **measurement**—used to estimate portal vein pressure.

WEDI (Workgroup for Electronic Data Interchange)—a standard-setting organization that addresses issues related to HIPAA and electronic privacy of healthcare information. *WEDI* may be pronounced as a word.

wee bag—urine collection bag.

Weerda distending operating laryngoscope.

Wegener granulomatosis—systemic vasculitis that can involve any organ system. A newly identified serologic marker, cytoplasmic pattern antineutrophil cytoplasmic autoantibody, makes possible the early diagnosis of Wegener granulomatosis.

Wehbe arm holder—for operating table.

Wehrs incus prosthesis—used in ear reconstructive surgery.

Weigert stain—see *elastic fibers stain*.

weightbearing, **nonweightbearing**—terms frequently used in orthopedic dictation (*nonweightbearing extremity*, *weightbearing crutches*), although they do not appear in medical dictionaries. Many ask whether they should be hyphenated. The trend in language is to combine words without hyphens after compound nouns become common. An architectural term comparable to *weightbearing* is *loadbearing*, and it is treated as one word. Some may wish to hyphenate, as *non-weightbearing*, *non-weight-bearing*, or *nonweight-bearing*, but it seems simpler and clearer to make *weightbearing* and *nonweightbearing* single words.

Weill sign—indicative of pneumonia in an infant. During respiration, the subclavicular space on the affected side shows no expansion.

Weir excisions—alar excisions of the nose.

Weiss fixed wing epidural needle.

Weitlaner retractor.

Welch Allyn ear wash system—an enclosed tap water-based ear wax removal system that has water temperature and pressure safety controls. Its technology eliminates the need for patient water-barrier gowns and cleanup of expelled wastewater.

weld—term applied to wound closure with Superglue or other tissue adhesive.

Wellcogen latex agglutination test.

Well operation for rectal prolapse.

well, pericardial—the space around the heart where iced saline slush is placed in coronary artery bypass graft surgery. *Not* pericardial wall.

wen—a sebaceous cyst or other bland swelling on, in, or under the skin.

Wenckebach cycle length (WBCL).

Werdnig-Hoffmann disease—infantile motor neuron disease.

Wernicke area of the brain (in the superior temporal gyrus)—important as the area involved in spoken language.

Wernicke disease—a vitamin B_1 deficiency disease that causes memory loss.

Wesolowski vascular prosthesis—fine-knit Dacron prosthesis. See *Microknit vascular prosthesis*.

WEST (Weinstein Enhanced Sensory Test)—tests various body parts to determine degree of diabetic neuropathy.

Westcott needle—a cutting biopsy needle.

Westergren test—for sedimentation rate.

Westerman-Jensen needle—used for bone marrow biopsy and aspiration.

Western blot (blotting) **electrotransfer test**—a second-line AIDS test, more sensitive, given as a backup when the ELISA test is positive.

WEST-foot—a sensory nerve tester using patented SofTip monofilaments.

West Nile virus—a mosquito-borne encephalitis spread from the northeast area of the United States by birds migrating south. Although most patients suffer only mild flu-like symptoms, the elderly and those with immune deficiencies are extremely vulnerable to more serious infection.

West nomogram—see *body surface area.*

wet age-related macular degeneration (ARMD) (Oph)—the more severe type of ARMD. The membrane underlying the retina thickens, then breaks. The oxygen supply to the macula is disrupted, and the body responds by growing new abnormal blood vessels. These begin to grow through the breaks in the membrane behind the retina toward the macula, often raising the retina. These abnormal blood vessels tend to be very fragile and often grow, leak, or bleed, causing scarring of the macula. The damage to the macula results in rapid central vision loss. Once the vision is destroyed, it cannot be restored.

wet field cautery *(not* Wetfield).

wet mount—a method of microscopic examination in which the specimen (a fluid or fluid suspension) is placed on a slide and then covered with a coverslip, rather than drying the specimen. Usage: "Wet mounts showed positive trichomoniasis."

wet prep (also *wet mount*). Usage: "Wet preps were taken, which were negative for yeast but positive for *Trichomonas*."

wet reading—a term describing a stat (immediate) radiograph film reading. When wet chemistry was in use, a radiologist read a freshly developed wet film in the darkroom when a fast result was needed. Dry chemicals have been used for many years in radiology darkrooms, but convention still calls a stat report a "wet reading."

wet sandpaper appearance of inflammatory bowel disease—a fine granular appearance of the mucosal surface of the colon or rectum in ulcerative colitis. The mucosa is friable and bleeds easily with minimal endoscopic trauma.

wet-to-dry dressings—sterile gauze is soaked in sterile normal saline, applied to a wound, and allowed to dry; when removed, it facilitates debridement.

whale tail—part of the Octopus tissue stabilizer from Medtronic, used in beating heart surgery.

Wharton tumor (and *duct*)—benign papillary cystadenoma of the submaxillary gland. Cf. *Warthin tumor*.

wheal *(not* wheel). If you scratch the skin of your forearm with your fingernail, you may find, after a few minutes, a raised area appearing where you made the scratch. It may also become erythematous and may or may not itch. This is a wheal. A wheal may represent a positive reaction in skin tests (such as the tine test for PPD), and the diameter of the wheal is measured to determine whether the response is positive or negative. In tuberculin testing, a wheal of 8 to 10 mm in diameter 48 to 72 hours after injection is considered positive. Cf. *wheal and flare reaction*.

wheal and flare reaction—reaction to a test administered via injection. See *wheal*.

wheat gliadins—dietary exposure to wheat gliadins has been found to

wheat *(cont.)*
contribute to celiac disease, which occurs in approximately 1 in 300 people. Treatment is to eliminate all wheat and gluten-containing foods.

Wheaton Pavlik harness—orthopedic brace for children.

wheat weevil disease—extrinsic allergic alveolitis caused by exposure to wheat flour and weevils.

wheelchair artifact (Radiol)—seen in patients x-rayed in their wheelchairs because they were too ill to lie flat for imaging.

wheelchairs and motorized personal transport systems (Rehab)
Action A4 sports chair
Affiniti Hoveround mobile chair
Amigo mobile chair
Barracuda sports chair
Chairman Corpus motorized chair
Convaid buggies
Cruiser Transport
EZ Rider chair
Hoveround HVR 100 power control programmable chair
Invacare chair
Iron Horse outdoor activity chair
Kid-EXB 2 child's chair for bus transport
Kuschall chair
Kusch'kin wheelchair
LaBac adjustable chair system
Mulholland Growth Guidance System
Paraglide chair
Quickie P210/Sunrise chair
Slam'R adjustable chair
Spirea adjustable foldable wheelchair
Supernova Xtreme sports chair
Tarsys tilt and recline system
Viper chair by Radius
Vision/Epic chair
Zippie P500

Wheeless method—for surgical construction of a J rectal pouch.

WHI (Women's Health Initiative).

whiplash technique—for repositioning a catheter with a trocar under fluoroscopy.

Whipple disease—intestinal lipodystrophy, a rare chronic inflammatory disease, and an intestinal disorder of malabsorption. It primarily affects the small intestine and the mesenteric lymph nodes, but it may affect other organs including the brain, spinal cord, and peripheral nerve plexuses. The onset is usually in middle age and occurs nine times more often in men than in women. Symptoms involve multisystems and may include ataxia, personality changes, seizures, memory deficits, ophthalmoplegia, and hearing loss.

Whipple pancreaticoduodenectomy—used for tumor of the distal common duct or when severe pancreatitis is confined to the head of the pancreas.

whistle-tip ureteral catheter.

Whitacre spinal needle.

White and Panjabi criteria—for cervical spine x-ray evaluation.

White classification—diabetes mellitus.

white clot—a clot with a platelet-rich core. See *red clot*.

white clot syndrome—spontaneous major arterial thrombosis in a patient receiving heparin therapy, usually preceded by thrombocytopenia (low platelet count).

white dot syndrome—see *multiple evanescent white dot syndrome*.

white limbal girdle of Vogt (Oph).

white line of Toldt—lateral reflection of posterior parietal pleura of abdomen over mesentery of ascending and descending colon.

Whiteside line—an arbitrary 3 to 4 degrees of external rotation and transepicondylar axis (TEA), accepted landmarks for determining femoral component rotation in total knee arthroplasty that include the posterior condyles.

whitlow, herpes—herpetic infection of the fingertips.

Whitnall ligament—one of the support structures of the eyelid.

Whittlestone Physiological Breast-milker, The—a breast pump that incorporates a thin-walled liner which gently and rhythmically compresses the nipple-areolar area to stimulate breast milk flow. It does not create the breast trauma that often results from use of vacuum-type breast pumps.

WHO (World Health Organization) **classification of papillary urothelial neoplasms of the bladder**.

WHO/ISUP (International Society of Urological Pathology) **classification of papillary urothelial neoplasms of the bladder.**

whole body hyperthermia—see *hyperthermia, whole body*.

whole body 29FDG scanning.

whole-field scotopic sensitivity screening (Oph)—field-based screening for glaucoma.

whole lung lavage (WLL).

Wholey ("wooley") **wire**—used in opening a stenosed vessel. Usage: "The subclavian stenosis was crossed with a Wholey wire and a 7F diagnostic catheter."

whorl—a circular swirl or vortex.

WHR (waist-to-hip ratio).

WHVP (wedged hepatic vein pressure) **measurement**.

Wiberg center edge (CE) **angle**—a point on the acetabulum, measured radiographically.

Wiberg classification of patellar types (I, II, III) in relation to shapes of the inferior surface of the patella, and in association with chondromalacia patellae.

wick (usually gauze)—used for drainage of a wound. Usage: "A large amount of liquid pus was drained from the wound. The wound was packed with 1/2" plain gauze. He is to have the wick removed in two days."

Wiener filter (MRI term)—recovers resolution and reduces image noise while improving quantification of regional myocardial perfusion with thallium-201 tomography.

Wiktor balloon expandable coronary stent (Cardio)—compressed stent made of tantalum wire which is inserted over the balloon of a coronary artery catheter and then expanded at the site of the angioplasty. Left in place, the stent remains expanded and prevents re-stenosis of the artery.

Wiktor GX—a coronary stent coated with Hepamed (heparin) to retard clotting. You may also hear it dictated as *Hepamed-coated Wiktor stent*.

Wilde incision (ENT).

wild type (Genetics)—used to designate a normally occurring allele or normal phenotype.

Williams-Beuren syndrome—idiopathic infantile hypercalcemia. Patients have elfin facies, failure to thrive, and sometimes supravalvular aortic stenosis and mental retardation.

Williams cardiac device.

Williams flexion exercises—involving flexion of the neck, trunk, pelvis, and legs. Designed to alleviate lower back pain by stretching the extensor muscles in the lower back and strengthening flexors, such as the

Williams *(cont.)*
rectus abdominis and gluteus maximus.

Williams vulvovaginoplasty.

Will Rogers phenomenon—a higher observed survival for every stage of disease without actually improving overall survival. Based on a comment by humorist Will Rogers, "When the Okies left Oklahoma and moved to California, they raised the average intelligence of both states!"

Wilmington—see *port of Wilmington*.

Wilson-Cook wire-guided sphincterotome (modified)—used in endoscopic procedures.

Wiltse approach—midline or bilateral paraspinal approach used in lumbosacral fusion.

Wiltse pedicle screw system—fixation system used for the treatment of severe spondylolisthesis of the L5-S1 vertebra, degenerative lumbar scoliosis, and spinal stenosis when decompression is required.

Wiltse rods—used with bone graft in correcting and stabilizing vertebrae in spondylolisthesis.

WinABP ambulatory blood pressure monitor—stores up to 120 hours of ambulatory BP readings and sends to a Windows-compatible printer in chart or graph form.

Winchester syndrome—rare disorder believed by some scientists to be closely related to hereditary lysosomal storage disorders. Major symptoms may include short stature, arthritis-like symptoms, and eye and skin abnormalities.

windlass effect—creates an intrinsic foot support system that counters the pronatory ground reactive forces on the forefoot during propulsion.

windowed balloon—a shaded balloon (the unshaded portion is the "window") used with photodynamic therapy to deliver laser radiation to a targeted area, such as a portion of the esophagus. See *photodynamic therapy*.

window period—a general term referring to an interval of time during which an expected change is not yet observable, especially the interval between the development of an infection (for example, with HIV) and the appearance of detectable antibody in serum.

winged scapula—caused by a stretching injury to the long thoracic nerve. This results in weakness of the serratus anterior, with "winging," or wing-like protrusion, of the scapula.

wing sutures.

wink—see *anal wink*.

WINS (Women's Initiative for Nonsmoking)—clinical trial designed to test the effectiveness of cognitive-behavioral, nurse-managed smoking cessation intervention.

Winston-Lutz linac (linear accelerator) **method**.

Winters shunt—corpus spongiosum to corpus cavernosum (for priapism).

Wirsung dilatation—dilatation of Wirsung duct. Usage: "There was no bile duct or Wirsung dilatation or vascular invasion." It is used on an abdominal CT report in pancreatic metastasis from renal cell carcinoma.

Wirt test—for assessing stereoscopic acuity.

Wise areola mastopexy breast augmentation (WAMBA).

Wise pattern—for reduction mammoplasty. Named for Dr. R. J. Wise.

Wishard catheter—a catheter with one hole at the end; used for diagnostic purposes.

wishbone retractor—see *Omni-Tract adjustable wishbone retractor*.

Wiskott-Aldrich syndrome—dysgammaglobulinemia.

Wissinger rod—to correct shoulder instability. Usage: "We inserted a Wissinger rod anteriorly, and we looked for the probe as it entered anteriorly."

WIT (water-induced thermotherapy).

Witzel duodenostomy.

Witzel tunnel—for feeding jejunostomy.

Wixson hip positioner—for total hip and revision hip surgery.

Wizard cardiac device.

Wizard microdebrider—self-irrigating debrider used in endoscopic sinus surgery.

WLL (whole lung lavage).

WNM system—an esophageal cancer staging alternative to the TNM system. It is based on wall penetration, nodal status, and distant metastasis.

Wobenzym—over-the-counter tablet containing proteolytic enzymes, touted as a treatment for "economy class syndrome," a condition in which blood clots form as a result of flying for long periods in cramped quarters.

wobble board—a physical therapy apparatus used for patient education of proprioception and balance.

Wolfe graft—used in hand surgery.

Wolfe mammographic parenchymal patterns.

Wolff-Parkinson-White syndrome.

Wolvek sternal approximation fixation instrument—used to close a sternotomy incision after cardiopulmonary bypass surgery.

Womack procedure—splenectomy, resection of superior half of the greater curvature of the stomach, devascularization, and transgastric suturing of the varices for portal hypertension-induced variceal bleeding.

Woman Abuse Screening Tool (WAST). Also, **WAST-Short** form.

Wong-Staal scissors—another innovative way to keep the AIDS virus from replicating, from scientist Flossie Wong-Staal. Working with Arnold Hempel, she fashioned a molecule that cuts up the genes of the virus which control its activities.

Wood light examination—of skin and hair for evidence of fungal infection.

wood pulp worker's lung disease—extrinsic allergic alveolitis caused by exposure to moldy logs.

Woodson and Hamilton Motor Activity Scale (MAS)—rates motor activity in infants on a scale from 0 to 5.

Woods screw maneuver (Ob-Gyn)—used in vaginal delivery to deliver the infant's shoulders, sometimes used in conjunction with other maneuvers.

Woods technique of follicular relocation—single hair follicle transplant microsurgery. In this technique, physicians transplant only the hair follicle itself, not the excess tissue attached to it that other techniques generate. This technique is minimally invasive, painless, and leads to hair restoration that is said to look and feel completely natural as compared to other hair transplant techniques that can be painful and cause unsightly scars and hair patterns.

Wooler-plasty (not Whooler-plasty).

word salad—mixture of words and phrases that lack comprehensive

word *(cont.)*
meaning or logical coherence, commonly seen in schizophrenic states.

Woringer-Kolopp disease—manifested in cutaneous lymphoma.

work hardening—an individualized program to return patient to previous work capacity.

Workhorse percutaneous transluminal angioplasty balloon catheter—used for PTA treatment of obstructive lesions of the iliac, femoral, and renal arteries or synthetic arteriovenous dialysis fistulae; catheters are not designed for use in coronary arteries.

workup—thorough diagnostic evaluation.

Woronoff rings—in psoriasis.

Worst gonioprism contact lens—a lens that allows the surgeon to directly examine synechiae (adhesions) which have formed around the haptics of an anterior chamber intraocular lens. The surgeon can then lyse these synechiae without having to cut the haptics of the intraocular lens. The intact intraocular lens can then be removed with less tissue trauma than if the haptics had been cut.

Worth 4-dot test (W4D) (Oph)—combined with stereopsis on the Titmus stereo test, used for evaluating the ability of the two eyes to perceive images simultaneously.

Woun'Dres hydrogel dressing.

wound cleansers—see *cleansers*.

Wound-Span Bridge II—trade name for a dressing that holds the ends of a wound together by spanning it rather than pressing on it.

Wound Stick measuring system—includes Wound Stick for measuring and marking the size and depth of a wound, and Wound Stick tunneler for probing the dimensions of an ulcer.

wrap-around ghosting artifact (Radiol)—see *aliasing artifact*. If the field of view (FOV) is too small, some of the radiographic image can wrap around and reappear on the other side of the image. The zebra artifact can occur with interference between the main image and the aliased part in gradient echo sequences.

WRAT ("rat") (Wide Range Achievement Test).

wreath pattern corneal infiltrates—the visual appearance of a keratitis caused by a fungal infection.

Wrightlock posterior fixation system—spinal fixation system used for correction of scoliosis and spine instability, consisting of a stainless steel rod and Morse taper locking mechanism.

Wright needle—used to fashion a fascia lata sling to repair ptosis.

Wright peak flow—a metered measurement used in testing pulmonary function. "The lungs are clear to percussion and auscultation. There is no wheezing. His Wright peak flow on three occasions was 525."

Wright stain—used in the diagnosis of *Pneumocystis carinii* pneumonia. See *GMS*, *Gomori or Grocotti methenamine silver*.

wringer wrap—see *aortomyoplasty*.

wrinkle artifact—see *kink artifact*.

wrinkle treatments—see *Artecoll, CosmoDerm (1 and 2) human-based collagen implant, Fibrel, Fraxel SR Laser, Hylaform gel, Hylaform Plus, Perlane, PlasmaGel, Restylane, Restylane Fine Lines injectable gel, Reviderm, Sculptra wrinkle filler*.

Wrisberg—see *nerve of Wrisberg*.

Wristaleve—a corrective wrist support to alleviate symptoms of carpal tunnel syndrome.

wrist drop—passive flexion of the wrist due to paralysis of extensor muscles.

Wroblewski method—of testing serum LDH.

WR-2721—see *ethiofos*.

WSCM (water-soluble contrast medium).

WSQ (wavelet scalar quantization).

W-stapled urinary reservoir (or ileal neobladder)—a procedure for providing post total cystectomy patients with an orthotopic neobladder (rather than ileal diversion). A portion of the ileum is removed for construction of the reservoir, and the ileum is anastomosed end-to-end. The removed portion is shaped into a W, using absorbable staples. The ureters are attached to the two upper limbs of the W, and the urethra is attached to the bottom of the W. The procedure can be performed quickly, in 12 to 21 minutes.

Wu bunionectomy—a modification of the Mitchell distal metatarsal osteotomy/bunionectomy. Uses a distal transverse first metatarsal osteotomy using Herbert bone screw fixation. Named for Dr. Kent K. Wu.

Wurzburg plating system—titanium craniomaxillofacial plate and screws.

WuScope system—combination laryngoscope and intubation device designed for both awake and anesthetized patient intubation via either the oral or nasal route.

Wylie carotid artery clamp.

X, x

Xanar 20 Ambulase CO_2 laser—used in dermatologic and gynecologic surgery.

xanthelasma—a flat or slightly raised yellowish tumor, found most frequently on the upper and lower lids, especially near the inner canthus.

xanthogranulomatous cholecystitis—a rare inflammatory condition of the gallbladder associated with marked proliferative fibrosis, which occasionally invades surrounding tissues such as the liver bed and porta hepatis. Unfortunately, this condition so closely mimics gallbladder carcinoma that an intraoperative biopsy is necessary to make a diagnosis. May also be referred to as *ceroid-like histiocytic granuloma* or *fibroxanthogranulomatous inflammation*.

X-body—see *Birbeck granule*.

Xcytrin ("ek-SIGH-trin") (motexafin gadolinium) **injection**—drug used for the treatment of cancer patients with brain metastases.

XeCl (xenon, chloride excimer) **laser**.

Xenaderm (trypsin, balsam, castor oil)—a prescription drug in ointment form to promote healing of pressure ulcers and provide protection from harmful irritants such as urine or feces.

XenoDerm graft—provides a suitable matrix for engraftment of cultured epidermal autografts to generate a reconstituted skin. They are processed porcine dermis, an animal-derived equivalent to LifeCell patented AlloDerm processed tissue grafts.

xenograft—a graft from a donor of one species to a host of a different species. See *graft*.

Xenomedica prosthetic valve.

xenon arc photocoagulator.

xenon 133 scan (^{133}Xe)—measures cerebral blood flow by isolating the internal carotid artery and injecting xenon 133. The cerebral blood flow is then calculated by automated cerebral blood flow analyzer.

Xenotech prosthetic valve.

xenotransplantation—any procedure that involves the transplantation, implantation, or infusion into a human recipient of either live cells, tissues, or organs from a nonhuman animal source, or human body fluids, cells,

xenotransplantation *(cont.)*
tissues, or organs that have had ex vivo contact with nonhuman animal cells, tissues or organs.

xenotransplantation product—live cells, tissues, or organs used in xenotransplantation.

xenotropic donor organisms—organisms originating in nonhuman animal tissue that pose the risk of infectious disease transmission through xenotransplantation.

xenozoonoses—animal diseases that may be transferred through xenotransplantation.

Xeroform ("zero-form") **gauze**.

Xillix LIFE-Lung system—GI fluorescence endoscopy imaging system for detection and localization of cancerous and precancerous lesions of the gastrointestinal tract. It is believed to be more effective than conventional white light bronchoscopy alone.

xiphoid ("zi′foid") **process** (Greek, sword-shaped)—the pointed cartilage and bone attached to the lower end of the sternum. Cf. *scyphoid*.

XKnife—software for stereotactic radiation therapy treatment planning. This software is used for the development of radiotherapy treatment plans to treat lesions in the brain, including tumors and vascular malformations.

XL (extra length).

X-linked—in genetics, referring to a trait, disease, or pattern of transmission involving one or more genes located on the X chromosome (the female sex chromosome). An X-linked trait, such as hemophilia A, is not transmitted from male parent to male offspring, but all female offspring of an affected male are heterozygous carriers of the trait and can transmit it to their male offspring. See *sex-linked*.

X-linked familial spastic paraparesis—a disease characterized by spastic gait and increased reflexes without other associated neurologic signs.

X-linked retinoschisis—a splitting of the retina that may be complicated by vitreous hemorrhage and retinal detachment.

X-linked SCID—severe combined immunodeficiency disease of unknown genetic origin.

XLnt (crosslinking nucleotides)—a technology for improving signal-to-background levels in nucleic acid hybridization-based assays.

XMG (x-ray mammogram).

XMMEN-OE5 monoclonal antibody—for patients in shock from a systemic gram-negative infection.

Xomed DCR (dacryocystorhinostomy) **drill**—a drill used in dacryocystorhinostomy procedures.

Xpeedior 60 catheter—used for removal of clots from dialysis grafts.

Xpeedior 100 catheter—for removal of lower extremity arterial clots. This catheter is part of the Angiojet rheolytic thrombectomy system for clot removal.

Xplorer—a filmless high-resolution digital radiography imaging system.

X-PRESS vascular closure system—a suture-based closure device designed to seal arterial access sites and permit early ambulation following catheterization procedures.

XPS Sculpture system—see *liposhaver*.

XPS StraightShot—a micro tissue resector system used in endoscopic sinus surgery.

XQ230 Olympus gastroscope.

x-ray *(not* X-ray)—roentgenogram or roentgen ray.

x-ray tomographic microscope (XTM) —originally invented to analyze ceramic components used in jet engines, this technology is now being used by dental researchers to observe structures in tooth dentin measuring as small as 2 micrometers, about the size of a human cell.

X-SCID (X-linked severe combined immunodeficiency disease).

XT cardiac device.

X-10 Crosslink plates—a spinal plate system that allows surgeons to convert a dual-rod construct into a frame to improve both axial and torsional stiffness, reduce motion at the bone-implant interface, and decrease the risk for fatigue breakage.

X-TEND-O knee flexer—provides patient-controlled flexion and extension exercises.

XTRAC—laser system for the treatment of vitiligo.

XT radiopaque coronary stent—developed by Bard, reportedly more flexible and easier to put in place than other coronary stents.

X-Trode—electrode catheter for intravenous insertion into a cavity of the heart.

xylol pulse indicator.

Y, y

YAG (yttrium-aluminum-garnet)—see *Nd:YAG laser.*

YagLazr system—used for treatment of a broad range of tattoo colors and epidermal lesions.

Yang-Monti ileovesicostomy—a technique that creates an efferent conduit from a transverse tubularized segment of ileum for bladder augmentation and continent urinary diversion. It preserves the appendix in the event of a MACE procedure. Related terms: *Yang-Monti conduit, Yang-Monti principle*.

Yankauer curette (curet).

Yasargil bayonet scissors.

YeastOne Colorimetric antifungal panel—a laboratory test for fungal susceptibility to antifungal agents.

Yellow IRIS—a workstation that performs blood cell counting in synovial and pericardial fluids and crystal examination in synovial fluid.

Yentl syndrome—refers to the fact that women's cardiac symptoms are often regarded less seriously than men's, with the male-dominated medical profession pursuing a less aggressive management approach to coronary artery disease in women than men, despite greater cardiac disability in women. ("Yentl" is from the story "Yentl, the Yeshiva Boy" by Isaac Bashevis Singer.)

Yeoman uterine biopsy forceps.

Yergason test—used in examining the shoulder to determine if subluxation of the long head of the biceps tendon is present.

Yersinia—genus of gram-negative rods. *Yersinia pestis* is the etiologic agent of plague.

Yoon rings—fallopian tube ligation rings.

"yoop-nee-ic"—phonetic rendering of *eupneic* (silent *e*) (breathing normally, without difficulty).

"yoo-pep"—phonetic for *UPEP* (urine protein electrophoresis).

York-Mason approach—posterior midsagittal transsphincteric approach for treatment of rectourethral fistula.

Young-Dees-Leadbetter bladder-neck reconstructive procedure—to create bladder outlet competence.

yo-yo syndrome—used to describe the practice of clinically severe obese people who "yo-yo" between weight loss and gain and cannot achieve long-term weight loss with dietary or behavioral modifications alone. Many turn to obesity surgery for treatment.

Yperwatch gamma control watch—measures exposure to radiation.

YPLL (years of potential life lost)—used in mortality studies.

Y-shaped graft.

Y stenting—an angioplasty technique that utilizes one or more intracoronary stents in an inverted Y configuration.

yttrium-aluminum-garnet (YAG)—see *Nd:YAG laser.*

Yunis-Varon syndrome—extremely rare inherited multisystem disorder with defects affecting the skeletal, ectodermal, and cardiorespiratory systems. It is characterized by growth retardation prior to and after birth; defective growth of the bones of the skull along with complete or partial absence of the shoulder blades; characteristic facial features; possible abnormalities of the fingers and/or toes; and, frequently, cardiomyopathy. The syndrome is thought to be inherited as an autosomal recessive genetic trait.

yuppie flu—see *chronic fatigue syndrome*; *myalgic encephalomyelitis*. Also, *postviral fatigue syndrome*.

Z, z

"Zabo"—phonetic for *Szabo-Berci.*

Zaditor (ketotifen fumarate)—drug that provides temporary relief from itching of the eye due to allergic conjunctivitis.

Zahn—see *line of Zahn.*

Zaidemberg technique—a method of creating a pedicled vascular bone graft.

Zancolli clawhand deformity repair.

Zandy bars, Zannies, Z-Bars—street slang for Xanax, fast becoming a drug of abuse in the college party scene. The 2-mg tablets are elongated and scored, hence the descriptive names. They are also called *footballs.*

Zanfel—a topical drug in cream form for treatment of poison ivy (urushiol), poison oak, or poison sumac, which is eliminated from the skin in 30 seconds.

Zang Fu differentiations—identifies disease entities and suggests acupuncture treatment by symptoms.

Zavanelli maneuver—returns the fetus into the pelvis during cesarean section for failed vaginal breech delivery.

ZD neurosurgical localizing unit—used in stereotactic biopsy and minimally invasive neurosurgery.

ZDV (zidovudine).

Zeavision—see *zeaxanthin.*

zeaxanthin—carotenoid found in some vegetables. There is some evidence that intake of carotenoids can reduce the risk of age-related macular degeneration and cataracts.

zebra artifact—see *wrap-around ghosting artifact.*

Zebra exchange guidewire—used with the SoloPass during endoscopic bile duct procedures.

ZEEP (zero end-expiratory pressure).

Zeiss—manufacturer of many ophthalmological instruments, cameras, and microscopes.

Zeiss EndoLive endoscope.

Zeiss Visulas 690s laser—for activation of Visudyne (verteporfin for injection) therapy to treat wet age-related macular degeneration.

Zelapar (selegiline HCl)—a drug formulation of selegiline, an MAO inhibitor, for the treatment of Parkinson disease.

Zelmac (tegaserod)—drug treatment for irritable bowel syndrome in patients whose primary symptom is constipation.

Zelnorm (tegaserod, "te-GAS-a-rod") —treatment for constipation-predominant irritable bowel syndrome in women. Diarrhea is a significant side effect of tegaserod.

Zelsmyr Cytobrush—used to obtain material from endocervical canal for Pap smear, Chlamydia screen, and other lab tests.

Zemaira (A_1-PI, alpha$_1$-proteinase inhibitor)—a drug therapy for emphysema.

Zenith AAA endovascular graft system—used for minimally invasive treatment of abdominal aortic aneurysm (AAA). Catheters are guided to the location of the AAA through the femoral arteries; once in position, the self-expanding, fabric-covered, metallic stent/graft is deployed to relieve pressure on the aneurysm.

Zenker diverticulum—see *Dohlman endoscopic repair of Zenker diverticulum.*

Zenker fixative—a mercury-containing solution used to harden and preserve tissue.

Zenotech—a biomaterial for synthetic ligaments.

zero diastolic blood pressure—a way of expressing blood pressure readings when the diastolic pressure drops down very low. For example, a recording of 80/0 in a gynecology patient who is hemorrhaging indicates she is going into shock because of reduced blood volume. In the upright position her systolic blood pressure (maximum pressure in arteries occurring with heartbeat) is so low that between beats of the heart, the diastolic pressure drops down to a point where it can't be measured by the standard cuff method. By this indirect method, vascular sounds can be heard in the compressed brachial artery all the way from 80 mmHg down to 0 mmHg; the way this is recorded is 80/0.

ZeroTip nitinol stone retrieval basket.

ZES (Zollinger-Ellison syndrome).

Zest Anchor Advanced Generation (ZAAG) bone anchoring system.

ZETA coronary stent—part of the Guidant Multi-Link stent line.

Zetia (ezetimibe)—used in combination with fenofibrate to reduce LDL cholesterol (LDL-C), non-high density lipoprotein cholesterol (non-HDL-C), and apo B1 in patients with mixed hyperlipidemia and high LDL cholesterol, when compared to fenofibrate alone.

zeugmatography—MRI term.

Zeus—computer- and voice-controlled robotic system that positions and maneuvers instruments in microsurgery, directed by a surgeon working at a Zeus workstation with video monitor.

Zeuss robot—used to assist in laparoscopic procedures.

Z-FAST trial of Femara and Zometa.

Zicam—over-the-counter nasal solution drug said to significantly reduce the severity of the common cold, including nasal congestion, sneezing, coughing, and sore throat.

ziconotide intrathecal infusion—see *Prialt*.

zidovudine—new name for *AZT* (azidothymidine).

Ziehl-Neelsen stain (Lab)—for acid-fast bacilli.

Zielke curette (curet).

Zielke instrumentation—used to correct thoracolumbar curvatures. It is composed of a threaded rod, bone screws, washers and nuts. Used with external bracing, it can stabilize a corrected thoracolumbar curvature until arthrodesis is considered to be solid.

"zi-foid"—phonetic for *xiphoid* (process).

ZIFT (zygote intrafallopian tube transfer)—used in cases of blocked fallopian tubes, to achieve pregnancy. This is a combination of techniques used in GIFT and IVF. In ZIFT, fertilization takes place in vitro (in a dish), and 18 hours later four of the zygotes that have formed are replaced in the fallopian tubes to work their way into the uterus. See *GIFT*, *IVF*, *zygote*.

zigzag wire technique (Cardio)—a technique in which 0.035-inch J-tip guidewire is reshaped manually at the distal 7-cm to 8-cm portion, including the flexible part and 2 cm to 3 cm of the stiff part, into zigzag shape for use in difficult cardiac catheterizations.

Zimmer CPT (collarless polished taper) **hip system**.

Zimycan—a medication for the treatment of Candida-associated diaper dermatitis in infants.

Zingg fractures (Oph/Plastic)—fractures of the zygomaticomaxillary complex classified as types A, B, and C. Type A injuries are at the zygomatic arch (type A1), the lateral orbital wall (type A2), and the inferior orbital rim (type A3). Type B fractures involve all four buttresses (classic tetrapod fracture). Type C injuries are complex fractures with comminution of the zygomatic bone itself.

Zinnanti Z-clamp.

Zipper Medical—hypoallergenic tracheostomy tube neck band.

zipper scar.

zipper sphincterotomy—incision into a sphincter performed in zipper fashion.

ziprasidone mesylate—drug for treatment of schizophrenia.

Zipzoc—stocking compression dressing and wrap.

Ziramic femoral head.

Zirconia orthopedic prosthetic heads—made of zirconium oxide ceramic.

Zirpursky regimen—low dose Ara-C (cytosine arabinoside) for transient myeloproliferative disorder, a transient leukemia associated with Down syndrome.

Z-lengthening of tendons and split tendon transfers.

Z line—an imaginary line indicating the squamocolumnar junction of the uterine cervix.

ZMC (zygomatic-malar complex) **fracture** (of the face).

Z-Med catheter—peripheral, high-pressure balloon catheter, low deflation profile, rapid inflation/deflation time.

ZMS intramedullary fixation system—a Zimmer fixation system that provides easy intramedullary passage over a guidewire through the fracture site without reaming.

ZODIAC (Ziprasidone Observational Study of Cardiac Outcomes) **study**.

"zo-med"—phonetic for *Xomed*.

Zoll defibrillator.

Zollinger-Ellison syndrome (ZES)—gastric hypersecretion, peptic ulceration, pancreatic tumor syndrome, ulcerogenic tumor of pancreas syndrome. See *apudoma*.

Zometa (zoledronic acid for injection) —drug for treatment of tumor-induced hypercalcemia, which often occurs as a complication of bone metastasis in patients with breast cancer, multiple myeloma, and non-small cell lung carcinoma (or cancer).

zona hamster egg test—used in male infertility to test the ability of spermatozoa to penetrate hamster ova, which approximate human ova.

zone
electric
Looser
triangle of doom
triangle of pain

Zone diet ("The Zone")—developed by Dr. Barry Sears, consisting of 40% carbohydrate, 30% protein, and 30% fat. Encourages intake of more fruits and vegetables, less grains and starches, substituting fish and poultry for red meat, and consuming more monounsaturated fats (olive oil, for example).

zone of lucency—finding on a radiograph that may surround a defect or lesion.

zone of partial preservation (ZPP)—in spinal cord injury.

Zone Specific II meniscal repair system—cannulas, needles, and rasps used for inside-out meniscal repair procedures.

zonula occludens—tight junction of endothelial cells.

zonulolysis—dissolution of the ciliary zonule by use of enzymes, to permit surgical removal of the lens.

zoom effect—created by the flexibility of the foldable intraocular lens implant when responding to changes in the ciliary body.

zoonosis—the transmission of an animal infectious disease to humans, a potential complication of xenotransplantation.

zoonotic retroviruses—retroviruses of animal origin that have the potential to incorporate in the genome of human cells and replicate.

Zorbtive (somatropin [rDNA origin] for injection)—a medication used for treatment of patients with short bowel syndrome, a condition which impairs the ability of the small intestine to absorb the nutrition a person needs from food.

zoster immune globulin vaccine.

Z-Pak—packaging form of the antibiotic drug Zithromax, 6 capsules.

ZPP (zone of partial preservation).

ZstatFlu—rapid diagnostic test for influenza A and B.

Z stent—a self-expanding stent for bile duct and esophageal stenosis. Its wires are crisscrossed in a Z pattern. Also, *Gianturco prosthesis*.

Z-stitch—used in percutaneous bladder neck stabilization procedure in women with stress urinary incontinence. The stabilization suture is attached at four points on the pubic bone in a Z configuration.

ZTT I and **ZTT II acetabular cups**.

Zucker and Myler cardiac device.

Zuckerkandl—see *tubercle of Zuckerkandl*.

Zuma guiding catheter—used in the coronary or peripheral vascular system to provide a pathway for the introduction of therapeutic devices.

ZUMI uterine manipulator.

Zung Depression Scale.

Zung Self-rating Anxiety Scale (SAS).

Zweymuller prosthesis—a cementless hip prosthesis.

Zyderm I, **Zyderm II**—collagen injections.

zygomycosis—see *mucormycosis*.

zygote—a one-celled pre-embryo.

zymogen cell (peptic cell) **of stomach**.

zymogen granule—cellular granules consisting of inactive digestive enzymes awaiting secretion.

zygosity—the mode of origin of a pair of twins, monozygotic vs dizygotic.

zygote—the diploid cell that results from the fertilization of an oocyte (ovum, egg) by a sperm cell.

Zyoptix Infinity laser—designed to provide individual customized laser vision correction.

Zyplast—collagen for thinner wrinkles.

Zywave aberrometer—an ophthalmology diagnostic device that uses wavefront technology, in which a beam of light is reflected off the retina to determine the unique features of each eye and identify abnormalities through the entire optical system. In eyes where there is an abnormality, the measurement of the variations between the actual direction of the outgoing beams of the light and their optimal positions determines the overall aberration of the eye.

Zzooties—therapeutic sleeping booties for adults.